ANNALS OF OTOLOGY, RHINOLOGY & LARYNGOLOGY

Founded in 1892

Volume 85

PUBLISHED BIMONTHLY
BY THE
ANNALS PUBLISHING COMPANY

ANNALS OF OTOLOGY, RHINOLOGY AND LARYNGOLOGY

VOL. 85 JULY - AUGUST, 1976 NO. 4

CONTENTS

PAGE

Second Daniel C. Baker, Jr. Memorial Lecture. Progress of Otolaryngology in Head and Neck Surgery. Joseph H. Ogura, MD 425

Etiology of Bilateral Abductor Vocal Cord Paralysis, A Review of 389 Cases. Lauren D. Holinger, MD, Paul C. Holinger, MD, Paul H. Holinger, MD 428

Bilateral Abductor Paralysis, 30 Years Experience with Arytenoidectomy. DeGraaf Woodman, MD, Claude L. Pennington, MD 437

Experience with Vocal Cord Injection. Robert B. Lewy, MD 440

Recurrent Laryngeal Nerve Section for Spastic Dysphonia. Herbert H. Dedo, MD 451

Fiber Components of the Recurrent Laryngeal Nerve in the Cat. Richard R. Gacek, MD, Michael J. Lyon, MA 460

An Implanted Electronic Laryngeal Prosthesis. Byron J. Bailey, MD, Ceri M. Griffiths, MD, Robert Everett, PhD 472

Otolaryngological Manifestations of Arthrogryposis Multiplex Congenita. Seymour R. Cohen, MD, Hart Isaacs Jr, MD 484

Congenital Laryngeal Defects in the Adult. William W. Montgomery, MD, Stephen A. Smith, MD 491

Mucus Gland Tumors of the Larynx and Laryngopharynx. Ronald H. Spiro, MD, John S. Lewis, MD, Steven I. Hajdu, MD, Elliot W. Strong, MD 498

Granular Cell Tumors of the Larynx. Harvey L. Coates, MD, Kenneth D. Devine, MD, Thomas J. McDonald, MD, Louis H. Weiland, MD 504

Recurrent Respiratory Papillomatosis, Management with the CO_2 Laser. M. Stuart Strong, MD, Charles W. Vaughan, MD, Sidney R. Cooperband, MD, Gerald B. Healy, MD, Manuel A. C. P. Clemente, MD 508

Dinitrochlorobenzene Skin Sensitization and Peripheral Lymphocyte Count: Predictors of Survival in Head and Neck Cancer. Robert H. Maisel, MD, Joseph H. Ogura, MD 517

Osteoplastic Frontal Sinusotomy: An Analysis of 250 Operations. James M. Hardy, MD, William W. Montgomery, MD 523

Laryngeal Suspension and Epiglottic Flap in Laryngopharyngeal Trauma. Nels R. Olson, MD 533

Verrucous Carcinoma of the Larynx: Management by Radiotherapy and Surgery. Hugh P. Burns, MB, A. W. Peter van Nostrand, MD, Douglas P. Bryce, MD 538

X-Ray of the Month: Mucopyocele of the Frontal Sinus. Alfred L. Weber, MD, B. Donald Sklansky, MD 544

Scanning Electron Microscopic Study of the Organ of Corti in Normal and Sound-Damaged Guinea Pigs. Eduard R. Soudijn, MD ..... Supplement No. 29

Obituary 546

Communication 547

Book Reviews 548

Abstracts from National and International Journals 550

Index to Advertisers 551

The "area under the curve" demonstrates the superior absorption of Larotid[T.M.] (amoxicillin)

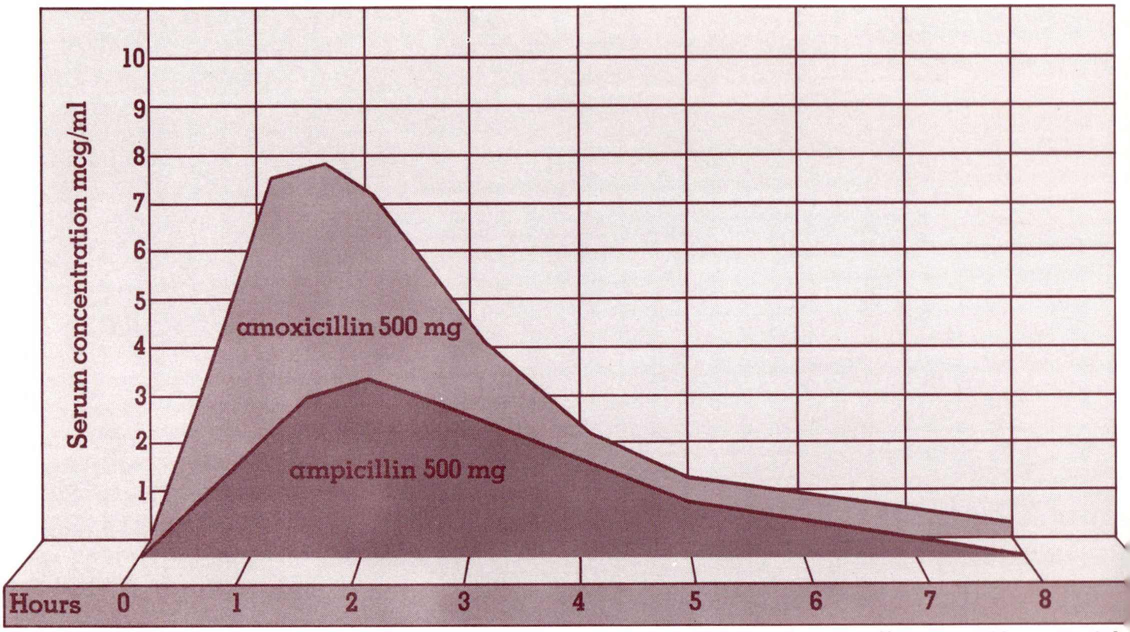

Mean serum concentrations and "area under the curve" for amoxicillin and ampicillin after 500-mg oral d in eight fasting subjects.[1]

In comparing the absorption of oral amoxicillin and oral ampicillin, the significantly greater absorption of amoxicillin was demonstrated not only by the higher average peak serum concentrations but also by the average "area under the curve," which was approximately double that of ampicillin. Expressed as a percentage, the area under the ampicillin serum concentration curve was 50.3% of the area under the amoxicillin curve.[1]

References: 1. Gordon RC, Regamy C, Kirby WMM: *Antimicrob Agents Chemother 1*:504-507, 1972. **2.** Data on file, Hoffmann-La Roche Inc., Nutley, New Jersey.

Of course, the critical test of antibiotic therap must always be clinical response. Larotid (amoxicillin) has now been administered to more than a million patients with a wide ran of infections due to susceptible bacteria. In a comprehensive series of clinical evaluations therapy was rated a "success" or "improvement" in 1266 of 1349 evaluable cases (93.8% based on a combination of clinical and bacteriologic criteria. (In strep throat and gonorrhea, only successes were included.) For the results by type of infection, see the table at right.[2] Please note that Larotid is contraindicated in patients with a history of penicillin hypersensitivity.

ANNALS OF OTOLOGY, RHINOLOGY AND LARYNGOLOGY

VOL. 85 SEPT - OCT, 1976 No. 5

CONTENTS

PAGE

Observations on Laryngeal Disease, Laryngeal Behavior and Voice. G. Paul Moore, PhD ... 553

Acute Epiglottitis in Infants and Children. Bruce Benjamin, Brian O'Reilly ... 565

Acquired and Congenital Subglottic Stenosis in the Infant. James L. Parkin, MD, Michael H. Stevens, MD, August L. Jung, MD ... 573

Tracheostenosis and Bronchial Abnormalities Associated with Pulmonary Artery Sling. Seymour R. Cohen, MD, Benjamin H. Landing, MD ... 582

Subglottic Stenosis in Infants and Children. Paul H. Holinger, MD, Steven L. Kutnick, MD, Joyce A. Schild, MD, Lauren D. Holinger, MD ... 591

Repair of Laryngeal Stenosis with Nasal Septal Grafts. Robert J. Toohill, MD, Dean L. Martinelli, MD, Michael C. Janowak, MD ... 600

Clinical Experience with the Tracheoesophageal Anastomosis for Intractable Aspiration. Roger C. Lindeman, MD, C. Thomas Yarington, Jr, MD, Dwight Sutton, PhD ... 609

Congenital Tracheoesophageal Fistulas in Adults. Robert W. Stephens, MD, Raleigh E. Lingeman, MD, Lawrence J. Lawson, MD ... 613

Tracing the Tracheostomy. Elizabeth A. M. Frost, MD ... 618

Laser Adapter for Tracheoscopy. Albert H. Andrews, Jr, MD, Larry L. Bailey, MD ... 625

Educational Training in Endoscopy. John E. Rayl, MD ... 627

Tracheal Resection and Mucociliary Clearance. Anthony Giordano, MD, Douglas S. Holsclaw, MD ... 631

Flexible Fiberoptic Nasopharyngolaryngoscope. Harvey D. Silberman, MD, Harold Wilf, MD, John A. Tucker, MD ... 640

Newer Techniques in Fiberoptic Bronchoscopy. Joseph P. Atkins, Jr, MD, Lee D. Rowe, MD, Bruce W. Jafek, MD ... 646

Percutaneous Jet Ventilation. Edward Carden, FRCP(C), Gary Becker, MD, Hassney Hamood, MD ... 652

Endotracheal Intubation and Venturi (Jet) Ventilation for Laser Microsurgery of the Larynx. Martin Lloyd Norton, MD, M. Stuart Strong, MD, Charles W. Vaughan, MD, John C. Snow, MD, Benjamin J. Kripke, MD ... 656

Tracheal Afferent Nerves. Roger M. Traxel, MD, William F. Prudlow, MD, John P. Kampine, MD, Robert L. Coon, PhD, Edward J. Zuperku, Phd ... 664

Transbronchoscopic Cryosurgery of Respiratory Structures: Experimental and Clinical Studies. Aryeh Gorenstein, MD, H. Bryan Neel III, MD, David R. Sanderson, MD ... 670

Test-Retest Reliability in Clinical Electrocochleography. L. M. Bergholtz, MD, R. E. Hooper, MD, D. C. Mehta, MD ... 679

Antihistamines: Guidelines and Implications. Anthony S. Krausen, MD ... 686

X-Ray of the Month: Ameloblastoma. Alfred L. Weber, MD, Walter Guralnick, DMD ... 692

Survey of the Development of Laryngeal Epithelium. John A. Tucker, MD, Branislav Vidic, SD, Gabriel F. Tucker, Jr, MD, Jeffrey Stead, BS ... Supplement No. 30

Fine Structures of the Normal Mucosa in Developing Rat Middle Ear. Shoichi Maeda, MD, Goro Mogi, MD, Motow Oh, MD ... Supplement No. 31

Spiral Migration Theory of Organ of Corti Development. William F. Marovitz, PhD, Joel M. A. Shugar, MDCM, Khalid M. Khan, MS ... Supplement No. 32

Book Reviews ... 694 Index to Advertisers ... 695

ANNALS OF OTOLOGY, RHINOLOGY AND LARYNGOLOGY

VOL. 85 NOV - DEC, 1976 NO. 6

CONTENTS

PAGE

Physiological Basis of Cochlear Transduction and Sensitivity. Vicente Honrubia, MD, David Strelioff, PhD, Stephan T. Sitko, PhD 697

Safe Level for Noise Exposure? Barbara A. Bohne, PhD 711

Degeneration Patterns in Human Ears Exposed to Noise. Lars G. Johnsson, MD, Joseph E. Hawkins, Jr., PhD 725

Ultrastructural Cochlear Changes Following Acoustic Hyperstimulation and Ototoxicity. David J. Lim, MD 740

Auditory-Nerve Activity in Cats Exposed to Ototoxic Drugs and High-Intensity Sounds. Nelson Y. S. Kiang, PhD, M. Charles Liberman, PhD, Robert A. Levine, MD 752

Sodium Loading of Inner Ear Fluids. Herbert Silverstein, MD, Tiero Takeda, MD.. 769

Hearing Loss in Patients with Dialysis and Renal Transplants. Cedric A. Quick, MD 776

Electron Microscopic Cochlear Observations in Bilateral Ménière's Disease. Robert S. Kimura, BA, Carol Y. Ota, BA, Harold F. Schuknecht, MD, Tadahiko Takahashi, MD 791

Histopathologic and Experimental Models for Sensory and Neural Deafness. Gershon J. Spector, MD 802

The Combined Correlated Audiohistogram, Incorporation of the Superior Ventral Cochlear Nucleus. William B. Dublin, MD 813

Masking Level Differences for Cochlear and Brain Stem Lesions. Wayne O. Olsen, PhD, Douglas Noffsinger, PhD 820

Hearing Loss of a Central Type Secondary to Anoxic Anoxia. Kazumi Makishima, MD, Roger B. Katz, MD, James B. Snow, Jr., MD 826

New Developments in Evaluating Central Auditory Mechanisms. Charles I. Berlin, PhD 833

Effects of Removal of the Statoacoustic Ganglion Complex upon the Growing Otocyst. Thomas R. Van De Water, PhD ..... Supplement No. 33

Some Unresolved Problems Concerning the Cochlear Nerve. R. Lorente de Nó, MD ..... Supplement No. 34

Obituary. Dean M. Lierle, MD 842

Report on First International Conference on Cholesteatoma 844

Communications 846

Book Reviews 848

Author Index 850

Subject Index 852

Information for Contributors 859

Statement of Ownership 860

Index to Advertisers 861

The "area under the curve" demonstrates the superior absorption of Larotid™ (amoxicillin).

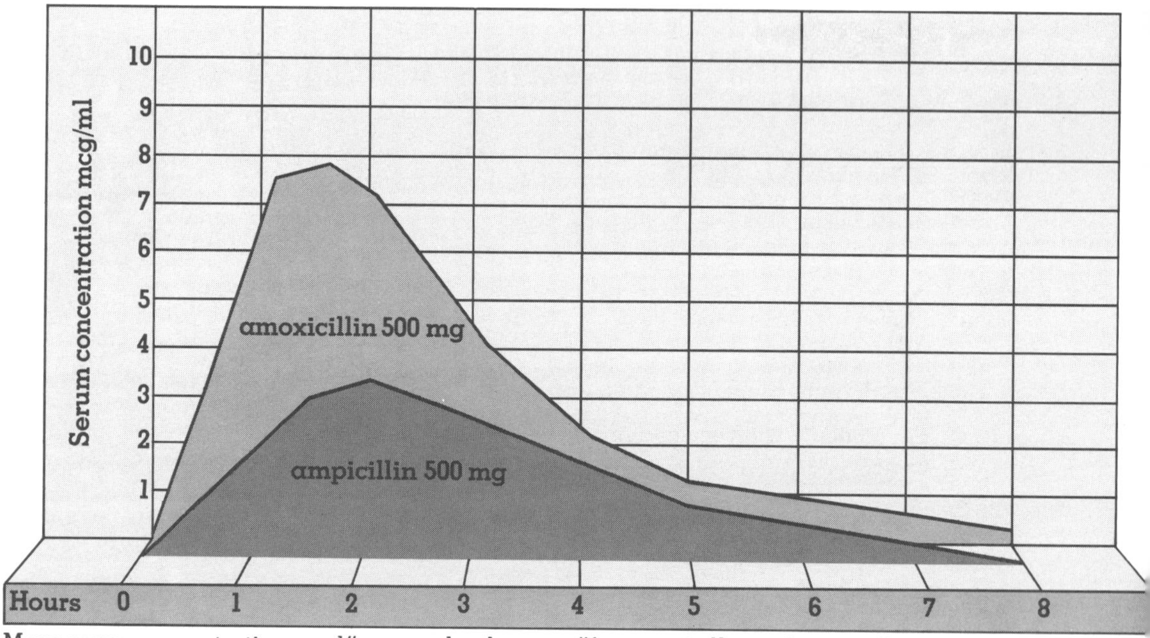

Mean serum concentrations and "area under the curve" for amoxicillin and ampicillin after 500-mg oral dose in eight fasting subjects.[1]

In comparing the absorption of oral amoxicillin and oral ampicillin, the significantly greater absorption of amoxicillin was demonstrated not only by the higher average peak serum concentrations but also by the average "area under the curve," which was approximately double that of ampicillin. Expressed as a percentage, the area under the ampicillin serum concentration curve was 50.3% of the area under the amoxicillin curve.[1]

References: 1. Gordon RC, Regamy C, Kirby WMM: *Antimicrob Agents Chemother* 1:504-507, 1972. **2.** Data on file, Hoffmann-La Roche Inc., Nutley, New Jersey.

Of course, the critical test of antibiotic therapy must always be clinical response. Larotid (amoxicillin) has now been administered to more than a million patients with a wide range of infections due to susceptible bacteria. In a comprehensive series of clinical evaluations, therapy was rated a "success" or "improvement" in 1266 of 1349 evaluable cases (93.8%), based on a combination of clinical and bacteriologic criteria. (In strep throat and gonorrhea, only successes were included.) For the results by type of infection, see the table at right.[2] Please note that Larotid is contraindicated in patients with a history of penicillin hypersensitivity.

SECOND DANIEL C. BAKER, JR.
MEMORIAL LECTURE

PROGRESS OF OTOLARYNGOLOGY IN HEAD AND NECK SURGERY

JOSEPH H. OGURA, MD

ST. LOUIS, MISSOURI

Over 100 years ago the first laryngectomy for cancer was performed by C. Billroth, although he was a general surgeon. It was a historical event. The surgical mortality rate from this operation was high for years and its progress was slow. But in 1878, another historical event took place. Twenty men under the presidency of Dr. H. Elsberry held the first meeting in New York City of the American Laryngological Association. The title of his first lecture was "Laryngology in America." It was a long address of 56 pages with a 100 page bibliography. Today, we accept laryngology as something we have been doing for years, but in New York in 1879 it was only ten years old. The frequency of infection of the larynx leading to serious or fatal consequence with respiratory and deglutition difficulties and the development of the laryngoscope for recognition of these problems led to the establishment of many departments of laryngology.

There was a long period of void in the evolution of surgery in laryngology, from the laryngofissure by C. Jackson in 1904 until 1928 when Dr. G. B. New described the two stage laryngectomy because of infectious complications and fistulas.

From the narrow field laryngectomy in 1938 we entered a period of irradiation alone or radical surgery in the treatment of laryngeal cancers. Because it was known that the lymphatics were separate above and below the true vocal cords, the basis for conservation surgery was formed. We are all familiar with the development of the subtotal operation so this really needs no comment. J. Alonso and others in America (J. Ogura and M. Som) further refined this technique. Early laryngeal cancer operations and many early head and neck cancers are treated by irradiation. Larger lesions are treated by radical surgery or by the addition of pre- or postoperative irradiation.

In the late forties with the return of veterans from the war, there was a brief period of excess of residents. The training period for residents was lengthened to three years, but there was a shortage of qualified applicants. This was also the period of ascendancy for ear surgery, but despite this, otolaryngology was in a period of great difficulty and decline.

Some 26 years ago D. Lierle addressed this association on the training of the resident. At that time, things were very bright. Most of the institutions were teaching basic sciences, giving residents experience in head and neck surgery, and otology. The papers were mostly philosophical, personal attitudes of management, and documentation of case reports. This is understand-

From the Department of Otolaryngology, Washington University School of Medicine, St. Louis, Missouri.

Presented at the meeting of the American Laryngological Association, Palm Beach, Florida, April 24-25, 1976.

able because sophisticated electronic or biochemical markers were not available. Clinical and basic research were minimal.

The advent of National Institutes of Health (NIH) training grants and research funds have increased and improved the research environment of many departments, thus improving greatly the clinical training available. You can see this today in the improved quality of our residents. Now it is not at all unusual that a candidate for Board certification has completed two years of general surgery and four years of otolaryngology. Better residents are making better young staff men and practitioners.

It is not possible for all residents to receive equal and uniform training, however, the American College of Surgeons in conjunction with the American Board of Otolaryngology and the Council of Medical Education of the AMA, has sponsored and passed the special Essentials of Otolaryngology. The Society of Head and Neck Surgeons and the American Society for Head and Neck Surgery have also been working to seek a solution to this problem for head and neck cancer. It is the hope to standardize training with options in providing training in head and neck surgery, plastic surgery of the head and neck, oncology, and immunology. However, it is likely that the number of head and neck surgeons to be certified as competent by certification will not be accomplished at this time.

Today's otolaryngologist has become an expert in the head and neck area. Because of this, the treatment of glomus vagale, carotid body, parotid, oral cavity, and esophageal tumors has often fallen his way. The use of flaps in reconstructive procedures has evolved into a great interest by many otolaryngologists in surgery of the head and neck. However, otology still has an active hold on others.

Finally, I would like to comment on the progress being made by the Head and Neck Cancer Cadre. This idea had its origin from the National Cancer Advisory Board of which I am its representative. To gain cooperation, confidence, assistance and security from the other disciplines, we made it purposely multidisciplinary over a few years. Through six subcommittees we have developed over the last two years a number of well-designed research protocols that can be implemented through a national program of treatment, cure, and control of cancers of the head and neck. However, it became evident last year that our basic science approach lacked a solid focus. A state of the art conference was suggested as the best forum for securing and disseminating the needed information and the National Cancer Institute (NCI) and the American Cancer Society agreed to cosponsor such a conference.

A steering committee that was selected from the Cadre membership and consultants drafted a conference goal and a program which would satisfy this goal.

The State of the Art Conference participants convened in New Orleans, February 16, 1976. This was of necessity a closed conference to get needed discussion from these experts. The conference consisted of five sections — Immunology; Pharmacology, Cell Kinetics and Radiation Biology; Epidemiology, Carcinogenesis and Virology; Natural History and Modification of Head and Neck Cancer; and Quality of Life. Clinical cooperation studies previously randomized were omitted.

Each of the five sections was chaired or guided by a steering committee member to insure achievement of the conference goal, with the participants of each section chosen for their competency in a given professional speciality.

The interdisciplinary cooperation and probing by the participants in their quest for the most interesting and demanding subjects for investigation gave us results beyond our expectations. Most of the presentations were varied and equally valuable.

The first morning was devoted to immunology. The afternoon section provided an overview for pharmacology, cell kinetics and radiation biology.

On the second morning, Section III, Epidemiology, Carcinogenesis and Virology met. Again, the examination of subject areas revealed many sources for future investigation. The Natural History and Modification of Head and Neck Cancer met that same afternoon. It was our heaviest scheduled section.

The last section on the third day was Quality of Life. This section brought within one spectrum medical professionals, paraprofessionals, and legal specialists needed to provide comprehensive and compassionate care prospectives.

This particular state of the art conference was a genuine success to all who attended and an overwhelming success as finally summarized by the NCI staff members, and from which a national program on head and neck cancer should evolve.

This I believe – the orderly, gradual development and evolution of laryngology is in head and neck surgery.

As I conclude this Daniel C. Baker Lecture, let me comment that it was indeed a great honor to deliver this lecture. To me, our growth has been spectacular, our future is secure, our platform very broad, firm, and indeed bright. If Dan Baker were here today I am sure he would be the first to agree with this.

OTOLOGY SEMINAR

The Otolaryngology Service at Madigan Army Medical Center will conduct an Otology Seminar September 9-11, 1976. Featured speakers will include Doctors Charles Bluestone, Robert Schindler, Robert Kohut, Francis Sooy and others.

Ann Otol 85: 1976

ETIOLOGY OF BILATERAL ABDUCTOR VOCAL CORD PARALYSIS

A REVIEW OF 389 CASES

LAUREN D. HOLINGER, MD

PAUL C. HOLINGER, MD PAUL H. HOLINGER, MD

CHICAGO, ILLINOIS

SUMMARY – The etiology of 389 cases of partial or complete bilateral abductor vocal cord paralysis has been determined and classified. One hundred and forty-nine were infants and children 12 years of age and under; 240 were adults, age 13 and older. In the infants and children the paralyses were congenital in 82 cases, of which 43 were associated with other congenital anomalies, and 39 were without associated anomalies. Fifty-nine cases were considered acquired, most being secondary to underlying congenital anomalies, particularly the associated findings of meningomyelocele, Arnold-Chiari malformation, and hydrocephalus. Eight cases of paralysis in this age group were of undetermined etiology. Of the 240 adult cases of bilateral vocal cord paralysis, 138 followed thyroidectomy. Fifty-two cases were associated with various neurologic disorders, including poliomyelitis, Parkinson's disease, cerebrovascular accident, Guillain-Barré syndrome, multiple sclerosis, neoplasm, and other miscellaneous neurologic conditions. Sixteen cases were due to malignant neoplasms of the neck and mediastinum. The remaining 34 cases constitute a miscellaneous group which includes foreign bodies, bilateral neck dissection, infection, congenital lesions, trauma, and idiopathic paralyses. The characteristic symptoms of bilateral abductor vocal cord paralysis include normal or near normal phonation with inspiratory stridor which may progress to complete respiratory obstruction. These symptoms are due to the stationary but flaccid midline position of the vocal cords which places them in a phonating position, where they both obstruct the airway and produce a fairly clear voice or cry. This paradoxical combination of symptoms was frequently found to be responsible for a failure or delay in diagnosis.

Bilateral abductor vocal cord paralysis is a distressing condition, often life-threatening, and not infrequently a direct cause of asphyxial death. Yet many times it is unrecognized clinically because the voice or cry of the patient with bilateral paralysis is quite normal and invariably better than that of the patient with unilateral paralysis. This paradox is due to the fact that in bilateral paralysis both cords remain weakly adducted, in which position they vibrate during expiration or phonation, passively but equally. In unilateral paralysis, on the other hand, differences in tension between the normal and the paralyzed cord result in a hoarse, aspirate voice. Patients with bilateral vocal cord paralysis have a limited airway and a persistent, soft, inspiratory stridor which may be barely audible or may increase to a loud, agonal, even terminal crow. Any additional edema of the cords results in extreme dyspnea, for which intubation or tracheotomy may become necessary. Failure to recognize the condition most often occurs in the thyroidectomized adult. Similarly, in the stridorous infant with a major central nervous system (CNS) defect, bilateral paralysis may remain undiagnosed because of a failure to examine the larynx routinely and without anesthesia.

From the Department of Otolaryngology, Abraham Lincoln School of Medicine of the University of Illinois; the Department of Psychiatry, Psychosomatic and Psychiatric Institute, Michael Reese Hospital and Medical Center; the Department of Bronchology, The Children's Memorial Hospital; and the Department of Otolaryngology and Bronchoesophagology, Rush/Presbyterian-St. Luke's Medical Center, Chicago, Illinois.

Presented at the meeting of The American Laryngological Association, Palm Beach, Florida, April 24-25, 1976.

TABLE I

ETIOLOGY OF BILATERAL ABDUCTOR VOCAL CORD PARALYSIS IN INFANTS AND CHILDREN

Congenital				
Without associated anomalies		39		
With associated anomalies				
Neurologic	21			
Laryngeal	10			
Cardiac	8			
Other	4			
		43		
	Total Congenital		82	(55%)
Acquired				
Secondary to congenital anomalies				
Meningomyelocele, A-CM, hydrocephalus	24			
Hydrocephalus unrelated to A-CM	6			
Postoperative for congenital lesion	11			
		41		
Secondary to acquired conditions				
Infectious	7			
Neoplasm	7			
Birth trauma	2			
Guillain-Barré syndrome	2			
		18		
	Total Acquired		59	(40%)
Undetermined		8	8	(5%)
	Total		149	(100%)

METHODS AND MATERIALS

This study reviews the etiology of 389 cases of partial or complete bilateral abductor vocal cord paralysis in infants and children 12 years of age and under, and adults age 13 or older. Diagnosis in all cases was confirmed by mirror or endoscopic examination. In infants, the diagnosis can be established only by direct laryngoscopic examination without anesthesia.[1] The spatulous tip of a standard Jackson pediatric laryngoscope is placed in the vallecula to lift the base of the tongue and epiglottis to evaluate vocal cord mobility. Care must be taken to avoid contact with the vocal cords or arytenoids, which would alter cord mobility. Passive mobility should be evaluated by palpation to rule out midline vocal cord fixation.[2] In adults the examination is made with the laryngeal mirror, not only during the phonation of "e-e-e-e," but especially during inspiration as well.

RESULTS

The data derived from this study are most informative when infants and children are evaluated separately from adults. Bilateral paralysis in infants is largely congenital in origin, or secondary to congenital anomalies of the CNS. In adults the great majority of cases are acquired. Unfortunately, the leading cause is surgical injury to the recurrent laryngeal nerves at thyroidectomy. Neurologic lesions are the second most common cause of bilateral paralysis in adults. A classification based on the two age groups is presented in Tables I and II.

Of the 389 cases, 149 (38%) were present in infants and children under 13 years of age; 240 (62%) were found in adults. There were 146 males and 243 females. Sex distribution was similar among the infants and children (80 males, 69 females), but among the adults there were 66 males and 174 females. This was due to a higher incidence of thyroid disease in females; of 138 cases of bilateral paralysis due to thyroidectomy, only 11 occurred in

TABLE II

ETIOLOGY OF BILATERAL ABDUCTOR VOCAL CORD PARALYSIS IN ADULTS

Thyroidectomy		138	(58%)
Neurologic			
Poliomyelitis	14		
Parkinson's disease	4		
Cerebrovascular accident	4		
Guillain-Barré syndrome	3		
Multiple sclerosis	3		
CNS neoplasm	3		
CNS infection	2		
Charcot-Marie-Tooth	2		
Other	17		
		52	(22%)
Malignancy of the neck		16	(6%)
Miscellaneous			
Foreign bodies	2		
Bilateral neck dissection	3		
Infection	3		
Congenital	3		
Trauma	2		
Substernal thyroid	2		
Idiopathic	8		
Other	3		
Undetermined	8		
		34	(14%)
Total		240	(100%)

males. Tracheotomy was required at some time during the patient's course in 199 cases (51%); 71 cases were in infants and children and 128 in adults; 48% of the infants and children required tracheotomy, as did 53% of adults.

DISCUSSION

Stridor is the most prominent symptom of bilateral abductor vocal cord paralysis. It varies from a soft, high-pitched, inspiratory sound to an extremely loud, distressing crow. Adult patients' families volunteer that often it is easily heard throughout the room or ward and even by neighbors if the windows are open in the summertime. Snoring is especially pronounced when the patient is relaxed during sleep. The voice and speech are somewhat abnormal; a peculiar monotone with long, hurried sentences is interrupted by a stridorous, inspiratory pause as the patient attempts to fill his lungs for continuation of his comment. Laughter is consciously suppressed to avoid the air loss which must be followed by distressing inspiration. Cough is desperately suppressed for the same reason. In infants, while the cry may be clear, stridor is high-pitched and not necessarily accompanied by acute respiratory distress, although marked indrawing of the suprasternal notch and epigastrium is usually apparent. With prolonged obstruction, however, fatigue becomes the major factor precipitating either intubation or tracheotomy.

The degree of aspiration, especially of liquids, helps localize the site of the lesion superior or inferior to the origin of the superior laryngeal nerve. While this should be a fairly accurate diagnostic criterion, patients with aspiration due to superior laryngeal nerve involvement soon learn to control coughing and choking, and the clinical significance of this diagnostic point is lost.

The most serious symptom, of course, is respiratory obstruction, which is evidenced by stridor, dyspnea, retraction, and nasal flaring. Since the airway through the larynx is limited, the least effort, activity, inflammation or edema may result in increasing dyspnea, and even psychiatric symptoms in adults. As obstruction increases, restlessness, the use of the accessory respiratory musculature, and eventually cyanosis become apparent. If unrelieved, total asphyxia follows. Many patients tolerate their condition for considerable lengths of time, remaining marginally compensated until a minimal change in their status renders the airway inadequate. Patients with postthyroidectomy bilateral paralysis usually adapt to a minimal airway over a period of years; yet eventually, even 10 to 20 years later, may require surgical intervention such as a tracheotomy or arytenoidectomy. This may be associated with myxedematous infiltration of the cords due to hypothyroidism or laryngeal spasm associated with the hypocalcemic tetany of hypoparathyroidism. Infants and children may remain stridorous but undiagnosed until an upper respiratory infection leads to obstruction, or a prolonged episode of croup, for which the child is ultimately referred for endoscopic evaluation. The importance of direct endoscopic examination of children with stridor or persistent episodes of croup cannot be overemphasized. In a recent review of subglottic stenosis in infants and children,[3] 34% of 115 cases of congenital subglottic stenosis presented with recurrent or persistent croup.

INFANTS AND CHILDREN

Congenital Paralysis. Vocal cord paralysis represents approximately 10% of all congenital anomalies of the larynx.[4] It is the second most common laryngeal anomaly; only laryngomalacia is seen more often. In this series, 82 of the 149 infants and children had congenital bilateral paralysis.

In 39 of the 82 congenital cases the paralysis was without associated anomalies, most of which tended to resolve spontaneously over a period of weeks or months; a closer study of this group is now under way to more accurately determine the outcome. In some of these infants, the arytenoids were observed to move in the absence of any mobility of the vocal cords, which were immobile in the median position. Palpation demonstrated the arytenoids could be moved with forceps.

Forty-three infants and children had other congenital anomalies associated with congenital bilateral paralysis. Twenty-one had associated neurologic lesions. The association between the paralysis and the neurologic disorders had greater etiologic significance in some cases than in others. Congenital bilateral paralysis was seen in six infants with cerebral agenesis, four infants with congenital cranial nerve palsies including X, and one infant with congenital nuclear hypoplasias including X. In these 11 cases the congenital bilateral vocal cord paralysis was apparently secondary to the neurologic lesions. In the remaining ten cases the relationship between the vocal cord paralysis and the neurologic disorder was less well defined. Three of these ten had benign congenital hypotonia, one had Werdnig-Hoffmann disease, another had leukodystrophy (Alexander's disease), and there was one child with scapuloperoneal muscular dystrophy. The exact nature of the neurologic lesion remained obscure in three cases. Congenital bilateral paralysis was found in one patient with Charcot-Marie-Tooth disease; the occurrence of congenital bilateral vocal cord paralysis in families has been documented and is discussed elsewhere.[5-8]

Ten infants and children had other laryngeal anomalies associated with their congenital bilateral vocal cord paralysis; subglottic stenosis was present in six; laryngomalacia in three and laryngocele in one. One of the infants with laryngomalacia had other congenital anomalies, including hypospadias and bilateral dysplasia of the hips; a chromosomal abnormality was documented with karyotype interpretation 46, XY, one of D chromosomes having a short arm.

A wide variety of cardiac anomalies occurred in eight infants and children with congenital bilateral paralysis; these included ventricular septal defect, three; coarctation of the aorta, two; transposition of the great vessels, two; and atrial septal defect, one. Two of these patients also had Down's syndrome.

A miscellaneous group of congenital anomalies comprised the other four cases associated with congenital bilateral paralysis. These included spontaneous pneumothorax, muscular hypertonia and tracheomalacia with a narrow right main bronchus.

Acquired Paralysis. In this series, 59 of the 149 infants and children had acquired bilateral paralysis. In 41, the acquired paralysis occurred secondary to underlying congenital anomalies or was secondary to the surgical treatment of such anomalies. Of these 41, 24 involved infants born with meningomyelocele.

The association of meningomyelocele with paralysis of the vocal cords was noted in 1932,[9] 1939,[10] 1941[11] and again 15 years later.[12,13] Investigators later identified the relationship in more extensive case reports,[14-17] and others have recently probed the pathogenesis of bilateral vocal cord paralysis when related to meningomyelocele.[18-22] Associated meningomyelocele, Arnold-Chiari malformation, and hydrocephalus, as well as the neurosurgical efforts to repair these abnormalities, may result in increased intracranial pressure with subsequent airway obstruction due to bilateral vocal cord paralysis. Arnold-Chiari malformation (Chiari II), documented in 9 of the 24 cases with meningomyelocele, is probably present to some degree in all of these cases.[23] It is a developmental disorder characterized particularly by varying degrees of herniation of the cerebellum and kinking of the medulla oblongata, the causes of which are debated, but for which there may be a genetic background.[24]

In this series, neurosurgical repair of the meningomyelocele was usually accomplished shortly after birth; increased intracranial pressure and hydrocephalus occurred at varying lengths of time thereafter. Shunting procedures were instituted to control the hydrocephalus. The increased intracranial pressure which preceded signs and symptoms of airway obstruction was most frequently associated with malfunctioning or infected shunts. Less frequently, the bilateral paralysis occurred following repair of the meningomyelocele but before a diagnosis of hydrocephalus was made. Some children were later readmitted when the stridor of bilateral paralysis developed as the first sign of increased intracranial pressure due to a malfunctioning or infected shunt. The clinical course and pathophysiology seen in these are reviewed in greater detail elsewhere.[22]

Six cases of infants with bilateral paralyses were seen with hydrocephalus secondary to tumor, meningitis, and other underlying conditions, but without meningomyelocele.

Signs and symptoms of increased intracranial pressure, particularly increased head size, bulging fontanelle, and vomiting, usually preceded evidence of airway obstruction. Stridor and respiratory distress were prominent among the signs and symptoms of the ensuing bilateral paralysis. While associated with increased intracranial pressure, the precise etiology of the bilateral vocal cord paralysis in these cases is uncertain and discussed in detail elsewhere.[21,22] Among the possible hypotheses are brain stem dysgenesis, mechanical compression of the vagus nerve by the herniated posterior fossa contents, stretching of the vagus nerve rootlets during herniation with resulting neuronal degeneration, and circulatory impairment of the brain stem.

Although the etiology of the bilateral vocal cord paralysis in these cases is uncertain, the resulting airway obstruction can be life-threatening, and an airway must be promptly secured by intubation. Subsequent direct laryngoscopy discloses the median or paramedian position of the cords; tracheotomy is frequently necessitated when extubation attempts are unsuccessful. At The Children's Memorial Hospital in Chicago, where nearly all of the infants and children were seen, the neurosurgical service has been acutely aware of the relationship between bilateral vocal cord paralysis and increased intracranial pressure for many years. When stridor develops in a child known to have a potential for increased intracranial pressure, *e.g.*, those with hydrocephalus and meningomyelocele, they are assumed to have bilateral paralysis on the basis of increasing pressure. An endotracheal tube is placed, the cause of the increased pressure treated (it is most often related to an infected or malfunctioning shunt) and the child extubated.

Eleven instances of acquired bilateral paralysis followed surgical repair of congenital lesions which were not related to the CNS. Six became apparent after repair of tracheoesophageal fistula, three following surgery for congenital heart disease. One was diagnosed following the excision of a congenital bronchial cyst and one following craniotomy for craniostenosis.

Eighteen of the 59 children with acquired bilateral paralysis had no associated congenital anomaly. Seven were due to infectious disease: meningitis, encephalitis and poliomyelitis. Neoplasms of the CNS caused the paralysis in six; a seventh patient had Hodgkin's disease of the mediastinum and suffered bilateral paralysis following radiation therapy. Birth trauma was implicated in two cases and Guillain-Barré syndrome in two.

Undetermined Paralysis. The etiology of bilateral abductor vocal cord paralysis was undetermined in 8 of the 149 infants and children.

ADULTS

Two hundred and forty of the patients with bilateral abductor vocal cord paralysis were adults 13 years of age and older. Unlike the infants and children, the overwhelming majority of adults had acquired paralyses. Only three were considered to have congenital paralyses, these on the basis of a history of stridor since infancy. None had ever been examined directly or indirectly until seen at ages 33, 59, and 70, when their obstruction became severe enough to necessitate investigation.

Postthyroidectomy. One hundred and thirty-eight of the acquired adult cases followed thyroidectomy. Many of these had no symptoms of upper airway obstruction until after their second or even third thyroidectomy, although they generally gave a history of voice change following the original operation. In addition to respiratory obstruction, many had signs and findings of hypothyroidism and hypoparathyroidism. The number of cases observed increased during the period of time a total thyroidectomy was recommended for certain cardiac conditions. Psychiatric symptoms associated with hypothyroidism and hypoparathyroidism were freqeunt in this group of 138, and included depression, psychomotor retardation, irritability, and other personality changes.

Hoarseness following thyroidectomy is most often the result of paralysis of one vocal cord, due to trauma to a recurrent laryngeal nerve. The voice is weak and breathy; aspiration is frequent. However, when both nerves are involved, the voice, which may be temporarily affected, soon returns to almost normal, punctuated only by varying degrees of stridor. On examination with a laryngeal mirror during the phonation of "e-e-e-e," the larynx appears quite normal. However, the patient is usually so dyspneic that attempts to watch for the separation of the cords during inspiration are often abandoned.

In a review of 63 cases of bilateral vocal cord paralysis following thyroidectomy reported in 1955,[25] 40% were found to be hypothyroid while 21% were hypoparathyroid. The symptoms are generally manifested by the progressive limitation of the individual's activity, resulting from pulmonary and circulatory involvement as well as the increasing airway obstruction. Bouts of acute respiratory obstruction may be noted after an episode of emotional stress or in association with respiratory tract infections to which these patients are particularly susceptible. When the obstruction becomes sufficiently severe, intubation or tracheotomy must be undertaken to relieve the hypoxia and to protect the circulation: anoxia with its depressant effect on the myocardium can create a circulatory crisis to the extent of precipitating congestive heart failure.

The signs and symptoms of hypothyroidism are readily recognized. The complacent attitude, slowness of response, dull facies, dry skin, marked pallor, coarse hair, and poor tolerance to cold are characteristic. These findings are emphasized to stress their significance in patients who have postthyroidectomy respiratory obstruction from bilateral vocal cord paralysis. The myxedema of hypothyroidism includes the vocal cords and the supporting tissues of the larynx, and thus increases the degree of obstruction. The correction of the laryngeal myxedema with proper thyroid replacement therapy is necessary before surgical intervention is considered, and may obviate the need for surgery.

The symptoms due to hypoparathyroidism may be masked by those of hypothyroidism, and the diagnosis overlooked for this reason. When symptoms of fatigue, muscular weakness, tetany and paresthesias are present in the thyroidectomized patient, hypoparathyroidism should be suspected. Depending upon the degree of hypocalcemia, there may be cramps of the extremities, carpopedal as well as laryngeal spasm; even generalized convulsions may occur. Not uncommonly, these symptoms may be misdiagnosed as psychogenic. Cardiac conduction disturbances relating to calcium metabolism may also be present.

Paralysis Associated with Other Neurological Disorders. The commonest neurologic disorder associated with bilateral paralysis in adults was found to be poliomyelitis. The frequency with which bilateral laryngeal paralysis was caused by bulbar polio has been well documented by Galloway and Seifert.[26] Their description of the life-threatening and fatal complications of not only respiratory obstruction but aspiration of pharyngeal secretions is classic. Similar concepts of management were employed by Ibsen during the great Copenhagen polio epidemic of 1952, through the use of cuffed endotracheal tube and positive pressure ventilation.[27] Our experience in the acute phase[28] is not as extensive as that of Galloway and Ibsen. The 14 cases recorded in this series were encountered during a later stage when the respiratory obstruction of bilatral paralysis was complicated by the atelectasis associated with diaphragmatic and intercostal paralysis. Pharyngeal and laryngeal sensory involvement was thought to complicate the motor paralysis contributing to patients' aspiration of food and fluids, thus increasing the respiratory embarrassment. The resulting respiratory difficulties became extreme and tracheotomy was urgently needed. Yet many physicians who treated poliomyelitis were apparently unaware of the fact that the patient with bilateral vocal cord paralysis is able to phonate without difficulty, although the airway may have been so obstructed that he lapsed into unconsciousness.

In addition to the 14 cases of polio, several other acquired neurologic disorders have been found complicated by bilateral vocal cord paralysis, most with dyspnea so severe that they required tracheotomy. These cases include Parkinson's disease (four), cerebrovascular accident (four), Guillain-Barré syndrome (three), multiple sclerosis (three), CNS tumors (three), encephalitis and meningitis (two), and others (bulbar and pseudobulbar palsies, 17). Also, two patients with Charcot-Marie-Tooth disease, a mother and her son, were both found to have an associated bilateral vocal cord paralysis.

Paralysis Associated with Malignancy of the Neck. Sixteen cases of malignant neoplasms of the thyroid, cervical esophagus, subglottic larynx, neck and upper mediastinum were found to be responsible for bilateral abductor paralysis by pressure or invasion of the vagus or its recurrent branches. Usually one side was affected first; later the dyspnea of bilateral involvement became unmistakable. Mirror laryngoscopy or x-ray studies of the larynx and trachea are necessary to distinguish this symptom from tracheal compression or invasion by the neoplasm.

Miscellaneous Etiology. The 34 remaining patients with bilateral paralysis were found to have a variety of disorders. Foreign bodies in the esophagus were responsible for two cases of bilateral paralysis of the larynx. One was a 2-year-old child who was admitted to the hospital with severe dysphagia and dyspnea. Roentgen studies revealed a large, nonopaque button in the cervical esophagus which the mother was able to identify as having been swallowed nine months previously. Following tracheotomy the button was removed from a bed of scar, granulation tissue, and pus. Laryngoscopy demonstrated the bilateral midline position of the vocal cords. Extensive ulceration of the esophageal walls with periesophageal inflammation, induration, and abscess accounted for the paralysis.[13] The paralysis was permanent and eventually required arytenoidectomy. The second case was an adult who had an extensive cervical mediastinitis following esophageal perforation by a chicken bone.

In three cases in the miscellaneous group the paralysis followed bilateral neck dissection. Three others developed their paralysis following respiratory tract infections. In another three cases discussed previously, the etiology was considered congenital. Two patients had bilateral paralysis due to cervical trauma, and in two others, substernal thyroids involved both recurrent nerves. There was one case each of arthritis, leukemia, and a lesion of the cervical esophagus.

Eight cases in this group of miscellaneous paralyses were seen once in consultation for verification of the diagnosis only, and the etiology was not determined.

Eight adult patients were studied extensively but the etiology of their bilateral vocal cord paralyses was not discovered; these are considered idiopathic. Diagnostic evaluation began with a thorough history, which in many instances led directly to the etiology. Patients were questioned specifically about trauma, previous surgery, the degree and onset of hoarseness, dysphagia, aspiration, stridor and pain. A history of infection or recent upper respiratory infection was sought. Others had had thyroidectomies decades previously with symptoms beginning only weeks or months prior to evaluation; many of these were found to be hypothyroid or hypoparathyroid.

Remaining patients had medical and neurologic evaluations and laboratory studies which usually consisted of CBC, urinalysis, fasting and two-hour postprandial blood glucose, serologic tests for syphilis (VDRL, FTA-abs), erythrocyte sedimentation rate, PBI, T3 and T4. When the etiology remained obscure, thorough head and neck physical examination was extended to include endoscopic evaluation of larynx, trachea, and cervical esophagus. When indicated, these were preceded by special roentgenographic examinations, such as tomography and contrast studies (barium esophagram). Further specialized tests were employed to define associated neurologic lesions.

CONCLUSIONS

The etiology of 389 cases of partial or complete bilateral abductor vocal cord paralysis has been analyzed. There were 149 cases of infants and children 12 years of age and under: in 82, the lesions were congenital in origin, in 59, the etiology was acquired, and in 8, the etiology was undetermined. Two hundred and forty of the patients were adults 13 years of age and older; in all but three the condition was acquired. One hundred and thirty-eight followed thyroidectomy, 52 were neurologic, 16 were due to malignancies of the neck, and 34 were miscellaneous, eight of which were considered idiopathic.

The diagnosis of bilateral vocal cord paralysis is obscured by the paradoxical association of a relatively clear voice or cry with varying degrees of respiratory obstruction. The diagnosis may be overlooked in stridorous infants and children with meningomyelocele, Arnold-Chiari malformation and hydrocephalus, because the larynx is not examined without anesthesia; in such infants the onset of stridor is most often due to bilateral cord paralysis precipitated by increasing intracranial pressure. In adults, mirror examination of the larynx must be made during both phonation and inspiration. While some thyroidectomized adults adapt to the compromised airway of bilateral paralysis, the additional insult of hypothyroid myxedema or hypoparathyroid tetany may upset their compensated state. Conservative management involves correction of the underlying metabolic abnormality before any surgical intervention is undertaken.

REFERENCES

1. Holinger PH: Clinical aspects of congenital anomalies of the larynx, trachea, bronchi and oesophagus. J Laryngol Otol 75:1-44, 1961

2. Cox DJ, Simmons FB: Midline vocal cord fixation in the newborn. Arch Otolaryngol 100:219, 1974

3. Holinger PH, Kutnick SL, Schild JA, *et al*: Subglottic stenosis in infants and children. Ann Otol Rhinol Laryngol, to be published.

4. Holinger PH, Brown WT: Congenital webs, cysts, laryngoceles and other congenital anomalies of the larynx. Ann Otol Rhinol Laryngol 76:744-752, 1967

5. Platt D: Congenital laryngeal – abductor paralysis due to nucleus ambiguus dysgenesis in three brothers. N Engl J Med 271: 593-597, 1964

6. Watters GV, Fitch N: Familial laryngeal abductor paralysis and psychomotor retardation. Clin Genet 4:429-433, 1973

7. Gacek RR: Hereditary abductor vocal cord paralysis. Ann Otol Rhinol Laryngol 85: 90-93, 1976

8. Holinger PC, Holinger LD, Vuckovich MD, *et al*: Familial bilateral abductor vocal cord paralysis in Charcot-Marie-Tooth disease, to be published.

9. New GB, Childrey JH: Paralysis of the vocal cords. Arch Otolaryngol 16:143-159, 1932

10. Heatly CA: The larynx in infancy: A study of chronic stridor. Arch Otolaryngol 29: 90-103, 1939

11. Work WP: Paralysis and paresis of the vocal cords: A statistical review. Arch Otolaryngol 34:267-280, 1941

12. Bigler JA, Holinger PH, Johnston KC, *et al*: Tracheotomy in infancy. Pediatrics 13: 476-486, 1954

13. Holinger PH, Johnston KC: Bilateral recurrent laryngeal nerve paralysis; medical and surgical aspects. Eye Digest 38-45, June 1956

14. Cavanagh F: Vocal cord palsies in children. J Laryngol Otol 69:399-418, 1955

15. Rullan A: Associated laryngeal paralysis. Arch Otolaryngol 64:207-212, 1956

16. Smith MEN: The association of laryngeal stridor with meningomyelocele. J Laryngol Otol 73:188-190, 1959

17. Graham MD: Bilateral vocal cord paralysis associated with meningomyelocele and the Arnold-Chiari malformation. Laryngoscope 73:85-92, 1963

18. Snow JB, Rogers KA Jr: Bilateral abductor paralysis of the vocal cords secondary to the Arnold-Chiari malformation and its management. Laryngoscope 75:316-321, 1965

19. Kirsch WM, Duncan BR, Black FO, *et al*: Laryngeal palsy in association with meningomyelocele, hydrocephalus, and the Arnold-Chiari malformation. J Neurosurg 218: 207-214, 1968

20. Sieben RL, Hamida MB, Shulman K: Multiple cranial nerve deficits associated with the Arnold-Chiari malformation. Neurology 21:673-680, 1971

21. Bluestone LD, Delerme HN, Samuelson GM: Airway obstruction due to vocal cord paralysis in infants with meningomyelocele and hydrocephalus. Ann Otol Rhinol Laryngol 81:778-783, 1972

22. Reichert TJ, Schild JA, Holinger PH: Respiratory obstruction in infants with meningomyelocele and hydrocephalus. Presented at the Third Annual Meeting of Society for Ear Nose and Throat Advances in Children, Mexico City, Mexico, November 8, 1975

23. Emery JL, MacKenzie N: Medullocervical dislocation deformity (Chiari II deformity) related to neurospinal dysraphism (meningomyelocele). Brain 96:155-162, 1973

24. Gardner E, O'Rahilly R, Prolo D: The Dandy-Walker and Arnold-Chiari malformations. Arch Neurol 32:393-407, 1975

25. Ranke EJ, Holinger PH: Paralysis of the vocal cords following thyroidectomy. JAMA 158:543-547, 1955

26. Galloway TC, Seifert MH: Bulbar poliomyelitis. Ann Otol Rhinol Laryngol 56:250-263, 1947

27. Ibsen B: Anesthetists' viewpoint on treatment of respiratory complications in poliomyelitis during the epidemic in Copenhagen in 1952. Proc R Soc Med 47:72-74, 1954

28. Holinger PH, Johnston KC: Tracheotomy in acute tracheobronchitis and poliomyelitis. Prog Ophthalmol Otolaryngol 1:590-597, 1952

REPRINTS—Lauren D. Holinger, MD, 700 N. Michigan Avenue, Chicago, IL 60611.

Ann Otol 85: 1976

BILATERAL ABDUCTOR PARALYSIS

30 YEARS EXPERIENCE WITH ARYTENOIDECTOMY

DeGraaf Woodman, MD

Easton, Maryland

Claude L. Pennington, MD

Macon, Georgia

SUMMARY – Modifications of the technique originally reported in 1946 are presented, which may help in improving the percentage of successful decannulations. The importance of a change in the level of the vocal cord by this procedure is emphasized. The ten cautions to be followed are reviewed in doing this procedure.

An excellent and detailed paper on arytenoidectomy was presented in 1975 by Newman and Work[1] in which successful decannulations were reported in 75% of the 23 cases. In 1953, we reported 521 cases by 90 different surgeons, with a better than 90% success rate of decannulation, when the operations were done on patients with no previous history of attempts at lateralizing surgery.[2]

We will now describe some of the modifications that have been done to the original method, some of which may help raise the success level.[3,4] One step in particular has been completely eliminated – that of placing a traction ligature around the arytenoid cartilage to aid in this dissection. We found this to be a handicap. The placement of the endotracheal tube holds the cartilage rather firmly, making the dissection of the attached muscles possible with the aid of a small suction tube. The tissues are then dissected free of the cartilage with a Freer septum knife (Fig. 1). When all muscular attachments are freed with particular attention to the interarytenoid muscle fibers, the arytenoid is removed by cutting across and leaving a sufficient nubbin of cartilage intimately associated with the vocal process around which the lateralizing sutures can be placed. Then, two single zero atraumatic sutures are used to include the vocal process and pass laterally, so as to include some of the vocalis and thyroarytenoideus muscle, and brought out laterally anterior to the inferior thyroid cornu. The second suture is placed just anterior to the first (Fig. 2).

Before tying either of these sutures around the inferior cornu, their traction ability is observed through the laryngoscope. Once assured of the lateralizing effect, they are tied. A second inspection is then made by the laryngoscope.

We have come to feel that it is a distinct advantage to have some change in the level of the lateralized cord. The tendency for retraction to occur later will still permit adequate airway due to the change of the level of the cord. We have examined many postoperative cases and wondered why there was sufficient airway. This is due to the fact that while the cords may appear in the midline, there is a change in the level permitting adequate airway (Fig. 3).

We also believe that if the cautions previously noted in our summary of 521 cases reported in 1953[2] are carefully observed and followed, the results today should be as good as those reported then by 90 different surgeons.

Presented at the meeting of the American Laryngological Association, Palm Beach, Florida, April 24-25, 1976.

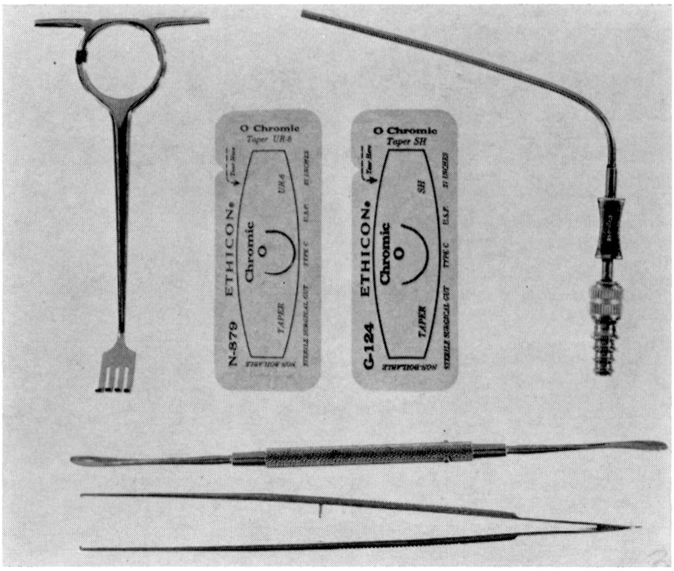

Fig. 1. Instrumentation which facilitates accurate dissection of the arytenoid and placement of the lateralizing suture. Left - Thyroid ala retractor. Right - No. 8 Frazier suction. Center - Lateralizing sutures. Below - Freer septum knife, Cushing forceps with teeth.

These cautions are:

1. In the selection of cases it is well to eliminate those in which there is localized laryngeal tuberculosis or cancer, or in which considerable irradiation has been given to laryngeal tissues. While ankylosis of the arytenoid is relatively rare, it should be thought of and checked as it makes a successful lateralization difficult.

2. A careful medical workup is essential, the serum calcium and phosphorus levels being noted. One should have the patient well stabilized as to the thyroid and parathyroid metabolic balance. In some of the hypoparathyroid patients, tetany and psychotic symptoms develop.

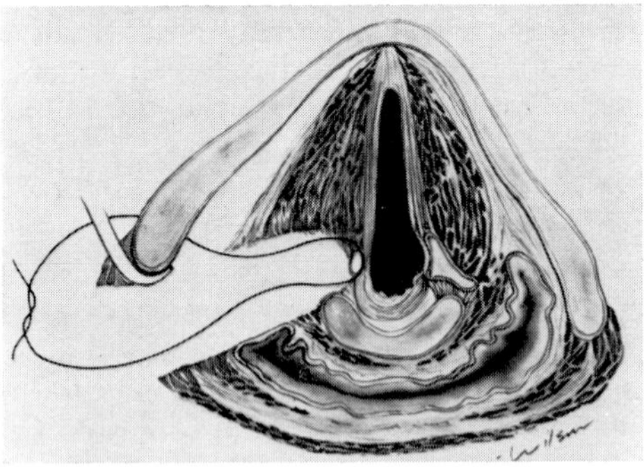

Fig. 2. A coronal section showing passage of the lateralizing suture around the nubbin of vocal process cartilage to include some of the vocalis and thyroarytenoideus muscles.

3. While many of these patients come to the surgeon with tracheotomy tube already placed, if a primary tracheotomy is to be done, it is better that it be done a week or ten days prior to any plastic operation, for the cough which accompanies the placement of a tube during the first week may help to dislodge the lateralized cord or loosen the lateralizing suture.

4. An endotracheal tube of medium size should always be placed down between the cords even though there is a tracheotomy tube in place. This procedure helps to hold the arytenoid in the field and offers some support for its dissection. Be sure to cut all interarytenoid fibers. The surgeon should also be sure to remove the endotracheal tube before placing the lateralizing sutures.

5. Exposure of the arytenoid can often be improved by cutting across the

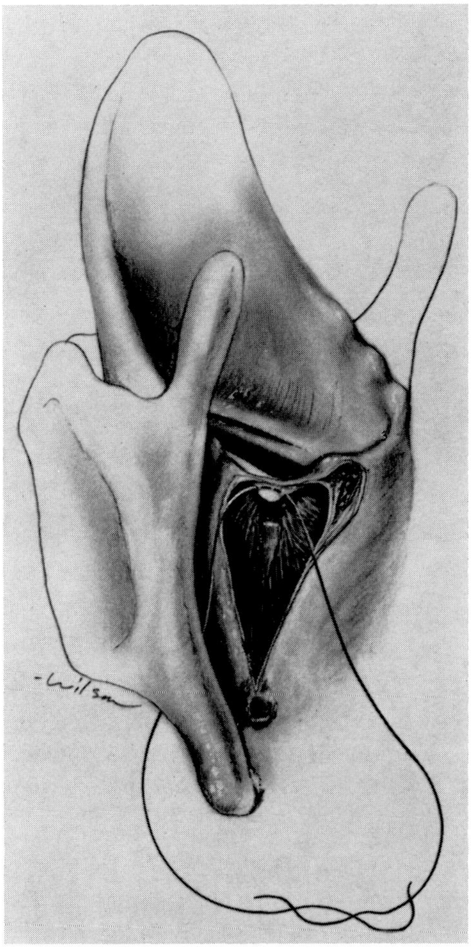

Fig. 3. An artist's concept of completed surgical procedure, showing the change in level on the vocal cord by the suture, as well as correct placement of the suture around the cartilaginous nubbin of the vocal process. The suture is secured around the inferior thyroid cornu.

superior cornu of the thyroid cartilage, thus giving greater mobility to the thyroid ala, permitting better rotation of the cartilage and increasing the size of the operated field.

6. As an extra assurance, two lateralizing sutures should be used. We prefer an atraumatic curved sharp needle with Single zero chromic suture.

7. Inspection should always be made by the laryngoscope after the sutures are placed but before they are anchored. This permits one to know that the suture has a hold on the vocal process and gives some idea as to how much lateralization tension is needed to obtain the desired glottic space. It is well to err by producing a wider space than needed as the tendency is towards later retraction.

8. The surgeon should never fail to leave in a drain for two or three days. This prevents the formation of any organized hematoma.

9. If we must operate on a patient who has had previous lateralization surgery without sufficient airway, it is recommended that one operate on the same side by a laryngofissure approach.[5] It is better not to operate on the other side if an operation can possibly be avoided, in order to preserve the full adductor powers of the other cord. These will be very helpful in stronger voice rehabilitation.

10. Finally, if speech therapy is available, it should be utilized. We have found marked improvement in the voices of all patients who have had the advantage of such training.

REFERENCES

1. Newman MH, Work WP: Arytenoidectomy revisited, presented April 8, 1975 at the national meeting of the Triological Society, Atlanta, Georgia. (To be published in Transactions of Triological, American Laryngological, Rhinological and Otological Society, Inc.)

2. Woodman D: Bilateral abductor paralysis: a survey of 521 cases of arytenoidectomy via the open approach as reported by ninety surgeons. Arch Otolaryngol 58:150-153, 1953

3. Woodman D: A modification of the extralaryngeal approach to arytenoidectomy for bilateral abductor paralysis. Arch Otolaryngol 43:63-65, 1946

4. Woodman D: The open approach to arytenoidectomy for bilateral abductor paralysis, with a report of twenty-three cases. Ann Otol Rhinol Laryngol 57:695, 1948

5. Woodman D: Laryngeal stenosis. Laryngoscope 63:714-720, 1953

Reprints—DeGraaf Woodman, MD, P.O. Box 560, Easton, MD 21601 and Claude L. Pennington, Jr., MD, 800 First St., Macon, GA 31201.

Ann Otol 85: 1976

EXPERIENCE WITH VOCAL CORD INJECTION

ROBERT B. LEWY, MD

CHICAGO, ILLINOIS

SUMMARY – For 14 years investigators accredited by the FDA have been injecting a Teflon® – glycerin mixture into lateral-lying, paralyzed vocal cords. This paper represents a summary of the work of this author, including successes, failures, and complications; it is the largest reported series, plus that of accredited investigators. The method described is exceptionally useful; it has restored voices, laughter, the ability to strain, and has prevented aspiration. A new surgical technique involving the injection of sterile glycerin into comparable vocal cords in acute new situations is also described. This is done by direct or indirect laryngoscopy, and has been used to eliminate some tracheotomy surgery by virtue of the immediately improved cough effectiveness.

The larynx should be regarded as a physiological valve that functions to make the process of breathing effective and efficient. If the glottis leaks, air cannot be held in the alveoli long enough for a sufficient oxygen interchange.

If one vocal cord is fixed and not in the midline, the voice loses its timbre and becomes hoarse and breathy. The valve closure function of the larynx also permits, by voluntary control, sudden explosive releases which permit the clearing of the lungs, a protection against pneumonia, foreign body, and irritants. Similarly, closure of the larynx acts to permit increased intraabdominal pressure for lifting and for straining. In a corresponding fashion, it functions to permit the greatest of human expressions, laughter.

With appropriate laryngeal function, there is obviously a greater efficiency of oxygen exchange at the alveolar interfaces and, therefore, better oxygenation of all body tissues. This permits more effective cardiac function, relieving the symptoms of the failing heart of angina pectoris (with oxygen deprivation to the myocardium).

Anything, therefore, which would cause a paralyzed lateral-lying vocal cord to be brought to the midline where it can work with its fellow, would improve the glottic functions of voice, laughter, straining ability, cough and offer protection against aspiration as well as better oxygenation. Many things have been noted in the past to do this; twisted positions of the neck, acute laryngitis, pressure against the side of the larynx, all of which would force one cord inward when it is otherwise fixed in a lateral, lying position.

In 1911, Brunings[1] corrected the problem by a peroral laryngoscopy injection, vocal cord augmentation technique. He used paraffn as the implant. His colleague, Killian, criticized the implant material, suggesting the risk of paraffinoma formation.

The method lingered within the scientific memory, but largely disappeared from view. Subsequent reports on occasional cases by various investigators suggested the use of plastics, cartilage, and a variety of other implant materials for this purpose. These usually required a laryngofissure approach to secure them into the vocal cord. If they were

----

From the Department of Otolaryngology, University of Illinois at the Medical Center.
This study was supported by research grant R01 NS 09891-01A1 CMS from the Department of Health, Education and Welfare.

Presented at the meeting of the American Laryngological Association, Palm Beach, Florida, April 24-25, 1976.

not absorbed, and if no foreign body reaction occurred, they benefited the patient.

Arnold,[2-4] Brunings' student, re-established the injection procedure. First he used ground-up tantalum, then went on to use ground particulate Teflon® mixed with equal parts of glycerin, injected into the vocal cord through a laryngoscope with a needle combined with a pistol type syringe. The process varied a little from Brunings' treatment in that though the technique was similar, the implant substance was different.

An early objective was to find a satisfactory substance which tissues would tolerate and with which there would be a minimal amount of foreign body response or rejection and maximum of safety and healing. This proved to be Teflon®.

Teflon®, itself, is a tradename for a polymer of tetrafluoroethylene. This substance was discovered by serendipity, a fortuitous accident and intelligent observation by a chemist working for the Manhattan Project for the Atomic Energy Commission. It was immediately recognized that the substance was most inert, and therefore it was used in the work on the atomic project.

Prior to its laryngeal application, it was determined that this substance would be well tolerated in human tissue. It had been used in thousands of cases to replace the stapes in a middle ear condition of deafness (otosclerosis). It had been used often as an artery substitute. It was not rejected by the host tissue and caused minimal foreign body response. Arnold,[4] earlier, and Kirchner *et al*[5] later, did animal tissue tolerance tests and found minimal reaction.

In 1973, Dedo[6] made a report before the American Laryngological Association of a successful series of 135 patients. Rubin,[7] in 1975, reported an occasional mild misadventure with misplaced Teflon®. He also reported high speed photographic studies of the vocal cord after Teflon® injection.

Our series includes principally Teflon®. Tantalum was used only in the first two cases of the series. Tantalum, incidentally, while found to be effective and nonreactive, was difficult to work with. It was very hard, and therefore its granules tended to freeze the glass syringes that were used at that time. Fresh sterile preparations had to be made for each individual case.

PURPOSE

The purpose of this retrospective study as stated in the request for the grant from the Department of Health, Education and Welfare, which made this study possible, follows:

> "To establish the clinical usefulness, the safety and evaluation of the results of the injection of a Teflon®* glycerin mixture into the lateral, lying paralyzed vocal cord. The objective is to offer substantive proof of both the long term and short term value of the injection of the Teflon®-glycerin mixture."

This investigator has published five articles relating to this problem.[8-12] These articles describe the instruments that have been developed for the procedure and the technique involved. They cover as well the etiology of vocal cord paralysis and the changes in the larynx before and after the procedure. They also describe the absence of migration of the foreign material and suggest the reasons for this.

All observations, across a period of 13 years, indicate a remarkable degree of success; therefore, it was considered highly desirable to evaluate long-term data. If favorable, the procedure could develop from a somewhat experimental technique to that of an accepted procedure for all appropriately trained laryngologists.

The central core of information in this paper is drawn from two sources. The first represents a statistical evaluation of the returns of 144 patients obtained from 218 cases who had Teflon® injection of the vocal cord performed by

----

* Mentor Division, Codman and Shurtleff, Inc., Randolph, MA.

TABLE I

SUMMARY OF RESEARCH DATA
(Author's Series of Patients from 1962-1974)

Male/Female ratio	Males	101
	Females	43
Age at time of injection	Youngest	9
	Oldest	83
	Median	55
Duration of laryngeal dysfunction	Minimum	5 wk
	Maximum	35 yr
	Median	1 yr
Primary presenting complaints Hoarse weak voice?	Yes	143
	No	1
Type of anesthesia	Local	132
	General	3
	Intravenous	4
Immediate results (24-hour impression of voice as determined by author)	Excellent	15
	Good	42
	Fair	1
	Poor	3
Second injection required?	Yes	18
	No	126
Current status	Living	118
	Deceased	26
Causes of death (when known)	Pneumonia	1
	Pulmonary embolus	1
	Stroke	1
	Congestive heart failure	2
	Carcinoma of lung	12
	Carcinoma of esophagus	4

this investigator (Table I). The second includes information from 38 accredited investigators throughout the country who performed 1139 procedures (Table II).

They reported the type of anesthesia used: local, general, or intravenous (combined with local), immediate complications within the first 48 hours, delayed complications, and success rate based upon the improvement of voice quality.

Corresponding studies are drawn from the questionnaires and voice tapes returned by those patients contacted.

The voice tapes form a permanent record, invaluable in evaluating results for legal protection and persuasion. Tapes however, have a disadvantage: they are not objective. Expert judges would vary in the interpretations of changes of voice quality.

The sonagram offers an excellent evaluation from visual record of voice quality. This has been used by von Leden *et al*,[13] as well as this author.[10] The visual record is persuasive and specific. Spectrographic studies obtained from voice tapes showing varied results are illustrated in this paper (Figs. 1-4).

Spectrography has been of value in voice studies and research in the physiology of the cough mechanism. Rontal *et al*[14] refer to three characteristics which can be recognized in the voice spectrograph. Excessive breathiness

TABLE II

QUESTIONNAIRE SUBMITTED TO THE INVESTIGATOR*

Where procedure was performed:		
Private office	0	0.0%
Hospital	1139	100.0%
Type of anesthesia:		
Local anesthesia	835	73.3%
General anesthesia	178	15.6%
Intravenous anesthesia	161	14.1%
Immediate complications:		
Severe edema	13	1.1%
Respiratory obstruction	13	1.1%
Drift or misplacement of Teflon®	22	1.9%
Excessive injection	65	5.7%
Other	17	1.4%
Long-term complications:		
Carcinoma of the vocal cord	1	<0.1%
Granuloma of the vocal cord	4	0.3%
Failure to improve voice	46	4.0%
Other	1	<0.1%
Success rate (indicated by no. of patients)		
Poor voice quality	39	3.4%
Fair voice quality	89	7.8%
Good voice quality	246	21.5%
Excellent voice quality	389	34.1%

* Note that not all questions were answered by the investigators.

(air wastage), aperiodicity of vocal cord movement, and poor formant structure. Our observations agree. We add an illustration of a cough sonagram before and after glycerin was injected to improve cough effectiveness (Figs. 5, 6).

Our data presents:

1. Male/female ratio
2. Age at time of injection
3. Duration of laryngeal dysfunction
4. Primary presenting complaints
5. Type of anesthesia
6. Immediate results (24-hour impression of voice)
7. Second injection required
8. Current status
9. Causes of death (when known)

We, therefore, offer a source of information which can be used as a reference background for the future of many workers in this vineyard, including those who may wish to modify or improve this procedure. It would be of value as a source of information to determine the appropriate expectations within a given case. The information acquired therefore becomes a substitute for experience to a new operator in this field.

RESEARCH DATA

Similarities and differences between the author's series and those of other investigators are of interest. Some can be accounted for by differences in the patient population group. An example is illustrative. In the author's series, 63 cases of a total of 218 were done at a veterans' hospital. This population is predominantly male, more elderly, heavy smoking, and therefore would have an expected higher incidence of carcinoma of the lung. Such indeed is

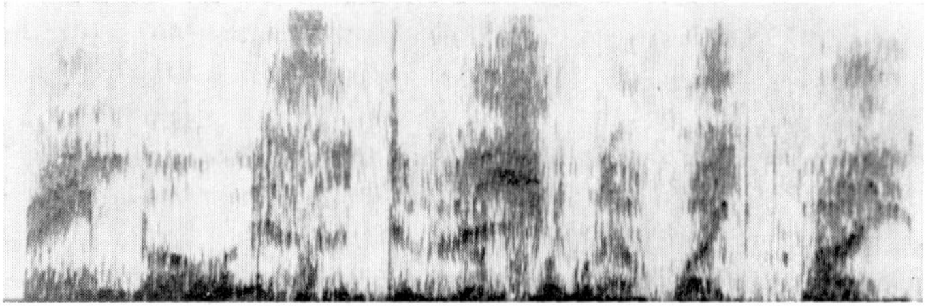

Fig. 1. Sonagram failure – postoperative.

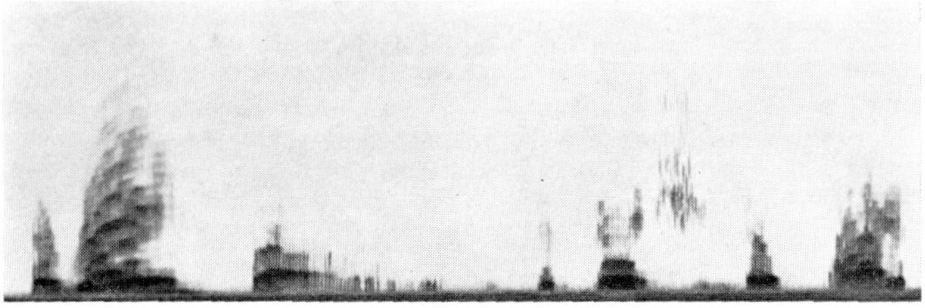

Fig. 2. Sonagram success – postoperative.

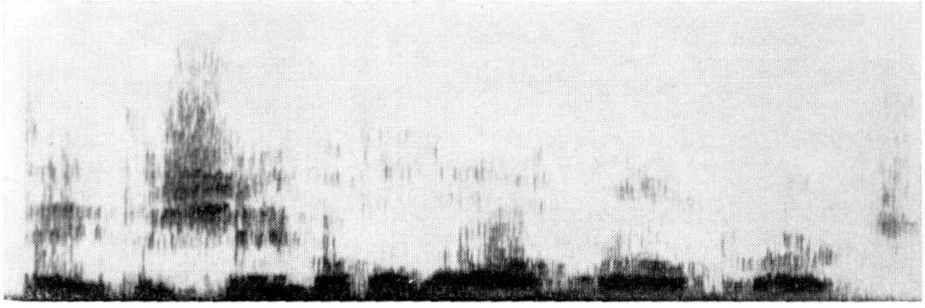

Fig. 3. Preoperative recording, wide band "takes the shape of a long, round arch." Note the lack of individual clarity of vibrations, formants and harmonics.

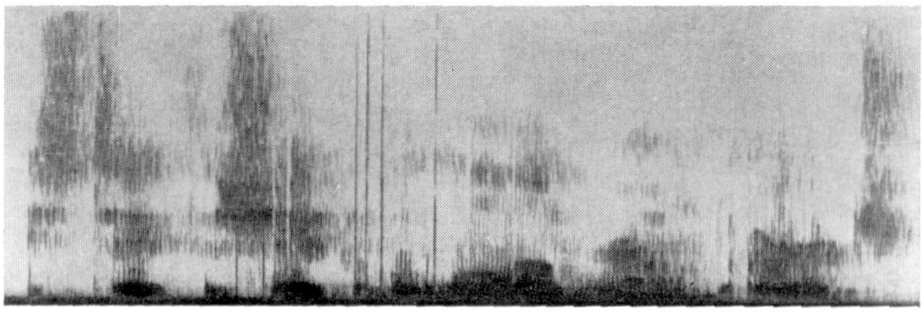

Fig. 4. Postoperative recording, wide band. "Takes the shape of a long, round arch." Note individual clarity of vibrations, formants and harmonics.

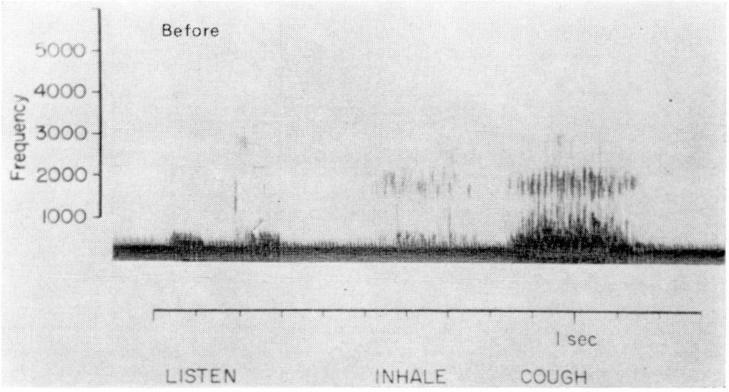

Fig. 5. Time measurement of cough *before* injection.

the case, 16.3% (author's series) as compared with 6.9% (other investigators' series). In idiopathic causes (viral?): the author's series led the list at 16.7%, other workers', 13.6%.

In both series, the commonest causes of the paralysis were the same: idiopathic, carcinoma of the lung, and thyroid surgery, with thyroid surgery as the commonest cause of recurrent laryngeal nerve paralysis in other investigators' series (Table III).

Of considerable interest are newer surgical procedures and diagnostic techniques, represented in incidence of mediastinal surgery, cardiac surgery and pacemaker implant procedures as causes.

The combined statistics disclose a total of 18 cases associated with mediastinal surgery, therefore, this is a standard risk of this procedure. The association with metastasis of carcinoma of the breast should be noted. Also noteworthy is the risk in surgery of diverticulum of the esophagus by transcervical approach (nine cases).

The risk to the recurrent laryngeal nerve (eight cases) in thoracic aortic aneurysm surgery is also very real. Thus, it is evident that some modern surgical procedures can contribute to the problem.

In the author's research, most of the figures speak for themselves and only an occasional comment seems in order. Male/female ratio was greater than two to one. This was perhaps because of higher incidence of carcinoma of the lung in the male. Age at time of injection varied from age 9 to 83. This is a tribute to the easy applicability of the procedure. Maximum duration of paralysis was 35 years, yet with excellent voice result.

The most frequent indication for in-

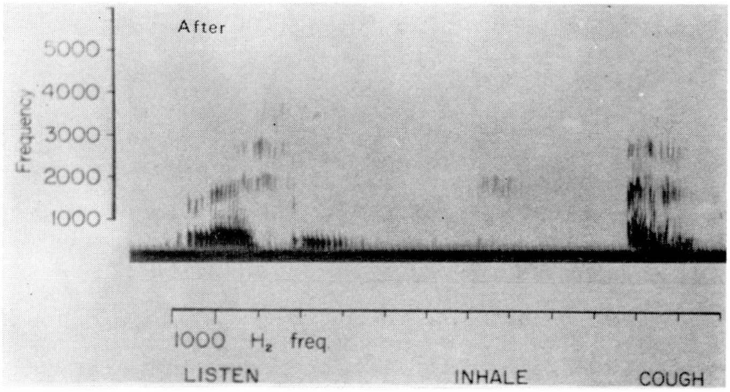

Fig. 6. Time measurement of cough *after* injection.

TABLE III

CAUSES OF VOCAL CORD DYSFUNCTION

Causes	*Author*		*Other Investigators*	
Head:				
Brain injury	4	2.1%	15	1.3%
Vascular accident	2	1.1%	9	0.7%
Neck:				
Thyroid surgery	24	13.0%	254	22.3%
Radical neck surgery	6	3.0%	23	2.0%
Diverticulum of esophagus surgery	2	1.1%	7	0.6%
Bowed cords (congenital or acquired)	8	4.1%	21	1.8%
Cordectomy	12	5.6%	34	1.8%
Gun-shot wound	1	0.5%	11	0.9%
Auto accident	10	5.4%	13	1.1%
Thyroid tumors	2	1.1%	6	0.5%
Neck trauma	4	2.2%	13	1.1%
Deformed cord	4	2.2%	7	0.6%
Carcinoma of esophagus	2	1.1%	7	0.6%
Chemodectoma	4	2.2%	4	0.3%
Carcinoma of vocal cord	4	2.2%	31	2.7%
Neurilemoma	2	1.1%	10	0.8%
Foreign body in larynx	1	0.5%	1	<0.1%
Chest:				
Mediastinal pathology	1	0.5%	6	0.5%
Sarcoidosis	2	1.1%	5	0.4%
Tuberculosis	1	0.5%	8	0.7%
Mediastinal surgery	2	1.1%	16	1.4%
Carcinoma of lung	30	16.3%	79	6.9%
Enlarged heart	2	1.1%	2	0.1%
Aortic aneurysm	3	1.6%	5	0.4%
Carcinoma of breast	4	2.2%	6	0.5%
Pneumonia	2	1.1%	0	0.0%
Lipoma of bronchus	3	1.6%	0	0.0%
Cardiac arrest and surgery	2	1.1%	5	0.4%
Chest crush	2	1.1%	0	0.0%
Pacemaker implant	2	1.1%	0	0.0%
Neurological:				
Poliomyelitis	2	1.1%	2	0.3%
Parkinson's disease	2	1.1%	0	0.0%
Meningitis	1	0.5%	1	<0.1%
Other Causes:				
Idiopathic	31	17.3%	156	13.6%

jection (143 cases to 1) was the hoarse, weak, breathy voice.

The anesthesia used is of note with the exception of one child and two other especially difficult cases. One hundred and thirty-two patients were operated upon, using a topical, local anesthesia, with Innovar®*, deliberately maintaining the patient's consciousness. This proved safe. The phonatory co-operation of the patient was invaluable in controlling the amount of injected

* McNeil Laboratories, Inc., Fort Washington, PA.

substance as well as the location of implant of the material.

Absolute precision was not always possible. This accounted for a series of 18 failures and subsequent second injections. However, a stabilized laryngoscope was used routinely.

All procedures of the author's series and the other investigators' series were performed in the hospital. Considering that direct laryngoscopy was the usual approach (Dedo's work[6] was the principal exception to this), this was logical. It was an essential safety factor in protecting against edema which challenged the airway.

The most frequent complication in the author's series and that of the other investigators was failure to improve the voice. In both, however, the success rate was above 90%. Any reasonable voice improvement was considered a success.

As for immediate results, the 24-hour impression of voice by author was excellent in 15 cases, good in 42 cases, fair in one case and poor in 3 cases. An occasional immediate result was almost perfect and lasted.

Within 24 hours, there was usually edema of the vocal cord, aryepiglottic fold, and the arytenoid on the injected side of the larynx. Therefore, it was impossible to make a prognosis on the basis of the immediate result. It was five days, on the average, before the edema subsided and the expected result could be evaluated. Infrequently, a longer wait was required.

Atrophy of the vocal cord, far-lateral position of the vocal cord, small larynx, marked hypertrophy of the false cords, were contributing factors of that group in which a second injection was required.

It could be fairly stated that the procedure shortened the life of no one and improved the life of more than 90%. It is believed that the patients' lives were lengthened, breathing efficiency was improved, and aspiration was prevented.

One of the excellent aspects of this study was the cooperation received from accredited investigators throughout the United States. There was a high correspondence in the results. It increased by 1139 cases, the number of cases in which information was obtained.

There are some differences. The other investigators had a higher percentage of general anesthesia. There is a frequent disagreement among otolaryngologists on this issue. The opinion depends in part upon the circumstances in which a physician was originally trained and conditioned.

The incidence and types of immediate complications, *i.e.,* severe edema, respiratory obstruction, drift, and misplacement, corresponded in both series. This author's series had no reports of excessive injection, but other investigators reported 65 cases, or 5.7%. There was, of course, a substantial failure to improve voice in 46 cases. This is only 4.0% of 1139 cases, therefore represents a 96% success rate.

Some patients reported that they were forced to change occupations temporarily; a teacher became a librarian, a cantor gave up his singing, a minister gave up his pulpit. All these and others returned to their previous occupations after augmentation therapy.

The most prominent of all symptoms was the inability to talk with ease. This had the corresponding difficulty of inability to be well heard and well understood. Outstanding too, was the inability to strain, inefficiency of breathing, inability to laugh, problems with swallowing food, including aspiration and cough.

The test of voice improvement is the accuracy of pronunciation of phrases and of sentences as a result of the implant. Using these criteria, a large group of tapes were studied by two research associates. Eighty-two before and after injection procedure voice tapes were evaluated. These were classified success, intermediate, or failure. This subjective analysis resulted in a 69% success rate.

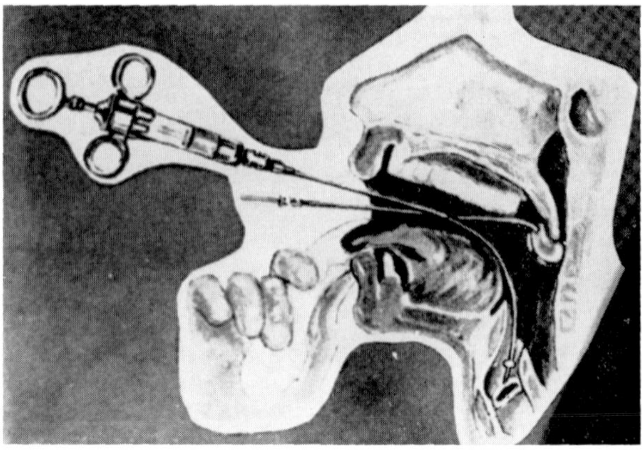

Fig. 8. Sagittal section indicating indirect method glycerin vocal cord injection.

COMPLICATIONS

One of the gratifying elements of this study was the low incidence of complications. The term, complications, requires some definition. We define complications as events that developed which required additional actions.

There were two immediate complications in our own series of 218 cases in which we found excessive swelling requiring a tracheotomy. There were two improper placements of material.

In the reports of the other investigators, there was one of carcinoma of the vocal cord, 22 cases of the Teflon® being misplaced, and 13 cases of respiratory obstruction.

There were no fatalities. The end results were excellent. All other problems were corrected by repeat procedure or by removal of granulations or the Teflon® granuloma palpable under the skin.

Of special note is the one reported carcinoma. It is clearly established that the patient had carcinoma of the larynx. There is substantial doubt that the carcinoma had any relationship to the Teflon®, itself, except that it occurred after the Teflon® injection. The patient was a heavy smoker and contrary to doctor's advice, continued to smoke. The carcinoma was found some distance from the Teflon® location. Progressive histopathologic tissue changes were evident on microscopic study but distant from the location of the implant material.

In another study, published by this author,[11] coronal sections were taken of a larynx in which Teflon® had been implanted 14 months earlier. The larynx was removed postmortem and studied by four pathologists whose opinions agreed. The tissues showed no signs of carcinogenesis. A healed, mild, inflammatory process, a very thin, marginal capsule, and a few giant cells in the substance of the vocalis muscle tissue plus the granular Teflon® could be observed (Fig. 7).

Of all cases reported, therefore, only one could be interpreted as having any neoplastic relationship to the result of the Teflon®.

Work,[15] in a statistical review of paralysis and paresis of the vocal cord, refers to three cases of unusual causation. One of the three cases was pneumonectomy because of a diagnosis of neoplasm of the lung. At the present time, pneumonectomy, partial pneumonectomy, or carcinoma of the lung, have become common causes of recurrent laryngeal nerve paralysis, the first two because of the great progress in thoracic surgery, the last because of tragedies subsequent to tobacco smoking and perhaps environmental pollution.

EXTENSION AND NEW IDEAS

With needle implantation of the Teflon®-glycerin mixture into the vocal

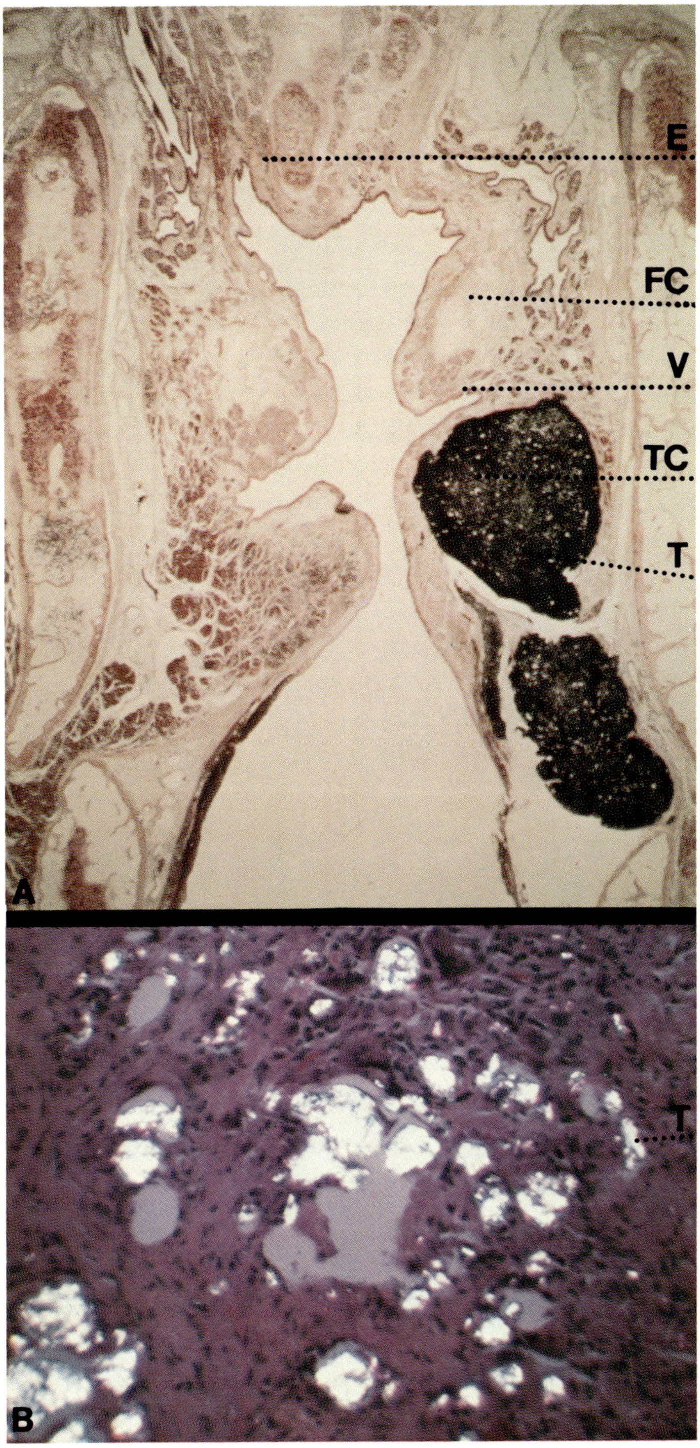

Fig. 7. A) Coronal section of larynx showing Teflon® *in situ*. E - Epiglottis. TC - True cord. FC - False cord. V - Ventricle. T - Teflon®. B) Teflon® granuloma under polarized light; bright particles are Teflon® granules.

cord as a basis, three additional useful procedures have developed (Fig. 8). Two are mentioned in passing. The first is the closure of the velopalatine gap in which there is air escapage. This is far simpler than pharyngeal surgery and it is equally or more effective.

The second procedure[16] is often helpful in Teflon® injection of the tubotubarious area for the problems associated with chronic, excessive patency of the Eustachian tube opening.

The third procedure reported by Lewy and Mathews[10] is the injection of sterile glycerin of a newly paralyzed vocal cord where the recurrent laryngeal nerve was sacrificed in chest surgery. This has, therefore, reduced the need for a protective cleansing type of tracheotomy. Occasionally, the paralyzed vocal cord has remained in the midline as a result of glycerin injection, and no further Teflon® implantation has been required.

This can be a bedside or a clinic procedure with a curved needle and indirect laryngoscopy. It can, when necessary, be done via the direct laryngoscopy. A three-ringed glass syringe is used, to give a good grip and to avoid glycerin leakage. Because of the lower viscosity of glycerin, the Brunings' syringe (pistol grip) is not desirable.

CONCLUSIONS

1. The combination of particulate Teflon® (tetrafluoroethylene polymer) and glycerin as an augmentation implant seems well established.

2. The procedure is usually not difficult. It is well tolerated by patients of any age, via direct laryngoscopy.

3. There is limited immediate foreign body tissue reaction.

4. Continuing long term residence of the implant *in situ* without cancerogenic responses is the rule.

5. There are minimal manageable complications on immediate or long-term basis.

6. Re-establishment of impaired voice quality and the other physiological functions of the laryngeal valve occurs in a very high percentage of cases.

7. Pulmonary protection from aspiration and improved oxygen utilization is the rule.

8. These statements are supported by statistical analysis of long-term patient reports and the parallel evaluation of results of other investigators.

REFERENCES

1. Brünings W: Über eine neue Behandlungsmethode der Rekurrenslähmung. Verhandl Ver Dtsch Laryngol 18:93-151, 1911

2. Arnold GE: Vocal rehabilitation of paralytic dysphonia. IX Technique of intrachordal injection. Arch Otolaryngol 76:358-368, 1962

3. Arnold GE: Vocal rehabilitation of paralytic dysphonia. X Functional results of intrachordal injection. Arch Otolaryngol 78: 179-186, 1963

4. Arnold GE: Alleviation of aphonia or dysphonia through intrachordal injection of teflon paste. Ann Otol Rhinol Laryngol 72: 384-395, 1963

5. Kirchner FR, Toledo PS, Svoboda DJ: Studies of the larynx after teflon injection. Arch Otolaryngol 83:350-354, 1966

6. Dedo HH, Urrea RD, Lawson L: Intrachordal injection of Teflon® in the treatment of 135 patients with dysphonia. Ann Otol Rhinol Laryngol 82:661-667, 1973

7. Rubin HJ: Misadventures with injectable polytef (teflon). Arch Otolaryngol 101: 114-116, 1975

8. Lewy RB: Glottic rehabilitation with teflon injection — the return of voice, cough and laughter. Acta Otolaryngol (Stockh) 58: 214-220, 1964

9. Lewy RB: Glottic reformation with voice rehabilitation in vocal cord paralysis: the injection of teflon and tantalum. Laryngoscope 73:547-555, 1963

10. Lewy RB, Mathews R: Immediate temporary restoration of glottic valve function. Laryngoscope 75:1348-1351, 1965

11. Lewy RB: Responses of laryngeal tissue to granular teflon in situ. Arch Otolaryngol 83:355-359, 1966

12. Lewy RB: Tracheotomy avoidance: glycerine vocal cord injection. Arch Otolaryngol 92:502-504, 1970

13. von Leden H, Yanagihara N, Werner-Kukuk E: Teflon in unilateral vocal cord paralysis: preoperative and postoperative function studies. Arch Otolaryngol 85:666-674, 1967

14. Rontal E, Rontal M, Rolnick MI: The use of spectrograms in the evaluation of vocal cord injection. Laryngoscope 85:47-56, 1975

15. Work WP: Paralysis and paresis of the vocal cords. Arch Otolaryngol 34:267-280, 1941

16. Pulec JL: Abnormally patent eustachian tubes: treatment with injection of polytetrafluoroethylene (teflon) paste. Laryngoscope 77:1543-1554, 1967

ACKNOWLEDGMENT—The author would like to thank Dr. A. J. Derbyshire, Gayle Burgess, Lee Hamilton, Charles Gerlach and Audio-visual Services, Department of Otolaryngology for their assistance in various aspects of this project.

REPRINTS—Robert B. Lewy, MD, 25 East Washington St., Chicago, IL 60602.

Ann Otol 85: 1976

RECURRENT LARYNGEAL NERVE SECTION FOR SPASTIC DYSPHONIA

HERBERT H. DEDO, MD

SAN FRANCISCO, CALIFORNIA

SUMMARY – Spastic dysphonia is a severe vocal disability in which a person speaks with excessively adducted vocal cords. The resulting weak phonation sounds tight, as if he were being strangled, and has also been described as laryngeal stutter. It is often accompanied by face and neck grimaces. In the past it has been regarded as psychoneurotic in origin and treated with speech therapy and psychotherapy with disappointing results. Because of laboratory and clinical observation that recurrent nerve paralysis retracts the involved vocal cord from the midline, it was proposed that deliberate section of the recurrent nerve would improve the vocal quality of patients with spastic dysphonia. In 34 patients the recurrent nerve was sectioned after Xylocaine® temporary paralysis showed significant improvement in vocal quality. Several patients have been advised against this operation because of the type of voice they developed with one vocal cord temporarily paralyzed. With nerve section plus postoperative speech therapy, approximately half of the patients have returned close to a "normal" but soft phonatory voice. The rest had varying degrees of improvement, but all, so far, have been pleased with the improvement in ease and quality of phonation and reduction or elimination of face and neck grimaces. Two men have a breathy component in their phonatory voices, and one woman has variable pitch.

The first description of a spastic form of psychogenic hoarseness was made by Traube[1] in 1871. Four years later the Viennese laryngologist, Schnitzler,[2] provided a detailed description of spastic dysphonia and coined the diagnostic term. Berendes[3] defined spastic dysphonia as a disorder of phonation which is characterized by a strained, creaking, and choked vocal attack, a tense and squeezed voice sound which is accompanied by extreme tension of the entire phonatory system. He noted that the stressed vowels may be broken into two portions and that the disorder disturbs primarily the communicative function of speech with variations in intensity. Often the patient can speak to himself, whisper, laugh, achieve a falsetto singing tone and sometimes phonate isolated vowels or whole sentences with a normal phonatory voice. During indirect laryngoscopy, the structure of the larynx and vocal cords appears normal. While silent respiration is normal, the frustrated vocal effort causes severe obstruction to expiration of air from the lungs causing aching fatigue of the upper anterior chest muscles.

Spastic dysphonia has been repeatedly described as "stuttering with vocal cords."[3] It is often accompanied by associated spastic or grimacing type contractions of the neck and facial muscles, causing complete closing of the eyes at times. In some people there is superimposed stuttering of the lips and tongue and palate as an extreme form of an already serious disability. It ordinarily starts in people over the age of 40 years, but one patient in our series had the onset in her 20s.

Virtually all of the contributors to this subject in the last hundred years have stated that spastic dysphonia is an expression of psychoneurosis. According to the early psychiatric teaching, such conditions were regarded as hysterical.[1] In a most exhaustive review by Ber-

----

From the Department of Otolaryngology, University of California, San Francisco, San Francisco, California.

Presented in part at the meeting of the American Laryngological Association, Palm Beach, Florida, April 24-25, 1976.

endes in 1939, spastic dysphonia was regarded as a typical neurosis without hysterical traits.[3] Robe *et al*[4] and Aronson *et al*[5,6] were among the exceptional authors who suggested that spastic dysphonia is due to some organic pathology of the nervous system, rather than hysteria or psychogenic disorder or reaction to stress. These investigators also were among the few who admitted the singular ineffectiveness of voice therapy and psychotherapy in spastic dysphonia.

Multiple treatments have been tried without achieving consistent permanent cure of vocal spasticity. Brodnitz comments that psychotherapy has not been too helpful.[7] It may help the patient to gain better insight into his psychological background but he still will exhibit a marked degree of dysphonia; only one of his patients improved "significantly." He adds that it is one of the characteristics of the disorder that many of the patients react violently to the suggestion of psychiatric counseling. One only has to give such advice to lose the patient immediately. Brodnitz further states that voice training alone has proved to be of only very limited value. Cooper reported that of 41 patients, 22 entered speech therapy and only 6 of them completed therapy with results described as excellent – one; good – three; and fair – one.[8] Even this much improvement required a minimum of 1½ years. Boone comments that with speech therapy "progress has been erratic and limited, with no one patient experiencing a permanent restoration of normal voice. The problem of spastic dysphonia still remains both a diagnostic and etiologic unknown, which, of course, makes the development of an effective therapeutic approach impossible."[9]

In the spring of 1975 I was asked to see M.Y. in consultation. I feel that because of the special nature of her problem, including the tenacity with which she continued to seek help after 17 years of disappointment, and her willingness to knowingly undergo experimental procedures, she and her husband deserve credit for participating in the discoveries which were made. She had treatment by more than 29 doctors, including laryngologists, speech therapists, psychiatrists, and hypnotists in the United States. She continued to be disabled by severe dysphonia which was accompanied by marked associated grimaces of the face and neck during her attempts to talk. Speech therapists confirmed that their modality could not offer her the chance to return to normal. Because of the disruption of her life caused by her being a vocal cripple, there was considerable encouragement to develop a new approach to help her. I proposed that we again try temporary topical and local paralysis of the internal branch of the superior laryngeal nerve which had earlier given her only partial, temporary relief and if this failed, to test the effects of paralysis of the recurrent nerve. Diligent review of the literature did not provide any support for such a proposal. In fact, the only report of surgery for this disorder was that of Rethi,[10] in which he reported some success in one patient with dividing the stylopharyngeus muscle, which is considerably different than deliberately paralyzing the recurrent laryngeal nerve (RLN).

RATIONALE

Laryngeal research in dogs and humans with electromyography and still and motion pictures has confirmed that paralysis of one recurrent laryngeal nerve in the normal individual not only paralyzes the vocal cord but sets it in the paramedian position so that the normal (unparalyzed) cord fails to reach it as firmly as usual, causing a breathy but often phonatory soft voice.[11] It has long been recognized that the voice can sound nearly normal, although soft in some persons, if the normal vocal cord can compensate by crossing the midline to reach a paralyzed vocal cord. In patients with Teflon®* injections of paralyzed vocal cords, many had a brief period of spas-

* Polytef paste for injection; Mentor Division, Codman & Shurtleff, Inc., Randolph, MA.

tic or tight phonation for a few moments after the injection before the mobile vocal cord quit compensating across the midline. It seemed possible that if a recurrent laryngeal nerve were paralyzed in a patient with spastic dysphonia, the other vocal cord might prove to be "precompensated" so that its excessively strong adduction would carry it across the midline to the deliberately paralyzed cord, giving a relatively normal phonation. After describing the above hypothesis, it was proposed to M.Y. that one recurrent laryngeal nerve be paralyzed temporarily with lidocaine since paralysis of the superior laryngeal nerve had temporarily improved her voice by only 10% or 15%. She and her husband agreed, and to our amazement and delight, once the recurrent nerve had been thoroughly paralyzed by the injection of 1% lidocaine, she was able to talk with a phonatory voice without vocal spasticity. Furthermore, as soon as she found she had a consistent phonatory sound, she was able to stop the neck and facial grimaces and special respiratory efforts. Although her voice at this point had a raspy or husky sound, Dr. Lucie Lawson, speech therapist, was rapidly able to help her raise the pitch and bring the sound "up in the front of her mouth," largely clearing the huskiness. Unfortunately, as soon as the lidocaine wore off, the spasticity of voice and face and neck returned. When this had been repeated four more times with identical results, she and her husband agreed to surgical section of the recurrent nerve to try to make the vocal improvement permanent, even though there was no guarantee what would happen to her voice or psyche. Although she did not appear hysterical or psychoneurotic when her vocal cord was temporarily paralyzed and she was able to phonate properly, there was some trepidation about whether she would develop hysterical phenomena such as paralysis or numbness of a limb, since the literature had stressed the psychiatric etiology of this disease for over a hundred years. However, when the right recurrent nerve was sectioned on September 9, 1975, she had an uneventful convalescence. Her speech and facial movements were dramatically better on awakening from the anesthetic. With speech therapy she regained an essentially normal voice within weeks, and she was able to stop the associated movements of her face or neck. She has now even resumed her political, radio, and television career after an 18-year hiatus.

TREATMENT TECHNIQUE

Diagnosis. There are several different types of spastic dysphonic speech. The basic type has a constant, very tight, hoarse, soft, barely phonatory sound which may vary slightly with fatigue and stress. Several have resorted to a stage whisper voice, inspiratory speech, or even the small buzzer* used by laryngectomees to talk, and when requested to phonate they can only produce a soft, harsh, tight sound low in the back of the throat. A second type has frequent breaks in the tight sound caused by momentary vocal cord abductions which produce a quavering, spastic dysphonic sound low in the back of the throat. Considerable variation in the spasticity can occur in one patient. Some are able to achieve a clear, normal phonatory voice with occasional single words, phrases or sentences. In one patient, within one sentence the voice went from a whisper through clear phonatory, to spastic phonatory, back through clear phonatory to a whisper. (Her spastic dysphonia had been present less than two years, and in the majority of patients who had had the disorder longer than this, the voice did not have such remarkable variability.) There is often throat clearing or groaning phonations made between words in an attempt to obtain a clear phonatory sound. Many of these patients can laugh and sing a falsetto musical note or phonate some vowels such as "e" and "o" with a clear phonatory sound. There is considerable variation between patients on the amount of associated grimacing

* Western Electric buzzer available through local telephone company.

movements of the face and neck and oral tics which they have, similar to that of a severe oral stutterer. Indirect laryngoscopy ordinarily shows that there are no lesions on the vocal cords. Naturally it is essential to rule out benign or malignant tumors of the vocal cords and unilateral or bilateral voice cord paralysis by indirect laryngoscopy before proceeding.

Two patients were noted to have mobile vocal cords which were bowed during phonation but created a spastic type of phonation. Although the initial reaction was that Teflon® injection was indicated as with previous patients with bowed mobile vocal cords and breathy voices,[12] it was found that paralysis of one recurrent laryngeal nerve with lidocaine dramatically improved the voice by clearing the spasticity. However, this made the voice worse in one patient with bowed mobile cords during phonation and a breathy voice. Therefore, it appears that patients with spastic dysphonia *and* bowed mobile vocal cords during phonation actually have adopted the technique of cricothyroid relaxation in their attempts to achieve a nonspastic voice. They can benefit by recurrent nerve section if indicated by lidocaine test paralysis. Teflon® injection of *one* vocal cord should be reserved for bowed mobile vocal cord with *breathy* phonation.[12]

Preoperative Evaluation. The voice is tape-recorded and evaluated by a speech therapist and the surgeon. Temporary paralysis is then achieved by injecting 1% lidocaine, 3-6 ml adjacent to the cricothyroid joint. Paralysis is then confirmed after two to four minutes by repeat indirect laryngoscopy. The risks of this lidocaine, of course, are explained to the patient. Although they are unlikely, they include the possibility of severing the nerve with the needle, entering the carotid artery or jugular vein or the trachea. The temporary paralysis wears off in 7 to 30 minutes, sometimes before the patient can break through the old speech therapy relaxation training and hear and feel the improvement.

The patient must be prepared to accept this voice as the minimum achievable voice after surgery in case speech therapy does not achieve maximum potential improvement. As soon as the recurrent nerve has been temporarily paralyzed, the voice is tape-recorded again and the speech therapist, the surgeon and the patient decide whether enough improvement has been obtained to justify permanent section of the recurrent laryngeal nerve. Ordinarily these procedures are performed on the right side because the laryngeal nerves and vocal cords are symmetrical and it is technically preferable on the right. Several patients have been refused recurrent nerve section because they or the surgeon were not satisfied they had achieved the typical and proper change in their voice. The voice change during lidocaine paralysis differs somewhat from that obtained after permanent recurrent nerve paralysis. This is because the adjacent external branch of the superior laryngeal nerve and therefore the right cricothyroid muscle is often paralyzed by the lidocaine but not the surgery. (This is shown by posterior rotation of the larynx to the left.) They often have a temporary Horner's syndrome and a "lump" sensation in the throat during lidocaine paralysis which disconcerts them during the usual 10 to 15 minutes they have to determine whether the recurrent laryngeal nerve paralysis should be made permanent. Thus, the temporary lidocaine paralysis only approximates the vocal improvement which can be obtained by recurrent nerve section. However, even though this has usually been exceeded by surgical division of one recurrent nerve, especially when supplemented by speech therapy, it is emphasized that the voice, while likely to be improved, will not necessarily be completely normal after permanent section.

Surgical Technique. Under general anesthesia a collar incision is made one finger-breadth below the cricoid cartilage. Dissection is carried down to the anterior surface of the trachea and around its right side to the tracheoesophageal groove. The recurrent nerve is identified ordinarily at the level of the inferior pole of the right thyroid gland 1 cm lateral to the trachea. It is sometimes necessary for adequate exposure to divide the isthmus and resect the upper portion of the thyroid gland off of the trachea with resultant extra bleeding. Direct laryngoscopy is then performed so that the right vocal cord can be observed while an assistant crushes the presumed recurrent nerve with a hemostat. If the vocal cord contracts abruptly at the instant of crushing, the structure is presumed to be the whole recurrent nerve and is ligated with a 2-0 silk ligature. A 1 cm segment is then removed adjacent to the inferior pole of the thyroid gland about 3 - 4 cm below the cricoid. Care needs to be taken to avoid injury to the trachea, thyroid gland, parathyroid glands, carotid artery, cervical esophagus, cervical sympathetics and, especially to the recurrent nerve on the other side. (It is possible to dissect through the party wall between the trachea and esophagus and reach the left recurrent laryngeal nerve.) It is *not* necessary or desirable to section both recurrent nerves. Care must also be taken to avoid injury to the innominate artery and vein which are nearby in the upper mediastinum in some patients.

The incision is closed with gut subcutaneous sutures and Steri-strips®* to the skin with a drain in place. A pressure dressing is installed. When the endotracheal tube is removed and the patient awakens, it is usually possible to hear marked improvement in the voice, even in the recovery room. One exception was a patient in whom a small amount of arytenoid and vocal cord edema resulted from the intubation or direct laryngoscopy so that an injection of cortisone was necessary, and improvement was delayed for several days.

RESULTS

We have now temporarily paralyzed the right recurrent laryngeal nerve in 41 patients and have surgically sectioned 34 recurrent laryngeal nerves. All of these patients have been pleased with the improvement (loss of spasticity) in their voices and decrease or clearance of associated tics and grimaces. However, several of the patients have spoken with a mild residual hoarseness (huskiness or raspiness or a soft low pitch), and one has had some intermittent mild spastic phonation and pitch variability after surgery. Two have breathy but phonatory voices when tired or they have to push their voices in a noisy environment. Although clarity of tone, good pitch control and elimination of associated face, neck and chest movements (grimaces, tics, oral stuttering, and chest muscle fatigue) have been achieved by some patients spontaneously after surgery, most have benefited by speech therapy varying from a few days to several weeks. So far there has been no reversion to the severe preoperative spastic dysphonia and no hysterical conversions. Three patients had been receiving psychotherapy, including one who had a complete nervous breakdown five months before surgery and two who had attempted suicide. They are reported by their psychiatrists as doing much better because the disability of spastic dysphonia had been causing or increasing their emotional disturbances, rather than the reverse situation which has generally been the one described in the literature.

DISCUSSION

Etiology. If the etiology for a disorder is unknown, it is ordinarily blamed on psychoneurotic reaction to stress, or on viruses, or on allergy. In the past, most authors stated that spastic dysphonia was caused by emotional stress.[13] This just increased the patient's problems and resentments because psychotherapy has been singularly ineffective in treating this disorder. Psychotherapy should be used, if necessary, for other emotional problems which may be present, but not in an attempt to treat the spastic dysphonic since it has not been useful in the past. It just adds to these patients' problems by suggesting they are benefiting from their terrible speech dis-

* 3M, Minnesota Mining and Manufacturing Co., St. Paul, MN.

ability and they can talk normally if they just will try.

The fanciful psychodynamics in the psychiatric reports sent with these patients is incredible. It is interesting that when Aronson[5,6] used the Minnesota Multiphasic Personality Test (MMPT) to evaluate patients with spastic dysphonia, he found a lower incidence of repressed anger and compulsive personality traits than were present in the general medical population at Mayo Clinic. This whole concept that spastic dysphonia was due to hysteria or psychoneurosis apparently was based on the clinical observation that even though these patients could get a clear phonatory sound with singing and laughing, they spoke with spastic dysphonia when required to talk "with emotional content."[1] Furthermore, the spasticity was variable and, in some, increased with stress or fatigue or seemed to start originally after some special stress. Therefore, it was assumed that this was a conscious attempt to penalize family members or coworkers and that all that was necessary was to trick or analyze the patient out of the problem. This was reinforced by occasional observations that spastic dysphonic patients could speak with a clear, phonatory voice while awakening from general anesthesia or if they were plied with enough alcohol to make them drunk. None of these are useful observations since it is not possible to remain in a drunken or drugged state from alcohol or general anesthetic agents and to continue to function with full effectiveness. In fact, in discussions with psychiatrists who were seeing three of these patients, they readily agreed that the spastic dysphonia had increased the emotional problems rather than the emotional problems being the cause of the spastic dysphonia.

Only a few authors have suggested that spastic dysphonia was caused by organic disorder of the neuromuscular system. Moore and his coworkers[4] found that 10 of 14 patients with spastic dysphonia had abnormal electroencephalograms. Aronson *et al*[5,6] then exhaustively reviewed 31 spastic dysphonia patients seen at Mayo Clinic. Of 27 patients given neurologic examinations, 20 had one or more neurologic signs, including tremor, hyperreflexia, reduced alternate motion rate and faciolingual asymmetries. (Only one of our patients has had organic neurologic defects elsewhere, and her spinocerebellar degeneration was far advanced before spastic dysphonia appeared.) These signs occurred with greater frequency than would be expected in normal population. They hypothesized that spastic dysphonia has a neurologic substrate and may be related to the essential tremor syndrome. Of the 29 patients given psychiatric interviews, 18 were judged to have some emotional problems, and 11 did not. Although as a group they gave the impression of being compulsive, of overcontrolling their anger, and of being quite unaggressive verbally, it is suggested that these traits are not exclusively characteristic of spastic dysphonia. It should be remembered that these traits are present in a vast number of people who show no signs of spastic dysphonia.

I would now like to suggest that this disease is caused by a disturbance in the proprioceptive control of the vocal cords. Specifically, it is proposed that neurotropic viral infection damages the a & c fibers either peripherally or in the central nervous system while sparing the larger diameter motor nerve fibers to the intrinsic laryngeal muscles. Neurotropic viral injury of the large motor nerve fibers is invoked for many cases of paralysis of the facial nerve causing Bell's palsy. Viral damage of the large motor nerve fibers unilaterally or bilaterally is given as the present best explanation of spontaneous recurrent laryngeal nerve paralysis. Proprioceptive control of the vocal cord muscles is poorly understood because even with electroneurophysiology techniques now available, it is difficult to study in the normal human and dog. Furthermore, there is no good animal model for spastic dysphonia. It is interesting that over half of these patients had a clinically apparent viral illness of the respiratory or gastrointestinal system at, or shortly before, the onset of spastic dysphonia. In fact, it was easier to elicit this than a history of specific stress at or about the time of onset. One patient had poliomyelitis some time before, and one had a temporary partial paralysis of the right facial nerve which started at the same time as the spastic dysphonia. An advantage of using this hypothesis is that there is no specific treatment for viral infection so the patient's money is not wasted on psychotherapy.

It is striking that these patients do not appear hysterical or emotionally disturbed after the recurrent laryngeal nerve has been cut and they are able to resume reasonably normal phonation. In every patient a control injection to test the Psychoneurotic Etiology Hypothesis was performed by injecting Xylocaine®* subcutaneously and beside the cricoid cartilage or for two to four minutes after placing it on the nerve sheath. There was no change in the voice even though the patient was unable to see precisely where the Xylocaine® was being placed. The spasticity left the voice only when the recurrent laryngeal nerve became fully paralyzed by the lidocaine, as confirmed by indirect laryngoscopy. Furthermore, the spasticity returned as soon as the lidocaine began to wear off, in spite of the fact that these patients did not know exactly how long the lidocaine effect would last. If their spastic dysphonia were on a voluntary or hysterical basis, at least some of them would have cleared with the combination of suggestion, and an injection of a powerful medicine in the neck or the improvement should have lasted after the lidocaine wore off. Only one patient has had an hysterical manifestation elsewhere in the body (a brief glove anesthesia of one hand one month before surgery). None have had postoperative hysterical conversion reactions or increase in emotional problems. In fact, there has been a striking decrease in manifestation of emotional disorders after their voices have returned to normal or to even near-normal status. Intensive speech therapy during temporary lidocaine paralysis of the vocal cord did not achieve permanent resolution of the spastic dysphonia in a single patient. Associated movements of the face, neck and throat, clearing of the throat, whisper voice, bowed mobile vocal cords during phonation, and even use of a W.E. Buzzer to achieve phonation were all caused by conscious attempts to achieve phonatory sound. When consistent, reliable glottic phonation became possible and apparent to these patients after lidocaine injections and later when recurrent laryngeal nerve section had repositioned the cord, these associated problems usually cleared rapidly. If the patient had really been trying to use the disease for psychological or social reasons, these voluntary manifestations would be expected to continue or to increase. Usually after section of the recurrent laryngeal nerve, the pitch is low "in the back of the throat," showing they were trying to relax the vocal cords before the paralysis.

There is no reliable clinical or experimental evidence for classifying spastic dysphonia as a psychoneurotic or hysterical disease. In fact, it just causes time and money to be wasted on psychotherapy, at least for the vocal disorder itself, and it increases the patient's guilt and emotional stress. Proprioceptive disturbance by neurotropic viral infection has as solid a theoretical and clinical basis as psychoneurosis and causes less expense (for ineffective psychotherapy) and less social opprobrium.

Treatment. Psychotherapy, allergy treatment, hypnosis, acupuncture, special diets, vitamins, cortisone and tranquilizers had all been tried repeatedly on these patients and have no place in the treatment of spastic dysphonia. Speech therapy before recurrent laryngeal nerve section had only helped *some* patients *partially* and then it took 1½ years or more at considerable cost and constant deliberate effort which always continued to be necessary.

---

* Astra Pharmaceutical Products, Inc., Worcester, MA.

The speech therapists who have seen this group of patients have now agreed that speech therapy is not useful or effective if spastic dysphonia has been present three months or more. In fact, we are still looking for an established spastic dysphonic who has been returned to a normal voice by speech therapy. Therefore, patients in whom spastic dysphonia has been present more than three months are advised to have the lidocaine paralysis test of the RLN, and if there is the typical improvement in the voice, a RLN section. The advantage of this approach is that the RLN can be paralyzed temporarily with lidocaine before the surgery so the patient and family can determine whether they wish to make it permanent. This kind of inexpensive diagnostic test is not possible with any of the other modalities, such as speech therapy alone, psychotherapy, hypnosis, acupuncture, special diets, tranquilizers, allergy treatment and cortisone shots. The surgery is a low risk, general anesthetic procedure and is rapidly effective in one or two hours, instead of one or more years. Postoperative speech therapy is provided when the patient is not able to spontaneously return to a relatively normal, clear, soft phonatory voice. The chest muscle fatigue (from pushing against the tightly closed glottis during phonation) is eliminated. Most importantly, these persons are able to stop being vocal cripples and even to forget about their voices and just proceed to talk. It is not necessary for them to make an enormous effort to learn to speak in an unnatural way. In fact, the biggest problem in resuming "normal" phonatory speech so far has been in the patients who have had the most effective preoperative speech therapy or who have developed a lot of associated movements in their desperate attempt to speak. Even the worst of these, however, were dramatically better within minutes after the lidocaine injection and within an hour after surgery (*i.e.*, as soon as they were awake enough to talk in the recovery room).

Theoretically, a vocal cord could also be repositioned slightly away from the midline and preserve the recurrent nerve by placing a silk suture between the arytenoid and the thyroid ala. Since there is a limit to how far the mobile cord can adduct, this would tie it back so the mobile one could just reach it at the end of its excursion, preventing the overtight closure and vocal spasticity. However, it is more difficult to reposition a cord in the ideal paramedian position with a tie-back suture than by sectioning a recurrent nerve. Furthermore, the suture would soon cut through the cartilage because of the strong persistent adduction, which is not present in the patients who require Woodman operations for bilateral recurrent nerve paralysis. Speech therapy has then improved the voice further when necessary. It is designed to get the patient to do three things:

1. Raise the pitch from the back of the throat ideally to a clear phonatory level (which may well not equal the prespastic dysphonic "normal"). This pitch adjustment is sometimes necessary to minimize or eliminate diplophonia, which is present in some of these patients postoperatively because of the slightly different vocal cord tension on the two sides. (The diplophonia can be minimized or eliminated by matching the mobile vocal cord frequency to that of the paralyzed vocal cord.)

2. Resume normal volume and pressure of air flow through the larynx.

3. Eliminate the associated face and neck movements and throat clearing, which all the patients so far have been able to do rapidly once they were able to achieve reliable, easy laryngeal phonation.

If the vocal cord were to atrophy and move too far from the midline, Teflon® injection could be used to reposition it. If the cord did not end up far enough lateral from the midline to prevent the other vocal cord from reaching it too tightly, a direct laryngoscopy and excision of some of the free edge of the vocal cord could be performed. So far neither of these secondary procedures has been necessary.

The main problem now is getting used to the idea of sectioning a recurrent nerve for a disease widely considered to be psychoneurotic. However, severing the facial nerve for blepharospasm must have been just as shocking initially.

Many of these people have had difficulty retaining jobs and friends and some have become recluses. The satisfying part of this surgical procedure, which has been as dramatic as with many patients after repair of severe hearing loss by stapedectomy, is seeing these patients resume normal, happy lives. Just as stapedectomy can provide a dramatic improvement in hearing and be successful without return to "normal" (0 dB), recurrent nerve section can dramatically improve a spastic dysphonic voice even when it does not return completely to "normal." However, deliberate surgical section to achieve permanent unilateral recurrent nerve paralysis is not yet standard treatment for even as disabling a disease as spastic dysphonia; it should not be done without careful preparation and evaluation.

REFERENCES

1. Traube, cited by Arnold GE: Spastic dysphonia: I. Changing interpretations of a persistent affliction. Logos 2:3-14, 1959

2. Schnitzler, cited by Arnold GE: Spastic dysphonia: I. Changing interpretations of a persistent affliction. Logos 2:3-14, 1959

3. Berendes, cited by Arnold GE: Spastic dysphonia: I. Changing interpretations of a persistent affliction. Logos 2.3-14, 1959

4. Robe E, Brumlik J, Moore P: A study of spastic dysphonia. Neurologic and electroencephalographic abnormalities. Laryngoscope 79:219-245, 1960

5. Aronson AW, Brown JR, Litin EM, *et al*: Spastic dysphonia. I. Voice, neurologic, and psychiatric aspects. J Speech Hear Dis 33:203-218, 1968

6. Aronson AW, Brown JR, Litin EM, *et al*: Spastic dysphonia. II. Comparison with essential (voice) tremor and other neurologic and psychogenic dysphonias. J Speech Hear Dis 33:219-231, 1968

7. Brodnitz FS: Spastic dysphonia. Ann Otol Rhinol Laryngol 85:210-214, 1976

8. Cooper M: *Modern Techniques of Vocal Rehabilitation*, ed 2. Springfield, Ill., Charles C. Thomas, 1974

9. Boone DR: *The Voice and Voice Therapy*. Englewood Cliffs, N.J., Prentice-Hall, Inc., 1971

10. Rethi A: Role des stylopharyngealen muskelsystems im Krankheitsbild der Taschenbandstimme und der dysphonia spastica. Folia Phoniatr (Basel) 4:201-216, 1952

11. Dedo HH: The paralyzed larynx: An electromyographic study in dogs and humans. Laryngoscope 80:1455-1517, 1970

12. Dedo HH, Urrea RD, Lawson L: Intracordal injection of Teflon® in the treatment of 135 patients with dysphonia. Ann Otol Rhinol Laryngol 82:661-667, 1973

13. Bloch P: Neuro-psychiatric aspects of spastic dysphonia. Folia Phoniatr (Basel) 17: 301-364, 1965

ACKNOWLEDGMENTS—The author wishes to express appreciation to Francis A Sooy, MD, Joseph H. Ogura, MD, Roger Boles, MD, and the Nationl Institutes of Health for providing the training, support, and milieu which made this work possible.

REPRINTS—Herbert H. Dedo, MD, Department of Otolaryngology, University of California, 400 Parnassus Ave., San Francisco, CA 94143.

Ann Otol 85: 1976

FIBER COMPONENTS OF THE RECURRENT LARYNGEAL NERVE IN THE CAT

Richard R. Gacek, MD
Michael J. Lyon, MA
Worcester, Massachusetts

SUMMARY — Experimental neuroanatomical methods were employed in 21 adult cats to determine 1) the number and size of myelinated motor and sensory fibers in the recurrent laryngeal nerve (RLN), and 2) the fiber components originating in the nucleus ambiguus (NA) and retrofacial nucleus (RFN) of the brain stem. Intracranial transection of the X and XI cranial nerves and selective destruction of the NA or RFN were the experimental lesions inflicted in order to obtain the following results. About 55% (312) of the right RLN (565 fibers) is composed of myelinated motor nerve fibers which measure 4 μ - 9 μ in diameter. Nine percent come from the RFN and are smaller (4-6 μ) than the 46% which emanate from the NA and measure 6-9 μ in diameter. The remaining 45% of the RLN is made up of sensory neurons which can be divided into three groups. 1)The largest numerical group (32%) is very small in caliber (1-3 μ) and supplies extralaryngeal regions (trachea, esophagus). 2) The intermediate size fiber group (4-9 μ) comprises 11% of the RLN and probably supplies the subglottic mucosa. 3) The smallest group (2%) of sensory fibers is the largest in diameter (10-15 μ) and may represent either the innervation of muscle spindles or afferents from the superior laryngeal nerve coursing down into the chest.

A need for morphological data on the fiber components of the recurrent laryngeal nerve (RLN) is indicated by the recent physiological[1] and anatomical[2] demonstrations of different types of motor units supplying intrinsic laryngeal muscles in the cat. Accurate description of the size and number of fibers associated with the functions served by the RLN is necessary before the physiology of laryngeal function can be fully understood. The ultimate purpose of such knowledge is its application in the understanding and treatment of disorders affecting the human larynx.

The present study represents an experimental anatomical demonstration of the motor and sensory fiber components of the cat's RLN. Major contributions of this report are: 1) the identification of the nerve fibers emanating from each of two brain stem nuclei (retrofacial nucleus [RFN] and nucleus ambiguus [NA]) responsible for laryngeal motor innervation, and 2) division of the myelinated fibers in the RLN into three categories according to diameter and functional components.

METHODS AND MATERIALS

Twenty-one adult cats were used in this study. Adult cats rather than kittens were chosen because the myelinization of nerve fibers is more complete in adult animals. This difference permits more accurate data on fiber sizes and also allows for a clear distinction between myelinated and unmyelinated fibers. Furthermore, since adult animals are the choice of many neurophysiological investigations, this anatomical information can be more directly related to physiological data. These animals were anesthetized with intraperitoneal sodium pentobarbital* (30 mg per kg of body weight) and the back of the head and neck were shaved and prepared for surgery. After a posterior fossa craniotomy was carried out, the cerebellopontine angle and the brain stem on the right side was carefully exposed. This

* Pentosol® 65 mg/ml. Burns-Biotec Lab., Inc., Oakland, CA.

From the Department of Otolaryngology, University of Massachusetts Medical School, Worcester, Massachusetts. This study was supported by Grant No. NS08451 NINCS. NIH, Bethesda, MD.

Presented at the meeting of the American Laryngological Association, Palm Beach, Florida, April 24-25, 1976.

exposure permitted a view of the cochlear nucleus and the IX, X, and XI nerve rootlets.

Two types of intracranial lesions were carried out. 1) Transection of the rootlets of the X and XI nerves between the brain stem and the base of the skull. This lesion was produced in order to determine the total number of motor and sensory fibers in the RLN. Since the ganglion cells of the sensory neurons are located extracranially, this intracranial transection of the nerve rootlets would cause wallerian degeneration of only the motor neurons whose cell bodies are located within the brain stem. 2) The second type of lesion was electrolytic destruction of each of the two brain stem nuclei (retrofacial nucleus and nucleus ambiguus) concerned with laryngeal motor innervation. The RFN was approached by inserting an electrode through the dorsal surface of the restiform body in the caudal brain stem. After the electrode was inserted in a vertical direction to a predetermined depth, a current of 20 ma was applied for five seconds. Location of the electrode within the retrofacial nucleus was monitored by the observation of facial muscle twitching from stimulation of the nearby facial nucleus. In order to produce a lesion in the NA, the electrode was moved progressively more caudally from the facial nucleus to a premeasured location and 20-50 ma of current were applied for ten seconds. The electrode was again moved progressively in a caudal direction and the current injury applied two additional times in order to destroy this extensive nucleus. The posterior cervical muscles and the skin incision were approximated with interrupted sutures. The postoperative course was usually benign in these animals; those animals with intracranial transection of the X and XI nerves and those with NA destruction were treated prophylactically with tracheostomy because of the possibility of airway obstruction from the complete unilateral vocal cord paralysis.

All the animals were allowed to survive a two-week period in order to allow sufficient time for complete wallerian degeneration of the transected axons. This interval was short enough to minimize the possibility of retrograde degeneration in sensory neurons in the RLN. Animals were sacrificed by first producing anesthesia with intraperitoneal sodium pentobarbital. Intracardiac perfusion was used to first infuse Ringer's solution, then the fixative solution. In those animals where the preparation of the RLN was to be carried out with the Sudan Black B stain, 10% buffered formalin was used as the fixative. Where electron microscopic evaluation was to be carried out on the RLN, the animals were perfused with a 2% glutaraldehyde and 2.5% paraformaldehyde solution as the fixative.

After a 24-hour period of immersion in the respective fixative solution, the brain stems were carefully removed from the cranial cavity and both RLN's were carefully dissected out under the operating microscope.* They were then placed separately in labeled bottles containing fixative. A 2 cm length of the RLN just proximal to its entrance inferior to the thyroid lamina was removed in each instance.

The RLN's were prepared in two ways: 1) Those nerves fixed in 10% formalin were stained by immersing them in 70% alcohol solution of Sudan Black B and then embedded in 15% gelatin solution. After this embedding medium had hardened in the refrigerator, frozen sections were cut at 10 μ. These sections were collected and mounted in glycerine on slides. Photographs were taken of the nerves and enlarged to a known magnification before constructing a montage about one-third of a meter in diameter. The fibers were then carefully counted and measured according to a previously determined scale which depended on the magnification used in the photography. 2) Those nerves which were immersed in the glutaraldehyde-paraformaldehyde fixative were stained with osmium and embedded in Epon 812®** for electron microscopic sectioning. Thin sections were cut on an ultra microtome*** and prepared for study under the electron microscope. Photographs were taken of the entire nerve cross-section through the transmission electron microscope and enlarged to a magnification of about 4,500 X. A montage was then constructed of these component photographs which usually extended about two-thirds of a meter in diameter. The nerve fibers were measured according to a predetermined scale and counted. Both myelinated and unmyelinated fibers were counted in nerves prepared in this manner.

The brain stems of all animals in which electrolytic lesions had been produced were blocked so that sections could be taken of the caudal brain stem. Horizontal sections were cut at 25 μ thickness and collected serially. These were stained with 1% cresyl violet to display neurons and mounted on slides. The brain stem sections were carefully evaluated under the light microscope and were reconstructed after projecting outline drawings of the lesions in these sections.

Those animals in which the electrolytic lesion intended for the RFN was not located in the nucleus were used as control animals. In almost all of these animals the lesion was placed in the facial nerve nucleus or its perimeter.

RESULTS

Control Nerves. A careful survey of the cat's RLN revealed that three major

----

* Carl Zeiss, Inc., N.Y., NY.

** Shell Chemical Co., N.Y., NY.

*** Sorvall MT2-B, Ivan Sorvall, Inc., Newtown, CT.

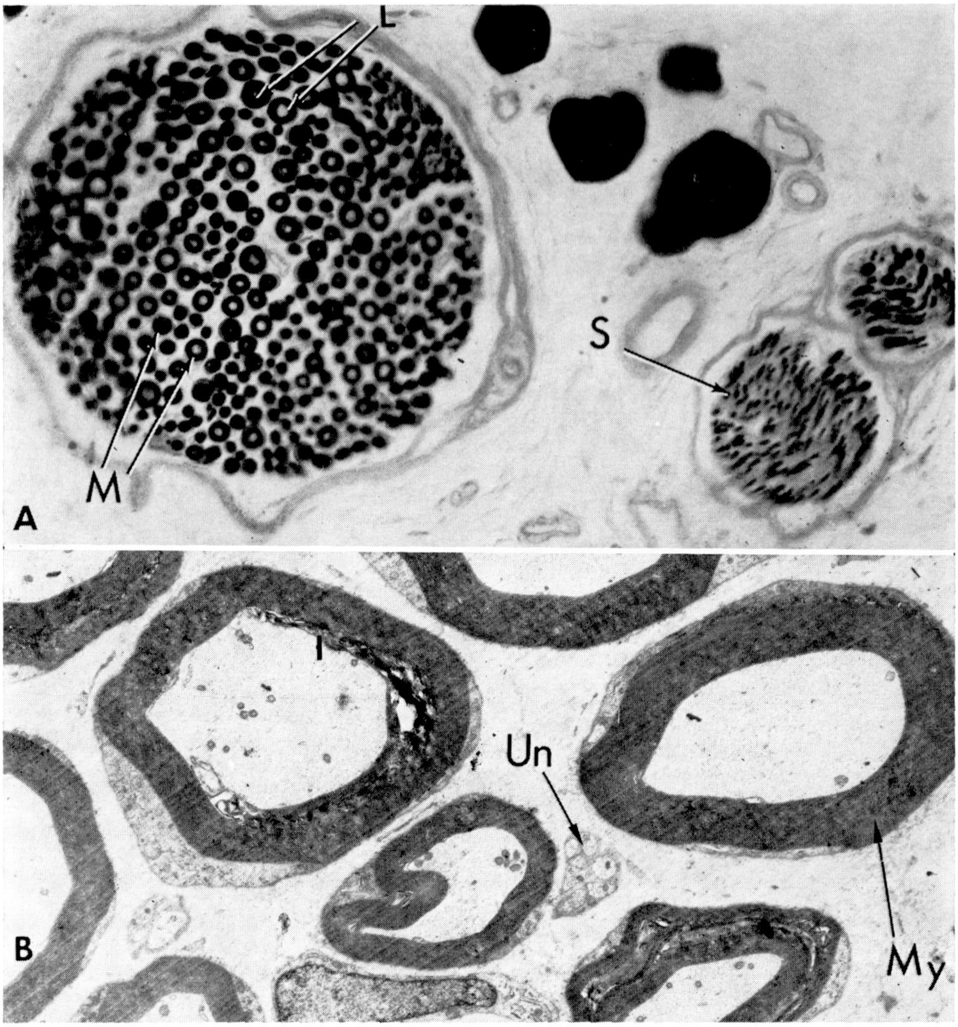

Fig. 1. A) Normal cat RLN stained with Sudan Black demonstrating small (S), medium (M), and large (L) myelinated fibers (X110). B) Electron micrograph of normal cat RLN showing myelinated (My) and unmyelinated fibers (Un). I - Irregularity due to fixation. (X5780).

groups of myelinated fiber sizes could be distinguished (Fig. 1). There are numerous small fibers 3.0 μ or less in diameter which either are grouped together within the main trunk of the RLN or comprise a separate small nerve bundle which accompanies the RLN. A second category of very large fibers measuring 10 μ - 15 μ in diameter which are few in number, are found scattered throughout the RLN. The third and most numerous group of fibers have diameters intermediate in size measuring 4 - 9 μ. Subsequent experimental animals indicated that all myelinated motor (efferent) fibers are contained in this intermediate fiber group.

Table I summarizes the results of nerve fiber counts and measurements in the right and left RLN of animals used as controls. This group of ten animals represents those in which attempted electrolytic destruction of the RFN was unsuccessful and resulted in a lesion which did not involve this nucleus.

Although in two animals, 7 and 8,

TABLE I

ANALYSIS OF MYELINATED FIBERS IN THE NORMAL RLN

Animal No.	Total Fibers	Small (1-3 μ)	Medium (4-9 μ)	Large (10-15 μ)
1	R 422	110	304	8
	L 539	199	318	22
2	R 568	165	386	17
	L 512	215	276	21
3	R 584	208	363	13
	L 421	75	339	7
4	R 470	128	329	13
	L 447	101	334	12
5	R 773	338	427	8
	L 671	244	418	9
6*	R 487	120	361	6
	L 460	118	335	7
7	R 728	349	357	22
	L –	–	–	–
8*	R 580	167	407	6
	L –	–	–	–
9	R 528	184	338	6
	L 499	176	314	9
10*	R 514	176	327	11
	L 306	15	287	4
Avg. N=10	R 565	195	360	11
N= 8	L 482	143	330	11

* Electron microscope evaluation

only the right RLN was counted because the left RLN was lost in preparation or removal, the nerves of both sides were analyzed in the remaining eight animals. In seven of these, the right RLN contained more fibers than the left RLN. The average total fiber count in ten right RLNs was 565 compared to 482 fibers in eight left RLNs. The number of left RLN fibers was not greatly changed when ten additional normal left RLNs from the experimental animals were also included in the averaging; the overall average fiber count in left RLNs from both the control and experimental animals was 499. Since all the experimental lesions were inflicted on the right side, separate analysis of the right and left RLN was important in order to determine a valid standard for numerical comparison of results in experimental animals. Therefore, the significantly higher figures of the right RLN were chosen as the normal standard against which the experimental right RLN counts were compared.

TABLE II

MYELINATED FIBER COUNTS IN RLN FOLLOWING TRANSECTION OF RIGHT X AND XI CRANIAL NERVES

Animal No.	Total Fibers	Small (1-3 μ)	Medium (4-9 μ)	Large (10-15 μ)
11	R 385	319	47	19
	L 448	137	293	18
12	R 218	184	25	9
	L 475	112	335	28
13*	R 426	346	74	6
	L 405	89	311	5
Avg.	R 342	283	48	11

* Electron microscope evaluation

Analysis of the three fiber categories indicated considerable numerical variation in the small and large fiber groups while the intermediate (medium) fiber group was relatively constant. The exceptionally low count of small fibers in the left RLN of animals 3 and 10 could be due to loss of an unrecognized small accessory nerve bundle during removal of the RLN.

Transection of X and XI Nerves. In three animals, 11, 12 and 13, intracranial transection of cranial nerves X and XI was performed, causing wallerian degeneration of all motor axons in the RLN (Fig. 2). Table II summarizes the results in these animals. Loss of fibers occurred in only the medium fiber group, demonstrating that the small and large fiber groups contain sensory nerve fibers only. However, 47, 25, and 74 fibers in the medium sized group were not degenerated in these three animals, indicating that a small portion of this group contains sensory neurons. Subtraction of the average number of intact fibers (48) in the medium category following this lesion from those in the control right RLN (360), indicates that there are about 312 motor nerve fibers in the right RLN.

In two animals which are not in-

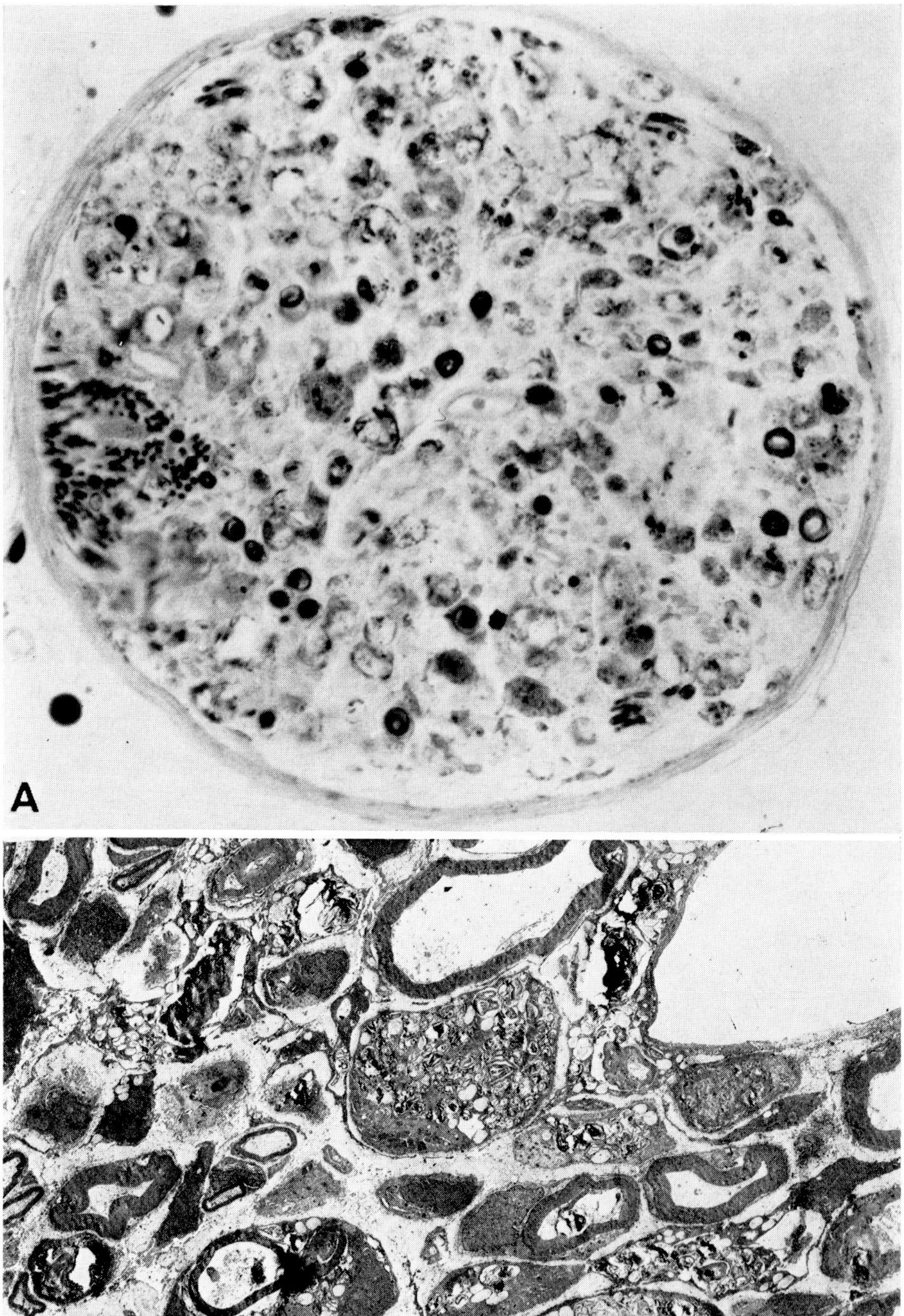

Fig. 2. A) Sudan Black preparation of RLN following intracranial transection of nerves X and XI in 12. Some large, medium, and small fibers remain intact although most of the nerve is degenerated. A separate bundle of intact small fibers has been omitted from the photograph. (X110) B) Electron micrograph of RLN from 13 also shows intact large, medium, and small fibers and various stages in degeneration of motor fibers in the nerve (X2030).

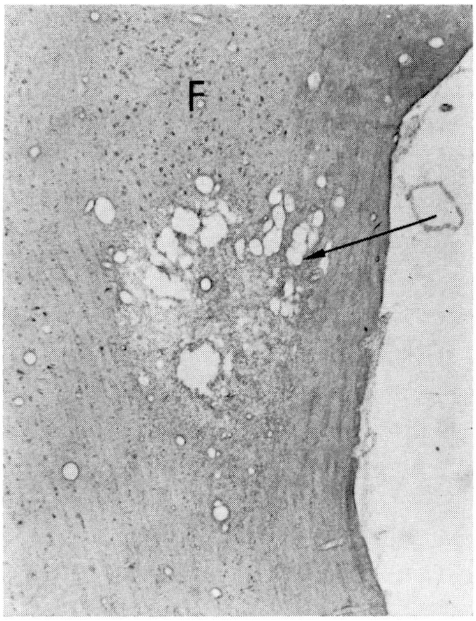

Fig.3. Horizontal brain stem section from animal 16 illustrating the selective destruction (arrow) of the RFN just caudal to the facial nerve nucleus (F) (X6).

cluded in this report, transection of only the most rostral one or two rootlets of the vagus nerve was carried out and resulted in almost as much degeneration in the RLN as complete transection of both the X and XI nerves. This indicates that most, if not all of the motor fibers to the RLN, travel in the rostral rootlets of the vagus nerve and the XI nerve contributes little to this fiber component.

Selective Destruction of RFN. In six animals successful selective destruction of only the RFN was accomplished (Fig. 3). The RLNs in three of these were evaluated by light microscopy while those in the other three were examined under the electron microscope. Although the decrease of fibers in the nerves evaluated by light microscopy was not great (Fig. 4A), a consistent pattern of fewer medium sized fibers in the right RLN than in the left RLN was seen (Table III). This suggestion of fiber loss was strengthened by the electron microscopical observation of numerous degenerating myelinated fibers measuring 4 - 6 μ in diameter in the right RLN of animals 16, 18 and 19 (Fig. 4B).

TABLE III

MYELINATED FIBER COUNTS IN RLN FOLLOWING DESTRUCTION OF RIGHT RETROFACIAL NUCLEUS

Animal No.	*Total Fibers*	*Small (1-3 μ)*	*Medium (4-9 μ)*	*Large (10-15 μ)*
14	R 469	172	269	28
	L 438	116	314	8
15	R 576	236	317	23
	L 652	255	390	7
16*	R 549	180	350	19
	L 679	293	369	17
17	R 549	256	282	11
	L —	—	—	—
18*	R 438	156	271	11
	L 481	221	252	8
19*	R 526	153	367	6
	L 392	41	336	15
Avg.	R 518	193	309	16

* Electron microscope evaluation

Since the average number of intact medium sized fibers following destruction of the RFN is 309, and those in the control right RLN is 360, the estimate of fibers arising from the RFN is 51 fibers.

Partial Destruction of NA. In two animals partial destruction of the NA was produced, one of these also extending to involve the RFN (Table IV). In four other animals an attempt was made to completely destroy the NA with extensive electrolytic means. However, these animals failed to survive, all of them expiring within the first 24 to 48 hours. Since no evidence of intracranial bleeding or respiratory tract obstruction was present, it is probable that extensive destruction in this part of the brain stem also injures the nearby respiratory center.

In both animals in which partial destruction of the NA was achieved, the fiber degeneration was also restricted to the medium size fiber category. The greater decrease of fibers in animal 20 was commensurate with the larger le-

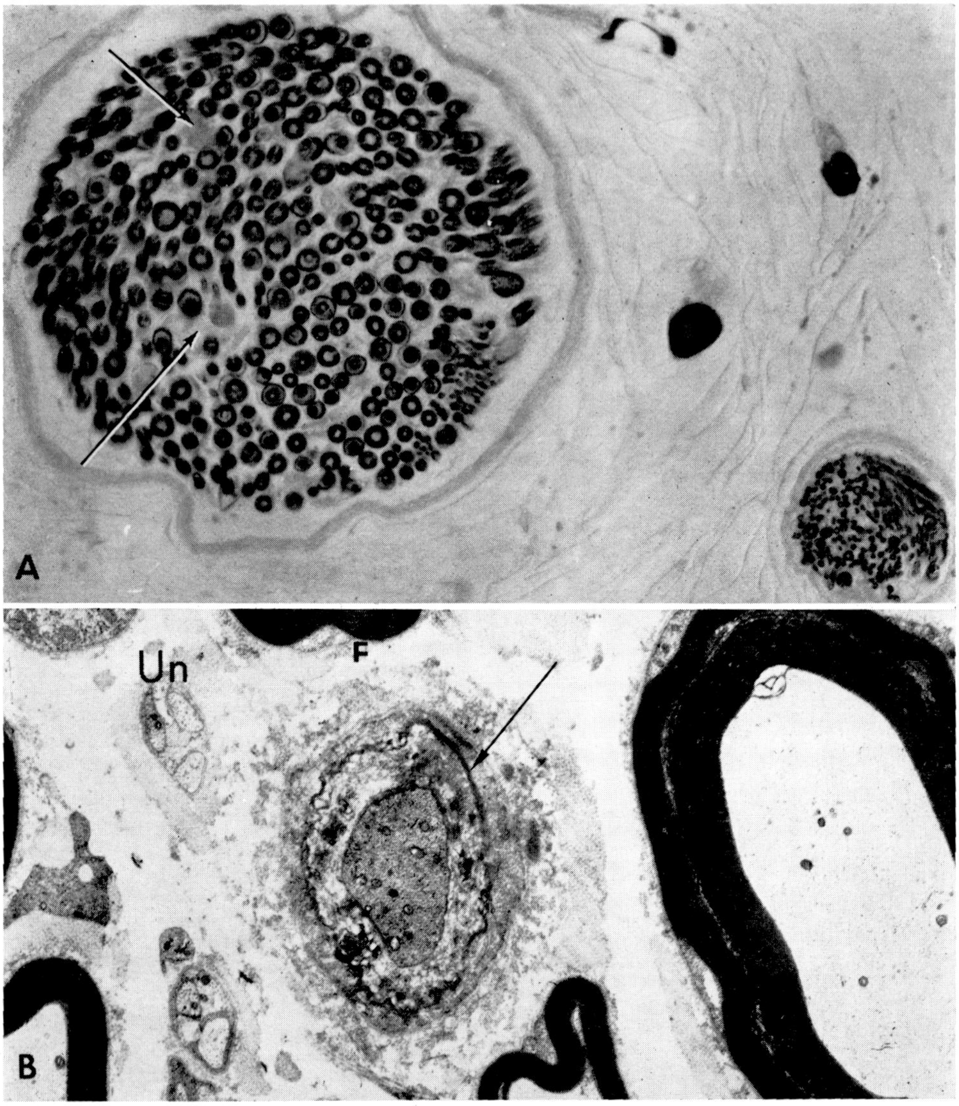

Fig. 4. A) Sudan Black preparation of RLN from animal 15 indicates a slight fiber loss (arrows) following selective lesion of RFN (X110). B) Electron micrograph of RLN in animal 16 where RFN was injured selectively. A degenerating myelinated fiber (arrow) is shown in the center of the field. Un-Unmyelinated fibers. (X8500)

sion which involved the RFN and about one-third of the NA (Fig. 5). In animal 21 only a small portion of the NA was destroyed by a small electrolytic lesion, resulting in less fiber degeneration in the medium size group.

Unmyelinated Fibers in the RLN. An analysis of unmyelinated fibers was performed in those nerves examined by electron microscopy. These nerves were taken from animals in the control, transection of nerves X and XI, and the RFN lesion groups. Table V summarizes the counts of unmyelinated fibers in each of these animals. Although the total unmyelinated fiber count varied greatly, from 399 in the left RLN of animal 13 to 1256 fibers in the right RLN of animal 16, there was no unmyelinated fiber loss in the right RLNs

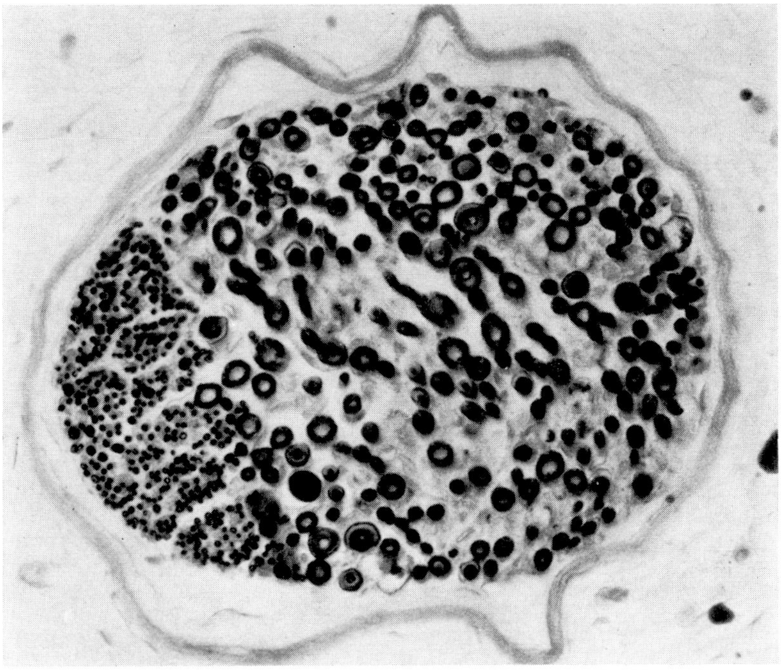

Fig. 5. RLN from animal 20 demonstrates a noticeable myelinated fiber loss following a lesion involving the RFN and part of NA. Note that the small fiber component is located within the main RLN rather than in a separate bundle as shown in Figures 1A and 4A. (X110)

in any of the lesioned animals. This indicates that the unmyelinated fibers do not represent axons of motor neurons within the brain stem. Instead, it seems likely that these unmyelinated fibers represent either cervical sympathetics entering the RLN in the neck or postganglionic parasympathetic fibers whose cell bodies lie in the vagus nerve near the base of the skull. A distinct preponderance of unmyelinated fibers in the right RLN over the left was observed in this series of six animals.

DISCUSSION

Control Nerves. The evaluation of this series of normal cat RLNs should provide valid data on the myelinated and unmyelinated fiber composition of this nerve since these nerves were eval-

TABLE IV

MYELINATED FIBER COUNTS IN RLN FOLLOWING PARTIAL DESTRUCTION OF RIGHT NUCLEUS AMBIGUUS

Lesion	*Animal No.*	*Total Fibers*	*Small (1-3 μ)*	*Medium (4-9 μ)*	*Large (10-15 μ)*
RFN and part of NA	20	R 620	438	156	26
		L 612	179	425	8
Small part of NA	21	R 403	161	234	8
		L 592	217	364	11
	Avg.	R 511	299	195	17

RFN - Retrofacial nucleus
NA - Nucleus ambiguus

TABLE V

UNMYELINATED FIBERS IN RLN

Animal No.	Lesion		Fiber Counts R	L
6	Control		565	645
10	Control		867	488
13	Transection X & XI		652	399
16	RFN		1256	1022
18	RFN		951	837
19	RFN		673	693
		Avg.	827	680

uated by both light microscopy and electron microscopy. The average total number of 565 fibers in the cat's right RLN and 482 in the left RLN compare well with total counts by Murray[3] (400-600 fibers in six nerves) and by Abo-El-Enein[4] (545 to 962 fibers in four nerves). However, Murtagh and Campbell[5] reported 1026 to 1456 fibers in three cat RLNs. The fiber diameter spectra found in this study also compare favorably with those found by Murray, Abo-El-Enein, and Murtagh and Campbell.

The tendency for the right RLN to have a significantly larger number of fibers than the left RLN was also reported by Abo-El Enein,[4] who analyzed two pairs of nerves. The present study demonstrates that this is true for both myelinated and unmyelinated fibers. An explanation for part of this difference may lie in the fact that the left RLN descends into the chest and some afferents from the vagus may terminate in the chest, whereas on the right side they continue on with the RLN into the regions of the larynx, trachea, and esophagus. Since the difference in number of medium sized fibers of the right and left RLN could be in the afferent component, it is not possible to say that there is a significant difference in the efferent component also. The answer to that question must come from degeneration studies of the left RLN.

The determination of the motor or efferent fibers in the RLN rests upon transection of the motor axons at a point proximal and far removed from the sensory neurons, which are contained in the nodose and jugular ganglia at the base of the skull. Intracranial transection of all of the rootlets of the X and XI cranial nerves at their emergence from the brain stem and before penetration of the dura at the jugular foramen was the point selected for carrying out this lesion. In this manner, wallerian degeneration of the motor neurons in the vagus nerve destined for the RLN will occur rapidly, while sensory neurons located in the vagal ganglia at the base of the skull remain intact. A two-week survival period was selected to allow sufficient time for complete wallerian degeneration, yet not long enough to permit significant retrograde degeneration of sensory neurons in the vagal ganglia. All rootlets of the X and XI cranial nerves were transected because of the possibility that motor neurons to the laryngeal muscles may be contributed by both cranial nerves exiting from the brain stem almost the entire length of the NA.

The results of the intracranial transection experiment indicate that all motor fibers are contained in the medium size fiber group (measuring 4 - 9 μ) which comprises more than one-half of the total fiber population of the RLN at a point approximately 2 cm below the thyroid cartilage. However, at this point the RLN also contains a numerous small fiber component which has been shown to contain afferents to the trachea and esophagus.[6] If one discounts this small fiber group as containing nonlaryngeal afferent fibers, the motor fibers could be regarded as making up over 80% of the RLN just prior to its entering the intrinsic larynx.

These motor nerve fibers represent the axons of neurons in the RFN and the NA located in the caudal brain stem. According to numerical estimates made from retrograde tracer studies in the kitten,[2] there are approximately 100 neurons in the RFN and about 285 neurons in the NA which project into the RLN. The total number of motor axons determined by the present experimental study is about 312 fibers. While this number is lower than the cell counts arrived at in the kitten, it should be noted that these RLN fiber counts were performed in adult cats so that neuron loss from aging could account for some, if not all, of the numerical difference. In addition, since these figures can only be regarded as estimates, this approximation may be considered to be in agreement.

Selective destruction of the RFN in six animals indicated that the myelinated fibers projecting from this nucleus are smaller than those from the NA. RFN axons measure 4 - 6 μ in diameter while those from the NA range from 6 - 9 μ in diameter. This difference in fiber size is not surprising since it is in keeping with the difference in neuron size, the retrofacial neurons being decidedly smaller than the large multipolar neurons which comprise the NA.[2] An estimate of the RFN fiber component in the RLN was 51 myelinated axons.

Although complete destruction of the NA was not possible because of the frequent involvement of the nearby respiratory centers, it is reasonable to assume that the remaining motor axons in the RLN belong to the NA motor neurons. This assumption rests upon retrograde tracer studies which show that only the NA and the RFN are responsible for the motor supply in the RLN.[2] Furthermore, the agreement of numerical estimates of the combined RFN and NA cell counts in the kitten and the RLN motor fiber counts in the adult cat supports this statement.

The demonstration of two separate motor neurons to intrinsic laryngeal muscles invites speculation on their respective roles. It has been shown[7-9] in other animals where there are two distinct groups of motor nerve fibers to skeletal muscles, that stimulation of small diameter (5 μ) myelinated nerve fibers causes slow, graded muscular contractions resulting in low amplitude muscle potentials of long duration. Stimulation of large myelinated nerve fibers (10 - 12 μ) produces fast motor unit twitches with rapidly propagated muscle potentials of short duration. The small motor nerves have been regarded as part of a neuromuscular system with a tonic function.

Since different motor units have been demonstrated physiologically in the posterior cricoarytenoid (PCA) muscle of the cat,[1] and the dual innervation from the RFN and NA are associated with the PCA and cricothyroid (CT) muscles,[2] a hypothesis of the role of these motor neurons could involve these muscles.

Morphologically, the smaller size of the retrofacial motor neuron could qualify it as the unit which produces a slow contraction of long duration. The larger motor neurons of the NA could then be responsible for the rapid contraction short-acting kinetic muscle activity in these laryngeal muscles. Such different roles for these two neural units might fit in with the dual actions of the PCA and CT muscles in both inspiration and phonation. For example, while the PCA muscle contracts rapidly in inspiration to abduct the vocal cords, the CT muscle also tenses and exerts a tonic pull on the cords to increase the anterior-posterior glottic dimension.[10] Conversely, while the CT muscle contracts to produce strong adduction of the vocal cords in phonation, the PCA muscle also is responsible for a steady tonic counterpull on the arytenoid to result in more effective adduction.

Another possible role for the dual innervation of these laryngeal muscles is to result in a smooth, coordinated and more effective muscle contraction. Such a contraction could represent the additive effect of neuromuscular units having long, short, and intermediate contraction times as demonstrated in the PCA muscle by Kirchner and his coworkers.[1]

The afferent myelinated fibers occupy all three of the fiber categories recognized in the RLN of the cat. The small fiber group (1 - 3 μ) is the most numerous (32% of RLN). These afferents have been shown by both morphological[3] and physiological[6] studies to supply the tracheal and esophageal mucosa. In a sense, these fibers may not be considered as truly laryngeal. The largest sensory fibers in the RLN are those measuring 10 - 15 μ in diameter and represent only 2% of the RLN. Since the sparse presence of muscle spindles and spiral receptors has been demonstrated within the intrinsic laryngeal muscles of animals[4] and the human,[11-14] it is possible that these fibers provide innervation to such structures.[15-17] Large size myelinated fibers are known to innervate spindles in other muscles of the body.[18] It is also possible however, that these large afferent fibers merely represent the extension of afferents from the superior laryngeal nerve through the ramus communicans into the RLN where they extend in a retrograde fashion into the thoracic cavity to innervate baroreceptors.[3] The medium sized fiber group also contains a variable number of afferent fibers which average approximately 48 fibers per nerve in the cat. These afferent fibers representing 11% of the RLN presumably supply the mucosa of the subglottic region.

Unmyelinated fibers in the RLN have not previously been carefully counted, primarily because the RLN has not been studied extensively under the electron microscope. Murray[3] counted 48 to 81 unmyelinated fibers in the cat RLN using a light microscopic technique. He also found that these did not diminish following transection of the vagus nerve high in the neck. Abo-El-Enein[4] and Murtagh and Campbell[5] did not evaluate unmyelinated fibers in the cat RLN. The present study shows that the RLN actually contains more unmyelinated than myelinated fibers. The tendency for the right RLN (average 827 fibers) to possess more unmyelinated fibers than the left RLN (average 680 fibers) parallels this relationship with regard to myelinated fibers. The number of unmyelinated fibers in the RLN was not diminished following destruction of the intracranial nuclei or nerve rootlets which contribute to the RLN. The logical conclusion is that the unmyelinated fiber component either represents sympathetic fibers from the cervical sympathetic chain which enter the RLN in the neck or that they represent postganglionic parasympathetic fibers whose cell bodies are located near the base of the skull. It seems likely that these autonomic nerve fibers travel along the RLN to enter the larynx where they provide the innervation for blood vessels and glandular structures in this region.

REFERENCES

1. Suzuki M, Kirchner JA: The posterior cricoarytenoid as an inspiratory muscle. Ann Otol Rhinol Laryngol 78:849-864, 1969

2. Gacek RR: Localization of laryngeal motor neurons in the kitten. Laryngoscope 85:1841-1861, 1975

3. Murray JG: Innervation of the intrinsic muscles of the cat's larynx by the recurrent laryngeal nerve: A unimodal nerve. J Physiol (Lond) 135:206-212, 1957

4. Abo-El-Enein: *Functional Anatomy of the Larynx*, Ph.D. thesis. University of London. Quoted by Bowden REM in, Wyke B (ed): *Ventilating and Phonatory Control Systems.* London, Oxford Univ Press, 1974, chap 22

5. Murtagh JA, Campbell CJ: The respiratory function of the larynx. III. The relation of fiber size to function in the recurrent laryngeal nerve. Laryngoscope 61:581-590, 1951

6. Suzuki M, Kirchner JA: Sensory fibers in the recurrent laryngeal nerve. Ann Otol Rhinol Laryngol 78:21-31, 1969

7. Kuffler SW, Hunt CC, Quilliam JP: Function of medullated small nerve fibers in mammalian ventral roots: efferent muscle spindle innervation. J Neurophysiol 14:29-54, 1951

8. Kuffler SW, Vaughan-Williams EM: Small-nerve junctional potentials. The distribution of small motor nerves to frog skeletal muscle, and the membrane characteristics of the fibers they innervate. J Physiol 121:289-317, 1953

9. Hunt CC, Kuffler SW: Motor innervation of skeletal muscle: Multiple innervation of individual muscle fibers and motor unit function. J Physiol 126:293-303, 1954

10. Suzuki M, Kirchner JA, Murakami Y: The cricothyroid as a respiratory muscle. Ann Otol Rhinol Laryngol 79:976-983, 1970

11. Goerttler R: Die anordnung, histologie und histogenese der quergestreiften muskulatur im meuschlichen stimmband. Z Anat Entwicklungesch 115:352-401, 1950

12. Paulsen R: Untersachungen uber das vorkommen und zahl von muskelspindeln im M. vocalis des menschen. Z Zellforsch Mikrosk Anat 47:363-366, 1958

13. Keene MF: Muscle spindles in human laryngeal muscles. J Anat 95:25-29, 1961

14. Bowden REM: Muscle spindles in the human foetus. Acta Biologica Med Ger 9 (fasc 1-4):35-59, 1963

15. Hunt CC: Relation of function to diameter in afferent fibers of muscle nerves. J Gen Physiol 38:117-131, 1954

16. Scheur JL: Fiber size frequency distribution in normal human laryngeal nerves. J Anat 98:99-104, 1964

17. Bowden REM: Innervation of intrinsic laryngeal muscles, in Wyke B (ed): *Ventilatory and Phonatory Control Systems.* London, Oxford Univ Press, 1974, chap 22

18. Barker D: The innervation of the muscle spindle. Q J Microsc Sci 89:143-186, 1948

REPRINTS—Richard R. Gacek, MD, Dept. of Otolaryngology, University of Massachusetts Medical School, 55 Lake Ave., North, Worcester, MA 01605.

SOCIETY FOR EAR, NOSE AND THROAT ADVANCES IN CHILDREN

The Society for Ear, Nose and Throat Advances in Children will be holding its Fourth Annual Meeting in New Orleans, Louisiana, Maison Dupuy Hotel, November 16-18, 1976. For further information, please contact B. Jazbi, MD, (Secretary-Treasurer) The Children's Mercy Hospital, 24th at Gillham Road, Kansas City, MO 64108.

Ann Otol 85: 1976

AN IMPLANTED ELECTRONIC LARYNGEAL PROSTHESIS

BYRON J. BAILEY, MD

GALVESTON, TEXAS

CERI M. GRIFFITHS, MD

GALVESTON, TEXAS

ROBERT EVERETT, PHD

HOUSTON, TEXAS

SUMMARY – The authors present a preliminary progress report on their investigations dealing with the development of an implanted electronic laryngeal prosthesis system. Their initial observations indicate success in the design and fabrication of the implantable, retropharyngeal transducer and secondary induction coil elements. The surgical procedure for implantation is described, and the complications encountered during the first thirteen procedures are reported. These complications included five seromas, one postoperative abscess, one partial wound breakdown secondary to animal-inflicted trauma, and two anesthetic deaths at the time of follow-up radiographic procedures. Additional observations are presented regarding the acoustical output of the transducer in air and after implantation. Projections are made concerning the use of this laryngeal prosthesis system in human patients for vocal rehabilitation after total laryngectomy.

Since the first report of esophageal speech by Reynaud in 1841,[1] physicians have been searching for better solutions to the problem of vocal rehabilitation of the patient whose voice has been lost through accident or surgery. The social, economic and psychological impact of laryngectomy has been observed on numerous occasions by almost all head and neck surgeons. Conversely, measures which can restore effective communication to these patients are of immeasurable value to the victim and his family.

The purposes of this paper are to review significant developments in this field, and to report our preliminary investigational observations regarding an implantable electronic laryngeal prosthesis.

HISTORICAL REVIEW

The period from 1859 to 1942 was characterized by a number of highly innovative attempts to develop procedures and devices which would assist the laryngectomized patient (Table I).[1-23] Limitations of surgical and mechanical technology were such that these efforts were only partially successful and were attempted in only a small number of patients.

The work of Briani between 1942 and 1952 ushered in the modern era of surgical procedures and prosthetic devices with which we are dealing today. This innovative Italian surgeon developed a functional external air bypass prosthesis which is fitted into a surgically-created, skin-lined, cervical-esophageal fistula. Working independently in this country, Conley reported his experiences with external and internal tracheopharyngeal shunts in 1958 and 1959. These reports were followed by important contributions from various head and neck surgeons in North America and England. The most widely accepted and utilized procedures have been those described by Asai, Montgomery, Calcaterra, Shedd, Komorn, Edwards, Taub, and Sisson and McConnel.

While most of the publications on

From the University of Texas Medical Branch, Galveston, Texas, and the University of Houston, Houston, Texas. This work was supported in part by NIH Research Grant CA 17961-01 from the NCI.

Presented at the meeting of the American Laryngological Association, Palm Beach, Florida, April 24-25, 1976.

TABLE I

SPEECH REHABILITATION AFTER TOTAL LARYNGECTOMY
CHRONOLOGY OF DEVELOPMENTS

Date	*Scientist Development*
1841	Reynaud[1] described esophageal speech. Followed by reports by Bourquet (1856), Sawyer (1856) and Bose (1865).
1859	Czermak[1-3] developed a reed-containing tube which passed externally from the trachea to the mouth.
1861	Bruns[1-3] a flexible metal tube (containing a rubber band) which was placed externally between the trachea and mouth.
1874	Gussenbauer[1-3] a tracheopharyngeal air bypass prosthesis with a reed required a pharyngeal fistula.
1887	Stoerk[1-3] devised a tracheooral tube with a whistle held between the teeth. Later modified to be powered by a hand-held bellows.
1925	Brown[4] reported the use of a pitch whistle and ear speculum inserted into a small pharyngeal fistula.
1927	Beck[2,5] presented a patient who had created a tracheopharyngeal fistula with an ice pick and had developed speech.
1928	Scuri[3] described a patient with speech after the spontaneous development of a tracheopharyngeal fistula.
1935	Guttman[3] reported three patients who had been able to speak following a tracheopharyngeal fistula created by a diathermy knife.
1942-1958	Briani[6] developed and reported speech rehabilitation employing a skin-lined cervical-esophageal fistula and an external air bypass prosthesis.
1958-1959	Conley[5,7] developed external and internal tracheoesophageal fistula techniques.
1962	Ogura, *et al*[8] described an experimental technique (in dogs) for creation of a tracheopharyngeal fistula.
1965	Asai[9] described a staged technique for creation of a tracheopharyngeal internal voice tunnel.
1965	Barton[10] reported a tracheooral speech tunnel technique.
1968	Montgomery and Toohill[10,11] developed tracheoesophageal and tracheopharyngeal fistula techniques.
1969	Goode[12] published his work on an external electronic laryngeal prosthesis which utilizes a pharyngeal fistula.
1970-1971	McGrail and Oldfield[13] reported the use of a deltopectoral flap to create a tracheopharyngeal fistula for speech.
1970	Kitamura[14] described a tracheopharyngeal fistula for speech rehabilitation.
1971	Calcaterra[8] reported his findings involving a tracheoesophageal fistula for speech.
1972	Shedd[15] developed an external reed-fistula prosthesis which utilizes a pharyngocutaneous fistula.
1973	Komorn[16,17] published his experience with a tracheoesophageal fistula technique.
1973	Edwards[18] described another form of tracheopharyngeal shunt using an air bypass prosthesis.
1973	Taub[19,20] reported his work with an esophageal fistula and an external air bypass prosthesis.
1974	Shedd[21] developed a second air bypass prosthesis which employs a higher pharyngeal fistula.
1975	Sisson and McConnel[22] published their technique which uses an external air bypass prosthesis and a pharyngeal fistula.
1975	Rogers, Frederickson and Bryce[23] described an implanted electronic laryngeal prosthesis which had been studied experimentally in dogs.

TABLE II

NONINVASIVE AIR-POWERED METHODS OF VOCAL REHABILITATION

	Air Source	*Vibrator*
Esophageal speech[1]	Esophageal reservoir	Pharyngeal mucosa
Czermak's device[1]	Pulmonary air	Rubber band
Bruns' device[3]	Pulmonary air	Rubber band
Stoerk's device[1]	Mechanical bellows	Whistle
Tokyo device[24]	Pulmonary air	Rubber band

vocal rehabilitation after total laryngectomy provide some historical material, two of the most comprehensive reviews on this subject are found in the articles by Hanson[2] and Arnold.[1]

CLASSIFICATION OF PROCEDURES AND DEVICES

The diversity of the theoretical, mechanical and surgical approaches which have been taken to this problem creates a need for an attempt at classification (Tables II,[1,3,24] III,[1,3-10,13-22,25] IV).[1,12,23,26,27]

Table II lists the major types of noninvasive, air-powered methods of vocal rehabilitation after total laryngectomy. These range from conventional esophageal speech to a recently reported modification of the Japanese (Tokyo) pneumatic speech aid. These rehabili-

TABLE III

INVASIVE PROCEDURES FOR PULMONARY AIR-POWERED VOCAL REHABILITATION

	Prosthesis Required	*External Fistula/ Internal Shunt*	*Fistula/ Shunt Location*	*Presumed Vibrator Sound Source*
Conley-I[5,7]	No	I	T-E	M & T
Conley-II[5,7]	Yes	E	T-E	M & T
Montgomery-I[10]	Yes	E	T-E	M & T
Calcaterra[8]	No	I	T-E	M & T
Komorn[16,17]	No	I	T-E	M & T
Taub[19,20]	Yes	E	T-E (? low pharyngeal)	M
Gussenbauer[1]	Yes	E	T-P (H)	Reed
Brown[4]	Yes	E	T-P (L)	Pitch Whistle
Guttman[3]	No	I	T-P (L)	M & T
Briani[6]	Yes	E	T-P (H)	M
Asai[25,9]	No	I	T-P (H)	T
Montgomery-II[10]	Yes/No	E	T-P (L)	M
McGrail[13]	Yes	I	T-P (H)	T
Kitamura[14]	No	I	T-P (H)	T
Shedd-I[15]	Yes	E	T-P (L)	Reed
Shedd-II[21]	Yes	E	T-P (H)	M
Edwards[18]	Yes	E	T-P (H)	T
Sisson[22]	Yes	E	T-P (H)	T O
Barton[10]	Yes	I	T-Oral	T O

E - External. I - Internal. T-E - Tracheoesophageal. T-P - Tracheopharyngeal. (H) - High. (L) - Low. M - Mucosa. T - Tunnel. T O - Tunnel Opening.

TABLE IV

ELECTRONIC POWERED DEVICES FOR VOCAL REHABILITATION

	Varieties of Devices
External transoral[1,26]	(Cooper-Rand, Tait, Ticchioni pipe)
External transcervical[1,26]	(Aurex, Kett, Electro-larynx)
Goode[12]	External sound source — Pharyngocutaneous fistula
Pichler[12]	Intraoral (dental) transducer with wireless transduction
Frederickson[23]	Implanted pharyngeal transducer with wireless transduction
Bailey[27]	Implanted pharyngeal transducer with wireless transduction

tative methods require no surgical procedures. The air source and vibrator mechanism for each of these methods are indicated.

The most extensive variety of vocal rehabilitative procedures are those which require an operative procedure (invasive techniques) and utilize expired pulmonary air for their power source.

Table III lists the invasive procedures for pulmonary air-powered vocal rehabilitation which are of historical relevance and current interest. Table III indicates whether it is necessary to employ a prosthetic device in conjunction with the surgical procedure, differentiates between those surgical procedures which employ the creation of an external fistula with a prosthetic device and those which consist of the construction of an internal (subdermal) air shunt, describes the anatomic location of the external fistula/internal shunt, and designates the presumed vibrating source which produces the air column necessary for speech.

More recently, efforts have been made to develop an electronic sound source for speech. Table IV lists the different varieties of electronic devices, and includes both noninvasive (external and nonsurgical) devices, and those which must be implanted behind the pharyngeal wall. Currently, the latter group are experimental but may become available for use in patients within the next two years.

Numerous studies from various major institutions presumed to have excellent speech pathology support indicate that one-third of the patients who undergo total laryngectomy do not develop satisfactory esophageal speech.[28] In patients over 60 years of age, approximately 50% may fail to develop adequate communicative ability with this method. It is estimated that 25,000 patients living in the United States have undergone total laryngectomy. Therefore, it is possible that from 8,000 to 10,000 patients in this country would benefit from the development of a satisfactory laryngeal prosthesis for speech.

The Western Electric Electro-larynx®* is the most popular device for solving this problem. Despite its usefulness in many patients, it has certain serious disadvantages, including monotonous speech, high noise to signal ratio and limited effectiveness in some patients.

Many of the surgical techniques listed in Table III are associated with technical problems and postoperative complications when employed in patients whose treatment has included irradiation therapy.

The prosthetic devices shown in Tables III and IV have several disadvantages. In some instances, they are not commercially available for widespread use. In other instances, they are extremely expensive. Most are quite visible, and, therefore, objectionable to the patient. Others restrict the patient's activity, limiting free use of both hands.

* Western Electric, New York, NY.

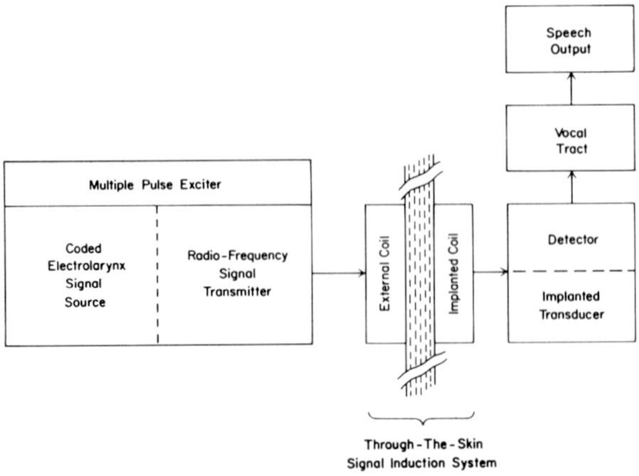

Fig. 1. Diagrammatic representation of the electronic laryngeal prosthesis system.

In addition, they require varying degrees of cleaning, maintenance and replacement.

Recent advances in electronic technology provide the opportunity to explore the possible development of a lightweight, durable, implanted electronic laryngeal voice prosthesis.

OBJECTIVES

The three specific objectives of our approach are: 1) To design and fabricate an electronic laryngeal prosthesis. This prosthesis will be implanted between the posterior pharyngeal wall and the cervical spine and will be a passive-type sound generator, deriving its power from an external signal source via transdermal transduction. 2) To evaluate the tissue acceptance, durability and sound generating capability of this device on the basis of careful animal experiments. 3) Ultimately, to evaluate the usefulness of an implantable electronic laryngeal prosthesis as a voice-producing mechanism for patients who have undergone laryngectomy.

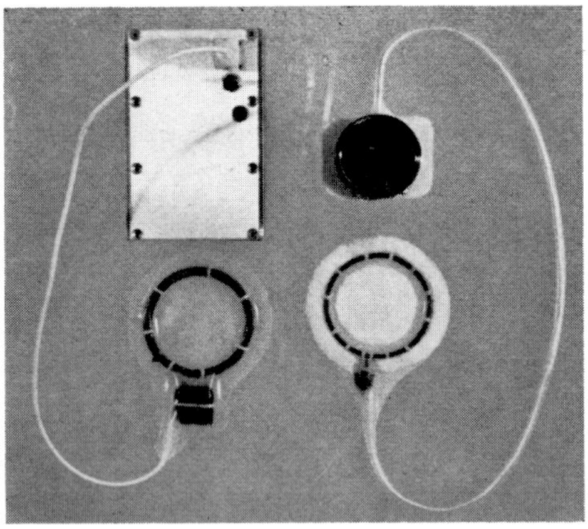

Fig. 2. The prosthetic system currently being investigated. The transducer and secondary induction coil are implanted, and the power supply/signal transmitter and primary coil are worn outside the animal.

DEVELOPMENTAL APPROACH AND PROGRESS

The focus of our experiments has been on the development and investigation of a two-part electronic laryngeal prosthesis system. The basic elements of this system and their relationship to the speech output are shown in Figure 1.

The external portion of the system, consisting of a multiple pulse exciter unit and power supply, will generate a radio frequency power source which drives an induction coil on the external body surface. This external induction coil creates a large magnetic field, inducing a voltage in a secondary coil which is implanted appropriately just under the surface of the skin. The purpose of this dual coil system is to eliminate the need for wired electrical connections through the skin. The implanted coil will be connected by a small coaxial cable to the electro-me-

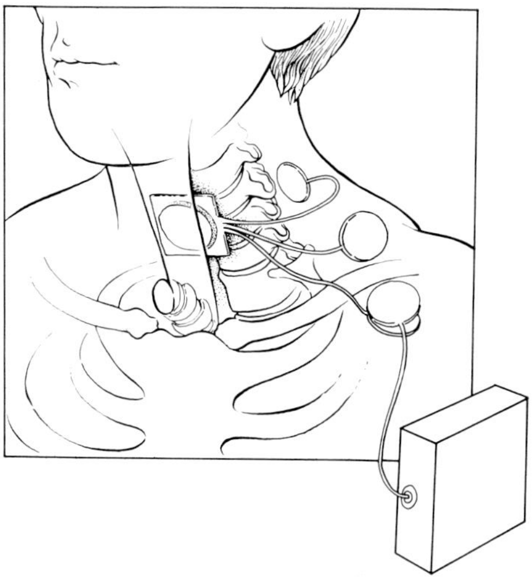

Fig. 3. Location for implantation of the transducer element and the various options available for placement of the subdermal secondary coil.

chanical transducer which has been implanted just behind the pharyngeal wall at the level of the fifth cervical vertebra. The inward and outward movements of the transducer diaphragm produce a moving column of pharyngeal air which is then formed and articulated into the vowels and consonants essential for intelligible speech.

The elements of this system which have been developed to date are shown in Figure 2.

The electro-mechanical transducer unit is the element which is central to all of our efforts and has received most of our initial attention. Factors relating to case design and biocompatibility have been studied. We have determined that adequate sound pressure levels can be generated by a transducer unit of stainless steel which houses all of the necessary standard electronic components and measures approximately 4.0 cm in diameter by 0.9 cm in thickness.

In our initial studies with dogs, we used a system which employs a hard-wired connection between the transducer and the pulse generator/power supply through the skin of the upper back of the dog. We are currently developing the two-coil, through-the-skin transdermal transduction element, and our observations have been favorable. The power transduction through-the-skin generates no excessive levels of heat and the power loss of this transduction system, as compared to the hard-wired connection through-the-skin, does not appear to be a significant problem.

A number of anatomic options exist for the placement of the two coils as shown in Figure 3.

The two superimposed coils utilized in the through-the-skin transduction system could be located in the posterior cervical area, the supraclavicular portion of the lateral neck or the lateral deltopectoral area (a common place for the implantation of subdermal cardiac pacemakers). The external coil would be housed in a lightweight plastic sheath which could be attached to the skin with adhesive paste. This coil would connect with the power supply/multiple pulse exciter unit which could be worn in a comfortable, lightweight chest halter.

The surgical procedure for implantation of the transducer unit is quite simple in the dog experiments and is within the technical ability of any head and neck surgeon. A lateral cervical incision, measuring approximately 8 cm, is made, and a combination of sharp and blunt dissection is used to develop a surgical plane which begins lateral to the carotid artery and internal jugular vein and passes deep to these structures and all of the significant neural elements of the midneck. The prevertebral fascia overlying the fifth cervical vertebra is exposed. The transducer unit is positioned exactly in the midline in this area and sutured to the fascia. The surgical steps for transducer implantation are shown in Figure 4B.

EXPERIMENTAL OBSERVATIONS

The Electro-mechanical Transducer Unit. Our initial objective was to design and build an electro-mechanical transducer which would meet the criteria of being a) biocompatible, b) of a size suitable for implantation in the retro-

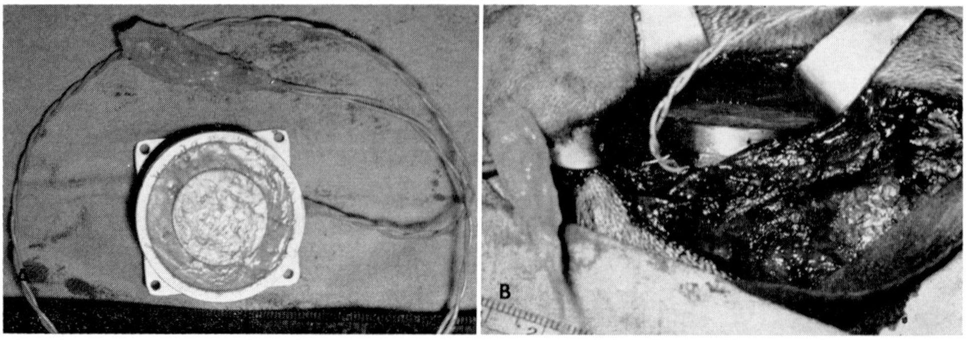

Fig. 4. A) The implantable early transducer and connecting wire. B) Creation of the retropharyngeal pouch at the level of the fifth cervical vertebra and implantation of the transducer into this pouch.

pharyngeal space, c) capable of producing sound pressure levels in excess of 85 dB, and d) capable of producing a periodic signal in the vocal tract which has the harmonic structure similar to that of the signal produced by the action of the vocal folds.

Our initial approach was to design a transducer which uses the principle of magnetic circuits. This is a transducer comprised of a magnetic circuit with a steady magnetic field bias derived from a permanent magnet, a magnetic field source comprised of a coil set for introducing control signals and a mobile diaphragm which would induce motion of the posterior pharyngeal wall. The principle of operation of this type of transducer is based on the fact that the steady field of the permanent magnetic field attraction on the diaphragm is against its spring action. Mechanical action is produced by the additive and subtractive magnetic field produced by currents in the coils of the magnetic circuit. During the early phase of our studies, we identified fourteen factors which required separate analysis. These were:

1. Transducer migration
2. Factors related to midline versus lateral placement
3. Performance factors related to the level of placement
4. Complications related to the surgical implantation procedure
5. Factors related to transducer size
6. Factors related to transducer weight
7. Transducer case design and fabrication
8. Diaphragm design and fabrication
9. Transducer magnets
10. Transducer electronic circuitry
11. Transducer backplate design
12. Transducer case-diaphragm seal
13. Transducer acoustical output tuning factors
14. Transducer-secondary coil connection

Though the limitations of space prohibit a detailed discussion of each of these areas, some summary statements are appropriate.

Transducer migration does not appear to be a significant problem with the perforated metal backplate, the stainless steel mesh backplate or the Dacron®* felt/Silastic®** sheeting backplate, because the transducer is anchored by local tissue ingrowth fairly soon after implantation.

Transducer acoustical output is maximal with midline placement of the

* E. I. DuPont de Nemours & Co., Inc., Wilmington, DE.
** Shell Chemical Co., N.Y., NY.

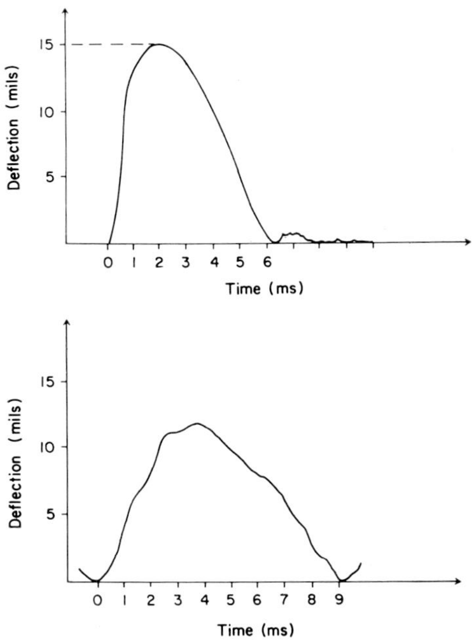

Fig. 5. A) Unloaded wave shape of the transducer diaphragm output. B) The deflection response of the loaded transducer.

transducer unit, but declines rather sharply if the transducer is implanted off-center or migrates laterally.

Our hypothesis is that the quality of the speech output will be superior when the transducer is located toward the inferior limit of the pharyngeal funnel. Extra-oral sound pressure level recordings have shown that acceptable sound pressure levels can be recorded at one meter from the dog's mouth, and it is presumed that this level of placement will maximize the ability of a patient to form and articulate the vibrating column of air into intelligible speech.

The size and weight of the transducer are of concern in terms of comfort when the electronic laryngeal prosthesis system is employed in patients. It is our impression that the transducer size (4.0 cm in diameter and 0.9 cm in thickness) which we have developed has been maximally miniaturized consistent with the desired levels of sound pressure output and the utilization of standard electronic components. We feel that this size and weight is consistent with general patient comfort and minimal impairment of swallowing.

The transducer units are bench-tested extensively in air and in a liquid medium with diaphragm loading to simulate the performance of the unit in the retropharyngeal space. The pulses generated by our latest series of transducers have the unloaded wave shape shown in Figure 5A.

This deflection pulse is the response of the transducer to a 2 msec maximal pulse. The small pulses of latency more than 6 msec are the result of the diaphragm bounding on a mechanical stop.

The tissue loading effects were simulated by placing the transducer unit in a bath of water and attaching a heavy viscous mass with properties similar to the pharyngeal tissues on the diaphragm. The measured pulse deflection under repetitious 100 pulses/sec excitation is shown in Figure 5B.

As shown, the principal effects of transducer loading are to diminish the amplitude response and to lengthen or smear out the unloaded response. The transducer diaphragm is acting as a ballistic device. An excitation pulse releases it, and the stored energy in the diaphragm pushes out the diaphragm and the associated tissue mass. When the pulse is discontinued, the magnetic force commences to pull the diaphragm in again. However, the diaphragm is only responding to determinate forces which have little to do with the exact excitation pulse.

The small irregularities on the pulse wave are mechanical oscillations induced by the loading mass and the spring constant of the diaphragm. The appearance of such oscillations introduces no particular difficulty.

Each transducer is individually fabricated to produce its optimal wave shape. This optimal wave shape corresponds closely with maximal sound pressure level output of the device. The sound pressure level output of the first two series of transducers which were produced is shown in Figure 6.

Sound transmitted from the open and

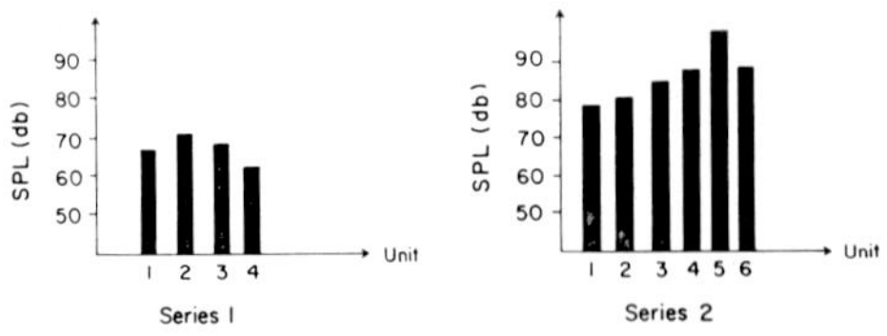

Fig. 6. Sound pressure level output from the transducer units. The transducers in Series 1 had a diaphragm diameter of approximately 28 mls, while those in Series 2 have a diaphragm of approximately 41 mls.

unobstructed oral cavity and pharynx of the dogs was measured after transducer implantation and excitation. Typical levels of such signals were 60 to 70 dB at a distance of one meter. Attenuation by the tissue of the pharyngeal wall and the vocal tract was calculated by subtracting the vocal tract transmitted sound pressure level from the free space radiated sound pressure level. We find that when the transducer remains centered over the midline of the posterior pharyngeal wall, the typical attenuations are only 3 to 5 dB. The best unit which we encountered had an original versus transmitted wave shape displayed in Figure 7.

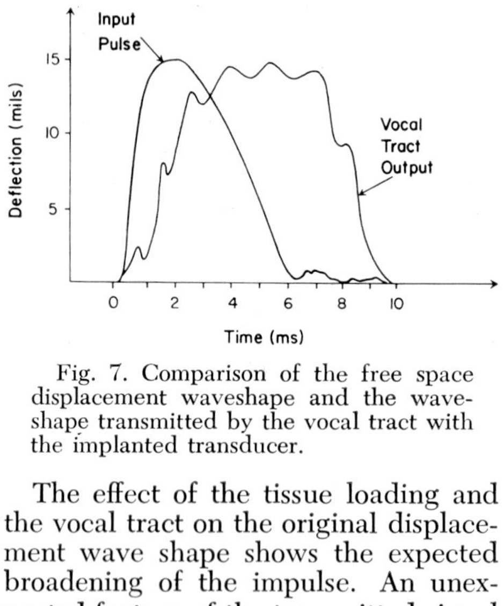

Fig. 7. Comparison of the free space displacement waveshape and the waveshape transmitted by the vocal tract with the implanted transducer.

The effect of the tissue loading and the vocal tract on the original displacement wave shape shows the expected broadening of the impulse. An unexpected feature of the transmitted signal was the rapidly falling trailing edge of the pressure wave.

When we have approximated typical glottal wave shapes with our transducer when it is *in situ*, if we find that tissue loading effects change with passage of time, the only way that we can effect the proper wave shape corrections is to modify the electronic drive currents. As it is, the standard transducer response that we use is the result of a short (1-2 ms) current pulse. For current pulses less than maximal and for current pulses longer than the standard period, the response of the device will be different.

In order to conserve driving power, both in the electronic system and in the transducer, it is desirable to use only rectangular pulses for excitation purposes. In the experiments carried out to date, with the transducer *in situ* or in free space conditions, it has been simple to observe the acoustical output wave shape of the transducer while varying the number, amplitudes and latencies of the driving pulse train so as to arrive at excellent approximations of the appropriate wave shape. For our device, in which care is taken to arrive at a reasonable approximation of the proper wave with a single pulse, any subsequent pulses introduce only minor modifications in the trajectory of the diaphragm and involve little expenditure of power.

Surgical Observations and Complications. The surgical procedure for implantation of the electro-mechanical transducer has been described. The first critical step in the procedure is to accomplish the dissection without injuring the important neurovascular structures of the upper and midneck. The second critical step is to accomplish the placement of the transducer element in the midline immediately over the fifth cervical vertebra. Our studies regarding transducer migration have been promising, particularly with the currently favored model in which the transducer unit is attached to a Dacron® felt/Silastic® sheeting backplate.

During the coming months, we will focus our attention on the local tissue response to the transducer unit. Our primary concern will be the biocompatibility between the transducer and the surrounding tissue in terms of the formation of both granulation tissue and a seroma around the foreign body. We will study this reaction with weighted "dummy" units and with chronically excited units. We anticipate more problems with the excited units in view of the effect of the acoustical energy of the transducer on the surrounding tissue.

As the sound pressure level output of our newer models will be above 90 dB, we will also include careful studies of the temporal bones in order to be certain that these units do not induce cochlear damage as a result of the sound pressure levels which will be generated.

In our first 13 experiments, we encountered difficulty with postoperative seroma in five dogs. These seromas responded to periodic aspiration when the swelling was visible, and they are probably to be expected in a situation where a large pocket is made and a nonconforming foreign body is introduced. It is technically impossible to close all of the dead space around the transducer unit. Though this complication has produced no serious problems, we are in the process of designing a tapered Silastic® transducer holder to be studied in future experiments.

Anesthetic deaths occurred in two instances during the early phase of our project when animals were anesthesized for routine radiographic studies. In the last six months, there have been no anesthetic deaths.

A postoperative wound abscess developed in one dog. This abscess responded to antibiotics, incision, and drainage without rejection or loss of the transducer unit.

We observed a partial breakdown of the healing surgical incision in one dog. This may have been related to trauma inflicted by the animal during the postoperative period and did not result in loss of the prosthesis or any other complications.

Analysis of our postoperative complications reveals no serious problems in terms of extrapolation of this procedure to the human patient. The seromas were all controlled by aspiration, and the other complications probably would not have occurred if these procedures were performed in a sterile hospital operating room using standard precautions.

PROJECTIONS FOR VOCAL REHABILITATION

We are cognizant of the giant step between the development of sophisticated, prosthetic hardware and the practical rehabilitation of the laryngectomized patient.

Putney[28] reviewed and analyzed 440 patients who had undergone total laryngectomy at Jefferson Hospital. He noted that 38% of these patients were unable to develop any esophageal speech. A small percentage of this group was satisfied to communicate with the Western Electric Electro-larynx®, but many of the patients failed to achieve any means of verbal communication.

In his excellent monograph on the scientific foundations for voice restoration, Snidecor[29] discusses several of the parameters which must be considered in the process of speech rehabilitation. During the design and early fabrication stage, we are addressing the issues of vocal tone, rate, loudness, pitch and quality. We believe that it is possible to produce electronic circuitry which can provide a speaking voice with programmed patterns of pitch and quality changes which will result in a more normal speaking voice than any current methods.[30] The speaker with a normal speech mechanism can produce approximately 12.5 words per breath, whereas the superior esophageal speaker can produce only four to five words per air charge. One definite advantage of the electronic laryngeal prosthesis is its capacity for prolonged speech without interruption.

At the Centennial Conference on Laryngeal Cancer in Toronto in May of 1974, Murry[31] reviewed the basic biophysical requirements for new and projected procedures and devices for voice rehabilitation after total laryngectomy. We were impressed by his distinction between speech intelligibility and speech acceptability. It is our objective to develop an electronic laryngeal prosthesis which will effectively address the issues which he raised and fulfill the requirements which he proposed.

In a recent publication,[27] one of the authors, BJ Bailey, proposed guidelines for the further progress of vocal rehabilitation after total laryngectomy. Any new procedure or device should meet the following criteria:

1. Use of newer procedures/devices should not compromise any phase of tumor management for cure.

2. Patients should first be encouraged to develop satisfactory esophageal or external electro-laryngeal voice.

3. Patients should decide if their communication ability is adequate to meet their personal needs.

4. *Informed consent* is essential if new procedures are to be employed. Patients must be aware of *all* risks and complications.

5. Patients should be offered several options and alternatives for vocal rehabilitation.

6. The use of new techniques in patients should be preceded by careful animal experimentation.

7. External prosthetic devices should be small, simple, durable and reasonably priced.

8. The ideal prosthetic voice device should leave both hands free and not require frequent adjustment in order to breathe, phonate or cough.

9. The ideal fistula should be placed so that it opposes salivary leakage, avoids major neck vessels, can be employed after irradiation therapy, and can be accomplished in one or two stages.

10. Patients must be selected carefully in terms of intellect, motivation, and freedom from the likelihood of cancer.

Our research plan is to pursue our objectives within the framework of the ten guidelines presented in the preceding paragraph. We hope that our initial progress will stimulate others to work in this important field, so that we may hasten the day when patients will be able to select from a variety of successful procedures and devices which can provide successful vocal rehabilitation after total laryngectomy.

REFERENCES

1. Arnold GE: Alleviation of alaryngeal aphonia with the modern artificial larynx: I. Evolution of artificial speech aids and their value for rehabilitation. Logos 3:55-67, 1960

2. Hanson WL: A new artificial larynx with a historical review. Ill Med J 7:483-486, 1940

3. Guttman MR: Tracheohypopharyngeal fistulization: a new procedure for speech production in the laryngectomized patient. Trans Am Laryngol Rhinol Otol Soc Inc, 1935, pp 219-226

4. Brown RG: A simple but effective artificial larynx. J Laryngol Otol 40:793-797, 1925

5. Conley JJ, DeAmesti F, Pierce MK: A new surgical technique for the vocal rehabilitation of the laryngectomized patient. Ann Otol Rhinol Laryngol 67:655-664, 1958

6. Briani AA: Riabilitazione fonetica di laringectomizzati a mezzo della corrente aerea espiratoria polmonare. Arch Ital Otol 63:469-475, 1952

7. Conley J: Surgical techniques for the vocal rehabilitation of the postlaryngectomized patient. Trans Am Acad Ophthalmol Otolaryngol 73:288-299, 1969

8. Calcaterra TC, Jafek BW: Tracheo-esophageal shunt for speech rehabilitation after total laryngectomy. Arch Otolaryngol 94:124-128, 1971

9. Asai R: Laryngoplasty after total laryngectomy. Arch Otolaryngol 95:114-119, 1972

10. Montgomery WW, Toohill RJ: Voice rehabilitation after laryngectomy. Arch Otolaryngol 88:499-506, 1968

11. Montgomery WW: Postlaryngectomy vocal rehabilitation. Arch Otolaryngol 95:76-83, 1972

12. Goode RL: The development of an improved artificial larynx. Trans Am Acad Ophthalmol Otolaryngol 73:279-287, 1969

13. McGrail JS, Oldfield DL: One-stage operation for vocal rehabilitation at laryngectomy. Trans Am Acad Ophthalmol Otolaryngol 75:510-512, 1971

14. Kitamura T, Kaneko T, Togawa K, *et al*: Supracricoid laryngectomy. A new technique for vocal rehabilitation. Laryngoscope 80:300-308, 1970

15. Shedd D, Bakamjian V, Sako K, *et al*:

Further appraisal of reed-fistula speech following pharyngolaryngectomy. Can J Otolaryngol 4:583-587, 1975

16. Komorn RM, Weycer JS, Sessions RB, *et al*: Vocal rehabilitation with a tracheoesophageal shunt. Arch Otolaryngol 97:303-305, 1973

17. Komorn RM: Vocal rehabilitation in the laryngectomized patient with a tracheoesophageal shunt. Ann Otol Rhinol Laryngol 83:445-451, 1974

18. Edwards N: Post-laryngectomy vocal rehabilitation using expired air and an external fistula method. Laryngoscope 85:690-699, 1975

19. Taub S, Bergner LH: Air bypass voice prosthesis for vocal rehabilitation of laryngectomees. Am J Surg 125:748-756, 1973

20. Taub S: Voice prosthesis for speech restoration laryngectomees. Trans Am Acad Ophthalmol Otolaryngol 78:287-288, 1974

21. Shedd DP, Bakamjian VY, Sako K, *et al*: Post-laryngectomy speech rehabilitation by a simplified, single-stage surgical method. Am J Surg 128:505-511, 1974

22. Sisson GA, McConnel FMS, Logemann JA, *et al*: Voice rehabilitation after laryngectomy: results with the use of a hypopharyngeal prosthesis. Arch Otolaryngol 101:178-181, 1975

23. Rodgers JH, Fredrickson JM, Bryce DP: New techniques for vocal rehabilitation. Can J Otolaryngol 4:595-604, 1975

24. Nelson IW, Parkin JL, Potter JF: The modified Tokyo larynx: an improved pneumatic speech aid. Arch Otolaryngol 101:107-108, 1975

25. Miller AH: Four years experience with the Asai technique for vocal rehabilitation for the laryngectomized patient. J Laryngol Otol 85:567-576, 1971

26. Goode RL: Artificial laryngeal devices in post-laryngectomy rehabilitation. Laryngoscope 85:677-689, 1975

27. Bailey BJ, Goode RL: New and projected procedures and devices for voice rehabilitation after total laryngectomy. Can J Otolaryngol 4:605-609, 1975

28. Putney FJ: Rehabilitation of the postlaryngectomized patient: specific discussion of failures, advanced and difficult technical problems. Ann Otol Rhinol Laryngol 69:544-549, 1958

29. Snidecor JC: Some scientific foundations for voice restoration. Laryngoscope 85: 640-648, 1975

30. Everett RL, Mitchell C, Yanowitz A: An electronic laryngeal prosthesis for the production of natural sounding speech, in *Proceedings of the 28th Annual Conference on Engineering in Medicine and Biology.* Chevy Chase, Md., Alliance for Engineering in Medicine and Biology, 1975, vol 17, p 202

31. Murry T: Biophysical requirements for new and projected procedures and devices for voice rehabilitation after total laryngectomy. Can J Otolaryngol 4:571-578, 1975

REPRINTS: Byron J. Bailey, MD, University of Texas Medical Branch, Galveston, TX 77550.

Ann Otol 85: 1976

OTOLARYNGOLOGICAL MANIFESTATIONS OF ARTHROGRYPOSIS MULTIPLEX CONGENITA

SEYMOUR R. COHEN, MD

HART ISAACS JR., MD

LOS ANGELES, CALIFORNIA

SUMMARY – The important otolaryngological manifestations of arthrogryposis multiplex congenita (AMC), which heretofore have not been described in otolaryngological and other specialty journals, are reviewed. Thirty-seven patients with AMC were studied. Nine of these patients with neurogenic AMC, had otolaryngological manifestations. Six of these had Pierre Robin-like syndromes. Seven patients had severe dysphagia and aspiration pneumonitis. Five patients had voice changes, and three of these required tracheotomy to relieve laryngeal obstruction and prevent aspiration. Two of these patients were aphonic and had laryngeal paralysis. Three of the nine patients who had laryngeal examination showed supraglottic narrowing similar to laryngomalacia. Six patients with otolaryngological problems were autopsied, and two had pharyngeal biopsies. The histological examination demonstrated normal laryngeal and pharyngeal musculature. The cricoarytenoid joints were found normal in all the larynges examined. Central nervous system dysfunction rather than simple muscle weakness, caused the dysphagia and respiratory difficulties in patients with neurogenic AMC. Dysphagia with aspiration was the single most important cause of death in approximately 20% of patients with AMC. A tracheotomy and feeding gastrostomy appears essential for successful management of the otolaryngological complications of AMC.

The important otolaryngological manifestations of arthrogryposis multiplex congenita (AMC) have heretofore not been described in the otolaryngological literature, and are rarely mentioned in other specialty journals. AMC is an uncommon congenital, and sometimes familial disorder, characterized by multiple fixed joint deformities, involving the upper and the lower extremities, and, less commonly, the spine and mandible. It may be associated with other congenital defects.

The purpose of this paper is to acquaint the otolaryngologist with the laryngeal and pharyngeal problems associated with this entity. Severe aspiration pneumonia and airway difficulties are frequently present. While the disease is well known to pediatricians, neurologists and orthopedic surgeons, the otolaryngologist is less frequently involved in the care of these patients.

REVIEW OF THE LITERATURE

AMC was originally described by Otto[1] in 1841. The patient he reported had rigidity of the limbs, which were fixed in bizarre positions. Since then, hundreds of cases have been described in the literature. Rosenkranz[2] in 1905, first applied the term "arthrogryposis," meaning curved joints, to this disease. Stern,[3] in 1923, named the syndrome arthrogryposis multiplex congenita. While Otto described this entity as a congenital myodystrophy, arthrogryposis now is generally considered a syndrome with several causes rather than a single disease. The orthopedic problems are characterized by club feet (equinovarus) deformity, torticollis, hip dislocations and vertebral joint involve-

From the Departments of Surgery (Division of Otolaryngology) and Pathology, Childrens Hospital of Los Angeles, and University of Southern California School of Medicine, Los Angeles, California.

Presented at the meeting of the American Laryngological Association, Palm Beach, Florida, April 24-25, 1976.

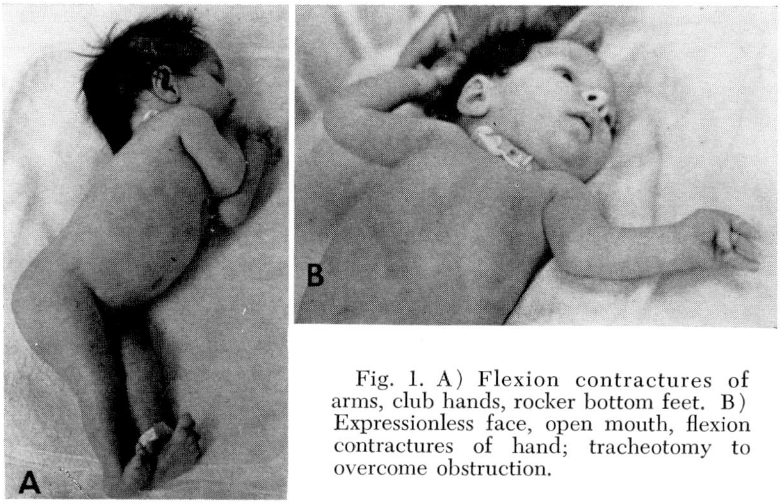

Fig. 1. A) Flexion contractures of arms, club hands, rocker bottom feet. B) Expressionless face, open mouth, flexion contractures of hand; tracheotomy to overcome obstruction.

ment. The wrist, hand and finger contractures (club hand) are either flexion or extension deformities.[4] The frequency of joint involvement increases from proximal to distal, and is more frequent in the lower than in the upper extremity. Temporomandibular joint involvement produces varying degrees of trismus. Facial diplegia (Möbius syndrome) occurs not infrequently. Pearson and Fowler[5] reported a 10-year-old boy with slurred speech, mushy voice, trismus, deformed tongue with inability to protrude it, and inability to whistle. Temporary marked difficulty in swallowing was noted at age three months. The patient's sister, also an arthrogrypotic, had only curling of the tongue, but none of the other ear, nose or throat anomalies. Sandbank and Cohen[6] report a case of tuberous sclerosis with AMC in a patient who had dysphagia, inspiratory stridor, costal retractions, and subsequently died of airway obstruction. No mention is made of laryngeal examination, and the tongue was not examined.

ETIOLOGY

Many causes of AMC have been proposed. Intrauterine problems, such as increased pressure on, or malposition and inactivity of the fetus, have been considered as mechanical etiologic factors. Arthrogryposis has been produced in animals by curarization of the fetus.[7] Central nervous system (CNS) abnormalities have been described, including dysplasia and/or degeneration of the anterior horn cells, meningoceles or myeloceles, involvement of the nuclei of the V and VII cranial nerves (Möbius syndrome), cortical atrophy, microgyria, and varying degrees of hydrocephalus. While most authorities question the role of heredity in this disorder, the myopathic type can clearly show an autosomal recessive genetic pattern.[8] AMC has occurred in twins, but in other instances, one twin was free of the disease. The condition also occurs in families with no previous family history of the disease, and other causes postulated include embryonic muscle abnormalities, abnormal tendon attachments, connective tissue abnormalities, prenatal viral disease, or intrauterine periarthritis.[9] An analysis of pathologic studies from muscle biopsies and autopsy material suggests there are at least two fundamental mechanisms for AMC: neurogenic and myogenic.[5]

CASE REPORTS

Case 1. C.B., a Caucasian female, was born February 11, 1967, and admitted to the Childrens Hospital of Los Angeles, at age 36 days. The purpose of her admission was for casting of her feet. This infant was the product of a traumatic birth, with leg fractures. She had had five episodes of apnea since birth. Arthrogryposis with a muscular disorder was the diagnosis (Figs. 1A, B). Examination revealed an infant in distress, cyanotic at room

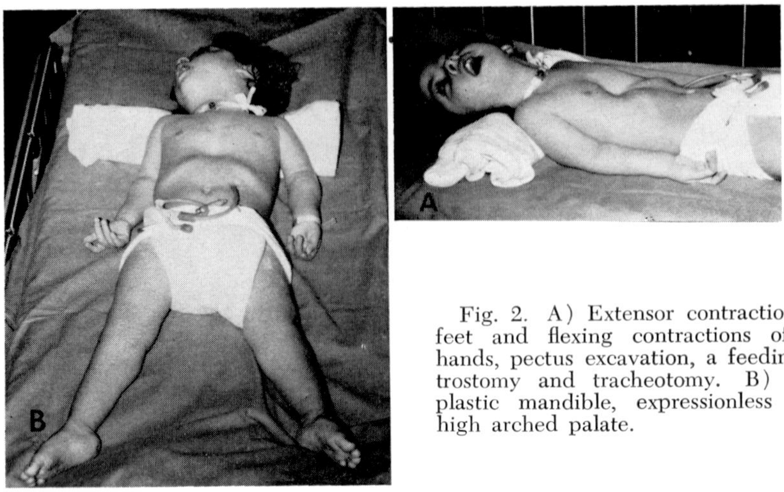

Fig. 2. A) Extensor contraction both feet and flexing contractions of both hands, pectus excavation, a feeding gastrostomy and tracheotomy. B) Hypoplastic mandible, expressionless facies, high arched palate.

air, but pink in oxygen, with an extremely weak voice. Retraction at the xiphoid with loud inspiratory stridor and pooling of saliva in the oropharynx and mouth were noted. The suck reflex was poor, and, because of severe dysphagia, gavage feedings were necessary. Respiratory distress progressed, and on March 21, 1967 laryngoscopy, bronchoscopy, and tracheotomy were performed. The sternocleidomastoid muscle was hypertrophied on the right, and almost absent on the left. The larynx was seen to be inflamed, with marked redundancy of all the superglottic structures. The pharynx was flat, and did not constrict with stimulation. The gag reflex was absent. Pooling of saliva was seen. Whereas the left vocal cord remained in the midline, the right vocal cord abducted 1 mm from the midline. Purulent secretion was seen in the tracheobronchial tree. With the tracheotomy in place she continued to require constant care. On April 10, 1967 biopsy of pharyngeal musculature showed a slight, focal increase in interstitial fibrous tissue, without evidence of either dystrophy or denervation atrophy. On May 17, 1967 direct laryngoscopy again showed superglottic collapse similar to laryngomalacia, the vocal cords were the same, and esophagoscopy revealed hypertrophy of the cricopharyngeus and upper esophagus. The lower esophagus was normal. On March 11, 1968 laryngoscopy again showed retention of saliva in the pharynx, with spilling into the larynx, plus superglottic collapse due to widespread relaxation of the musculature and loss of tone. The vocal cords moved poorly, with loss of tension, and poor adduction. Spasmodic closure of the larynx was absent, accounting for aspiration. The child expired on January 2, 1969 following a rapidly spreading pulmonary infection and *Salmonella gastroenteritis*. An autopsy was not permitted.

Case 2. J.D.G. was admitted to the hospital age 10 hours, because of multiple congenital anomalies. This child was the product of a 30-year-old mother with two healthy children. Presentation and delivery were double footling breech. The mother had a respiratory infection during the first trimester of pregnancy. The child was born at full term. Examination showed multiple joint contractures, a high arched palate, and severe arthrogrypotic involvement of the mandible, which hampered examination of the mouth and throat. The jaw was ankylosed and hypoplastic (micrognathia). The course in the hospital was one of serious feeding difficulty, with resultant aspiration bronchopneumonia. The child was gavage fed, but gradually the course was downhill, and the child died one month after admission. Postmortem examination revealed focal cortical neurone deficiency and heterotopic grey matter nodules in the arachnoid. Skeletal muscle fibers were uniformly small, but showed no other abnormality.

Case 3. B.B.T., a 3-hour-old Caucasian male, was admitted to the hospital on May 11, 1967 in moderately severe distress, cyanotic, and unresponsive. The product of a pregnancy of unknown gestational period, the child required immediate resuscitation at birth. Multiple congenital anomalies were noted. A cleft palate, single umbilical artery, rudimentary left thumb, omphalocele and contractures of the feet bilaterally were noted. The suck reflex was poor. Moro and grasp reflexes were depressed. A spinal tap was normal. The patient was intubated after a cardiorespiratory arrest, but could not be resuscitated. Death occurred three hours after admission. At autopsy esophageal, diaphragm, intercostal, psoas and cervical muscle fibers were uniformly small in diameter. Other than immaturity, the brain and spinal cord were not remarkable.

Case 4. B.G.P., a female Caucasian infant, was admitted to the hospital on February 1, 1964, immediately after her birth. She was

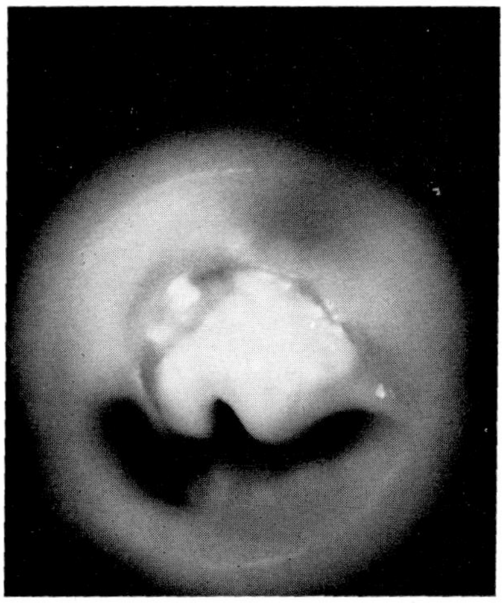

Fig. 3. Marked enlarged thickened, inflamed, and swollen epiglottis and aryepiglottic folds.

three weeks premature. Her mother had "flu" in the first trimester of pregnancy. Delivery was normal. The child was noted to be asphyxiated at birth, required oxygen, and was transferred to the hospital with a diagnosis of tracheoesophageal fistula. The infant was severely depressed, with pooling of saliva in the mouth. In addition, she had severe aspiration pneumonitis, a ureteral vaginal fistula, pectus carinatum, and Potter's facies. In spite of therapy for severe pneumonitis, the patient expired on the ninth hospital day. At autopsy, laryngeal and cervical skeletal muscle fibers were uniformly small in diameter, but otherwise unremarkable. Central nervous system exhibited no diagnostic abnormality.

Case 5. D.W., a Caucasian female, born June 5, 1973, was admitted to the hospital on September 5, 1973. The child was transferred

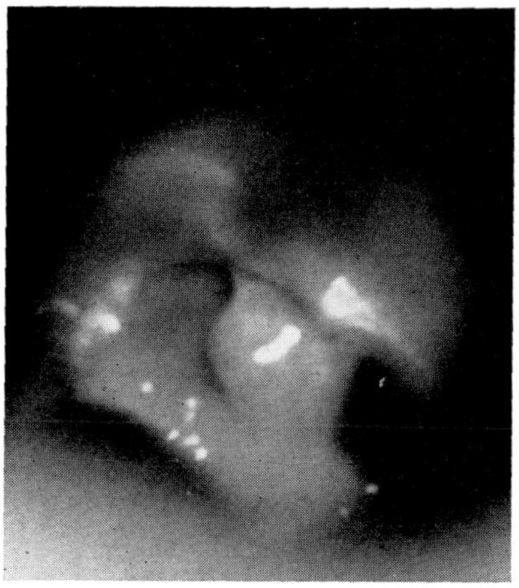

Fig. 4. Swollen displaced right arytenoid and swollen short aryepiglottic folds.

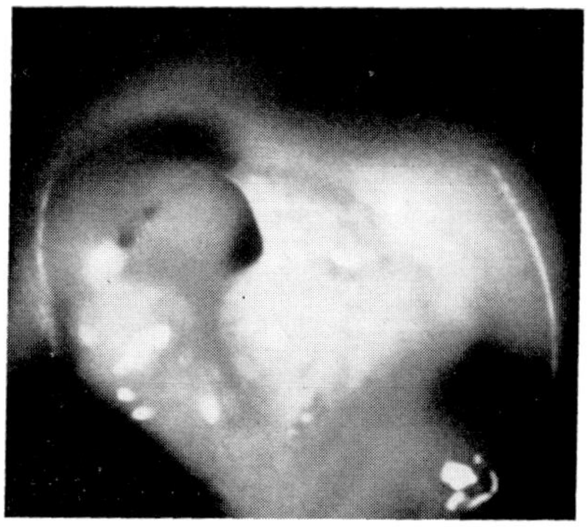

Fig. 5. Bulbous arytenoids, anterior and medial displaced right arytenoid, poor closure mechanism.

from another hospital with a diagnosis of AMC, multiple anomalies and pneumonitis. Born by frank breech presentation, she required continued hospitalization because of severe apneic spells. Recurrent pulmonary problems persisted, necessitating continuous oxygen and suctioning. She could not take oral feedings and required intravenous fluids. Examination revealed a Caucasian female with multiple orthopedic anomalies (Figs. 2A, B), severe pallor with periods of cyanosis, and irregular respirations. Both upper and lower extremities were involved by contractures. X-ray of the chest showed bilateral pulmonary infiltrates. An esophogram with an indwelling tube showed the esophagus to be normal. She required resuscitation with respirator aid during severe periods of respiratory difficulty, and was transferred to the hospital at age three months. On admission to the hospital, she was taken to the operating room where direct laryngoscopy, bronchoscopy and a tracheotomy were performed. The findings were those of severe micrognathia, glossoptosis, and a high arched palate without a cleft. The pharynx was filled with secretions. The cough reflex was intact, and purulent secretion filled the tracheobronchial tree. The larynx was difficult to visualize because of the small hypopharynx. The supraglottic structures were inflamed and hypertrophic (Fig. 3). The right vocal cord remained in the midline, with the right arytenoid anteriorly and medially displaced (Fig. 4). The left vocal cord moved only into the paramedian position. Spasmodic closure was faulty (Fig. 4). Neither a cleft of the larynx, nor a tracheoesophageal fistula were found. Bronchoscopy showed the tracheobronchial tree to be normal, but flooded with secretions. A tracheotomy was performed. The infant continued to aspirate secretions and required constant tracheal suctioning. A feeding gastrostomy was performed. During the next two-and-a-half years, the patient had numerous admissions to the hospital, for splinting and casting of her extremities, and repeated

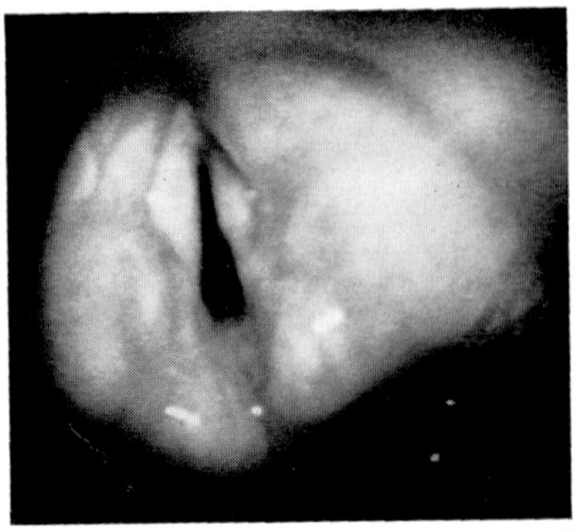

Fig. 6. Faulty adductor spasmodic closure; right vocal cord in paramedian position.

laryngeal examinations showed persistent, poor spasmodic closure of the vocal cords, but abduction of vocal cords has improved. On July 14, 1975 and on subsequent examinations, the epiglottis was extremely thickened (Fig. 3) and diffusely inflamed. The arytenoids were bulbous and the right was anteriorly and medially displaced (Fig. 5). The vocal cords appeared to abduct normally but adduction was faulty (Fig. 6). The pharynx was filled with secretion. Esophagoscopy showed the cricopharyngeus to be hypertrophic with folds which filled the esophageal lumen. The lower portion of the esophagus was not examined. On December 29, 1975 a hypopharyngeal muscle biopsy was performed, but showed no diagnostic abnormality. Only mild focal fibrosis was seen. However, sections of gastrocnemius, and quadriceps femoris skeletal muscle biopsies, on the other hand, revealed muscle atrophy consistent with late denervation atrophy. The child as of this date is still tracheotomized, and requires gastrostomy

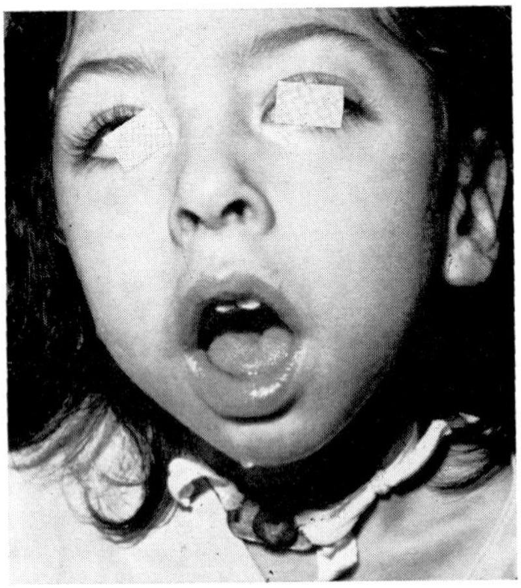

Fig. 7. Typical facies, expressionless drooling, curled tongue, and slightly hypoplastic mandible.

feedings. Her face remains expressionless and drooling persists (Fig. 7).

Case 6. M.W., a Caucasian male infant, was admitted to the hospital at age four months on April 7, 1958. He was a full term infant, the product of an uncomplicated pregnancy and normal delivery. A sibling died at age four months of congenital heart disease. The mother and grandfather had club feet. His admitting diagnosis was multiple congenital anomalies—micrognathia, glossoptosis, and bilateral club feet. His course in the hospital was one of failure to gain weight, poor suck reflex, constant aspiration and pneumonitis. It was impossible to maintain his airway. The child expired on July 27, 1958. Autopsy revealed a Pierre Robin-like syndrome without cleft palate. Significant findings included cerebral hypoplasia, flooded tracheobronchial secretions and pneumonitis, AMC, and congenital absence of the right kidney. Histologically, the tongue and skeletal muscles demonstrated uniformly small fibers. In addition, the tongue showed a hyperkeratotic epithelial surface which cascaded upon itself. Spinal cord anterior horn cells were reduced in number. The brain was histologically immature.

Case 7. F.R., a four-month-old Caucasian male, was admitted to the hospital on June 17, 1972 with severe respiratory distress, fever and dysphagia. A diagnosis of Werdnig-Hoffmann disease with arthrogryposis had been made one month prior to admission. The infant was floppy, drooled and was unable to handle excessive saliva. Physical examination showed absent deep tendon reflexes, and Moro reflexes were absent. The patient responded to pain. The course was rapidly downhill and he expired on June 19, 1972. Postmortem findings included neurogenic muscular atrophy involving most skeletal muscles. The musculature of the tongue, esophagus and diaphragm were spared. Anterior horn cells of spinal cord and XI and XII cranial nerve nuclei showed neuronal "ballooning degeneration" and nerve cell loss.

Case 8. H.H., a female Caucasian infant, was admitted to the hospital at age 17 days because of "failure to thrive" and excessive salivation. The infant had been born prematurely during the 35th week of gestation and weighed 2 kg. She was the product of a breech delivery following eight hours of labor. The patient was apparently doing well until age three days when she developed fever and was found to have pneumonia. She was treated for a week with antibiotics and apparently recovered from the pneumonia. However, from that time the infant progressively lost weight, and on admission to the hospital weighed only 1.6 kg. Physical examination on admission revealed a poorly developed infant with multiple skeletal anomalies and stigmata of the Pierre Robin syndrome. She had a small mouth and a high arched palate. There were flexion contractures of the wrists and fingers with hypermobility of both wrists. The fingers as well as the toes were elongated. She had bilateral congenital dislocations of the hips and genu valgus deformities of both knees. A mass was palpable in the right flank which was thought to be the right kidney. The heart and lungs were clear. While in the hospital, the patient was gavage fed. It was felt that some congenital anomaly of her genitourinary system was present as well as multiple musculo-skeletal abnormalities (AMC). She was doing relatively well until the day prior to death when she developed marked respiratory distress. Physical examination was suggestive of a high airway obstruction. She was taken to surgery for a tracheotomy, at which time direct laryngoscopy and bronchoscopy revealed laryngomalacia (supraglottic collapse). Following the tracheotomy, she improved somewhat, but expired the following day. Postmortem examination showed early bronchopneumonia and right hydronephrosis with double collecting systems. The CNS exhibited no diagnostic abnormality other than immaturity. Skeletal muscle fibers were uniformly small in diameter, but not otherwise remarkable.

Case 9. C.O., a Caucasian female infant, was admitted to the hospital at four days of age on January 31, 1963 with inability to feed. Mother's pregnancy was uncomplicated. The infant was born by breech delivery and was noted to have only a squeaky cry, a weak suck reflex and a hypoplastic mandible facies. Acrocyanosis was observed with a slow respiratory rate and paroxysmal abdominal movements. A tensilon test and lumbar puncture were normal. Because of aspiration of feedings, she was gavage fed. A muscle biopsy showed uniformly small fibers. Neither dystrophic nor inflammatory changes were evident. Histology was consistent with disuse atrophy. Clinical diagnosis was AMC with spinal cord lesion other than Werdnig-Hoffmann disease. Her second admission was on March 5, 1963 for treatment of pneumonia. Chest x-ray revealed a right upper and right lower lobe pneumonia. Her ability to feed improved, and she was followed until 1968. Her mental development was normal and her dysphagia subsided. While diabetes mellitus developed, the patient at present is living and well.

PATHOLOGY

Postmortem and biopsy material of nine infants and children with AMC were reviewed. The larynx, pharynx, esophagus, skeletal muscles and CNS were studied. Two patients had pharyngeal biopsies and two extremity muscle biopsies (D.W. and C.O.).

One infant (F.R.) had AMC associated with Werdnig-Hoffman disease. Most of the skeletal muscles showed severe neuromuscular atrophy, but the diaphragm, larynx and tongue musculature were spared. The spinal cord and caudal medulla exhibited nerve cell loss and "balloon cell" degeneration.

In the other five autopsied patients, skeletal muscles, including the larynx, showed no diagnostic abnormality. In addition to H. and E., trichrome and PTAH stains were used to study skeletal muscle morphology. Skeletal muscles were essentially normal except that the muscle fibers tended to be uniformly small in diameter in all muscle groups sampled. In one patient (M.W.), a decreased number of anterior motor neurons was noted in the cervical spinal cord, but neuromuscular atrophy was not observed. Microscopic examination of the CNS of the other four patients showed immaturity without other abnormalities.

A three-year-old girl (D.W.), one of the two presently living children with laryngeal problems, had biopsies of pharyngeal, gastrocnemius and quadriceps femoris muscles. Pharyngeal biopsy showed normal muscle fibers with mild focal interstitial fibrosis, but the extremity muscles exhibited striking changes consistent with late denervation atrophy.

The pharyngeal muscle biopsy of the other surgical patient (C.B.) revealed essentially normal fibers with mild focal interstitial fibrosis.

SUMMARY AND CONCLUSIONS

The clinical courses of 37 patients (20 male, 17 female) with arthrogryposis multiplex congenita (AMC) were reviewed. Nine patients, all with neurogenic AMC, had otolaryngological manifestations. Six of these had Pierre-Robin syndrome (or a similar disorder with two of the three criteria for this entity). Seven of the nine patients had severe dysphagia and aspiration pneumonitis. One patient, with hypoplastic mandible and severe dysphagia, had temporomandibular joint disease with trismus severe enough to prevent adequate examination of the oropharynx. Five of the patients, all of whom had severe aspiration problems, had voice changes; three of these required tracheotomy to relieve laryngeal obstruction and prevent aspiration.

Two patients had expressionless facies, pharyngeal paralysis, and absent gag reflexes. They could not protrude the tongue, were aphonic, and had laryngeal paralysis with displaced bulky arytenoids. At first these two patients had midline vocal cord paralysis, but later developed defective adductor closure mechanisms. The supraglottic structures were thickened and inflamed. Only three of the nine patients had laryngeal examination, each showing supraglottic narrowing similar to that of "laryngomalacia." In two patients esophagoscopy revealed marked hypertrophy of the cricopharyngeus and upper one-third of the esophagus.

Of the nine patients with otolaryngological problems only two are alive, and one of these has severe CNS disease. Six of these patients with otolaryngological problems were autopsied, and two had pharyngeal muscle biopsies. Autopsy and muscle biopsies demonstrated normal laryngeal and pharyngeal musculature even in one infant with advanced Werdnig-Hoffmann disease and AMC. In all larynges studied, the cricoarytenoid joints were normal.

Central nervous system dysfunction rather than simple muscle weakness thus appears to be an important cause of dysphagia and respiratory difficulty in patients with neurologic AMC, as a result of dysfunction of pharynx, palate, tongue and larynx. Since the resultant severe dysphagia with aspiration pneumonitis can be fatal, a tracheotomy and feeding gastrostomy appear essential for successful management of the otolaryngological complications of AMC.

Although otolaryngologic difficulties caused the death of approximately 20% of patients with AMC in this study, and were the single most important cause of death in these patients, other significant lesions may also reduce survival in AMC. Additional disorders present in patients in this series included optic atrophy, imperforate anus, cryptorchidism, genitourinary system anomalies, cardiomyopathy, and congenital heart disease.

REFERENCES

1. Otto AW: Monstrorum sexcentorum descriptio anatomica in Uratislaviae Museum. *Anatomico-Pathologicum Vratislaviaevise*: 1841

2. Rosenkranz E: Uber Kongenitale Kontrakturen der oberen Extremital. Z Orthop Chir 14:52-93, 1905

3. Stern WG: Arthrogryposis multiplex congenita. JAMA 81:1507-1510, 1923

4. Swinyard CA: Congenital contractures (arthrogryposis), Nature of the syndrome and hereditary considerations. Neurology 15:1397-1398, 1974

5. Pearson CM, Fowler WG Jr: Hereditary non-progressive muscular atrophy inducing arthrogryposis syndrome. Brain 86:75-88, 1974

6. Sandbank V, Cohen L: Arthrogryposis multiplex congenita associated with tuberous sclerosis. Pediat 64:571-574, 1964

7. Drachman DB, Coulombre AJ: Experimental clubfoot and arthrogryposis multiplex congenita. Lancet 2:523-526, 1962

8. Lebenthal E, Schochet SB, Adam A, *et al*: Arthrogryposis multiplex congenita 23 cases in an Arab kindred. Pediat 46:191-199, 1970

9. Friedlander HL, Westin GW, Wood WL Jr: Arthrogryposis multiplex congenita. J Bone J Surg 50:89-112, 1968

ACKNOWLEDGMENTS—The authors are grateful to Benjamin H. Landing, MD, Chairman of the Department of Pathology, Childrens Hospital of Los Angeles, and Professor of Pathology and Pediatrics at the University of Southern California School of Medicine, for his help with the final review of the paper.

REPRINTS—S. R. Cohen, MD, 1300 North Vermont Avenue, Los Angeles, CA 90027.

Ann Otol 85: 1976

CONGENITAL LARYNGEAL DEFECTS IN THE ADULT

WILLIAM W. MONTGOMERY, MD

STEPHEN A. SMITH, MD

BOSTON, MASSACHUSETTS

SUMMARY – Two types of congenital laryngeal defects in the adult are presented. The first case is a patient with a laryngeal cleft who became symptomatic at 42 years of age. Dysphagia, dyspnea, hoarseness and aspiration progressed in severity until surgery was necessary at the age of 48 years. The second case presented is a 21-year-old male with nonfusion of the thyroid laminae. He was asymptomatic except for persistence of a high-pitched voice after puberty. The case histories and radiographic studies are reviewed, emphasizing that the diagnosis of these defects was more difficult than their management. The surgical repair is described and illustrated. Briefly, this involved repair of the laryngeal cleft using techniques similar to those of a herniorrhaphy. The nonfusion of the thyroid laminae and resultant defective anterior glottis was repaired using bipedicled muscle flaps and a silicone keel.

Congenital laryngeal defects in the newborn and infant are rarely encountered. Congenital laryngeal defects which clinically manifest for the first time in adulthood are even more rare. Two such defects are the subject of this paper. The first is a posterior laryngeal cleft and the second is an anterior nonfusion of the thyroid cartilages.

Posterior laryngeal cleft in the newborn should be suspected when the symptoms of dysphagia, aspiration, abnormal cry, and respiratory distress are present. The primary diagnostic examination is fluoroscopy. Contrast material is introduced through a catheter which is gradually withdrawn from the stomach and esophagus to search for a tracheoesophageal fistula. Following this, a swallowing cine-esophagram with thin contrast material is carefully performed, with attention focused on the hypopharynx and larynx. The congenital defect is then confirmed by endoscopy. Several excellent reviews of the congenital posterior laryngeal cleft in the neonatal and pediatric age groups have been published.[1-20]

Dysphagia, aspiration, hoarseness, and dyspnea can also be symptoms of posterior laryngeal cleft in the adult. To make the diagnosis prior to endoscopy or exploratory surgery is a noteworthy accomplishment.

CASE REPORTS

Case 1. Posterior Laryngeal Cleft. A 48-year-old white woman presented with a history of six years of progressive dysphagia and one year of slowly progressive hoarseness and dyspnea. A complete review of her medical history revealed that she was the product of an uncomplicated pregnancy and delivery. Birth weight was 3.6 kg and there were no neonatal respiratory or feeding difficulties. However, she had three episodes of pneumonia between the ages of 1 and 15 years, and two more as an adult. The family history was unremarkable.

At the age of 42, she was admitted to the hospital for removal of a foreign body in the esophagus. No abnormalities of the larynx or esophagus were noted at esophagoscopy.

Five years later she was evaluated by the same otolaryngologist with complaints of increasing dyspnea on exertion, progressive hoarseness, and aspira-

---

From the Massachusetts Eye and Ear Infirmary, Boston, Massachusetts.

Presented at the meeting of the American Laryngological Association, Palm Beach, Florida, April 24-25, 1976.

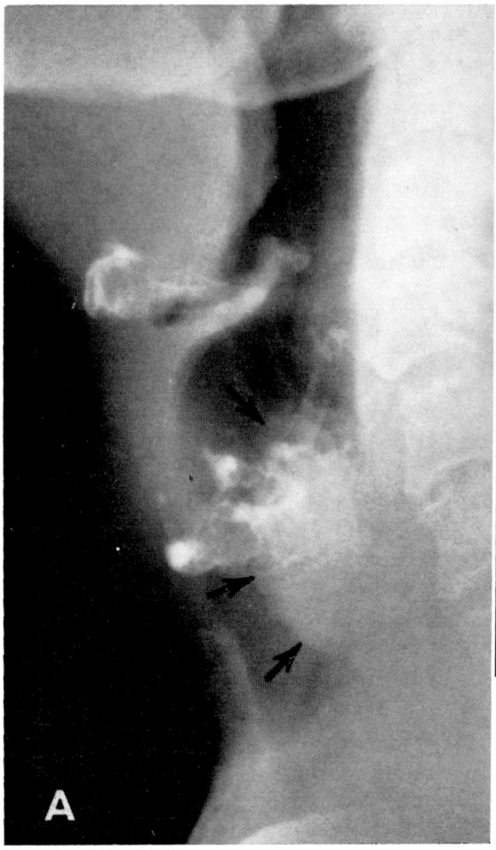

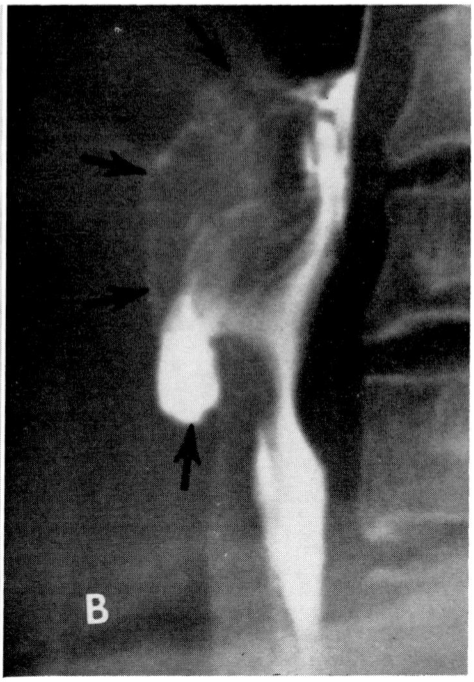

Fig. 1. a) The arrows point to a mass in the posterior laryngeal lumen extending from the level of the arytenoids to the subglottic region. At this point the diagnosis of posterior laryngeal cleft was not suspected. b) The upper three arrows again outline the mass. In the posterior larynx the lower arrow points to the pouch of the cervical esophagus which herniates into the subglottic lumen. The diagnosis of posterior laryngeal cleft was added to the differential diagnosis.

tion with cough. Direct laryngoscopy at that time revealed a large "mass" involving the posterior larynx, and biopsy of this mass demonstrated "normal epithelium."

At the Infirmary, indirect laryngoscopy revealed a large "tumor" mass involving the posterior commissure and projecting anteriorly into the glottic and subglottic regions. The glottic airway was limited to a narrow passage anteriorly. Both arytenoids appeared to function normally; the true vocal cords were obscured posteriorly and were normal anteriorly.

Plane films demonstrated a large mass involving the posterior larynx and extending 2 cm below the glottis. Barium swallow (Fig. 1) revealed a pouch extending into the glottic and subglottic lumen from the postcricoid region.

Direct laryngoscopy under general anesthesia revealed a "floppy" soft tissue mass in the interarytenoid space, extending well into the glottic and subglottic spaces. The mass was easily compressible, unlike a tumor. The esophageal inlet appeared normal, and the esophagus was easily entered. No defect in the posterior cricoid lamina was detected.

Following endoscopy, the larynx was exposed by way of an anterior thyrotomy. The defect in the posterior cricoid lamina became immediately apparent, the "tumor" mass representing esophageal herniation anteriorly into

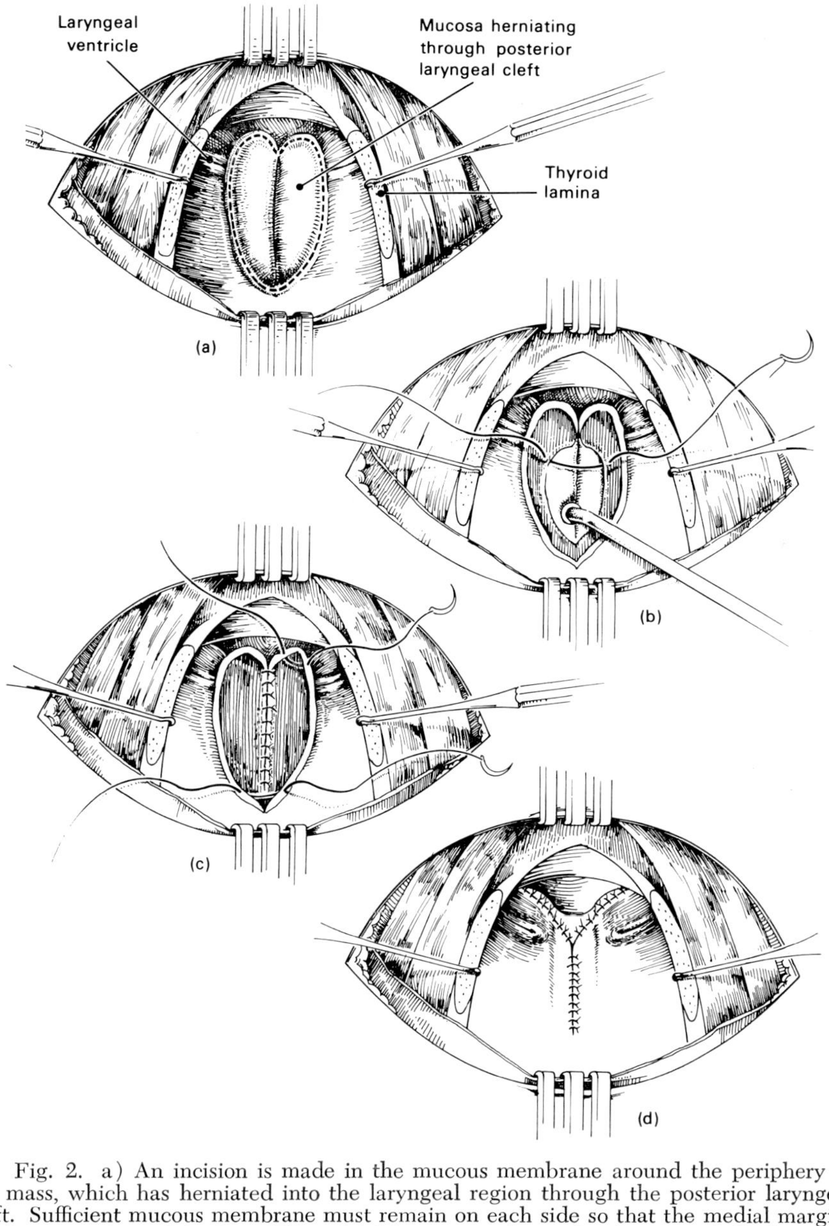

Fig. 2. a) An incision is made in the mucous membrane around the periphery of the mass, which has herniated into the laryngeal region through the posterior laryngeal cleft. Sufficient mucous membrane must remain on each side so that the medial margins can be approximated in the midline. b) Mucous membrane has been carefully dissected from the anterior aspect of the mass, which herniated from the esophagus through the posterior laryngeal cleft. The defect in the postcricoid region is repaired with 3-0 chromic catgut suture material. The herniating esophageal mucous membrane must be pushed posteriorly as this repair is accomplished. c) The first layer of closure has been accomplished. Two sutures have been applied to the postcricoid mucous membrane, which is also repaired using interrupted 3-0 chromic catgut sutures. d) The closure is complete. The normal structures of the larynx can be much more readily visualized. The thyrotomy is closed in the usual fashion. No stent or keel is necessary.

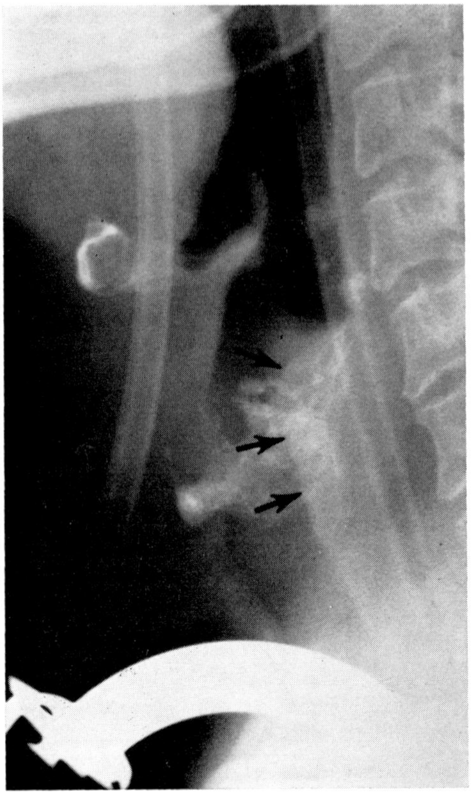

Fig. 3. A postoperative x-ray demonstrating the absence of the mass and pouch.

the larynx and subglottic region. The diagnosis of congenital laryngeal cleft was confirmed and the defect was repaired as illustrated in Figure 2.

A postoperative x-ray (Fig. 3) demonstrates the absence of the mass which was previously present in the larynx and the subglottic regions. The tracheotomy tube was removed two weeks following the surgery. The patient has had no difficulty with deglutition, and her voice and airway are normal three years postoperatively.

Comments. We assume that this patient's recurrent pneumonias were early evidence of this malformation, and that the cleft facilitated the lodging of a foreign body in the cervical esophagus. It was only in the patient's fourth decade that soft tissue support bolstering the cleft became sufficiently weakened to permit progressive herniation of postcricoid tissue through the cleft. Symptoms referable to this herniation ultimately led her to seek relief.

If the diagnosis is considered during endoscopy, the cleft can be explored with a laryngeal spatula. The large mass of herniated tissue in the present case would have made this difficult, however.

The embryology of this malformation is well-described in the literature.[3-5,9-11] Over 40 cases have been reported to date, many with multiple anomalies. The rate at which new cases are published is accelerating. Unlike tracheoesophageal fistula and esophageal atresia, a familial tendency has been documented in this condition.[1,7,18,21]

In the past, successful repairs have been effected in children via lateral pharyngotomy.[4,12,13,15,16,19,20] Haguenauer's[16] excellent experiences with three thyrotracheotomies in children refute the theoretical concerns of laryngeal damage from the procedure. Indeed, this was a direct and ideal approach for our adult patient. Notably, some patients may respond well to careful observation, avoidance of low viscosity diet as soon as possible, and supportive gastrostomy and/or tracheotomy.[20] How many patients managed this way will become symptomatic as adults, like our patient, is a question for the future.

Case 2. Anterior Laryngeal Defect. A normal appearing 17-year-old boy first consulted an otolaryngologist in 1970 complaining of a high-pitched voice. Short, but normally functioning vocal cords were noted during indirect laryngoscopy (Fig. 4a). Flattening and widening of the larynx were reported as part of the neck examination. The patient was referred to a second otolaryngologist who advised vocal therapy. There was no improvement. Endocrine evaluation was normal at that time.

At the age of 21, the patient was first examined at the Infirmary. By external palpation it was apparent that the thyroid notch was absent and the larynx

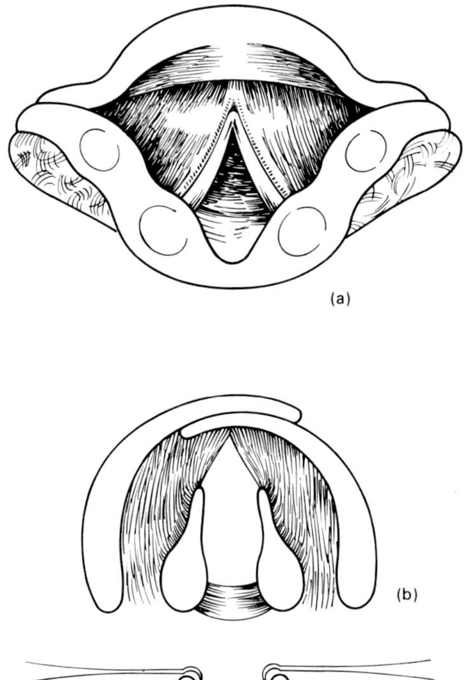

Fig. 4. a) A sketch of the mirror view showing a shortening of the anteroposterior dimension in Case 2. b) A horizontal sketch through the larynx showing nonfusion and overlapping of the anterior thyroid laminae which resulted in shortening of the vocal cords. c) The thyroid laminae have been dissected free and retracted laterally. The anterior half of the true and false vocal cords along with the immediate supraglottic regions are absent.

was flat and wide. It was thus suspected that the thyroid laminae were not fused anteriorly. The vocal cords functioned normally, but were quite short and produced a feminine-type voice.

X-ray evaluation added nothing to establish a positive clinical diagnosis

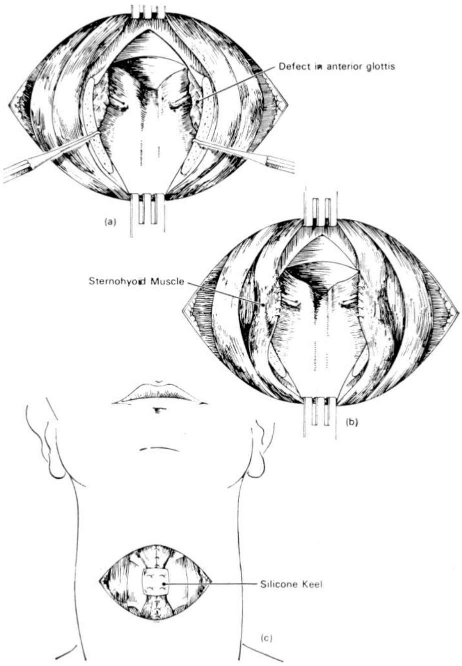

Fig. 5. a) The defect in the anterior glottis is illustrated. b) The sternohyoid muscles and fascia are used as bipedicled flaps to repair the defect of the anterior larynx. c) A silicone keel is sutured in place between the sternohyoid muscles and thyroid laminae.

other than confirmation of the short antero-posterior dimension of the larynx.

In November, 1974, the larynx was exposed by way of a horizontal anterior cervical skin incision at the midlaryngeal level. After performing a tracheotomy, the thyroid laminae were exposed and found not to be fused anteriorly, but were more curved than usual and overlapped to produce the flattening and widening of the larynx as well as the shortening of the vocal cords (Fig. 4b).

The thyroid laminae were separated from one another and retracted laterally with a resultant defect of the anterior half of the glottis (Figs. 4c, 5a). In other words, the soft tissues of the anterior half of the vocal cords and immediate supraglottic and subglottic regions were absent. It was necessary to score the thyroid laminae vertically in order to break the spring of their ab-

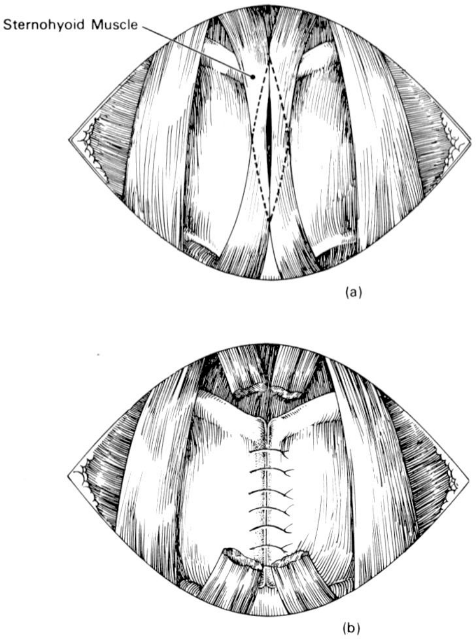

Fig. 6. a) The silicone keel has been removed. The superior and inferior portions of the sternohyoid muscles not used for the repair are transected (broken line) so that the newly constructed anterior commissure can be closed. b) The thyroid laminae have been approximated anteriorly.

normal curvature and retract them laterally.

The sternohyoid muscles with their fascia were carefully dissected so that they could be reflected into the larynx in order to supply tissue for the anterior half of each side of the glottis (Fig. 5b). This repair was accomplished using 4-0 catgut suture material.

A silicone keel[22] was inserted between the sternohyoid muscles inside the larynx and sutured in place with 3-0 polyethylene suture material (Fig. 5c). Three weeks postoperatively the silicone keel was removed as an office procedure. The tracheotomy tube was removed one week later.

After two months his voice was definitely at a lower pitch, but not satisfactory to either the patient or surgeon. It became apparent that the thyroid laminae had not united because of the presence of the laryngeal keel.

Ten months postoperatively the thyroid laminae were again exposed. The superior and inferior portions of the sternohyoid muscle, which were external to the laryngeal lumen and not used as part of the repair, were incised so that the anterior margin of each thyroid lamina could be visualized (Fig. 6a). The thyroid laminae were carefully approximated in the midline with nonabsorbable suture material (Fig. 6b). The airway was not entered, and no tracheotomy was necessary. The result was excellent. Shortly thereafter he enjoyed a normal airway and the voice of a normal adult male.

Comments. In this case the second stage operation was clearly necessary, but possibly could have been performed at the time the keel was removed. Perhaps the thyroid laminae could have been more securely approximated anteriorly above and below the silicone keel at the first operation, making the second operation unnecessary.

Polytomography of the larynx in a vertical plane was not done. This would have demonstrated the overlapping of the nonfused thyroid laminae. Had the thyroid laminae been ossified, the reconstruction would have been much more difficult.

Interestingly, we have found no reported significant anomalies of the thyroid cartilage compatible with life. From an evolutionary standpoint, the thyroid cartilage is the newest feature of the laryngeal skeleton.[23,24] It is peculiar to placental mammals, the more primitive hyobranchial apparatus of vertebrates consisting primarily of a hyoid-cricoid framework.

The thyroid cartilage is represented in the embryo, at the end of the fourth week, as a cell mass situated immediately anterior to the fourth arch and cleft. The thyroid mass is continuous with the primordium of the greater cornu of the hyoid bone in the 9.5 mm embryo, sixth week. A week later, chrondrification is underway; the alae are markedly convex and widely separated superiorly. The inferior cornu begins to develop, and in the middle of the third month (the 35 mm embryo) the inferior cornu makes contact with the thyroid cartilage. The thyroid alae join ventrally first at the lower ends.[25]

During puberty in boys, as the larynx grows rapidly, the vocal cords normally become about 1 cm longer, contributing to the normal lowering of pitch which occurs at this time.[26] In our patient, as the laryngeal skeleton enlarged at puberty, nonfusion and overlapping of the thyroid laminae precluded the normal lengthening of the vocal cords and left him with his high-pitched voice.

Possibly if a diagnosis of anterior nonfusion of the thyroid laminae is kept in mind, a few more males will not be called "Miss" on the telephone.

REFERENCES

1. Finlay HVL: Familial congenital stridor. Arch Dis Child 24:219-233, 1949
2. Palmer HD: Clinicopathologic conference: congenital cricoid cartilage defect. Q Med Bull Children's Hosp, Denver, 3:168-181, 1951
3. Holinger PH, Brown WT: Congenital webs, cysts, laryngoceles and other anomalies of the larynx. Ann Otol Rhinol Laryngol 76: 744-752, 1967
4. Pettersson G: Inhibited separation of the larynx and the upper part of the trachea from esophagus in a newborn. Acta Chem Scand 110:250-254, 1955
5. Triboletti E: Unusual congenital anomaly involving the larynx, trachea, and esophagus. N Engl J Med 258:1002-1003, 1958
6. Fisher JH: Extensive tracheoesophageal communication. Bronches 19:105-109, 1961
7. Zachary RB, Emery JL: Failure of separation of larynx and trachea from esophagus: persistent esophagotrachea. Surgery 49: 525-529, 1961
8. Cameron AH, Williams TC: Cleft larynx: a cause of laryngeal obstruction and incompetence. J Laryngol Otol 76:381-387, 1962
9. Blumberg JB, Stevenson JK, Lemire RJ, *et al*: Laryngotracheoesophageal cleft, the embryologic implications: review of the literature. Surgery 57:559-566, 1965
10. Harrison HS, Fuqua EB, Griffin RB: Congenital laryngeal cleft: report of a case. Am J Dis Child 110:556-558, 1965
11. Griscom NT: Persistent esophagotrachea, the most severe degree of laryngotracheoesophageal cleft. Amer J Roentgenol Radium Ther Nucl Med 97:211-215, 1966
12. Shapiro MJ, Falla A: Congenital posterior cleft larynx (laryngotracheoesophageal cleft): report of a case. Ann Otol Rhinol Laryngol 75:961-967, 1966
13. Jahrsdoerfer RA, Kirchner JA, Thaler SU: Cleft larynx. Arch Otolaryngol 86:108-113, 1967
14. Delahunty JE, Cherry J: Congenital laryngeal cleft. Ann Otol Rhinol Laryngol 78: 96-106, 1969
15. Imbrie JD, Doyle PJ: Laryngotracheoesophageal cleft: report of a case and review of the literature. Laryngoscope 79:1252-1274, 1969
16. Haguenauer JP, Berdal P: Le diasteure larynge congenital: a propos de 6 observations. Ann Otolaryngol Chir Cervicofac 87:651-662, 1970
17. Donahoe PK, Hendren WH: The surgical management of laryngotracheoesophageal cleft with tracheoesophageal fistula and esophageal atresia. Surgery 71:363-368, 1972
18. Phelan PD, Stocks JG, Williams HE, *et al*: Familial occurrence of congenital laryngeal clefts. Arch Dis Child 48:275-278, 1973
19. Pracy R, Stell PM: Laryngeal cleft: diagnosis and management. J Laryngol Otol 88:483-486, 1974
20. Cohen SR: Cleft larynx: a report of seven cases. Ann Otol Rhinol Laryngol 84: 747-756, 1975
21. Crooks J: Noninflammatory laryngeal stridor in infancy. Arch Dis Child 29:381, 1954
22. Montgomery WW: *Surgery of the Upper Respiratory System.* Philadelphia, Lea & Febiger, 1973, vol 2, chap 8, p 570
23. Goodrich ES: *Studies on the Structure and Development of Vertebrates.* New York, Dover, 1958
24. Hyman LH: *Comparative Vertebrate Anatomy.* Chicago, University of Chicago Press, 1942
25. Myerson MC: *The Human Larynx.* Baltimore, CC Thomas, 1964
26. Pressman JJ, Keleman G: Kirchner JA (rev): *Physiology of the Larynx. Continuing Education Manual.* Rochester, Am Acad Ophthalmol Otolaryngol, 1970

Reprints—William W. Montgomery, MD, Massachusetts Eye and Ear Infirmary, 243 Charles Street, Boston, MA 02114.

Ann Otol 85: 1976

MUCUS GLAND TUMORS OF THE LARYNX AND LARYNGOPHARYNX

RONALD H. SPIRO, MD
JOHN S. LEWIS, MD
STEVEN I. HAJDU, MD
ELLIOT W. STRONG, MD

NEW YORK, NEW YORK

SUMMARY – During the 30-year period from 1939 through 1968, 20 patients were seen who had "minor salivary" tumors arising in the mucus glands of the larynx or laryngopharynx. This group comprised about 3% of more than 600 patients with mucus gland tumors of the upper aerodigestive tract treated at Memorial Sloan-Kettering Cancer Center during the same interval. In each instance the tumor was malignant, and all but three of these patients were men. Location and histology of these uncommon tumors is described. Only 2 of 18 treated cases were "cured." Uncontrolled cervical lymph node involvement or distant metastasis was more often the reason for treatment failure, rather than local recurrence at the primary site.

It is well known that mucus glands beneath the epithelium of the upper respiratory and digestive tract may occasionally give rise to tumors histologically identical to those occurring in the major, or paired salivary glands. In most instances, these so-called minor salivary neoplasms are found in the mouth, usually in the palate. At times, the nasal cavity or paranasal sinuses may be involved. In this report we direct attention to the larynx and laryngopharynx as a most unusual site for salivary type neoplasms.

During the years 1939 through 1968, 21 patients who had a salivary neoplasm arising in the larynx or laryngopharynx were seen at Memorial Sloan-Kettering Cancer Center. This group comprised only 3% of more than 600 patients with minor salivary gland tumors, or 0.8% of 2,793 patients with cancer of the larynx seen during the same 30-year interval.[1] As reported previously from our hospital, most nonepidermoid carcinomas of the larynx proved to be of mucus gland origin.[2]

HISTOPATHOLOGY

All of the patients in this series had malignant tumors, but other reports suggest that any type of salivary neoplasms, whether benign or malignant, may occur in the larynx or laryngopharynx.[3-8] One exception seems to be acinic cell carcinoma, which only rarely occurs in mucus glands.[1] No histologic material is available in one patient who was treated elsewhere, and this case has been excluded.

Using a classification which is a modification of that originally proposed by Foote and Frazell,[9] the tumor proved to be an adenocarcinoma in 13 patients. Most of these were of the solid variety and showed a striking resemblance to mammary carcinoma in some instances. These tumors infiltrated the submucosal connective tissue in cell cords and clusters; a minimal connective tissue stroma was present between the tumor cells. Reactive histiocytes and lymphocytes were seen in many tissues sections, but necrosis of the tumor was rare (Fig. 1). Others showed a small cell pattern with features suggestive of carcinoid tumors. Mucus production was conspicuous in one patient who had an adenocarcinoma, and another had a most unusual tumor with Pagetoid changes in the overlying mucous membrane (Fig. 2).

From the Head and Neck Service, Department of Surgery, and the Department of Pathology, Memorial Sloan-Kettering Cancer Center, New York, New York.

Presented at the meeting of the American Laryngological Association, Palm Beach, Florida, April 24-25, 1976.

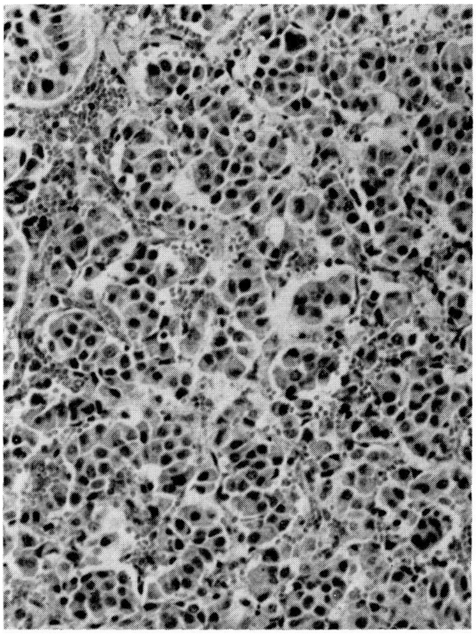

Fig. 1. Adenocarcinoma of solid duct cell type (H & E X170).

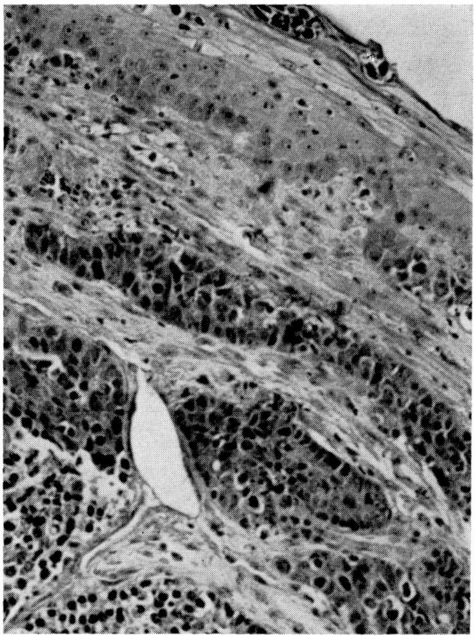

Fig. 2. Adenocarcinoma in the submucosa and areas of Pagetoid change in the surface mucosa (H & E X170).

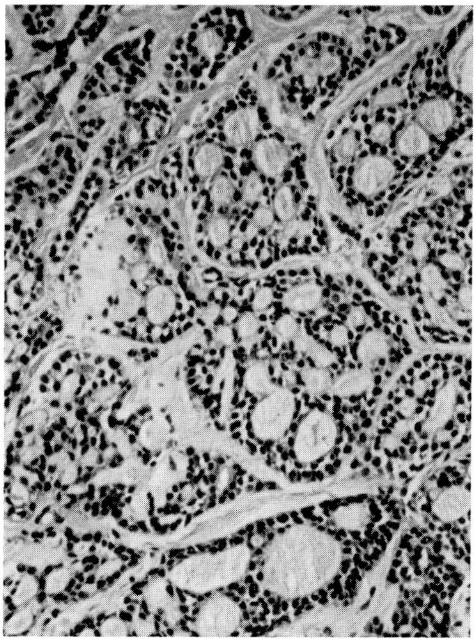

Fig. 3. Adenoid cystic carcinoma. Note transition from a low grade, glandular appearance on the right, to cord-like structures suggestive of a higher grade tumor on the left (H & E X170).

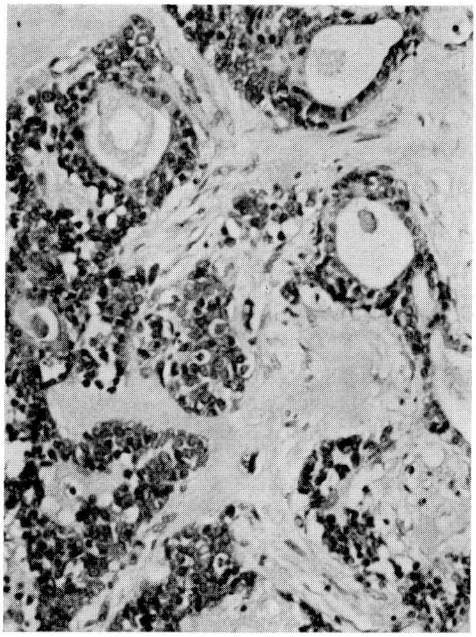

Fig. 4. Mucoepidermoid carcinoma, histologic Stage II (H & E X170).

TABLE I

HISTOPATHOLOGY AS RELATED TO SITE OF ORIGIN

	Adeno-carcinoma	*Adenoid Cystic Carcinoma*	*Muco-epidermoid Carcinoma*	*Anaplastic Carcinoma (oat cell)*	*Total*
Glottic	2	1	1	—	4
Supraglottic					
Epiglottis	2	2	1	1	6
Ventricular band	4	—	—	—	4
Aryepiglottic fold	4	—	1	—	5
Pyriform	1	—	—	—	1
Total	13	3	3	1	20

Adenoid cystic carcinoma was the diagnosis in three patients whose tumors showed features ranging from glandular arrangement to cell clusters or cell cord formation (Fig. 3). Gland formation with mucinous material in the lumen and areas composed of poorly differentiated cells helped to identify the tumor as mucoepidermoid carcinoma in three others (Fig. 4). One patient had an anaplastic carcinoma which closely resembled oat cell carcinoma of the lung.[10] Distribution of the various histologic types according to the site of origin is given in Table I.

OBSERVATIONS

The patients ranged in age from 38 through 79 years (median 59 years) and all but three were men. Symptoms varied in duration from one month to four years and hoarseness was the usual presenting complaint (12 patients). Sore throat (five patients), dysphagia (four patients), cough (three patients), and the sensation of a foreign body in the throat (three patients) were also noted. In three instances, a lump in the neck was the main reason the patient sought medical attention. Treatment had previously been given elsewhere in four patients.

TABLE II

CLINICAL STAGE ACCORDING TO SITE IN 16 PREVIOUSLY UNTREATED PATIENTS

	Stage I	*Stage II*	*Stage III*	*Stage IV*
Glottis	1	1	1	1
Epiglottis	—	2	3	—
Ventricular band	—	—	3	—
Aryepiglottic fold	—	—	3	—
Pyriform fossa	1	—	—	—
Total	2	3	10	1

The tumor involved the supraglottic larynx in 15 patients, 6 of whom had lesions in the epiglottis. Aryepiglottic folds or ventricular bands were the site of origin in five and four instances, respectively. The lesion involved the glottic larynx in four patients and one had a tumor located in the pyriform fossa.

With few exceptions, these patients had sizeable exophytic or ulcerated growths which were thought to be epidermoid carcinoma. The examining physician suspected that the tumor was unusual in one patient who had intact mucous membrane over a swelling involving a ventricular band, and in two others who had a pedunculated lesion on the medial wall of the pyriform fossa and aryepiglottic fold, respectively.

Most had tumors which were locally advanced by the time they were first seen. Moreover, cervical lymph nodes were initially involved in seven instances, including one patient who had bilateral metastases. According to the criteria proposed by the American Joint Committee on Staging,[11] 10 of 16 previously untreated patients had Stage III lesions, whereas three had Stage II, two

TABLE III

RESULTS IN 18 TREATED PATIENTS

Age Sex	*Primary Histology Clinical Stage*	*Iniitial Treatment*	*Result*	*Comment*
50 M	Glottic Adenocarcinoma Stage IV	Laryngectomy	DOD 1 yr, 3 mo	Lung and visceral metastases
53 M	Glottic Adenocarcinoma Stage III	Laryngectomy	DOC 1 yr	Neck recurrence
57 M	Glottic Adenoid cystic Stage II	Laryngectomy	DOD 2 yr	Carcinomatosis
55 M	Glottic Mucoepidermoid Stage I	Laryngectomy	NED 10 yr	Small commissure lesion
59 M	Epiglottis Mucoepidermoid Stage III	Laryngectomy and neck dissection	DOD 7 mo	Neck recurrence and bone metastases
70 F	Epiglottis Adenoid cystic Stage III	External irradiation	DOD 6 yr, 5 mo	Local recurrence
38 M	Epiglottis Adenoid cystic Stage II	External irradiation	DOC 6 mo	Hemorrhage due to radionecrosis
79 M	Epiglottis Anaplastic Stage III	Epiglottectomy and neck dissection	DOD 6 mo	Carcinomatosis
51 F	Epiglottis Adenocarcinoma (Prev. treated)	Chemotherapy	DOD 3 mo	Metastases present initially
64 M	Ventricular band Adenocarcinoma Stage III	Laryngectomy	DOC 9 mo	Tumor incompletely excised
70 M	Ventricular band Adenocarcinoma Stage III	Laryngectomy and neck dissection	DOD 5 mo	Neck recurrence
65 M	Ventricular band Adenocarcinoma (Prev. treated)	Laryngectomy, bilateral neck dissection	Postoperative death	Cerebrovascular accident
77 M	Ventricular band Adenocarcinoma Stage III	Laryngectomy	DOC 4 yr, 3 mo	Neck recurrence and distant metastases
41 M	Aryepiglottic fold Adenocarcinoma (Prev. treated)	Laryngectomy and neck dissection	DOD 4 yr	Neck recurrence lung metastases
70 M	Aryepiglottic fold Adenocarcinoma Stage III	Laryngectomy	DOD 1 yr, 6 mo	Local and neck recurrence and bone metastases
50 F	Aryepiglottic fold Adenocarcinoma Stage III	Laryngofissure excision and radical neck	DOD 3 yr, 7 mo	Local and neck recurrence
72 M	Aryepiglottic fold Adenocarcinoma (Prev. treated)	Laryngectomy and neck dissection	DOD 5 yr, 9 mo	Lung and brain metastases
57 M	Pyriform fossa Adenocarcinoma Stage I	Laryngectomy and neck dissection	NED 11 yr	Small pedunculated lesion

DOD - Died of disease; DOC - Died of other causes; NED - No evidence of disease

TABLE IV

CERVICAL LYMPH NODE INVOLVEMENT IN 18 TREATED PATIENTS

	No. of Patients	*Involved Initially*	*Involved Subsequently*	*Never Involved*
Adenocarcinoma	12	5*	4	3
Adenoidcystic carcinoma	3	—	1	2
Mucoepidermoid carcinoma	2	1	—	1
Anaplastic carcinoma	1	1	—	—
Total	18	7	5	6

* Bilateral involvement in one patient.

had Stage I and one had Stage IV disease, respectively (Table II).

TREATMENT AND RESULTS

No treatment was given in one patient who had an extensive primary, as well as a synchronous adenocarcinoma of the prostate, and another who refused laryngectomy and went elsewhere. Of the remaining 18 patients, irradiation was the only treatment in 2, both of whom were seen in the early years of this study. Laryngectomy was required in 13 patients, one had an epiglottectomy and another had local excision of a recurrence through a laryngofissure approach. Radical neck dissection was performed initially in nine patients, seven of whom had clinical evidence of cervical lymph node involvement. Chemotherapy alone was the treatment in one patient who presented with disseminated metastatic disease after irradiation elsewhere.

Postoperative death occurred in the one patient who had simultaneous bilateral radical neck dissection. In 11 patients, uncontrolled or metastatic mucus gland carcinoma was directly responsible for death, with survival ranging from seven months to 6½ years. One other patient died elsewhere within six months and is presumed to have been a treatment failure. Death due to other causes was recorded within nine months to four years in three additional patients who also had evidence of tumor recurrence. One patient who had a small, pedunculated adenocarcinoma in the pyriform fossa remains alive and well 14 years after total laryngectomy and radical neck dissection. Another remained free of disease ten years after laryngectomy for a small, glottic mucoepidermoid carcinoma and was then lost to follow-up (Table III).

Information about treatment failure was available in 14 of the 15 patients who survived initial treatment and subsequently died of or with disease. Local recurrence was documented in only four patients, one of whom had incomplete excision of an extensive primary tumor at the time of laryngectomy. Failure to control cervical lymph node metastasis, noted in nine instances, was a more frequent problem. In all, 12 of the 18 treated patients had evidence of cervical lymph node involvement at some time during the course of the disease (Table IV).

Including one patient who died postoperatively and was found to have unsuspected disseminated metastases on postmortem examination, a total of nine treated patients had distant metastasis (50%). This propensity for distant dissemination was evident for each histologic variety of tumor, and multiple sites were usually involved.

SUMMARY AND CONCLUSIONS

On rare occasion, mucus glands of the larynx and laryngopharynx may give rise to typical salivary type neoplasms. Twenty such cases are reported which comprise about 3% of our total minor salivary gland tumor experience during a 30-year period. The neoplasm in each instance was malignant and was usually extensive when most of these patients were initially examined. The preferred treatment was surgical, but only 2 of 18 treated patients were long term "cures." Uncontrolled cervical node metastasis or distant dissemination of tumor was more often the reason for treatment failure than local recurrence. Our experience suggests that the results might possibly have been improved if regional lymph nodes had been treated more aggressively, either by more liberal use of elective radical neck dissection or by combinations of radiation therapy and surgery.

REFERENCES

1. Spiro RH, Koss LG, Hajdu SI, *et al*: Tumors of minor salivary origin, a clinicopathologic study of 492 cases. Cancer 31:117-129, 1973
2. Cady B, Rippey JH, Frazell EL: Nonepidermoid cancer of the larynx. Ann Surg 167:116-120, 1968
3. Ahued SV: Cylindroma of the epiglottis. Arch Otolaryngol 63:366-371, 1956
4. Donald PJ, Krause CJ: Papillary cystadenoma of the larynx. Laryngoscope 83:2024-2028, 1973
5. Jokinen K, Seppala A, Palva A: Laryngeal pleomorphic adenoma. J Laryngol Otol 88:1131-1134, 1974
6. New GB, Erich JB: Adenocarcinoma of the larynx. Ann Otol Rhinol Laryngol 50:706-712, 1941
7. Olofsson J, van Nostrand AWP: Anaplastic small cell carcinoma of the larynx. Ann Otol Rhinol Laryngol 81:284-287, 1967
8. Sabri JA, Hajjar MA: Malignant mixed tumor of the vocal cord. Arch Otolaryngol 85:118-120, 1967
9. Foote FW Jr, Frazell EL: Tumors of the major salivary glands. Cancer 6:1065-1133, 1953
10. Koss LG, Spiro RH, Hajdu SI: Small cell (oat cell) carcinoma of minor salivary gland origin. Cancer 30:737-741, 1972
11. *Clinical Staging System for Carcinoma of the Larynx, Revision.* Chicago, American Joint Committee for Cancer Staging and End Results Reporting, 1972, pp 1-16

REPRINTS—Ronald H. Spiro, MD, Memorial Sloan-Kettering Cancer Center, 1275 York Ave., New York, NY 10021.

INTERNATIONAL CONGRESS ON THE EDUCATION OF THE DEAF

The International Congress on the Education of the Deaf voted in August 1975 to establish an International Congress Committee on the Education of the Deaf with the aim of creating a mechanism to insure a more orderly continuity in the congresses. For information write to Dr. S. Richard Silverman, Chairman, International Congress Committee on the Education of the Deaf, 818 South Euclid Avenue, St. Louis, MO 63110, U.S.A.

Ann Otol 85: 1976

GRANULAR CELL TUMORS OF THE LARYNX

HARVEY L. COATES, MB THOMAS J. MCDONALD, MD
KENNETH D. DEVINE, MD LOUIS H. WEILAND, MD
ROCHESTER, MINNESOTA

SUMMARY — Granular cell tumors of the larynx are relatively uncommon, always benign, and most commonly located in the posterior portion of the larynx. They are easily identified and should be differentiated from other lesions. A possible problem in the differential diagnosis is the presence of pseudoepitheliomatous hyperplasia, which overlies the granular cell tumor and which may mimic squamous cell carcinoma. Careful histopathologic differentiation is important because the laryngeal granular cell lesion should be managed conservatively, with transoral local excision usually being adequate. The histogenesis of these lesions remains in doubt, with a neural or epithelial derivation being the most likely possibility.

Granular cell tumors are uncommon benign lesions distributed mainly in mucous membranes of the head and neck.* Differentiation from squamous cell carcinoma is important because granular cell tumors are treated conservatively. Confusion and inappropriate treatment occur when pseudoepitheliomatous hyperplasia, which frequently overlies granular cell tumors, is misinterpreted as squamous cell carcinoma.

We present 12 new cases to stress the clinical and histopathologic features that differentiate these lesions from others occurring in the larynx, especially squamous cell cancers. In addition, current concepts on the histogenesis of this lesion are reviewed.

OBSERVATIONS

Clinical Features. The series included 12 patients with histologically proved granular cell tumors. Eight were men and four were women; at the time of diagnosis, their ages ranged from 23 to 64 years (Table I). All patients had smoked the equivalent of one or more packages of cigarettes daily. Five of the patients had their lesions noted on routine indirect laryngoscopy, and five others had their lesions noted during examination for hoarseness and throat discomfort.

One unexpected finding was that 2 of the 12 patients had coexisting squamous cell carcinoma and presented with symptoms — pain and hemoptysis — caused by their cancers. In one of the patients, the preoperatively noted granular cell tumor was situated on the posterior portion of the true vocal cord, separate from the coexisting supraglottic squamous cell carcinoma. In the other patient, a large squamous cell cancer involved the base of the epiglottis, anterior commissure, and false cords. In this patient, the previously unsuspected granular cell lesion was situated on the left side of the laryngeal surface of the epiglottis, apart from the squamous cell cancer. In 11 of 12 cases, the granular cell tumors occurred in the posterior portion of the vocal cord in the region of the arytenoid process.

Morphologic Features. The tumors are usually described as small (0.2 to 0.8 cm), gray to yellow, and subepithelial. All had an intact but distinctly attached overlying epithelial layer. One of the tumors was pedunculated. Microscopically, the tumors feature cells that have given rise to their descriptive name

* Weiland LH, Ryan RE Jr, McDonald TJ: Unpublished data.

From the Mayo Clinic and Mayo Foundation, Rochester, Minnesota.

Presented at the meeting of the American Laryngological Association, Palm Beach, Florida, April 24-25, 1976.

TABLE I

CLINICAL FEATURES OF 12 PATIENTS WITH GRANULAR CELL TUMORS OF THE LARYNX

Case	Sex and age, yr	Symptoms	Site	Characteristics	Diameter of tumor (cm)	Treatment	Other
1	M 58	Sore throat, hemoptysis	Post V.C.†	Gray lesion	10 x 2 x 2	Removed in laryng.	1½ PPD
2	F 45	Hoarseness	Interaryt. region	Granulomatous mass	8	Laryngofissure	1 PPD
3	F 49	None, routine exam	Aryt. region	Gray lesion	6	T.e.	1 PPD; SCC biopsied
4	M 39	None, routine exam	Aryt. region	Pink matchhead appearance	2	T.e.	2 PPD; Also SCC of lip
5	M 36	Hoarseness	Post. V.C.	White-gray cyst	5	T.e.	2 PPD
6	M 51	None, routine exam	Post. V.C.	White-yellow tumor	3	T.e.	1 PPD
7	M 23	None, routine exam	Post. V.C.	Pedunculated lesion	4	T.e.	1 PPD
8	M 45	None, routine exam	Post. V.C.	Not mentioned	Not mentioned	T.e.	1 PPD
9	F 32	Sore throat	Aryt. region	Gritty gray appearance	4	T.e.	1 PPD; SCC diagnosed
10	F 42	Soreness	Interaryt. region	Yellow lesion	5	T.e.	1 PPD
11	M 64	Hoarseness	Aryt. region	Firm mass	6	T.e.	1 PPD
12	M 57	Dysphagia, otalgia	Epiglottis‡	Not mentioned	Not mentioned	Laryng.	2 PPD

Post. V.C. - Posterior vocal cord. † - Associated with supraglottic and laryngeal squamous cell carcinoma. Interaryt. - Interarytenoid. Aryt. - Arytenoid. ‡ - Associated with squamous cell carcinoma of the base of the epiglottis, anterior commissure, and false cords. Laryng. - Laryngectomy. T.e. - Transoral excision. PPD - Packages of cigarettes smoked per day. SCC - Squamous cell carcinoma.

(Fig. 1). The cells are large, have abundant granular eosinophilic cytoplasm, and have relatively small and inconspicuous nuclei. Because cytoplasmic borders are indistinct, there is a resulting syncytium of cells without any semblance of encapsulation. The cells do not have malignant features, but the closely adjacent squamous epithelium may undergo hyperplasia. With inadequate biopsy and lack of awareness, this may lead to an erroneous diagnosis of carcinoma.

Treatment. The two patients with coexisting squamous cell cancers underwent laryngectomy. One patient underwent laryngofissure for removal of the tumor; the remaining nine patients had transoral excision of the lesion. There were no recurrences.

DISCUSSION

The term "granular cell myoblastoma" was coined by Abrikossoff[1] in 1926.

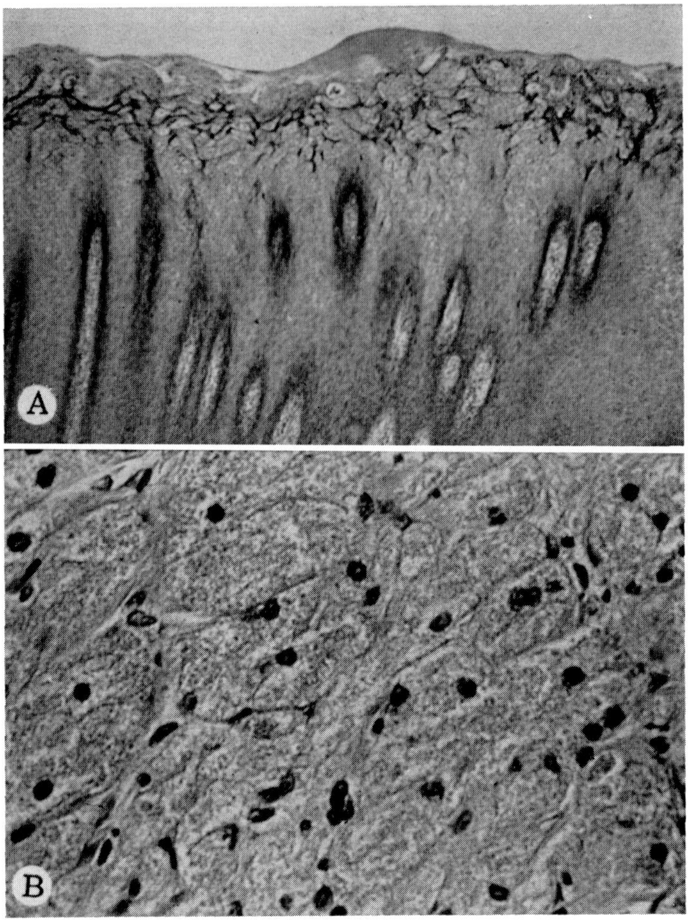

Fig. 1. Granular cell tumor. A) Pseudoepitheliomatous hyperplasia (H&E X50). B) Showing typical appearance (H&E X500).

Several reports before his had described an identical lesion.[2] The choice of this term was based on the theory that the granular cells which typified these tumors were derived from striated cells of embryonic muscle, the myoblasts. Numerous isolated reports and small reviews on the subject have followed.[3-5] In addition to the skeletal muscle cell as the possible cell of origin, the derivation of the granular cell also has been ascribed to histiocytes,[6] fibroblasts,[7] nerve sheath cells,[8] and mesenchymal cells.[9] Current studies strongly support a neurogenic origin, whereas some believe cells of diverse origin can become granular cells.

Granular cell tumors have been frequently noted in the head and neck region[4,5] and are especially common on the tongue.[9] In 1970, Booth and Osborn[10] reviewed 69 cases of laryngeal granular cell tumors. Our review of the literature includes 15 additional cases.[11-14] With the present 12 cases, the total number of cases involving granular cell tumors of the larynx is now 96.

The characteristics of the laryngeal lesions in the present 12 cases are similar to those reported by others.[4,5,10] A possible problem in the differential diagnosis concerns pseudoepitheliomatous hyperplasia and squamous cell carcinoma. The need for a close working relationship between the pathologist and the clinician is obvious. We have found that frozen-section diagnosis in granular cell tumors is both reliable and convenient.

Granular cell tumors of the larynx are "silent" lesions. The patient is usually seen by the otolaryngologist not because of complaints relative to the lesion but because of symptoms due to other causes, such as smoking. The granular cell tumor is usually detected incidentally. Relatively few patients present with hoarseness, perhaps because of the posterior location of the tumors on the vocal cord and the absence of ulceration. Chronic irritation has been indicated by some authors as a possible cause and may explain the interarytenoid location.[5]

In 1949, Fust and Custer[8] suggested a neural origin. This was later supported by Fisher and Wechsler[3] in 1962. More recently, Frable and Fischer[5] reported results of ultrastructure study of a congenital myoblastoma from a 1-hour-old female patient. They found no neural elements, but they noted junctional complexes between the granular cells, which suggested to them an epithelial origin.

The 12 cases of laryngeal granular cell tumors in the present series are part of approximately 90 cases, the total number of granular cell tumors in the Mayo Clinic files. None of the 90 lesions showed malignant change. Review of the lesions designated as malignant indicated that placement into one of the known categories of soft-tissue malignancies would have been more accurate.

The coexistence of the granular cell lesion with squamous cell carcinoma in two cases in our series was most unusual; this association has been reported only once before.[12] The obvious importance of this association is that the presence of one does not exclude the concomitant presence of the other.

Our study of these 12 laryngeal lesions and the 90 patients from which this series was extracted supports the concept that the embryonal muscle cell is not necessarily the cell of origin for this tumor. Until further work delineates the exact cell of origin, the term "granular cell tumor" is preferable to the probably erroneous term "granular cell myoblastoma."

REFERENCES

1. Abrikossoff A: Über Myome, ausgehend von der quergestreiften willkürlichen Muskulatur. Virchows Arch Pathol Anat Physiol 260:215-233, 1926

2. Murphy GH, Dockerty MB, Broders AC: Myoblastoma. Am J Pathol 25:1157-1181, 1949

3. Fisher ER, Wechsler H: Granular cell myoblastoma – a misnomer: electron microscopic and histochemical evidence concerning its Schwann cell derivation and nature (granular cell schwannoma). Cancer 15:936-954, 1962

4. Canalis RF, Cohn AM: Granular cell myoblastoma of the larynx. Arch Otolaryngol 91:125-127, 1970

5. Frable MA, Fischer RA: Granular cell myoblastomas. Laryngoscope 86:36-42, 1976

6. Whitten JB: The fine structure of an intraoral granular-cell myoblastoma. Oral Surg 26:202-213, 1968

7. Pearse AGE: The histogenesis of granular-cell myoblastoma (? granular-cell perineural fibroblastoma). J Pathol Bacteriol 62: 351-362, 1950

8. Fust JA, Custer RP: On the neurogenesis of so-called granular cell myoblastoma. Am J Clin Pathol 19:522-535, 1949

9. Aparicio SR, Lumsden CE: Light- and electron-microscope studies on the granular cell myoblastoma of the tongue. J Pathol 97: 339-355, 1969

10. Booth JB, Osborn DA: Granular cell myoblastoma of the larynx. Acta Otolaryngol (Stockh) 70:279-293, 1970

11. Bhatnagar HN, Schwarz HJ: Granular cell myoblastoma of larynx with papillary adenocarcinoma of thyroid. Arch Otolaryngol 90:156-158, 1969

12. Goldstein A, Thaler S, Rozycki D: Granular cell myoblastoma and carcinoma of the larynx. Arch Otolaryngol 94:366-368, 1971

13. Miglets AW, Gebhart DE, Gregg LO: Airway obstruction due to a large laryngeal granular cell myoblastoma. Laryngoscope 81: 971-978, 1971

14. Thawley SE, Ogura JH: Granular cell myoblastoma of the head and neck. South Med J 67:1020-1024, 1974

REPRINTS—Section of Publications, Mayo Clinic, Rochester, MN 55901.

Ann Otol 85: 1976

RECURRENT RESPIRATORY PAPILLOMATOSIS

MANAGEMENT WITH THE CO_2 LASER

M. Stuart Strong, MD

Charles W. Vaughan, MD Gerald B. Healy, MD

Sidney R. Cooperband, MD Manuel A. C. P. Clemente, MD

Boston, Massachusetts

SUMMARY – Recurrent respiratory papillomatosis is most common in childhood but it affects all age groups; it represents a diathesis of the aerodigestive tract so that lesions may develop at various sites – the nares, lips, pharynx, nasopharynx, larynx, tracheobronchial tree, and the lungs. Ablation of all visible papillomas with the surgical laser achieved remissions in approximately one-third of patients for one year or more; since relapses may occasionally occur 2 to 20 years later, cure can never be assumed. At the present time, management is directed towards total ablation of all visible papilloma consistent with preservation of the airway and voice; reduction of the tumor burden to minimal proportions is thought to allow the maximum opportunity for remission. As the host-papilloma relationship is unraveled, it may be possible in the future to provoke an immune response so that remissions can be predicted and produced consistently.

Recurrent papillomas, occurring in the larynx and related areas, have been a vexing problem for many decades in the United States and elsewhere. One hundred years ago, MacKenzie[1] found papillomas to be the most common benign tumor of the larynx. The myriad of treatments that have been used attest to the frustration of generations of otolaryngologists throughout the world.

When the CO_2 surgical laser became available for clinical usage in 1971, it was natural that it should be given a trial in the management of recurrent papillomas. The precision of laser surgery and the lack of bleeding occurring during laser dissection suggested that the laser might be an ideal instrument for ablation of laryngeal papillomas; the technique would provide for removal of all visible lesions and allow for preservation of important structures, such as laryngeal cartilage, vocalis muscle, and uninvolved mucosa.

During the years 1972 to 1975, 110 patients with recurrent papillomas were examined and operated upon with the surgical laser at the University Hospital and the Boston Veterans Administration Hospital. This experience has made it possible to draw conclusions regarding the complex nature of the disease, the role of the CO_2 laser in the management of recurrent papillomas and the need for investigation of the papilloma-host relationship. It appears that something more than total ablation under microscopic control will be needed before papillomas can be eradicated consistently and permanently.

METHODS AND MATERIALS

The CO_2 surgical lasers used in this study were standard 50 watt and 80 watt prototype instruments designed by American Optical Corporation. For the treatment of papillomas the laser was coupled to the Zeiss operating microscope and controlled with the micromanipulator.[2] All patients were operated upon under general anesthesia using a small bore endotracheal tube protected with aluminum tape; in the event that exposure of the interarytenoid space was inadequate (especially in children), the endotracheal tube was withdrawn and the patient was then ventilated using a Venturi system. Various combinations

Presented at the meeting of the American Laryngological Association, Palm Beach, Florida, April 25-26, 1976.

of nonflammable anesthetic gasses, sedatives, narcotics and muscle relaxants were used, most often nitrous oxide, oxygen, halothane or enflurane and succinyl choline. In patients with tracheobronchial disease, the laser was coupled to a standard ventilating bronchoscope via the laser endoscopic attachment.[3]

One hundred and two patients were treated at University Hospital and eight at the Boston Veterans Administration Hospital; a few patients came from the Boston area, but many came from other parts of Massachusetts and the United States. Five patients came from overseas.

The patients were admitted to the hospital the day before operation, and almost invariably were discharged the day after surgery. No restrictions were imposed with regard to diet or talking after surgery except that patients with laryngeal disease were advised to talk softly. During the operation, patients requiring prolonged intralaryngeal manipulation were administered 40 mg of methylprednisolone intravenously. Although the interaction between the laser and soft tissue is not associated with visible postoperative edema, extensive manipulation with probes, suction tips, retractors and the laryngoscope tip may produce postoperative swelling; this sequela can be minimized by intravenous administration of steroids.

The larynx was most often exposed with a Jako-Pilling wide bore laryngoscope of appropriate size, but occasionally a difficult patient required the use of the Dedo-Pilling anterior commissure laryngoscope.

After the distribution of the papillomas had been determined, a biopsy was taken for light microscopy; 20 patients had biopsies taken of papillomas and adjacent mucosa for electron microscopy. The lesions were then ablated, often exposing submucosa, perichondrium or muscle of various parts of the larynx. If papillomas involved the anterior commissure, a fragment of papilloma was purposely left on one cord to discourage web formation; in favorable situations this residual fragment was excised at an operation four to six weeks later. After initial laser excision, patients were usually reoperated upon promptly in four to six weeks in order to reduce the tumor burden to nonvisible proportions, so that the patient would have the maximum opportunity for remission. In the event of recurrence reoperation was advised at sufficient intervals to avoid the need for tracheostomy.

Patients with tracheobronchial disease were examined with a ventilating bronchoscope and the papillomas were destroyed with the laser directed through the bronchoscope. Bronchoscopy and laser destruction were repeated often enough to preserve the lower airway if two excisions did not suggest the possibility of early remission. In some patients with massive recurrences in the larynx, attention was concentrated on preserving the patency of the tracheobronchial tree only.

Lesions in the nares, oral cavity, or nasopharynx were excised using suitable retractors or gags; to reach the vault of the nasopharynx or dorsum of the soft palate, stainless steel mirrors were used to view the lesions and reflect the laser beam onto them.

After laser surgery patients were followed as their symptoms demanded. If symptom free they were followed in the office every four months; children who could not be examined with a mirror had direct microscopic laryngoscopy under anesthesia at 6 and 12 months after the last recurrence before it was assumed that they had gone into remission.

In addition to the usual history and physical examination in the office and in the hospital prior to operation, 25 patients were tested for evidence of a cutaneous delayed hypersensitivity reaction to tuberculin, candida, streptokinase, streptodornase and trichophyton; these tests were performed at least two weeks before or two weeks after a general anesthetic and operation. The standard intradermal injections were made into the volar aspects of each forearm, two on each side, and the results were read 48 hours later.

TABLE I

AREAS OF RESPIRATORY TRACT INVOLVED IN 110 PATIENTS

Nasal vestibule	2
Lips	2
Gingiva	1
Palate	13
Nasopharynx	3
Larynx	103
Tracheobronchial tree	22
Lungs	3

RESULTS

General Features of the Disease

Study of these 64 male and 46 female patients quickly revealed that recurrent papillomatosis has a predilection for a wide variety of sites within the oral cavity and the respiratory tract (Table I); the larynx was by far the predominant site (103 patients) but the tracheobronchial tree and the palate were involved in 22 and 13 instances respectively. In the nasal vestibules the lesions were found to be growing on the mucosa near the mucocutaneous junction. One patient presented with multiple recurrent papillomas of the lips, the upper and lower gingivae, the palate, tonsil fossa, nasopharynx, larynx and tracheobronchial tree! A history of skin warts was present in 4 out of 53 patients under the age of 16, and in 19 out of 57 patients over the age of 16 years, including 4 patients with perineal warts. In several patients, during the course of managing their respiratory tract papillomas, their cutaneous warts disappeared spontaneously. This, however, was not correlated with a similar disappearance of the mucosal lesions.

It was apparent that the disease has a worldwide distribution; patients came from Iran, Italy, East Africa, the Caribbean, Canada and all regions of the United States. From this experience it does not appear that the disease is significantly more common in warm climates than cold, although it would appear from the origin of many of these patients that the disease is particularly prevalent in Kentucky, Tennessee, Georgia and the Carolinas.

The influence of *socioeconomic status* was not apparent in the study; the patients were from all levels of society. It was noted, however, that 9 of 36 children below the age of five years had been adopted by their parents; a history of the circumstances of their births was therefore not available. Some of the patients showed evidence of poor personal hygiene and neglect while others showed no such traits.

Antigen responses were studied in 24 patients with severe recurrent disease. Eleven out of 24 patients when tested produced no response to intradermal injections of tuberculin, candida, streptokinase, streptodornase or trichophyton, 48 hours after injection; all but one of the 11 have continued to produce recurrences of papilloma relentlessly. Two patients who did react to one or more of the antigens, however, presented with the most advanced stage of the disease, namely, involvement of the lung parenchyma.

The *histology* of all these lesions was one of benign squamous papilloma; in a few specimens varying degrees of cellular atypia were noted but in no instance was malignancy suspected. None of these multiple recurrent lesions was seen to be keratinizing so that there was no confusion with solitary papillary keratoses occurring in older patients or with verrucous carcinoma. Scanning and transmission electron microscopy was carried out on 20 specimens by Incze *et al*,[4] whose findings are being reported in detail elsewhere. Papova-like virus particles were seen in 20% of cases. It was also noted that papilloma cells have an abnormal number of microvilli and desmosomes upon their surface; similarly, the surface epithelial cells of mucosa taken from an area immediately adjacent to papilloma presented with an abnormal number of microvilli and desmosomes. This finding suggests a gross abnormality of the microstructure of epithelial cells covering apparently normal appearing mucosa adjacent to a papilloma.

The *reservoir of recurrent respiratory papillomatosis appears to be condylomata acuminata.* Of 36 patients under the age of five years, 18 or 50% were born of mothers who had vaginal warts at the time of delivery; if a history could have been obtained from the natural mothers of nine adopted children, the proportion might have been higher. Four patients who acquired their disease after the age of 20 years volunteered a history of oral-genital contact with an infected partner; a history of such contact was solicited from only a few of the remaining 33 patients whose age of onset was 16 to 50 years (Fig. 1).

Natural History of the Disease

Age of Onset. In children this information was obtained from the parents and probably is accurate, even though nine children were adopted. In adults it was often difficult for the patients to recall exactly when the diagnosis was first made, but they were certain as to whether it was in childhood or adult life. While the disease was most commonly diagnosed before the age of five years (66%), it was apparent that there is another important age of onset be-

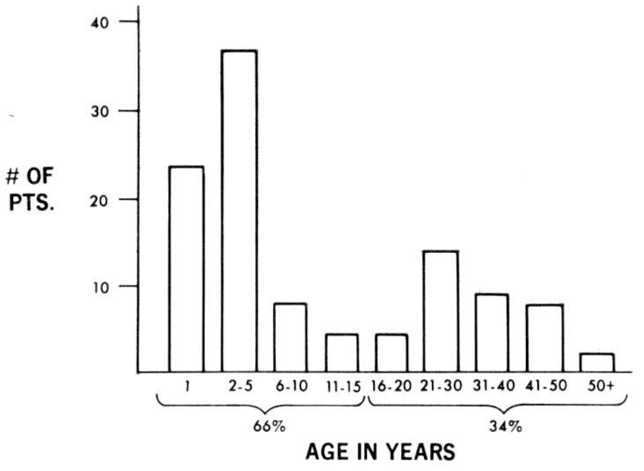

Fig. 1. Age of onset of papillomata. While the greatest number of patients dated the onset in childhood, one-third had no symptoms until age 16 years or older.

tween 16 and 50 years (34%) (Fig. 1). One patient developed hoarseness due to papilloma at the age of 68!

Age at Presentation. It was a surprise to find that more than 50% of patients who presented for further treatment were 16 years of age or older (Fig. 2). Referred patients of course are highly selected; those patients with refractory disease tended to be referred because of the long duration of their condition.

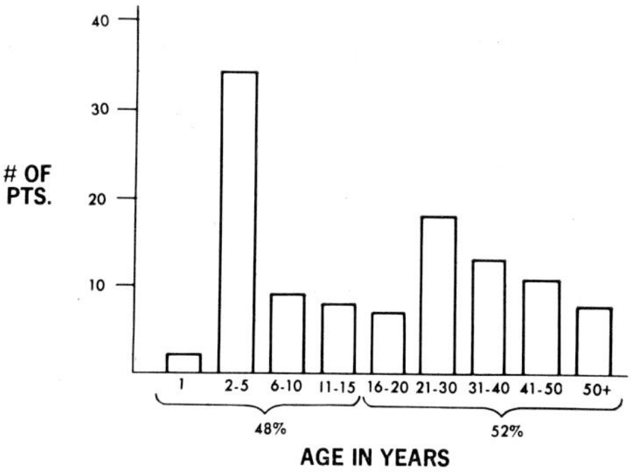

Fig. 2. Age at presentation. The higher proportion of patients aged 16 years or more reflects the referral of some patients who had their disease for many years and had not responded to other forms of treatment.

Prior Treatment. The number of procedures that patients had prior to undergoing laser excision varied greatly (Fig. 3). Sixteen patients had a simple biopsy or excisional biopsy and one patient had a history of 137 operations.

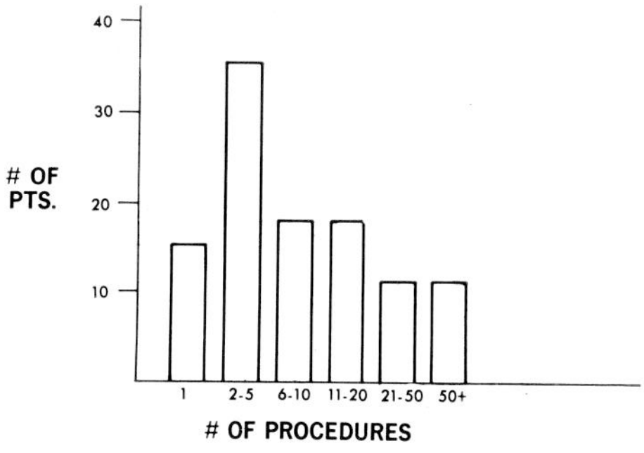

Fig. 3. The number of prior procedures indicate the refractory nature of the disease.

Several patients had lost count after 100 operations!

In addition to surgical excision, five patients had been treated with cryosurgery, two of them on seven occasions. Two patients had surgical excision combined with ultrasound irradiation, one of them on 15 occasions. Three patients had received autogenous vaccine prior to being treated by laser excision.

Remissions. It was impossible to predict when the disease might become arrested. On some occasions the amount of recurrent disease that was excised was very small and yet in six months another recurrence appeared at the same or a different site. On other occasions, after many rapid recurrences of bulky lesions, quite unexpectedly the recurrence rate slowed down and the disease vanished after one or two more excisions.

In this series of 110 patients, 11 patients were lost to follow-up; no answer could be elicited from their last known address. Of the remaining 99 patients, 76 had been in this study for a year or more and hence were at risk of undergoing remission. Remission was defined as no evidence of visible disease for one year or more by mirror examination in older children and adults or by direct microlaryngoscopy in small children. There were 47 patients less than 16 years of age and 29 patients greater than 16 years of age who were followed for one year or more (Fig. 4).

Of the 76 patients under follow-up

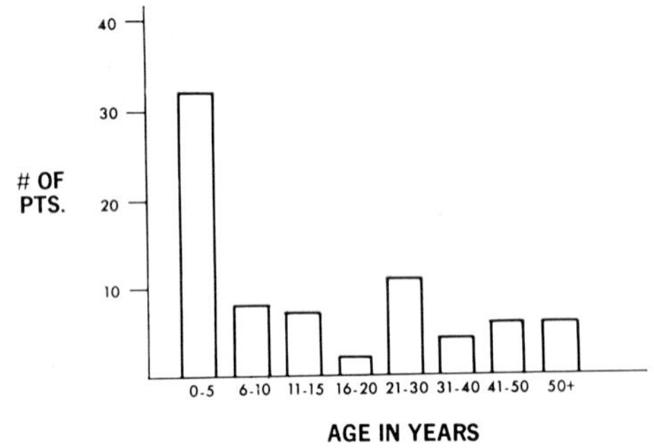

Fig. 4. Age of 76 patients in follow-up for one year or more. In addition to the group of children under 5 years of age, an opportunity for remission was present in 29 patients over 16 years of age.

for one year or more, 26 patients stayed in remission for one year or more (34%). Figure 5 shows the age of patients when remission was achieved. The table indicates that remission can occur at any time, but is most predictable after age 40 years. By referring to Figures 4 and 5 it can be seen that of 47 patients less than 16 years of age, 12 patients underwent remission (25%) and of 29 patients 16 years of age and over, 14 underwent remission (50%). This suggests that the change of remission occurring increases slightly with age, but is lowest between the ages of 16 and 40 years – 3 out of 17 patients. There were 18 patients with laryngeal and tracheobronchial disease; only three of these achieved total remission after multiple laser excisions.

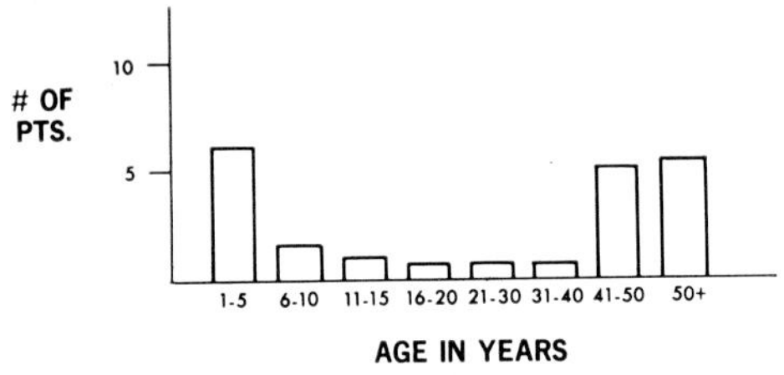

Fig. 5. Age of onset of remission in 26 patients. The paucity of remissions between age 11 and 40 years is very striking.

The number of prior procedures was not related to the possibility of laser excision promoting a remission; some of the patients who had more than 50 previous operations went into remission as some of those did who had only one

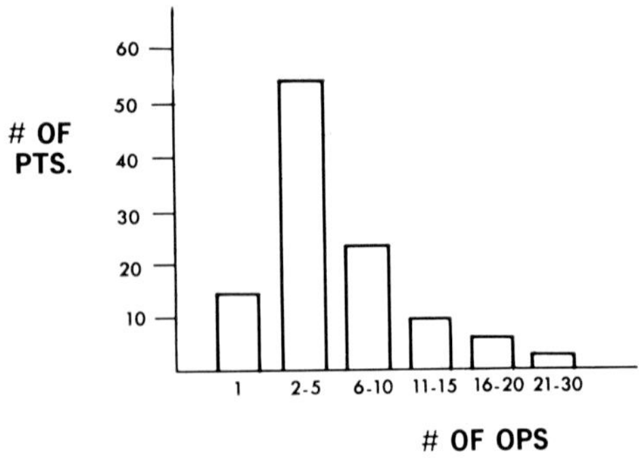

Fig. 6. Number of laser excisions. Most of the patients requiring more than 15 operations have tracheobronchial papillomas.

or two procedures. Only two of the five patients previously treated by cryosurgery went into remission and none of those who had received ultrasound irradiation or autogenous vaccine responded to laser excision.

The number of laser excisions performed is shown in Figure 6 and although 18 patients have undergone more than 11 laser operations, no remission was encountered if more than 10 operations were required. Operations in excess of ten served to maintain the airway and/or a voice.

Although remission of one year should augur well for the future, four patients were encountered in the series who suffered delayed recurrences. One 8-year-old male was free of disease at two years, but had a recurrence after 2½ years of follow-up; a 58-year-old male was free of disease for 1½ years but had a recurrence after two years. Two other patients, aged 31 and 32 years, had documented laryngeal disease 25 and 19 years before respectively. These patients illustrate the tenuous nature of remission and that recurrence may occasionally appear even decades later.

Incidence of Tracheobronchial Disease and Tracheostomy. In nine patients over 16 years of age who presented with a history of having had a previous tracheostomy and since removed, four had residual papillomas in the trachea and five had no tracheal disease. Eighteen patients presented with a tracheostomy tube in place; of 15 patients less than 16 years, 11 had tracheobronchial papillomas and of 3 greater than 16 years, all had tracheal lesions. If two long-term tracheostomies in patients operated upon with the laser (one of whom developed tracheal papillomas) are included, the incidence of tracheal "seeding" and tracheostomy was 19 out of 29 patients or 65%.

Complications. Postlaser excision tracheostomy was required in three patients. In one 3-year-old patient, the rate of recurrence of papillomas in the larynx was so great that it became impractical to remove the lesions as frequently as every ten days; to preserve the airway a tracheostomy was done. Within a month there was extensive involvement of the trachea with papillomas requiring bronchoscopic removal every two months. A second 2-year-old male had a tracheostomy because the mother had become pregnant and felt she would not be able to bring the child back for several months. A third 4-year-old boy required tracheostomy for three days because of edema secondary to excessive intralaryngeal manipulation. The incidence of tracheostomy in 53 children less than 16 years of age was three or 6%. Tracheostomy was not needed in any patient over 16 years.

Laryngeal webs were present in nine patients, with anterior commissure webbing of 20% or more, secondary to multiple previous excisions. Three patients presented with posterior webs between the apices of the arytenoid cartilages. Seven patients developed webs of 20% or more following laser excision of papillomas in the anterior commissure; three of these were severe and involved 50% of the membranous portion of the cords. These patients were treated early in this series before it was realized that excision, even with a laser, must not be carried out simultaneously on each cord in the area of the anterior commissure.

Laryngoceles developed in two patients with extensive involvement of the false cords and ventricle. After laser excisions on several occasions, the laryngoceles subsided spontaneously as obstruction of the ventricle was relieved.

Pulmonary papillomatosis was present in three patients at the time of presentation in two 14-year-old males and one 26-year-old female. The 2 to 3 cm cystic lesions could be clearly seen on routine chest x-ray involving several of the lobes of the lung. In one patient the cysts presented with an air-fluid level.

Malignant degeneration was encountered in only one patient who presented as a laryngectomee. She had received x-radiation at the age of 12 for laryngeal papillomas and developed cancer of the larynx at age 31. Following laryngectomy the patient continued to produce obstructive masses of papillomas in the lower trachea and bronchi.

Near asphyxiation developed in a 5-year-old girl who had a tracheostomy since two years of age. Her tracheobronchial tree had cleared following laser excision, but the larynx required operation every four months to maintain a voice; she was found unconscious with cardiopulmonary arrest at school due to obstruction of the inner cannula of her tracheostomy tube by inspissated mucus. Resuscitation was accomplished by the rescue squad but the child did not regain consciousness. Repeat bronchoscopy revealed no tracheobronchial papillomas but the child has remained in coma.

DISCUSSION

The nomenclature of this disease has been a source of confusion in the past. There appears to be no difference in the microstructure or biologic behavior of papillomas that occur in the nares or the larynx, or in those that occur in children or adults.[5] Papillomas may first appear in any area of the aerodigestive tract and at any age; the lesions are both multiple and recurrent. This being the case, the qualifying prefixes "juvenile" and "laryngeal" are redundant when describing recurring papillomas. It appears that the solitary, pedunculated papilloma commonly seen on the uvula or tonsil pillars may be a different disease; although they have a similar histologic appearance, they do not tend to recur. Solitary papillary lesions occurring in the adult larynx most often present a degree of keratinization which distinguishes them from recurrent respiratory papillomatosis. A keratinizing papillary lesion of the larynx or oral cavity may, of course, represent an early stage of verrucous carcinoma.

Evidence that recurrent respiratory papillomatosis is of viral origin is convincing although proof is not as yet available. Papova-like viruses were seen in this study[4] and in others.[6] It is presumed that the particles are visible only in a small proportion of cells because the remainder of the cells are in the transformed state. Solisch *et al*[7] not only saw papovavirus particles in some specimens but were able to culture viruses from many specimens. The clinical behavior of the disease, its transmission, remissions and recurrences, are certainly compatible with a disease of viral origin. It is most probable that the reservoir of recurrent respiratory papillomatosis is genital warts;[8] the concept was reinforced by this series. Transmission to the child during passage through the birth canal is most likely. Appearance of the disease for the first time in an adult is more difficult to explain; either the disease was transmitted at birth and lay dormant until later years or it was acquired secondarily during the years of sexual activity. The prevalence of oral-genital practices and the documentation of incidents where patients had contact with infected partners, are most suggestive that this is an alternate method of transmission. We have no idea as to the infectivity of the disease, but it is probably low. We know of no siblings with the disease, and mothers who have recovered from condyloma have had further children without problems. However, we would advise an infected mother to be delivered by cesarean section. The incidence of this disease is not known. It has been suggested that it is on the increase in certain areas.[9] Since there has been an explosive increase in the incidence of condylomata acuminata, especially among young adults, it is quite possible that there will be an increase in the incidence of respiratory tract papillomatosis.

The disease appears to have sites of predeliction but how and why it appears at more than one site is a mystery. The frequent "spread" of papillomas from the larynx to the tracheobronchial tree after tracheostomy suggests seeding onto the traumatized area of mucosa. However, multiple papillomas have been encountered in the tracheobronchial tree in the absence of laryngeal disease[10] so it is possible that the cells of tracheal epithelium have already been infected, and the trauma of the tracheostomy tube merely activates the dormant viral infection resulting in the production of a papilloma. Invasion of the lung parenchyma defies explanation;[11] it has been encountered only in patients with laryngeal disease requiring tracheostomy.

The occurrence of disease at extralaryngeal sites – the nares, lips, gums, and nasopharynx is interesting; these are sites of airway constriction (as well as the larynx) where air flow rates and consequent cooling from evaporation are high. It is known that cell mediated immune response can be temperature related;[12] perhaps both local cooling and the trauma associated with drying and crusting play a role in the development of papillomas in these sites of predeliction. Perhaps the beneficial effect, if any, of ultrasound (which is known to raise the tissue temperatures 1.1 C) is related to elevation of the cell mediated immune response.[13]

The significance of cellular immunity in respiratory papillomatosis is not known; the finding of 11 out of 24 patients with severe disease to be nonreactive to any of four common skin antigens suggests an anergic background. As this part of the study progresses, it will be possible to determine whether or not there is any correlation between the presence or absence of anergy and the occurrence of remission.

Remission in respiratory papillomatosis is most unpredictable. So far it

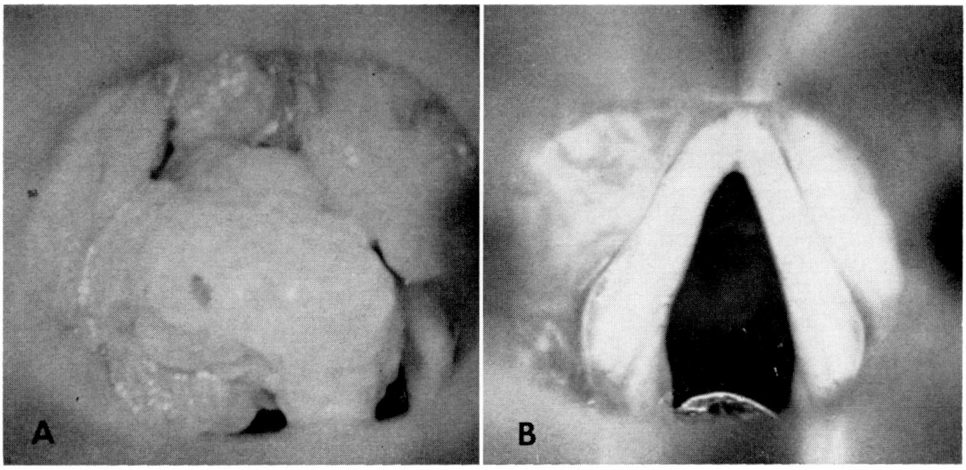

Fig. 7. A) Multiple papillomas in the larynx of an 11-year-old girl requiring excision twice a year. B) The larynx as seen in A after two laser excisions. Note the healthy mucosa and absence of visible scarring.

has not been possible to predict when it is going to occur or how long it will last. It is highest below 10 years of age[14] and lowest between 20 to 40 years of age as seen in this series. The onset of puberty did not appear to have an influence on the age of remission in this series. While a remission of one year bodes well for the future, there is no assurance that the remission will be maintained. Since recurrences can occur years later,[15] it is probable that we cannot speak of "cure" in this disease any more than we can speak of cure in herpes labialis; because relapses are not unusual one and two years later, only three-year remissions should be considered when comparing the efficacy of various methods of management.

The *origin of the recurrence* remains a mystery. After laser excision of a localized papilloma of the vocal cord down to the underlying muscle and including a margin of surrounding mucosa, the lesion may vanish and not recur, or in three months a papilloma may reform just as if the lesion had never been removed! Were the "seeds" of a new papilloma within the muscle or were fragments of papilloma seeded into the wound? Neither possibility is likely. A more plausible suggestion is that the origin of the new papilloma is in the cells of the surrounding normal appearing mucosa; the surrounding margin of epithelium may contain transformed cells which, when stimulated to regenerate a new epithelial covering of the wound, may be stimulated into producing a new papilloma. This may explain the apparent success of decortication of the vocal cord and resurfacing with vein graft after excision of vocal cord papilloma. The vein graft survives as a viable graft so that epithelial migration does not occur.[16] Electron microscopy studies of the epithelium surrounding a papilloma support this concept. Unfortunately, total excision of all the laryngeal epithelium and replacement with a new covering is not a practical consideration.

Total ablation of all visible papilloma reduces the tumor burden to invisible proportions; the best that can be hoped for is that the immune response of the host will be sufficient to contend with the invisible residue and promote a remission. There is no question that the surgical laser is the optimal method of papilloma removal; all visible papilloma can be removed at the expense of minimal damage to supporting structures such as the vocal cords, *etc* (Fig. 7 A, B). However, at the present time no method of tissue destruction by surgical removal, cautery, ultrasound irradiation, cryosurgery or laser, can be expected on its own to promote permanent remissions consistently.

The *present goals* of management are:

1. To maintain the airway and voice and to avoid tracheostomy whenever possible.

2. To reduce the tumor burden to minimal proportions and provide the best chance of remission.

3. In the presence of tracheostomy, to maintain the patency of the tracheobronchial airway by bronchoscopy and to use the shortest tracheostomy tube possible.

Future goals do not call for a method of papilloma removal more ideal than the surgical laser; they do call for elucidation of the subtleties of the papilloma-host relationship. When this relationship is understood, then perhaps it will be possible to manipulate the immune response of the host and produce remissions in all patients.

REFERENCES

1. MacKenzie M: *Diseases of the Pharynx, Larynx and Trachea.* New York, William Wood and Company, 1880, p 226

2. Strong MS, Vaughan CW, Polanyi TG, *et al*: Laser surgery in the aero-digestive tract. Am J Surg 126:529-533, 1973

3. Strong MS, Vaughan CW, Polanyi TG, *et al*: Bronchoscopic CO_2 laser surgery. Ann Otol Rhinol Laryngol 83:769-776, 1974

4. Incze JS, Lui PS, Strong MS, *et al*: The morphology of human papillomas of the upper respiratory tract. To be published

5. Kleinsasser O, Oliviera EG: Juvenile and adult laryngeal papillomas. HNO 21:97-100, 1973

6. Boyle WF, Riggs JL, Oshiro LS, *et al*: Electron microscopic identification of papova virus in laryngeal papilloma. Laryngoscope 83:1102-1107, 1973

7. Solisch T, Hannefeld H, Brandt RH: Zur papova virus ëtiology des menschlicken laryngopapilloma. Z Erkr Atmungsorgane 138: 379-384, 1973

8. Cook TA, Cohn AM, Brunschwig PS, *et al*: Laryngeal papillomas: etiologic and therapeutic considerations. Ann Otol Rhinol Laryngol 82:649-655, 1973

9. Dekelboum AM: Papillomas of the larynx. Arch Otolaryngol 81:390-397, 1965

10. Al-Saleem T, Peale AR, Norris CN: Multiple papillomatosis of the lower respiratory tract. Cancer 22:1173-1184, 1968

11. Smith L, Gooding C: Pulmonary involvement in laryngeal papillomatosis. Pediatr Radiology 2:161-164, 1974

12. Portilo DT, Walsh GP, Storrs EE, *et al*: The impact of cool temperature on transformation of human and armadillo lymphocytes as related to leprosy. Nature 248:450-452, 1974

13. Birck HG, Manhart HE: Ultrasound for juvenile laryngeal papillomatosis. Arch Otolaryngol 77:603-608, 1963

14. Majoras M, Parkhill EM, DeVine KD: Papilloma of the larynx in children. Am J Surg 108:470-475, 1964

15. Klos J: Clinical course of laryngeal papillomatosis in children. Ann Otol Rhinol Laryngol 79:1132-1138, 1970

16. Tabb HG, Kirk RL: Vein grafts in the management of laryngeal papillomas. Laryngoscope 72:1228-1238, 1962

Reprints—M. Stuart Strong, MD, 75 E. Newton St., Boston, MA 02118.

Ann Otol 85: 1976

DINITROCHLOROBENZENE SKIN SENSITIZATION AND PERIPHERAL LYMPHOCYTE COUNT: PREDICTORS OF SURVIVAL IN HEAD AND NECK CANCER

ROBERT H. MAISEL, MD

MINNEAPOLIS, MINNESOTA

JOSEPH H. OGURA, MD

ST. LOUIS, MISSOURI

SUMMARY – Dinitrochlorobenzene (DNCB) is a simple chemical useful to evaluate both afferent (sensitizing) and efferent (reacting) limbs of the delayed, cell-mediated immune system. This system invokes the small lymphocyte (T cell) and is apparently part of the host defense against cancer. Seventy-two patients with new primary squamous cell carcinomas of the larynx, hypopharynx and oropharynx were sensitized to DNCB by contact application, and delayed cutaneous hypersensitivity tested. The T cells were also assessed in this study by lymphocyte count. All patients were treated for cure. Ninety-one percent of DNCB reactors were alive and tumor-free at two years. Forty-five percent of negative reactors had recurrent tumor and died of carcinoma. Cases grouped by site among glottic, supraglottic and inferior hypopharynx showed identical results. Lymphocyte counts showed a trend in the same direction. On statistical analysis, all differences were significant. Eighty-five percent of recurrent tumors occurred in patients who were nonresponders. The present data suggest DNCB reactivity is helpful in predicting outcome after surgery, or combined radiation and surgery, for mucosal squamous carcinoma of the head and neck.

Malignant epithelial tumors of the head and neck are amenable to careful mapping by tumor site and size because these tumors are palpable, visible, and relatively easily accessible. Analysis of treatment regimens based on tumor size and precise location has been done for many years.[1-3] Patients with carcinoma have been suspected of being immune deficient. Recently, studies on host response to the tumors have begun. Eilber and Morton,[4] Eilber *et al*[5] and Morton *et al*[6] were among the first to evaluate prognostically the immune system in clinical neoplasia, and others have followed their lead.[7] Many of these studies are based on large tumor clinic populations where the head and neck sample is small and poorly defined. These patients often are evaluated after primary cancer therapy is accomplished and recurrent or progressive disease is evident.[8]

The host response to foreign protein is a precisely tailored mechanism which protects against bacteria, virus, and neoplasia. In humans the system is mediated through a B cell line which comprises stationary immune cells including plasma cells. This humoral system functions via circulating immunoglobulins or antibodies which interact with antigens or foreign protein to effect their destruction, removal and dispersal.

The T cell or thymus derived system is manifest as small circulating lymphocytes. These are in deep cortical areas of the lymph node and in the spleen from where they can enter the blood stream.

All recent evidence suggests the small

From the Department of Otolaryngology, University of Minnesota Medical School, Minneapolis, Minnesota, and the Department of Otolaryngology, Washington University, St. Louis, Missouri. This study was supported in part by NIH Grant 5 T01 NSO 5190.

Presented at the meeting of the American Laryngological Association, Palm Beach, Florida, April 24-25, 1976.

lymphocyte is integral in delayed hypersensitivity, protects the internal environment from fungal infection, inhibits homograft transplant, and performs the immune surveillance which seeks and destroys the multiple neoplastic cells hypothesized to be created daily within all living vertebrates.[9] Using this information, many students of cancer and immunology have assessed delayed hypersensitivity reactions looking for group differences between normal and tumor populations.

One nitro 2-4 dichlorobenzene (DNCB) is a simple compound with disinfectant properties which until recently had a limited industrial application. (More recently, this chemical has been used in swimming pool cleansers in Europe). Thus in the past, few people have had exposure to this chemical, which like several other chemicals (including Dinitroflorobenzene), acts as a hapten by forming covalent bonds with lysine in skin proteins.[10,11] The complex interacts with the defense mechanism to sensitize a lymphocyte population which develops a "memory" for the complex. This event occurs in regional nodes and utilizes the small (T) lymphocytes.[12,13] Such lymphocytes, once sensitized, react at any subsequent encounter in a hypersensitive manner, thus demonstrating an intact immune arc. Sensitization requires 7 to 21 days and is a delayed cutaneous hypersensitivity reaction (DCH). This is distinguised by the time sequence from the initial irritative reaction of sensitization which occurs in the first 24 to 72 hours after application, and by histologic characteristics of delayed hypersensitivity.

This clinical test of immune competence used in humans for over 20 years is more valuable than introducing bacterial or fungal antigens, since it assesses the afferent (sensitizing) and efferent (hyperreacting) loops of the system.

If immune deficiency in the cancer patient is due to failure of sensitization of the small lymphocyte to the malignant cell, as well as failure to sensitize to any other "foreign" protein (DNCB plus skin hapten), the DNCB test will be unreactive and will discover this failure. Stimulating a new response to previously unencountered protein requires the entire system to be functional. This will be perceived when testing this delayed cutaneous response. Unlike tuberculosis antigens (PPD), this test makes no presumption of previous antigen contact. Clinical work suggesting the preservation of the efferent loop in the cancer patient furthers the importance of assessing the complete circuit *in vivo* by DNCB.

Since the small lymphocyte is felt to be integral to the delayed hypersensitivity reaction, several investigations of cancer immunology have assayed this cell. Many methods of DNCB testing and interpretation have been used. Eilber and Morton[4] described a simple repeatable method which we have followed.

Other investigators have felt that the cancer patient has a loss of ability to mount a histamine response. They have measured response to croton oil (an irritant), and have found patients unresponsive to this are often also DNCB negative.[14] Roth *et al*[15] recently have refuted the purported value of croton oil irritation. Dermatologists have biopsied the sensitization and challenge sites and have described histologic characteristics of DCH.[13] Despite these sophistications the method we follow continues to be widely used clinically.[14,16]

Our sample was selected on a consecutive basis among new untreated patients clinically diagnosed to have squamous carcinoma of the oral cavity, larynx, or pharynx. All patients were evaluated on their first office visit and as part of the examination had a DNCB sensitization dose of 2000 μg applied to the left volar antebrachium. A 100 μg dose was applied to the right arm in an identical location to insure no previous sensitivity was operant. A decision at the first office visit was made that these patients were amenable to primary therapy either via surgery alone or preoperative irradiation in combina-

TABLE I

PERCENTAGE OF DNCB REACTORS IN CONTROL AND CANCER PATIENTS

	DNCB +	*DNCB −*	*% Reactors*
Control	26	5	84
Cancer Patients	32	40	44

tion with surgery. All patients were tested before institution of radiotherapy, and no patients had received chemotherapy. No patients had undergone surgery in the two weeks prior to testing. Several patients did have a short surgical procedure (biopsy) within a week subsequent to application of the DNCB. Fourteen to 21 days after the sensitizing test, a test dose of 100 μg DNCB was applied to the left arm 3 inches distal to the original 2000 μg dose. Complete blood cell count and differential was obtained at the first office visit or on hospital admission.

Our hypothesis was that cancer patients would have a lower incidence of reactivity to DNCB and would have a lower absolute lymphocyte count than age-matched controls. We further predicted that the subgroup who survived the usual treatment protocol tumor-free would contain more positive skin reactors regardless of stage or site of tumor than the treatment failure group.

RESULTS

We have completed all studies on 72 patients with squamous cell carcinoma and have followed all patients 24 months or longer. Twelve patients who entered the study were disqualified, because despite a clinical presentation compatible with squamous cell carcinoma, their biopsy revealed other malignant histology (lymphoma, adenocarcinoma). Three patients were dropped from the series because of early postoperative death. All 72 patients had the prescribed DNCB and lymphocyte count. Many of them had mumps antigen and PPD application. Our control population was drawn from the orthopedic ward and included patients 40 to 70 years old, none with a history of previous carcinoma. Eighty-four percent of these controls were DNCB reactors while 44% of the cancer patients reacted (Table I).

TABLE II

PERCENTAGE OF DNCB REACTORS AMONG TUMOR FREE PATIENTS COMPARED TO PATIENTS WITH RECURRENT CARCINOMA

	DNCB +	*DNCB −*
Tumor Free	29	22
Recurrent	3	18
	91%	55%

Increased tumor-free survival of positive reactors. T test significant statistically. $P<0.01$.

We have described the results in Table II. Ninety-one percent of positive DNCB reactors survived greater than two years tumor free. Twenty-two of 40 patients (55%) who were nonresponders were tumor free at two years. This group difference is statistically significant at the 0.01 level.

Table III divides the patients into groups by two measures of delayed hypersensitivity. Fifteen of 24 patients with lymphocytopenia (<1500 (lymphocytes/cm^3) survived tumor free two years, as did 36 of 48 patients with normal lymphocyte counts. This shows a trend to decreased survival with lymphocytopenia, but it is not statistically significant. Table IV shows that 20 of 21 patients (95%) with both normal DNCB reaction and normal lymphocyte counts were free of disease at two years. Analysis of the data shows this is significant to the 0.01 level.

The cancers were divided by location into four groups to assess the validity of the DNCB test in different regions and sites in the head and neck (Table

TABLE III

RELATIVE LYMPHOCYTOPENIA AND ITS RELATION TO RECURRENT TUMOR

	WBC >1500	*WBC <1500*
No Recurrence	36	15
Recurrent Tumor	12	9

TABLE IV

DINITROCHLOROBENZENE SKIN REACTIVITY AND LYMPHOCYTOPENIA RELATIONSHIP TO RECURRENT TUMOR

	DNCB +		*DNCB −*	
	WBC > 1500	< 1500	WBC > 1500	< 1500
No Recurrence	20	9	16	6
Recurrent Tumor	1	2	11	7

Absolute lymphocyte count and DNCB reactivity. Statistical significance 0.01; $P < 0.01$.

V). Bulky laryngeal lesions are classified by considering the center of the tumor mass the named site of origin. Fifty-two percent of the patients with glottic lesions reacted to the DNCB. This group included large T_4 lesions as well as small lesions amenable to vertical hemilaryngectomy. Twelve of 17 supraglottic lesions were in people who were skin test positive (71%). Thirteen patients with pyriform sinus lesions were studied and four were DNCB positive (30%). The other 17 lesions included several anatomic areas (tongue base, tonsil, floor of mouth) and these are not included in Table V.

As noted in Table V, for laryngeal and pyriform lesions 27 of 29 patients (93%) who manifested DCH survived. The nonresponders showed a 39% recurrence rate.

DISCUSSION

Our results show DNCB reactors almost unfailingly (91%) survived two years. This two-year result agrees with the short-term follow-up of Morton *et al*,[6] and confirms our previous work.[17] In view of the conclusions of Session[18] and Fletcher,[19] that 85 to 90% of recurrences occur within two years, our results suggest the long-term prognosis for DNCB reactors is excellent.

DNCB skin testing can predict, at a statistically significant level, the outcome for patients with squamous cell carcinoma primary to the head and neck. Lymphocytopenia dims the prognosis, but not to a statistically significant degree.

DNCB skin testing is now a well-accepted part of the evaluation of a new patient in a major cancer treatment center. Its importance and value to planning cancer therapy is not yet clear. This series of 72 patients with regional cancer of the head and neck is the first to admit only patients whose tumor and general health uniformly

TABLE V

DINITROCHLOROBENZENE SKIN REACTIVITY GROUPED BY ANATOMIC LOCATION OF THE PRIMARY CARCINOMA

	Recurrence	*DNCB +*	*DNCB −*	*Total*
Glottic	No	13	9	25
	Yes	—	3	
Supraglottic	No	11	3	17
	Yes	1	2	
Pyriform sinus	No	3	4	13
Extrinsic larynx	Yes	1	5	
	2 yr tumor free	27/29	16/26	

Positive reactors with fewer recurrences than negative DNCB reactors.

allows a planned curative treatment program. All patients were treated for cure, and none received chemotherapy. The DNCB test is a valuable adjunct in an initial evaluation of the patient with cancer. Small vocal cord cancers will almost uniformly respond to treatment.[2] Three of 25 in this subseries suffered recurrence (one salvaged by laryngectomy). All three were nonresponders. The same holds in larger and more dangerous tumors of the pharynx and oral cavity. Of 21 recurrent tumors in this series, only three had normal skin reactivity (15%).

We feel DNCB testing holds an advantage over *in vitro* tests as a functional measure of delayed hypersensitivity. This simply performed, easily interpreted clinical measure is a valid predictor of survival from squamous carcinoma of the head and neck. It holds true for two-year survival which is sufficient time under good clinical follow-up for tumor regrowth to occur and be discovered. In our series, it differentiates with reliability, and to a statistically significant level, the patients whose tumor will recur from those in whom the usual therapy will be successful.

From our data, failure of patients to respond, implies about a 45% chance of recurrent tumor, with the likelihood of dying from the cancer. The DNCB test does not differentiate potential failures but does forecast an excellent incidence of tumor cure when positive.

For laryngeal and inferior hypopharyngeal lesions, 27 or 29 DNCB positive reactors survived two years (93%). Sixteen of 26 nonresponders were tumor-free after two years (61%). This further shows the sharp predictive value of *in vivo* double-limbed (afferent and efferent) DCH measure. The results are similar for each site, but statistical analysis was not performed because of the scarcity of cases within each site in the oral cavity and superior hypopharynx.

We have evaluated this test only once on each patient. We intend to expand our study, to measure as Krant[16] did, if recurrent tumor can convert a responder to negative, and we plan to elucidate the gross parameters which associate with failure of immune surveillance. Our present study comprises a two-year clinical follow-up at several institutions and includes other noninvasive measures of delayed hypersensitivity (keyhole lampert cyanin, phytohemagglutinin, and T cell rosette) as well as histologic exam of neck lymph nodes from patients operated by radical neck dissection for lymphocyte depletion pattern.

The clinical application of the DNCB test as a predictor in survival remains in the large tumor which, by location and size alone (T_3T_4), offers a poor survival prospect. A positive skin test in such a lesion suggests a favorable outcome and implies aggressive therapy to irradicate these tumors is advisable. Contrarily, a negative test implies a generally less favorable prognosis despite clear surgical margins. It may mean adjunctive immuno-and chemotherapy has merit in such a patient. It may also suggest that aggressive surgical radiotherapeutic measures are not advisable since the chances for a successful outcome are dim, and palliative therapy may be the recommended method of treatment. This information is not yet forthcoming.

REFERENCES

1. Ogura JH, Biller HF: Conservation surgery in cancer of the head and neck. Otolaryngol Clin North Am 3:641-665, 1969

2. Biller HF, Ogura JH, Pratt LL: Hemilaryngectomy for T_2 glottic carcinoma. Arch Otolaryngol 93:238-243, 1971

3. Krause CJ, Lee JG, McCabe BJ: Carcinoma of the oral cavity. Arch Otolaryngol 97:354-358, 1973

4. Eilber FR, Morton DL: Impaired immunologic reactivity and recurrence following cancer surgery. Cancer 25:362-367, 1970

5. Eilber FR, Nizze JA, Morton DL: Sequential evaluation of general immune competence in cancer patients: correlation of clinical course. Cancer 35:660-665, 1975

6. Morton DL, Holmes EC, Eilber FR, *et al*: Immunological aspects of neoplasia: a

rational basis for immunotherapy. Ann Intern Med 74:587-604, 1971

7. Mandel MA, Kiehn CL: The prognostic significance of delayed cutaneous reactivity in head and neck cancer patients. Plast Reconst Surg 53:72-76, 1974

8. Parker R, Alexander S, Shaheen OH, *et al*: On the immunology of head and neck cancer – prognostic index. Preliminary communication. J Otol Laryngol 89:687-695, 1975

9. Craddock CG, Longmire R, McMillan R: Lymphocytes and immune response. N Engl J Med 285:324-331, 1971

10. Eisen HN, Orris L, Belman S: Excitation of delayed allergic skin reactions with haptens: the dependence of elicitation of hapten combination with protein. J Exp Med 95: 473-487, 1952

11. Eisen HN, Tabachnick M: Elicitation of allergic contact dermatitis in the guinea pig: the distribution of bound dinitrobenzene groups within the skin and quantitative determination of the extent of combination of 2, 4 dinitrochlorobenzene with epidermal protein *in vivo*. J Exp Med 108:773-796, 1958

12. Catalona WJ, Cretien PB: Abnormalities of quantitative dinitrochlorobenzene sensitization in cancer patients: correlation with tumor stage and histology. Cancer 31:353-356, 1971

13. Catalona WJ, Taylor PT, Rabson AS, *et al*: A method for dinitrochlorobenzene contact sensitization. A clinicopathological study. N Engl J Med 286:399-402, 1972

14. Johnson NW, Mailback HI, Salmon SE: Skin reactivity in patients with cancer. Impaired delayed hypersensitivity or faulty inflammatory response. N Engl J Med 284: 1255-1257, 1971

15. Roth JA, Eilber FR, Nizze JA *et al*: Skin reactivity to DNCB and croton oil in patients with cancer. N Engl J Med 293:388-389, 1975

16. Krant MJ, Manekopf G, Brandrup CS, *et al*: Immunologic alterations in bronchogenic cancer. Cancer 21:623-631, 1968

17. Maisel RH, Ogura JH: Abnormal dinitrochlorobenzene skin sensitization: a prognostic sign of survival in head and neck squamous cell carcinoma. Laryngoscope 83:2012-2019, 1973

18. Sessions DB: Cancer of the head and neck. Laryngoscope 85:1960-1976, 1975

19. Fletcher GH, Lindberg RD, Hamberger A, *et al*: Reasons for radiation failure in squamous cell carcinoma of the larynx. Laryngoscope 85:987-1003, 1975

Acknowledgments—Ms Caroline Bradley, Registrar of the Washington University ENT Cancer Registry, was instrumental in obtaining data on the patients studied. The help of Ms. Toy Lin Lee, Otolaryngology Department Secretary, Hennepin County Medical Center, is gratefully acknowledged.

Reprints—Robert H. Maisel, MD, Hennepin County Medical Center, 701 Park Avenue, Minneapolis, MN 55415.

Ann Otol 85: 1976

OSTEOPLASTIC FRONTAL SINUSOTOMY

AN ANALYSIS OF 250 OPERATIONS

JAMES M. HARDY, MD

WILLIAM W. MONTGOMERY, MD

BOSTON, MASSACHUSETTS

SUMMARY – The operative approach and findings of 250 osteoplastic frontal sinusotomy operations performed from 1956 through 1972 at the Massachusetts Eye and Ear Infirmary are reviewed. Indications for surgery were symptomatic and/or complicated disease of the frontal sinus, including primary chronic sinusitis and osteoma or trauma with or without associated infection. Immediate postoperative complications were minor. Follow-up of at least three years was obtained in 83% of the patients, and 93% of these have no significant symptoms to date. A distressing problem of persistent postoperative frontal pain is discussed in detail. Revision surgery has been performed in 6% of patients due to recurrent frontal sinus infection. The reasons for failure are analyzed, and recommendations are made to minimize the possibility of recurrence.

June 19, 1976 marks the 20th anniversary of the first osteoplastic frontal sinusotomy done at the Massachusetts Eye and Ear Infirmary. On that date this method was used to revise a patient who had a mucocele recur one year after a Lynch frontoethmoidectomy. In spite of admonitions that such radical surgery would never be as successful, nor would it ever replace the Lynch sinusotomy, the osteoplastic operation soon became the standard procedure at this institution for all chronic symptomatic diseases of the frontal sinus except malignant disease.* Since the first 100 operations were reported in 1966,[1] considerably more experience has been accumulated. It is the purpose of this paper to review 250 patients treated by this method with attention to operative indications, findings at surgery, and postoperative results including revision surgery.

Two hundred and fifty-five consecutive osteoplastic frontal sinusotomy operations performed from 1956 through 1972 were identified. Five hospital charts were lost, thus 250 records were reviewed. Sixty-five procedures were performed by residents and 185 by 29 members of the Attending Staff. Follow-up was obtained on 208 patients (83%), 129 by examination, and 79 by questionnaire. Median follow-up was 8 years, but ranged from 3 to 19 years. Eighty-four patients were followed for more than ten years.

The etiologies of frontal sinus disease leading to surgery are broken down into four categories: chronic infection, osteoma, trauma, and miscellaneous (Table I).

One hundred and ninety patients (76%) had chronic infection as the etiology for surgery. Of these patients, 61% had mucoceles or pyoceles, and 39% had chronic infection without mucocele or pyocele. Sixty percent had unilateral disease.

Twenty-five patients (10%) were operated on for osteoma or its related complications. Thirteen of these patients had secondary chronic infection

* Goodale, RL. Personal communication.

From the Department of Otolaryngology, Harvard Medical School, and the Massachusetts Eye and Ear Infirmary, Boston, Massachusetts.

Presented at the meeting of the American Laryngological Association, Palm Beach, Florida, April 24-25, 1976.

TABLE I

OSTEOPLASTIC FRONTAL SINUSOTOMY

Etiologies		*No. Patients*	*%*
Chronic infection		190	76
Osteoma			
with infection	13		
without infection	12		
Total		25	10
Trauma			
with infection	15		
acute without infection	10		
Total		25	10
Miscellaneous		10	4
Total		250	100%

with or without mucocele or pyocele. Unilateral osteomata were present in 19 patients.

Twenty-five patients (10%) had surgery due to trauma or its sequelae in the frontal sinus. In 15 of these patients there was associated chronic sinusitis, which generally followed from violation of the sinus or its nasofrontal duct by fracture, or by foreign body secondary to trauma or neurosurgery. Acute trauma was present in ten patients. Three patients had cerebrospinal fluid (CSF) leak, two with secondary meningitis. The CSF leaks had been present for 16 days, one month and 16 years respectively.

Ten patients (4%) had miscellaneous indications for sinusotomy. Eight were related to neoplastic disease including three with mucoceles secondary to nasal inverted papilloma, two with mucoceles associated with fibrous dysplasia of the sinus, one with meningioma invading the sinus, one with reticulum cell sarcoma, and one with Wegener's granulomatosis.

ANALYSIS

Of the 250 total patients, 154 (62%) were male and 96 (38%) were female. The youngest was age 10 years and the oldest 84 (Table II). Sixty-four percent of the patients were between the ages of 31 and 60. The median postoperative hospitalization was six days, with a range of 2 to 40 days.

TABLE II

OSTEOPLASTIC FRONTAL SINUSOTOMY

1956-1972	*250 Consecutive Operations*	
62% M	Age	83% Follow-up
38% F	10-84	(from 3 to 19 yr)

Allergy

Respiratory tract allergy was present in 59 (24%) of 250 patients. Chronic infection was the only primary etiology leading to sinusotomy in which allergy may have played a role since 28% of these patients had associated allergy.

Previous Surgery

One hundred and four of 250 patients (42%) had previous frontal surgery: 46 Lynch operations, 37 trephines, eight duct probings, six Riedel procedures, five osteoplastic sinusotomies performed at other institutions, and two operations of unknown type. Several patients had histories of multiple frontal procedures. These operations were performed from four days to 43 years prior to definitive sinusotomy, the median time being eight years. Seventy-four patients (30%) had 145 previous nasal and sinus procedures other than on the frontal sinus.

Presenting Signs and Symptoms

Frontal pain or headache was the chief complaint in 61% of all patients, forehead or periorbital swelling in 27%, draining fistulae in 5%, diplopia in 4%, and miscellaneous in 3%. Symptom duration ranged from one day to 40 years. In 40% of patients, symptoms were present for more than one year (average 7.7 years).

Seventy-eight patients (27%) had normal physical examination except for decreased or absent transillumination. Forty-five had proptosis, 43 had masses in the superior medial canthal region, 42 had frontal or lid edema, 31 had tenderness, 16 had purulent rhinorrhea, 13 had depression of the frontal bone due to previous trauma or surgery, 10 had "Pott's Puffy Tumor" associated with chronic disease, and 6 demonstrated decreased extraocular motion.

Of special interest are 28 patients (11%) who had painless swelling of the forehead or upper lid region, or had painless proptosis as their only presenting symptom. Swelling had been present for a median of six months duration. Examination revealed proptosis and/or nontender mass of the supraorbital area or superior medial canthal region. This group included patients with chronic infection alone, osteoma with or without infection, trauma with infection, fibrous dysplasia with mucoceles and reticulum cell sarcoma. All patients but two with osteoma had erosion of the bony walls of the sinus, including six patients with erosion of the posterior wall with exposed dura. Thus, these patients had rather frighteningly extensive disease in light of the paucity of symptoms.

Regional Complications

Thirty-one patients (12%) presented with regional complications of frontal sinusitis, the primary etiologies being chronic infection alone or chronic infection associated with osteoma or trauma. Four patients had meningitis; six, brain abscess; nine, periorbital cellulitis; four, periorbital abscess; and, eight, osteomyelitis of the frontal bone. All but one of the nine patients with central nervous system (CNS) complications of meningitis or brain abscess had erosion of the posterior wall of the sinus with exposed dura.

Patients with regional complications rarely had a past history of symptoms compatible with frontal sinus disease. In about 80% of CNS and orbital complications, the presenting picture was that of the complication rather than of the primary chronic frontal sinus disease.

The brain and the periorbital abscesses were drained four to six weeks before the sinusotomy. *Staphylococcus aureus* was cultured in the majority of cases. There were no ophthalmologic sequelae. Eight of ten patients with CNS complications had no sequelae.

All patients with osteomyelitis of the frontal bone had significant residual deformity due to erosion of bone or debridement. This deformity was unrelated to the osteoplastic operation. Several subsequently have had cranioplasty to correct the defect.

Incision

One hundred and eighty-seven patients (75%) had brow incisions, 60% being unilateral. Sixty had coronal incisions, and 3 had incisions via previous scar. Average blood loss was 250 cc for unilateral brow incision, 350 cc for bilateral incision, and 650 cc for coronal incision.

TABLE III

OSTEOPLASTIC BONE FLAP

Operation	*Patients*
Unilateral flap	124
Bilateral flap	126
32 unilateral disease	
94 bilateral disease	

Bone Flaps

One hundred and twenty-four patients (50%) had unilateral bone flaps for approach to unilateral sinus disease, 32 (13%) had bilateral bone flaps for approach to unilateral disease, and 94 (37%) had bilateral bone flaps for approach to bilateral disease (Table III). In eight patients, the bone cuts were inadvertently made outside the confines of the frontal sinus. Seven of these eight had exposure of dura, and three had dural lacerations which were small, easily controlled, and without sequelae. One flap was inadvertently fractured into three pieces during elevation. The periosteum was kept intact between the pieces and the final cosmesis was good. There were no instances of necrosis or osteomyelitis of a bone flap.

Wall Erosion

Bony wall erosion occurred in 118 patients (47%). Seventy patients had exposed periorbita, 51 had exposed dura (8 with CNS complications), 20 had interfrontal septum erosion, and 12 had front wall erosion. Several had erosion of more than one wall. Thirty-two of the 70 patients with exposed periorbita had proptosis (46%). Twenty-seven had a palpable mass in the superior medial canthal region. Only three had periorbital cellulitis or abscess. Eight of the 51 patients with exposed dura (16%) had history of meningitis or frontal lobe abscess.

Culture

One hundred and eighty-four culture reports were available for analysis. Of these, 75 showed no growth and 38 grew only *Staphylococcus albus*. These reports were obtained from patients who were on preoperative antibiotics, or from cases with no associated infection. Seventy-one patients had pathogens isolated. There were 61 Gram positive organisms including 46 with *S. aureus*, six pneumococci, five alpha streptococci, and four beta streptococci. There were ten Gram negatives including four *Escherichia coli*, two Proteus, two Pseudomonas, one Klebsiella and one Bacteroides.

Fat Obliteration

Eighty-three percent of the osteoplastic frontal sinusotomies (208 patients) were obliterated with fat after meticulous removal of all mucous membrane and the inner cortical lining of the sinus. Seventeen percent (42 patients) did not have fat obliteration.

The median follow-up of those with no obliteration is 12 years, indicating that most were done in the early years of experience with this procedure. Ten percent of the patients who did not have fat obliteration required revision surgery because of recurrent frontal sinus infection. Likewise, 4% of those who had fat obliteration were revised.

Supraorbital Ethmoid

Supraorbital ethmoid cells located between the floor of the frontal sinus and the roof of the orbit were recognized in 29 patients (12%). Twenty-two were obliterated with fat after converting them into a common cavity with the frontal sinus, and none required revision. In seven patients the supraorbital ethmoid was not obliterated. In one of these, an unrecognized pyocele led to revision surgery two months later.

Deep Posterior Extension of the Frontal Sinus

This condition was present in 11 patients and often extended as a slit-like pseudopod for two or more centimeters posteriorly between the roof of the orbit and the anterior cranial fossa. Nine were obliterated with fat and remain uncomplicated. There has been one revision of the two cases not obliterated.

TABLE IV

OPERATIVE AND POSTOPERATIVE COMPLICATIONS

47 of 250 Patients (18%)	
Abdominal wound	13
Frontal wound	14
6 hematoma or seroma	
8 abscess (6 required revision)	
Bone cuts outside confines of sinus	8
Dural laceration	7
Miscellaneous	5

Operative Complications

Forty-seven patients (18%) had complications related to the frontal sinus surgery (Table IV).

Abdominal Wound. Thirteen patients had abdominal wound complications. There were 11 hematoma or seroma, and two abscesses, one due to *S. aureus* and one to *E. coli.* All were drained appropriately and added little to the morbidity or duration of hospitalization.

Frontal Wound. Six patients were complicated by uninfected hematoma or seroma, which were drained by removing a few sutures, inserting a rubber drain and applying a pressure dressing. Eight additional patients had abscess of the frontal wound, (five *S. aureus*, one *E. coli*, and two nonpathogens). In six of these, revision surgery was necessary.

Osteoplastic Flap Made Outside the Confines of the Frontal Sinus. Seven patients had exposure of dura, of which three had small dural lacerations. In one patient the bone cut extended into the opposite normal sinus without consequence.

Dura Laceration. Seven patients had inadvertent dura lacerations. Three were due to bone cuts outside the frontal sinus, and four occurred while stripping mucous membrane from dura exposed by disease. Five of these lacerations were small and were controlled by the adipose obliteration. Two lacerations were large. One was an avulsion which required fascia for repair, and one was repaired with silk sutures. There were no CNS sequelae, and all of these patients remain asymptomatic.

Nasal Skin Necrosis. This complication occurred in two patients secondary to the pressure dressing. In each there was a 2 cm depressed linear scar on the dorsum of the nose. One patient has had revision of the scar.

Other. Three patients had other complications:

1. total anosmia.
2. temporary ptosis which resolved in two months.
3. temporary loss of unilateral frontalis muscle function which resolved in six months.

TABLE V

FOLLOW-UP SYMPTOMS

(208 Patients)	
No significant symptoms	93%
Persistent postoperative pain	6%
Persistent neuralgia	1%

FOLLOW-UP SYMPTOMS

No Significant Symptoms. Of the 208 patients with follow-up (Table V), 193 (93%) have no significant symptoms with median follow-up of eight years. This includes those patients now asymptomatic after revision surgery.

Severe Persistent Frontal Pain or Headache. Twelve of the 208 patients with follow-up (6%) have persistent moderate or severe frontal pain or headache, 3 to 13 years postoperatively. This pain or headache does not have the characteristics of neuralgia. There is no relation to allergy, type of incision, fat obliteration or lack of, bony wall erosion, previous frontal surgery, presence or absence of infection at the sinusotomy or to the primary etiologies leading to surgery.

There does seem to be a significant relationship to the existence of chronic moderate or severe preoperative pain or headache. Eleven of these 12 patients had such preoperative symptoms, and in 8, the symptoms had been present for more than two years preoperatively.

Eleven of the 12 patients have no evidence of frontal sinus disease on examination or serial x-ray. Most have had antibiotic treatment in an effort to prove or disprove recurrent infection. All have had extensive negative neurological examination and laboratory studies. Four patients had revision osteoplastic sinusotomies, and no evidence of frontal sinus disease was found at surgery. One patient has had a recommendation for revision surgery at another institution.

Seven of these 12 patients have x-ray evidence of chronic sinusitis in sinuses other than the frontal sinus. One patient is to undergo surgery for an ethmoid mucocele. Five, by x-ray, had no evidence of disease in other sinuses.

Two patients have had neurectomies without relief of symptoms. One had a supraorbital nerve neurectomy, and one a sphenopalatine ganglionectomy. Two patients had a history of psychiatric disorder. One had a history of conversion reaction, and the other, drug addiction.

Neuralgia. Three of 208 patients with follow-up have had persistent frontal neuralgia for up to ten years postoperatively. These patients had brow incisions with the necessary severance of the supraorbital nerves, which probably is causative. They have been treated with repeated local anesthetic and alcohol injections of the supraorbital nerves without permanent relief. An additional patient had severe neuralgia completely relieved after alcohol injections six months postoperatively. Several other patients with brow incisions had temporary neuralgia in the first few months after surgery.

Persistent Abnormal Forehead Sensation. Almost 100% of patients with brow incisions, and the majority with coronal incisions, had temporary distorted forehead sensation described as numbness, pruritis, tightness, crawling paresthesias, and pins and needles paresthesias. In 65% of these patients, symptoms disappeared in six to twelve months. However, in 35% the abnormal sensation is persistent, though no patient described the symptoms as more than a minor annoyance. There was no significant difference in the percentage of patients who had brow or coronal incisions when considering the persistent anesthesia and paresthesias. However, those with brow incisions generally stated that the symptoms were more annoying.

TABLE VI

COSMESIS

Scar		
Good or excellent		88%
Fair or poor		12%
Bony forehead contour		
Good or excellent		79%
Fair or poor		21%
Defect existed preoperatively	75%	
Elevated or depressed bone flap	25%*	

* 6% of all patients

Cosmesis

Evaluation of cosmetic result was divided into appearance of the scar, and appearance of the bony forehead contour (Table VI). These observations were the subjective opinion of the examining physician.

Scars. Eighty-eight percent of all scars, brow and coronal, were considered good or excellent. Fair or poor coronal scars were due to exposure of the scar by natural balding in two males. Fair or poor brow scars resulted when the incision was made too high above the brow, when incisions from previous surgery were reincised, or when the incision between the brows did not extend to the deepest recess of the glabella.

Bony Contour. Seventy-nine percent of all forehead contour cosmesis was considered excellent or good (89% of coronal, 74% of brow). In three-fourths of those with fair or poor forehead contour, the deformity was secondary to a previous surgical defect, or to anterior sinus wall erosion due to disease. Thus in 6% of all patients was the bone flap cosmesis considered fair or poor, secondary to depression or elevation of the flap. Relatively more of these were associated with brow incisions rather than coronal, particularly unilateral brow incisions. This may be due to the more difficult exposure with the unilateral brow incision which can produce difficulty in beveling the superior bone cuts. There were no permanent floating osteoplastic flaps due to nonunion.

Twelve patients had surgery to correct cosmetic defects. Two patients had scar revision, and ten had cranioplasty or bone grafting to correct the bony depressions. Nine of these defects were due to previous surgery or anterior wall erosion by disease. One was related to a depressed flap following osteoplastic operation.

X-ray

Initial x-ray evaluation was extremely accurate in predicting the extent and etiology of disease even in the prepolytomography era. The most frequent error of omission, without polytomography, was not being able to predict wall erosion. With polytomography, the surgeon can accurately be advised as to wall erosion and the presence of supraorbital ethmoid cells, or deep posterior extensions of the frontal sinuses.

Serial postoperative x-rays of the frontals have been of great value in determining whether or not recurrent infection of the sinus is present. In three instances, such serial radiographs ruled out recurrent mucoceles which were thought to be present on initial postoperative x-rays. Subsequent films have shown no change in the lucencies

TABLE VII

REVISION FRONTAL SURGERY

20 of 208 Patients with Follow-up		*Patients*
Short-term revisions		6
Acute wound infection and fat necrosis	5	
Acute wound infection due to unrecognized supraorbital ethmoid pyocele	1	
Long-term revisions		14
Negative exploration for persistent pain	4	
Osteomyelitis outside normal sinus	2	
Recurrent chronic sinus infection	7	
Recurrent fibrous dysplasia with infection	1	
	Total	20

after several years. In one patient, serial studies revealed an expanding mucocele in an otherwise asymptomatic patient.

Initial x-rays in 115 of 190 patients with chronic infection (61%) indicated involvement of other sinuses in addition to the frontals. Ethmoid involvement was more common than antral or sphenoid. Only 17% of patients with osteoma, trauma, and miscellaneous etiologies showed sinusitis in other than the frontals, and all of these had secondary chronic infection of the frontals. Thirty-five percent of those patients with evidence of ethmoid, sphenoid or maxillary sinusitis on preoperative x-ray had complete clearing of the sinuses on follow-up radiography. Conversely, 10% of those with no evidence of disease in other sinuses preoperatively did have such sinusitis on follow-up films.

REVISION FRONTAL SURGERY

Twenty patients of 208 with follow-up (9.5%) have had revision frontal surgery from four days to 14 years (median two years) following the initial procedure (Table VII). Four of these cases were performed initially on the Resident Service (6.5% of 61 cases with follow-up). Sixteen of the revisions were initially done by nine members of the Attending Staff (11% of 147 cases with follow-up).

Short-Term Revisions

Six revisions were done in the first few days or months after the original surgery because of persistent purulent drainage via a fistula following acute wound infection. All had fat obliteration at the first sinusotomy, and the operative findings in each, at revision, was acute infection with fat necrosis. However, in one of these the initial procedure failed because a supraorbital ethmoid pyocele was unrecognized. These six patients represent 3% of all those who had fat obliteration at the first operation.

At revision two patients had fresh fat obliteration, the wounds were closed primarily, and specific antibiotics instituted. Four did not have obliteration; two had Riedel procedures, one had the wound packed open due to allergy to appropriate antibiotics, and in the fourth, no reason was given for not re-obliterating. The last patient developed another wound infection, and was re-explored a second time. The other five patients are asymptomatic to date.

Long-Term Revisions

Fourteen patients had revision a median of five years after the original surgery; the longest interval was after fourteen years. Eight of the patients were found to have recurrent infection in the frontal sinus, whereas six were found to have no infection in the sinus. Of the latter, four had negative reexplorations for persistent postoperative pain, and two developed frontal bone osteomyelitis at sites of previous trauma outside the sinus.

Of the eight patients with recurrent

chronic infection within the frontal sinus, all but one presented with acute gross findings of complicated chronic disease: swelling, proptosis, forehead abscess, fistulae or tenderness. The other patient had evidence of enlarging mucocele on serial radiographs, though his examination was unremarkable. This is in contrast to no evidence of recurrent disease on exam or x-ray in the four reexplored for persistent pain.

The reasons for failure in the eight patients with recurrent chronic sinus infection were evident in all but one:

1. Three did not have removal of all mucous membrane at the first operation according to the operative records. Two of these had fat obliteration.
2. Three were not obliterated with fat, possibly allowing regrowth of mucous membrane from the nasal cavity.
3. One patient had recurrent fibrous dysplasia plus chronic infection.

Excluding the patient with fibrous dysplasia, seven patients, or 3% of 208 with follow-up, had long-term failure with recurrent chronic frontal sinus infection.

TABLE VIII

REVISION DUE TO RECURRENT SINUS INFECTION

Of 208 Patients with Follow-up	
Acute infection	6 (3%)
Chronic infection	7 (3%)
Total	13 (6%)

Discussion of Revisions with Recurrent Infection

Thirteen patients, or 6% of 208 with follow-up, had revision due to acute infection or recurrent chronic infection within the frontal sinus (Table VIII). There was an equal revision rate for each initial etiology. Fifty-four percent had associated allergy (versus 24% of all patients). Seventy percent had bony wall erosion by the original disease (versus 47% of all patients). Four percent (9 of 208) who had original fat obliteration were later revised, whereas 10% (4 of 42) of those who did not have fat obliteration, had revision. In comparison to the total patient population, there was no correlation of the revision surgery in reference to types of incisions used at initial surgery, whether the initial disease was unilateral or bilateral, culture at original sinusotomy, presence of associated systemic disease, or history of frontal sinus surgery prior to the initial osteoplastic procedure.

It should be mentioned that 13 patients had fat obliteration at revision surgery, and none have evidence of disease to date. Conversely, four of seven patients with no fat obliteration subsequently had a second revision.

CONCLUSIONS

1. The osteoplastic frontal sinusotomy is the procedure of choice for treating all chronic complicated diseases of the frontal sinus except malignant disease. Adipose obliteration should be accomplished in all cases, regardless of etiology, unless unsuspected malignant disease is encountered.

2. Subcutaneous fat should be obtained with atraumatic technique just before insertion into the prepared sinus. Two patients with acute postoperative wound infection and fat necrosis had fat obtained at the beginning of the procedure, possibly allowing drying and necrosis before insertion into the sinus.

3. Specific antibiotic therapy should be instituted preoperatively in all cases associated with chronic infection. Until culture and sensitivity reports are available, coverage for *S. aureus* is recommended.

4. The patient should be crossmatched for blood replacement.

5. The coronal incision is ideal for females, and also for males who have demonstrated no tendency for balding. It offers better cosmesis and exposure than the brow incision at the expense of increased blood loss. No patient with the coronal incision had postoperative neuralgia.

6. Bilateral bone flap approach for unilateral disease can be technically easier, and can offer better exposure than a unilateral flap.

7. Supraorbital ethmoid cells should be converted into a common cavity with the frontal sinuses, and obliterated. Likewise, deep posterior extensions of the frontal sinus sould be included with fat obliteration. Removal of the inner cortical lining often requires the smallest diamond burr, and an operating microscope may be necessary.

8. Treatment of osteomyelitis associated with chronic frontal sinus disease should include preoperative antibiotics, surgery with a combination of osteoplastic adipose obliteration and debridement of necrotic bone, and postoperative antibiotics for six weeks. Most cases of osteomyelitis associated with an initial acute frontal sinusitis will respond to antibiotic treatment only. Occasionally, trephination can be used in addition to antibiotics.

9. Operative complications have generally been minor and of no permanent consequence. There have been no operative deaths, nor CNS or ophthalmologic complications.

10. Thirteen patients had revision due to recurrent frontal sinus infection. This is a 6% failure rate. Six patients (3%) had short-term revisions due to acute postoperative wound infection and fat necrosis. One of these had an unrecognized supraorbital ethmoid pyocele. Postoperative frontal wound infections should be treated aggressively with specific antibiotics and drainage. If infection persists, the sinus should be reexplored, the necrotic fat removed, and fresh fat obliteration accomplished. Seven patients (3%) had long-term revisions due to recurrent chronic infection. All had gross physical or x-ray findings of recurrent disease. All patients who came to revision, except one with osteoma, had chronic infection evident at the first operation. Associated allergy and bony wall erosion was significantly higher in patients who had revision.

11. After discharge from the hospital, postoperative follow-up care, patient inconvenience, and discomfort are usually minimal. This is in contrast with most other radical frontal sinus procedures. The patient should have postoperative x-rays three weeks after surgery, after one year, and serially thereafter if symptomatic.

12. Six percent of patients have moderate to severe persistent frontal pain or headache postoperatively with no evidence of recurrent disease. Those with chronic severe preoperative pain or headache seem most likely to develop this distressing symptom. Reexploration is rarely indicated if extensive otolaryngologic, neurologic, and serial radiologic work-up is negative in these patients.

13. Thirty-five percent of all patients have persistent anesthesia or paresthesia of the forehead after surgery.

14. Though cosmesis after the osteoplastic procedure is generally far superior to other radical frontal operations, unpleasant results can occur. Properly placed incisions and meticulous closure can minimize scar deformity. Beveled bone incisions and meticulous closure of periosteum can avoid osteoplastic flap elevation or depression. If there is any question concerning the stability of the bone flap, drill holes and wiring are indicated.

15. While it is believed that the osteoplastic sinusotomy with fat obliteration is far superior to other frontal operations in regards to disease eradication, cosmesis, minimal postoperative care, and patient discomfort, it must be reiterated that frontal sinus disease can be insidious. Follow-up in this study is nineteen years, whereas recurrent disease has become evident up to forty-three years after other types of frontal surgery.

REFERENCES

1. Zonis RD, Montgomery WW, Goodale RL: Frontal sinus disease: 100 cases treated by osteoplastic operation. Laryngoscope 56: 1816-1825, 1966

ACKNOWLEDGMENTS—The authors thank the members of the Massachusetts Eye and Ear Infirmary Staff for allowing use to include their patients in this study. We particularly thank Robert L. Goodale, MD, for his kind advice. Follow-up radiology was interpreted by Alfred L. Weber, MD. Special acknowledgment is due Mary Ellen Doyle, Patricia Egan and Pauline Hardy for their technical assistance.

REPRINTS—James M. Hardy, MD, 1127 North Boulevard, East, Leesburg, FL 32748.

XV INTERNATIONAL CONGRESS OF BRONCHOESOPHAGOLOGY

The XV International Congress of Bronchoesophagology will be held in Sao Paulo, Brazil, March 24-26, 1977, following the II World Congress of Otolaryngology in Buenos Aires. For information write: Dr. Plinio de Mattos Barretto, President of the Congress, Rua Cons. Torres Homem, 371, 01432, Sao Paulo, Brazil.

Ann Otol 85: 1976

LARYNGEAL SUSPENSION AND EPIGLOTTIC FLAP IN LARYNGOPHARYNGEAL TRAUMA

NELS R. OLSON, MD

ANN ARBOR, MICHIGAN

SUMMARY – Physicians treating laryngeal trauma are still looking for ways to improve results. Severe disruption of the supporting structures between hyoid and trachea may allow stretching and narrowing of the laryngeal lumen during the healing period. This can easily be prevented by placing wires across the disrupted zone. In addition, loss of the epithelial lining of the larynx is a serious cause of stenosis. By dissecting out the epiglottic cartilage, one can create a sizeable, useful flap of mucous membrane based in the vallecula to use in relining of the anterior larynx.

The search continues for the best ways to prevent stenosis in repair of blunt laryngeal injuries. In two recent cases I have treated, I have utilized two techniques which have not been reported previously, to my knowledge. One of these techniques I call laryngeal suspension. It involves wiring between the hyoid and the larynx to support structural weakness and prevent stretching and narrowing of the lumen. The other is the use of a flap of mucosa developed by dissecting out the epiglottis to help reline the larynx, thereby promoting primary healing.

CASE REPORTS

Case 1. A male, aged 25, struck his neck on the steering wheel of his car in an accident on February 26, 1974. Soon thereafter, he underwent open reduction, suture of mucosal lacerations and placement of a silicone stent (Montgomery's type). Two weeks later the repair had broken down and the stent was exposed anteriorly and surrounded by granulation tissue. The wound was reopened, using a "T" incision. Granulation tissue was excised from the larynx. A vallecula-based flap was developed by dissecting out the epiglottic cartilage. The larynx was stented with a skin graft sutured raw side out around a sponge covered with finger cots. The epiglottic flap was placed in the anterior larynx where mucosa had been lost. Wires were then placed between

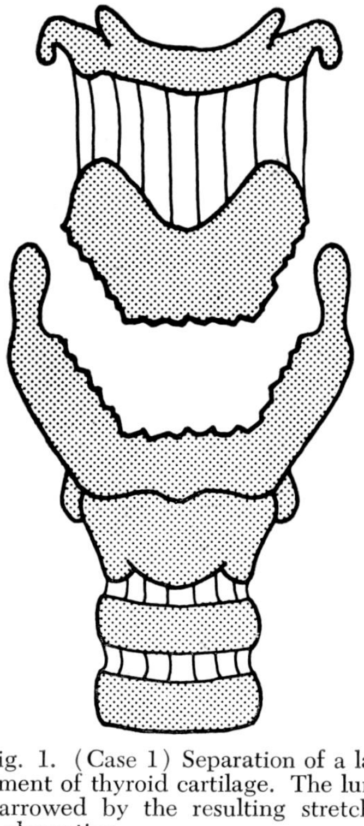

Fig. 1. (Case 1) Separation of a large fragment of thyroid cartilage. The lumen is narrowed by the resulting stretching and elongation.

From the University of Michigan Medical School and Ann Arbor Veterans Administration Hospital, Ann Arbor, Michigan.

Presented at the meeting of the American Laryngological Association, Palm Beach, Florida, April 24-25, 1976.

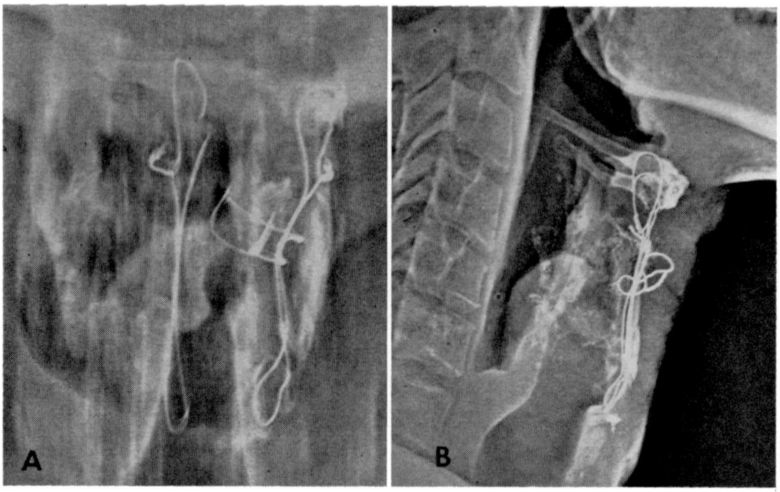

Fig. 2. A) (Case 1) Suspension wires placed from hyoid to cricoid. Direct wiring of the loose fragment of thyroid cartilage. B) (Case 1) Lateral view of repair.

the hyoid and the cricoid on each side and the elongated laryngopharynx was drawn together (Figs. 1 - 2B). This resulted in 2 cm of shortening between hyoid and cricoid. A segment of thyroid cartilage which had been severed in the original injury was wired into place. Eighteen days later the sponge stent was removed. At this time healing was by primary intention and no granulation was seen in the larynx. Two months after that, the tracheotomy tube was removed. The patient had a breathy voice because of an abducted, immobile right vocal cord and in March of 1975, about one year after his initial injury, he had a Teflon® paste injection of the right vocal cord to improve the voice quality. Currently, he has some dyspnea on exertion and a fair voice. He is working full time.

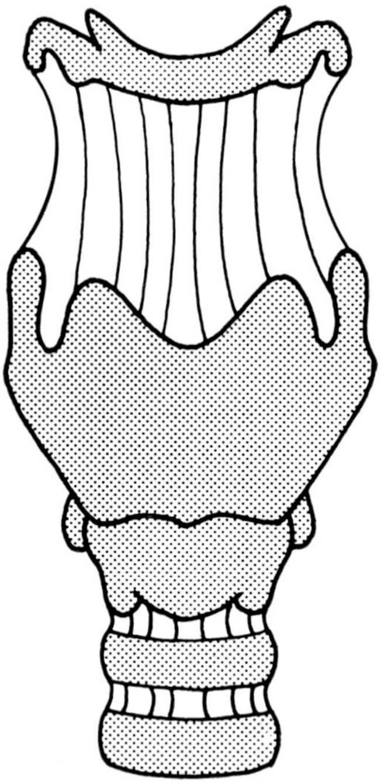

Fig. 3. (Case 2) Scarf injury has destroyed support between hyoid bone and thyroid cartilage, resulting in elongation and narrowing of the lumen.

Case 2. On March 18, 1972, this 9-year-old boy backed into a lathe, catching both ends of a scarf he was wearing in the turning machinery. Fortunately, the machine was stopped quickly. He was hospitalized with stiff neck, skin abrasions, subcutaneous emphysema and dysphagia. There was no airway problem at first. Initial treatment consisted of antibiotics, steam, steroids, bedrest, voice rest, oxygen. Thirteen days later he was still unable to swallow and a direct laryngoscopy was done. Circular granulations were seen just above the true cords and extending around the entire pharyngeal wall. He was discharged on tube feedings. Gradually, airway obstruction developed and on April 12, 1972, 26 days after injury,

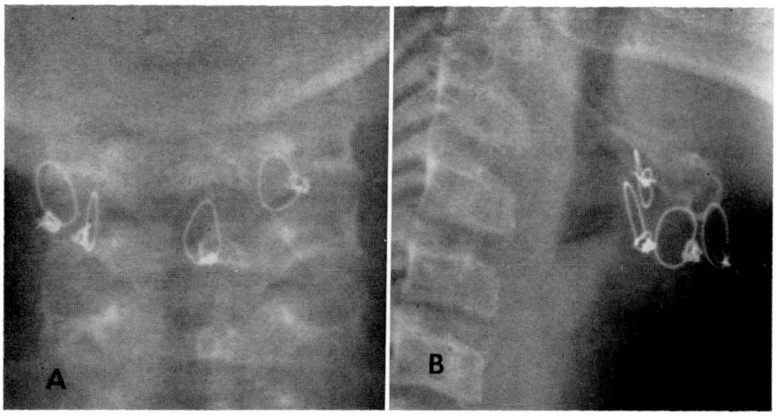

Fig. 4. A) (Case 2) Suspension wires placed between hyoid bone and thyroid cartilage. B) (Case 2) Lateral view of repair.

a tracheotomy was performed. Shortly thereafter the area of injury closed completely except for the feeding tube.

On June 16, 1972 he underwent pharyngotomy, excision of some scar tissue, and skin grafting of the pharynx. This operation succeeded to the extent that he could swallow liquids and some soft solids, but he still had to wear his tracheotomy tube.

Three years later, on June 19, 1975 he underwent another procedure. This time he had circumferential resection of scar tissue, sparing the mucosa. Additional mucosa was obtained by dissecting out the epiglottic cartilage. The gap between the hyoid bone and thyroid cartilage which had been produced by the injury was closed, using wires to draw these structures together (Figs. 3 - 4B). Placement of the wires resulted in 2 cm of shortening between hyoid bone and thyroid cartilage. The mucosa was carefully sutured. No stent was used. Two months later, he was eating

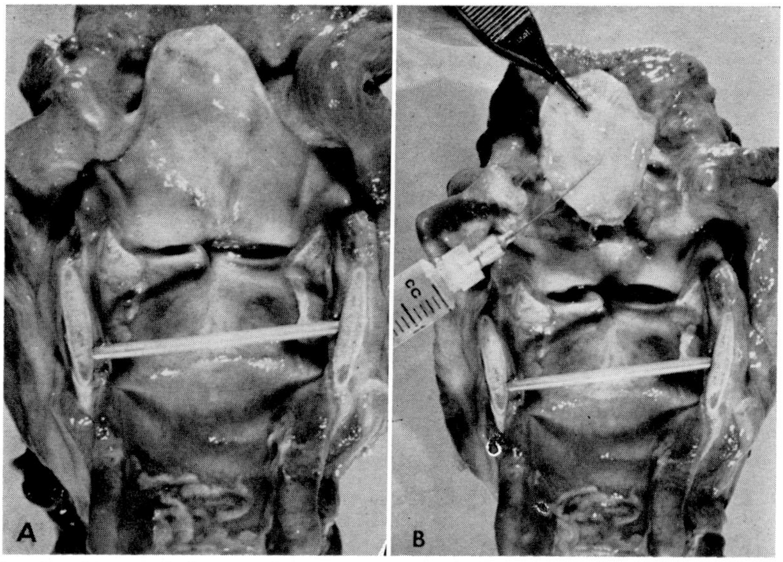

Fig. 5. A) Fresh laryngeal specimen, posterior-anterior view of epiglottis. B) Incision from vallecula through aryepiglottic fold around petiolus of epiglottis, through contralateral aryepiglottic fold and ending in contralateral vallecula. Injection of saline beneath mucosa aids elevation.

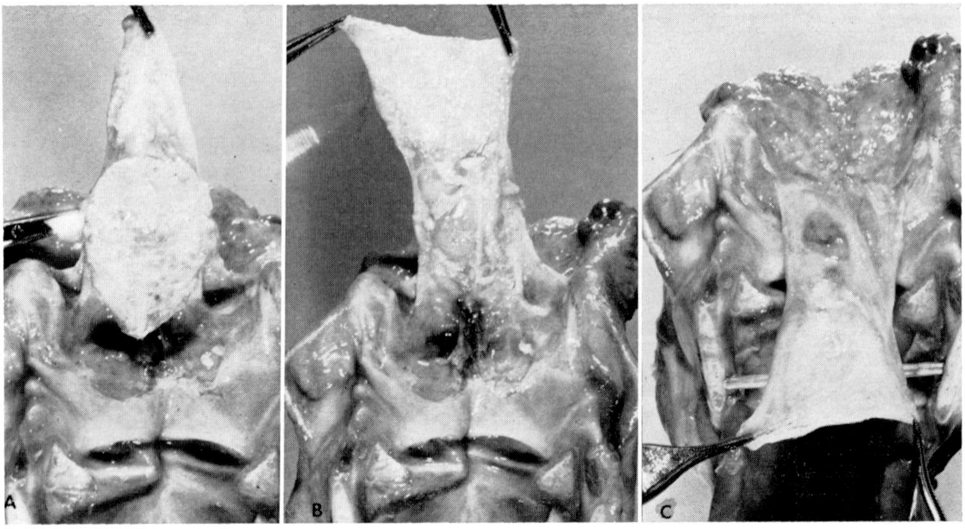

Fig. 6. A) Laryngeal surface of epiglottis dissected completely. B) Epiglottic cartilage removed. C) Flap easily reaches from vallecula to upper trachea.

with ease, gaining weight and could be decannulated. He has functioned normally since.

DISCUSSION

Laryngeal Suspension. With each swallow, there is forcible elevation of the hyoid bone, larynx, and trachea by contraction of the mylohyoid muscle. The supporting elements which transmit this force through the larynx to the treachea are the thyroid cartilage, thyrohyoid muscle, thyrohyoid membrane and associated ligaments. With crushing or disruption of some of these structures, the upward pull of the mylohyoid will stretch and elongate the soft tissues in the area of injury. This will lead to narrowing analagous to the drawing out of a heated glass tube.

Wiring across the area of injury ("laryngeal suspension") has these advantages:

1. The wiring of weakened structure prevents elongation and narrowing of the lumen.

2. By drawing the wires quite snug one can overcorrect slightly, hoping thereby to widen the lumen of the larynx or pharynx a little.

3. The wiring eliminates all motion between the wired parts, putting the unit at rest and promoting healing. This is especially important when a flap or graft has been placed in the lumen or the mucosa has been sutured.

Epiglottic Flap. One of the important principles in repair of the crushed larynx is to create conditions which will result in primary healing. The goal is to prevent granulation and fibrosis. I have used a skin graft in the lumen whenever there has been disruption of the mucosa, as added insurance against granulation and fibrosis in case sutured mucosal lacerations break down.

In Case 1, the epiglottis and part of the thyroid cartilage were separated from the rest of the larynx. There was considerable loss of anterior laryngeal mucosa. It was therefore decided that the epiglottis should be dissected out in such a way that a flap of mucosa based in the vallecula would be formed (Figs. 5, 6). It appears that such a flap will be useful in many cases of laryngeal injury because of the high priority of the anterior commissure region and the ease with which this area can be reepithelialized by this method.

SUMMARY

I have described two adjuncts to treatment of laryngopharyngeal injuries.

One, laryngeal suspension, is designed to prevent or correct elongation and narrowing of the lumen by upward motion of the hyoid with swallowing. The other, the epiglottic flap, is a way of providing epithelial lining for the anterior part of the larynx when necessary.

Reprints—Nels R. Olson, MD, University of Michigan Medical Center, Ann Arbor, MI 48104.

XV PAN-AMERICAN CONGRESS OF OTOLARYNGOLOGY AND BRONCHOESOPHAGOLOGY

The XV Pan-American Congress of Otolaryngology and Bronchoesophagology will be held in New Orleans, Louisiana, November 4-11, 1976. For further information write: Creative Associates, 5005 Newport Dr., Rolling Meadows, IL 60008. Anyone desiring to present a free paper write: Dr. Irving M. Blatt, Secretary-General, Pan-Am Otocongress, P.O. Box 52378, New Orleans, LA 70152.

Ann Otol 85: 1976

VERRUCOUS CARCINOMA OF THE LARYNX
MANAGEMENT BY RADIOTHERAPY AND SURGERY

HUGH P. BURNS, MB

A. W. PETER VAN NOSTRAND, MD DOUGLAS P. BRYCE, MD

TORONTO, CANADA

SUMMARY – Verrucous carcinoma is an unusual and distinct variant of well differentiated squamous cell carcinoma, and accounts for approximately 1 to 2% of all primary squamous cell carcinomas of the larynx. There has been considerable controversy regarding the role of radiotherapy in the management of these tumors, as they are said to be radioresistant, and in a number of instances "anaplastic transformation" has apparently occurred following such therapy. We have reviewed 18 patients with verrucous carcinoma of the larynx in which eight received surgical therapy alone, eight received radiotherapy alone, and two received combined therapy. We conclude that radiotherapy and surgery are equally effective in eradicating the disease. "Anaplastic transformation" of these tumors represents a small but nevertheless real risk following radiotherapy. Accordingly, our current therapeutic policy is to treat by surgical excision those smaller tumors which can be removed by conservation laryngectomy procedures, reserving radiotherapy for those large tumors which would require total laryngectomy if treated surgically.

Verrucous carcinoma is a distinct variant of well differentiated squamous cell carcinoma. Ackerman[1] first coined the term "verrucous carcinoma" in 1948, and delineated the interesting and peculiar, clinical and pathological characteristics of this group of neoplasms.

Ackerman emphasized the following features: Most lesions occur in elderly men, usually on the buccal mucosa and lower gingiva. Tobacco chewing may be of etiologic significance. The lesions have a warty, papillomatous appearance, tend to grow slowly, but may be very extensive and tend to invade local structures, for example, bone structures. With coexisting infection, the regional lymph nodes are often enlarged and tender, but metastasis to local lymph nodes is very unusual, and distant metastasis has not been documented. Microscopically, these lesions are extremely well differentiated, and have papillary surface projections and downgrowth of club-shaped, finger-like processes of squamous epithelium. Hyperkeratosis is a prominent feature. The advancing margin of the tumor has pushing borders associated with a prominent chronic inflammatory infiltrate.

The oral cavity is the most common site. Other sites include the larynx, external genitalia, nasal fossa, and esophagus. Verrucous carcinoma may account for up to 10% of all squamous cell carcinomas of the buccal mucosa. One to 2% of all squamous cell carcinomas of the larynx are of the verrucous variety.[2]

There has been considerable controversy regarding the role of radiotherapy in the management of these tumors, as they are said to be radioresistant, and in a number of instances, "anaplastic transformation" has apparently occurred following such therapy. In their review of 105 cases, Kraus and Perez-Mesa[3] indicated that radiotherapy was employed in 17 patients, and failed to control the lesion in all instances. In 4 of the 17 patients a sudden alteration in the character of the lesion to an anaplastic pattern occurred. These lesions

From the Departments of Otolaryngology and Pathology, University of Toronto, and Toronto General Hospital, Toronto, Canada. This work has been supported in part by the Charlie Conacher Cancer Research Fund.

Presented at the meeting of the American Laryngological Association, Palm Beach, Florida, April 24-25, 1976.

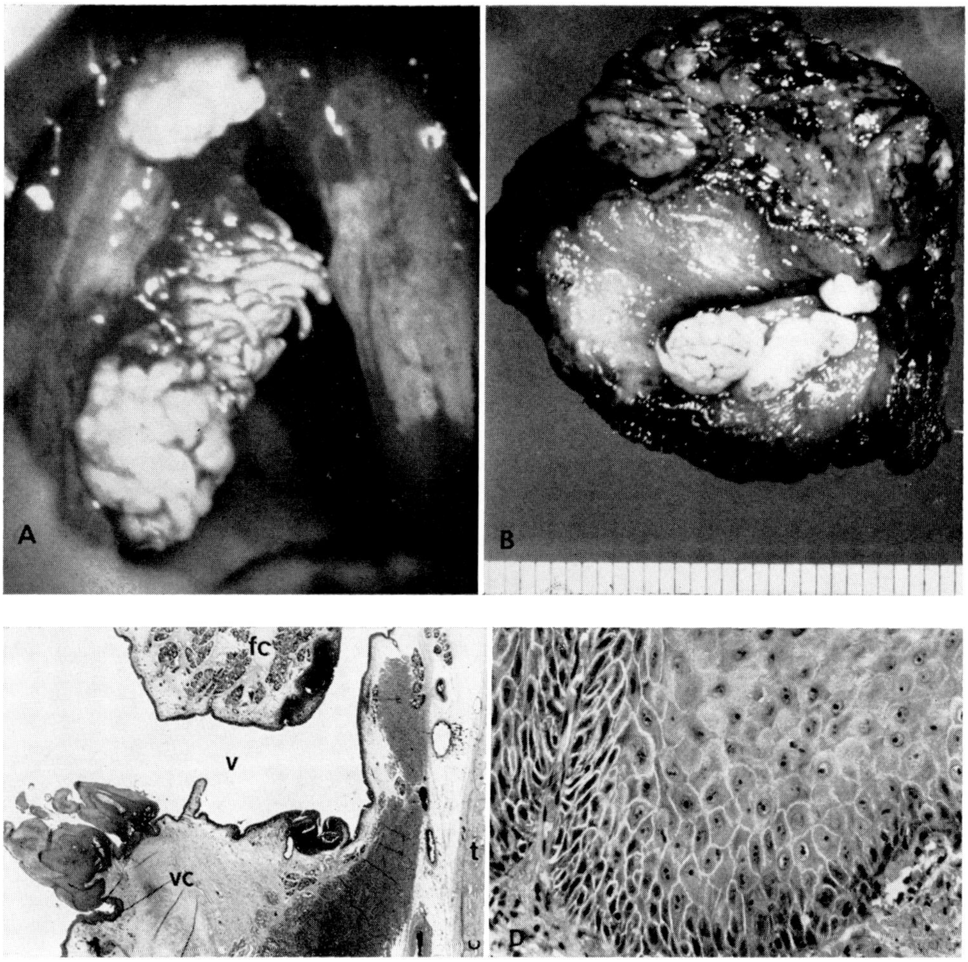

Fig. 1. (Case 6) A) Endoscopic view of a multifocal papillary lesion confined to the left vocal cord of a 53-year-old male. B) Gross photograph of the left vertical hemilaryngectomy specimen illustrating the multifocal nature of the lesions and emphasizing the white warty appearance. C) Low power photomicrograph of the hemilaryngectomy specimen. The papillary verrucous tumor is confined to the mucosa and submucosa of the free margin of the vocal cord (vc) (H & E X 15). fc - False vocal cord. t - Thyroid ala. v - Laryngeal ventricle. D) Photomicrograph of the advancing margin of the tumor. The "pushing" border and well differentiated nature of the neoplasm are clearly shown (H & E X 375).

grew rapidly, with distant metastases, and death attributable to the tumor rapidly followed in three patients.[3,4] Five additional cases having similar transformation have been reported.[2,5,6]

The purpose of this paper is to review the results of therapy in 18 patients with verrucous carcinoma of the larynx. We are currently conducting a similar study of 36 cases of verrucous carcinoma originating in the oral cavity.[7]

METHODS AND MATERIALS

In the Toronto area, virtually all new patients with head and neck carcinoma are referred to the Princess Margaret Hospital (a radiotherapy center) for assessment prior to therapy. In the 15 year period 1960 - 1975, of a total of approximately 1,300 cases of laryngeal carcinoma seen, 18 new cases (1.4%) of verrucous carcinoma of the larynx were diagnosed.

The clinical charts, x-rays, photographs, pathological reports and microscopic slides were examined in all instances. We adhered

TABLE I

VERRUCOUS CARCINOMA OF THE LARYNX
RESULTS OF THERAPY

Case	*Age/Sex*	*Site*	*Treatment*	*Follow-up*
1	61 M	T_{1A} G	VH	A & W 6 yr
2	77 F	T_{1B} SG	Horiz. SG. Later, TL for aspiration	A & W 1 yr
3	65 M	T_{1A} G	Cordectomy	A & W 4 yr
4	39 M	T_{1B} G	TL	A & W 13 yr
5	61 M	T_2 G	TL	A & W 14 yr
6	53 M	T_{1A} G	VH	A & W 1 yr
7	61 M	T_2 G	VH	A & W 9 mo
8	58 M	T_2 G	VH	Died with multiple separate primaries (larynx clear) - 2 yr later
9	52 F	T_3 G	Co60 5500 R/5 wk	A & W 6 yr
10	58 M	T_2 SG	Co60 4500 R/3 wk	A & W 4 yr
11	66 F	T_{1B} SG	Co60 5500 R/5 wk	A & W 2 yr
12	77 M	T_2 G	Co60 5500 R/5 wk	A & W 5 yr
13	34 F	T_2 G	Co60 5500 R/6 wk	A & W 9 yr
14	83 M	T_2 SG	Co60 5500 R/5 wk	A & W 9 mo
15	76 M	T_2 SG	Betatron 5000 R/3 wk	Died unrelated causes - 5 yr later
16	69 F	R. Ary. Ep. fold	Co60 5500 R/7 wk	Died with disseminated malignancy ("anaplastic transformation") 10 mo later
17	58 M	T_2 G	Co60 5500 R/5 wk Pos. biopsy 6/52 later TL specimen negative	A & W 7 yr
18	65 M	T_{1B} G	Co60 5500 R/5 wk for SCC - developed verrucous ca 3½ yr later, treated by TL	A & W 9 yr

G - Glottic; SG - Supra-glottic; R. Ary. Ep. - Right aryepiglottic; VH - Vertical hemilaryngectomy; TL - Total laryngectomy; Co60 - Cobalt-60; A & W - Alive and well.

to the diagnostic criteria laid down by Ackerman,[1] and amplified by Kraus and Perez-Mesa,[4] and others.[2]

The details of the clinical features, treatment and follow-up of the 18 laryngeal cases are provided in Table I. Twelve of the 18 laryngeal cases were of glottic origin, and presented with voice disturbance. The remaining six cases were of supraglottic origin and presented with dysphagia, discomfort in the throat and/or sore throat. The average age was 62 years, with a range of from 34 to 85 years.

RESULTS

Of the 18 patients, 8 were treated by surgery alone. Six patients had a partial laryngectomy performed (Fig. 1) and two patients had a total laryngectomy. Follow-up revealed seven patients to be alive and well from nine

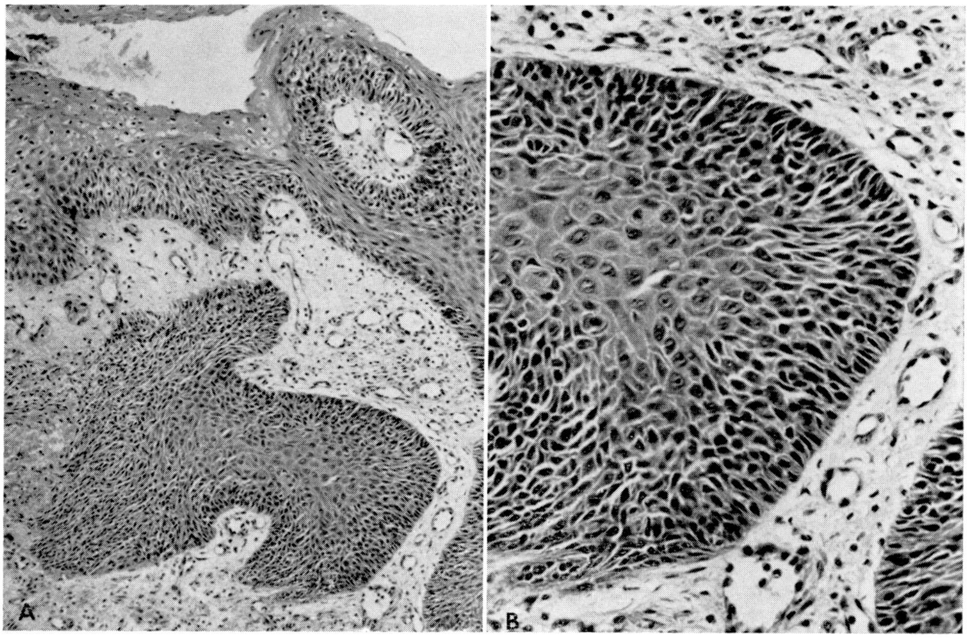

Fig. 2. (Case 10) Photomicrographs of the laryngeal biopsy specimen from a 58-year-old male with a T_2 supraglottic tumor. This patient received radiotherapy and is free of disease four years following treatment. A) A low power view illustrating the keratinization of the surface of the lesion (top) and the islands of tumor in the vascular submucosa (H & E X 60). B) The same field under greater magnification. The normal maturation sequence of the squamous cells and the well defined margins of the tumor are readily evident (H & E X 375).

months to 14 years following treatment. One patient died two years later of multiple, separate primaries (stomach, lung, thyroid) without evidence of recurrent or residual disease in the larynx.

Eight patients were treated with radiotherapy alone (Figs. 2, 3). Cobalt-60, 4500 - 5000 rads was administered over a three to seven week period. Follow-up reveals six patients to be alive and well from nine months to eight years following completion of therapy. One patient died five years later from unrelated disease (ischemic heart disease). One patient died ten months later of "anaplastic change" resulting in widespread distant metastases.

Two patients received combined therapy. Both deserve special mention. The first patient had a T_2 glottic lesion treated with cobalt-60, 5500 rads over five weeks, with a positive biopsy some six weeks later. A total laryngectomy was performed 12 weeks after completion of the course of radiotherapy, and the laryngectomy specimen was negative for tumor. This patient is alive and well seven years following treatment. The second patient had a squamous cell carcinoma of the larynx, staged as T_{1B} glottic, treated with cobalt-60, 5500 rads over five weeks. The lesion regressed, but 3½ years later, at the same site, another tumor arose which had the typical gross and microscopic features of a verrucous carcinoma. This man was treated by total laryngectomy, and is alive and well nine years later.

CONCLUSIONS

Contrary to previous reviews, verrucous carcinoma, at least when it occurs in the larynx, can be successfully treated by radiotherapy alone. In our material, the results of treatment by radiotherapy alone are equally as good as by surgery alone.

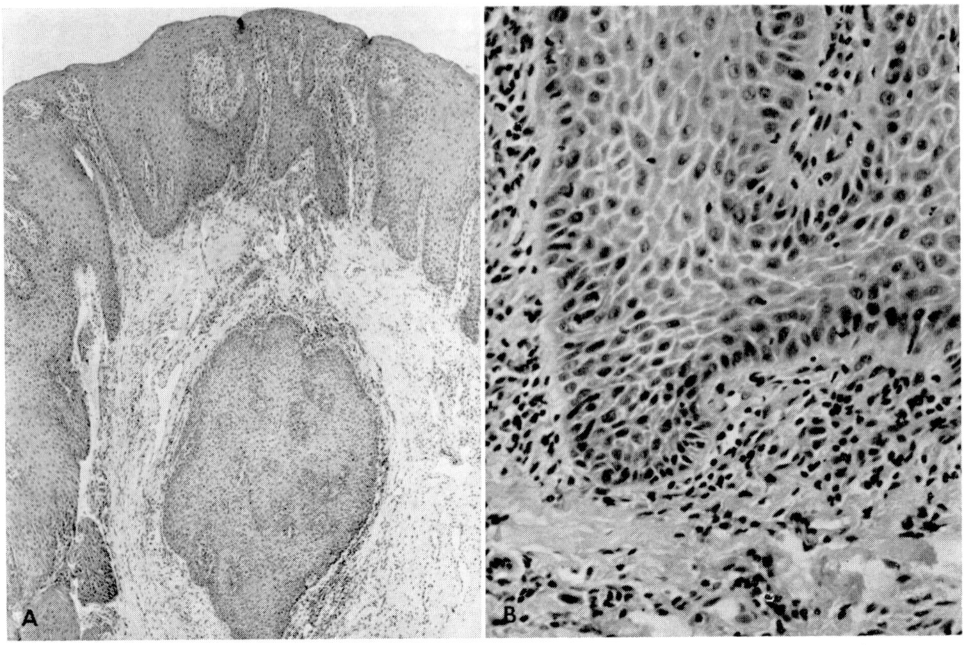

Fig. 3. (Case 11) Photomicrographs of the laryngeal biopsy specimen from a 66-year-old female with a T_{1B} supraglottic tumor. This patient received radiotherapy and is free of disease two years following treatment. A) Low power view showing the well differentiated nature of the lesion and prominent inflammatory halo adjacent to the advancing margin of the tumor (H & E X 60). B) Another portion of the same biopsy specimen under higher magnification. The halo of lymphocytes is clearly seen in the submucosa adjacent to the tumor. Close cooperation between the clinician and the pathologist is essential in order to establish the diagnosis in such cases (H & E X 375).

"Anaplastic transformation" occurred in one of our ten cases of verrucous carcinoma treated by radiotherapy. This patient received 5500 rads of cobalt-60 over seven weeks for a "supraglottic" tumor, occupying the right aryepiglottic fold; this had the typical gross and microscopic appearance of a verrucous carcinoma. Less than five months later the tumor had enlarged, and a biopsy showed anaplastic tumor. This lady died ten months after radiotherapy, with a clinical diagnosis of disseminated malignancy, although permission for autopsy could not be obtained. While the interval between the completion of radiotherapy and the appearance of the anaplastic tumor would appear to be rather short (five months), this interval is similar to that recorded in the eight cases previously reported in the literature (two to seven months).[3-6] The risk of such transformation occurring is difficult to assess, but does appear to be a real one. We have not encountered a similar transformation in 30 cases of oral cavity lesions receiving radiotherapy.[7]

It is from an analysis of these results that our current therapeutic policy has evolved. At the present time, surgery alone is used on those tumors that are small enough and localized enough to be removed by "voice conserving" partial laryngectomy procedures. Radiotherapy alone is used for those tumors sufficiently large to require a total laryngectomy, if treated surgically.

REFERENCES

1. Ackerman LV: Verrucous carcinoma of the oral cavity. Surgery 23:670-678, 1948

2. van Nostrand AWP, Olofsson J: Verrucous carcinoma of the larynx. A clinical and pathologic study of 10 cases. Cancer 30:691-702, 1972

3. Kraus FT, Perez-Mesa C: Verrucous carcinoma. Clinical and pathologic study of

105 cases involving oral cavity, larynx and genitalia. Cancer 19:26-38, 1966

4. Perez CA, Kraus FT, Evans JC, *et al*: Anaplastic transformation in verrucous carcinoma of the oral cavity after radiation therapy. Radiology 86:108-115, 1966

5. Fonts EA, Greenlaw RH, Rush BF, *et al*: Verrucous squamous cell carcinoma of the oral cavity. Cancer 23:152-160, 1969

6. Proffit SD, Spooner TR, Kosek JC: Origin of undifferentiated neoplasm from verrucous epidermal carcinoma of oral cavity following irradiation. Cancer 26:389-393, 1970

7. Burns HP, van Nostrand AWP, Palmer J: Verrucous carcinoma of the oral cavity. Management by radiotherapy and surgery, to be published.

ACKNOWLEDGMENTS—The laryngeal sectioning was performed by Kenneth Ekem and Janice Etty. Jean Cetkovski typed the manuscript.

REPRINTS—A. W. Peter van Nostrand, MD, Department of Pathology, Banting Institute, 100 College Street, Toronto, Canada, M5G IL5.

X-RAY OF THE MONTH

MUCOPYOCELE OF THE FRONTAL SINUS

Alfred L. Weber, MD
B. Donald Sklansky, MD
Boston, Massachusetts

PATIENT

A 60-year-old Caucasian male presented in August of 1975 with bilateral cystic supramedial canthal masses of seven months' duration. There were no other symptoms or signs, such as headaches, fever, rhinorrhea, nasal obstruction, and allergies. The patient had extensive soft tissue facial trauma at age four, but the past history was otherwise not significant.

On August 25, 1975, the patient was taken to the operating room and an osteoplastic frontal flap was elevated. A large mucopyocele containing approximately 50 cc of purulent material was found which had eroded the posterior wall and part of the floor of both frontal sinuses and extended into both ethmoids. The wall of the mucopyocele was removed from the dura. The frontal sinuses were obliterated with adipose tissue after complete removal of the mucous membrane. The patient made an uneventful recovery.

DIAGNOSIS

The radiographic findings are diagnostic of a frontal sinus mucopyocele.

DISCUSSION

The radiographic signs of a mucocele[1,2] depend on its size and location. In the early stage there is increased density of the sinus cavity from retained fluid. When bony attenuation or destruction takes place, an oval or round radiotranslucency is demonstrated. There may be a variable degree of marginal sclerosis, secondary to osteitis, reflecting proliferative new bone formation. Normal marginal scalloping found in the frontal sinus is lost throughout the entire sinus or within one of its compartments. Further expansion of the mucocele leads to depression of the roof of the orbit and lateral expansion of the lamina papyracea. The latter may be seen as a very thin curvilinear density, projecting into the orbital cavity. In large lesions there is erosion of the posterior wall of the frontal sinus and marked posterior displacement into the anterior cranial cavity. The displacement of the posterior wall may approach the level of the planum sphenoidale.[3] There may be thinning of the anterior wall of the frontal sinus and in extreme cases complete erosion. Fluid levels are rarely seen in these mucoceles. In about 5% of the cases a variable amount of calcification is seen in the wall of the mucocele, simulating an osteoma when extensive. In the differential diagnosis the following lesions should be considered:

1. Nonscalloped, nonseptate oval to round normal frontal sinus;
2. Frontal meningocele (usually a midline lesion);
3. Inflammatory lesions in the frontal sinus;
4. Epidermoid cyst either arising within the sinus or extending into the sinus from adjacent frontal bone;
5. Frontal sinus carcinoma.[4]

REFERENCES

1. Palubinskas AJ, Davies H: Roentgen features of nasal accessory sinus mucoceles. Radiology 72:576-584, 1959

2. Wigh R: Mucoceles of the fronto-ethmoidal sinuses. Radiology 54:579-590, 1950

3. Smith GW, Chavez M: Giant mucocele of the frontal sinus. J Neurol Neurosurg Psychiatry 23:179-181, 1960

4. Robinson JM: Frontal sinus cancer manifested as a frontal mucocele. Arch Otolaryngol 101:718-721, 1975

From the Department of Radiology, Massachusetts Eye & Ear Infirmary, Boston, Massachusetts.

RADIOGRAPHS

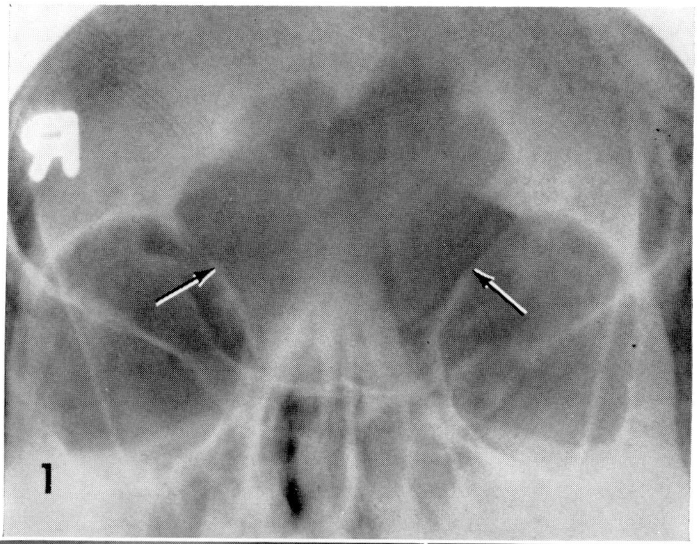

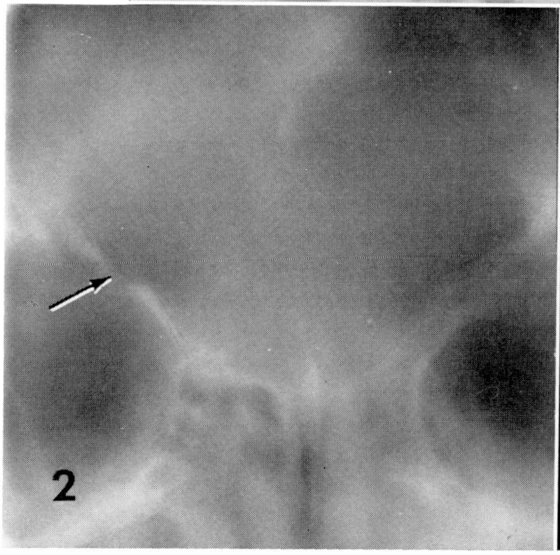

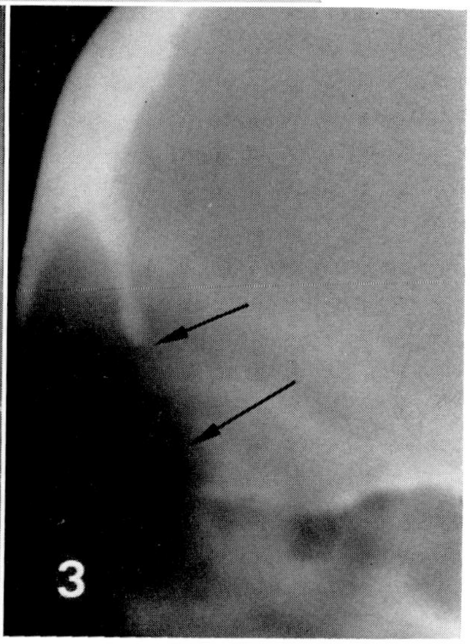

Fig. 1. A Caldwell view demonstrates enlargement of the frontal sinus with loss of normal scalloping, septation and marginal osteitis (sclerosis). There is slight lateral displacement of the upper medial wall of both orbits and depression of the adjacent roof (arrows).

Fig. 2. AP laminagram gives a detailed outline of the mucocele and more clearly demonstrates the marked attenuation (arrow) of the displaced walls of the left and right orbits.

Fig. 3. Lateral laminagraphic section demonstrates dehiscence of the posterior wall of the frontal sinus (arrows). There was also marked thinning of the anterior wall.

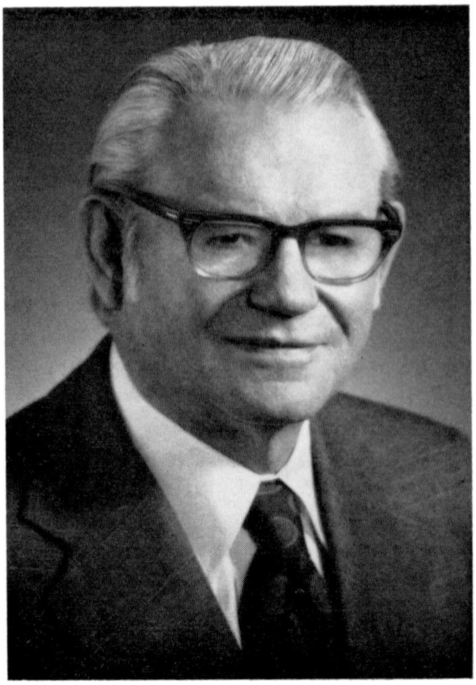

RAYMOND CARHART, PhD

1912 - 1975

Raymond Carhart established the first academic program in audiology in the United States. From that beginning until his death he continued to exert a significant influence on the development of his field, holding chairmanships, trusteeships and consultantships in literally dozens of organizations. Among his many honors, those he cherished most were his Associate Fellowship in the American Laryngological, Rhinological and Otological Society and his fellowships in the Acoustical Society of America and the American Speech and Hearing Association.

Carhart's status as a clinical researcher was recognized in 1963 when the National Institutes of Health granted him a Research Career Award. He was the only audiologist ever so honored, and the seriousness with which he accepted that award is reflected by the fact that almost half of his total number of publications appeared during the 11½ years that he held it.

Though Ray Carhart's influence touched countless individuals, those who knew him as a teacher will probably remember him best. He was a superb teacher and part of his success surely resulted from his abiding respect for his students as individuals. He personally led 45 of them to the successful completion of doctoral or postdoctoral study.

In 1972, Ray's former students presented a portrait of their teacher to his department for display in its new quarters. The inscription on that portrait accurately characterizes the man. It reads simply, "Raymond Carhart, Teacher, Scholar, and Friend. From his students."

Tom W. Tillman, PhD

COMMUNICATIONS

TUBERCULOSIS OF THE LARYNX MASQUERADING AS CARCINOMA

SIRUS NARAQI, MD
MANFRED W. RAISER, MD
N. MARK RICHARDS, MD
BURTON R. ANDERSEN, MD
CHICAGO, ILLINOIS

SUMMARY – A patient with laryngeal and pulmonary tuberculosis is described. The similarity between the clinical presentation and gross appearance of laryngeal carcinoma and tuberculosis in this patient and others reported in the literature is emphasized. Laryngeal biopsy is necessary to establish the correct diagnosis, but this must be done only after the proper precautions are taken to reduce the risk of infection to the physician performing the biopsy. Examination of the chest x-ray and acid-fast stain of the sputum are rapid and highly reliable screening tests for laryngeal tuberculosis.

Over the past 15 years, laryngeal tuberculosis has been given little attention in the English language literature.[1,2] Awareness of this disease is important because it is highly infectious[3] and is frequently misdiagnosed as carcinoma of the larynx.[1,4] Nedwicki[4] described two patients who underwent direct laryngoscopy and biopsy for presumed carcinoma and were found to have tuberculosis. The two physicians who performed the laryngoscopy and biopsy subsequently had conversion of their tuberculin reactions and later developed evidence of active pulmonary tuberculosis. Out of ten patients with laryngeal tuberculosis reported by Bull,[1] seven had the appearance of a carcinomatous lesion. Six were raised and granular and one was ulcerated. Only three patients had edema and hyperemia of the larynx, usually seen in chronic laryngitis. We describe a patient with laryngeal tuberculosis who had very few of the systemic complaints usually associated with this disease, and a laryngeal lesion with the gross appearance of carcinoma.

CASE REPORT

A 59-year-old male Caucasian was referred to University of Illinois Hospital for the evaluation of a laryngeal lesion. He complained of persistent dysphagia, sore throat and hoarseness for two months and 6.75 kg weight loss. He also complained of dyspnea, but denied fever, chills, night sweats, cough, sputum, hemoptysis, chest pain, or exposure to persons with tuberculosis.

Physical examination revealed a well-developed man in no distress who did not look chronically ill. Blood pressure was 110/70 mm Hg., respiratory rate 20/min, pulse 92/min and temperature 37 C. Examination of the throat was negative. A nontender, firm and freely movable enlarged lymph node was felt in the left submandibular area. Fine moist rales and tubular breath sounds were heard over the upper chest posteriorly, more pronounced on the left side. Bilateral palmar erythema was noted.

Initial laboratory tests showed that the hemoglobin was 13.5 g/100 ml and hematocrit 44%. White cell count was 8600/cu mm with 85% neutrophils, 7% lymphocytes, 7% monocytes and 1% eosinophils.

Chest x-rays showed thin-walled large cavities with extensive surrounding infiltration throughout both upper lung field and hilar regions, minimal pleural thickening in both apices and blunting of left costophrenic angle (Fig. 1). X-ray of the sinuses was normal. A barium swallow did not show any abnormality in the esophagus. A lateral roentgenogram of the larynx was negative.

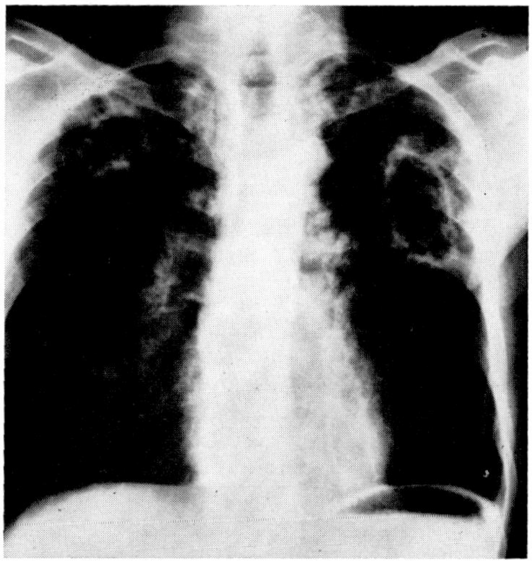

Fig. 1. Admission chest x-ray showing bilateral apical cavities.

At laryngoscopy, the pharynx, tonsils and epiglottis were normal. An exophytic mass was present on the false vocal cord on the left side which involved the anterior half of the true cord. Both cords were mobile and the anterior commissure appeared to be free.

Histologic examination of biopsied material revealed a caseating granuloma with acid-fast bacilli seen on Ziehl-Neelsen stain. Smears and cultures of sputum, tracheal secretions, and biopsied tissue were all positive for *Mycobacterium tuberculosis* and negative for fungi. No malignant cells were found in the biopsy.

He remained afebrile and his general condition was unchanged during the hospital course. On the 11th hospital day, he was

From the Section of Infectious Diseases, Department of Medicine, University of Illinois at the Medical Center, Chicago, Illinois.

transferred to a tuberculosis sanitarium for completion of his treatment.

DISCUSSION

The clinical presentation of patients with tuberculosis and carcinoma of the larynx may be similar and includes cough, pharyngitis, hoarseness, and weight loss. In patients with tuberculosis, the chest x-ray is usually abnormal and commonly shows apical cavitary disease associated with bilateral nodular infiltrates.[2] The patient described in this report was presumed to have carcinoma because of the absence of systemic symptoms, such as fever, chills, and the night sweats usually associated with tuberculosis, and the gross appearance of the laryngeal lesion. His chest x-ray, however, was compatible with pulmonary tuberculosis, but because of strong suspicion of malignancy, biopsy was performed.

Tuberculosis of the larynx is usually secondary to cavitary pulmonary tuberculosis. Therefore, it is important that chest films be evaluated prior to laryngoscopy and if suspicious for tuberculosis, acid-fast smears of sputum should be obtained. Rarely, it is associated with miliary tuberculosis.[5] Direct extension of lesions from the oronasal cavity is another possible, but uncommon source. It is generally accepted that tuberculosis of the larynx is the most infectious form of tuberculosis.[6] The high degree of infectivity is due to suspension of the bacteria in small water droplets by the vocal cords during phonation. Riley *et al*[3] studied the infectiousness of tuberculosis for guinea pigs by exposing them to air from a tuberculosis ward. Sixty-three animals were infected during a two-year period. Fifteen of them became infected during the three-day stay of a patient with laryngeal tuberculosis on the ward. Development of pulmonary tuberculosis in two physicians, shortly after performing laryngoscopy and biopsy of the larynx on two unsuspected cases of laryngeal tuberculosis,[4] seems to confirm Riley's findings.

Rohwedder,[2] in his report suggested that the cervical and submandibular lymphadenopathy are not prominent in laryngeal tuberculosis, but are commonly found in carcinoma of the larynx. Our patient is an exception to this rule and we think that lymph node enlargement is not helpful in the diagnosis of these conditions.

Lesions caused by fungi, syphilis and other granulomatous diseases must also be differentiated from tuberculosis of the larynx.[7,8] This differentiation can usually be made by special cultures and serology.

Carcinoma of the larynx seems to be the major problem in the differential diagnosis of laryngeal tuberculosis.[1,2,4,9] Abnormal chest x-ray, acid-fast smears of sputum, lateral x-ray of the larynx, and laryngeal tomograms are all helpful in making the diagnosis, but definitive diagnosis can only be made by biopsy, because both entities may coexist in the same patient.[10] The biopsy, however, must only be done with necessary precautions and isolation measures in order to minimize the risk of infection of the physician performing the biopsy and other involved medical personnel.

REFERENCES

1. Bull TR: Tuberculosis of the larynx. Br Med J 2:991-992, 1966

2. Rohwedder JJ: Upper respiratory tract tuberculosis. Sixteen cases in a general hospital. Ann Intern Med 80:708-713, 1974

3. Riley RJ, Mills CC, O'Grady F, *et al*: Infectiousness of air from a tuberculosis ward. Ultraviolet irradiation of infected air: Comparative infectiousness of different patients. Am Rev Resp Dis 85:511-525, 1962

4. Nedwicki EG: Laryngeal tuberculosis simulating carcinoma of the larynx. Med Times 98:181-187, 1970

5. Oatway WH: Laryngeal changes in acute hematogenous tuberculosis. Am Rev Tuberc 40:378-388, 1939

6. Weidman WH, Campbell HB: Laryngeal tuberculosis. Am Rev Tuberc 40:85-89, 1939

7. Lyons GD: Mycotic diseases of the larynx. Ann Otol Rhinol Laryngol 75:162-175, 1966

8. Maloney WH: Laryngeal manifestations of systemic diseases. Ann Otol Rhinol Laryngol 69:421-426, 1960

9. Maran AG, Stewart LA: Laryngeal tuberculosis. Br Med J 2:775, 1971

10. Morse JO: Laryngeal tuberculosis or tumor. Ann Intern Med 81:711-712, 1974

REPRINTS—Burton R. Andersen, MD, VA West Side Hospital, 2079 West Ogden Ave., Chicago, IL 60612.

BOOK REVIEWS

Atlas Der Pathologischen Anatomie

By *Von Wilhelm Doerr, Gerhild Schumann, Gunter Ule.* One volume, 874 illustrations in color, 312 pp. George Thieme Verlag, Stuttgart, Germany, 1975, in German. Price DM 240

This is a beautifully illustrated atlas presented by major organ-systems. A balanced spectrum of lesions is depicted ranging from the very common to the rare and unusual. The authors have exercised great skill in the choice of gross specimens and photomicrographs in demonstrating the characteristic anatomical findings. In many instances both the gross and the photomicrographs are juxtaposed to communicate features not possible by either one alone. Photographic excellence and an artistic eye is evident in the use of clean, sharply focused, appropriately arranged tissues on suitable backgrounds. Especially creative is the use of special stains and low power photomicrographs that provide visual dramatization of the topographical features of important lesions. The balance of colors, textures, closeups, and layout combine to make this very enjoyable to use and study. Each illustration is accompanied by a short descriptive text (in German) which mentions diagnostic terms or synonyms that will be easily recognizable to the American reader. The scanty description or the German text should not detract much for the reader familiar with some of the basic diagnostic terms; the illustrative material speaks for itself in beautiful descriptive language understood by all.

It is unfortunate, however, that only a minor portion of the material deals with the head and neck region. There are approximately 50 illustrations of interest to the head and neck specialist or trainee. This cannot be construed as a valid criticism of the atlas because it was not intended to deal with a specific specialty. The book may find limited usefulness among those primarily interested in the ear, nose and throat area; but it also demonstrates what could be done.

Walter C. Bauer, MD

Pathologies of Speech Systems

By *Edward D. Mysak*, PhD. Soft cover, indexed by subject and author, referenced, black and white line drawings, 297 pp, 1976. The Williams & Wilkins Company, 428 East Preston Street, Baltimore, MD 21202. Price $11.95

This text is written primarily for the speech pathologist and audiologist, although, according to the author, it is intended also as a source of information for physicians and other health related professionals.

The material is organized by what the author calls "systems"; some examples are the receptor system, the transmitter system, the higher-order integrator system, and so forth. Hence, peripheral disturbances of the auditory mechanism are discussed in the section on the speech receptor system, while certain voice disorders are considered in the material on the speech effector system.

In my opinion, this somewhat unorthodox organization of material makes interesting and stimulating reading for the professional communication specialist, but can be confusing for the nonspecialist who is looking for a quick, easy reference about a specific communication disorder.

Clearly, Mysak has an excellent feeling for the complexity of the communication process and that point of view is very well made throughout the book.

On occasion, his very elaborate terminology (most of which is not used with much frequency in contemporary writings in the field of communication disorders) serves to impair reading comprehension. Some examples of such terms are: palilia, pedolalia, embolophrasia, logophobia, kinetic and tonal paralanguage, and phonasthenia. Many readers will be able to figure out his meanings, but the total impact of such specialized language makes reading many sections of the book very difficult.

In general, it is a fascinating textbook, with many stimulating notions, but is most suitable for the speech pathologist and audiologist, and not for other health related professionals.

Hughlett L. Morris, PhD

The Year Book of Drug Therapy: 1975

Edited by *Dale G. Friend*, M.D. Hard cover, line drawings, indexed by subject and author, 425 pp. Year Book Medical Publishers, Inc., Chicago, 1975. Price $20.00

The 1975 Year Book of Drug Therapy is one of the Year Book series which provides an annual compilation of abstracts of the preceding year's literature. Each abstract is accompanied by editorial comment and includes the bibliographic reference to the original paper.

In the present volume Friend has covered the literature on drug therapy through October 1974. The volume includes approximately 500 papers. The abstracts are concise and factual; importantly, they give the reader sufficient pertinent information to allow him to decide whether or not to consult the original paper.

Although the eye, ear, nose and throat section includes only eight papers, there are abstracts of interest in the sections on allergy, infection, neoplastic disease, surgery, and drug action. Residents and practitioners may find this a useful reference source for up-to-date information on an area of growing complexity and concern.

Frank E. Lucente, MD

Auditory Assessment of the Difficult-to-Test

By *Robert T. Fulton* and *Lyle L. Lloyd*. Hard cover, indexed and referenced, illustrated in black and white, 297 pp. Williams & Wilkins Company, Baltimore, MD 21202. Price $15.75

This book is primarily a review of the literature in many areas of auditory measurement. The several authors cover their subjects quite adequately, touching lightly on each area in broad terms with many references. The book should be a good reference work for those who must attempt to assess auditory function in the child and mentally retarded.

William F. Carver, PhD

NATIONAL AND INTERNATIONAL JOURNALS
ABSTRACTS FROM

Carotid-Cavernous Sinus Fistula Occurring After A Rhinoplasty

Song IC, Bromberg BE: Plast Reconstr Surg 55:92-96, 1975

The authors present an interesting case report of the immediate development of a carotid-cavernous sinus fistula following an otherwise routine rhinoplasty. The frequency of occurrence, diagnosis and management of the problem are discussed. That surgeons operating in this area should be aware of the possibility of this rare complication is stressed.

Three figures and 18 references are included.

PAYNE

T-Cell Deficiency in Patients with Squamous Cell Cancer of the Head and Neck

Wanebo HJ, Jun MY, Strong EW, et al: Am J Surg 130:445-451, 1975

T-cell levels (lymphocytes associated with cellular immunity), B-cell levels (lymphocytes associated with humoral immunity), and *in vivo* and *in vitro* lymphocyte stimulability were determined and correlated with stage of disease.

T-cell counts were significantly lower in patients with carcinoma than in controls or in patients with benign disease of the head and neck. There was a progressive reduction in absolute T-cell counts with an increase in the stage of the lesion. B-cell counts did not show this.

In vivo (skin testing with DNCB) and *in vitro* lymphocyte activity (stimulation of lymphocytes with mitogens) were depressed. This depression was greater with increasing stage of lesion, and maximal depression was noted in patients with large fixed nodal metastases.

Immunological evaluation may become an important supplement to the present TMN classification in determining prognosis and selecting the most appropriate course of therapy.

KATZ

The Epstein-Barr Virus and Neoplasia

Klein G: New Engl J Med 293:1353-1355, 1975

Dr. Klein reviews current research on Epstein-Barr virus (EBV) and its association with Burkitt's lymphoma and poorly differentiated nasopharyngeal carcinoma.

EBV alter chromosomal proteins in B-lymphocytes *in vitro* allowing permanent cell lines to proliferate. These cells when injected into animals have malignant properties. The virus also has oncogenic activity in certain primates without *in vitro* transformation.

Burkitt's lymphoma is the only lymphoproliferative disease demonstrating an association with EBV positive serologies. The finding of chromosomal differences between normal and lymphoma cell lines supports the fact that a specific or altered genetic constitution may have to exist in the host before viral transformation can occur.

The EBV genome has also been regularly found in poorly differentiated nasopharyngeal carcinoma. The virus is present in the anaplastic cell, and not in tumor infiltrating lymphocytes as was previously reported. It appears that host genetic differences or differences in regulatory mechanisms are required for the pathogenesis of the fully autonomous nasopharyngeal carcinomas in persons harboring the Epstein-Barr virus.

GANTZ

Reconstructive Surgery In Chronic Otitis Media

Pfaltz CR, Pfaltz R, Schmid P: ORL 37:257-270, 1975

The anatomical and functional results of 440 cases of tympanoplasty followed for two to ten years are presented. Factors such as the condition of the tympanic membrane and ossicular chain, Eustachian tube patency, condition of middle ear mucosa, middle ear pathology, and type of tympanoplasty are correlated with postoperative hearing adequacy, and incidence of postoperative drainage, persistent perforation, and recurrent cholesteatoma. Of the 28 cases of secondary perforation, 24 of these had an active otitis media at the time of surgery and 18 had demonstrated impaired tubal function. Active otitis media decreased the chance of postoperative hearing improvement by about one-third. The postoperative hearing improvement was found to be significantly lower (35% vs 62%) with cholesteatoma or tympanosclerosis, as compared to uncomplicated suppurative otitis media; this was due to the more frequent impairment of the ossicular chain.

DREYER

Ann Otol 85: 1976

OBSERVATIONS ON LARYNGEAL DISEASE, LARYNGEAL BEHAVIOR AND VOICE

G. PAUL MOORE, PHD

GAINESVILLE, FLORIDA

SUMMARY – This discussion accepted the hypothesis that every laryngeal sound is produced by its unique type of vocal cord vibration. The production of vocal sound is not capricious, it follows certain laws many of which are not known. Research into the behavior of the larynx has produced some interesting and perhaps, useful findings. It was the intention of this paper to describe some of the features of laryngeal behavior as they relate to both phonation and laryngeal disorders in the belief that such knowledge lends itself to the more efficient management of certain vocal and laryngeal problems. The central theme has been that it is laryngeal behavior and not laryngeal disease itself that determines vocal deviation.

Conversations with laryngologists have led me to the conclusion that the recognition and diagnosis of laryngeal disease, structural anomalies and physiological disorders do not constitute major problems for this specialty. The laryngeal conditions are usually visible and are amenable to such evaluative procedures as biopsy, endocrine assessment, respiratory study, allergin evaluation, and the like. Furthermore, the disorders respond more or less adequately to surgery, irradiation or medication. In contrast, major problems in diagnosis and behavioral assessment often do exist in the relationships between voice disorders and associated laryngeal conditions.

If the strictly medical problems and the protection of the thoracic airway were the only concerns of the laryngologist and broncho-esophagologist there would be little justification for the presentation of this paper. However, the fact is generally recognized that the larynx and associated respiratory system together have a significant role in the communication process. Fortunately, the modern laryngologist does not limit his concerns strictly to medical problems; he has become increasingly involved with behavioral and psychological deviations as they are expressed in communicative disorders. Laryngologists appear to be relatively confident about the appropriateness of the medical therapy they select, but most are uncertain about the prognosis for voice and the behavioral sequelae of their therapeutic procedures. Apparently much more is known about the management of laryngeal disease and anomalies than about the behavior of the larynx in the production of voice. It is logical to believe that increased understanding of the factors that determine both normal and abnormal voice will lead to improvement in the treatment of laryngeal disorders. When there are elective decisions about the advisability of surgery, or when choices exist among surgical procedures, an understanding of phonatory behavior may provide the basis for rational decision.

From the Department of Speech, College of Arts and Sciences, University of Florida, Gainesville, Florida. This research has been supported primarily by grants awarded by NINCDS.

Presented at the meeting of the American Broncho-Esophagological Association, Palm Beach, Florida, April 27-28, 1976.

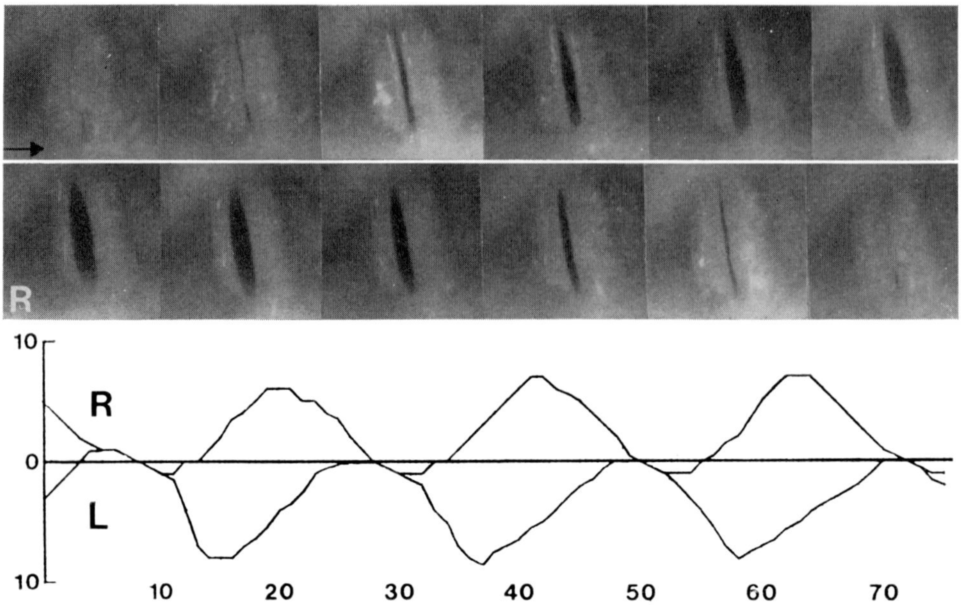

Fig. 1. (Upper section, left to right) Sequence of images from ultraspeed film of a normal female larynx showing one cycle of phonation at 196 Hz, low intensity. Alternate film frames were omitted to conserve space. (Lower section) Graphic presentation of motion approximately at the anterior-posterior midpoints of the membranous portions of the vocal cords. The upper curve indicates excursions of the right cord (R) in relation to an arbitrary median sagittal plane represented by the zero line. The motions of the left vocal cord (L) are below the line. Time is measured in film frames. The phase differences between the two vocal cords and their lateral shift while in contact are not unusual in the normal larynx. All laryngeal photographs used in this paper present indirect, mirrored images.

Of course, the laryngologist is not always confronted with a structural anomaly or disease. He is often required to advise singers, actors, public speakers or ordinary citizens who have noted some adverse change in the pitch, loudness, or quality of the voice. Frequently, there is no evident reason to account for the voice problem. This does not mean that an abnormality in behavior is not present, it just indicates that the abnormality has not been detected. This observation leads to the generally accepted hypothesis that, whenever there is vocal sound that is recognized as hoarse, that is, rough, harsh, breathy, *etc.*, there is a corresponding form of laryngeal behavior. The search for this behavior has been the focus of considerable research over the years, and although there is much more to be learned, valuable information has been obtained about the association of laryngeal behavior, laryngeal disorders and voice. This occasion presents an appropriate opportunity to report on some of this research and at the same time to acknowledge the foresighted interest of Chevalier Jackson, MD, in the communicative role of the larynx.

Basic Characteristics of Normal and Abnormal Vocal Fold Vibration. Vibratory patterns of the vocal folds which produce normal voice have been described in the literature[1,2] and undoubtedly, the features of such vibration are known. They can be reviewed in the upper part of Figure 1, which presents a sequence of images from a section of ultraslow motion film of a normal female larynx producing a low pitched tone at relatively low intensity. (When this paper was presented it was accompanied by illustrative, ultraspeed motion pictures of laryngeal behavior.) Normal vibration is characterized by an

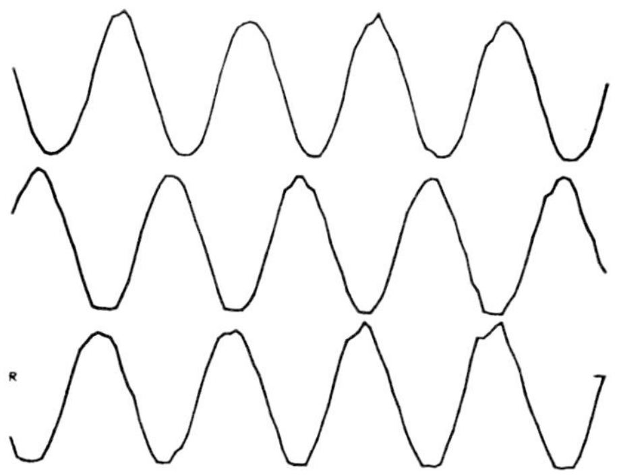

Fig. 2. Area function of 13 consecutive cycles from the film of the larynx presented in Figure 1. The curve was produced by computer following determination of the glottal area from sonic pen tracings of projected film images. The curve is continuous from left to right with each of the lower sections following the one immediately above. The regularity of both the time and amplitude changes probably determines the normality of the voice despite the phase differences shown in Figure 1.

opening phase in which the vocal cords move laterally to open the glottis, a closing phase in which the direction of motion is essentially reversed, and a closed phase in which the vocal folds are in contact with each other. These vibratory phases are traditionally represented graphically as presented in the lower portion of Figure 1. The movements of the anterior-posterior midpoint of the membranous portion of the right vocal fold are shown above the zero line, which denotes an arbitrary median sagittal plane. The corresponding motions of the left fold are below the line.

Recognition should be made of the fact that the opening and closing excursions of the vocal cords also contain vertical components which, in combination with the lateral movements, cause the vibration of the glottal borders to be somewhat ellipsoidal. Recent research by Baer[3] demonstrates these complex movements. In the normal pattern the relative time occupied by each vibratory phase can vary even when maintaining the total period, *i.e.*, the same frequency. The ratio between the times occupied by the opening and closing phases is represented by the speed quotient (SQ). The third or closed phase of the cycle may vary from three-fourths or more of the total period to an instantaneous contact between the folds. The relationship between the length of the closed phase and the period of glottal opening can be determined from the open quotient (OQ) which expresses the ratio between the time the glottis is open and the total vibratory period. The vibratory sequence in a normal female larynx, presented in the graph of Figure 1, reveals that the vocal folds shifted across the median plane during the closed phase and that the movements of the two cords were partly out of phase. This type of phase difference occurs frequently and suggests some type of imbalance which is probably not uncommon.[4]

The second feature of normal vibration is that the cycle repeats itself regularly with essentially the same time period when the pitch is held constant. The area function of the larynx that is represented in Figure 1 is shown in Figure 2. It is regular and uniform, which accounts for the normalcy of the sound despite the slight asymmetries of the movements of the vocal cords. In contrast, it may be postulated that any time the length of the vibratory cycle or the area of the glottis varies randomly in successive cycles, the voice sounds rough or hoarse. Furthermore, if glottal closure is not complete during the vibratory cycle, the voice may be perceived as breathy. There are many possible combinations of these cyclic and phase aberrations that can occur in either the normal or abnormal larynx which provide the bases for the great variety of vocal deviations.

Physical and Physiological Factors that Influence Vocal Fold Vibration. The larynx has been described traditionally as though it contained a single vibrator and unitary sound source. This concept recognizes the fact that the vocal folds have approximately the same length, mass and elasticity, are activated by a single air supply, usually vibrate at the same frequency, and tend to

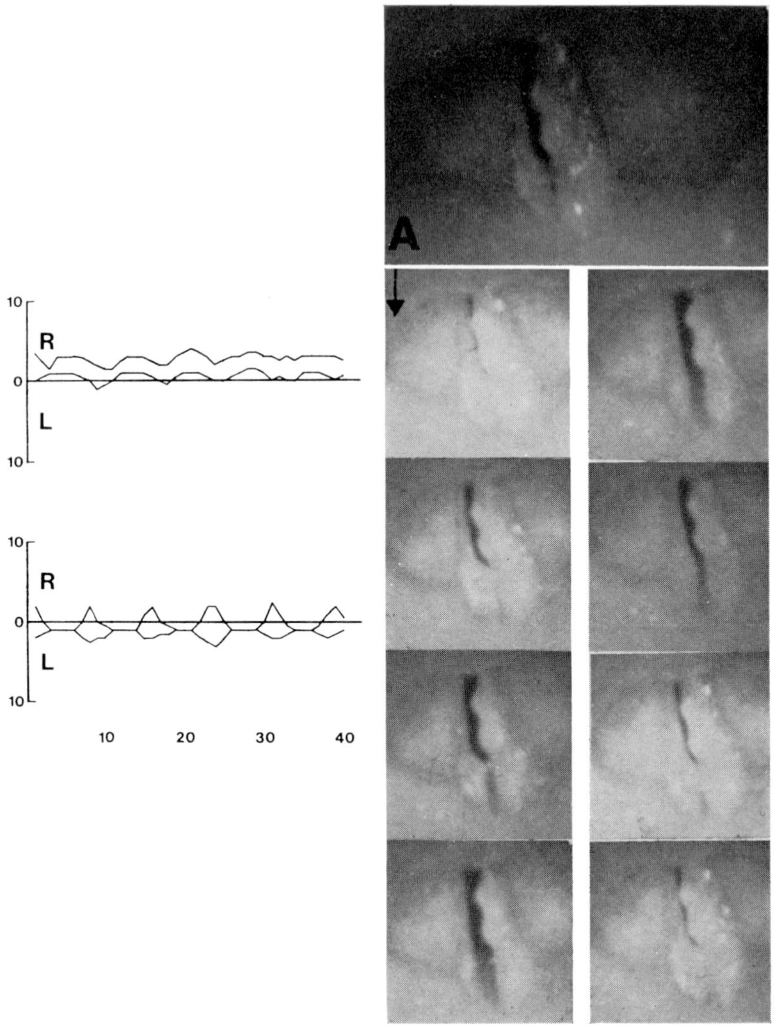

Fig. 3. The photographs picture a benign tumor on the left vocal cord, which fits into a lesion on the right caused by the removal of another tumor and underlying tissue. The larger photograph (A) reveals anatomical details; the series of smaller photographs picture a vibratory cycle. The image sequence progresses downward from the upper photograph in the left column and follows in the same direction on the right. The upper pair of curves represent vibratory motions of the right and left vocal cords at the indentation between the protruberances of the tumor. The lower curves demonstrate movements of the posterior segments.

move simultaneously and in phase. Their frequency is regulated primarily by their length, elasticity and mass; their amplitude at any selected frequency is determined by the volume-velocity of the air flow; their vibrational complexity, which provides vocal quality, is associated with many factors, including the relative proximity of the folds and their elasticity, stiffness, compliance, and mass as these may exist independently in each vocal cord.

The traditional concept of laryngeal function is somewhat incomplete; it fails to include the possible effect on sound generation of the vertical components of the movements as these combine with the lateral to release the breath pressure.[3] More importantly, the traditional fails to recognize the potential

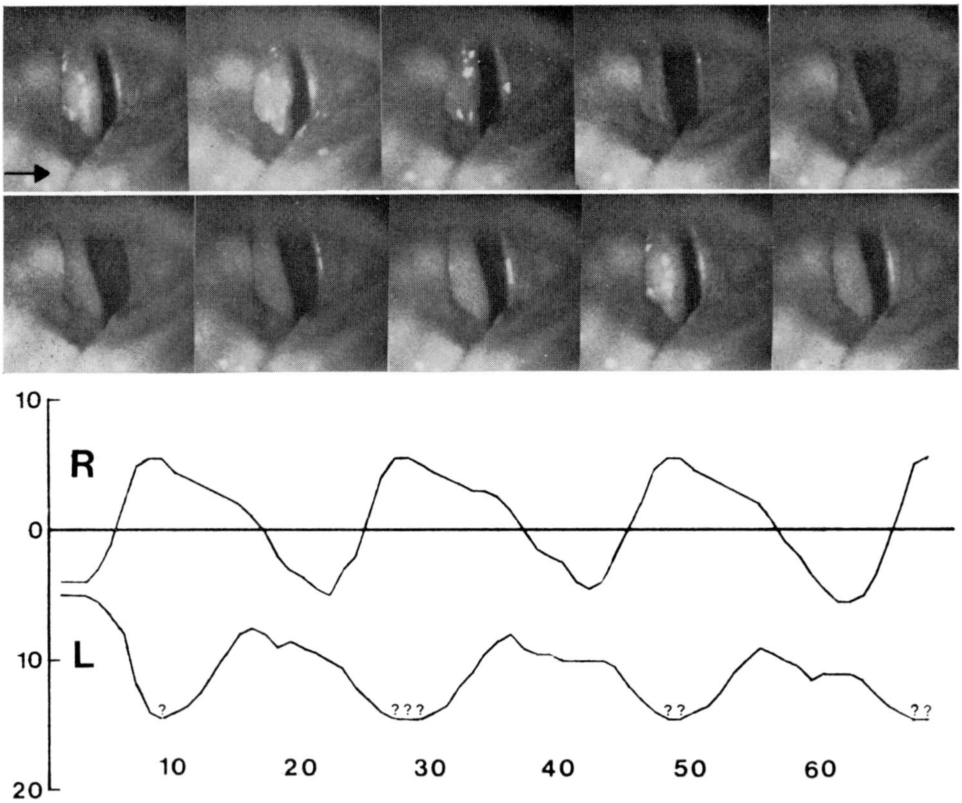

Fig. 4. Male larynx with paralysis of the left vocal cord. The sequence of photographs progresses from left to right in the top row followed by the same order in the second row. The graph illustrates the motions of the approximate anterior-posterior midpoints of the glottal borders and demonstrates the absence of glottal closure, the crossing of an arbitrary median sagittal plane by the healthy vocal cord, the start of the lateral movements of the paralyzed vocal cord before the normal cord reaches its medial limit, and vibrations of both cords at the same frequency.

significance of the vibratory rest positions of the folds.[5,6] The rest position is the posture the folds assume when they are adjusted for phonation prior to activation. There are many possible vibratory rest positions, any of which many exert a unique influence on vibration, but for this discussion, they have been generalized into three categories. The first is present when the medial edges of the folds are in contact, thereby causing vibration to develop from a closed glottis. One of the significant features of vibration with this position is that the vocal folds meet forcefully and press tightly against each other as they attempt to swing medially past their positions of rest. Their amplitude, rate of movement, and degree of flaccidity determine the degree of compression and consequently, both the period of glottal occlusion and the size of the area of contact.

The second rest position differs maximally from the first and is present when the folds are abducted enough to allow vibration to occur without any contact between the glottal edges. This adjustment allows the air to flow continuously in greater and lesser amounts and emphasizes the fact that the folds are potentially independent vibrators.

The third position of rest discussed here is an intermediate adjustment in which the folds are separated enough to permit independent or quasi-independent motion, and where the medial

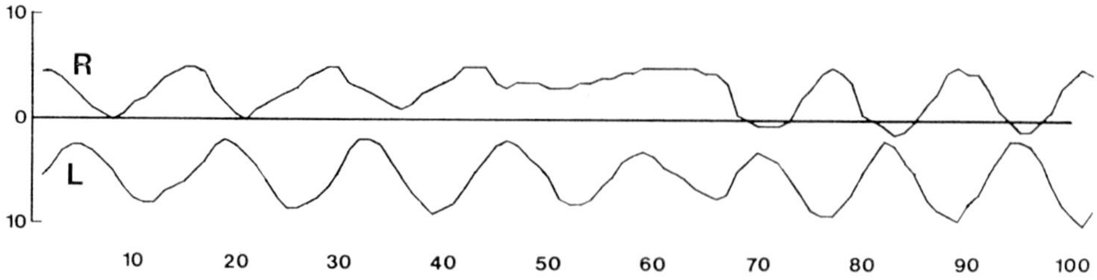

Fig. 5. Graphic representation of vibratory patterns in a female larynx with left vocal cord paralysis. Four characteristics of vibration observed in Figure 4 are also present here and, in addition, the upper curve of this graph reveals a period of approximately two cycles during which the healthy right cord stopped vibrating, apparently to make an adjustment which produced a higher frequency in both vocal cords when vibration resumed.

vibratory excursions are capable of achieving vocal fold contact even though this does not always occur.

Vibration When the Vocal Folds are in Contact at Their Rest Positions. When the glottis is closed before vibration begins and the vocal folds make complete or essentially complete contact regularly in each vibratory cycle, a normal vocal sound is almost always produced. By following this line of reasoning, it would be expected that a normal sound would be generated even in an abnormal larynx when periodic vibratory opening and closing occurs.

The photographs in Figure 3 picture a benign tumor on the left vocal fold fitting into a defect in the opposite member in such a way that closure is essentially complete. The lesion in the right cord remained after the removal of a benign tumor and some of the underlying tissue. The pathology alone predicts a serious vocal deviation, but the unique anatomic contours provide a nearly regular pulsatile flow of air that generates an almost normal, slightly hoarse voice. After the attending laryngologist observed the behavior of the larynx in high speed film, he elected to leave the lesion on the left cord intact on the presumption that its removal would accomplish no essential benefit to health and probably would create a more serious voice defect.

Attention is drawn to the vibration at the region of the tumor and also posteriorly as revealed respectively in the upper and lower pairs of curves in Figure 3. In both locations the amplitudes are small and in the anterior region the movements of the tumor are often out of phase with the opposite fold. The posterior segment of the right fold and its opposite part vibrate regularly. Figure 3 demonstrates the small amplitude of movement, the anterior phase differences and the regularity of the posterior vibration. It is probable that the three-phase, periodic movements of the posterior segments are responsible for the relatively normal sound.

Vibration Without Glottal Closure. The second vibratory rest position referred to previously permits vibration without contact between the folds. This adjustment usually accompanies unilateral laryngeal paralysis when the paralyzed cord lies in an intermediate or lateral position. The sequence of high speed photographs in Figure 4 shows the customary vibratory characteristics of unilateral paralysis when there is wide separation between the folds. The major features are presented by the graph in Figure 4 and may be listed as follows: an absence of vibratory contact, the healthy cord appears to swing across the median plane (however, this plane could not be located accurately in this film); the paralyzed fold usually begins its lateral motion before the normal fold reaches its medial limit; and both folds vibrate at the same frequency.

Since the presumption is usually made that there are differences in elasticity, mass, and contour between para-

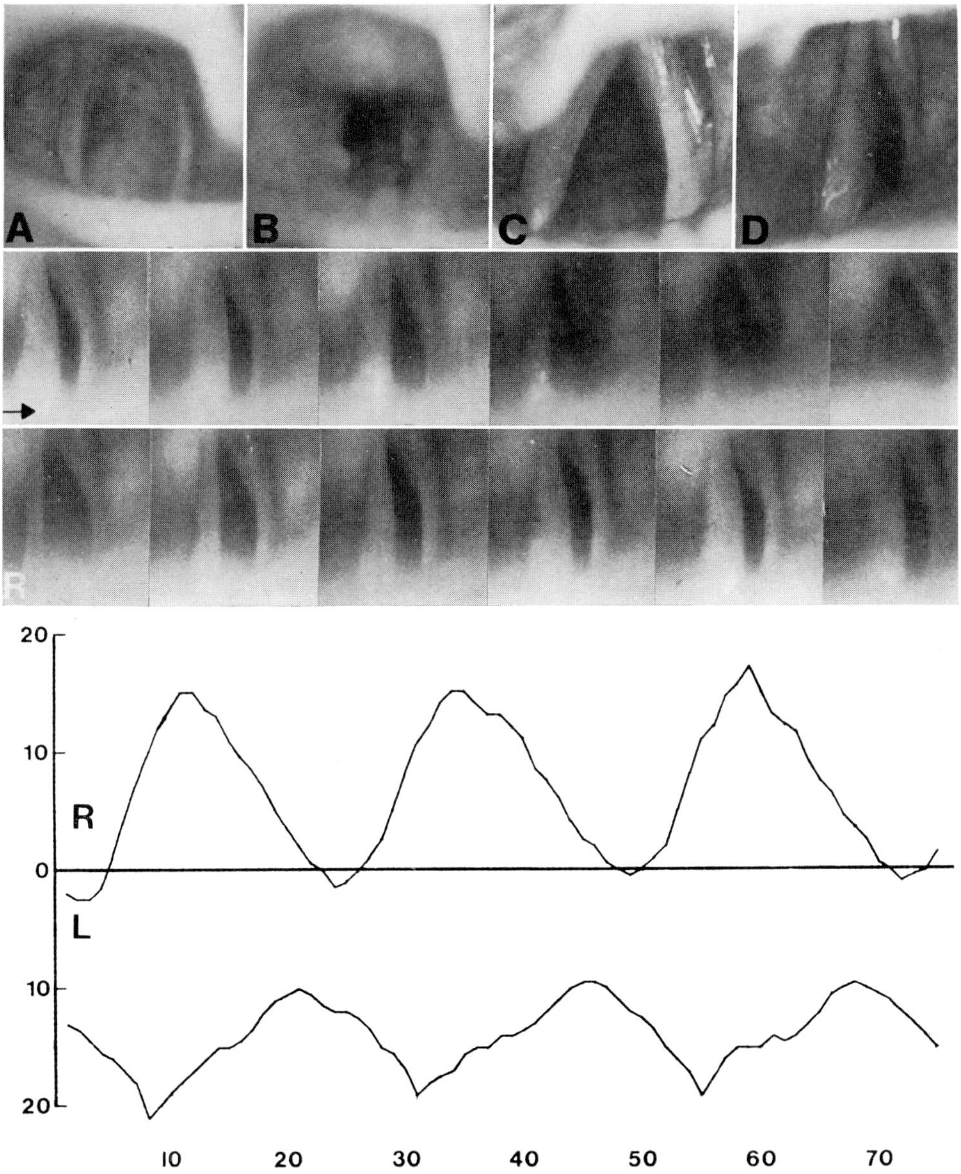

Fig. 6. (Top row). A) View of adult, male larynx approximately six months after traumatic injury. B) Maximum adduction at the same time. The voice was completely aphonic. C) Same larynx in full abduction two years later. D) Maximum adduction for phonation; right vocal cord completely recovered; voice breathy. (Middle two rows). The series of images representing a cycle of vibration progresses from left to right in the top row and continues in the same order in the second row. The graph demonstrates vibratory characteristics of unilateral paralysis.

lyzed and nonparalyzed vocal folds, some explanation is needed to account particularly for the observation that such folds vibrate at the same frequency. The hypothesis that seems to satisfy most of the observed conditions is that the paralyzed fold is a slave to the healthy fold. This concept is based on the following considerations: paralyzed vocal cords are obviously capable

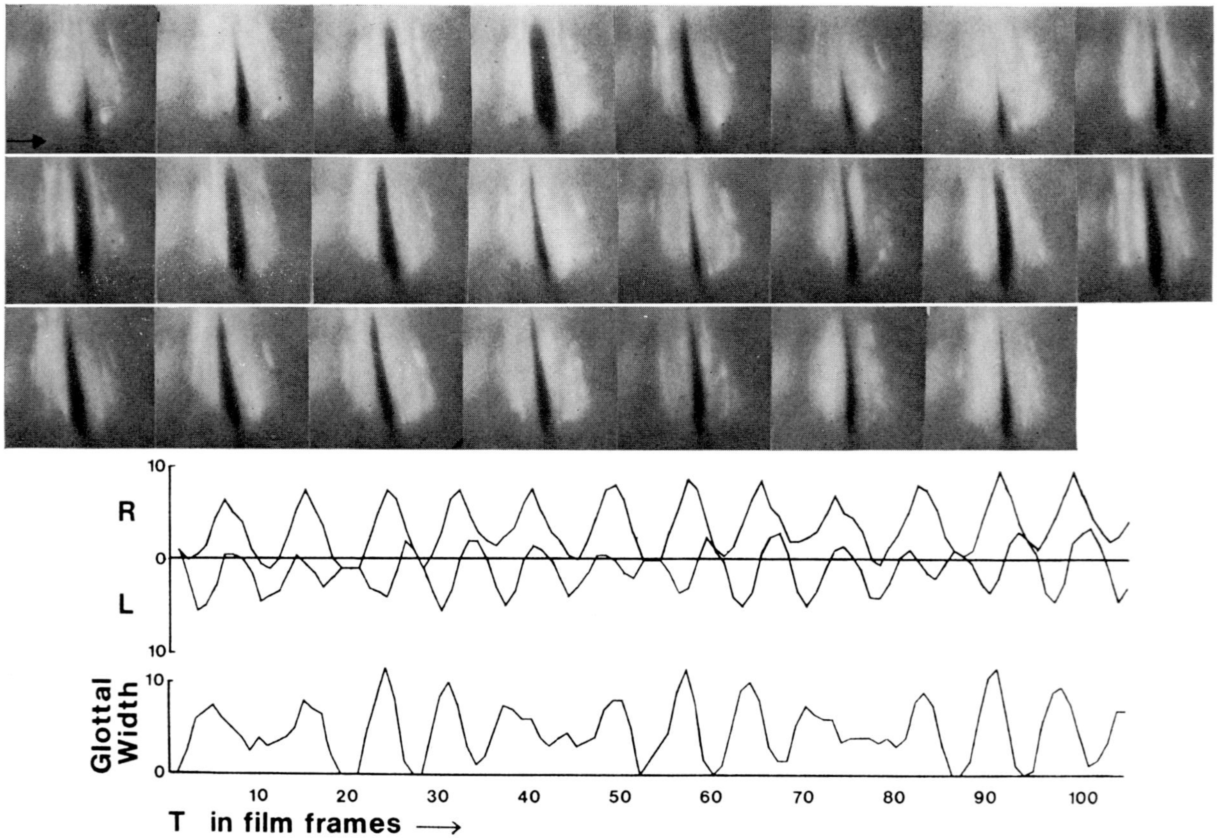

Fig. 7. Voluntary diplophonia. The series of 23 high-speed photographs progresses from left to right and from the top row downward. The movements shown in the photographic series can be related to the pair of curves marked R and L by identifying frame 20 on the graph as photograph number one and following the graphic and photographic sequence. Vibratory differences between the vocal cords are apparent in frequency, amplitude and phase. The single curve at the bottom of the graph represents the progressive changes in glottal width. Zero on this section of the graph indicates glottal closure at the point of measurement.

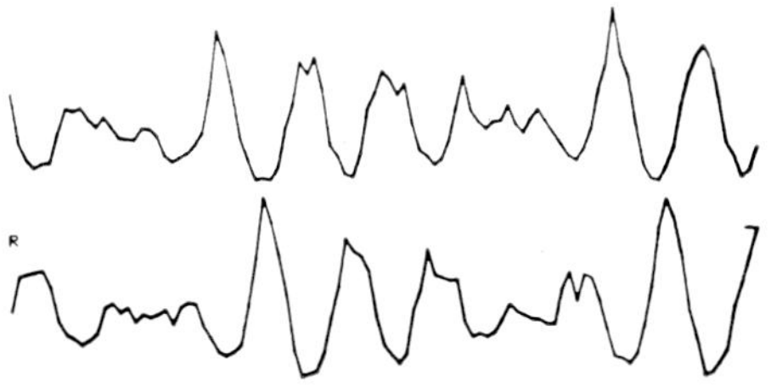

Fig. 8. Area function of the glottis in voluntary diplophonia. The curve was produced by computer from sonic pen tracings of projected individual frames of ultraspeed film. The curves read from left to right and the lower tracing is a continuation of the upper. The general similarity between glottal area and glottal width as shown in Figure 7 is apparent.

of being vibrated by the air stream; in unilateral paralysis muscular adjustments can be made in the healthy fold to cause it to vibrate at the desired frequency; vibration regularly begins on the unimpaired side; it is presumed that as the normal fold moves medially in its vibratory cycle the subglottal air pressure increases progressively and the air stream is diverted toward the paralyzed fold.[7] The combination of flow and pressure pushes the paralyzed fold from its position of rest and will do so repeatedly each time the healthy fold goes through its cycle. When the involved fold is in a paramedian position, the presence or absence of glottal closure during vibration often depends upon the pitch and loudness of the voice. That is, when the folds are elongated for phonation at high pitch, the glottis is narrowed, and if a loud sound is attempted concurrently, the increased amplitude of both folds combined with the Bernoulli effect may accomplish closure.

The female larynx represented graphically in Figure 5 contains a paralyzed left vocal cord. The voice was usually produced at the upper portions of the range because the sound was louder, less breathy, and relatively less hoarse. The figure illustrates the four vibratory characteristics of unilaterally paralyzed vocal cords that were noted in Figure 4, and in addition, reveals a mechanism of frequency adjustment. The section of high speed film that was measured contains a segment in which the healthy right vocal cord stopped vibrating for approximately two cycles, apparently to make an adjustment before resuming vibration at a slightly higher frequency. It is probably significant that the healthy cord made the adjustment. The amplitude of the paralyzed fold decreased during the interval and resumed full vibration at a higher frequency concurrently with the healthy fold.

Laryngeal trauma may create lesions and vocal problems that improve in contradiction to reasonable prognosis. A young male motorcyclist injured his larynx severely when he collided with a chain hung across a trail at neck height. A stent supported the laryngeal structures during the recovery period. After a few months the voice remained completely aphonic and adduction of the vocal folds did not occur with coughing or any other function. Photographs A and B of Figure 6 show the larynx in abduction and maximum adduction respectively at that early period. Two years later the larynx appeared as in Photographs C and D, and in the associated series of images representing one vibratory cycle. The function was regained in the right fold, but the left remained in a lateral position. The vibratory pattern as displayed in the graph of Figure 6 is similar to that seen in other unilateral paralyses. As would be expected, the voice is breathy but serviceable for conversational purposes.

Vibration With an Intermediate Rest Position. The intermediate vibratory rest position encompasses a great variety of laryngeal adjustments and organic problems. The potential complexity of such vibration is infinite. Isshiki and several associates[5] recently conducted a study in which the vibratory rest positions of vocal cords were regulated in excised larynges. Vibration was activated by air through the trachea and vocal fold tension was systematically varied unilaterally. The conditions of the study simulated unilateral paralysis of the cricothyroid muscle. When the

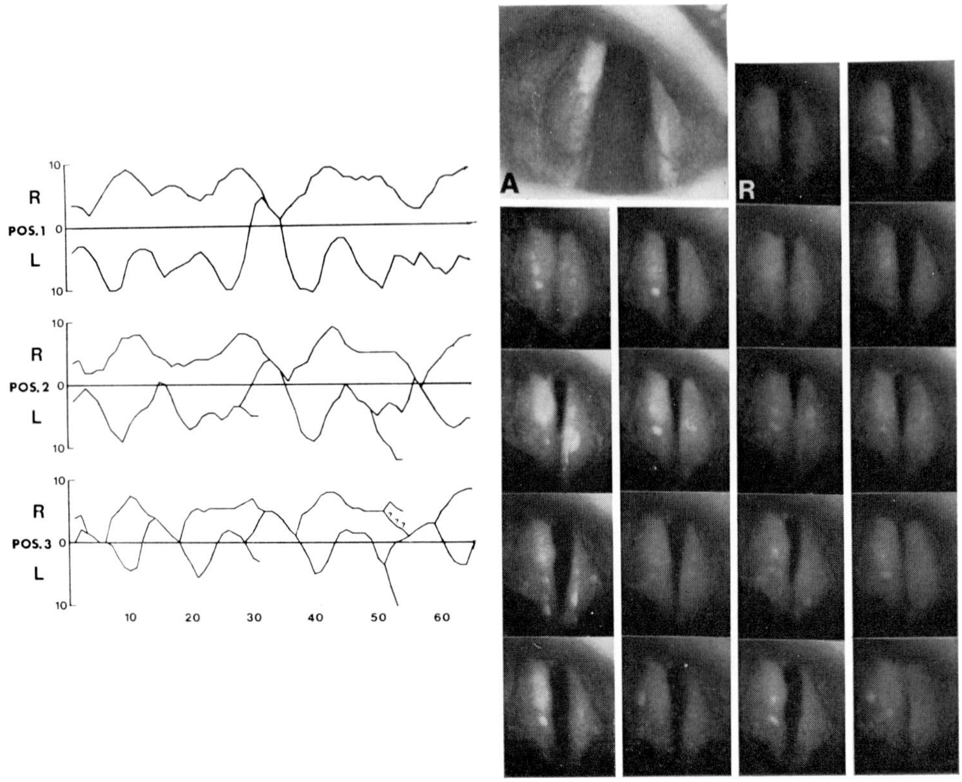

Fig. 9. Photograph A shows a male larynx with acute laryngitis and edema, particularly on the right vocal cord. The associated series of photographs from ultraspeed film begins at the upper left and reads downward progressively in each column. Alternate frames have been omitted to conserve space. The three sets of curves in the graph represent simultaneous vocal cord motions at three glottal locations: Position 2, approximately at the anterior-posterior midpoint; Position 1, halfway between Position 2 and the anterior commissure; and Position 3, halfway between Position 2 and the posterior commissure. The zero line approximates the median sagittal plane. Random, almost chaotic vibration associated with extreme hoarseness is evident.

tension in one fold was greater than in the other they tended to vibrate at different frequencies and complexity of motion. However, the vibration was influenced by the position of rest; that is, when the folds made firm contact they maintained the same frequencies except when the tension imbalance was very large. When an intermediate vibratory position of rest was maintained, differences in the complexity of motion occurred. This report made the further observation that changes in subglottal pressure could alter vibratory patterns when other factors were held constant. These investigators also noted that slight variations in vibratory rest positions, fold tension, damping ratio and stiffness often caused a change in vibratory pattern.

The report by Isshiki and his associates leads to interesting speculation about the information provided by laryngeal photography. The first subject presented above in this paper produced a normal voice and was a singer, but her vocal folds vibrated slightly out of phase and shifted laterally during the closed phase. Does she have some as yet unrecognized impairment?

Further speculation may be made about a larynx whose owner can voluntarily produce either normal or diplophonic voice. When such a larynx phonates normally the vocal folds maintain a position of rest in which they are in contact, causing the vibration to follow the customary three-phase pattern. In contrast, as revealed in the sequence of images in Figure 7, which pictures the voluntary production of diplophonia, the folds are separated slightly to an intermediate position of rest, they vibrate quasi-independently and each has its own frequency. Some readers may recall that the laryngeal image presented here was used previously in a motion picture produced by Ward and associates.[8] The frequencies of the two folds and the amplitude variations during the production of diplophonic voice are displayed in the upper curves of Figure 7. The corresponding glottal width is represented in the lower curve. It is apparent that the vocal folds vibrated at different frequencies; in this portion of the film they maintained a frequency ratio of approximately 5:4. The area function of the glottis as measured by an electronic pen associated with a computer is displayed in Figure 8. The glottal areas were calculated from tracings of single frame images projected from 16 mm high-speed film. The lower curve in the figure is a continuation of the upper.

If normal larynges contained only one vocal fold which intermittently occluded the airway by contact with a fixed area or shelf instead of another movable member, the sound produced probably would be quite normal. All of the conditions necessary for normal phonation would exist, but not those for diplophonia. When two vocal folds are present and one vibrates at a frequency different from the other, each will contribute to the pressure changes at the glottis, and together they will produce a complex sound wave that will be perceived as a double voice. The ear hears the sound as though it were coming from separate sound sources. When each vibrator maintains a relatively regular, repetitive pattern the sounds will be musical and can be harmonic or inharmonic as they would be also from independent sources. However, when one or both vibratory sequences becomes randomly variable, the ear is stimulated irregularly in time or amplitude and the sound is heard as rough. Current theory postulates that phonatory sound results from the pulsatile flow of air through the glottis and not the motions of the folds themselves. That is, if the vocal folds could be vibrated mechanically, independent of an air stream, they probably would not generate much sound. In diplophonia the separate vocal fold motions combine at the glottis to produce a complex sequence of air pressure changes which, when they reach the ear of the listener, stimulate the auditory mechanism as though they were two pressure waves from independent sources.

When edema of the vocal folds is present, the factors of mass, contour, and what might be called surface viscosity must be added to such other considerations as elasticity, length, and air flow to account for vibratory patterns. Since edema may not be expressed uniformly over the surface of the folds, its distribution also becomes a possible influencing factor. Figure 9 shows a male larynx with an acute upper respiratory infection that produced a rough sounding, hoarse vioce. Photograph A suggests the condition of the larynx, and reveals the extensive edema of the right vocal cord. The left cord remained more flexible than the right.

The sequence of film frames from ultraspeed film reveals random vibration in both folds, and different patterns of motion in each fold including simultaneous movements in different directions in the same fold. There does not seem to be any satisfactory way to display the details of this extremely complex movement short of actual projection of the film. However, some suggestion of the vibratory detail can be obtained from the three sets of curves in Figure 9 which represent simultaneous movements at three locations along the glottis: Position 2 is approximately at the anterior-posterior midpoint and Positions 1 and 3 half-way toward the anterior and posterior commissures respectively. The general impression is of chaotic vibration, but it is presumed that additional study with computer assistance will offer a means for correlating vocal cord behavior and the sound produced.

This paper has attempted to support the concept that vocal sounds are directly related to specific patterns of vocal cord vibration. These patterns may be modified voluntarily or by disease but it is the vibration and not the disease itself that determines the sound. This is another way of saying that a laryngeal disease cannot be diagnosed on the basis of the sound produced, or that laryngeal disease does not reveal itself in the vocal sound until it alters vocal cord vibration.

REFERENCES

1. Timcke R, von Leden H, Moore GP: Laryngeal vibrations: measurement of the glottic wave. Part I, the normal vibratory cycle. Arch Otolaryngol 68:1-19,1958

2. Moore GP, von Leden H: Dynamic variations of the vibratory pattern in the normal larynx. Folia Phoniatr (Basel) 10:205-238, 1958

3. Baer T: *Investigation of Phonation Using Excised Larynges,* dissertation. Massachusetts Institute of Technology, Boston, 1975

4. Hildebrand BH: *Vibratory Patterns of the Human Vocal Cords During Variations in Frequency and Intensity,* dissertation. University of Florida, Gainesville, 1976

5. Isshiki N, Tenabe M, Ishizaka K, *et al*: Clinical significance of asymmetrical vocal cord tension. Ann Otol Rhinol Laryngol. In press

6. Moore GP: *Organic Voice Disorders.* Englewood Cliffs, NJ, Prentice Hall Inc, 1971

7. von Leden H, Moore GP: Vibratory patterns of the vocal cords in unilateral laryngeal paralysis. Acta Otolaryngol (Stockh) 53:493-506, 1966

8. Ward PH, Sanders JW, Goldman R, *et al*: Diplophonia. Ann Otol Rhinol Laryngol 78:771-777, 1969

REPRINTS–G. Paul Moore, PhD, 2234 NW 6th Place, Gainesville, FL 32603.

PLASTIC SURGERY RESEARCH AWARDS

The American Academy of Facial Plastic and Reconstructive Surgery invites entries in its annual competition for original research in head and neck plastic surgery.

The Ira J. Tresley Research Award consists of a $500 prize and is open to any physician who has been board certified for three years or longer.

The Benjamin Shuster Memorial Awards open to residents and fellows in otolaryngology offer $250 to the first place winner and $100 to the second place winner. Papers submitted during the first year after completion of residency will be considered provided the research was performed during the author's residency program.

Only original, non-published papers will be considered. The winning authors will present their papers at the Academy's annual scientific meeting May 7-14, 1977 in Boston.

Notification of intent to enter the competitions must be sent to the Academy no later than November 30, 1976. Deadline for final papers is January 31, 1977. Notice and papers should be sent to Robert L. Simons, MD, 16800 NW Second Avenue, North Miami Beach, Fl 33162.

Ann Otol 85: 1976

ACUTE EPIGLOTTITIS IN INFANTS AND CHILDREN

BRUCE BENJAMIN

BRIAN O'REILLY

SYDNEY, AUSTRALIA

SUMMARY — Sixty-one cases of acute epiglottitis at the Royal Alexandra Hospital for Children, Sydney, from July 1968 to December 1974 are reviewed. The average age of 2.7 years is lower than previously reported. The average time from the initial symptom to arrival at the hospital was 14 hours. The average time from arrival to performance of tracheotomy was two hours. The diagnosis was made when first seen and assessed in 50 of the 61 cases. There were eight respiratory arrests in the Casualty and five of these were successfully resuscitated. We believe that an artificial airway is necessary in most cases, and in this series, tracheotomy was performed, with minimal complications. Particular emphasis is given to diagnosis from the history, and a detailed description is given of physical examination of the oropharynx. Although x-ray examination is usually unnecessary when the diagnosis is in doubt, a plain lateral x-ray may be useful, with due precaution not to increase the respiratory obstruction. We consider that a patient with acute epiglottitis should be transferred immediately to a major pediatric hospital, and that in almost every case an artificial airway should be established.

Early this century laryngeal diphtheria was the main cause of acute infectious laryngeal obstruction in children, and only later were nondiphtheritic infections considered separately. As the incidence of diphtheria declined, clinicians clearly documented acute laryngotracheitis or "croup" as a separate category.

In 1900 Thiesen[1] recorded three cases of a condition which he referred to as "angina epiglottidea anterior." Although he described the clinical features of acute infectious epiglottitis and stated that the condition was first mentioned in 1871, there was little further reference to the disease for some 40 years.

In the 1940's,[2,3] acute epiglottitis became more widely recognized as a definite clinical entity. Sinclair,[4] in 1941, reported ten patients with acute obstructive laryngitis where *Haemophilus influenzae* type B had been grown from the blood culture. Alexander,[5] in 1942, described a similar consistent clinical pattern, again in ten patients, in whom *H. influenzae* type B had been isolated.

In 1949, Miller[6] clearly outlined the important clinical features of acute epiglottitis, and emphasized the distinction between acute inflammatory airway obstruction in children caused by the subglottic and supraglottic types of laryngeal inflammation. Many publications have appeared since then, confirming that the disease of acute epiglottitis is a clearly demarcated clinical and pathological entity.

Jones and Camps,[7] in 1959, reported 26 deaths in 29 patients, a high mortality rate, whereas Vetto,[8] in 1960, reported only three deaths in 37 patients. In recent years there have been many series where the mortality has been low.

This paper reviews 61 patients with acute epiglottitis admitted to the hospital in the last 6½ years. Particular

---

From the Ear, Nose and Throat Department, Royal Alexandra Hospital for Children, Sydney, Australia.

Presented at the meeting of the American Broncho-Esophagological Association, Palm Beach, Florida, April 27-28, 1976.

emphasis is given to the age distribution and to the time elapsed between the initial symptom and the arrival at the hospital. The clinical features are discussed, and a detailed description of the clinical examination of the oropharynx and epiglottis is emphasized. The need for provision of an artificial airway in most cases is stressed, and in this series tracheotomy was used.

CLINICAL SERIES

The patients reported in this series cover the period July 1968 to December 1974. During this 6½ years there were 61 children with a diagnosis of acute epiglottitis and of these 37 were males and 24 females. The average age was 2.7 years. The youngest patient was six months and the oldest patient five years six months (Fig. 1).

The time which had elapsed from the first symptom to arrival at the hospital was estimated, although this was difficult to assess because of uncertainty about the onset of the initial symptom. The average time was 14 hours (Fig. 2).

The average time which elapsed from arrival at the Casualty Department to performance of the tracheotomy was two hours. The average time the tracheotomy was in place and until its removal was five days. In a single patient pernasal endotracheal intubation was performed, and the tube was left in place without complication for 59 hours, the Pediatrician in charge preferring that no tracheotomy be performed.

The throat swab for *H. influenzae* was positive in 11 patients, negative in 34 patients, and was not done in 16 patients. The blood culture for *H. influenzae* was positive in 36 patients, negative in 15 patients and was not done in 10 patients.

Of 61 patients, the diagnosis in 50 was made in the Casualty, *i.e.*, when first seen and assessed. Of the remainder: Three patients were misdiagnosed as acute laryngotracheitis, the correct diagnosis being made after three hours in one and after eight hours in the other two. One patient was seen in Casualty and sent home with a diagnosis of viral upper respiratory tract infection, but he returned four hours later and the correct diagnosis was made. Seven patients were first seen in other hospitals; one was referred with the tracheotomy in place; four were referred with an endotracheal tube in place; one died on the way to the hospital with an endotracheal tube in place, and one was referred without either endotracheal tube or tracheotomy.

There were eight respiratory arrests in the Casualty, and five were successfully resuscitated. Of the three who died: in one, intubation was unsuccessful; in the other two, intubation was successful and was followed by tracheotomy but without recovery, the cause of death being cerebral hypoxia.

Pleural effusion with right upper lobe collapse was found in one patient and "septic arthritis" occurred in one patient in the right ankle, but the effusion showed no growth. Nonspecific radiological changes were seen in the chest x-ray in almost every patient, *e.g.*, areas of segmental collapse or increased pulmonary markings.

The following complications occurred following tracheotomy: mediastinal emphysema in three patients, bilateral pneumothorax in one patient (the tracheotomy having been performed in another hospital), granulation tissue formation at the site of the tracheotomy in three patients, with removal at bronchoscopy prior to decannulation.

In summary we have found that the diagnosis was made promptly in most cases in the Casualty Department, although eight of the 61 patients had respiratory arrest due to laryngeal obstruction in the Casualty Department itself and three of the eight died.

Incidence. The condition is uncommon and has been said to account for approximately one in 1000 hospital admissions. Fearon[9] reviewed 4,148 patients with acute obstructive laryngitis admitted to the Hospital for Sick Children in Toronto, from 1952 to 1959, of whom only 78 had acute epiglottis.

As shown in our series the diagnosis

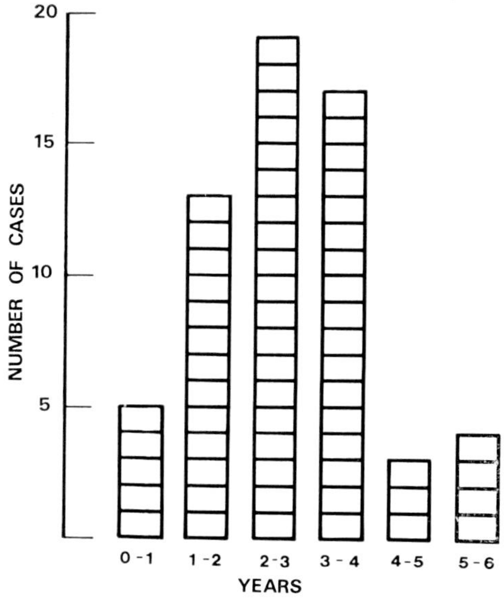

Fig. 1. Age distribution of chidren with acute epiglottitis (av. age – 2.7 yrs).

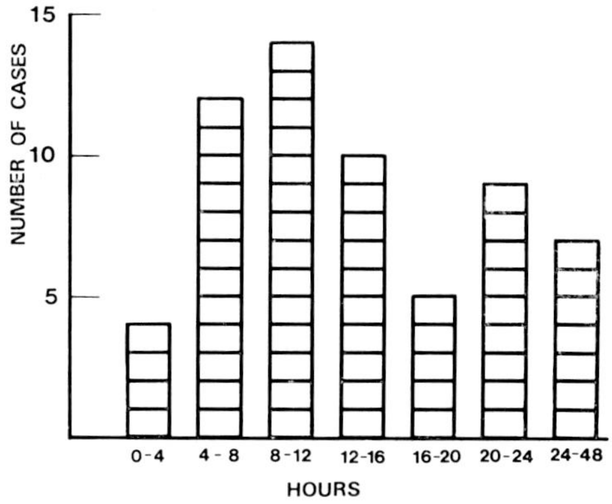

Fig. 2. Duration of patients' symptoms prior to arrival at the hospital (av. time – 14 hrs).

is seldom made before the child is admitted to a pediatric hospital; in fact, the diagnosis may be entirely missed during life and found only at postmortem examination.

Although more common in winter, acute epiglottitis may occur at any time of the year. There is quite a variation in the yearly incidence so that cases appear to occur in groups. There is no known reason for the increased incidence in males as compared to females.

The condition has been reported at all ages from the second month of life to adulthood and the peak incidence has generally been considered to be between three and six years of age. However, in our series the peak incidence is in younger children, the average age being 2.7 years (Fig. 1).

Etiology. H. influenzae is an important bacterial species producing serious clinical infections in children.[10] Although its exact etiological role in diseases in man is not fully understood, it is clear that it acts as etiological agent in septicemia which may become localized as meningitis, acute epiglottitis, pneumonia, pyarthrosis, osteomyelitis, or cellulitis. Most of these serious infections have been attributed to encapsulated, typable strains, principally type B.

Most authors agree that *H. influenzae* type B is the causal agent in acute epiglottitis, but some point out that other bacteria may be implicated. It seems doubtful that pneumococci, streptococci or staphylococci have any significance when grown from the throat swab of a child with "croup" or acute epiglottitis, as throat swabs or swabs from the epiglottis are unreliable. Blood culture should be obtained routinely, before antibiotic treatment is given, and it then probably gives a truer picture of the causative organism.

Pathology. The pathological changes in the supraglottic structures affect mainly the loosely attached mucous membrane. Edema and acute inflammatory swelling involves the laryngeal structures above the vocal cords – the ventricular bands, the arytenoids, the aryepiglottic folds, and the epiglottis. The pharynx, true cords, subglottic region, and trachea are never directly involved, but the reason for this curious anatomic specificity is unknown.

Clinical Features. Acute epiglottitis is an acute fulminating infection characterized by rapid, relentless progression to severe respiratory obstruction within 6 to 24 hours (Fig. 2). The onset may be sudden, unexpected and abrupt.

TABLE I

FEATURES DISTINGUISHING ACUTE LARYNGOTRACHEITIS FROM ACUTE EPIGLOTTITIS

Acute Laryngotracheitis	*Acute Epiglottitis*
More common in males.	Males and females approximately equal.
Usually occurs below the age of five and often recurs. Severe airway obstruction takes from one to several days to occur, with a variable clinical course. There is a firm indurated pink subglottic swelling.	Occurs at any age from infancy to adulthood and "never" recurs. Severe airway obstruction occurs within 6 to 24 hours with a relentlessly progressive clinical course. An acute inflammatory fulminating swelling in the supraglottic laryngeal tissues.
There is little toxemia or generalized effect as the etiology is almost certainly a localized viral infection.	There is severe toxemia and prostration from septicemia due to *H. influenzae* type B.
Cool moist air is the main therapy and steroids are probably beneficial, antibiotics being used only for secondary bacterial infection.	Parenteral antibiotics always necessary and steroids probably of little benefit.
Very seldom requires tracheotomy.	Usually requires tracheotomy.

More often the child develops vague prodromata suggesting an impending upper respiratory tract infection and these features are rapidly followed by sore throat, pain on swallowing, and refusal to eat or drink.

The voice may be relatively unaffected early but is usually somewhat muffled and thick later. There is little cough.

The child is acutely ill, with a variable degree of fever, ashen pallor, prostration and anxiety. In infants, exhaustion may occur due to the airway obstruction and the severe toxemia from the *H. influenzae* septicemia. The older child characteristically sits up, hands propping him steady with the mouth wide open, jaw forward, head extended and an anxious expression on his face. He may drool his saliva and refuse to drink. Older children do not struggle to breathe but find that quiet respirations serve them better, and despite the relatively poor air entry heard on auscultation of the chest, respiratory stridor may not be a prominent feature. As hypoxia, hypercarbia and acidosis progress, irritability, restlessness and disorientation are likely to occur. If spontaneous or therapeutic improvement does not occur, cyanosis, respiratory arrest and cardiac arrest complete the relentless and fatal sequence of clinical events.

The oropharynx is best examined with an angled, metal tongue depressor while the child sits opposite the examiner. The tongue is depressed firmly but without undue force and classically the suspected diagnosis is confirmed when a very swollen, fiery red, acutely inflamed epiglottis protrudes briefly above the base of the tongue. If the examination is done quickly and skillfully, there is only a momentary increase in dyspnea. However, occasionally, in advanced cases with impending obstruction, complete airway obstruction may be precipitated by inept, repeated or prolonged attempts to examine the epiglottis. Examination in the supine position may also precipitate terminal asphyxia. The examination should not be attempted in such circumstances unless facilities to provide an artificial airway by immediate endotracheal intubation or tracheotomy are readily at hand. Once an experienced clinician has adequately observed the pharynx and diagnosed the condition, reexamination is neither necessary nor warranted.

It is important to stress that occasionally the epiglottis itself is only minimally involved, the edema and inflammatory swelling being confined to the other supraglottic structures, namely the false cords, the arytenoids and the aryepiglottic folds, but causing equally severe airway obstruction. In such cases the features of the history and general physical examination should alert the clinician to the possibility of acute epiglottitis in a child with progressive airway obstruction. Reexamination at intervals may be rewarded and the diagnosis made with certainty when the epiglottis is seen to become enlarged. In these cases a lateral x-ray of the upper airway may confirm the diagnosis.

Differential Diagnosis. Deaths occur from failure to consider the diagnosis and recognize the potential danger.[11] There is usually little difficulty in making the diagnosis once the possibility has been suspected. However, in some situations the clinical picture may be clouded by other events, *e.g.*, pneumonia or septicemia, or there may be no history available in the first instance. It may be necessary to provide an artificial airway to overcome severe upper airway obstruction before a diagnosis has been made.

In uncomplicated cases, however, the condition must be differentiated from:

1. Acute laryngotracheitis. This is the most common clinical problem and Table I shows the distinguishing features.[12]

2. Foreign body in the pharynx, larynx, trachea or upper esophagus. Although a sudden choking attack may have been observed, there is frequently no history. Foreign body should be considered where laryngospasm, husky voice, stridor or inspiratory wheeze dominate the clinical picture. An upper esophageal foreign body may develop periesophageal swelling and cause tracheal compression.

3. Laryngopharyngeal diphtheria. This remains a relatively rare but important cause of acute respiratory obstruction. The child is seldom properly immunized. There may be evidence, during a minor epidemic, of contact with other known cases of diphtheria, the child is toxic and a diphtheritic membrane may or may may not be seen in the oropharynx.

4. Gross hypertrophy of the tonsils and adenoids. Serious airway obstruction with or without cardiac failure due to chronic or acute enlargement of the tonsils and adenoids is now easily recognized. There are variations of the syndrome and the diagnosis is confirmed by inspection of the oropharynx.

5. Acute bacterial abscess of the pharyngeal area. This includes peritonsillar abscess, retropharyngeal abscess, pharyngomaxillary space abscess and parapharyngeal abscess. There are usually features of a preceding infection of the tonsils or pharynx, then persistent high fever, irritability, enlarged cervical lymph nodes and airway obstruction. Respiratory obstruction may be especially serious in infants with a retropharyngeal abscess.

Radiological Examination. In most cases the diagnosis of acute epiglottitis is established with reasonable certainty by the clinical findings. X-rays are then unnecessary and may delay the institution of therapy. At times, however, the condition presents a confusing clinical picture and when examination of the oropharynx is difficult or the diagnosis is in doubt, for instance where the epiglottis itself is not significantly involved by swelling, x-rays are useful.

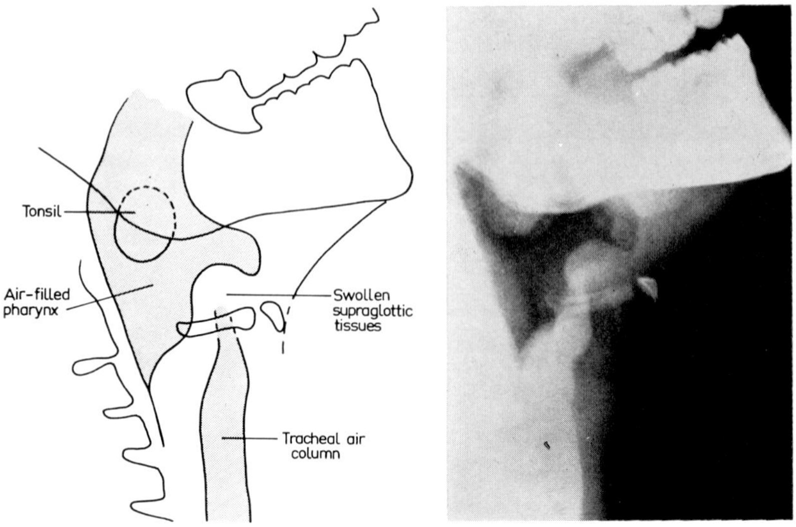

Fig. 3. Line drawing and lateral x-ray showing swollen supraglottic tissues.

The disease is recognized easily radiologically by an experienced pediatric radiologist.[13,14] It must be emphasized that during exposure of the film, while the child's neck is positioned in extension, all unnecessary manipulation must be avoided or respiratory obstruction will be made worse.

We rely on a lateral film of the upper airway and an attempt is made to take the film during inspiration. Swelling of the epiglottis and aryepiglottic folds almost fills the hypopharynx and above this swelling, there is ballooning of the pharyngeal airway indicating inspiratory obstruction (Fig. 3). These changes contrast with those in acute laryngotracheitis where there is subglottic swelling with a localized narrowing of the airway below the vocal cords.

TREATMENT

Acute epiglottitis, with appropriate therapy administered before irreversible changes have occurred, is a self-limiting disease with improvement occurring about 72 hours from the onset. Deaths occur from failure to recognize and adequately treat the disease or, very occasionally, from complications of the treatment itself.

A patient with a suspected diagnosis of acute epiglottitis should be transferred immediately to a hospital, preferably a major pediatric hospital. During transportation, in advanced cases, oxygen may be given as supportive therapy, if necessary with assisted ventilation by mask and bag. However, in other cases the use of oxygen is best avoided as it may obscure the signs of increasing respiratory obstruction.

Where total laryngeal obstruction occurs, in an emergency situation, providing a laryngoscope and a suitable endotracheal tube or a bronchoscope is available, swift intubation, even by a relatively inexperienced person is preferable to attempting emergency tracheotomy. Where facilities for intubation are not available or where intubation fails, emergency tracheotomy may be a lifesaving last resort.

As soon as a diagnosis of acute epiglottitis has been made it is our practice at the hospital to make arrangements for tracheotomy, although in an occasional mild or early case it is possible to continue close observation.

Conservative management has been advocated initially by some authors and may be successful in isolated cases, but the results are uncertain. Treatment using antibiotics and/or corticosteroids have been reported as having isolated successes but again the results are unpredictable. We firmly believe that to rely only on such treatment is to invite disaster. In most cases it is safer to provide an artificial airway for several days while appropriate medical treatment controls the infection. Johnson *et al*[15] reviewed 248 patients from the literature, 184 received tracheotomy with a mortality of just over 1%, while 64 received "observation," with a mortality of approximately 8%.

Relief of airway obstruction by provision of an artificial airway is usually necessary as soon as the diagnosis is confirmed. Prolonged pernasal endotracheal intubation has been used successfully in many centers[16-19] as an alternative to tracheotomy with comparable results. However, we have continued to perform tracheotomy although our policy is reviewed regularly.

The tracheotomy is carried out under general anesthetic induced using halothane and oxygen with atropine (15-20 μg/kg given intravenously. An endotracheal tube* with a suitable, atraumatic metal introducer is generally preferred. Intubation requires considerable experience, and it is often made difficult by the distortion and swelling of the supraglottic structures.

A proper surgical technique will minimize the potential complications of tracheotomy in infants and small children.[20] A vertical skin incision is recommended and a minimum of blunt dissection only is used to avoid unnecessary opening of tissue planes in the neck. The incision into the trachea is situated lower than is usually recommended for adults and should be at least at or below the fourth tracheal ring. There should be no excision of tracheal cartilage.

Dehydration is probably the most important single factor causing crusting of exudate. Intravenous fluids are necessary and the child is always nursed in a cool, moist atmosphere for at least 48 hours, but added oxygen is not necessary in uncomplicated cases. The adequacy of humidification is often neglected or underestimated. The lower respiratory tract is denied the normal nasal function once the nose is bypassed and the physiological action of nasal breathing no longer preserves the mucociliary mechanism of the normal lower respiratory tract. Moistening of the inspired air goes part way towards correcting this deficiency.

Ampicillin is the antibiotic of choice, 200 to 400 mg/kg of body weight per 24 hours is administered in divided doses, intravenously initially and then orally.

Removal of the tracheotomy tube is usually possible in three to five days, and the child is generally well enough to be discharged about two days later.

In this series, tracheotomy has proved a satisfactory means of providing an artificial airway in the treatment of acute epiglottitis, there being no mortality from the tracheotomy itself and very small morbidity.

* Portex Division, Smith Industries Inc., Wilmington, DE.

REFERENCES

1. Theisen DF: Angina epiglottidea anterior: Report of three cases. Albany Med Ann 21:395-405, 1900

2. Miller AH: Hemophilus influenzae type b epiglottitis or acute supraglottic laryngitis in children. Laryngoscope 58:514-526, 1948

3. Davison FW: Acute laryngotracheo bronchitis. Arch Otolaryngol 47:455-464

4. Sinclair SE: Hemophilus influenzae type b and acute laryngitis with bacteremia. JAMA 117:170-173, 1941

5. Alexander HE, Ellis C, Leidy C: Treatment of type-specific hemophilus influenzae infections in infancy and childhood. J Pediatr 20:673-698, 1942

6. Miller AH: Acute epiglottitis. Acute obstructive laryngitis in small children, caused by Haemophilus Influenzae Type b. Trans Am Acad Ophthalmol Otolaryngol 53:519-526, 1949

7. Jones HM, Camps FE: Acute epiglottitis. Practitioner 178:223-239, 1957

8. Vetto RR: Epiglottitis: Report of thirty seven cases. JAMA 173:990-994, 1960

9. Fearon B: Acute laryngotracheo-bronchitis in infancy and childhood. Pediatr Clin

North Am 9:1095-1112, 1972

10. Sell SHW: The clinical importance of hemophilus influenzae infections in children. Pediatr Clin North Am 17:415-426, 1970

11. Fearon BW, Bell RD: Acute epiglottitis: a potential killer. Can Med Assoc 112: 760-766, 1975

12. Benjamin BN: Acute inflammatory airway obstruction in infants and children. Med J Aust 2:1254-1257, 1970

13. Poole CA, Altman DH: Acute epiglottitis in children. Radiology 80:798-805, 1963

14. Capitanio MA, Kirkpatrick JA: Upper respiratory tract obstruction in infants and children. Radiol Clin North Am 6:265-277, 1968

15. Johnson GK, Sullivan JL, Bishop LA: Acute epiglottitis. Arch Otolaryngol 100:333-337, 1974

16. Mc Donald AH, Stocks JG: Prolonged nasotracheal intubation. Br J Anaesth 37:161-173, 1965

17. Geraci RP: Acute epiglottitis — management with prolonged naso-tracheal intubation. Pediatrics 41:143-144, 1968

18. Allen TH, Steven IM: Prolonged endotracheal intubation in infants and children. Brit J Anaesth 37:566-573, 1965

19. Sweeny DW, Allen TH, Steven IM: Acute epiglottitis — management by intubation. Anaesth Intensive Care 1:526-528, 1973

20. Benjamin BN: Tracheotomy in infants and children. J Otolaryngol Soc Aust 3:254-259, 1971

Reprints—Bruce Benjamin, 229 Macquarie Street, Sydney. 2000 Australia.

PSYCHOSOCIAL CARE OF THE DYING PATIENT

A postgraduate course in Psychosocial Care of the Dying Patient will be presented June 3-4, 1977 by the Cancer Research Institute and Extended Programs in Medical Education, University of California School of Medicine, San Francisco, CA.

Ann Otol 85: 1976

ACQUIRED AND CONGENITAL SUBGLOTTIC STENOSIS IN THE INFANT

James L. Parkin, MD

Michael H. Stevens, MD August L. Jung, MD

Salt Lake City, Utah

SUMMARY – During the calendar year of 1974, the Intermountain Newborn Intensive Care Center at the University of Utah Medical Center had 603 admissions. A representative group of 293 charts were reviewed which indicated that 44% of these children were intubated from hours to weeks. The overall mortality rate for the 293 children was 29%. Eighteen of the 603 children were diagnosed as having subglottic stenosis. Fifteen of these children appeared to have acquired subglottic stenosis secondary to endotracheal intubation. Three children had congenital subglottic stenosis. Tracheostomy was necessary in the management of 15 patients. Ten of the 18 patients have survived and two of these patients still have tracheostomy tubes in place. The survival and thickness of the stenotic area are inversely proportional to the birth weight and the duration of intubation. Endoscopic excision, dilatation and stenting were techniques utilized in the treatment of these stenotic lesions. The extubation technique utilized is described. The factors involved in the production of acquired subglottic stenosis are presented along with suggestions to decrease the incidence of this problem in the intubated child.

Assisted ventilation with various respirator machines and techniques has become a common practice in the care of the newborn with respiratory dysfunction. Maintenance of a closed system is necessary for the performance of such ventilatory assistance. The indwelling endotracheal tube is usually the initial technique by which this closed system is achieved. Much attention in recent years has been focused on the problems associated with such intubation. This paper reviews the experience with a group of newborn patients who demonstrated narrowing of the subglottic airway as seen in a newborn intensive care unit. The relationship of endotracheal intubation in the etiology and treatment of this problem will be discussed.

METHODS AND MATERIALS

During the calendar year of 1974, 18 infants with subglottic stenosis were evaluated and treated in the Intermountain Newborn Intensive Care Center (INICC) at the University of Utah Medical Center. The experience with these infants was reviewed retrospectively and forms the basis for this clinical study. The total number of children admitted during this period was 603. The charts of 293 consecutive admissions from July 1 to December 31, 1974, were studied to determine incidence of endotracheal intubation, development of subglottic stenosis and mortality in this group of newborns.

All patients with a diagnosis of subglottic stenosis have now had a one to two-year follow-up. The infants who otherwise were patients of the Newborn Intensive Care Center received follow-up only until their death or discharge from the INICC.

In all infants receiving closed system ventilatory assistance, endotracheal intubation was performed by pediatric house staff and specialized INICC nurses. Uncuffed, Murphy type endotracheal tubes were utilized. Tubes were not reused. The tubes were changed on an average of every three to five days or more frequently if secretions were copious, thick, or obstructive. All tracheobronchial endoscopies and tracheostomies were performed by the otolaryngology service under the direct supervision of the authors.

From the Department of Surgery, Division of Otolaryngology, and the Department of Pediatrics, University of Utah College of Medicine, Salt Lake City, Utah.

Presented at the meeting of the American Broncho-Esophagological Association, Palm Beach, Florida, April 27-28, 1976.

TABLE I

INTUBATION, TRACHEOSTOMY AND MORTALITY IN 293 CONSECUTIVE NEWBORN INTENSIVE CARE PATIENTS

	Intubated	*Tracheostomy*	*Expired*
No. of patients	128	7	86
Total patients	293	293	293
Percent	44%	2.4%	29%

The tracheostomies were done over an endotracheal tube or bronchoscope. Horizontal skin incisions were utilized and the tracheal incision performed was either a lazy "H" or an inferiorly based anterior tracheal wall flap incorporating two adjacent tracheal rings.

During the first three days, a gauze or net tracheostomy dressing was used to allow the escape of free air around the tube. This is important in the prevention of subcutaneous cervical emphysema and pneumomediastinum. The first tracheostomy tube change was accomplished at 48 to 72 hours. Silk or nylon traction sutures (5-0) were placed in the trachea at the time of tracheostomy to facilitate the initial tube change. These traction sutures were removed at the first or second tube change. The tracheostomy tubes were then changed at three-day intervals. Franklin or Shiley pediatric tracheostomy tubes were utilized in all patients. Extubation techniques will be covered in the discussion section.

The INICC services a large geographic area. The majority of patients referred to the INICC have respiratory distress syndromes with or without other associated congenital problems. Those patients being transferred from other medical facilities are transported by a specialized air-transport team equipped to provide ventilatory as well as other supportive care while in transit.

TABLE II

TRACHEOSTOMY, ACQUIRED SUBGLOTTIC STENOSIS AND MORTALITY IN INTUBATED INFANTS

	Tracheostomy	*Acquired Subglottic Stenosis*	*Expired*
No. of patients	7	7	62
Total intubated patients	128	128	128
Percent	5%	5%	48%

TABLE III

INCIDENCE OF SUBGLOTTIC STENOSIS

	All Cases of Stenosis	*Congenital Stenosis*	*Acquired Stenosis*
Number	18	3	15
Total patients	603	603	603
Percent	3%	0.5%	2.5%

RESULTS

The review of charts from 293 consecutive patients admitted to the INICC revealed an overall mortality of 86 or 29% (Table I). The number of patients who required endotracheal intubation was 128 of these 293 or 44%. Of the 128 intubated patients, 62 died, giving a 48% mortality rate among the intubated infants (Table II). Deaths occurred in 24 patients who were not intubated. It would be expected that the death rate would be higher in the intubated patients as they were generally the more seriously ill.

Subglottic stenosis was diagnosed in 10 of the 128 intubated patients. The stenosis was considered to be congenital in three patients and acquired in seven patients. No subglottic stenosis was diagnosed in the nonintubated group of patients. Tracheostomy was necessary in seven patients. The subglottic stenosis was managed without tracheostomy in three patients. The incidence of acquired subglottic stenosis in this total group of 293 patients was 2.4%. The incidence of acquired subglottic stenosis in the intubated group was 5%.

During the entire year of 1974, acquired subglottic stenosis was diagnosed in 15 of 603 patients for an incidence of 2.5% (Table III). Congenital subglottic stenosis was diagnosed in three of 603 patients for an incidence of 0.5%. All three of these patients received endotracheal intubation during their initial airway management. One of these patients required tracheostomy and was successfully extubated. The other two patients were managed without tracheostomy. All three patients are alive and well with good airway function.

TABLE IV

SUBGLOTTIC STENOSIS

Sex		*Stenosis Type*		*Stenosis Etiology*	
Male	*Female*	*Thick*	*Thin*	*Acquired*	*Congenital*
9	9	11	7	15	3

Tracheostomy		*Tracheostomy Extubated*		*Expired*		*Alive*	
Yes	*No*	*Yes*	*No*	*Yes*	*No*	*With Trach*	*Without Trach*
15	3	5	10	8	10	2	8

The remainder of the results will be from the evaluation of the 18 patients with diagnosed subglottic stenosis managed in 1974 (Tables IV and V). Of the 18 patients, nine were male and nine were female. Acquired stenosis was present in 15 patients. All 18 patients had endotracheal tube placement and 16 patients required respirators. Tracheostomy was required in the management of 15 patients. The type of stenosis was considered thin if the length of subglottic involvement was less than 4 mm. If greater than 4 mm, the stenosis was typed as thick. Thin stenosis was seen in 7 patients and thick stenosis was seen in 11 patients. All congenital subglottic stenoses were of the thin type.

Death occurred in eight patients. Five of these patients were discharged from the INICC with tracheostomies in place and died at home or at other medical facilities. The tracheostomy was probably a factor in one death. This patient developed tracheal granulomata below the tracheostomy site near the carina. These were periodically removed endoscopically. The patient died at home with a pulmonary infection and at autopsy there was compromise of the right main stem bronchus by the granuloma. All other children died because of their underlying illnesses. None of the expired children were extubated prior to death.

Sixteen of the 18 patients were premature by weight or gestation time or both. Respiratory distress syndrome was present as hyaline membrane disease, Wilson-Mikity syndrome or bronchopulmonary dysplasia in 16 patients. Significant cardiovascular disease was also seen in 12 patients with patent

TABLE V

SUMMARY OF 18 SUBGLOTTIC STENOSIS PATIENTS

	RS	*JC*	*SC*	*JJ*	*AD*	*BE*	*BF*	*PM*	*BF*	*JP*	*GJ*	*MK*	*AH*	*MM*	*SV*	*GS*	*BW*	*HT*
Birth weight in kilograms	1.2	2.8	.96	1.1	2.3	1.0	2.3	2.4	.68	2.5	2.7	1.9	1.7	1.1	.93	.74	2.0	.93
Days of intubation	60	10	56	31	36	20	6	10	45	7	3	4	24	29	34	29	10	41
Acquired or congenital stenosis	A	A	A	A	A	A	C	A	A	C	C	A	A	A	A	A	A	A
Thick or thin stenosis	Tn	Tk	Tk	Tk	Tk	Tk	Tn	Tn	Tk	Tn	Tn	Tn	Tk	Tk	Tk	Tk	Tn	Tk
Tracheostomy	+	+	+	+	+	+	−	−	+	−	+	+	+	+	+	+	+	+
Tracheostomy extubation	+	−	−	+	−	−			−		+	+	−	−	−	−	+	−
Survival	+	+	−	+	−	−	+	+	−	+	+	+	−	−	+	−	+	−

ductus arteriosus and congestive heart failure being most common. One patient had a bilateral vocal cord paralysis of uncertain etiology. He was intubated for 10 days and subsequently underwent tracheostomy with spontaneous improvement in vocal cord function. Extubation was accomplished but repeat tracheostomy was necessary because of progressive airway obstruction. Endoscopy at the time of repeat tracheostomy revealed a thick subglottic stenosis.

The mothers of six newborns had significant health problems at the time of delivery. Two mothers had sepsis, one was a heroin addict, and two had severe diabetes. Of the two diabetic mothers, one had polyhydramnios. These five newborns were premature and developed acquired subglottic stenosis. The sixth mother had myasthenia gravis in poor control. Her daughter had immediate airway distress at birth and was intubated. A peculiarity of the larynx was noted and the child was referred to the INICC. The endotracheal tube was removed three days later and an anterior glottic web was excised. In addition, a posterior and lateral subglottic thin web-like stenosis was discovered which had been partially avulsed by the endotracheal tube. The glottic web and the subglottic stenosis were excised and a nasotracheal tube placed. Extubation was accomplished but in the ensuing 72 hours the patient developed inspiratory stridor and repeat endoscopy was performed, revealing subglottic and glottic granuloma which were excised. Tracheostomy was performed. A soft stent was fashioned and secured in the larynx. The stent was removed and the child extubated ten days later with no additional airway problems.

Five patients were diagnosed as having subglottic stenosis three days to 12 weeks following the removal of the endotracheal tube. All five of these patients had thin subglottic stenosis and were intubated ten days or less. Two of these patients were diagnosed as having congenital subglottic stenosis. The stenotic area was dilated in one patient and excised in the second. Tracheostomy was not required in either patient. The other three patients were thought to have acquired stenosis. Two of these patients required tracheostomy. The stenotic area was excised in the third patient without tracheostomy. All five of these patients were discharged from the INICC with good airway function.

The prognosis for survival was poorer and the incidence of thick subglottic stenosis was greater as the time of intubation increased and the birth weight of the child decreased. The correlation of birth weight and intubation time with survival and stenosis type are seen in Tables VI and VII.

In addition to the subglottic narrowing, 11 of the patients had vocal cord abnormalities at the time of tracheostomy. The most common glottic finding was posterior intubation granulo-

TABLE VI

BIRTH WEIGHT RELATED TO STENOSIS TYPE AND SURVIVAL

Birth Wt. in Kilograms	*No. of Patients*	*Survival Alive*	*Survival Dead*	*Stenosis Type Thick*	*Stenosis Type Thin*
0.5-1.0	5	1	4	5	0
1.0-1.5	4	2	2	3	1
1.5-2.0	2	1	1	1	1
2.0-2.5	4	3	1	1	3
> 2.5	3	3	0	1	2
Total	18	10	8	11	7

TABLE VII

DURATION OF ENDOTRACHEAL INTUBATION RELATED TO STENOSIS TYPE AND SURVIVAL

Duration of Intubation in Days	*No. of Patients*	*Survival Alive*	*Survival Dead*	*Stenosis Type Thick*	*Stenosis Type Thin*
< 7	4	4	0	0	4
8-21	4	3	1	2	2
22-35	5	1	4	5	0
36-49	2	0	2	2	0
> 49	3	2	1	2	1
Total	18	10	8	11	7

mas. One vocal cord laceration was seen and vocal cord ulcerations were also noted. As mentioned above, two patients had congenital vocal cord pathologies, *i.e.*, bilateral vocal cord paralysis and an anterior glottic web.

Of the seven patients with thin type subglottic stenosis, all were discharged with good airway function and all are living. Three of these patients did not require tracheostomy. The stenotic area was endoscopically excised in three patients and dilated in four. Eleven patients had thick stenosis and only one of these patients has been extubated after serial dilatations over a 15-month period. This patient was extubated at seven months of age but required repeat tracheostomy three weeks later because of progressive stridor. He was re-extubated at 21 months of age and has done well for three months since then. Two of these 11 patients are alive with the tracheostomy in place. Both of these patients have undergone repeated dilatations and seem to be near final extubation. Eight patients with thick stenosis died with their tracheostomies in place.

Extubation was accomplished in the tracheostomized child by first endoscopically confirming the presence of an anatomically patent airway. The tracheostomy tube was removed at the time of endoscopy and a nasotracheal tube was reinserted for 24 to 48 hours. Six hours prior to removal of the endotracheal tube, the child was given intramuscular Decadron®* 0.25 mg/kg. One half of the initial Decadron® dose was then repeated every six hours for 24 to 48 hours. The patients also received IPPB with racemic epinephrine every two to four hours. The patient's heart rate, respiratory rate, and blood gases were all monitored. Our experience has found this to be the best decannulation technique.

Two of the 15 patients who underwent tracheostomy developed complications related to the tracheostomy placement. One patient was accidentally extubated 24 hours after her tracheostomy. The tube was reinserted and the patient received assisted ventilation. She failed to improve and an otolaryngology resident was called in who discovered that the tracheostomy tube had been replaced paratracheal. The tube was reinserted into the trachea with immediate respiratory improvement. Bilateral subcutaneous cervical emphysema and pneumomediastinum were diagnosed and managed uneventfully. The second patient developed tracheal granulomas below the level of the tracheostomy requiring repeated endoscopic excision. These were probably a contributing factor in the patient's subsequent death with a respiratory infection.

DISCUSSION

As the skills of the neonatologist increase and improved techniques become available to him, an increased survival of the more critically ill and smaller premature children will be achieved. Obvious factors in the reduction of mortality in the newborn child with respiratory distress syndromes are the efficiency and skills of the pediatric intensive care transport team. The air transport service which is operational at the University of Utah Medical Center makes possible the safe transport of critically ill newborns from rural areas to the Intermountain Newborn Intensive Care Center. A high percentage of these newborns require assisted ventilation, many utilizing a closed system with an endotracheal or tracheostomy tube.

Subglottic stenosis carries a much more serious prognosis for the surgical re-establishment of normal airway function. Unlike tracheal stenosis where excision and end-to-end anastomosis have provided satisfactory results in a large percentage of patients, the surgical control of subglottic stenosis has been less satisfactory. Many patients, particularly those with the thick type subglottic stenosis, will be discharged from the hospital with a tracheostomy

*Merck Sharp and Dohme, West Point, PA.

tube in place. Fearon and Cotton reviewed their experience with 25 consecutive cases of severe subglottic stenosis in children and reported a 24% mortality rate among children with tracheostomy in place.[1]. These authors presented a surgical approach to the correction of this problem which appears to have promise.

Endotracheal intubation with assisted ventilation has become a more frequent occurrence as evidenced by the 44% of patients admitted to the INICC experiencing this procedure. Endotracheal intubation has been promoted as a replacement for tracheostomy in acute inflammatory disease of the upper airway in children.[2-4] Injuries to the supraglottic, glottic, and subglottic laryngeal area as well as tracheal injuries have been described from acute as well as long-term endotracheal intubation.[5,6] Since it is apparent that prolonged endotracheal intubation can cause permanent airway damage with subglottic stenosis being a difficult pathological entity to manage, the question then becomes what constitutes prolonged intubation. There is no consensus of opinion on this matter. Recommendations for tracheostomy as a replacement of endotracheal intubation in children range from six days to never.[6-9] Komorn *et al*[10] emphasized that laryngotracheal damage can occur at the time of intubation as well as during the presence of the tube in the airway. Hence the skill and technique utilized in initial intubation and at subsequent tube changes are very important. Mucosal ulceration with exposure of the cartilaginous framework and secondary infection resulting in cicatrix formation are probably basic in the etiology of subglottic stenosis. Utilization of endotracheal tubes which are too large can lead to pressure necrosis of the mucosa and cartilage exposure.[11] Tube shape as well as tube size have been suggested as an important factor in the production of laryngotracheal injury.[6] Another important factor is the piston action developed by the respirator attached to the endotracheal or tracheostomy tube.

Humidification is an important factor.

TABLE VIII

FACTORS IN THE PRODUCTION OF LARYNGOTRACHEAL DAMAGE

1.	Physical trauma during intubation
2.	Endotracheal tube size
3.	Endotracheal tube shape
4.	Humidification
5.	Piston action of respirator
6.	Physiologic activity of larynx and trachea
7.	Infection
8.	Underlying systemic disease
9.	Duration of intubation

One author (JLP) was called to see an infant in severe respiratory distress with a pCO_2 of 124 and marked cyanosis. The child had an endotracheal tube in place. The humidifier apparatus had malfunctioned for an unknown period of time leaving the child with no supplemental humidity. Bronchoscopy was performed and a heavy fibrinous pseudomembrane of the entire tracheobronchial tree was encountered. Brisk lavage and removal of the majority of the visible pseudomembrane was accomplished. The child had rapid improvement in her respiratory status and blood gases with eventual uneventful recovery. This experience re-emphasized the importance of constant humidity in the assisted ventilation situations.

The duration of endotracheal intubation is an important but inconstant factor. Joshi *et al*[5] reviewed 172 infants with respiratory distress syndrome and demonstrated severe lesions in 15.8% of their cases. They correlated the severity of the changes with the duration of intubation. Our results also support this concept as our more severe thick subglottic stenoses were seen in the cases of more prolonged intubation. Ferlic,[7] however, reported prolonged intubation in infants without significant laryngotracheal injury. Table VIII outlines the important factors in the production of laryngotracheal injury during assisted ventilation.

Prevention of laryngotracheal damage results from conscientious efforts to control the factors mentioned in Table VIII. When dealing with the premature infant with respiratory distress it is not often possible to use the next smaller size endotracheal tube. It is advisable in these infants to use a 0.5 mm smaller tube than a tube that fits too snugly. Hengerer *et al*[6] suggested a modification of tube shape to prevent laryngeal injury. This suggestion would possibly help if the tube could be secured so that no physiologic motion of the larynx or transmitted motion of the respirator occurred. It would seem that transmitted motion would transform a triangular shaped tube into a laryngotracheal Roto-Rooter® with an increased damage risk. With any tube it is important to attach the respirator in such a way as to minimize transmitted motion. Adequate humidification is extremely important in prevention of crusting and tube occlusion by viscous secretions. Periodic tracheal lavage with normal saline has also been found to be a helpful additional therapy.

The determination of prolonged intubation in an individual patient is difficult. Endoscopy has been performed at three to five weeks of intubation and if subglottic ulcerations or narrowing is encountered, tracheostomy is advised. Subglottic narrowing is difficult to assess as the endotracheal tube acts as a stent and the subglottic area needs to be observed for narrowing over several minutes after removal of the endotracheal tube. If no evidence of severe laryngotracheal damage is present, the endotracheal tube is replaced. This method is not foolproof. We have recently seen two patients; one had large vocal cord granulomas and unilateral subglottic ulcerations, and the other child had concentric thin subglottic narrowing. Both children were extubated prior to tracheostomy. The child with vocal cord granulomas was subjected to endoscopy two weeks later without evidence of subglottic stenosis and with marked reduction in the granulomas. The other child has not been endoscoped since extubation but functions well without a tube five weeks later. Definite criteria for prolonged intubation are difficult to define.

Two of the 15 patients tracheostomized in this study developed tracheostomy related complications. If tracheostomy is performed, prevention of complications is very important. A higher complication rate has been reported in pediatric relative to adult tracheostomies.[12] The pediatric tracheostomy should be performed with an endotracheal tube or bronchoscope in place to give the trachea rigidity and facilitate identification. This also minimizes the amount of dissection necessary. The tracheal incision has been shown to be an important factor. We now utilize mainly an inverted U tracheal flap incision as described by Lulenski.[13] Tracheal traction ties are routinely placed at the time of tracheostomy to facilitate replacement of the tracheostomy tube if accidentally dislodged prior to the establishment of a mature tracheocutaneous fistula. It is also important during this time not to use an occlusive tracheal dressing. There is frequently an air leak around the tracheostomy tube and if an occlusive dressing is present this air is forced into the cervical or thoracic tissue to cause cervical emphysema or pneumothorax or pneunomediastinum.

As with the endotracheal tube, the tracheostomy tube should be attached to the respirator in such a way as to diminish transmitted respirator motion. In the premature infant, the standard pediatric tracheostomy tubes are too long. Radiographs should be obtained to assess tube length and shortening of the standard tube is frequently necessary. If accidental extubation occurs, a small suction catheter can be threaded into the trachea and used as a guide for the replacement of the tracheostomy tube, which is slid over the catheter followed by removal of the catheter when the tracheostomy tube is in place.

What is the best technique for the treatment of subglottic stenosis when it is encountered in the infant? We have had best results with endoscopic excision or serial dilatations of the thin type stenosis. However, with the thick stenosis, excision endoscopically has not been successful. Serial dilatations have been moderately successful. Intralesion steroid injections do not seem to add much benefit in our experience. An endolaryngeal stent was successfully utilized in the treatment of one patient with congenital glottic and subglottic stenosis where simple excision did not solve the problem. We have not utilized open surgical procedures in the young children of this series. Fearon and Cotton have reported promising results with the surgical treatment of subglottic stenosis and noted no effect on the developing larynx of the monkey subjected to their procedure.[1,14,15] Prolonged endotracheal intubation with siliconized endotracheal tubes has also been reported as a successful way to treat subglottic stenosis.[16,17] We have not had experience with this technique.

The extubation or decannulation technique which we utilize has previously been described under the Results section. The endotracheal tube is utilized as a temporary stent for extubation.[18,19] Systemic steroids are given prior to and following decannulation to decrease laryngotracheal edema.[20] Positive pressure ventilating assistance by mask with recemic epinephrine is also used following extubation to decrease laryngotracheal edema.[21] Attempted decannulation is always preceded by endoscopic assessment of the anatomic patency of the airway. This technique has been most satisfactory in our experience. Decannulation should be performed as early as possible because prolonged tracheostomy may affect the growth and development of the laryngotracheal airway.[22]

CONCLUSION

Subglottic stenosis is a serious management problem in the infant. Prevention should be attempted by diminishing the factors leading to its production. The duration of intubation is an important factor but is inconstant in its effect and difficult to individualize. Thin subglottic stenosis should be excised and/or dilated with establishment of airway function. Thick subglottic stenosis is more difficult to treat. Serial dilatations and tracheostomy are currently being used pending the success of reported surgical correction techniques.

REFERENCES

1. Fearon B, Cotton R: Surgical correction of subglottic stenosis in infants and children. Ann Otol Rhinol Laryngol 83:428-431, 1974

2. Tos M: Nasotracheal intubation instead of tracheostomy in acute epiglottitis in children. Acta Otolaryngol (Stockh) 75:382-383, 1973

3. Heldtander P, Lee P: Treatment of acute epiglottitis in children by long-term intubation. Acta Otolaryngol (Stock) 75:379-381, 1973

4. Schuller DE, Berck HG: The safety of intubation in croup and epiglottitis: an eight year follow-up. Laryngoscope 85:33-46, 1975

5. Joshi VV, Mandavia SG, Stern L, *et al*: Acute lesions induced by endotracheal intubation. Am J Dis Child 124:646-649, 1972

6. Hengerer AS, Strome M, Jaffe BF: Injuries to the neonatal larynx from long-term endotracheal tube intubation and suggested tube modification for prevention. Ann Otol Rhinol Laryngol 84:764-770, 1975

7. Ferlic RM: Tracheostomy or endotracheal intubation. Ann Otol Rhinol Laryngol 83:739-743, 1974

8. Lindholm CD: Prolonged endotracheal intubation. Acta Anesthesiol Scand (Suppl) 33, 1969

9. Johnsen S: What is prolonged intubation. Acta Otolaryngol (Stockh) 75:377-378, 1973

10. Komorn RM, Smith CP, Erwin JR: Acute laryngeal injury with short term endotracheal anesthesia. Laryngoscope 83:683-690, 1973

11. Strome E, Ferguson CF: Multiple postintubation complications. Ann Otol Rhinol Laryngol 83:432-438, 1974

12. Chew JY, Cantrell RW: Tracheostomy: complications and their management. Arch Otolaryngol 96:538-545, 1972

13. Lulenski GC, Batsakis JG: Tracheal incision as a contributing factor to tracheal stenosis. Ann Otol Rhinol Laryngol 84:781-786, 1975

14. Fearon B, Cotton R: Subglottic stenosis in infants and children: the clinical problem and experimental correction. Can J Otolaryngol 1:281-289, 1972

15. Fearon B, Cotton R: Surgical correction of subglottic stenosis of the larynx. Ann Otol Rhinol Laryngol 81;1-6, 1972

16. Bos CE, Berkovits RNP, Struben WH: Wider application of prolonged nasotracheal intubation. J Laryngol Otol 87:263-279, 1973

17. Andersen HC, Elbrond O, Geisen O: Treatment of tracheal stenosis. J Laryngol Otol 88:615-624, 1974

18. Greenberg LM, Davenport HT, Shimo G: Method for difficult decannulations in children. Arch Otolaryngol 81:72-76, 1965

19. Crysdale WS: Nasotracheal intubation in management of delayed decannulation. Ann Otol Rhinol Laryngol 83:802-809, 1974

20. Biller HF, Bone RC, Harvey JE, *et al*: Laryngeal edema: an experimental study. Laryngoscope 70:1084-1087, 1970

21. Jordan WS, Graves CL, Elwyn RA: New therapy for postintubation laryngeal edema and tracheitis in children. JAMA 212: 585-588, 1970

22. Freeland AP, Wright JLW, Ardan GM: Developmental influences of infant tracheostomy. J Laryngol Otol 88:927-936, 1974

REPRINTS—James L. Parkin, MD, Division of Otolaryngology, University of Utah College of Medicine, Salt Lake City, UT 84112.

ESSAY CONTEST

Ann Otol 85: 1976

TRACHEOSTENOSIS AND BRONCHIAL ABNORMALITIES ASSOCIATED WITH PULMONARY ARTERY SLING

Seymour R. Cohen, MD

Benjamin H. Landing, MD

Los Angeles, California

SUMMARY – Three patients with aberrant left pulmonary artery (sling artery) are reported to illustrate associated tracheobronchial abnormalities. The clinical picture was that of severe episodic or progressive respiratory distress without dysphagia in early infancy. Striking narrowing of the trachea by complete "ring cartilages," unrelated to compression by the abnormal pulmonary artery, was present. Tracheotomy and intubation failed to relieve the obstruction. In one patient the bronchi and bronchial segmentation pattern were normal, but in the other two patients, bronchial abnormalities included wide irregular cartilages in the main bronchi, forming more complete rings than is normal. In both, the right main bronchus was relatively longer than normal, and the bronchus intermedius showed poor cartilage ring formation and was relatively short compared to the main bronchus. This discrepancy did not appear to be due to distal displacement of the right upper lobe bronchus. In these two patients the left main bronchus was relatively short and wide with reduced number of cartilage rings (five-six vs usual normal number of nine), so that the right and left main bronchi were almost of equal length. However, the branch patterns of the lobar bronchi were within normal range. Bronchoscopy seems essential to demonstrate such ring tracheal cartilages (absence of the pars membranacea of the trachea), which when found should alert the examiner to the possible presence of an abnormal left pulmonary artery. Since surgical correction of tracheal stenosis of this type is not possible at present, the ultimate prognosis of patients with sling artery may depend more on the severity of the tracheal anomaly rather than on success of surgical correction of the abnormal left pulmonary arterial course. Although aberrant (sling) left pulmonary artery can occur in patients without respiratory tract symptoms, tracheal stenosis due to ring tracheal cartilages occurs in a significant fraction of patients with this arterial anomaly. Bronchoscopic study of the trachea, and possibly air or contrast bronchography of right and left main bronchi, can be of aid in diagnosis of this complex.

Three patients with aberrant left pulmonary artery (pulmonary artery sling) are reported to illustrate the tracheobronchial abnormalities which frequently occur in association with this condition. All three patients had diffuse tracheal stenosis from complete cartilage rings, with absence of the pars membranacea of the trachea. Bronchial ring cartilages, and other abnormalities of bronchial anatomy were also present. In only one of the patients was the sling or retrotracheal left pulmonary artery diagnosed clinically, and none had surgical correction of the arterial defect. The airway obstruction secondary to the tracheal cartilage anomaly was so severe as to preclude successful relief by surgery on the artery, and the obstructive phenomena were not relieved, in any of the three patients, by intubation or tracheotomy. Although airway obstruction associated with congenital abnormalities of the aortic arch and associated arteries is well known to otolaryngologists, pediatricians, and cardiovascular surgeons, the rarer pulmonary artery sling has not been reported in the otolaryngologic literature, although extensively reviewed in other

---

From the Departments of Surgery (Division of Otolaryngology) and Pathology, Childrens Hospital of Los Angeles, and University of Southern California School of Medicine, Los Angeles, California. Funding of the technical assistance was received from Childrens Hospital of Los Angeles General Research Support Grant.

Presented at the meeting of the American Broncho-Esophagological Association, Palm Beach, Florida, April 27-28, 1976.

specialty journals. These patients with tracheal stenosis and sling left pulmonary artery are reported to alert the otolaryngologists to this association. The findings of a stenotic trachea, with complete cartilaginous rings, should alert the endoscopist to the possibility of pulmonary artery sling, and may indicate a poor prognosis despite surgical correction of the arterial defect.

The anatomy of the pulmonary artery sling has been described in detail, but not so well known are the tracheobronchial abnormalities which can be associated with this vascular anomaly, and which may make correction of the arterial defect disappointing.

REVIEW OF LITERATURE

The first description of retrotracheal course of the left pulmonary artery was by Glaevecke and Doehle, in 1897.[1] Wolman[2] in 1941 reported a patient with congenital tracheal stenosis due to ring tracheal cartilages. An oblique groove seen just above the bifurcation, typical of that seen with anomalous left pulmonary artery, was ascribed by the author to a left pulmonary vein. A tracheotomy had failed to relieve obstruction in this patient. Wolman stated that the major bronchi possessed the normal pattern but were unusually narrow. Contro *et al*, in 1958[3] coined the term "vascular sling," rather than "vascular ring," to avoid confusion with more common systemic arterial malformations, causing constriction of the trachea and esophagus.

In 1975 66 patients with sling artery were reviewed by Koopot *et al.*[4] Nineteen survived surgery, 27 died during or after surgery, and 13 were diagnosed at autopsy. Seven with pulmonary artery sling diagnosed angiographically did not undergo surgical treatment, because of the mild character of their symptoms. Jue *et al*,[5] reviewing 23 necropsied patients, found that one-half had died by six months of age, and 85% before the age of one year. In contrast to other vascular anomalies (rings, not slings), where the prognosis with early diagnosis and surgical repair is excellent, the outcome of sling pulmonary artery is uncertain even with early surgical intervention, in good part because of the tracheobronchial abnormalities.

EMBRYOLOGY

Controversy and speculation surround the embryology of the anomalous retrotracheal left pulmonary artery.[5-7] Anomalies of arterial vessels may result from persistence of vessels which normally recede in fetal life.

The fetal lung bud, at the 4-5 mm stage, separates from the foregut. At this time, the sixth pair of branchial arch arteries appears on a level with the cranial portion of the lung bud. An artery plexus then develops around the foregut and the lung bud, and the tracheoesophageal septum appears on each side at the 5-8 mm stage. It is difficult to imagine how the left sixth arch artery, or its descending pulmonic branch, could develop to the right of the trachea. It appears more reasonable to assume that the pulmonary artery branch from the left sixth aortic arch failed to develop, or having formed, became obliterated at an early stage. The anomalous left pulmonary artery then develops from collateral vessels from the fetal mediastinal arterial plexus connecting the two lung hila. This may account for the course of the artery between the trachea and esophagus, which has been interpreted as origin of the left pulmonary artery from the right.[5-7] It is possible that the abnormalities of the trachea and bronchi can be explained by abnormality of their fetal blood supply. The exact cause of the abnormal development of the airways and the left pulmonary artery requires further embryological study.

CLINICAL DESCRIPTION

The symptoms of an aberrant left pulmonary artery are dependent on the extent of compression or tenting of the trachea and bronchi, on the severity of tracheal stenosis when it is present, and perhaps at times on bronchial abnormality. Symptoms usually start in the immediate neonatal period, with episodic respiratory distress, often precipitated by upper respiratory infection. Inspiratory and expiratory stridor can be heard with severe dyspnea, and periods of cyanosis, suprasternal and xyphoid retractions, and wheezing, with prolongation of the expiratory phase of respiration, may occur. When tracheal stenosis is severe, bilateral air-trapping may be a presenting finding, and when the right bronchus is tented or compressed without tracheal stenosis, the right lung may be hyperresonant, or there may be diminished aeration and pneumonia. With pulmonary infection, rales, rhonchi, and systemic signs of infection occur. The episodic course usually increases in severity as the child grows older. In contrast to vascular rings, dysphagia from esophageal obstruction is not a symptom of sling artery.

PATHOLOGY

Characteristically, the aberrant left pulmonary artery arises from the right pulmonary artery, turns backward over the right mainstem bronchus, and passes posteriorly between the trachea and esophagus to the left. Compression of the tracheobronchial tree occurs, and there is indentation of the anterior wall of the esophagus. This indentation is essentially characteristic of this abnormality. Although passage of an anomalous subclavian artery between the trachea and esophagus is reported,[8] this must be extremely rare, and vascular rings do not produce anterior indentation of the esophagus.

ROENTGENOGRAPHIC FINDINGS

The esophagram reveals anterior indentation of the esophagus, above the level of the carina, in many cases. Obstructive emphysema of one or both lungs depends on the degrees of tracheal compression and tracheobronchial abnormality. Right main bronchus compression may cause obstructive emphysema of all or part of the right lung. Angiocardiograms can demonstrate the course of the anomalous left pulmonary artery, and lateral views of the airway will frequently demonstrate the narrowed trachea. The trachea and esophagus may be separated by an apparent mass, at the level of, or just above, the tracheal bifurcation. The mediastinum may be shifted if differential air-trapping occurs, and unilateral or bilateral pulmonary infiltrates may be present.

ENDOSCOPY

Bronchoscopy shows tracheal stenosis and the abnormal "ring" cartilages. When the stenosis is severe, the bronchoscope cannot be passed to the level of the carina. When the trachea is normal, compression of the right main stem bronchus may be noted. Bronchoscopy must be carried out with great caution, and a bronchoscope should not be passed through a trachea with stenosis due to absence of the pars membranacea, unless a tracheotomy is planned.

CASE REPORTS

Case 1. On her first admission to the hospital at nine months of age, on December 19, 1974, this Caucasian female had a history of having wheezed all her life, and of having numerous cyanotic episodes, between which stridorous breathing, made worse by stress, was present. She was the product of a full term, uncomplicated pregnancy; delivery was normal, and there were no neonatal complications. She had fed well, but had failed to gain weight, weighing 6.5 kg at the time of admission. She had been hospitalized elsewhere, at four months of age, when she was treated with positive pressure breathing and antibiotics.

On admission, the child was alert, but in moderately severe distress, with prolonged inspiration, deep intercostal and sternal retractions, and to-and-fro stridor. The remainder of her examination was completely normal. Review of x-rays taken at a second hospitalization elsewhere showed hyperlucency of the left lung, with normal heart and mediastinal structures. Faint infiltrates were seen in the right perihilar region. Multiple spot films from an esophagram showed good esophageal distention, with no evidences of compression or displacement. Lateral views of the chest showed the tracheal air column to be markedly narrowed inferiorly.

Direct laryngoscopy, performed on the day of her admission, showed the larynx to be moderately inflamed, with slight subglottic swelling. Through the laryngoscope severe tracheal stenosis could be seen, starting at the laryngotracheal junction, with the lumen of the trachea funneling down and showing a concentric narrowing, suggesting ring tracheal cartilages. Bronchoscopy was not performed to avoid increasing her airway obstruction. Decadron®*, antibiotics, and humidification cleared her airway obstruction remarkably, and direct larnygoscopy on December 23, 1974, showed improvement of the inflammatory process, but persistence of the tracheal stenosis. She was discharged on December 24, 1974, and was again hospitalized on January 31, 1975 because of severe airway obstruction. X-rays of the chest revealed bilateral pneumonia involving the right lower and left upper lung fields. By February 3, 1975, clearing of the pneumonia had occurred, but, on lateral view, the tracheal air column continued to be narrowed and slightly lobulated. There was a suggestion of slight anterior displacement of the trachea just above the level of the carina, but no mass lesion was seen. She was readmitted to Childrens Hospital on February 7, 1975, with persistence of respiratory obstructive disease. An elective tracheotomy was planned on February 10, 1975. A 3 mm bronchoscope would not pass beyond the level of the third tracheal ring, and complete ring stenosis and severely hypoplastic trachea were noted. A tracheotomy was performed, but only a 3-0 Holinger tube could be passed into the markedly stenotic trachea. The airway was barely adequate, but she did well for a number of hours, when respiratory assistance became necessary. With the high pressures necessary, pneumomediastinum and pneumothorax developed. These were relieved by a chest tube, but respiratory acidosis developed, and the child expired in cardiopulmonary arrest on February 14, 1975.

Autopsy showed the left pulmonary artery to arise from the trunk farther to the right than normal, and to pass posterior to the lower trachea, between the trachea and esophagus, to the left lung (sling left pulmonary artery). The trachea showed diffuse absence of the pars membranacea (complete cartilage rings), with diffuse narrowing of the lumen, more severely so inferiorly; a tracheostomy had been performed. Additional findings included an anomalous left superior vena cava, a Meckel's diverticulum of the small intestine, and fatty metamorphosis of the liver.

Case 2. A 2-month-old Caucasian male was admitted on September 24, 1963 with gradually increasing respiratory distress and stridor. Birth had been complicated by a frank breech delivery. Respiratory distress in the immediate neonatal period cleared with removal of secretions, but three weeks prior to admission, respiratory distress, gasping cough, and cyanosis developed, and he was admitted for treatment of a suspected mediastinal tumor. On admission he was a well-developed child with marked sternal retractions, inspiratory and expiratory stridor, and respiratory distress. He fed well, but slowly. The remainder of his physical examination and the laboratory findings were all normal. X-rays of the chest and esophagus revealed displacement of the trachea and esophagus to the right, and posteriorly. No masses were visualized, but a mediastinal mass was suspected, and on September 25, 1963 exploratory thoracotomy was performed. A persistent left superior vena cava was found and the aorta descended in the midline rather than on the left. A large ligamentum arteriosum, with a small lumen, was divided. When the superior mediastinum was opened the trachea was noted to be quite small, and to be attached to the esophagus by a fibrous band. The band was divided, and the trachea was left free in the mediastinum. No obstructing vascular struc-

* Merck Sharp & Dohme, West Point, PA.

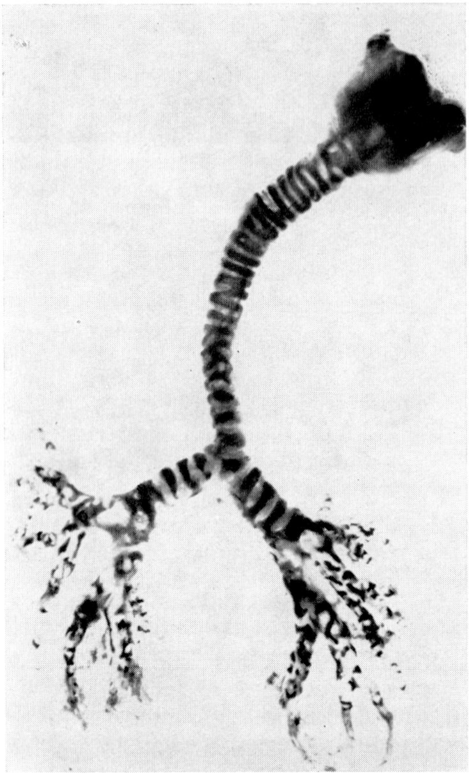

Fig. 1. Dissected, stained and cleared tracheobronchial specimen from patient No. 1, showing narrow trachea, from diffuse stenosis due to ring tracheal cartilages (absence of the pars membranacea of the trachea), and essentially equal length of right and left main bronchi, due to increased number of large widely-spaced cartilage rings in the right main bronchus, and reduced number of cartilages in the left main bronchus. The pattern of the lobar bronchi is normal. (Compare to Fig. 4.)

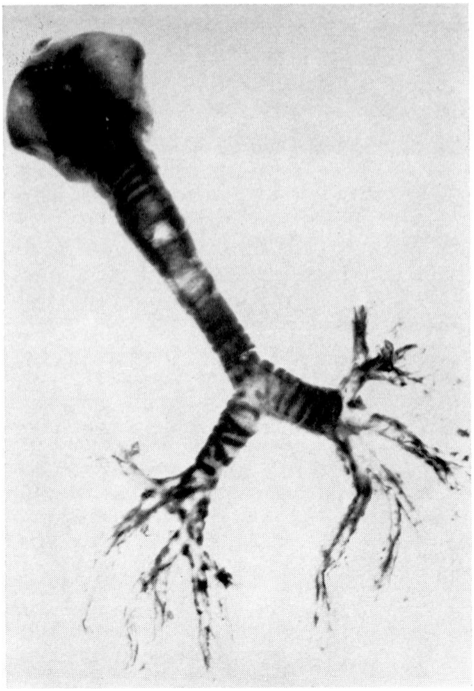

Fig. 2. Dissected, stained and cleared tracheobronchial specimen from patient No. 3, showing equal length of right and left main bronchi, the former being longer than normal and the latter shorter (compare to Fig. 4). The trachea shows narrowing from above downward, due to stenosis from ring cartilages. Lobar bronchial branch pattern is normal.

tures or mediastinal masses could be found. Postoperatively the child continued to have distress, and bronchoscopy was performed by the thoracic surgeon, who found the right main stem bronchus to be normal, while the left could not be visualized. A tracheotomy was performed, after intubation was necessary to relieve the severe obstruction and an episode of cardiopulmonary arrest. The airway obstruction was not relieved and progressive respiratory acidosis followed. The patient expired on September 27, 1963.

Autopsy showed a sling left pulmonary artery, and diffuse tracheal stenosis with complete cartilage rings and absence of the pars membranacea. A tracheotomy had been performed, and a patent ductus arteriosus had been ligated. The lungs showed chronic pneumonitis, and focal pulmonary hemorrhage. The brain was edematous, and there was an early Cushing's ulcer of the duodenum. An anomalous left superior vena cava was present.

Case 3. A white male was first admitted, age 12 hours, for evaluation of a firm, oval 3 x 4 cm right abdominal mass. Excretory urogram showed multiple cystic structures, with a faint superior rim of calcification, on the right, and moderate left hydronephrosis due to uretero-vesical obstruction. Right nephrectomy was performed at age three days; the kidney showed medul-

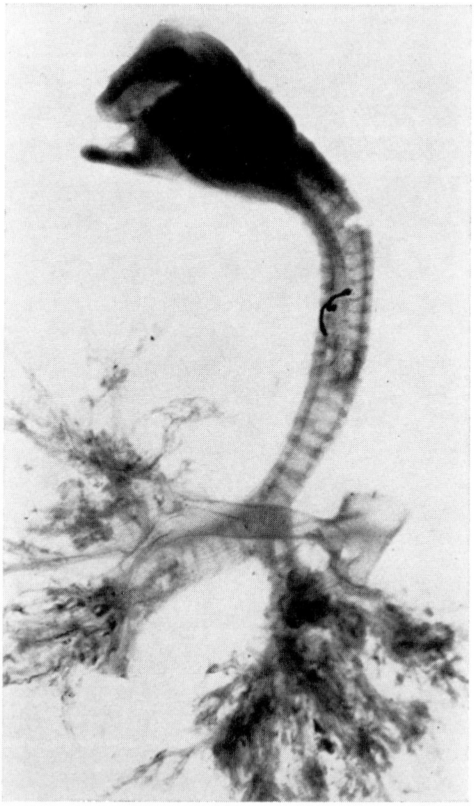

Fig. 3. Dissected and cleared tracheobronchial tree of patient No. 2, showing narrow trachea from stenosis due to ring tracheal cartilages. Proportions of right and left main bronchi, and bronchial branch patterns, are normal. The left pulmonary artery can be seen running behind the carina, from the right to the hilum of the left lung.

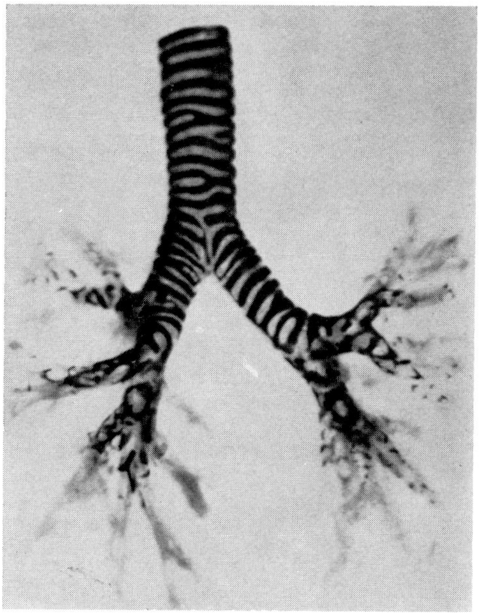

Fig. 4. Dissected, stained and cleared tracheobronchial specimen of newborn infant, showing normal anatomy of right and left main bronchi, and of trachea.

lary and cortical dysplasia, and multiple caliceal cysts. Postoperatively, he had oral thrush, and an episode of wound infection. Chest x-ray at this time showed overexpansion of the left lung, with mediastinal shift to the right. Cystogram showed right ureteral reflux with fistula-formation, and partial ureteral resection, urethral dilatation, and suprapubic cystotomy were performed. Laryngoscopy, performed for respiratory distress, was interpreted as showing a subglottic laryngeal web, but the respiratory distress subsided after several days and he was discharged aged four weeks. He was readmitted ten days later because of obstruction of the suprapubic catheter, but then did well for four months. At this time, respiratory difficulty for 24 hours was followed by cardiorespiratory arrest. He was resuscitated in the emergency room, and given epinephrine, sodium bicarbonate and calcium chloride; cardiac rhythm was restored, but respiratory effort was not, and he was placed on a respirator, with difficulty on intubation. He had poor air exchange, with diminished breath sounds; x-rays showed atelectasis of the right lower lobe, and overexpansion of the left lung. Bronchoscopy was attempted, but was unsuccessful because of tracheal stenosis, and tracheotomy was performed. However, coma persisted despite mannitol infusion, and the day after admission, alkalosis, elevated blood urea nitrogen and potassium levels, and isoelectric EEG were followed by cardiac arrest.

Autopsy showed a sling left pulmonary artery, and diffuse tracheal stenosis, with absence of the pars membranacea. The right kidney and adrenal had been removed surgically, and a tracheostomy had been performed. The

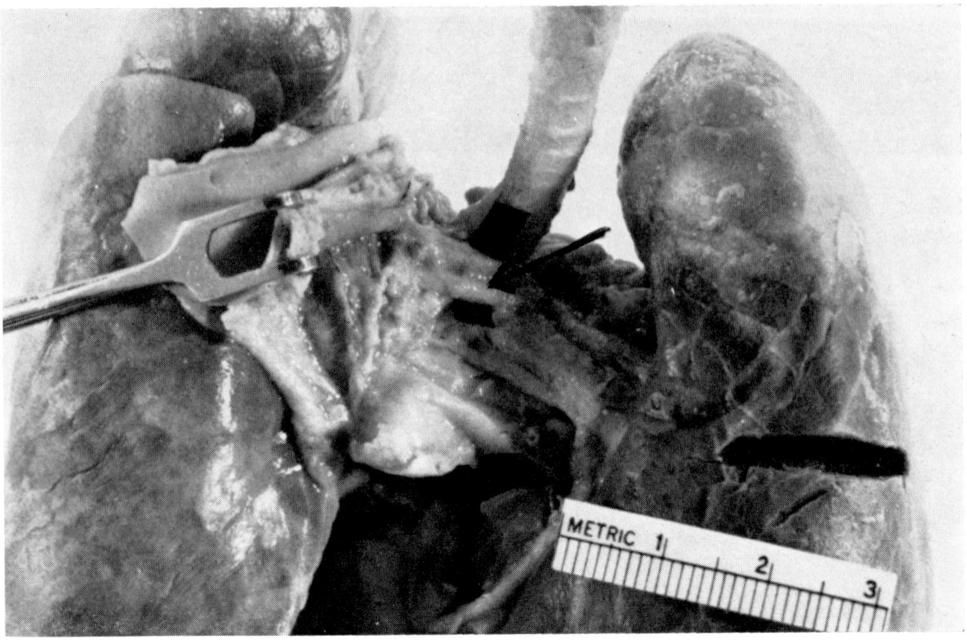

Fig. 5. Posterior view of autopsy specimen showing the right pulmonary artery passing behind the trachea (arrow). The esophagus is retracted.

lungs showed diffuse acute bronchopneumonia, as well as chronic aspiration pneumonitis. The left kidney showed hydroureter and hydronephrosis, and there was a Meckel's diverticulum of the small intestine. The brain showed diffuse severe ischemic neuronal necrosis.

PATHOLOGIC STUDIES

The tracheobronchial trees of the three patients were dissected (Figs. 1-3), and the two for which preservation was appropriate (the specimen had been kept in formalin less than three years) were stained with toluidine blue and cleared (Figs. 1, 2); the third was cleared without staining. This third specimen (from patient No. 2) showed normal bronchial branch pattern, with a normally long left main bronchus, and with the normally short right main bronchus giving rise to the eparterial bronchus to the right upper lobe, and to the intermediate bronchus, which in turn gave origin to the right middle and lower lobe bronchi (Fig. 3). The specimens from patients 1 and 3, however, showed similar abnormalities, with wide relatively irregular cartilages in the main bronchi (Figs. 1, 2); these cartilages formed more complete rings than is normal for main bronchi, so that the deficiency of pars membranacea seen in the tracheas also affected the main bronchi. In both these patients the right main bronchus was relatively long, with five rings (the most common number in normal patients is four), the relatively increased length of this segment also resulting from the wide spaces between the cartilages (compared to Fig. 4). In both specimens also, the bronchus intermedius showed poor cartilage ring-formation, and was relatively short compared to the right main bronchus, but this discrepancy in proportion did not appear to be due to distal displacement of the origin of the right upper lobe bronchus. In both patients, the left main bronchus was relatively short and wide, with reduced number of cartilage rings (five and six versus usual normal number of nine), so that right and left main bronchi were almost equal in length. However, in both, the branch patterns of the lobar bronchi were within normal range. This bronchial pattern, with right and left main bronchi more equal in size and length than normal, but with normal lobar bronchial branch pattern, has not been described before, to our knowledge. It differs from the symmetrical bronchial pattern, with bilaterally short main bronchi (pulmonary isomerism of right lung type; "bilateral right lung") seen in the Ivemark asplenia syndrome and in m-anisosplenia,[9] and from the symmetrical bronchial pattern with long main bronchi (pulmonary somerism of left-lung type; "bilateral left lung") seen in the polysplenia syndrome and in f-anisosplenia.[9] It also differs from the pattern found in the scimitar syndrome, where the eparterial right upper lobe bronchus may be absent, and from the pattern found in a patient reported by Landing and Wells,[10] who had a hyparterial right upper lobe bronchus and absence of the right middle lobe.

DISCUSSION

The high frequency of association of diffuse tracheal stenosis due to ring tracheal cartilages (absence of the pars membranacea of the trachea) with sling left pulmonary artery (also called "origin of the left pulmonary artery from the right") has been noted previously. The additional bronchial anomalies found in some patients with this complex, as reported here, may be of importance from two aspects:

1. Implications as regards surgical treatment of diffuse tracheal stenosis. That some patients with the complex of diffuse tracheal stenosis due to ring tracheal cartilage and sling left pulmonary artery improve little, if at all, following surgical correction of the anomalous retrotracheal course of the left main pulmonary artery, it has been noted by others, and it has been proposed that this poor response results from the fact that the tracheal stenosis may be more the result of the abnormal cartilages than of pressure on the lower trachea and carinal region by the abnormal artery. Surgical treatment of such tracheal stenosis is theoretically, even if not at present technically, possible. Bronchial stenosis, from the more complete cartilage rings in the main bronchi than normal, may possibly also occur in such patients, and be a cause of continued respiratory tract obstruction after successful enlargement of the tracheal lumen. On the other hand, in the specimens from both patients 1 and 3 described above, the calibers of the right and left main bronchi, at least externally, look more normal than does the caliber of the lower trachea.

2. Diagnostic implications. Although sling left pulmonary artery is ordinarily recognizable by x-ray, the course of the vessel between the lower trachea and the esophagus being demonstrable in lateral x-rays, this is not always the case (patients 2 and 3 above). Demonstration that a patient with tracheal stenosis has such an abnormal artery is thus of value, in indicating that the patient probably has diffuse tracheal stenosis due to ring tracheal cartilages, and thereby influencing both surgical and nonsurgical treatment. The "pseudoisomerism" of the main bronchi described in this paper, with the relatively long right and relatively short left main bronchi giving a more symmetrical bronchial pattern than normal, can theoretically be of aid, in suggesting the basic diagnosis in a patient with sling left pulmonary artery and tracheal stenosis due to ring tracheal cartilages. Establishment of the practicability of demonstration of this pattern by air or contrast bronchography, and determination of the exact frequency of this bronchial pattern in patients with the syndrome under discussion will require further experience.

REFERENCES

1. Glaevecke H, Doehle H: Uber eine selte angeborne Anomalie der Pulmonalartsie. Munchen Med Wochenschr 44:950-951, 1897

2. Wolman IJ: Congenital stenosis of the trachea. Am J Dis Child 61:1263-1271, 1941

3. Contro S, Miller RA, White H, *et al*: Bronchial obstruction due to pulmonary artery anomalies. I. Vascular sling. Circulation 17: 418, 1958

4. Koopot R, Nikaidoh H, Idriss FS: Sur-

gical management of anomalous left pulmonary artery causing tracheobronchial obstruction. J Thorac Cardiovasc Surg 69:239-246, 1975

5. Jue KL, Raghib G, Arnplatz K, *et al*: Anomalous origin of the left pulmonary from the right pulmonary artery. Am J Roentgenol Radium Ther Nucl Med 95:598-610, 1965

6. Wittenborg MH, Tantiwongsi T, Rosenberg BF: Anomalous course of left pulmonary artery with respiratory obstruction. Radiology 67:339-345, 1956

7. Quist-Hanssen SV: Mutual compression of the right main bronchus and an abnormal left pulmonary artery as causes for death of a 7 week old child. Acta Paediatr Scand 37: 87-94, 1949

8. Beabout JW, Stewart JR, Kincaid OW: Aberrant right subclavian artery: Dispute of commonly accepted concepts. Am J Roentgenol Radium Ther Nucl Med 92:855-858, 1964

9. Landing BH, Lawrence TYK, Payne VC, *et al*: Bronchial anatomy in syndromes with abnormal visceral situs, abnormal spleen and congenital heart disease. Am J Cardiol 28:456-462, 1971

10. Landing BH, Wells TR: Tracheobronchial anomalies in children, in Rosenberg HS, Bolande RP (eds): *Perspectives in Pediatric Pathology*. Chicago, Year Book Medical Publishers: 1973, pp 1-32

ACKNOWLEDGMENT—The authors wish to thank Lianne G. Dixon, HT (ASCP) for her technical assistance.

REPRINTS—S. R. Cohen, MD, 1300 North Vermont Ave., Los Angeles, CA 90027.

PEDIATRIC OTOLARYNGIC PATHOLOGY SEMINAR

The Armed Forces Institute of Pathology, Washington, D.C. in conjunction with the Committee on Otolaryngic Pathology, AAOO, will sponsor a seminar in Pediatric Otolaryngic Pathology, December 6-8, 1976.

The purpose of this course is to update information in the fields of embryology, congenital diseases, inflammatory and neoplastic pathology of the pediatric otolaryngic area.

Requests for further information and for course applications should be directed to: The Director, Armed Forces Institute of Pathology, ATTN: AFIP-EDZ, Washington, DC 20306.

Ann Otol 85: 1976

SUBGLOTTIC STENOSIS IN INFANTS AND CHILDREN

PAUL H. HOLINGER, MD STEVEN L. KUTNICK, MD

JOYCE A. SCHILD, MD LAUREN D. HOLINGER, MD

CHICAGO, ILLINOIS

SUMMARY – Of 158 cases of subglottic stenosis 115 were congenital and 43 acquired. Current follow-up has been obtained in 146 (92%) which constitutes the determinate group. Although stridor was the most common presenting symptom of the congenital group, 34% presented with recurrent or prolonged episodes of croup. Tracheotomy was required in 47 of the 107 determinate cases (44%). Further management of the congenital cases was based on the experience that children outgrow this disorder; periodic dilatation may augment the natural process. Of those infants and children tracheotomized, all but five have been decannulated, and there was one death – a mortality rate of 2.1%. Acquired subglottic stenosis proved to be a more difficult management problem. Tracheotomy was necessary in 38 of the 39 determinate cases (97%). Repeated active dilatations for prolonged periods were usually required as well as endoscopic removal of granulation tissue. Of those infants and children tracheotomized, all but eight have been decannulated. There were nine deaths; five were due to unrelated underlying disease; four were attributable to complications of long-term tracheostomy. Thus, in the entire series, 85 infants and children required tracheotomy and five deaths may be attributable to long-term tracheostomy complications – a mortality rate of 5.9%.

Subglottic stenosis in infants and children may be congenital or acquired. Congenital subglottic stenosis is the third most common congenital laryngeal anomaly; only laryngomalacia and recurrent laryngeal nerve paralysis are seen more often.[1] It is the most common congenital laryngeal lesion that produces serious respiratory distress and constitutes the largest single group of anomalies requiring tracheotomy under one year of age.[2,3] As neonatal survival has improved in the newly developed pediatric intensive care units, more cases of acquired subglottic stenosis are being recognized. This study was undertaken in order to better define this condition and to evaluate its management and prognosis.

METHODS AND MATERIALS

One hundred fifty-eight consecutive cases of subglottic stenosis were evaluated at The Children's Memorial Hospital Division of Bronchology during the ten-year period from January 1, 1965 through December 31, 1974. Infants and children with subglottic edema following one acute episode of croup or endotracheal intubation were excluded from the study. The diagnosis was confirmed endoscopically in all cases; by definition subglottic stenosis was considered present when a 3 mm infant bronchoscope could not pass easily through the subglottic region. Current follow-up has been obtained in 146 patients (92%), which constitute the determinate group.

CONGENITAL SUBGLOTTIC STENOSIS

Subglottic stenosis was considered to be congenital in the absence of a history of prolonged endotracheal intubation or other apparent cause. This diagnosis was made in 115 infants and children during the ten-year period, and current follow-up is available in 107 cases (93%).

The symptoms of congenital subglottic stenosis were not always present at birth or in the neonatal period, but they usually became evident during the first few weeks or months of life. Stridor, the most common initial symptom, was present in 49 infants and children (43% of the cases). This was often associated

---

From the Department of Bronchology, The Children's Memorial Hospital, and the Department of Otolaryngology and Maxillofacial Surgery, Northwestern University Medical School, Chicago, Illinois.

Presented at the meeting of the American Broncho-Esophagological Association, Palm Beach, Florida, April 27-28, 1976.

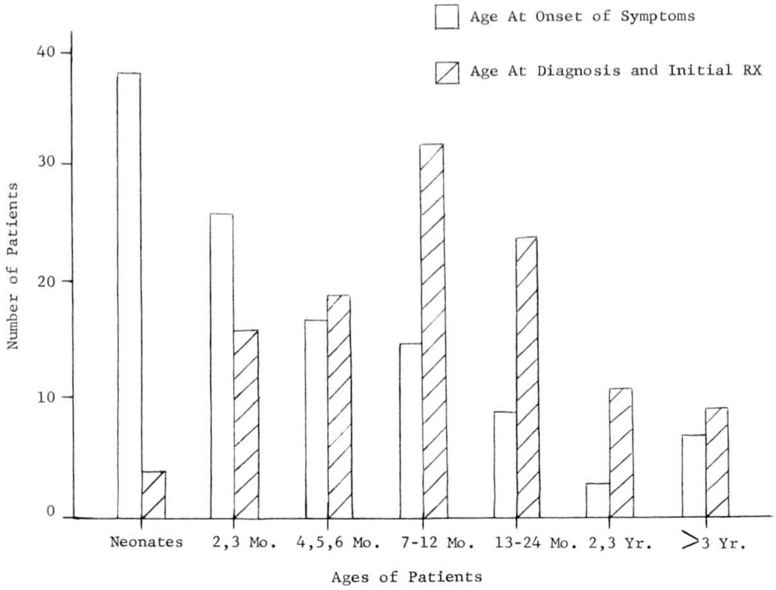

Fig. 1. Congenital subglottic stenosis (115 cases).

with dyspnea, a barking or brassy cough, or hoarseness. The stridor usually had an expiratory as well as inspiratory component. A prolonged episode of croup was the initial manifestation in 21 patients (18%); 19 others (17%) had recurrent episodes of croup. Eleven (9.6%) presented with a history of one or several episodes of pneumonitis or atelectasis. Eight patients (7%) had persistent, postextubation stridor following a short general anesthetic for elective surgery of less than three hours duration; interestingly, five of these eight had a history of previous episodes of croup, implying a preexisting congenital lesion. Three infants (2.6%) presented with episodes of cyanosis. Noisy breathing, a barking cough, or a hoarse cry without obstructive symptoms were present in another four children (3.5%).

The age of onset of symptoms ranged from the neonatal period up to ten years of age (Fig. 1). Symptoms generally began in the first few months of life. The age at diagnosis and initial treatment usually followed the age of onset of symptoms by several months. Males predominated in this series two to one; there were 77 males and 38 females. Sixty percent of these infants and children were white, 25% were black and 15% were of Latin origin.

Associated laryngeal and tracheobronchial pathologic findings were present in 15 patients: five had laryngomalacia; three had an anterior glottic web; two had tracheomalacia; two had a concomitant tracheal stenosis; two had tracheoesophageal fistulae; and one had a right cord paralysis.

Congenital defects not related to the larynx, trachea, or esophagus were present in 14 patients. There were five cases of imperforate anus; two cases of cleft palate; one each of congenital rubella, congenital hypothyroidism, cystic fibrosis, hydrocephalus, meningomyelocele, familial neutropenia, and craniosynostosis.

The diagnosis was confirmed endoscopically in all cases. Instrumentation of the subglottic region was avoided if the airway was marginal and a tracheotomy was not planned. The most frequent endoscopic finding was a circumferential subglottic stenosis which occurred in 94 patients (82% of the congenital cases). This usually appeared as a soft tissue narrowing that

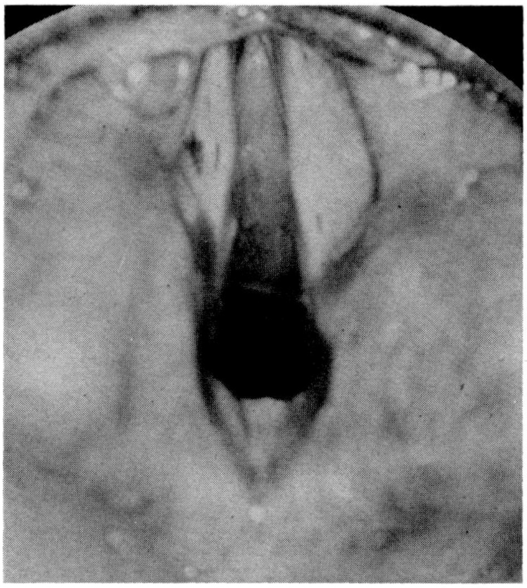

Fig. 2. Congenital subglottic stenosis — anterior narrowing.

extended approximately from the level of the cords to the cricoid area (Fig. 2). The point of greatest obstruction was generally 2-3 mm below the superior surface of the true vocal cords. An isolated anterior wall or posterior wall prominence was present in six cases each, and an oval anterior-posterior slit in five. The left subglottic area was prominent in three cases and the right in one. The subglottic narrowing was generally quite firm, but on occasion soft and easy to dilate. It is possible that in the six cases of anterior wall prominence the subglottic stenosis may have represented an abnormal cricoid cartilage.[2]

Management was based on the experience that children outgrow congenital subglottic stenosis. Progress was evaluated by direct laryngoscopy at three to four month intervals. Gentle periodic dilatation was often helpful; well lubricated, round standard tracheal dilators were employed. Only 37 patients (32%) needed more than one dilatation. Tracheotomy was required in 47 patients in the determinate group (44%). The smallest tracheostomy tube that would permit adequate ventilation was used to allow preservation of the function of the larynx and to permit the development of speech. In those children requiring tracheotomy prior to 1974 (40 cases), all but one has been decannulated, and in the entire group (47 cases) all but five have been decannulated. The one child with long-term tracheostomy is mentally retarded and needs frequent aspiration of secretions because of paralysis of cranial nerves IX and X. Tracheostomy was required for an average of 18 months and decannulation was usually achieved by age three or four.

There was one death in this group of congenital subglottic stenosis during the ten-year period. This infant developed stridor and cyanosis during the first week of life, and had a tracheotomy at 12 days of age for a severe circumferential subglottic stenosis. There had been no problems with the tracheostomy or its management, but at eight weeks of age the infant was found dead in his crib.

Discussion of Congenital Subglottic Stenosis. Theories regarding the origin of congenital subglottic stenosis should be firmly based on the embryology of the larynx, and a brief review is necessary. The larynx develops between the fourth and tenth weeks of fetal life. A longitudinal groove develops in the midventral wall of the primitive pharynx in the 3 mm embryo (26 days). This gives rise to a tubular outgrowth which is the anlage of the entire respiratory tract.[4] The larynx develops as a differentiation of the mesoderm surrounding the upper end of this respiratory primordium.[5,6] At five to six weeks the early epiglottis lies anteriorly and the anlage of the arytenoid cartilages lie laterally, forming a T-shaped primitive glottis. In the seven-week embryo there is marked epithelial proliferation around the glottis, obliterating the lumen for a short time. At nine weeks, recanalization occurs, and the lumen is reestablished. Failure to recanalize completely may result in atresia, webs, or stenosis in the larynx and trachea.[7] An increased incidence of associated laryngotracheal abnormalities might be expected when one area is affected. In this series, congenital subglottic stenosis was associated with three cases of anterior glottic webs, two cases of tracheal stenosis, and two cases of tracheoesophageal fistula.

The subglottic region of the larynx is formed by the conus elasticus and the rigid circumferential cricoid ring. The conus elasticus is bounded by the free edge of the true cords above and the upper border of the cricoid cartilage below. The submucosal structures are composed of loose areolar tissue which is lined by respiratory epithelium. The normal size of the subglottic lumen in a full term newborn has been studied repeatedly. In 1932, Tucker[8] determined the normal diameter to be 6 mm. He considered 5 mm small but compatible with life, and 4 mm a definite stenosis. In 1953, Wilson[9] noted that 4.5-5 mm was the normal range. In 1972, a study of autopsy material at the University of Toronto[10] indicated that the normal cartilaginous diameter was 5.5 mm, and the effective or intramucosal diameter 4.5 mm. It was also determined that the anterior-posterior dimension is often slightly longer than the lateral dimension. For the purposes of this study, subglottic stenosis was considered present in a full-term newborn when a 3 mm infant bronchoscope could not pass readily through the subglottic region. This bronchoscope has an inner diameter (ID) of 3 mm; the tip is oval in cross-section with outer diameter (OD) of 4 mm x 4.5 mm.

Subglottic stenosis is the most common laryngeal lesion in this age group that can cause serious respiratory distress. Obstruction may develop with alarming rapidity when the edema of a respiratory infection is superimposed upon the already compromised airway in subglottic stenosis. The airway which had been marginal becomes inadequate. Minimal laryngeal inflammation can precipitate the need for a tracheotomy since the limiting cricoid cartilage does not permit swelling of tissues other than inward at the expense of the airway.[11] One mm of edema in the subglottic region of the newborn will reduce the airway to 32% of its former area.

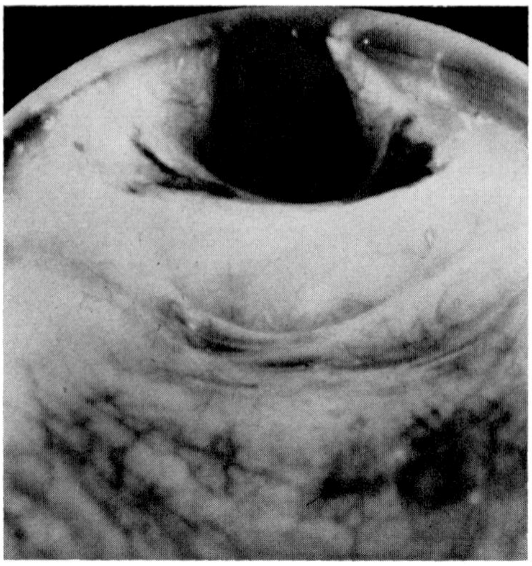

Fig. 3. Acquired subglottic stenosis – associated posterior glottic web.

ACQUIRED SUBGLOTTIC STENOSIS

Acquired subglottic stenosis was found in 43 cases and current follow-up is available in 39 (91%). The age at diagnosis and initial treatment ranged from two weeks to 10 years. Twenty-three (53%) were infants less than 12 months of age, nine (21%) were 12 to 24 months, and the remainder (28%) were scattered at ages up to ten years.

Endotracheal intubation was responsible for the development of subglottic stenosis in 37 cases (86%). In this group, 13 were intubated for eight days or longer; 15 from four to seven days; five from 48 to 72 hours; and two less than 48 hours; two children were referred following intubation of unknown duration. High tracheotomy caused the subglottic stenosis in two children (ages two and three years) and external neck trauma in two others (ages three and ten years). A laryngeal burn in a two-year-old and extrinsic compression secondary to a neurofibroma in the neck accounted for two other cases.

The severity of the underlying conditions that necessitated intubation made this a poor risk group. Of the 43 children with acquired subglottic stenosis, ten had respiratory distress syndrome, seven had central nervous system disorders, and five had congenital heart

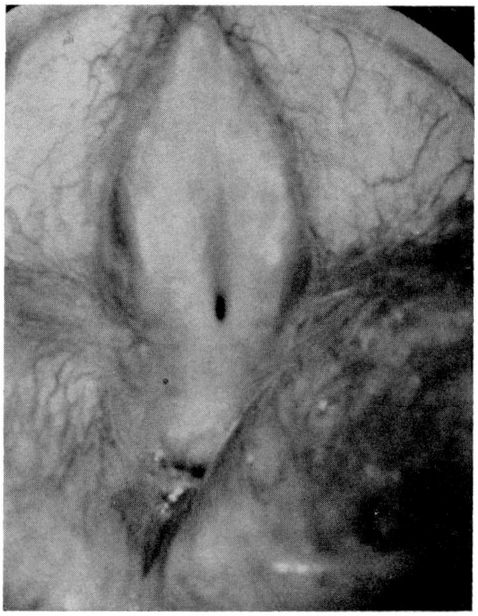

Fig. 4. Acquired subglottic stenosis – with concomitant glottic stenosis.

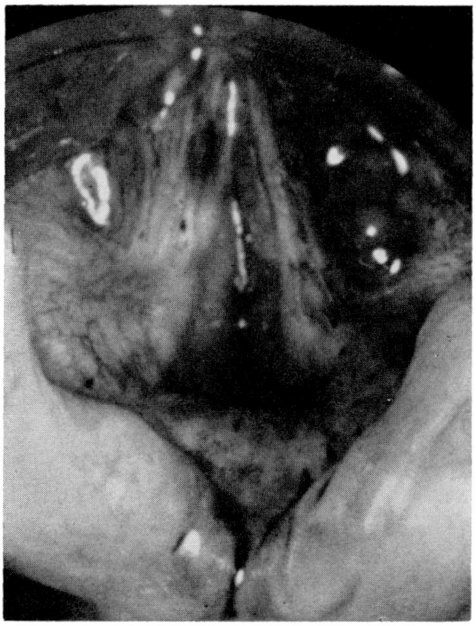

Fig. 5. Acquired subglottic stenosis – complete stenosis of subglottic area.

disease. There were four with respiratory failure due to severe pneumonitis; two children had drug overdose, two had tracheoesophageal fistula and one newborn had neonatal tetanus.

Invariably endoscopic findings were more severe in this group than in those with congenital stenoses. Circumferential subglottic stenosis with a concomitant glottic web, band or stenosis was the most common finding (Figs. 3, 4) and was present in 15 infants and children. An isolated circumferential subglottic stenosis, which was the most common finding in the congenital cases, was present in 14 cases. Complete stenosis of the subglottic area with concomitant glottic stenosis occurred in infants two and five months of age and in a five-year-old child. An isolated complete stenosis of the subglottic area was present in one three-week-old and one 13-month-old (Fig. 5). Edema and granulation tissue were the only findings in four cases. Anterior wall compression was present in three patients. One case had an oval anterior-posterior slit and another had a posterior compression. Bilateral cord paralysis was present in three cases, right cord paralysis in two, and a left cord paralysis in one.

Tracheotomy was required in 38 of the 39 cases in the determinate group (97%). Further management consisted of repeated dilatation and endoscopic removal of granulation tissue. Eighteen patients (46%) have required more than two dilatations and five (13%) had more than ten dilatations. Two children, each five years of age, have had endoscopic placement of laryngeal stents. In neither did the stent prevent restenosis.

Of those children with acquired subglottic stenosis who required tracheotomy (38 cases), all but eight have been decannulated. There have been nine deaths among the 38 infants and children over the ten-year period. Five of these deaths were due to unrelated underlying disease and not directly related to the tracheostomy or the subglottic stenosis. One died of hydrocephalus; a second had a cardiac arrest following surgery for an atrioseptal defect. Another died of cardiac disease 18 months following decannulation. Two patients died of pneumonia, one of whom had been taken from the hospital against medical advice. The deaths of four were related directly or indirectly to the acquired subglottic stenosis and long-term tracheostomy; obstruction by a mucus plug was documented in two cases.

Discussion of Acquired Subglottic Stenosis. The subglottic region is lined by a columnar respiratory epithelium which does not well tolerate constant irritation and is susceptible to slight trauma. The submucosal structures are made up of loose areolar tissue prone to inflammatory edema and completely surrounded by the rigid cricoid cartilage. Since this region is the narrowest part of the upper airway, it is therefore most susceptible to injury by an indwelling endotracheal tube. The pathogenesis of acquired subglottic stenosis begins with mucosal edema and hyperemia. If the trauma persists, ulceration and local infection develop with growth of granulation tissue. Further progression of this process leads to destruction of the cricoid ring and its cartilaginous support of the subglottic lumen. When the source of the trauma is ultimately removed, the denuded wall attempts healing by collagen production, and the resulting scar tissue contracts circumferentially as it matures, producing a stricture and, in some cases, complete stenosis.

Many factors contribute to the development of subglottic stenosis due to endotracheal intubation. The duration of intubation as a factor is controversial. Abbott[12] found that "permanent scarring is less common when the tube has been in place less than seven days." Johnsen[13] found no cases of laryngotracheal stenosis in children intubated less than five to six days, but a high incidence in those children intubated for longer periods; he defines prolonged endotracheal intubation as being in excess of six to seven days. Fearon[14] and others have reported severe laryngeal damage occurring after as little as 72 hours of intubation. In the series reported herein, seven cases of subglottic stenosis developed after less than 72 hours of intubation; these stenoses developed during the first several years of the study. Tracheotomy is strongly recommended after five to seven days of intubation if at the end of that time extubation cannot be accomplished. Tracheotomy should be performed earlier if it becomes apparent that prolonged ventilatory assistance will be necessary.

Other factors influencing the potential for stenosis include the size of the tube in relation to the size of the patient; the material of the tube – whether rubber or plastic; its sterilization – whether by chemicals or gas; the degree of trauma associated with intubation and tube maintenance; and the number of tube changes required.[15] Some authors report subglottic stenosis following intubation for upper airway inflammatory disease was found to be more frequent and more severe than stenosis following intubation for respiratory failure or lower respiratory tract disease.[16] In this series, however, not one of the 43 cases of acquired subglottic stenosis was found related to an upper respiratory tract infection, such as acute epiglottitis or acute laryngotracheobronchitis.

Controversy surrounds the management of acquired subglottic stenosis. The prevailing attitude of otolaryngologists is to wait for the growth of the larynx. Traditional teaching and experience indicates that extensive surgery of the immature larynx interferes with its normal growth and should be avoided;[17,18] others dispute this.[19,20] Most children do well with conservative management, as has been the experience at The Children's Memorial Hospital in Chicago. In this series, tracheotomy was required in 38 of the 39 cases of acquired subglottic stenosis in the determinate group (97%). Further management consisted of repeated dilatations and endoscopic removal of granulation tissue. Most of these patients responded well and could be decannulated after one or two years of this regimen, due to the expected growth of the larynx. This is, however, the group with high morbidity and mortality. Many months of hospitalization were required in several cases, usually because of severe underlying illnesses, but in some cases, because of the unsatisfactory home situation which did not permit adequate tracheostomy home care.

Alternative methods of management are few. The use of laryngeal stents following dilatation in two of these cases was not successful; restenosis quickly followed stent removal. Waggoner[21] has recommended weekly steroid injections into the subglottic region followed by gentle dilatation until a normal airway is maintained. Grahne[22,23] and his associates had little success with long-term bouginage in acquired subglottic stenosis; they now advocate the external surgical approach introduced by Aboulker.[24] Through an extended thyrotomy incision the subglottic scar tissue is excised and the cricoid cartilage divided posteriorly. The new lumen is maintained with a hollow Teflon® prosthesis for four months. All seven patients reported in Grahne's 1971 series have been decannulated. Evans[25] has employed laryngotracheoplasty in the successful treatment of subglottic lesions. His technique involves division of the thyroid, cricoid, and upper tracheal cartilages, submucosal excision of the lesion, and placement of a rolled Silastic® stent for six weeks.

Fearon[26] has reported a mortality rate of 24% in children with severe subglottic stenosis and has demonstrated the feasibility of correcting subglottic stenosis in infant primates without interfering with the subsequent growth of the larynx. The surgical technique involves dividing the cricoid cartilage and upper trachea anteriorly and interposing autogenous cartilage. Scar tissue is left in place and endolaryngeal stenting is not used. Selected children with severe subglottic stenosis have now undergone this procedure with significant success and no mortality.

CONCLUSIONS

Subglottic stenosis in infants and children may be congenital or acquired. In the absence of a history of prolonged intubation, other laryngeal trauma, or extrinsic compression, a specific case of subglottic stenosis was considered to be congenital. From this review of the presenting symptoms, endoscopic findings, management, and long-term prognosis of 158 infants and children with subglottic stenosis, it is apparent that the two groups vary considerably. The outlook for congenital subglottic stenosis is more favorable and the morbidity and mortality are less than in the acquired cases.

The most common presenting symptom in congenital subglottic stenosis was stridor usually accompanied by dyspnea, a barking or brassy cough, or hoarseness. A prolonged bout of croup or repeated episodes of croup was a frequent presentation. Prolonged postextubation stridor following a short general anesthetic, repeated episodes of pneumonitis or atelectasis, and apneic spells were also commonly seen. The acquired stenoses followed prolonged endotracheal intubation in 86%, although high tracheotomy, external trauma and extrinsic compression were also causes. None was related to intubation for an acute upper airway inflammatory process.

In congenital subglottic stenosis, there is a marked soft tissue narrowing greatest 2-3 mm below the superior surface of the true cords. At times the lumen is eccentric with greater involvement of the anterior, posterior or lateral walls. The endoscopic findings in the acquired cases were more severe. Complete atresia was not uncommon and the fibrosis often extended to the glottic level.

Management in the congenital cases was based on the experience that the process of growth aids in the correction of this disorder more than any other factor. Gentle periodic dilatations were thought to be helpful. Tracheotomy was required in 44% of the patients in the determinate group. Growth of the airway usually permitted decannulation by age three or four. In acquired subglottic stenosis, repeated active dilatations for prolonged periods were usually required; granulation tissue was removed endoscopically when present. Tracheotomy was required in 97% of the cases of acquired subglottic stenosis in the determinate group.

Of the entire 146 cases in the determinate group 85 (58%) required tracheotomy. In those infants and children requiring tracheotomy, 62 have been decannulated, 10 have died and 13 still require their tracheostomy. Five of these children succumbed to their underlying illness. The deaths of the other five patients in the determinate group may have been indirectly related to mucus plugging of the tracheostomy tube in the presence of an inadequate laryngeal airway. In those children requiring tracheotomy for their subglottic stenosis the mortality rate was 5.9% and in the entire determinate group (146 cases) the mortality rate was 3.4%.

The great majority of infants and children with subglottic stenosis have responded to conservative management, been decannulated, and have done well. Those patients with a severe or complete stenosis which have not responded to dilatations may require prolonged hospitalization and have a significant incidence of complications. The rationale for the conservative management of subglottic stenosis of the larynx has been based upon three premises: first, that as the larynx increases in size with maturation, the patient will outgrow the problem; second, that potential complications of external laryngeal surgery in the newborn and infant are avoided; and third, this analysis confirms the experience[27,28] that the great majority of these infants and children respond to conservative management and are decannulated.

REFERENCES

1. Holinger PH, Brown WT: Congenital webs, cysts, laryngoceles and other anomalies of the larynx. Ann Otol Rhinol Laryngol 76: 744-752, 1967

2. Holinger PH: Clinical aspects of congenital anomalies of the larynx, trachea, bronchi, and esophagus. J Laryngol Otol 65:1-44, 1961

3. Holinger PH, Schiller F, Johnston KC: Congenital anomalies of the larynx. Ann Otol Rhinol Laryngol 63:581-607, 1954

4. Ferguson CF: Congenital abnormalities of the infant larynx. Otolaryngol Clin North Am 3:185-200, 1970

5. Davies J: Embryology and anatomy of the larynx, respiratory apparatus, diaphragm and esophagus, in Paparella MM, Shumrick DA (eds): *Otolaryngology: Basic Sciences and Related Disciplines.* Philadelphia, W B Saunders Co, 1973, vol 1, pp 179-185

6. Hast MH: The developmental anatomy of the larynx. Otolaryngol Clin North Am 3: 413-437, 1968

7. McMillan WG, Duvall AJ III: Congenital subglottic stenosis. Arch Otolaryngol 87: 70-76, 1968

8. Tucker G: The infant larynx: Direct laryngoscopic observations. JAMA 99: 1899-1902, 1932

9. Wilson TG: Some observations on the infantile larynx. Acta Otolaryngol (Stockh) 43:95-99, 1953

10. Fearon B, Cotton R: Subglottic stenosis in infants and children: The clinical problem and experimental surgical correction. Can J Otolaryngol 1:281-289, 1972

11. Holinger PH, Schild JA, Weprin L: Pediatric laryngology. Otolaryngol Clin North Am 3:625-637, 1970

12. Abbott TR: Complications of prolonged nasotracheal intubation in children. Br J Anaesth 40:347-353, 1968

13. Johnsen S: What is prolonged intubation? Acta Otolaryngol (Stockh) 75:377-378, 1973

14. Fearon B, MacDonald RE, Smith C, *et al*: Airway problems in children following prolonged endotracheal intubation. Ann Otol Rhinol Laryngol 75:975-986, 1966

15. Mattila MAK, Suutarinen T, Sulamaa M: Prolonged endotracheal intubation or tracheostomy in infants and children. J Pediatr Surg 4:674-681, 1969

16. Striker TW, Stool S, Downes JJ: Prolonged nasotracheal intubation in infants and children. Arch Otolaryngol 85:106-109, 1967

17. Jackson C, Jackson CL: *The Larynx and Its Diseases.* Philadelphia, W. B. Saunders Co, 1937, p 188

18. Lederer FL: *Diseases of the Ear, Nose and Throat.* Philadelphia, FA Davis Co, 1943, p 657

19. Calcaterra TC, McClure R, Ward PH: The effect of laryngofissure on the developing canine larynx. Ann Otol Rhinol Laryngol 83: 810-813, 1974

20. Fearon B, Cotton R: Surgical correction of subglottic stenosis of the larynx: prelimi-

nary report of an experimental surgical technique. Ann Otol Rhinol Laryngol 81:508-513, 1972

21. Waggoner LG, Belenky WM, Clark CE: Treatment of acquired subglottic stenosis. Ann Otol Rhinol Laryngol 82:822-826, 1973

22. Grahne B: Operative treatment of severe chronic traumatic laryngeal stenosis in infants up to three years old. Acta Otolaryngol (Stockh) 72:134-137, 1971

23. Louhimo I, Grahne B, Pasila M, *et al*: Laryngotracheal stenosis in children. J Pediatr Surg 6:730-737, 1971

24. Aboulker P: Traitement des sténoses trachéales. Probl Actuels Otorhinolaryngol 1968, p 275

25. Evans JNG: Larnygeal disorders in children, in Wilkinson AW (ed): *Recent Advances in Paediatric Surgery.* New York, Churchill Livingstone, 1975, pp 174-182

26. Fearon B, Cotton R: Surgical correction of subglottic stenosis of the larynx in infants and children: A progress report. Ann Otol Rhinol Laryngol 83:428-431, 1974

27. Bigler JA, Holinger PH, Johnston KC, *et al*: Tracheotomy in infancy. Pediatrics 13: 476-486, 1954

28. Markus NJ, Schild JA, Holinger PH: Tracheostomy in the first year of life. Trans Am Acad Ophthalmol Otolaryngol 1976, to be published

Reprints—Paul H. Holinger, MD, Suite 401, 700 North Michigan Ave., Chicago, IL 60611.

ESSAY CONTEST

The American Broncho-Esophagological Association is offering an award of $200 for the best original paper on a subject related to research in clinical broncho-esophagology or physiology, or pathology of the larynx, tracheo-bronchial tree, or esophagus written by a Resident or Fellow in Training. A $50 award will be given for the second best paper.

The writer of the winning paper will be invited to present his work at the spring meeting of The American Broncho-Esophagological Association, May 9-10, 1977, Boston, Massachusetts. The travel expenses of the winner will not be paid by The American Broncho-Esophagological Association. Winners will be notified prior to February 1, 1977.

The paper will be published in the Transactions of the Association and The Annals of Otology, Rhinology and Laryngology. The manuscript must be submitted, double spaced, not later than September 1, 1976 to: M. Stuart Strong, MD, 720 Harrison Avenue, Boston, MA 02118.

Ann Otol 85: 1976

REPAIR OF LARYNGEAL STENOSIS WITH NASAL SEPTAL GRAFTS

ROBERT J. TOOHILL, MD

DEAN L. MARTINELLI, MD MICHAEL C. JANOWAK, MD

MILWAUKEE, WISCONSIN

SUMMARY – Autogenous nasal septal grafts were utilized in 18 dogs. The availability, method of transfer, placement, take, stability and long-term survival of these grafts are presented. Transfer of septal cartilage or composite grafts of nasal mucosa and cartilage to surgically created defects of cricoid and thyroid cartilage was performed on eight animals. Ten animals had composite grafts three months after stenosing procedures. Results were excellent in all grafts to the cricoid and subglottic areas. Grafts to the thyroid and glottic regions were characterized by severe resorption of cartilage and fibrosis. Composite grafts to the glottic area were successful in improving the airway. Results are documented by microlaryngeal photographs and histologic sections. A literature review accompanies the presentation with emphasis on clinical utilization of composite nasal septal grafts. Twelve previously reported cases of repair by this method for laryngeal and upper tracheal stenosis are discussed. A patient with severe traumatic laryngeal stenosis successfully rehabilitated is added to this list and details the clinical value of these grafts.

Rehabilitation of the patient with chronic laryngeal stenosis has been a difficult problem. Stenosis occurs as a complication of endotracheal intubation, high tracheotomy, neoplasm and granulomatous disease. External trauma to the larynx from crushing injuries, gunshot wounds, and stabbing have also contributed to the increased incidence of stenosis. Conservation procedures for carcinoma of the larynx may also be associated with this complication.

Supraglottic stenosis is frequently amenable to resection with excellent results.[1] The glottic lesions have been successfully treated with a variety of surgical procedures,[1-3] but subglottic stenosis is the more severe problem. Membranous subglottic stenoses have been removed by microlaryngoscopy with repeated dilations.[4] Grafting or stenting and steroid injections have been recommended for the more severe stenoses.[4-7] Surgical resections have been attempted in patients refractory to these conservative measures.[1,5] The incidence of restenosis is high following surgical intervention. Limitations of tissue resected and postoperative inflammatory responses with subsequent scarring and resorption of cartilage are the causes.

Recent approaches to this problem, particularly subglottic stenosis, have advocated surgical enlargement of the defect without further resection or sacrifice of tissue. Homograft cricoid arch transplantations with hyoid bone in dogs have been reported with good initial results, but later complicated by bone resorption.[8,9] In humans, there is the lack of suitable donor tissue and the possibility of graft rejection. Autografts of the hyoid bone have been utilized successfully in both dogs and humans.[10,11] Muscle pedicle grafts of the hyoid bone and clavicle have recently been used in similar fashion.[12,13]

From the Otolaryngology Section, Surgical Service, Veterans Administration Center, Wood (Milwaukee), Wisconsin and the Department of Otolaryngology, The Medical College of Wisconsin, Milwaukee, Wisconsin. This study was supported by Veterans Administration approved research project No. 8410-01.

Presented at the meeting of the American Broncho-Esophagological Association, Palm Beach, Florida, April 27-28, 1976

TABLE I

RESULTS OF DIRECT TRANSFER GRAFTS

Procedure	Dog No.	Size of Graft (cm)	Anterior Stenosis Subglottic (mm)	Glottic	Histologic Findings Epithelium	Cartilage Fibrosis
A	1	2.5 x 1.5	2	0	Respiratory	Intact
	2	2.5 x 2.0	2	0	—	—
B	3	2.0 x 2.5	6	0	Respiratory	50%
	4	1.5 x 1.2	4	0	Respiratory	Intact
C	5	1.5 x 1.0	3	2 mm web	Strat. squam.	20%
	6	2.1 x 1.1	2	7 mm web	Strat. squam.	50%
D	7	3.0 x 2.2	5	10 mm web	Pseudostrat. without cilia	100%
	8	2.5 x 1.5	5	10 mm web	Pseudostrat. without cilia	90%

Strat. - Stratified
Squam. - Squamous

Autogenous nasal septal cartilage with intact mucosa has been investigated and successfully employed as a grafting material in the trachea. Drettner and Lindholm[14] repaired window defects of the trachea in five dogs with composite grafts and theorized as to their clinical value. These results were confirmed in a larger series of dogs by Furstoss and Toohill,[15] who found excellent preservation of the cartilage at one year postoperatively.

The thin, less rigid wall of the trachea seems to be an ideal site for repair of defects, as the nasal septal cartilage is strong enough to provide the needed external support for the trachea. The thyroid and cricoid cartilages have greater strength and thickness than septal cartilage. This study was undertaken to investigate the effect of nasal septal grafts in stenosis of the glottic and subglottic regions in dogs.

METHODS AND MATERIALS

Eighteen adult mongrel dogs varying in weight from 15 to 30 kg were anesthetized with sodium pentothal (25 mg/kg) supplemented with 1% xylocaine, with epinephrine injected locally into the nasal dorsum. The dogs were intubated with an oral endotracheal tube and maintained on a respirator,* delivering 40% O_2. Dorsal rhinotomy was utilized to obtain the nasal septal grafts.[15]

Direct septal transfer grafts were utilized in the first eight animals with four different procedures performed. Eight animals had surgery, two in each of the following procedures: A) subperichondral removal of the anterior one-third of the cricoid cartilage with replacement of a similar sized septal cartilage; B) composite removal of the anterior one-third of the cricoid cartilage, perichondrium and subglottic mucosa and replacement with a composite septal graft consisting of cartilage and mucoperichondrium on the underside; C) subperichondrial removal of the anterior one-third of the thyroid cartilage followed by replacement with nasal septal cartilage; and D) composite removal of the anterior one-third of the thyroid cartilage, perichondrium, and the anterior one-half of the true and false cords by replacement with a composite nasal septal graft, having mucoperichondrium on the underside.

The second portion of the study consisted of creating defects in ten dogs and utilizing five different stenosing procedures.[16] The stenosis credited in each animal was documented

* Model Mark 7. Bird Corp., Palm Springs, CA.

TABLE II

RESULTS OF REPAIR OF LARYNGEAL STENOSIS

Pro-cedure	*Dog No.*	*Anterior Stenosis* *Glottic*	*Anterior Stenosis* *Subglottic (mm)*	*Size of Graft (cm)*	*Repair Stenosis* *Glottic*	*Repair Stenosis* *Subglottic (mm)*	*Histologic Findings* *Epithelium*	*Histologic Findings* *Cartilage Fibrosis*
I	9	None	6	3.0 x 2.0	None	None	Respiratory	Intact
	10	None	4	2.5 x 2.0	None	None	None	None
II	11	Flac. of TVC	8	2.5 x 3.5	Mild flac. of TVC	4	Respiratory	Intact
	12	None	6	3.0 x 2.5	None	2	Respiratory	20%
III	13	None	9	2.7 x 2.0	None	3	Moderate loss of cilia	75%
	14	None	7	3.0 x 2.0	None	None	Pseudostrat. occ. cilia	80%
IV	15	Severe coll. of ant. 2/3 of TVC	7	3.0 x 2.2	Severe coll. of TVC as preop.	2	Respiratory* Pseudostrat.**	90% 100%
	16	Mod. coll. of ant. 2/3 of TVC, 2 mm web	4	2.6 x 2.5	No coll. 4 mm web	None	None* Pseudostrat.**	None 75%
V	17	10 mm web	8	3.5 x 2.5	3 mm web	None	Respiratory* Pseudostrat.**	75% 100%
	18	10 mm web	9	3.0 x 2.5	5 mm web	4	Respiratory* Pseudostrat. occ. cilia**	60% 100%

Flac. - Flaccidity; Mod. - Moderate; Coll. - Collapse; Ant. - Anterior
*Cricoid **larynx

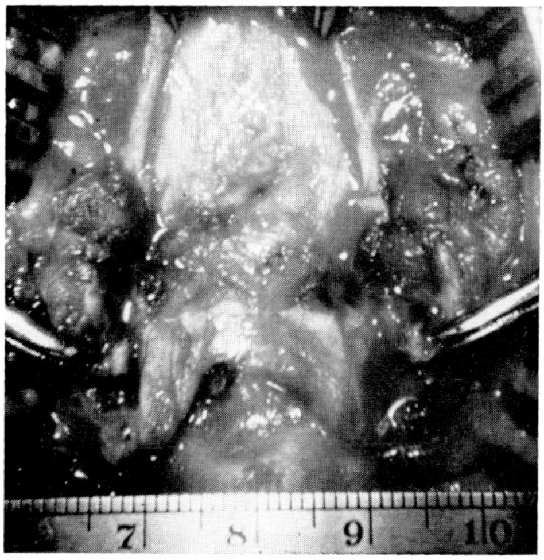

Fig. 1. External thyroid and cricoid stenosis from procedure V (No. 17).

and recorded at three months and then repaired by a wedge technique utilizing composite nasal septal grafts. The stenosing procedures performed were: I) subperichondrial removal of the anterior one-third of the cricoid cartilage; II) subperichondrial removal of the anterior two-thirds of the cricoid cartilage; III) composite removal of the anterior one-third of the cricoid cartilage, perichondrium and subglottic mucosa; IV) subperichondrial removal of the anterior one-third of the cricoid and thyroid cartilages; and V) composite removal of the anterior one-third of the cricoid and thyroid cartilages and the anterior one-half of the true and false cords along with subglottic mucosa.

In the four animals having direct transfer cartilage grafts, perichondrial closure with 3-0 chromic catgut was used to secure the grafts. Prolene®* interrupted sutures (3-0) placed

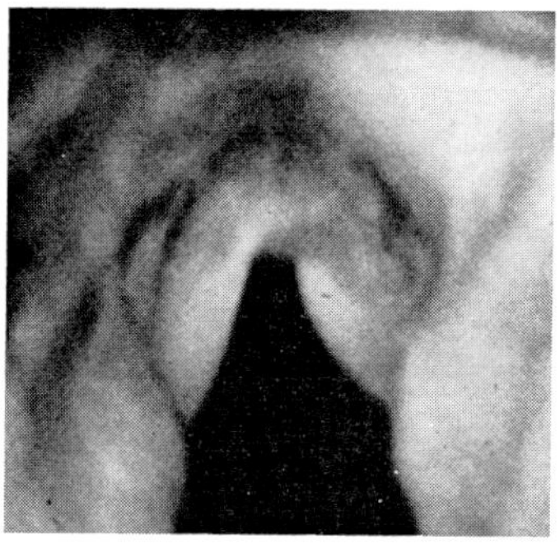

Fig. 2. Anterior stenosis (10 mm) of the vocal cords (No. 17).

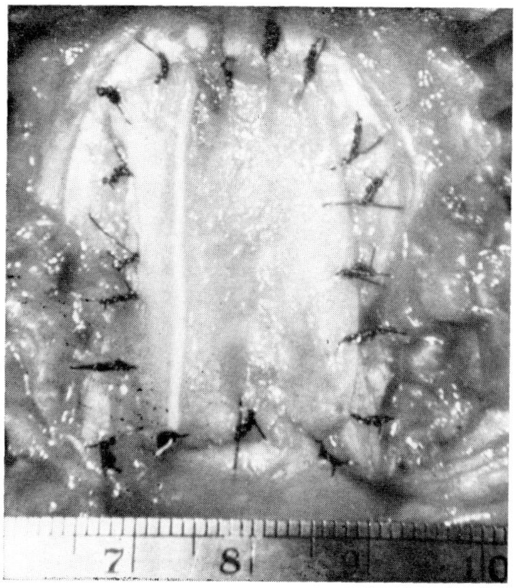

Fig. 3. Graft wedged anteriorly (No. 17).

submucosally were utilized on the 14 dogs with composite grafts. These grafts were sutured into position with the mucoperichondrial surface facing the laryngeal lumen. In general, the posterior portion of the composite graft was placed upward and the anterior portion downward toward the trachea in an effort to duplicate the ciliary flow of the normal animal.

No stents, steroids or tracheotomies were used, and all animals were extubated immediately postoperatively. All dogs were kept in an enclosed cage with high humidity and O_2 for 24 hours after surgery. They were given a regular diet within 48 hours. Antibiotic therapy consisted of Combiotic®**, b.i.d. for five days. All animals had suspension microlaryngoscopy performed at 6 and 12 weeks follow-

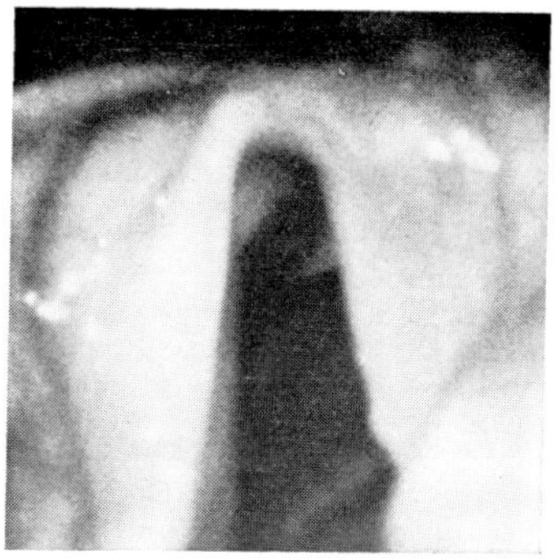

Fig. 4. Anterior stenosis (3 mm) post-repair (No. 17).

* Ethicon Laboratories, Somerville, NJ.
** Pfizer, Inc., Hoffman Estates, IL.

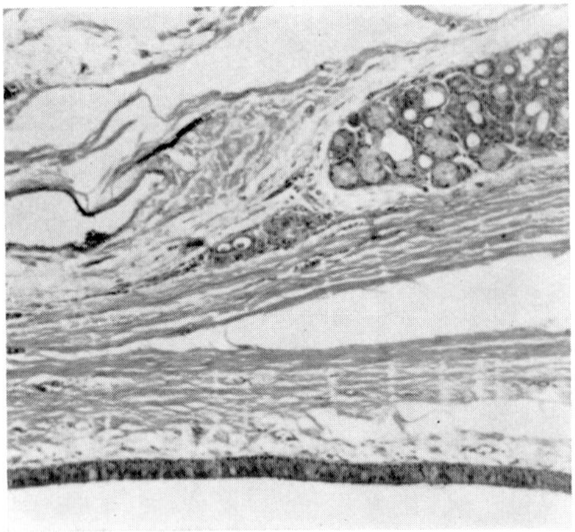

Fig. 5. Grafted cricoid portion showing intact respiratory epithelium (X50) (No. 17).

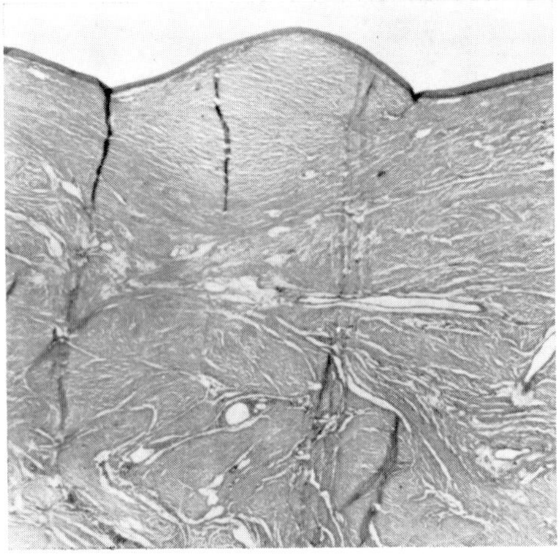

Fig. 6. Glottic portion of graft with fibrosis and pseudostratified epithelium (X10) (No. 17).

ing grafting. The relative size of each anterior luminal stenosis was estimated with the aid of microlaryngeal rulers developed for this study. The appearance of the graft and presence or absence of granulations were noted. The quality of breathing and bark were recorded at regular intervals. Photographs of the stenotic lesions were taken prior to grafting, and all animals were photographed prior to sacrifice. After three months, all animals were sacrificed, and the larynges were removed for serial sections and photomicrographs.

RESULTS

The studies of direct transfer grafts are summarized in Table I. The septal cartilage and composite replacements to the cricoid showed little resorption and intact respiratory epithelium. There was little diminution in the subglottic lumen, with minimal anterior flattening noted in each of the four animals.

The laryngeal grafts all had anterior commissure webs that varied in size from 2 to 10 mm. The composite replacement grafts showed almost complete resorption of cartilage, but the septal cartilage was partially preserved in the two dogs with procedure C.

All ten animals in the second portion of the study developed some degree of stenosis following their initial procedures (Table II, Figs. 1, 2).[16] Following repair with composite nasal septal wedge grafts all showed improvement in lumen diameter (Figs. 3, 4). The subglottic grafts in procedures I and II maintained respiratory epithelium with minimal cartilage resorption. Despite scarring and cartilage resorption in procedure III, correction of the stenosis was excellent.

The larger defects of combined glottic and subglottic stenosis in procedures IV and V also responded well to the grafts, with the exception of one. Although the subglottic lumen was improved in this animal, collapse and flaccidity of the true cords persisted. Like the direct transfer grafts, there was almost total resorption of cartilage.

Epithelial changes show an interesting pattern. The lower subglottic portions of these grafts had excellent ciliation. The glottic area, however, showed little evidence of cilia formation. Pseudostratified epithelium appeared to be undergoing a transition to stratified squamous epithelium (Figs. 5, 6).

In the subglottic grafts, all animals maintained arytenoid and vocal cord mobility with essentially normal bark. The laryngeal grafts had adequate arytenoid and posterior cordal mobility, but the bark was of a hoarse quality.

DISCUSSION

Composite nasal septal grafts for defects of the trachea have definite advantages over other grafts,[14,15] probably

TABLE III

COMPOSITE NASAL SEPTAL GRAFTS

Author	*Year*	*No. of Cases*	*Etiology*	*Location of Stenosis*
Kleinsasser[4]	1971	2	Intub.	Subglottic
Wilflingseder[21]	1972	6	Intub. & Trach.	Subglottic
Krizek & Kirchner[20]	1972	1	Trauma	Cricoid & upper tracheal
Furstoss & Toohill[15]	1973	2	1. Trach. 2. Intub.	1. Trach. site 2. Subglottic & upper tracheal
Strome & Ferguson[22]	1974	1	Intub.	Subglottic & upper tracheal
Toohill *et al*	1976	1	Trauma	Glottic & subgl.

Intub. - Intubation
Trach. - Tracheotomy

due to the similarities of the tissues in each area. This study has confirmed that these grafts can be placed in cricoid defects with assurance of success. With certain limitations, they can likewise be utilized in laryngeal stenosis. The resorption of cartilage with the glottic procedures is of some concern. The functionally active intrinsic and extrinsic laryngeal musculature may exert pressure on the wedge grafts contributing to cartilage resorption and subsequent fibrosis.

The fibrosis is of less concern on a long-term basis. Improved airways were consistently noted despite its development. This finding has been noted by others[12,14,15,17,18] where the initial graft

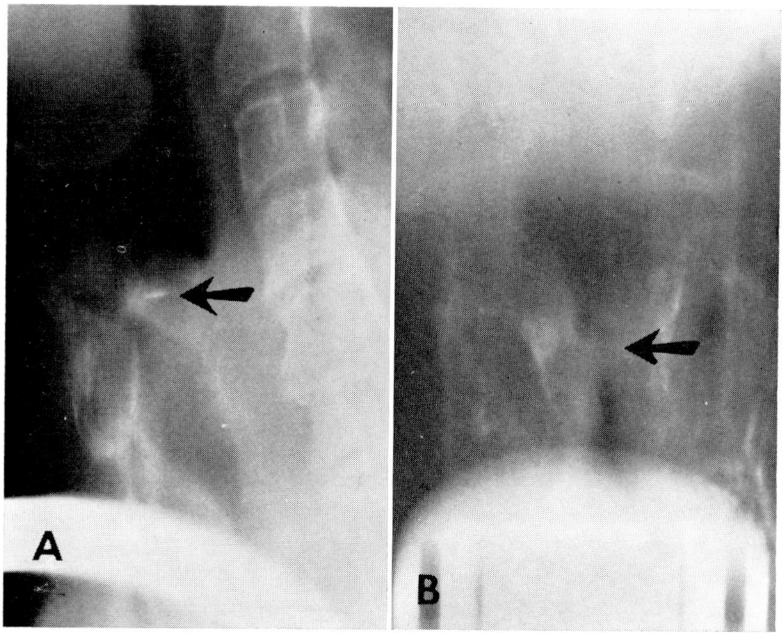

Fig. 7. Lateral tomogram showing severe laryngeal stenosis with thyroid and cricoid fractures. B) PA tomogram of stenosis.

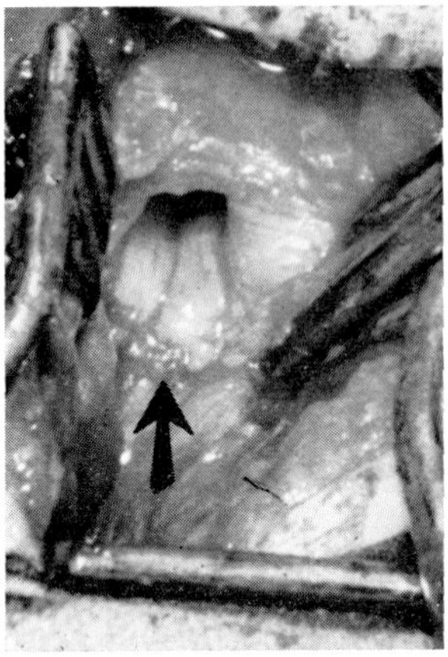

Fig. 8. Thyrotomy showing glottic stenosis below the arytenoids (arrow).

appears to act as a stent until sufficient stable fibrous tissue develops.

The anterior flattening of the grafted areas that occurred in this study also was previously noted.[14,15] Currently, attention is being directed to the interlocking stresses of cartilage[19] and new procedures to prevent this problem in the future.

The clinical utilization of composite nasal septal grafts has shown definite promise (Table III). Kleinsasser,[4] in 1971, reported repair of two cases of cricoid stenosis with composite grafts. His second case was a severe postintubation subglottic stenosis in a 5-year-old male, and at the time of the report had not been decannulated. Krizek and Kirchner[20] described subglottic and tracheal reconstruction in one case, and Wilflingseder[21] related his experience with six subglottic lesions in 1972. Furstoss and Toohill[15] added one successful tracheal stenosis repair in 1973. They also reported a combined subglottic and tracheal defect which showed improved airway after grafting but has not been decannulated because of severe lateral upper tracheal flaccidity and lack of external support. A muscle-bone pedicle graft of clavicle or hyoid bone is presently being considered on this patient. Strome and Ferguson[22] also reported a successful repair of a severe subglottic-tracheal stenosis with this technique in 1974.

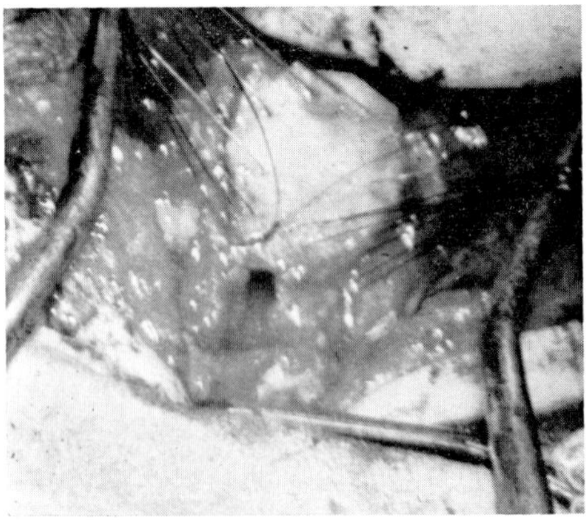

Fig. 9. Graft wedged anteriorly.

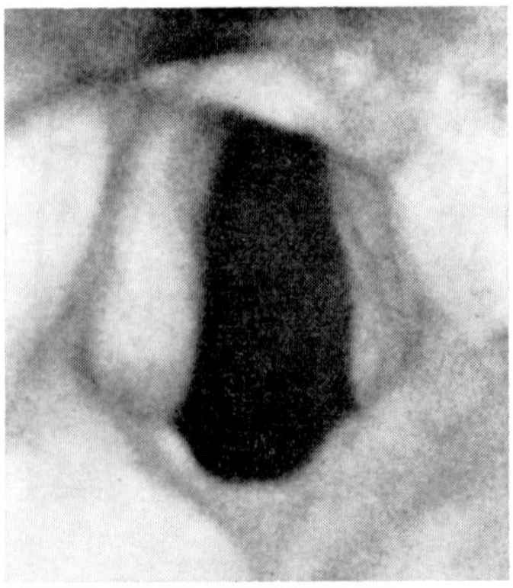

Fig. 10. Postrepair glottic airway with anterior flattening from graft.

Our recent experience in an additional case of severe laryngeal stenosis will be described in detail.

CASE REPORT

A 65-year-old female was seen in October of 1974, 15 months following a severe automobile accident in which she struck the dashboard with her anterior neck. There was immediate stridor and respiratory distress which necessitated insertion of a nasotracheal tube. Six days after injury a tracheotomy was done and the nasotracheal tube removed. Direct laryngoscopy at that time revealed a severe laryngeal collapse with evidence of denuded cartilaginous fragments in the lumen. Tomography confirmed severe comminuted fractures of the thyroid and cricoid cartilages.

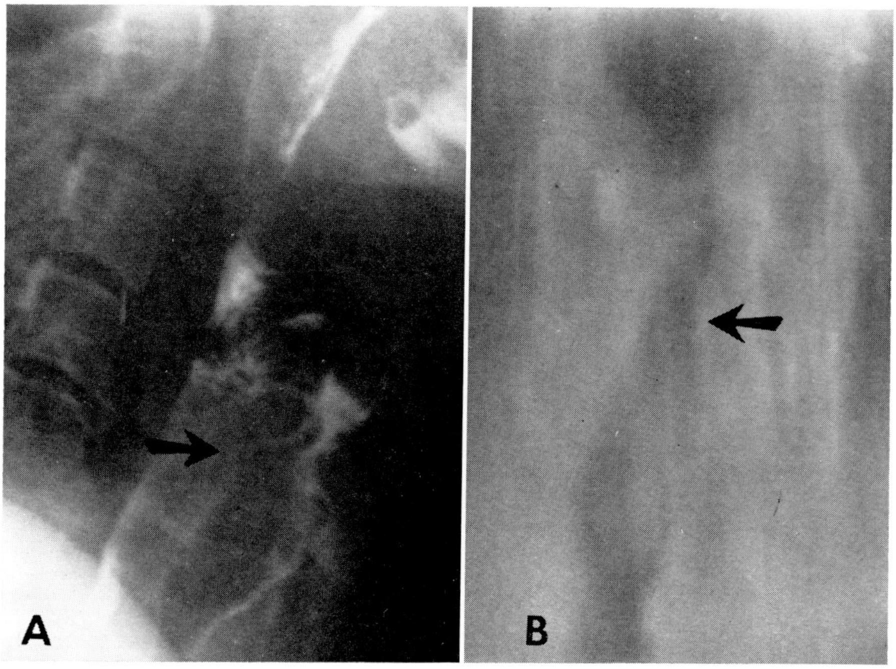

Fig. 11. A) Laryngogram four months postoperative. B) PA tomogram four months postoperative.

Thirteen days after injury a thyrotomy was performed and a silastic stent inserted. Over the next 15 months, the stent was reinserted, and the patient had multiple laryngeal dilatations without success. Laryngeal findings and tomography (Fig. 7) indicated a severe laryngeal and subglottic stenosis with a 1 mm airway and poor phonation. Twenty-one months following injury a 2.5 x 3.0 cm composite nasal septal graft was wedged into the anterior glottic and subglottic regions with submucosal excision of the posterior scar tissue (Figs. 8, 9). The nasal septal defect was repaired with the aid of a dermal graft.

The postoperative course was uneventful. Direct laryngoscopy (Fig. 10) and x-ray studies indicated remarkable improvement of the laryngeal airway (Fig. 11). The patient was decannulated four months later and has an improved voice but with a harsh, hoarse quality. A minor revision of a small persistent tracheocutaneous fistula was required at the tracheotomy site. The patient is now one year postoperative with an adequate laryngeal airway.

SUMMARY AND CONCLUSIONS

Primary therapy for stenosis of the larynx and upper trachea has been well described and the effectiveness of these procedures has been documented.[1-7] Many patients, however, do not respond to these methods. Current concepts for the treatment of these cases include the following: 1) avoidance of further resection or destruction of external supportive tissue; 2) prevention of damage to the recurrent or superior laryngeal nerves; 3) utilization of autogenous grafts that provide external supportive tissue similar to the area, *i.e.*, bone or cartilage; 4) assurance of a mucosal lining that will not inhibit vocal and respiratory rehabilitation; and 5) enlargement of the stenotic area by wedging of grafts into the defect.

An increasing number of successful autogenous grafts have been reported recently.[4,8-15,20-22] The composite nasal septal graft can be added in this list and should be considered when there is a need to rehabilitate the patient with severe laryngeal or upper tracheal stenosis.

REFERENCES

1. Ogura JH, Biller HF: Reconstruction of the larynx following blunt trauma. Ann Otol Rhinol Laryngol 80:492-506, 1971

2. Quinn HJ: Glottic reconstruction after hemilaryngectomy. Laryngoscope 80:599-609, 1970

3. Montgomery WW: Posterior and complete laryngeal (glottic) stenosis. Arch Otolaryngol 98:170-175, 1973

4. Kleinsasser O: Narbenstenosen des Kehlkopfes und der Trachea. HNO 19:294-302, 1971

5. Conley JJ: Reconstruction of the subglottic air passage. Ann Otol Rhinol Laryngol 62:477-495, 1953

6. Fearon B, Cotton R: Surgical corrections of subglottic stenosis of the larynx in infants and children. Ann Otol Rhinol Laryngol 83:428-431, 1974

7. Waggoner LG, Belenky WM, Clark CE: Treatment of acquired subglottic stenosis. Ann Otol Rhinol Laryngol 82:822-826, 1973

8. Delahunty JE, Alonso WA, Bordley JE: Cricoid arch transplantation. Laryngoscope 80: 137-144, 1970

9. Alonso WA, Bridger GP, Youngblood J, *et al*: Cricoid arch transplantation – long-term follow-up. Laryngoscope 81:1968-1970, 1971

10. Alonso WA, Druck NS, Griffiths CM, *et al*: Cricoid arch replacement in dogs. Arch Otolaryngol 101:42-45, 1975

11. Druck NS, Alonso WA, Ogura JH: Hyoid arch transposition. Trans Am Acad Ophthalmol Otolaryngol 82:175-187, 1976

12. Finnegan DA, Wong ML, Kashima HK: Hyoid autograft repair of chronic subglottic stenosis. Ann Otol Rhinol Laryngol 84:643-649, 1975

13. Work WP, Coulthard SW: The injured larynx: A new surgical procedure for repair. Presented at the Scientific Session of the Section of Otolaryngology, The Annual Meeting of the American Academy of Ophthalmology and Otolaryngology, Dallas, Texas, September 22, 1975

14. Drettner B, Lindholm CE: Experimental tracheal reconstruction with composite graft from nasal septum. Acta Otolaryngol (Stockh) 70:401-407, 1970

15. Furstoss JA, Toohill RJ: Composite nasal septal autografts of the trachea. Ann Otol Rhinol Laryngol 82:831-837, 1973

16. Martinelli DL, Toohill RJ: Experimental laryngeal stenosis. Presented at the Program of the Committee for Research in Otolaryngology, The Annual Meeting of the American Academy of Ophthalmology and Otolaryngology, Dallas, Texas, October 5, 1974

17. Flemming I, Hommerich KW: Tierexperimentelle Untersuchungen zur Rekonstruktion der vorderen Trachealwand bei begrenzten Luft röhrenver engerungen. Z Laryngol Rhinol Otol 47:336-339, 1968

18. Pearson FG, Goldberg M, daSilva AJ: Tracheal stenosis complicating tracheostomy with cuffed tubes. Arch Surg 97:380-394, 1968

19. Fry HJH: Interlocked stresses in human nasal septal cartilage. Br J Plast Surg 19:276-278, 1966

20. Krizek TJ, Kirchner JA: Tracheal reconstruction with an autogenous mucochondrial graft. Plast Reconstr Surg 50:123-130, 1972

21. Wilflingseder VP: Rekonstruktion der Trachea durch ein Segmenttransplantat vom Nasen septum. Wien Klin Wochenschr 84: 226-229, 1972

22. Strome M, Ferguson CF: Multiple post-intubation complications. Ann Otol Rhinol Laryngol 83:432-438, 1974

Acknowledgment—The animal facilities of the Allen-Bradley Medical Science Laboratory of the Medical College of Wisconsin were utilized for this study.

Reprints—Robert J. Toohill, MD, 5757 West Oklahoma Ave., Milwaukee, WI 53219.

Ann Otol 85: 1976

CLINICAL EXPERIENCE WITH THE TRACHEOESOPHAGEAL ANASTOMOSIS FOR INTRACTABLE ASPIRATION

ROGER C. LINDEMAN, MD

C. THOMAS YARINGTON, JR., MD DWIGHT SUTTON, PHD

SEATTLE, WASHINGTON

SUMMARY – Clinical experience in six patients in whom the tracheoesophageal diversion procedure or a modification thereof has been performed is presented. Two of these patients have been reconstructed with resulting normal laryngeal and esophageal function. Three of the patients have successfully undergone tracheoesophageal anastomosis and are candidates for reconstruction. One patient in whom the tracheoesophageal anastomosis has been present for 2½ years may never demonstrate neurological return sufficient for reversal of the procedure. On the basis of these six cases, we consider the tracheoesophageal anastomosis to be an effective, yet reversible, procedure for intractable aspiration.

The use of a tracheostomy has long been accepted as a primary means of isolating the lower respiratory tract from the upper respiratory tract and alimentary tract. Indeed, in a recent comprehensive review on tracheostomy,[1] the prevention of aspiration was considered one of the primary indications. Endotracheal intubation also can achieve this end, but its prolonged use has been open to question due to concern over the delayed complication of subglottic stenosis secondary to prolonged cuff inflation. A similar complication is of concern following tracheostomy however, and it is generally accepted that the use of a long-term endotracheal cuff for prevention of aspiration is hazardous.[2]

The threat of aspiration, when the mechanical coordination necessary for deglutition is absent or when the guarding mechanisms of the larynx are lacking, is no less a problem than the delayed complications of a long-term inflated cuff. Aspiration of toxic fluids, pathogenic bacteria or inert substances constitutes the triple threat of aspiration pneumonia.[3] Because of the danger produced by persistent aspiration and the risks of the use of a long-term endotracheal cuff as the sole prevention of these problems, other procedures have been devised for the management of intractable aspiration.

Double-barreled tracheostomies, pharyngostomas and laryngeal stents have been suggested, but have been unsatisfactory solutions to the problem.

An epiglottic flap procedure was described by Habel and Murray in 1972,[4] in which the epiglottis was sutured to the aryepiglottic folds and the arytenoid cartilages. Montgomery recently described a glottic closure procedure in which the vocal cords are stripped and sutured together.[5] These procedures are apparently effective, but necessarily result in intrinsic laryngeal damage. Reversibility is therefore limited.

A tracheoesophageal anastomosis (Fig. 1A) performed first in a series of mongrel dogs, was described by Lindeman in January of 1975 as a reversible procedure for intractable aspiration.[6]

From the Department of Otolaryngology and Facial Plastic Surgery, Mason Clinic, and the Laryngeal Research Laboratory, Virginia Mason Research Center, Seattle, Washington.
This work was supported in part by a grant from the Simpson Timber Company.

Presented at the meeting of the American Broncho-Esophagological Association, Palm Beach, Florida, April 27-28, 1976.

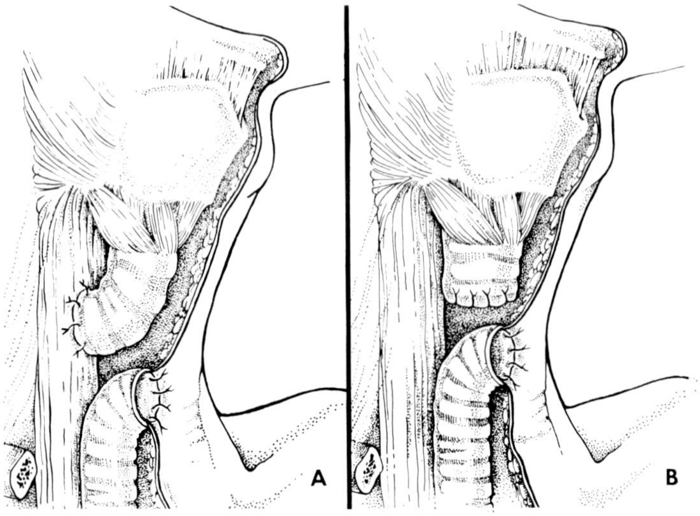

Fig. 1. A) Standard diversion procedure performed as originally described. B) Modified diversion with blind-end closure of proximal trachea when a high tracheostomy precludes tracheoesophageal anastomosis.

The goal of that research effort was to find a means by which the lungs could be totally, dependably, and consistently protected from aspiration for an indefinite period of time without in any way damaging the malfunctioning larynx; a procedure as dependable as total laryngectomy, yet reversible so that should recovery occur, the larynx could function once again.

The purpose of this report is to present the experience gained over the past three years with the tracheoesophageal anastomosis procedure and the results observed when the procedure has been reversed.

CASE REPORTS

Case 1. A 59-year-old female was admitted with a very large posterior fossa tumor in May of 1973. An infratentorial craniectomy was performed with total excision of the acoustic neuroma, but with resultant extensive lower cranial nerve deficit. Her hospital course was complicated by intractable aspiration and the resultant fulminant pneumonia. In June of 1973, a tracheoesophageal anastomosis procedure was performed, and aspiration was thus prevented. She ate a soft diet on the fourth postoperative day and progressed to a regular diet in one week.

Her chest x-ray gradually cleared and she suffered no further episodes of aspiration pneumonia. Antibiotics were discontinued. Her strength improved rapidly and she was discharged 3½ weeks after the anastomosis was performed.

During the ensuing year, recovery was monitored by indirect laryngoscopy and barium swallow. We noted improvement in vocal cord motion, lack of pooling of saliva in the hypopharynx, and a change in the barium swallow from marked aspiration to no aspiration at all.

One year after the original tracheoesophageal anastomosis, she was admitted for reversal of the procedure. The anastomosis was taken down, the defect in the esophagus was repaired, and tracheal continuity was restored by end-to-end anastomosis. The reconstruction procedure was well tolerated and she developed no aspiration problems. Breathing and swallowing are normal and her voice is strong.

Case 2. A 54-year-old female was initially admitted in August, 1973, suffering from a metabolic encephalopathy. At that time, she was diagnosed as having a medullary infarction due to occlusion of the left vertebral artery. A tracheostomy was performed in August of 1973, but she continued to aspirate around the inflated cuff. In September of 1973, due to intractable aspiration pneumonia, a tracheoesophageal anastomosis was performed. The procedure went without incident, and there was no subsequent problem with aspiration. She was readmitted in January of 1975, with tracheitis and some narrowing of her tracheostome. This was treated conservatively. Her neurological status has improved very slowly over the ensuing year, but not to the point where we can consider reconstruction. Vocal cord motion, although improved, is still poor, there is continued pooling of

TABLE I

SUMMARY OF CASE REPORTS

Pt	*Age Sex*	*Diagnosis*	*Procedure*	*Recon-struction*	*Result*
1	59 F	Brain tumor	D June 1973	Feb 1974	Normal function
2	54 F	CVA	D Sept 1973		Slow CNS improv.
3	29 F	Brain tumor	D Nov 1974	June 1975	Normal function
4	27 F	Brain tumor	D Feb 1976		Slow CNS improv.
5	59 M	CVA	MD Jan 1975		Slow CNS improv.
6	50 M	Brain tumor	MD Dec 1975		CNS death Jan 1976

CVA - Cardiovascular accident; D - Diversion; MD - Modified diversion; Improv. - Improvement.

saliva in the hypopharynx, and barium swallow still indicates a significant degree of aspiration. The anastomosis has remained functional for these 2½ years. There may never be adequate neurological return to allow reversal of the procedure.

Case 3. A 29-year-old housewife was admitted for resection of a cerebellar hemangioblastoma in August of 1974. Because of a problem with intractable aspiration, she underwent tracheoesophageal anastomosis one month following her neurosurgical procedure. This was accomplished without incident. During the ensuing year, she slowly achieved considerable neurological improvement as monitored by indirect laryngoscopy and barium swallow. She was readmitted to the hospital in June of 1975, and a reconstruction of her trachea was performed with primary closure of the esophageal opening. Following minimal aspiration of clear fluids and water immediately following the procedure, she demonstrated normal swallowing function, a good normal voice and was discharged on the seventh postoperative day. Some ten months following surgery, she now continues to have normal swallowing function, a normal airway, a good voice, and adequate motion of both vocal cords.

Case 4. A 27-year-old female underwent the neurosurgical removal of multiple intracranial neurofibromas in December of 1975. Lower cranial nerve deficit resulted in a chronic aspiration problem. As a result, in February of 1976, she underwent a tracheoesophageal anastomosis. The aspiration problem was eliminated and she has been discharged to an extended care facility where she is showing gradual improvement.

Case 5. A 59-year-old male was admitted in December of 1974, with central nervous system (CNS) deterioration following intracranial aneurysm with hemorrhage, which has been treated surgically and followed by residual left hemiparesis. A secondary thrombotic episode caused a right hemiparesis. He was admitted in this status from another hospital because of deteriorating CNS problems and aspiration pneumonia. A tracheostomy was performed early in the hospital course, but continued complications due to aspiration were noted. A tracheoesophageal anastomosis procedure was planned, but because of the high position of the previous tracheostomy, the anastomosis was not feasible and thus a blind pouch was created of the upper tracheal segment with a permanent tracheostomy being performed distally as usual (Fig. 1B). At the time of surgery, we were not particularly pleased with this alternative, fearing pooling of secretions in the blind pouch. Nevertheless, the procedure was effective and his pulmonary status improved markedly. He was fed by gastrostomy and later orally, and was discharged in March of 1975. He was subsequently admitted briefly in April of 1975, for gastritis. He has resumed ambulation with help and has developed slow but normal oral intake. Swallowing efforts, however, continue to demonstrate some aspiration and his larynx remains incompetent. However, in December of 1975, fibroptic tracheoscopy was performed and upon examination, it was noted that laryngeal guarding reflexes appeared much improved and there was notable progress in tongue protrusion and swallowing efforts. A decreased amount of laryngeal aspiration during barium swallow was noted as well. He remains under consideration for reconstruction.

Case 6. A 50-year-old male was admitted with a possible brain tumor, and subsequently underwent a suboccipital craniotomy with gross subtotal removal of a tumor of the fourth ventricle in October of 1975. This tumor proved to be a medulloblastoma and the patient subsequently deteriorated neurologically and required a tracheostomy some four days after the procedure. He continued with degenerating CNS and cranial nerve function as well as peripheral neuropathies, but with continuous nursing care was maintained on artificial ventilation. Approximately one month following the procedure, considerable intractable aspiration and the increasing danger of potentially fatal aspiration pneumonia became increasingly apparent and in early December, 1975, a tracheoesophageal anastomosis was scheduled. At the time of the procedure, the anastomosis could not be accomplished, due again to insufficient length of the superior segment of the trachea above the previously accomplished tracheostomy. Therefore, blind closure of the trachea was performed superiorly and a permanent tracheostomy provided inferiorly. Subsequently, the patient was able to be ventilated without the use of a tight cuff and aspiration was eliminated. He continued to suffer neurologic deterioration and finally succumbed approximately six weeks later. At the time of autopsy, his lungs were in remarkably good condition without signs of aspiration. (See Table I for summary of these cases.)

DISCUSSION

Our experience with these cases would suggest the following points. First, the tracheoesophageal diversion procedure can be performed in the human patient with the predictable result of eliminating intractable aspiration. Second, the procedure is reversible and restoration of function can be accomplished when the patient has otherwise recovered neurologically. Third, if adequate neurological recovery does not occur, the anastomosis can apparently be left intact perhaps indefinitely.

In addition, some patients may not be suitable for the standard diversion procedure due to the presence of a high tracheostomy which may preclude the standard tracheoesophageal anastomosis. In these cases, a modified procedure may be accomplished, creating a blind closure of the proximal trachea. We have not yet reconstructed a patient in whom the modified procedure has been performed, but evaluation of the autopsy specimen in one such case leads us to believe that reconstruction would present no significant problem.

Our experience would also suggest some words of caution. We acknowledge danger to the recurrent laryngeal nerves, both initially and in the reconstruction and can only suggest meticulous care in dissection, maintaining a plane very close to the tracheal wall in the diversion procedure and very close to the anastomotic site when resecting it in the reconstruction. It would be absolutely ideal if the tracheoesophageal anastomosis could be performed as a primary procedure in a suitable patient who is certain to have a prolonged recovery period rather than performing the operation on a patient who already has had a cuffed tracheostomy tube in place and has been aspirating around it for several months. Tissue planes will be infinitely better and the chances for damage to the recurrent nerves greatly lessened.

Also, if a tracheostomy is being performed on a patient in whom the tracheoesophageal anastomosis may later be appropriate, consideration must be given to avoiding an abnormally high tracheostomy which would later render a tracheoesophageal anastomosis impossible.

REFERENCES

1. Salmon LFW: Tracheostomy. Proc R Soc Med 68:347-356, 1975

2. Yarington CT Jr: Tracheostomy or endotracheal intubation. Emergency Med Service 4:25-73, 1975

3. Bartlett JG, Gorbach SL: The triple threat of aspiration pneumonia. Chest 68:560-566, 1975

4. Habel MB, Murray JE: Surgical treatment of life endangering chronic aspiration pneumonia. Plast Reconstr Surg 49:305-311, 1972

5. Montgomery WW: Surgery to prevent aspiration. Arch Otolaryngol 101:679-682, 1975

6. Lindeman RC: Diverting the paralyzed larynx: A reversible procedure for intractable aspiration. Laryngoscope 85:157-180, 1975

REPRINTS—Roger C. Lindeman, MD, 1118 Ninth Avenue, Seattle, WA 98101.

Ann Otol 85: 1976

CONGENITAL TRACHEOESOPHAGEAL FISTULAS IN ADULTS

ROBERT W. STEPHENS, MD

INDIANAPOLIS, INDIANA

RALEIGH E. LINGEMAN, MD

INDIANAPOLIS, INDIANA

LAWRENCE J. LAWSON, MD

MUNCIE, INDIANA

SUMMARY – Congenital tracheoesophageal fistula without esophageal atresia is commonly known as "H" type. This is an extremely rare anomaly in infants and accounts for approximately 1½ - 4% of all congenital tracheoesophageal malformations. An anomaly should be described by its anatomical defect, not by a number or letter. There are five main anatomical categories with 85-95% being of the esophageal atresia and distal tracheoesophageal fistula type. About 1½% are of the "H" type. Although today tracheoesophageal fistula is a well-recognized entity, a few of the "H" type have passed through the pediatric period without diagnosis. Those undetected fistulas have successfully masqueraded as chronic lung disease of unknown etiology. Congenital "H" type tracheoesophageal fistulas assume an oblique orientation with the growth of the host to adulthood. This helps to explain the difficulty in diagnosis plus the ability of the host to survive to adult life. Treatment is surgical, consisting of simple ligation via cervical or thoracic approach depending upon location. The 12 previously reported cases in the English literature are reviewed, and a 13th case has been added.

Congenital tracheoesophageal (TE) fistula without esophageal atresia, commonly known as "H" type, is a rare anomaly in infants, accounting for only 1½ to 4% of all congenital tracheoesophageal malformations.[1-3] Although today TE fistula is a well recognized entity, certain of the rare varieties may not be diagnosed during the pediatric period. Those fistulas that do persist to adult life masquerade as chronic lung disease of unknown etiology.

Many classifications of esophageal atresia and tracheoesophageal fistula have been proposed. These include those by Vogt,[4] Ladd,[5] Swenson,[6] Gross,[7] Koop,[8] and Haight.[9] Regardless of the classification used, there are five main categories as demonstrated in Figure 1: 1) esophageal atresia without TE fistula; 2) esophageal atresia with proximal TE fistula, 3) esophageal atresia with distal TE fistula, 4) esophageal atresia with tracheoesophageal fistula, both distal and proximal, and 5) TE fistula without atresia. Major studies to date have shown that 85 to 95% of the anomalies of the esophageal atresia-TE fistula category are of the type with esophageal atresia and distal TE fistula. This type is also known as the Vogt 3B, Ladd type 3, or Gross C type.[4,5,7] At present, there is no single theory of development which can satisfactorily explain the occurrence of all variants of congenital tracheoesophageal anomalies.[10-14]

CASE REPORT

A 26-year-old-male truck driver was referred for evaluation of abdominal pain. The symptoms of generalized painful abdominal cramping had been present intermittently for six weeks prior to admission. The pain was associated with hematemesis on occasion, and was not relieved by food ingestion. When the symptoms first occurred the patient was referred to a local hospital in another state and underwent a radiologic upper gastrointestinal examina-

---

From the Department of Otology and Head and Neck Surgery, Indiana University Medical Center, Indianapolis, Indiana, and the Department of Surgery, Ball Memorial Hospital, Muncie, Indiana.

Presented at the meeting of the American Broncho-Esophagological Association, Palm Beach, Florida, April 27-28, 1976.

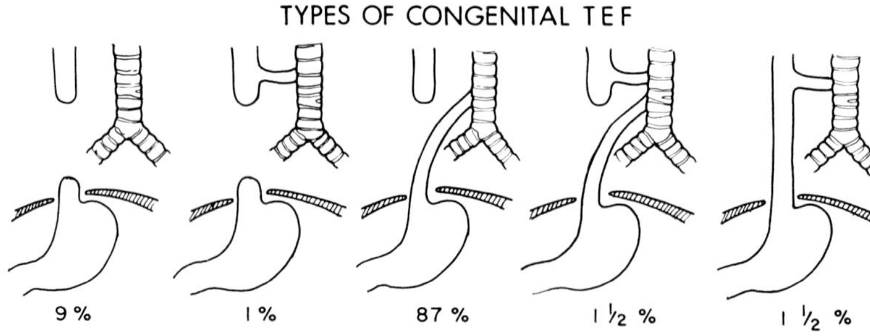

Fig. 1. Classification of tracheoesophageal fistulas by anatomic characteristics with percentages based on Waterston *et al.*[1]

tion. He was told his x-ray was normal except that he had "aspirated some of the barium into his lungs." The patient left that hospital and returned to his local physician who treated him for gastritis. When the symptoms continued, the patient was referred for definitive diagnosis.

The past history was significant in that the patient had suffered repeated episodes of bronchitis and pneumonia. The first episode occurred at age one month, with regular bouts at least annually thereafter. The patient was evaluated for his "chronic lung condition"

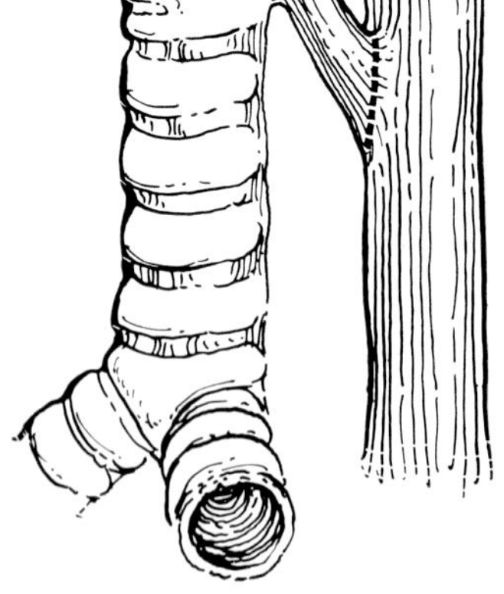

Fig. 2. Representation of resulting orientation of fistula in adult following differential growth of esophagus and trachea.

on at least two occasions at large teaching institutions with endoscopy and roentgenography. The past surgical history consisted of an appendectomy and Meckel's diverticulectomy at age 15.

Evaluation of his "chronic lung condition" was again initiated. A fiberoptic bronchoscope was utilized, and a midline circular defect was noted in the posterior tracheal wall approximately 5-6 cm inferior to the glottis. This defect opened and closed with respiration. During evaluation of the upper gastrointestinal tract with barium, including cineradiography, a fistulous tract was not visualized. However, the esophagus was noted to be dilated and demonstrated minimal peristalsis. In addition, it was noted the patient had again "aspirated" contrast media. Instillation of an iodized oil into the trachea via a tracheal catheter did not delineate a fistula. Under general anesthesia, rigid-tube esophagoscopy was performed, and anesthetic gas was noted in the esophagus. With each assisted respiration gas was expressed through the esophagus. No fistula could be visualized. A rigid 7 mm x 40 cm bronchoscope was then passed, and the previously described defect was seen. A No. 16 lumen finder was passed with ease through the defect which coursed inferiorly and into the esophagus. This confirmed the presumptive diagnosis of TE fistula.

The patient underwent a right thoracotomy and "H" type TE fistula was identified. The fistulous tract coursed obliquely from a more superiorly placed

TABLE I

SUMMARY OF REPORTED CASES OF CONGENITAL TRACHEOESOPHAGEAL FISTULAS IN ADULTS

Author	*Age Sex*	*Symptoms*	*X-ray*	*Endoscopy*	*Treatment*
Negus 1929	45 M	?	N	N	N, Died Ca lung
McKinney 1933	58 F	PC	+	+B −E	N
Krausey 1958	38 F	Vague	N	N	N, DAP
Caldwell 1954	54 M	RP	+	N	N, DAP
Mathey & Lemoine 1954	16 F	RP	+	+B	SL
Demong et al 1959	15 F	CC	N	+B	Ligation plus pneumonectomy
Ferguson & Schoemperlen 1959	23 F	CC	N	+B	SL
Lansden & Falor 1960	63 F	PC	—	+B −E	SL
Tenta & Ford 1967	16 M	CC	+	+B	SL
Zack & Owens 1967	32 M	RP	+	−B −E	SL
Bertelsen 1970	48 M	CB	+	+B +E	SL
Acosta & Battersby 1974	48 M	CP	+	−B −E	SL
Present Case	26 M	RP	—	+B +E	SL

PC - Postprandial cough; RP - Recurrent pneumonia; CC - Chronic cough; CB - Chronic bronchitis; CP - Chronic pneumonia; N - None; + - Positive findings; — - Negative findings; B - Bronch; E - Esoph; DAP - Died aspiration pneumonia; SL - Simple ligation.

tracheal stoma 8 cm above the carina to a more inferiorly placed esophageal stoma. The fistulous tract was ligated and sectioned. The patient had an uneventful postoperative course and has had no recurrence of respiratory tract problems to date.

DISCUSSION

Tracheoesophageal fistula without esophageal atresia is a difficult diagnosis to establish in spite of a high index of suspicion. Congenital TE fistula rarely is so innocuous as to permit the host to survive to adult life without the diagnosis being made. One would expect the size of the fistula to be related to the frequency and severity of symptoms. Considering the type of TE fistula, the "H" type is the variant which one would logically expect to see in the adult group as it is most compatible with prolonged survival. In fact, all congenital TE fistulas in adults reported to date have been the "H" type. Whether or not the number of patients with undiagnosed congenital TE fistula who reach adult life will increase remains to be seen. Certainly the widespread use of antibiotics should decrease mortality and morbidity in those patients in whom the diagnosis is yet to be made. Concomitantly, the number of patients undergoing bronchoscopy is certainly on the rise. Internists interested in pulmonary disease account for the greatest part of this rise as they are utilizing the fiberoptic bronchoscope to its fullest potential.

The diagnostic work-up should include PA and lateral chest x-rays, radiographic evaluation of the esophagus utilizing contrast media, including cineradiography when available and finally, endoscopic evaluation of the esophagus and trachea.

On the routine chest x-ray, a pneumoesophagram may be seen which should immediately call for a complete evaluation if the clinical history is suggestive. The contrast media utilized in adults may be iodized oil or thin barium. However, a fistulous tract will not be demonstrated radiographically when the esophagus is studied in many cases. This is due to the collapsible nature of the esophageal stoma and in some cases the presence of a mucosal tag which acts as a valve. In these cases it is easier to demonstrate the fistulous tract by injecting small amounts of iodized oil into the tracheal tree.

One must remember that the tracheal stoma of a congenital fistula is quite cephalad and the fistulous tract itself tends to course distally to the esophageal stoma. Thus, the mistake of looking too distal for the fistula can be made. Although no tract is demonstrated on esophageal evaluation, any evidence of "aspirated" contrast media should be considered as suggestive of the presence of a fistulous tract. Also, one must not forget that an esophagus which has been dilated periodically with air for many years tends to show abnormal motility. In fact, the radiologic picture of scleroderma or achalasia may be seen with a dilated adynamic esophagus which is actually the long term sequela of a TE fistula. Finally, in addition to the classic history which accompanies TE fistula, adults complain often of a large amount of flatus secondary to the involuntary aerophagia.

Treatment consists of simple division of the fistula and suturing of the esophagus and trachea. Depending upon the level of the fistula, the approach may be either cervical or through a right thoracotomy. Congenital TE fistulas, in which other anomalies of the esophagus are not involved, characteristically show a considerably higher location of the fistula in the trachea than that occurring with esophageal atresia.[9] As stated before, the opening in the trachea is usually situated in a more cephalad position than the opening into the esophagus. This obliquity is increased with age into adult life because of the differential growth rates of the esophagus and trachea (Fig. 2). This explains the difficulty in demonstrating the fistula radiographically, plus the paucity of morbidity seen in these patients for long periods of time.

In conclusion, the present case report brings the number reported in the English literature to 13.[14-25] Table I summarizes all thirteen cases as to author, age and sex of patient, presenting symptom(s), radiographic findings, findings at endoscopy if performed, and treatment. The ages of patients ranged from 15 years to 63 years. There were seven males and six females with the initial report of the entity by Negus in 1929.

REFERENCES

1. Waterston DJ, Carter REB, Aberdeen E: Oesophageal atresia, tracheoesophageal fistula: A study of survival in 218 infants. Lancet 1:819-822, 1962

2. Ware GW, Hall A: Congenital tracheoesophageal fistula in the adult. J Thorac Surg 36:58-62, 1958

3. Holder TM, Cloud DT, Lewis, JE Jr, *et al*: Esophageal atresia and tracheoesophageal fistula. A survey of its members by the surgical section of the American Academy of Pediatrics. Pediatrics 34:542-549, 1964

4. Vogt EC: Congenital esophageal atresia. Am J Roentgenol Radium Ther Nucl Med 22: 463-465, 1929

5. Ladd WE: The surgical treatment of esophageal atresia and tracheoesophageal fistulas. N Eng J Med 230:625-637, 1944

6. Swenson O: The diagnosis and treatment of atresia of the esophagus and tracheoesophageal fistula. Pediatrics 1:195-204, 1948

7. Gross RE: *The Surgery of Infancy and Childhood.* Philadelphia, WB Saunders Co, 1953, p 76

8. Koop CE, Kiesewetter WB, Johnson J: Surg Gynecol Obstet 98:687-692, 1954

9. Haight C: Some observations on esophageal atresias and tracheoesophageal fistulas of congenital origin. J Thorac Surg 34:141-172, 1957

10. Wayson E, Garnjobst W, Chandler JJ, *et al*: Esophageal atresia with tracheoesophageal fistula. Am J Surg 110:162-167, 1960

11. Humphreys G, Hogg B, Ferrer J: Congenital atresia of the esophagus. J Thorac Surg 32:334-346, 1956

12. Lober P: *Otolaryngology.* Paparella M, Shumrick D (eds), Philadelphia, WB Saunders Company, 1973, vol 1, chap 20

13. Smith E: *The Early Development of the Trachea and Esophagus, in Contributions to Embryology.* Washington, Carnegie Institute of Washington, 1957, vol 36, p 41

14. Tenta LT, Ford LH: Congenital TE fistula in a young adult. Arch Otolaryngol 85: 675-679, 1967

15. Negus VE: Esophagus from a middle aged man, showing a congenital opening into the trachea. J Laryngol Otol 44:184, 1929

16. McKinney R: Tracheo-esophageal fistula, probably congenital, in a woman 58 years of age. Ann Otol Rhinol Laryngol 42:1237-1239, 1933

17. Krausey B: Congenital tracheoesophageal fistula without oesophageal atresia with resultant asphyxial death. Br Med J 1:1433, 1953

18. Caldwell KPS: Congenital tracheoesophageal fistula in the adult. J Int Coll Surg 22: 387-390, 1954

19. Mathey J, Lemoine A: Tracheal diverticulum and congenital oesophagotracheal fistula without oesophageal atresia. Thorax 9: 106-111, 1954

20. Demong CV, Grown JB, Heitzman GC: Congenital tracheoesophageal fistula without atresia of the esophagus. Am Surg 25:156-162, 1959

21. Ferguson CC, Schoemperlin CB: Congenital tracheoesophageal fistula in an adult. Ann Surg 149:582-585, 1959

22. Lansden FT, Falor WA: Congenital esophagorespiratory fistula in the adult. J Thorac Cardiovasc Surg 39:246-251, 1960

23. Zack BJ, Owen MP: Congenital tracheoesophageal fistula in the adult. Arch Surg 95: 674-677, 1967

24. Bertelson S: Congenital oesophageal-tracheal fistulas in the adult. Scand J Thorac Cardiovasc Surg 4:80-82, 1970

25. Acosta JL, Battersby JS: Congenital tracheoesophageal fistula in the adult. Ann Thorac Surg 17:51-57, 1974

REPRINTS—Robert W. Stephens, MD, Department of Otorhinolaryngology and Bronchoesophagology, Indiana University School of Medicine, 1100 West Michigan St., Indianapolis, IN 46202.

INTERNATIONAL CONGRESS ON THE EDUCATION OF THE DEAF

The International Congress on the Education of the Deaf voted in August 1975 to establish an International Congress Committee on the Education of the Deaf with the aim of creating a mechanism to insure a more orderly continuity in the congresses. For information write to Dr. S. Richard Silverman, Chairman, International Congress Committee on the Education of the Deaf, 818 South Euclid Avenue, St. Louis, MO 63110, U.S.A.

Ann Otol 85: 1976

TRACING THE TRACHEOSTOMY

ELIZABETH A. M. FROST, MD

BRONX, NEW YORK

SUMMARY – The evolution of tracheostomy can be divided into five stages. The first and longest period (covering roughly 3,000 years from 1500 BC to 1500 AD) begins with references to incisions into the "wind pipe" in the Ebers Papyrus and the Rig Veda. However, Alexander the Great, Asclepiades, Aretaeus and Galen are all recorded as having used this operation. Between 1546 with the writings of Brassarolo until 1883, the procedure was considered futile and irresponsible and few surgeons had the courage to perform it. The third period starts with Trousseau's report of 200 cases in the therapy of diphtheria in 1833. Tracheostomy became a highly dramatized operation for asphyxia and acute respiratory obstruction. In 1932 Wilson suggested its prophylactic and therapeutic use in poliomyelitis. Tracheostomy was then recommended for a large variety of assorted maladies. This started a tremendous period of enthusiasm. Finally, the present era starting in 1965 comes as a period of rationalization. Complications, indications and interrelation with endotracheal intubation are clearly outlined. Tracheostomy has found its place.

Tracheostomy, derived from two Greek words meaning, "I cut the trachea," has probably been known for about 3,500 years.

In looking at the history of this operation, we can see that it falls roughly into five stages.

The first and by far the longest period covers approximately 3,000 years, from 1500 BC to AD 1500, and may be referred to as a time of legend as the exact interpretation of many of the writings is really a matter of opinion.

Of the three oldest known medical works, reference to opening the windpipe is found, certainly, in two of them. The sacred book of Hindu medicine, the Rig Veda,[1] which was written between 2000 and 1000 BC, mentions "the bountiful one who, without a ligature, can cause the windpipe to re-unite when the cervical cartilages are cut across, provided they are not entirely severed." Joachim's[2] translation of the Eber's Papyrus (another ancient medical reference dating about 1550 BC) describes an "incision of a fatty tumor in the throat, taking care of the vessels." The third medical tome, the ancient Chinese "Huang Ti Nei Ching Sû Wen," contains no reference to surgery of any kind.[3] It was taught that the superiority of Chinese internal medicine made surgery unnecessary and the Confucian tenets of the sacredness of the body countered any tendency to develop anatomical studies or surgical procedures. The companion reference to the Nei Ching Sû Wen, the Ling Shu, (or the book of acupuncture), graphically describes the effects of respiratory obstruction (that is, a cutting off of the energy of the great Yin meridians) . . . "as the face turns black, the patient is bound to die."[4]

A few hundred years later, Homer,[5] in the eighth century BC, is said to have referred to the operation of relieving choking persons by cutting open the trachea.

Legend also claimed that Hippocrates, in the fourth century BC, advocated tracheal cannulation but recent, careful translation of his writings does not bear this out. Instead of tracheostomy for quinsy, for instance, he

----

From the Department of Anesthesiology, Albert Einstein College of Medicine, Bronx, New York.

Presented at the meeting of the American Broncho-Esophagological Association, Palm Beach, Florida, April 27-28, 1976.

wrote — "spontaneous determination to the external parts of the neck is vital to recovery."[6] In modern language this may be interpreted to mean that a counter-irritant should be used to promote ulceration and drainage of the abscess through the neck.

Also in the fourth century BC, Alexander the Great is reported to have "punctured the trachea of a soldier with the point of his sword when he saw the man choking from a bone lodged in his throat."[5]

It would appear that Asclepiades of Bithynia, around 100 BC, was the first surgeon to perform elective tracheostomy. The operation and Asclepiades' technique was described by Galen,[7] writing towards the end of the second century AD. Aretaeus, in the same century, in his textbook "The Therapeutics of Acute Diseases,"[8] confirmed the work of Asclepiades but condemned the operation on the grounds that wounds of cartilages cannot heal — a point also made by Coelius Aurelianus[9] in the fifth century AD, who further remarked that it was "a fantastic operation" and "a futile and irresponsible idea set forth by Asclepiades."

Paulus Aegineta in the seventh century repeatedly seems to have opened the trachea and he also described the work of Antyllus of Rome (AD 340) who made a transverse incision into the trachea between the third and fourth rings, drew the cartilages apart with hooks and sewed the edges of the wound together again when the patient breathed more freely.[10]

At about the same time, in Arabian texts, tracheostomy was referred to by Abu'l Kasem and Ebn Zohr more as a possibility than as a reality.[10]

The barbarism of the Dark Ages eclipsed the world of science as it did that of literature. Little was heard of any type of surgery until the 15th century.

For around 300 years, from the beginning of the 16th century until 1833, frequent references to tracheostomy were made. But the operation was considered not only useless but dangerous. This period may best be categorized as one of fear. Many modifications of the procedure were suggested but promptly discarded amid violent criticism. During this time, reports of only 28 successful operations have been found in the literature.[11] A Florentine physician, Benivieni, reported a single operation at the beginning of the 16th century. At about the same time, Gulielmo de Saliceto[12] reported the successful use of tracheostomy in a case of angina. Of course, this is hardly the treatment of choice for this condition by anyone's standards. Rolandi, in Bologna, used a permanent tracheostomy to relieve a tracheal stenosis caused by a laryngeal abscess. In 1546, Musa Brassarolo of Ferrara, performed the operation and described his technique. Sanatorius in 1590 used a trocar for the first time and left a cannula in place for three days. In France, Ambroise Paré described opening the trachea with a transverse incision, again for angina.

In the laboratory some interesting animal experiments were performed by Robert Hooke in 1667.[13] These experiments were similar to, but more detailed than those described by Vesalius[14] in 1543 and consisted of maintaining the life of a dog by inflating the lungs through the bound distal end of its transected trachea after the ribs, diaphragm and pericardium had been cut away. Thus he demonstrated that life could be maintained through the severed cartilages of a trachea using a cannula connected to bellows for inflation.

At the beginning of the 17th century, Fabricius ab Aquapendente wrote, "the terrified surgeons of our times have not dared to exercise this surgery and I also have never performed it. Even the mention of this operation terrifies the surgeons; hence it is called a scandal."[15] Later, Fabricius modified his feelings a little and operated successfully in several cases of foreign body impaction in the larynx. He also incised the trachea "when that tube was clogged with viscid mucus." He used a vertical incision and introduced a cannula with wings. His pupil, Casserius, introduced a curved cannula with tapes to tie it in position. The improvement in the shape of the tube was quickly forgotten and the straight tube remained for many years.

In 1650 Theophilus Bonetus, the great pathological anatomist, recommended the use of a tracheostomy for a 7-year-old boy who had aspirated a piece of bone. He was overruled by the internist in accordance with the times and the child died. Naturally, he published the case in detail.[16]

Two other cases from the 17th century are worthy of mention. Nicholas Habicot, the surgeon to the Hôtel Dieu of Paris, performed a tracheostomy on a young man as a means of draining blood resulting from a penetrating wound of the larynx. He had previously opened the trachea of a youth, who, in an attempt to protect his possessions from robbers, had swallowed and aspirated several coins. Habicot also suggested that the operation might be of use for inflammatory conditions of the larynx.[17]

Towards the end of the 17th century several other physicians wrote warily of possible uses for tracheostomy. Among them were Severinus and Renatus Moreau who suggested its use in mumps. Scultetus,[18] Dionnis,[19] and Garengeot[20] made several suggestions as to possible but not very probable uses for tracheostomy. Dekkerus[21] of Leyden recommended a cutting trocar, an advance quickly forgotten, but re-described some years later by Bauchot.

One of the first detailed case reports was published in *Surgical Pathology* in 1717 by Verduc.[22] He described the extraction of a bone fragment through a free incision in the trachea.

Heister, who was the first actually to use the term "tracheotomy"[23] described the operation in 1739 and remarked rather boldly that it had been neglected by modern surgeons (*i.e.*, his contemporaries). He used a straight tube and trocar.

Professor Wendt[24] of Erlangen around 1760 described tracheotomy for removal of an acorn in a young girl. He opened the trachea by dividing the first three rings and separating the edges of the wound with blunt hooks.

A double cannula was introduced by George Martin[25] in 1770 – another important advance, also quickly discarded.

A widely used handbook for the physician, written by William Buchan in 1770, devoted a chapter to the care of the drowned person.[26] Detharting[27] had already advised bronchotomy for drowning but Buchan, although he described mouth to mouth resuscitation, counter chest pressure and mechanical nasal and oral airways, was most wary of advocating opening the trachea.

M. Louis presented his second memoire on bronchotomy to the Royal Academy of Surgery of Paris in April 1759.[28] His advocacy of tracheostomy, especially for the extraction of foreign bodies, was most judicious, but many practitioners opposed the operation as very dangerous. Among the more vocal antagonists were Van Swieten[29] and Sharp,[30] both celebrated surgeons of the times.

P. J. Desault, who enjoyed the grand title of "Surgeon in Chief of the Great Hospital of Humanity, Paris," insisted initially on the value of laryngotomy for aspiration. Later he wrote that the passage of a small naso-tracheal tube was to be preferred as it secured an airway and provoked coughing.[31]

Favier, also from Paris, described more laboratory experiments with dogs.[32] He introduced foreign bodies into the trachea of the animal and then performed laryngotomy. With the incision the pebbles were ejected by the coughing that ensued. Favier concluded that the difficulty of finding and extracting foreign bodies was a mere pretext put forward by timid practitioners opposed to bronchotomy.

In 1765 a Scottish physician, Francis Home,[33] described an upper airway inflammation which he called croup, an old Scottish word for a sore throat accompanied by harsh breathing. He recommended tracheostomy to alleviate the distress of children suffering from this disease.

"Croup" was prevalent also in the United States in the 19th century, particularly in the New York and Philadelphia areas where it was often called "cynanche trachealis" from two Greek words: Chyn (doglike) and archein (to choke). The medical thinking of Great Britain and the fear of tracheostomy had infiltrated this country. Therefore, when Dr. Elisha C. Dick recommended tracheostomy for a patient, Drs. James Craig and Gustavus Brown did not concur. And on December 14, 1799, George Washington died of an acute upper airway obstruction.

It was not until the beginning of the 19th century did tracheostomy in fact, come to be cautiously used in croup by such surgeons as Crawford,[34], Chaussier,[35] Schvilgue,[36] Vicq d' Azyr,[37] and Fourcroy,[38] who described cricothyroid laryngotomy as better management. In 1826, Pierre Bretonneau published his account of the disease and named it diphtheria.[30]

The third stage in the development of tracheostomy started around 1830. McKenzie in his textbook, *Diseases of the Pharynx, Larynx and Trachea,* summarized the general feeling of the time: "the question always arises in the mind of the young surgeon whether the symptoms are sufficiently urgent to render the operation necessary."[40] It was a time of dramatization. Tracheostomy was an operation for life and death situations. As Malgaigne cautioned, one should always be ready to use one's own mouth to suck out blood from a hemorrhaging tracheostomy wound.[41] Trousseau[42] reported, "I have now performed the operation in more than 200 cases of diphtheria and I have had the satisfaction of knowing that one-fourth of these operations were successful." (Actually, the figures were 47 survivors out of 215).

Tracheostomy came to be used for obstruction of the upper airway by croup, diphtheria, foreign bodies and trauma. It was also used to rest the larynx in chronic tuberculosis or syphilis. The medical literature became filled with violent arguments over such things as technique, postoperative complications, high versus low tracheostomy, and dangers of general anesthesia associated with acute respiratory obstruction. Millord, Chassaignac, Malgaigne, Kuhn, Thompson, Pitha, Ulrich, Hueter, Bardeleben, Fuller, March, Planchon, and Durham[43] were just a few of the surgeons who suggested modifications of the tube or its uses. The 1860 year book of the New Sydenham Society alone contained over 38 papers devoted to techniques and indications for tracheostomy. A definitive text reviewing the controversies was published by Dr. Max Schuller in 1880.[44]

In 1869, Dr. Erichsen[45] wrote, "In this country (Britain) the operation seldom succeeds because it is almost never resorted to except in hopeless cases." (A statement heartily endorsed by Henriette.[46]) Erichsen warned that the initial incision might cause death but the surgery should be completed as the patient might be resuscitated if a large silver tube were used. He advised the use of chloroform in children, but no anesthesia should be used for adults. He recognized four difficulties: 1) exposing the air tube; 2) hemorrhage; 3) opening the air passage; and 4) placing the tracheostomy tube. A tracheostomy was to be used in children and laryngotomy in adults. The tube was to be cleaned with feathers or a sponge on a stick with a solution of silver nitrate.

Sir William Jenner recommended tracheostomy in diphtheria because it saved the patient from the terrible death caused by asphyxia. He observed that patients might still die but in a less distressing manner.[45] Evans Conway, writing on croup and diphtheria in the Edinburgh Medical Journal in 1860, pointed out that the mortality in France where tracheostomy was used was only 68%[47] and with these figures, strongly recommended the more liberal use of the procedure in Scotland.

Resolution of many of the highly debated issues began probably with Chevalier Jackson.[48] From extensive experience, he did much to clarify the problems. He emphasized a long incision, avoidance of high cartilage dissection, slow and deliberate surgery and he advocated cutting the thyroid isthmus. He also designed many instruments both for laryngotomy and bronchotomy.

Another life saving use of tracheostomy was in the administration of general anesthesia. This had been advocated by Snow[49] and Trendelenburg[50] as the only means of securing an airway. However, endotracheal intubation was performed by Sir William MacEwan in 1878[51] and popularized by Bartholomy and Dufor[52] in 1907, and by Kelly in 1912.[53] Thus, one of the dramatic uses of the operation disappeared.

Early in the 20th century diphtheria was controlled by immunization. The discovery of the sulfonamides helped curb upper respiratory infections. The need for the emergency tracheostomy became a rarity.

The age of drama was waning.

The fourth stage in the development of tracheostomy, a time of almost uncontrolled enthusiasm, began in 1932 with Wilson's[54] suggestion of its use in poliomyelitis to prophylactically prevent pulmonary infection.

It was quickly advocated that tracheostomy would be advantageous in the management of tetanus, all head and chest injuries, drug overdose, after neurological and thoracic surgery and, in fact, all major surgery, as well as in many other diseases. The medical world became tracheostomy oriented.

Two important developments were evidenced during this time. Carte and Guiseppi[55] realized that tracheostomy reduced the volume of dead space and from this developed the use of this procedure in the treatment of chronic bronchitis, emphysema and pneumonia. The second development was intermittent positive pressure ventilation through a tracheostomy, described with simultaneous nebulization for the treatment of pulmonary disease in 1948 by Motley, Rang and Gordon. During the poliomyelitis epidemic in Europe, Ibsen further developed the use of continuous and intermittent ventilation through a tracheostomy tube. The success evidenced by this therapy revolutionized the managemnt of all forms of severe respiratory insufficiency. But like diphtheria, poliomyelitis also subsided with the worldwide use of the Salk vaccine. In addition, the rate of complications during and after tracheostomy, although much reduced, remained high.

By 1965, it became apparent that nasal or oral intubation could be performed quicker, more safely, and with a much lower complication rate in almost all situations. The modern era of tracheostomy-justification and rationalization was born.

Over the past ten years, the indications for tracheostomy and the techniques of the procedure have been strictly outlined and evaluated. Changes in design of the tube have allowed for reduced pressures, ease of cleaning or changing, minimal tissue reactivity, and firm placement in the stoma.

In summary, over a 3,000 year span, tracheostomy has developed from a straight reed thrust over the point of a sword into a choking soldier on the battlefield, to the meticulous aseptic insertion of a curved, nonreactive tube with a low pressure cuff into an anesthetized patient whose airway has already been secured by endotracheal intubation.

One could be reminded of the slogan, "You've come a long way, baby."

REFERENCES

1. McClelland RMA. *Progress in Anaesthesiology. Proceedings of the 4th World Congress of Anaesthesiologists.* Amsterdam, Excerpta Medica, 1970, pp 195-196

2. Wright J: *A History of Laryngology and Rhinology,* ed 2. Philadelphia, Lea and Febiger, 1914, pp 23, 29

3. Veith I: *Huang Ti Nei Ching Sû Wen.* University of California Press, 1966, p 3

4. Lu HC: *The Yellow Emperor's Book of*

Acupuncture. Vancouver, B.C., Academy of Oriental Heritage, 1973, p 119

5. Gordon BL: *The Romance of Medicine*. Philadelphia, FA Davis, 1947, p 461

6. Adam F: *The Genuine Works of Hippocrates, Translated from the Greek with a Preliminary Discourse and Annotations*. New York, W Wood and Co (undated)

7. Galen: *Introductio Seu Medicus*. CG Kuhn (trans) Leipzig, 1827, vol 14, p 734

8. Aretaeus: *The Therapeutics of Acute Diseases*. F Adam (trans), London, The Sydenham Society, 1856, chap 7, p 406

9. Aurelianus C: *De Morb. Acut*. (Circa 5th century A.D.) Book 53, chap 4

10. McKenzie M: *Diseases of the Pharynx, Larynx and Trachea*. New York, W Wood and Co, 1880, p 397

11. Goodall EW: The story of tracheotomy. Br J Child Dis 31:167-176; 253-272, 1934

12. Linhart W: *Compendium der Chirurg. Operation Lehre*. Vienna, 1877

13. Hooke R: An account of an experiment made by M Hook of preserving animals alive by blowing through their lungs with bellows. Phil Trans R Soc 2:539-540, 1667

14. Vesalius A: *De Humani Corporis Fabrica Libri Septem*. Basel, Oporinus, 1543, p 658

15. Fabricius H: *Opera Chirurgica*, vol VI, Frankfurt, 1660, para 1, cap 44, p 155

16. Bonetus T: *Sepulchetum Sive Anatomica Practica*. t.i. lib. 2 De Respiratione Laesa, Obs. i, Geneva, 1700 p 483

17. Habicot N: *Sur La Bronchotomie, Vulgairement Dicte Laryngotomie, ou Perforation De Flute Au Tuyau Du Poulman*. Paris, 1620

18. Scultetus J: *Armamentarium Chirurgicum*. Amsterdam, 1672, p 127

19. Dionnis P: *Operat. de Chirurg*. Paris, 1703, p 221

20. Garengeot: *Operat. de Chirurg*. Paris, 1720, vol 1, p 491

21. Dekkerus of Leyden: *Exercitat. Pract*. Lug. d. Bat., 1694, p 241

22. Verduc, cited by Gross SD: *On Foreign Bodies in the Air Passages. History of Bronchotomy, Section II*. Philadelphia, Blanchard and Lea, 1954, p 226

23. Heister L: *General System of Surgery*, ed 8. London, 1768, vol 2, p 52

24. Wendt A: *Historia Tracheotomiae nuperrimé Administratae*, in 8 vo. Vratislaviae, 1774

25. Martin G: Philosophical Trans. Vol 6. 1671, cited by McKenzie M in, *Diseases of the Pharynx, Larynx and Trachea*. New York, W Wood and Co, 1880, p 398

26. Buchan W: *Domestic Medicine*, ed 20. London (Edin Printer) T Cadell *et al*, 1807, p 596

27. Von Haller A: *Diss. Chirurg*. Berlin, 1750, vol 2, pp 438-439

28. Louis M: 2eMémoire sur la bronchotomie. Presented before the Royal Academy of Surgery, Paris, April 1759

29. Van Swieten G: *Commentar in Hermann Boerharii Aphorism*. Aph 813, 1741, p 42

30. Sharp J: *A Treatise of the Operations of Surgery*, ed 4. London, 1761, p 187

31. Bichat X: *The Surgical Works, or State of the Doctrine and Practice of P.J. Desault*. Philadelphia, Thos Dolson, 1814, vol 1, pp 229-234

32.. Favier M: *Memoires de l'Académie Royale de Chirurgie*. t.v. Paris, 1819, p 356

33. Home F: *An Enquiry into the Natural Causes and Cure of Croup*. Edinburgh, Kincaid and Bell, 1765

34. Crawford J: *Dissertation de Cynanche Stridula*. Edinburgh, 1771

35. Chaussier: Cited by McKenzie M, in *Diseases of the Pharynx, Larynx and Trachea*. New York, W Wood and Co, 1880, p 398

36. Schvilgue M: *Recueil d'Observation et de Faits Relat. au Croup*. Paris, 1808

37. d'Azyr V: *Mem. sur la laryngotomie*. Paris, Soc Roy de Med, T.i., 1776

38. de Fourcroy AF: *De Nova Laryngotomiae Methodo*. Paris, 1779

39. Bretonneau P: *Des Inflammations Speciales du tissu muquex et en particulier de la diphterite, ou inflammation pelliculaire, connue - sous le nom de croup, d'angine maligne, d'angine gangreneuse, etc*. Paris, Crevot, 1826

40. McKenzie M: *Diseases of the Pharynx, Larynx and Trachea*. New York, W Wood and Co, 1880, p 400

41. Malgaigne JF: *Manual of Operative Surgery*. Brittan F (trans), London, Henry Renshaw, 1846, pp 373-376

42. Trousseau A: *Lectures on Clinical Medicine*. JR Cormack (trans), London, The New Sydenham Society, 1869, Vol 2, p 598

43. McKenzie M: *Diseases of the Pharynx, Larynx and Trachea*. New York, W Wood and Co, 1880, p 399

44. Billroth H, Luecke: *Deutsche Chirurgie; Die Tracheotomie, Laryngotomie und Extirpation des Kehlkopfes*. Stuttgart, 1880

45. Erichsen JE: *The Science and Art of Surgery*. Philadelphia, Henry C Lea, 1869, p 919

46. Henriette M: *On Tracheotomy in Croup*. Presse Med Belge 34 Med. Times and Gaz., Sept. 8, 1860, p 274

47. Conway E: On tracheotomy in croup. Edinburgh Med J, Jan. and May, 1860

48. Jackson C: Tracheotomy. Laryngoscope 19:285-290, 1909

49. Snow J: *On Chloroform and other Anaesthetics*. London, J. Churchill, 1858, p 117

50. Trendelenburg F: Tamponode de trachea. Arch Klin Chir 12:121, 1871

51. MacEwan W: Clinical observations of introduction of tracheal tubes by mouth instead of performing a tracheotomy. Br Med J, 2:122-124, 163-165, 1880

52. Bartholomy, Dufor X: L'Anesthesie dans la Chirurgie de la Face. Presse Med, 15: 474, 1907

53. Kelly RE: Anesthesia by intratracheal insufflation of ether. Br Med J 2:112, 1912

54. Wilson JL: Acute anterior poliomyelitis treatment of bulbar and high spinal types. N Engl J Med 206:887, 1932

55. Carte BN, Guiseppi J: Tracheotomy, a useful procedure in thoracic surgery with particular reference to its employment in crushing injuries of the thorax. J Thorac Surg, 21:495, 1951

REPRINTS—Elizabeth A. M. Frost, MD, Department of Anesthesiology, Albert Einstein College of Medicine, 1300 Morris Park Avenue, Bronx, New York 10461.

XV INTERNATIONAL CONGRESS OF BRONCHOESOPHAGOLOGY

The XV International Congress of Bronchoesophagology will be held in Sao Paulo, Brazil, March 24-26, 1977, following the II World Congress of Otolaryngology in Buenos Aires. For information write: Dr. Plinio de Mattos Barretto, President of the Congress, Rua Cons. Torres Homem, 371, 01432, Sao Paulo, Brazil.

Ann Otol 85: 1976

LASER ADAPTER FOR TRACHEOSCOPY

ALBERT H. ANDREWS, JR., MD

LARRY L. BAILEY, MD

CHICAGO, ILLINOIS

SUMMARY — This adapter makes it possible for the operating microscope to be used monocularly, to see axially down the CO_2 laser beam, to use the aiming light and its joy stick control. This makes the laser useful for upper tracheal lesions through a tracheoscope.

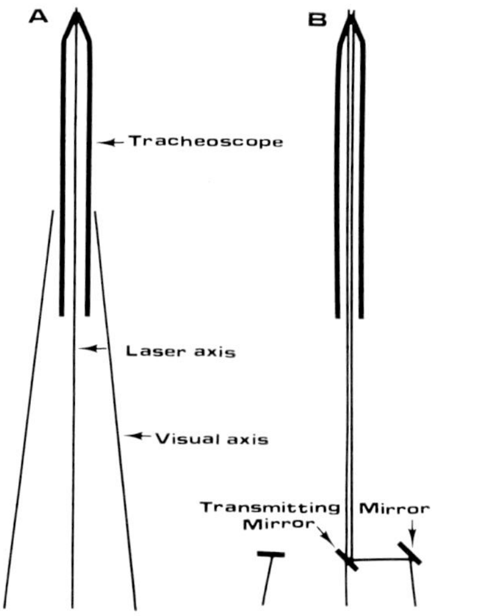

Fig. 1. Diagrammatic representation showing how A) the long, narrow tracheoscope blocks vision with the binocular operating microscope; B) the transmitting mirror passes the laser beam and reflects the visual beam to the second mirror and into the microscope.

Granulomas, papillomas, tracheal strictures and neoplasms may be best approached by the use of the tracheoscope. Laser therapy through the tracheoscope is not feasible because the angle of the visual beams of the operating microscope* prevents adequate vision through the tracheoscope (Fig. 1A). Utilizing the principle of the bronchoscopic adapter described by Strong *et al*,[1] the germanium transmitting mirror** passes the 10.6μ laser beam and reflects visual light onto the front surface mirror and into one visual axis of the microscope. Vision, axial with the laser beam is obtained plus the accurate control of the area of ablation with the joy stick and aiming light of the micromanipulator*** (Fig. 1B).

In use, the micromanipulator (Fig. 2) is adjusted for exact coincidence of the aiming light and laser burn. The adapter is locked in place and coincidence is again established by vertical and horizontal controls of the adapter. The microscope is lined up accurately with the tracheoscope, and the area of burn coincides with the aiming light. Moist gauze is placed around the tracheoscope to prevent inadvertent burn of the lips. Because of the short space between the tracheoscope and the adapter it may be necessary to move the microscope for insertion of instruments.

---

* Zeiss, Carl, Inc., New York, NY.

** Servo Corporation of America, Hicksville, NY.

*** American Optical Corp., Buffalo, NY.

From the Department of Otolaryngology, Abraham Lincoln School of Medicine, College of Medicine of the University of Illinois and the University of Illinois Hospital Eye and Ear Infirmary, Chicago, Illinois.

Presented at the meetng of the American Broncho-Esophagological Association, Palm Beach, Florida, April 27-28, 1976.

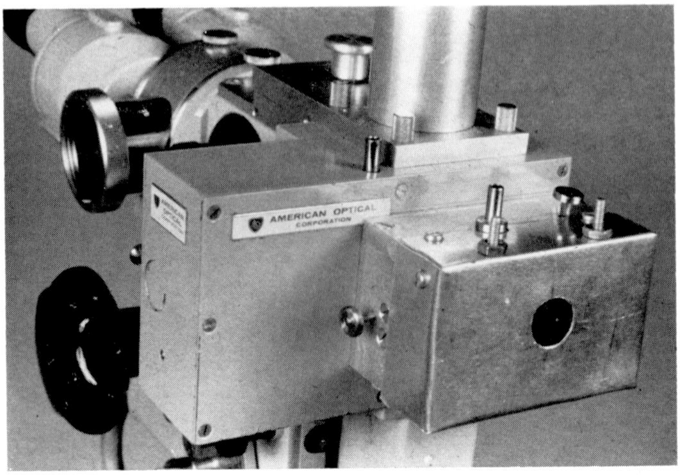

Fig. 2. The adapter attached to the micromanipulator and operating microscope.

REFERENCES

1. Strong MS, Vaughan CW, Polanyi T, *et al*: Bronchoscopic laser surgery. Ann Otol Rhinol Laryngol 83:769-776, 1974

Reprints—A. H. Andrews, Jr., MD, Dept. of Otolaryngology, Abraham Lincoln School of Medicine, 1855 W. Taylor St., Chicago, IL 60612.

EDUCATIONAL TRAINING IN ENDOSCOPY

JOHN E. RAYL, MD
LAKE CITY, FLORIDA

SUMMARY – An educational training need has developed as a result of the recent rapidly increasing acquisition of endoscopes. This acquisition has been occurring at a rate faster than training programs can acquaint physicians with their use. A Veterans Administration (VA) feasibility study has determined that color television-endoscopy can provide the type of instructional materials that could be used to assist a larger number of physicians in acquiring skills in endoscopy. Since the budget requirements for television-endoscopy are substantial, it seemed expedient for the VA to establish a Center for Endoscopic Programs (VACEP). The purpose of this Center is to prepare instructional materials that will enhance educational training in endoscopy. We believe that the provision of self-instructional and teaching supplement types of audiovisual materials are essential to the accomplishment of VACEP's educational objectives. Our society today is video oriented, and we believe very strongly in the value of the television medium as an educational adjunct in teaching endoscopy.

The field of endoscopy has changed so rapidly in the past six years that it has unexpectedly developed "growing pains." These changes are due to the introduction of many new endoscopes with a marked increase in the acquisition of these instruments by physicians. Correction of this apparently new "malady" will require a maximum effort in developing additional methods for educational training. This communication describes a type of educational training need in endoscopy; the applied educational research in endoscopy that has been completed at the (VA) Hospital in Lake City, Florida; and, finally, the plans of the VA to provide instructional materials for physicians who perform or teach endoscopy, as well as, to nursing personnel who care for this equipment.

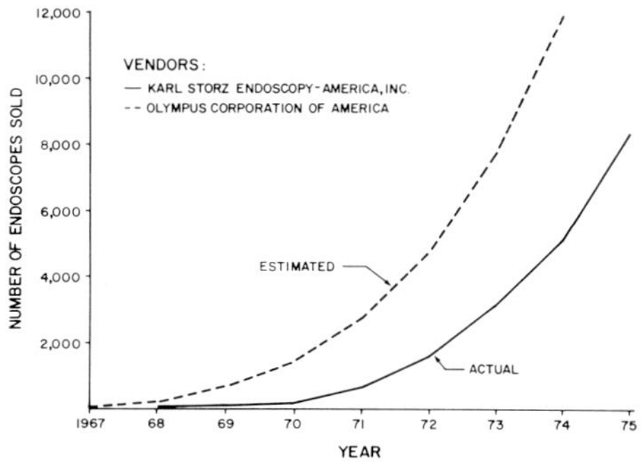

Fig. 1. Accumulated sales of endoscopes in the United States by two leading vendors. The solid line indicates the actual sales of Hopkins-Storz endoscopes. The dotted line indicates estimated sales of Olympus endoscopes.

EDUCATIONAL AND TRAINING NEED

New endoscopes are now being acquired by physicians faster than training programs can acquaint them with their use. Evidence of this rapid acquisition is shown in a review of the accumulated sales of these instruments in the United States by two leading vendors (Fig. 1). Following the introduction of Hopkins rigid endoscopes* in 1968, more than 8,000 of these instruments had been sold by the end of 1975. The policy of the Olympus Corporation would not permit them to divulge the actual number of flexible endoscopes** sold in the United States. However, they did furnish a graph of their annual

* Karl Storz Endoscopy-America, Inc., Los Angeles, CA.
** Olympus Corp. of America, New Hyde Park, NY.

From the Veterans Administration Center for Endoscopic Programs, Veterans Administration Hospital, Lake City, Florida.
Presented at the meeting of the American Broncho-Esophagological Association, Palm Beach, Florida, April 27-28, 1976.

sales omitting the numbers, from which we have estimated their accumulated sales (Fig. 1). If this estimation is correct and some Olympus personnel have said that it is close, the total number of sales reached more than 12,000 endoscopes from 1967 through 1974.

You might then ask, "Is there an educational training need associated with this rapid increase in use of endoscopes?"

An opinion in a letter dated May 2, 1975, from Milton M. Rubin, Karl Storz Endoscopy — America, states: "Although endoscopy is now part of some training curricula in major teaching institutions, the great majority of the physicians who have been in practive five years or more have not been academically trained in endoscopy. A few, scattered seminars are being offered in the various specialties, but no real training programs are available (except in the few teaching institutions mentioned above) nor is specific training required legally or by the medical profession before any physician can perform an endoscopic procedure." In the same letter, Mr. Rubin describes their educational effort by explaining: "We now have 19 films and approximately 41 reprints that are either loaned (films) or given (reprints) to physicians in the United States requesting such material. Unfortunately, the films are only 16 to 18 minutes in length and, as are the reprints, really for orientation and treat but do not teach endoscopy."

In a letter dated April 29, 1975, Mr. William C. Kofoed of Olympus Corporation of America expresses his opinion regarding endoscopic training programs: "Much of what is taught in doctors' offices, clinics, or medical schools could be taught by audiovisual aids, without the need of full-time instruction. It is sad to report that there are only seven known films or cassettes in English in the entire world on flexible endoscopy. To add to that dismay, most of this material is too broad and tries to cover an entire procedure in too short a time."

These opinions suggest that an educational training need is associated with the recent rapid acquisition of endoscopes, and that one need is for the development of instructional materials in endoscopy that can assist physicians in acquiring skills that will assure that all endoscopic examinations will be performed in a manner most beneficial to the patient.

APPLIED EDUCATIONAL RESEARCH COMPLETED

The recognition of the need to develop instructional materials in endoscopy led the Exchange of Medical In-Formation Review Group, the Special Medical Advisory Group, and the Chief Medical Director of the VA to support a three-year Exchange of Medical Information Project to investigate the feasibility of using color television as an instructional method in endoscopy. The objectives of this project, beginning on July 1, 1972, were to determine if television-endoscopy: 1) would be a feasible approach for improving the training of physicians, and 2) if it would enhance the clinical care of the patient.

Our experience with the use of closed-circuit color television in endoscopy has conclusively demonstrated that this application is an excellent clinical and educational tool with the following advantages:

1. Prior orientation of the resident with videotape improves his initial performance during clinical examination of patients.

2. Immediate replay of videotapes permits reevaluation and demonstration of endoscopic findings to physicians.

3. Simultaneous viewing increases the interest and participation in endoscopy and increases the number of physicians receiving training.

4. Magnified image aids in performing delicate endoscopic maneuvers and executing some precise techniques.

5. Permanent record on videotape can be used for education and clinical information purposes.

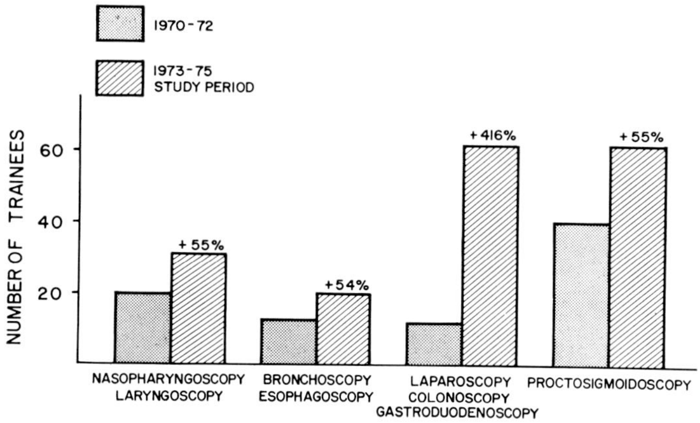

Fig. 2. Comparison of the number of residents training in endoscopy at the VA Hospital, Lake City, Florida, during the three-year period (1970-72) and the three-year period of the feasibility study (1973-75).

The two advantages, listed in No. 3 above, related to simultaneous viewing can be described in more detail:

1. A great deal of interest in endoscopy was created by employing color television at our hospital. This has been demonstrated by frequently finding as many as eight people in the small endoscopic suite during some examinations. Of course, each of these observers is learning endoscopic anatomy and pathology as they watch the television monitor. By introducing each junior resident to endoscopy in this manner, he becomes better prepared to do the same type of examination in his own patients.

2. The number of interns and residents trained in endoscopy during the three-year period (1972-1975) was compared with the number of trainees during the previous three-year period (Fig. 2). In the fields of nasopharyngoscopy and laryngoscopy, there was a 55% increase; and in bronchoscopy and esophagoscopy, there was a 54% increase. This increase in number of trainees in bronchoesophagoscopy was not associated with a proportional increase in number of patient examinations. However, the use of television expanded the clinical experience of these residents to such an extent that we have been able to compress the same training into shorter periods of time. The large increase in number of residents receiving training in laparoscopy, colonoscopy and gastroduodenoscopy, was associated with a corresponding increase in patient examination.

The results of our feasibility study have shown that closed-circuit color television is an excellent educational tool that can enhance endoscopic training and at the same time provide invaluable instructional materials that can be used to assist a greater number of physicians in acquiring skills in endoscopy.

PLANS TO PROVIDE INSTRUCTIONAL MATERIALS

Although the Exchange of Medical Information Project had found that it was feasible to utilize television as an instructional aid for endoscopy, the budget required for this application was substantial. It was therefore realized that every medical facility could not afford a comparable television-endoscopy program. For this reason, the Exchange of Medical Information Review Group, the Special Medical Advisory Group and the Chief Medical Director agreed that a VACEP should be established at our facility. As described in the letter of approval, the objectives of this Center are "the creation of a system and technical center to produce video and film endoscopy training and instructional materials for general VA use, and to make these available to the medical community."

On July 1, 1975, VACEP was established at the VA Hospital in Lake City, Florida. We are now adding additional facilities that will allow the development of endoscopic programs for distribution on videotape and motion picture formats. It is our intention that endoscopic anatomy and pathology demonstrated in these programs will have the same quality that would be seen by the trainee if he were looking directly through the endoscope himself.

We are now preparing for a national survey of the medical community to determine the needs for endoscopic programs. This survey will answer questions concerning: 1) the endoscopic specialties interested in programs, 2) the topics or subjects of endoscopic programs requested, 3) the intended audience, 4) the instructional method preferred, such as, self-instructional or teaching supplemental types, and 5) the media preference, whether videotape or motion picture formats.

Self-instructional courses will be designed to furnish basic techniques in the care of endoscopic equipment for nurses or nursing assistants, or preclinical training to the physician providing him with a working knowledge of endoscopic technique, anatomy, pathology, *etc.* In this way, these programs will prepare the physician for his first clinical experience with his teaching staff member. The clinical training phase of endoscopy will then be a hands-on experience during which he can apply the knowledge he has gained. His clinical training will then be more valuable to him, less time consuming to the teaching staff, and certainly less hazardous to his patients.

Endoscopic programs of the teaching supplementary type will be designed as continuing educational courses for the physicians already experienced in endoscopy. These courses will be used by individuals or in scientific programs, conferences, and seminars. Seminars in various fields of endoscopy will be conducted at VACEP on an annual or biannual basis through the cooperation of the VA Regional Medical Education Center in Birmingham, Alabama, and the Division of Postgraduate Medical Education at the University of Florida College of Medicine. According to our experience with the First VACEP Endoscopy Seminar on Flexible Bronchoscopy, these postgraduate seminars provide an excellent opportunity for exchange of educational ideas and information, as well as, the dissemination of instructional materials.

In addition to the educational programs in endoscopy that are produced by our staff, physicians in other hospitals who have become experts in some phase of endoscopy will be invited to VACEP to demonstrate their special skills so that recordings of these examinations can be made on videotape. Our staff will then assist these physicians in preparing educational programs that will demonstrate their new or improved endoscopic techniques, methods, *etc.*

REPRINTS—John E. Rayl, MD, VACEP, VA Hospital, Lake City, FL 32055.

Ann Otol 85: 1976

TRACHEAL RESECTION AND MUCOCILIARY CLEARANCE

ANTHONY GIORDANO, MD

MINNEAPOLIS, MINNESOTA

DOUGLAS S. HOLSCLAW, MD

PHILADELPHIA, PENNSYLVANIA

SUMMARY – Mucociliary transport following tracheal resection and end-to-end anastomosis was evaluated in beagle dogs, using the movement of ^{99M}TC labeled sodium pertechnetate solution as a marker. Preoperatively, mucociliary clearance was stable, but a three-fold decrease in tracheal mucus movement was found three days postoperatively. Clearance rates had returned to normal by 31 days postoperatively and remained stable over a ten week period of observation. By histological examination, normal ciliated epithelium was seen within six months following resection and anastomosis. Since up to 25% (4 cm or seven tracheal rings) of tracheal length was removed, significant longitudinal loss can take place without functional impairment of mucociliary clearance. Circumferential narrowing, however, was associated with a significant decrease in clearance.

Tracheal stenosis and its repair have been reported in the literature for the past 100 years.[1] Many methods have been utilized in the repair of tracheal stenosis, including circumferential resection with primary anastomosis,[2-5] endoscopic resection,[6,7] and resection with the use of a prosthesis.[8-11] Circumferential resection with primary anastomosis has become the most effective corrective procedure in most cases of tracheal stenosis.[2-5,12-15] The first successful resection and anastomosis was performed by Kuester in 1884.[1] Other investigators at the turn of the century reported successful resections and anastomoses of segments up to 4 cm.[1] More recently, investigators have reported that one of the limiting factors in determining success or failure was the tension at the suture line.[1,9,12,13] In dogs, primary anastomosis is 100% successful provided the suture line tension is below 1700 gm.[1,13] In humans, defects requiring more than 30% resection (3-4 cm) can be repaired end-to-end only after a procedure to decrease suture line tension, such as extreme neck flexion,[2,15-18] substernal methods of pulmonary freeing,[2,5,12,15-19] or laryngeal release[20-22] is performed. These methods either alone or in combination have made possible resections in humans of up to 7 cm (ten tracheal rings).

Resection with primary anastomosis restores the lumen of the trachea to an anatomically acceptable caliber. However, effects of the procedure on the more subtle aspects of tracheal function such as mucociliary clearance are unknown.

Mucostasis has long been thought to predispose to tracheobronchial infections. The trauma and anatomical break in the tracheal mucosa postanastomosis may cause a slowing of the mucus clearance with a resultant accumulation of secretions and increased possibility of infection. These, in turn, may hinder healing at the anastomotic site. Thus it is desirous to have information about the return of mucociliary clearance after the surgical procedure.

From the Department of Pediatrics, Section of Pediatric Pulmonary Disease, Hahnemann Medical College and Hospital, Philadelphia; and Department of Radiation Biology and Biophysics, University of Rochester, New York. Supported by NIH Research grant AM-17771 and Pulmonary Academic Award No. K07-HL-70832 (DSH).

Presented at the meeting of the American Broncho-Esophagological Association, Palm Beach, Florida, April 27-28, 1976.

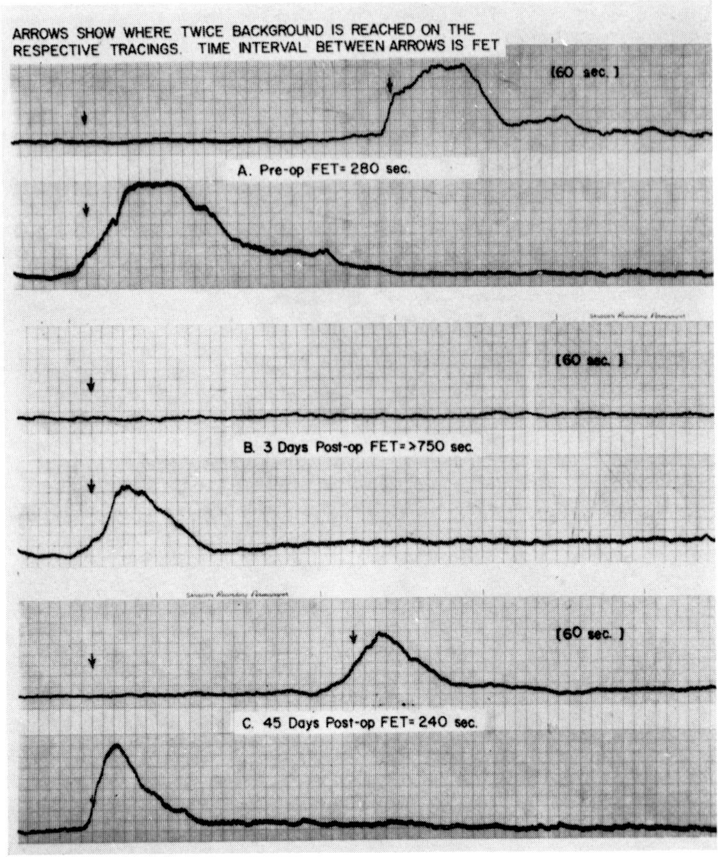

Fig. 1. Typical chart recordings. Top tracings on each of the sets are from cephalad detector, bottom tracings are from caudal detector. FET - First edge time.

We have studied the effects on tracheal mucociliary clearance of tracheal resection with subsequent end-to-end anastomosis at clinically acceptable suture line tensions. Histologic studies of the anastomotic sites were used to monitor the return of normal tracheal epithelium and to relate these observations to the physiologic function of mucociliary clearance.

METHODS AND MATERIALS

Two groups of dogs were studied.

Group A. Five conditioned adult mongrel dogs (6-10 kg) underwent tracheal resection and primary anastomosis. These dogs were sacrificed four to six months postoperatively, and the anastomotic site removed for gross and histological evaluation.

Group B. Seven adult purebred female beagles (6-10 kg), of whom six were subjected to preoperative tracheal mucus clearance measurements, underwent tracheal resection and primary anastomosis. Clearance measurements were repeated on the third postoperative day, and then repeated every two weeks for ten weeks. Two of these dogs also underwent bronchoscopy and tracheography. The remaining dog was the unoperated control and had only mucus clearance studies performed.

Surgical Procedure. The technique employed was similar to that reported by Wardell *et al.*[23] Intravenous pentobarbital sodium (40-50 mg/kg) was used for anesthesia. The ventral neck area was aseptically prepared, and a midline cervical incision made from just anterior to the cricoid cartilage to the suprasternal notch. The trachea was exposed from the cricoid cartilage to the 14th ring (7-10 cm) and the nerves and blood vessels blunt dissected at the areas where the trachea was to be transected. Medial 000 silk sutures were placed at the transection sites. Lateral 000 silk sutures were placed between rings 4 and either 13 or 14. The trachea was then transected first below the 11th or 12th ring caudad and then just below the fifth ring cephalad. The transected tracheal piece was moved to the

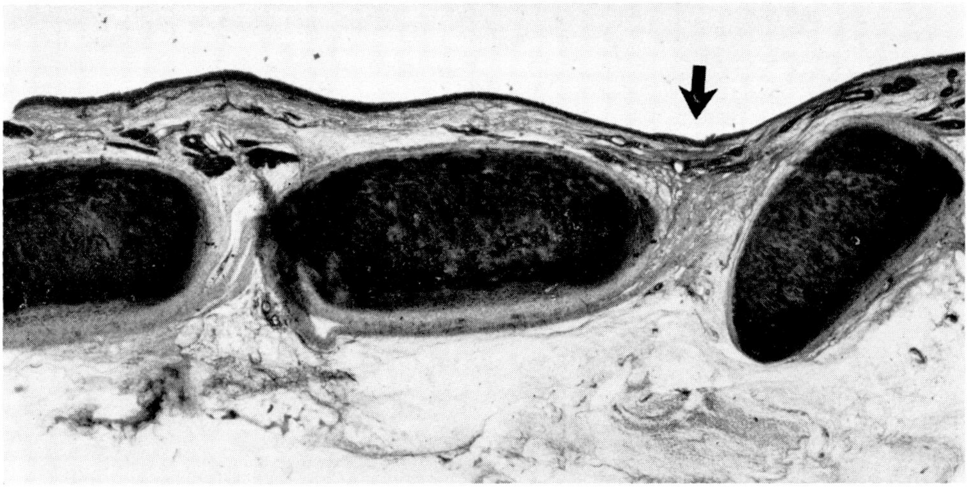

Fig. 2. Tracheal section. Arrow indicates malalignment of cartilaginous rings at what is thought to be the anastomotic site. Note proper alignment of cartilaginous rings to the left. (X20)

side, and the lateral silk retention sutures were tightened to bring the tracheal ends within 2 cm of each other. Ten to 14 interrupted 000 chromic sutures on an atraumatic needle were used for the anastomosis, entrapping one cartilaginous ring from each end. All knots were outside the lumen. The transected section of six to seven rings was allowed to remain beside the intact trachea. This was done to insure continuity of the vasculature below and innervation above the transection site, as well as allow a tracheal pouch to be formed for mucus collections involved in a separate study. A continuous locked 00 chromic suture was used to approximate the sternohyoid muscles in the midline. Then 4-000 interrupted chromic sutures were placed on each side to tack the subcutaneous tissues to the sternohyoid and sternothyroid muscles. Twelve to 16 00 silk double mattress sutures were used to close the skin. The dog was allowed glucose in water until the first postoperative clearance measurement was made on postoperative day three.

Clearance. Clearance was measured in the supine pentothal anesthetized dog by a previously described radioisotope method.[24] Five μl of a ^{99M}TC labeled Na-pertechnetate solution, a γ emitter, was injected into a percutaneous tracheal pilot needle.. Three cubic centimeters of air were then blown through the injection needle depositing the isotope on the tracheal mucosa. The movement of the pertechnetate solution from one 3 mm cross section of trachea to another section 35 mm more cephalad was the marker for mucociliary transport. This movement was followed by two NaI crystal scintillation detectors* connected to count rate meters** and chart recorders*** which provided the records from which mucus transport times and velocities were determined. Transport time was expressed as a "First Edge Time" (FET), which was the time interval for the mucus to move 35 mm. Rectal temperatures ranged between 37-39 C and only one clearance measurement per dog was made on a test day. Figure 1 shows typical tracings recorded at various pre- and postoperative times.

RESULTS

Group A. All dogs survived the resection and anastomosis. None showed signs of upper airway distress or obstruction. At sacrifice four to six months postoperatively, all five dogs showed cervical tracheal adhesions. On gross inspection of both the external and luminal tracheal surfaces, it was difficult to determine the anastomotic site. Only one dog had noticeable intratracheal stenosis. This was confined mainly to the posterior wall and caused less than a 20% reduction in tracheal cross-sectional area. On histologic inspection, slight malalignment of the cartilaginous rings aided in localizing the anastomotic site (Fig. 2). The mucosa itself gave no indication of the transection. In some anastomotic areas, the mucosa was

* No. 6S4/1.5 "Integral Line Assembly." Harshaw Chemical Co, Solon, OH.
** Nuclear Chicago 1620. Searle Analytic, Inc, Des Plaines, IL.
*** Sanborn Twin-Viso 60-1300. Sanborn Co, Cambridge, MA.

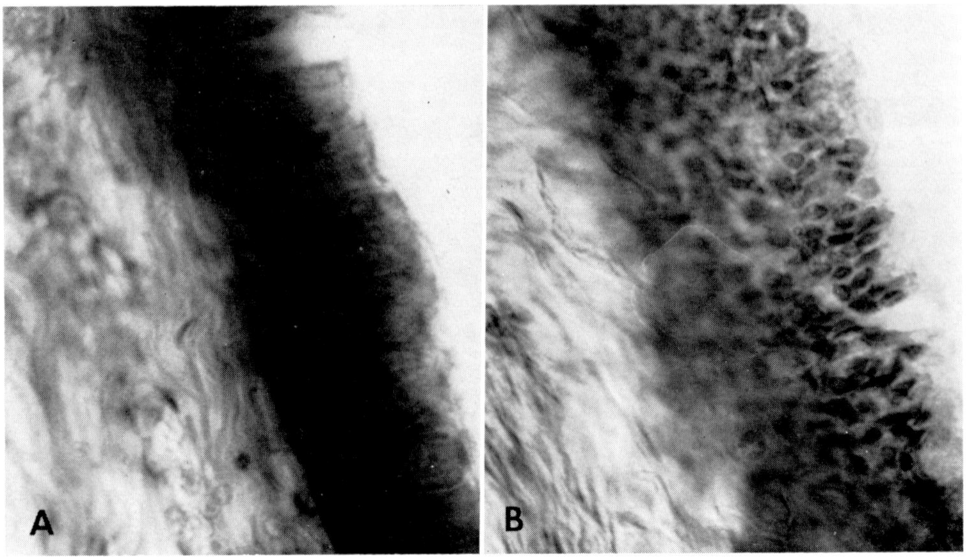

Fig. 3. A) Normal trachea. Uniformity of epithelial layer is outstanding characteristic. B) Anastomotic site. Disorganization and increased thickness of epithelial layer is present. (X800)

thicker, and the basal layer more disorganized but the ciliated outer layer was continuous, making it difficult to distinguish normal from anastomotic mucosa (Figs. 3, 4).

Group B. The control dog (No. 7) exhibited a consistent mucociliary clearance pattern throughout the entire study (Table I). The FET over the four-month period was 284±36 sec (mean ± Standard Deviation of Mean) and the clearance velocity 7.5±1.1 mm/min.

In the preoperative dogs, mucociliary clearance was also found to be relatively stable. The variations in individual clearance velocities and times for any one dog were less than the variations in measurements between two dogs. Thus, each dog was used as its own control. The FET was 231±80 sec and the clearance velocity 10.1±3.2 mm/min preoperatively. All dogs survived the surgery and had six postoperative clearance studies. Three days after surgery there was a three-fold or greater decrease in mucociliary clearance when compared to the slowest preoperative measurement ($p<.02$). Within 31 days, clearance returned to normal preoperative levels in all dogs. From 31 days on, as a group, the FET was 235±135 sec and clearance velocity 10.4±3.1 mm/min. Three of the dogs had postoperative clearance rates which increased 19, 41 and 86% over their preoperative measurements. The other three had rates which decreased 7, 16 and 38% from their respective preoperative values. Once baseline preoperative clearance rates were reached postoperatively, all dogs except one (No. 6) exhibited a similar degree of internal consistency as they had in the preoperative condition.

Approximately two months postoperative, the clearance rates of one of the dogs (No. 6) began to decrease. Two measurements over the next month indicated that the mucociliary clearance which had apparently returned to normal within 31 days was now depressed to only 30-40% of normal. Also, this dog had a wheeze when excited. It was felt that possible stenosis at the anastomotic site was responsible. Bronchoscopy and tracheography were performed on this dog as well as on a dog (No. 1) who maintained normal clearance function during the 2½ month postoperative period.

Bronchoscopy in both dogs revealed

TABLE I

PRE- AND POSTOPERATIVE FIRST EDGE TIME AND VELOCITY STUDIES

	Preoperative day					*Postoperative day*						
Dog	49	35	21	7	Mean± S.D.	3	17	31	45	59	73	Mean± S.D.****
					First time edge in seconds							
1	220	280	210	180	222±42	>750	280	160	240	160	200	190±38
2	190	160	140	170	165±21	>600	150	150	200	250	140	185±51
3	180	180	230	200	197±24	>750	460	200	340	200	230	242±67
4	310	380	410	350	362±43	>1800	260	170	210	160	250	198±41
5	220	310	350	250	282±59	>1050	300	160	210	190	250	202±38
6*	200	120	170	150	160±34	>600	250	180	140	600	660	393±273
			Average**		231±80			170±18				235±130
7***	210	330	280	310	282±53	280	300	310	250	310	260	282±32
					Velocity in mm/min.							
1	9.2	7.5	10.0	11.7	9.6±1.7	<2.8	7.5	13.1	8.8	13.1	10.5	11.4±2.1
2	11.1	13.1	15.0	12.4	12.9±1.6	<3.5	14.0	14.0	10.5	8.4	15.0	12.0±3.1
3	11.7	11.7	9.1	10.5	10.8±1.2	<2.8	4.6	10.5	6.2	10.5	9.1	9.1±2.0
4	6.8	5.5	5.2	6.0	5.9±0.7	<1.2	8.1	12.4	10.0	13.1	8.4	11.0±2.0
5	9.2	6.8	6.0	8.4	7.6±1.5	<2.0	7.0	13.1	10.0	11.1	8.4	10.7±2.0
6	10.5	17.5	12.4	14.0	13.6±3.0	<3.5	8.4	11.7	15.0	3.5	3.2	8.4±5.9
			Average		10.1±3.2			12.5±1.2				10.4±3.1
7	10.0	6.4	7.5	6.8	7.7±1.6	7.5	7.0	6.8	8.4	6.8	8.1	7.5±0.8

* Developed signs of stenosis two months postoperative.
** All dogs except control.
*** Unoperated control.
**** Postoperative days 31-73 only (4 measurements).

a well-healed mucosal surface at the anastomotic site approximately 4.5 cm from the vocal cords. In dog No. 6 there was a 20% reduction of the lumen due to a web-like protrusion primarily at the posterior wall which was not present in dog No. 1. These findings were supported by tracheography (Fig. 5).

DISCUSSION

There are two basic ways in which mucociliary clearance can be studied: 1) aerosol retention, and 2) recording of mucus movement with an applied marker. The first utilizes the percentage retention of an inhaled or deposited radioactive material as a determinant of mucus movement. By plotting these retention percentages as a function of time one can draw a clearance curve. The curve oftentimes can best be described by equations that contain two or more exponentials.[25] When the scanning measurements are begun immediately after deposition, the curves indicate a rapid initial phase (minutes to hours), a much slower second phase, (days to weeks), and sometimes even slower phases of clearance (months to years). The fastest phase of this clearance is attributed to mucus transport and the half time of this phase is considered to be an assessment of how well the mucus escalator is operating. However, factors such as rapid absorption of the radioactive material through the lining epithelia can contribute to this early phase and make mucus movement

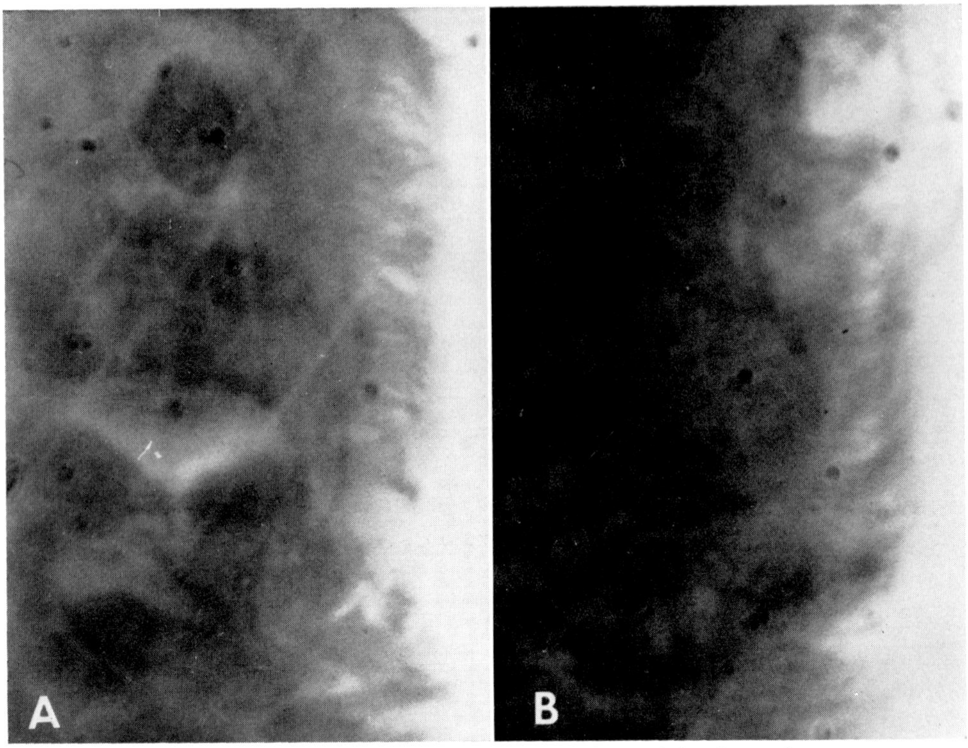

Fig. 4. A) Normal trachea. 6-8μ cilia seen at luminal border. B) Anastomotic site. 6-8μ cilia seen at luminal border. (X5000)

appear falsely better. When one is solely interested in how efficiently or fast the mucus escalator is functioning in a specific area, the direct marker methods are superior. Agents such as India ink, Teflon®* discs, radioactive solutions or particles, *etc*, have been used as markers in these studies.[24,26-29] The movement of these markers can be observed with the naked eye, through a bronchoscope or with radiation detection equipment.

The use of radioactive Na-pertechnetate solutions or tagged particles for the measurement of mucociliary clearance *in vivo* is now well established. These methods provide results similar to those obtained by other methods.[23-30] Our results are in good agreement with those in the literature (Table II).

The present study of repeated measurement of mucociliary clearance in dogs over a four-month period shows that mucus transport is an easily measurable and reproducible function of the healthy dog. Our studies indicate that tracheal mucociliary clearance after a seven tracheal ring resection (4 cm) returns to normal preoperative levels within 31 days. The only previous

TABLE II

CONTROL MUCOCILIARY TRANSPORT RATES IN DOGS

Investigator	*Preparation*	*mm/min Rate*
Marin and Morrow[26]	*in vivo*	16.1
Asmundsson and Kilburn[27]	*in vitro*	12.6
Sakakura and Proctor[28]	*in vivo*	10.5
Wanner *et al*[29]	*in vivo*	13.7
Hilding[30]	*in vivo*	14.5
Giordano and Holsclaw	*in vivo*	10.1

* Ethicon Laboratories, Somerville, NJ.

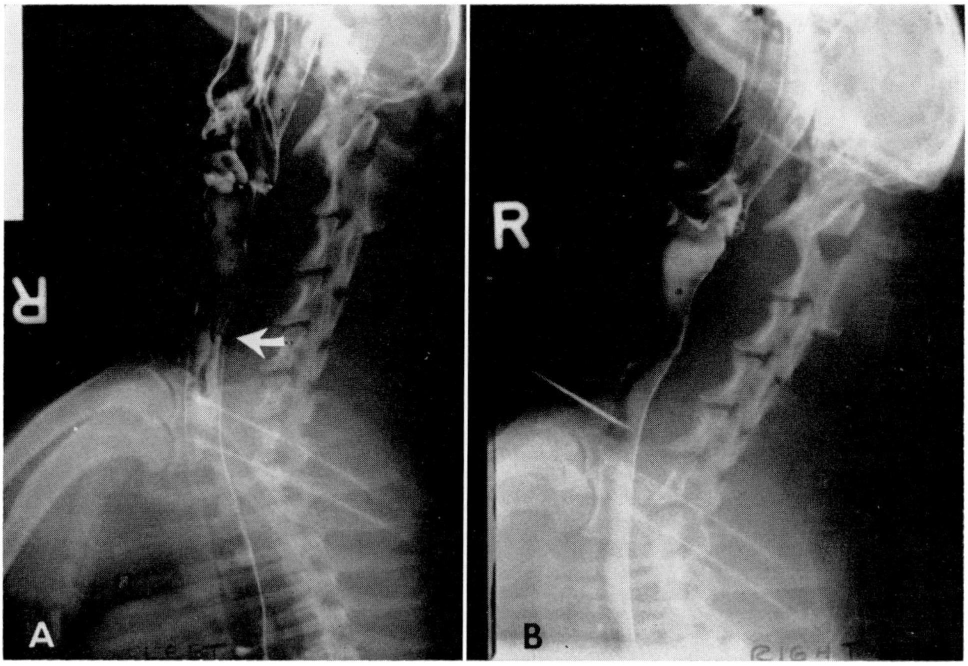

Fig. 5. Right lateral tracheogram. A) Dog No. 6; arrow indicates stenosis in trachea. B) Dog No. 1.

studies which are remotely similar are concerned with retention studies pre- and postoperative simple transection.[31-33] These authors found that a one-month period was significant for normal function to return. However, their studies did not involve the removal of a 3-4 cm section of trachea or bronchus, nor did they measure clearance directly across the anastomosis. From the clinical standpoint, resection studies are of more significance than those using transection, as currently the only procedure that would employ the latter would be lung transplants, and these are experimental at best.

Following primary anastomosis, a continuous unciliated epithelium is regenerated within one to three weeks.[13,34] This parallels the return of normal mucociliary clearance seen in this study. Within six months, a continuous ciliated epithelium has developed. Whether this regeneration of cilia was complete simultaneous with the initial return of normal mucus clearance is unknown. Even if anastomotic site epithelium was unciliated, mucus clearance can be normal, as it is recognized that due to its viscoelastic properties, the mucus layer can be transported across areas void of functional cilia provided there are sufficient normally functioning cilia in adjacent areas.[35] Another possible explanation for the quick return of normal mucus clearance while the epithelia is not totally reciliated is that provided by Hill who found that transport rates across stretched mucosa were faster than those across unstretched mucosa.[36] In some instances, transport over 4 cm of a stretched piece took only as long as transport over 2 cm of an unstretched piece of trachea. Thus in this study, where there is approximately a 20-25% stretching of the mucosa after the 4 cm resection, clearance over the stretched intact mucosa may compensate for any slowing of mucus flow which might occur at the unciliated anastomotic area. Even including data from the atypical dog (No. 6), postoperative clearance is slightly faster than preoperative clearance. Data over a much longer period of time would be needed to show if clearance was statistically better postoperatively and thus if stretching plays a role in *in vivo* clearance rates.

The mucociliary clearance system can compensate in many ways to insure that an efficient flow of mucus occurs. Our results bear this out. The one dog who did show a clearance response different from the average did so approximately 45-60 days postoperatively. This is in the time period when tracheal stenosis postanastomosis may be expected to occur. This clearance change from normal to a rate only 35% of normal and the development of a wheeze with exertion were the only abnormal findings. Tracheography and bronchoscopy both indicated a mild degree of stenosis in the dog with depressed clearance compared to a random dog similarly studied with normal clearance. This latter finding shows that the tracheal resection and anastomosis can result in a normal caliber lumen with no signs of stenosis or physiologic impairment. The findings in the dog with depressed clearance rates are of interest because the diagnostic procedures employed indicated about a 20% decrease in tracheal cross-sectional area. This is considered to be an acceptable result from the surgical standpoint, and no clinical signs of difficulty would be expected. Functionally, however, with these findings of mild stenosis, there is a severe degree of impairment of mucociliary transport.

SUMMARY

1. For an individual dog, mucociliary clearance is a reproducible function. Variability among dogs is greater than the variability within each dog.

2. Mucociliary clearance rates returned to normal within one month after tracheal resection of up to 25% (six to seven tracheal rings) with primary anastomosis in adult beagle dogs.

3. Stretching of the tracheal mucosa secondary to the resection may compensate for any slowing of mucus movement at the unciliated anastomotic area with the net result of making clearance normal.

4. Normal ciliated epithelium was seen within six months following resection and anastomosis.

5. Simultaneous with a mild degree of tracheal stenosis, severe impairment of mucociliary clearance was seen.

REFERENCES

1. Ferguson DJ, Wild JJ, Wangensteen OH: Experimental resection of the trachea. Surgery 28:597-619, 1950

2. Grillo HC: Reconstruction of the trachea. Thorax 28:667-679, 1973

3. Naef AP: Tracheobronchial reconstruction. Ann Thorac Surg 15:301-312, 1973

4. Mathey J, Binet JP, Galery JJ, *et al*: Tracheal and tracheobronchial resections. J Thorac Cardiovasc Surg 51:1-13, 1966

5. Barclay RS, McSwan N, Welsh TM: Tracheal reconstruction without the use of grafts. Thorax 12:177-180, 1957

6. Coulson AS, Rossiter SJ, Guernsey JM: Progressive tracheal obstruction. J Thorac Cardiovasc Surg 67:733-743, 1974

7. Lefemine AA, MacDonnell K, Moon HS: Tracheal stenosis following cuffed tube tracheostomy: anatomical variation and selected treatment. Ann Thorac Surg 15:456-462, 1973

8. Longmire WP: The repair of large defects of the trachea. Ann Otol Rhinol Laryngol 57:875-883, 1948

9. Belsey R: Resection and reconstruction of the intrathoracic trachea. Br J Surg 38:200-205, 1950

10. Clagett OT, Moersch HJ, Grindlay JH: Intrathoracic tracheal tumors: development of surgical techniques for their removal. Ann Surg 135:520-530, 1952

11. Beall AC, Harrington OB, Greenberg SD, *et al*: Tracheal reconstruction with heavy marlex mesh. Arch Surg 86:970-978, 1963

12. Miscall L, McKittrick JB, Giordano RP, *et al*: Stenosis of trachea: resection and end-to-end anastomosis. Arch Surg 87:726-731, 1963

13. Cantrell JR, Folse JR: The repair of circumferential defects of the trachea by direct anastomosis: Experimental evaluation. J Thorac Cardiovasc Surg 42:589-598, 1961

14. Nach RL, Rothman M: Injuries to the larynx and trachea. Surg Gynecol Obstet 16:614-622, 1943

15. Grillo HC: Obstructive lesions of the trachea. Ann Otol Rhinol Laryngol 82:770-777, 1973

16. Mulliken JB, Grillo HC: The limits of tracheal resection with primary anastomosis:

further anatomical studies in man. J Thorac Cardiovasc Surg 55:418-421, 1968

17. Gazzaniga AB, Rappaport I, Stemmer EA: Extended tracheal resection with end-to-end anastomosis. Arch Surg 102:589-591, 1971

18. Grillo HC, Dignan EF, Miura T: Extensive resection and reconstruction of mediastinal trachea without prosthesis or graft: an anatomical study in man. J Thorac Cardiovasc Surg 48:741-749, 1964

19. Naef AP: Extensive tracheal resection and tracheobronchial reconstruction. Ann Thorac Surg 8:391-400, 1969

20. Ogura JH, Roper CL: Surgical correction of traumatic stenosis of larynx and pharynx. Laryngoscope 72:468-480, 1962

21. Dedo HH, Fishman NH: Laryngeal release and sleeve resection for tracheal stenosis. Ann Otol Rhinol Laryngol 78:285-295, 1969

22. Dedo HH, Fishman NJ: The results of laryngeal release, tracheal mobilization and resection for tracheal stenosis in 19 patients. Laryngoscope 83:1204-1210, 1973

23. Wardell JR, Chakrin LW, Payne BJ: The canine tracheal pouch: a model for use in respiratory mucus research. Am Rev Respir Dis 101:741-754, 1970

24. Giordano AM, Morrow PE: Chronic low-level nitrogen dioxide exposure and mucociliary clearance. Arch Environ Health 25: 443-449, 1972

25. Morrow PE, Gibb FR, Gazioglu K: The clearance of dust from the lower respiratory tract of man: An experimental study, in Davies CN (ed): *Inhaled Particles and Vapours II*. New York, Pergamon Press, 1966, pp 351-359

26. Marin MG, Morrow PE: Effect of changing inspired O_2 and CO_2 levels on tracheal mucociliary transport rate. J Appl Physiol 27:385-388, 1969

27. Asmundsson T, Kilburn KH: Mucociliary clearance rates at various levels in dogs lungs. Am Rev Respir Dis 102:388-397, 1970

28. Sakakura Y, Procter DF: The effects of various conditions on tracheal mucociliary transport in dogs. Proc Soc Exp Biol Med 140:870-879, 1972

29. Wanner A, Hirsch JA, Greeneltch DE, *et al*: Tracheal mucous velocity in beagles after chronic exposure to cigarette smoke. Arch Environ Health 27:370-371, 1973

30. Hilding AC: Ciliary streaming in the bronchial tree and the time element in carcinogenesis. N Engl J Med 256:634-640, 1957

31. Morinari H, Shimada K, Taplin GV, *et al*: Bronchial mucus after lung autotransplantation in dogs. J Thorac Cardiovasc Surg 67: 484-490, 1974

32. Edmunds LH, Stallone RJ, Graf PD, *et al*: Mucus transport in transplanted lungs of dogs. Surgery 66:15-22, 1969

33. Brody JS, Klempfner G, Staum MM, *et al*: Mucociliary clearance after lung denervation and bronchial transection. J Appl Physiol 32:160-164, 1972

34. Maisel B, Dingwall JA: Primary suture of the divided cervical trachea: a preliminary experimental study. Surgery 27: 726-729, 1950

35. Ryander R: Current techniques to measure alterations in the ciliary activity of intact respiratory epithelium. Am Rev Respir Dis 93:67-72, 1966

36. Hill L: The ciliary movement of the trachea studied *in vitro*. Lancet 215:802-805, 1928

37. Couraud L, Massard JF, Bruneteau A, *et al*: Notre experience des resections anastomoses de la trachee et des bronches souches. Poumon Coeur 28:185-188, 1972

38. Carcassonne M, Dor V, Aubert J, *et al*: Tracheal resection with primary anastomosis in children. J Pediatr Surg 8:1-8, 1973

ACKNOWLEDGMENTS—We gratefully acknowledge the invaluable technical assistance of Ms Dianna McGookey, Robert Wilson, and Dr. Henry Schneider. Dr. John Tucker aided with the endoscopy. Mary Lou Gregory and Jeffrey Stead helped with the photo micrographs. Dr. Mitchell Litt and Paul Morrow helped with the preparation of the manuscript.

REPRINTS—Douglas Holsclaw, MD, Department of Pediatrics, Hahnemann Medical College and Hospital, Philadelphia, PA 19102.

Ann Otol 85: 1976

FLEXIBLE FIBEROPTIC NASOPHARYNGOLARYNGOSCOPE

HARVEY D. SILBERMAN, MD

HAROLD WILF, MD JOHN A. TUCKER, MD

PHILADELPHIA, PENNSYLVANIA

SUMMARY – A new practical flexible fiberoptic nasopharyngolaryngoscope is introduced. This instrument allows for a completeness of examination heretofore not totally possible in all cases as an office or bedside procedure. The ease of examination and patient tolerance make for a superior new clinical tool.

For many years we have recognized the difficulties with the routine methods of examining the nasopharynx and larynx. In 1970 our endoscopic armamentarium was broadened with the use of the flexible fiberoptic bronchoscope. As our techniques mainly utilized transnasal introduction, it became evident that the flexible bronchoscope afforded an examination of the nasopharynx and larynx with little discomfort or stimulation of the gag reflex. This led to the occasional use in the office of the flexible bronchoscope for nasopharyngoscopy and laryngoscopy. It was particularly reassuring in being able to view the larynx in those patients whose laryngeal mirror examination was inadequate. Others have had a similar experience.[1,2] Thus it was unnecessary to expose the patient's larynx with a rigid laryngoscope in a hospital setting. The same was true for those patients in whom the nasopharynx was not adequately accessible to the small nasopharyngeal mirror or the nasopharyngoscope.

The flexible bronchoscope not only allowed an excellent view but was more comfortable than the standard methods. Simple topical anesthesia was quite sufficient for a more than adequate examination of the nasopharynx and larynx.

The main drawbacks of using the flexible fiberoptic bronchoscope for this examination were the length, diameter and weight of the instrument. To clean thoroughly the bronchoscope between patients was also cumbersome in the office. Multiple procedures were time consuming.

Approximately 2½ years ago, a flexible fiberoptic laryngoscope designed for anesthesia intubation,* became commercially available.[3] This instrument was quite inexpensive. It was 49 cm long (effective length not including controls) and 6.25 mm in diameter. It had a controllable tip with a total tip deflection of 120°. The field view was 60° and the depth of focus was 5 mm to 30 mm. The total length of the instrument was 67 cm.

After an extensive clinical trial of this instrument for a six-month period, it proved unsatisfactory. It was much too large (6.25 mm) with poor optics. It was awkward to work with and in short, not practical for the accurate diagnosis necessary in otolaryngology. It was, however, quite adequate for intubation. Another flexible scope had also been designed in 1972 for anesthesia needs but again was too wide for otolaryngology's needs.[4]

It was apparent that the need existed for a scope primarily designed for otolaryngology. A Japanese instrument company with expertise in the field of

---

* American Optical Corp., Southbridge, MA.

Presented at the meeting of the American Broncho-Esophagological Association, Palm Beach, Florida, April 27-28, 1976.

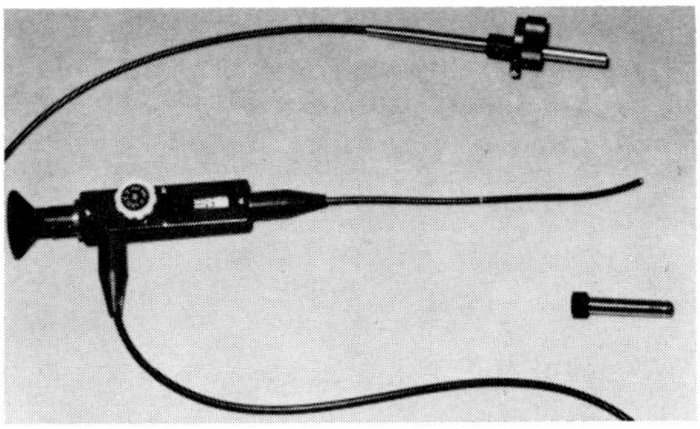

Fig. 1. The prototype scope, 20 cm long, and adapted to fit both Machida and Olympus light sources.

flexible fiberoptics aided us in the development and production of such an instrument.* They had previously produced one of the first flexible fiberoptic bronchoscopes, in 1966, for Dr. Shigeto Ikeda.[5] A prototype instrument underwent clinical trial in May, 1975 and by December, 1975, the prototype model had been used in over 1000 patients in both the office and hospital (Fig. 1). The prototype scope weighed approximately 0.2 kg and was 20 cm long (effective length). The diameter was 3.9 mm. The diameter must be kept below 4 mm in diameter (12 fr), to allow passage through the nasal cavity from newborn to adult age.

This diameter limits the flexibility of the tip to 90° in the downward direction, but is quite adequate. This lightweight, highly flexible and relatively short scope allows for 360° rotation in any direction without patient discomfort. Biopsy of the larynx through a flexible instrument is difficult, undependable and could in an office be quite dangerous. This view has not been shared by others who are using the flexible bronchoscope for laryngeal surgery.[1] Under controlled conditions, we have applied this modality and found it extremely inferior compared to modern microsurgical techniques of the larynx. It must be kept in mind that biopsying the larynx through the flexible instrument is extremely difficult because the larynx is a dynamic organ, highly reflexic, and is constantly in movement, as is the flexible scope. Therefore, barring fixation of the larynx, accurate and adequate biopsy is difficult.

A suction channel was judged unnecessary in view of the ease of topical anesthesia application in the nasopharyngeal-laryngeal area and the ability of the patient to clear mucus in the nose and throat by merely sniffing, blowing his nose and swallowing.

The prototype length was 20 cm. However, subsequent models were increased to 25 cm as in larger patients the vocal cords may not be reached. Twenty-five centimeters has proven short enough not to be cumbersome in use. The overall, effective length, that is including the control portion, is 45 cm (Model US 25*). Weight has been held to a minimum 0.2 kg. This allows extreme ease of handling and manipulation. The control knob is so situated to permit tip angulation by simply moving one's thumb.

Despite the decrease in diameter of the scope, the optical bundle has been doubled in size in comparison to the standard flexible bronchoscope of the same make. The resulting image is, therefore, superior to the flexible bronchoscope. When compared to rigid nasopharyngoscopes and laryngoscopes designed for similar purposes, the flexible nasopharyngolaryngoscope fares quite well, especially with a field of vision of 70° and the depth of focus 5 mm to 50 mm.

CLINICAL APPLICATIONS

The nasopharyngolaryngoscope was designed as an adjunct, not a replacement, for our routine methods of examining the nasopharynx and larynx. This instrument allows one to examine completely all patients, including those in whom the routine methods are not adequate. The instrument is routinely introduced transnasally. It is by far the most comfortable method for the patient and permits complete examination of the nasopharynx and larynx with one introduction.

* Machida America Inc., Closter, NJ.

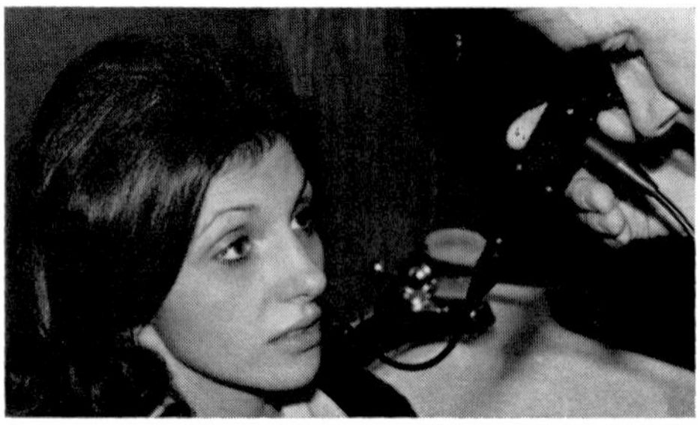

Fig. 2. The nasopharyngolaryngoscope is slid easily along the floor of the nose with no discomfort to the patient. The scope is lightweight, highly flexible and relatively short.

In the adult, the nose is anesthetized by means of applicator sticks dipped in 10% cocaine. The applicators are placed on the floor of the nose and progressively advanced towards the nasopharynx. Usually the oropharynx is sprayed with Cetacaine®.* There is often so little stimulation of the gag reflex that even the anesthetic can be omitted.

After the applicators are removed, the scope is slid along the floor of the nose. Examination of the nasal chambers is greatly facilitated with the nasopharyngolaryngoscope. One is able to inspect beneath each turbinate and high into the sphenoethmoidal recess. Visualization of the sphenoid ostia is readily accomplished. We routinely are able to examine the interior of the maxillary sinuses in patients with postsurgical nasoantral windows, following Caldwell-Luc procedures (Fig. 2).

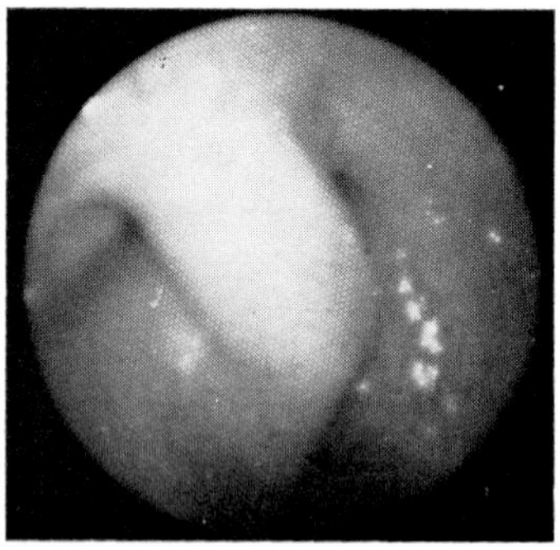

Fig. 3. An excellent view of the nasopharynx. Here is the right torus tubarius, to the left is the Eustachian tubal orifice. The fossa of Rosenmuller behind and to the right of the torus is clearly seen.

The nasopharynx and Eustachian orifice come shortly into view. Upon reaching the posterior edge of the septum, the scope is turned on its side and the tip angled to allow one to visualize the contralateral Eustachian tube orifice. Virtually all anatomical areas of the nasopharynx including the fossa of Rosenmuller are well visualized (Fig. 3).

Biopsy of the nasopharynx is accomplished with a degree of comfort and accuracy not previously possible. Unlike the larynx, this area is fixed and does not move freely. The technique consists of passing the scope, under topical anesthesia, locating the lesion and then passing the biopsy forceps through the ipsilateral or contralateral nares. Surprisingly, it is quite easy to pass the biopsy forceps alongside the nasopharyngoscope. The lesion is then biopsied under direct visualization. If bleeding should ensue, this area can be easily cauterized electrically or chemically under direct visualization.

After examination of the nose and nasopharynx, the patient is instructed to breathe through his nose. This allows the soft palate to fall away from the posterior nasopharyngeal wall. With the palate relaxed, the posterior aspect of the soft palate and uvula can be examined. This also allows for inspection of velopharyngeal incompetence.

Almost immediately the base of the tongue, vallecula, epiglottis, and larynx come into view. The scope is advanced to the level of the epiglottis. One is immediately impressed by the virtual lack of stimulation of the gag reflex by this route of introduction.

The shape of the epiglottis and the presence of anatomical abnormalities are in no way a problem. Thus far, no larynx has been examined in which the entire laryngeal area could not be seen. Certainly this cannot be said of the

* Cetylite Industries, Inc., Long Island City, NY.

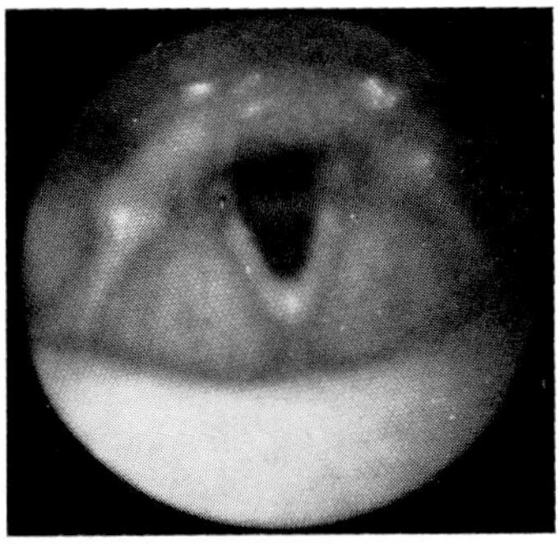

Fig. 4. The larynx is well visualized with an excellent view of the anterior commissure. The laryngeal surface of the epiglottis can be examined with great accuracy.

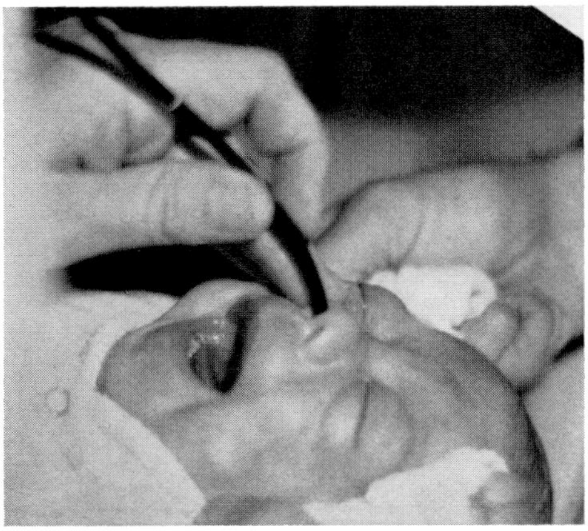

Fig. 5. The use of the nasopharyngolaryngoscope in the pediatric patient.

laryngeal mirror. Any mucus that may accumulate on the tip of the instrument can be simply cleared by having the patient swallow and using the epiglottis "as a windshield wiper."

Once the larynx is in view it is possible to see the laryngeal surface of the epiglottis and anterior commissure (Fig. 4). Without discomfort to the patient one is able to observe the larynx for an extended length of time, watching swallowing and coughing without need to remove the scope. Observation to this degree was not previously available in the office.

The scope being 25 cm in length allows us to advance to the level of the cords and pyriform sinuses. The scope could easily be advanced through the glottis, but in the office this is not advocated because of possible laryngospasm. In the operating room this has been done under topical anesthesia and allows examination of the under surface of the vocal cords, laryngeal ventricles and subglottic larynx.

Despite our expertise with the laryngeal mirror we have all had an occasional patient requiring direct rigid laryngoscopy. This is no longer necessary.

SPECIAL USES

Hospital Use (Bedside Laryngoscopy). Examination of the larynx in a bedridden patient has often been a problem. Cooperation from an elderly or comatose patient can frequently be impossible. With the flexible nasopharyngolaryngoscope this examination is as easy as an otoscopic examination. One merely requires the scope, a light source and a small amount of topical anesthesia. Cooperation from the patient is only a secondary need.

Inability to Open the Mouth. Not infrequently one is faced with patients who cannot open their mouths despite the fact that they are cooperative. Two examples are: a patient developed hoarseness following wiring of the mandible for facial fractures; and a woman with a floor of the mouth malignancy who also developed hoarseness, but because of radiation, her swollen tongue made it impossible for her to open her mouth. Neither of these patients presented any problem with evaluation of the larynges since we were able to bypass their oral cavities.

Photography. Photography is easily accomplished through the flexible nasopharyngolaryngoscope. At present, we are using the excellent Machida xenon light source* with built-in strobe light. Our camera is a specially constructed instamatic single lens reflex.* This unique camera is one of the very few single lens reflexes available in this rela-

* Model RN-300F. Kowa 110. Machida America, Inc., Closter, NJ.

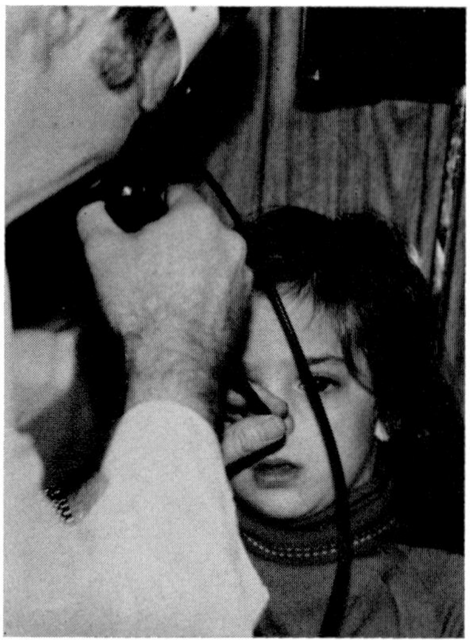

Fig. 6. Most children allow passage of the nasopharyngolaryngoscope, which makes possible an excellent view of the adenoids and larynx in school age children.

tively new format. The camera has a built-in light meter which automatically controls exposure and allows for perfect pictures. Photographs are invaluable. They are useable for teaching purposes and to explain graphically a patient's problem to him. The 110 format though smaller than existing 35 mm systems results in a much larger negative size than most flexible endoscopic photographic systems.

Pediatric Use. The use of this instrument in the pediatric patient is one of its most exciting aspects. It has been found that the 3.9 mm diameter will fit most full term newborn nasal chambers. The flexible scope allows us to rule out choanal atresia and at the same time perform laryngoscopy (Fig. 5).

Examination of the pediatric larynx with this instrument allows a rather unique examination. The larynx is in a "natural" state, not artificially suspended by the blade of a laryngoscope, nor are swallowing or cough reflexes stimulated unless one desires to do so.

Flexible examination of newborns with stridorous respirations has been found to be unusually easy. One can easily observe the floppy epiglottis or other pathologic lesions in the larynx which may exist.

One extremely valuable aspect of this instrument is its use in nasopharyngeal and laryngeal examination of school age children. It is well recognized there is a great difficulty in examining the nasopharynx and larynx in this age group. No longer do we have to depend upon x-ray or digital examination of the nasopharynx nor must we rely on an occasionally unreliable mirror examination of the larynx (Fig. 6).

Cooperative school age children will allow passage of the nasopharyngolaryngoscope under topical anesthesia, allowing us an excellent view of the adenoids and vocal cords. There is virtually no discomfort to the patient and greater accuracy is now provided.

Sinoscopy. In those patients who have had maxillary sinus surgery where a nasoantral window has been made, one is able to routinely examine the interior of the maxillary sinus. Obviously one can examine any area within the nose if you are able to get the scope to or into the area.

Tracheoscopy. The flexible scope can be passed through most tracheotomy tubes. We are more and more frequently doing routine examinations of the tracheotomy tube and the trachea following tracheotomy to insure an adequate airway.

Position of Endotracheal Tubes. Due to the small diameter of the scope, passage can be carried out through endotracheal tubes of 4.5 mm inside diameter and larger. This allows a quick check for position of endotracheal tubes. This was especially helpful in a recent case in which a four-year-old who was in respiratory arrest was brought to the emergency room. Crash intubation by an anesthesiologist was carried out and a tentative diagnosis of epiglottitis was made. When we first saw the child she was on a respirator and required assistant ventilation. We were safely able to confirm the diagnosis of epiglottitis following transnasal introduction of the nasopharyngolaryngoscope. We then passed the scope down the endotracheal tube to check its position.

REFERENCES

1. Davidson TM, Bone RC, Nahum AM: Flexible fiberoptic laryngobronchoscopy. Laryngoscope 84:1876-1882, 1974

2. Dellon AL, Hall CA, Chretien PB: Fiberoptic endoscopy in the head and neck region. Plast Reconstr Surg 55:466-471, 1975

3. Davis NJ: A new fiberoptic laryngoscope for nasal intubation. J Anesth Anal 52: 807-808, 1973

4. Stiles CM, Stiles QR, Denson JS: A flexible fiber optic laryngoscope. JAMA 221: 1246-1247, 1972

5. Ikeda S, Yanai N, Ishikawa S: Flexible bronchofiberscope. Keio J Med 17:1-16, 1968

Reprints—Harvey D. Silberman, MD, 156 Serrill Road, Elkins Park, PA 19117.

XV PAN-AMERICAN CONGRESS OF OTOLARYNGOLOGY AND BRONCHOESOPHAGOLOGY

The XV Pan-American Congress of Otolaryngology and Bronchoesophagology will be held in New Orleans, Louisiana, November 4-11, 1976. For further information write: Creative Associates, 5005 Newport Dr., Rolling Meadows, IL 60008. Anyone desiring to present a free paper write: Dr. Irving M. Blatt, Secretary-General, Pan-Am Otocongress, P.O. Box 52378, New Orleans, LA 70152.

Ann Otol 85: 1976

NEWER TECHNIQUES IN FIBEROPTIC BRONCHOSCOPY

JOSEPH P. ATKINS, JR., MD
LEE D. ROWE, MD   BRUCE W. JAFEK, MD
PHILADELPHIA, PENNSYLVANIA

SUMMARY – Flexible fiberoptic bronchoscopy has assumed a major role in the diagnosis and management of upper respiratory tract and pulmonary diseases. A new technique, utilizing a C-arm fluoroscopic control with an image intensification system, for the localization of peripheral lung lesions and subsegmental parenchymal infiltrates, is described. This method has proved useful in the early histologic and cytologic diagnosis of nonendoscopically visible bronchogenic carcinoma and in the drainage of lung abscesses. By employing a transendotracheal tube route with a ventilating, side-arm adaptor, continuous airway control and a selected inspired oxygen or anesthetic content is maintained. In addition, the problems of arterial hypoxemia, airway resistance, and ventilation-perfusion abnormalities are minimized. Several representative cases are discussed.

Flexible fiberoptic bronchoscopy, as originally introduced by Ikeda *et al* in 1968, was designed primarily for visualization of pathological changes within the trachea and bronchial tree. Emphasis was placed upon the early diagnosis of carcinoma of the lung.[1] As it has become commercially available, fiberoptic bronchoscopy has assumed a major role in the diagnosis and management of upper respiratory tract and pulmonary diseases.[2,3] This is particularly true with the rising frequency of primary carcinoma of the lung. Because many early lesions of carcinoma of the lung originate as epithelial changes in areas not visible with the rigid bronchoscope and migrate toward larger bronchi, flexible fiberoptic bronchoscopy is a valuable aid to the bronchoscopist.[4] Invasion and development of an endobronchial mass represent a much later stage of the disease, and has significantly poorer prognosis with respect to survival.[5]

Initially, exfoliative cytology was utilized in the early diagnosis of carcinoma of the lung. Christensen *et al* concluded that bronchial lavage alone had little diagnostic value in pulmonary carcinoma. In reviewing 396 patients proven to have malignant tumors of the lung, only 18% had positive cytologic washings. In only two patients, (0.5%), was examination of the cytology the sole criterion for establishment of a diagnosis of a malignant lesion of the lung.[6]

Fennessy described advancing a brush via a catheter fluoroscopically into the subsegmental bronchi. This technique had a yield of 67% for primary carcinoma of all types but a lower yield for metastatic carcinoma or malignant lymphoma.[7] The ease of passing a nylon brush through the inner channel of the bronchofiberscope led to a marked increase in the yield of positive cytologic specimens for malignancy. The placement of a brush through the fiberoptic bronchoscope for visible malignancies gave positive results in Richardson's group in 94% of cases and 78% of the peripheral carcinomas brushed with fluoroscopic control.[8]

Because many early lesions of carcinoma of the lung originate in areas not visible endoscopically, the addition of a fluoroscopic system is a beneficial aid to the bronchoscopist.[9] In addition, Marsh *et al* and Sanderson *et al* have developed specific protocols for the detection and localization of early bronchogenic carcinomas.[4,10]

From the Department of Otorhinolaryngology and Human Communication, University of Pennsylvania School of Medicine, Philadelphia, Pennsylvania.

Presented at the meeting of the American Broncho-Esophagological Association, Palm Beach, Florida, April 27-28, 1976.

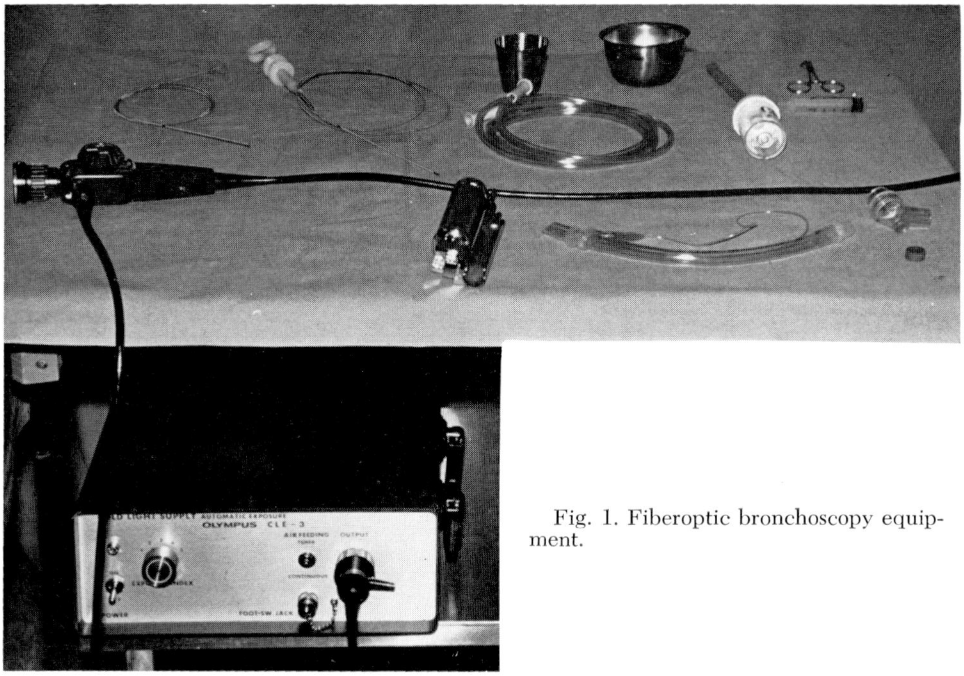

Fig. 1. Fiberoptic bronchoscopy equipment.

We present a newer technique, utilizing a C-arm, multiplanar fluoroscopic control with an image intensification system, for the localization of peripheral lung lesions and subsegmental parenchymal infiltrates.

This method has proved useful in the early histologic and cytologic diagnosis of nonendoscopically visible bronchogenic carcinomas and in the drainage of lung abscesses. Also, it has facilitated the placement of brush or biopsy forceps in tuberculous or bacterial pneumonias, mycetomas, cysts, and in transbronchial biopsy of diffuse lung disease.

By employing a transendotracheal tube route with a ventilating side-arm adaptor, continuous airway control and a selected inspired oxygen or anesthetic content is maintained. In addition, the problems of arterial hypoxemia, airway resistance, and ventilation-perfusion abnormalities are minimized.

TECHNIQUE

Following the identification of a peripheral lung lesion or subsegmental parenchymal infiltrate on chest roentgenogram, tomograms are obtained where further delineation of the lesion is indicated. In those patients with preexisting coronary artery disease or chronic obstructive lung disease, room air arterial blood gases and pulmonary function tests are obtained preoperatively.

Premedication, given 60 minutes prior to the procedure, combines a narcotic analgesic, meperidine hydrochloride 50-100 mg IM, with hydroxyzine hydrochloride 25-50 mg IM or diazepam 5-10 mg IM, and an anticholinergic, atropine 0.4-0.6 mg IM.

If a general anesthetic is desired, Innovar®* neuroleptanalgesia induction with 60% nitrous oxide — 40% oxygen and succinylcholine chloride is used. A greater than 50% inspired oxygen content is maintained where preoperative pulmonary function is marginal and arterial hypoxemia is present (a PaO_2 less than 70 mm Hg while breathing room air).

Where a general anesthetic is contraindicated because of poor pulmonary re-

* McNeil Laboratories, Inc., Fort Washington, PA.

serve or severe ischemic heart disease, a regional anesthetic technique is employed. Bilateral superior laryngeal nerve blocks, each using 2 cc of 2% lidocaine, are placed with a 22 gauge needle 1 cm anterior to the superior cornu of the thyroid cartilage in a line drawn midway between the hyoid bone and thyroid cartilage. Five cubic centimeters of 2% lidocaine is slowly instilled into the trachea through the cricothyroid membrane. Using indirect mirror laryngoscopy and a sprayer,* the oropharynx and hypopharynx are topically anesthetized with 1 cc of 10% cocaine. Electrocardiographic monitoring is maintained throughout the procedure.

Figure 1 indicates the arrangement of equipment used in performing the procedure. The patient is intubated with a 9.0 mm inside diameter cuffed endotracheal tube.** This is placed 20 cm below the inferior alveolar ridge in adult males and 18 mm in females, assuring location of the tube above the level of the carina. After inflation of the cuff, a swivel tracheostomy adaptor*** with a rubber adaptor† is attached to the proximal end of the endotracheal tube. This allows easy connection with the anesthesiologist's Y-piece assembly. A closed system is maintained by introducing the bronchofiberscope, lubricated with viscous lidocaine, through the 5 mm opening in the adaptor.

A bronchofiberscope†† with a 2 mm multipurpose suction channel and an angle of rotation of 130° up and 130° down, is primarily used. Light is supplied by a cold light source.††

The tracheobronchial tree is systematically examined. Using intermittent suctioning and small aliquots (5 cc) of normal saline, bronchial washings are collected in a specimen trap. The material is routinely sent for bacterial culture and sensitivity, acid fast smear and culture, fungus culture, and cytologic cell block.

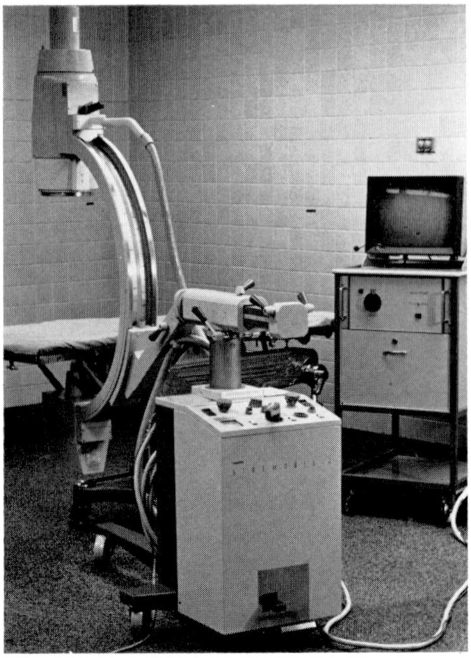

Fig. 2. C-arm multiplanar, fluoroscopic control with image intensification system.

Under direct endoscopic vision and utilizing a portable multiplanar fluoroscopic control with image intensification system‡ (Fig. 2), the fiberoptic bronchoscope is placed within a subsegmental bronchus. A nylon brush‡‡ with markings at 5 cm intervals on the proximal end, is advanced beyond the tip of the bronchofiberscope. Continuous multiplanar views are obtained fluoroscopically, confirming the intralesional placement of the instrument, and are stored within a memory storage unit for recall and photography.

Brushings are immediately smeared in standard microscope slides, and fixed.

---

* Carabelli sprayer, Pilling Co., Fort Washington, PA.
** Model 9.0 mm. Shiley Labs., Santa Ana, CA.
*** Harlake 57-00700. Harris Lake Co., Cleveland, OH.
† Wolf Co., Rosemont, IL.
†† Model 5.2 mm BF-B2. Model CLE-3. Olympus Corp., New Hyde Park, NY.
‡ Siemens Corp., Erlangan, Germany.
‡‡ 5 mm length, 2 mm diameter. Olympus Corp., New Hyde Park, NY.

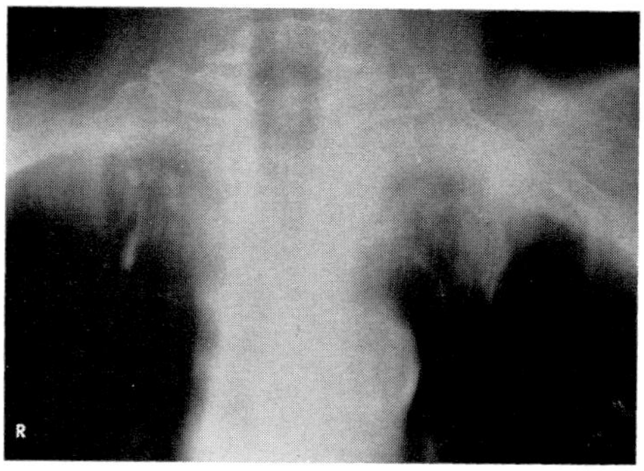

Fig. 3. Apical tomograms demonstrating a cavity within the apex of the left lung.

Biopsies are obtained with a cupped biopsy forcep* under continuous fluoroscopic control, and placed on filter paper with a 21 gauge needle to avoid inducing further crush artifact. In all cases the fiberoptic bronchoscope is withdrawn from the endotracheal tube with the instrument remaining beyond the tip of the bronchofiberscope to prevent crushing of tissue.

Lung abscesses are located in a similar fashion fluoroscopically, and a fine .047 inch radio-opaque, angiographic catheter is advanced inside the wall of the abscess. After instillation of Hypaque®** and the recording of multiplanar fluoroscopic images, the cavity is drained and irrigated with copious amounts of normal saline. After the completion of the procedure, the flexible fiberoptic bronchoscope is rapidly sterilized with Betadine®*** and 70% ethanol.

CASE REPORTS

Case No. 1. A 65-year-old Caucasian male was admitted to the Pennsylvania Hospital because of syncopal episodes. An extensive neurological evaluation including brain scan, EMI scan,† electroencephalogram and lumbar puncture were within normal limits. A chest film revealed bilateral apical scarring and evidence of a mass in the apical posterior segment of the left upper lobe. Apical tomograms demonstrated a cavity with a mass in the left apex of the lung (Fig. 3). He denied any history of fever, chills, night sweats, or weight loss. There was no history of arthralgias, hemoptysis, or skin eruptions.

Past medical history was positive for a partial gastrectomy and pulmonary tuberculosis treated with isoniazid ten years prior to admission. An intermediate strength PPD was positive and the erythrocyte sedimentation rate was elevated to 32 mm/hr. Under multiplanar fluoroscopic control the anterior subsegment of the apical posterior segment of the left upper lobe was brushed and biopsied. A grey-white material which was obtained, revealed on microscopic section a densely matted aggregate of branching septate hyphae, characteristic of an aspergilloma. Routine bacterial cultures and sensitivities, acid fast bacillus smears and cultures were negative, and washings yielded a Class 1 cytology. The patient was discharged on no medications.

Case No. 2. A 45-year-old Negro female with a history of chronic alcohol abuse, Laënnec's cirrhosis, aspiration pneumonia, adult-onset diabetes mellitus, and folate and iron-deficiency anemia was admitted to the hospital. At the time of admission, the patient was febrile to 39.4 C with a cough productive of yellow, purulent sputum.

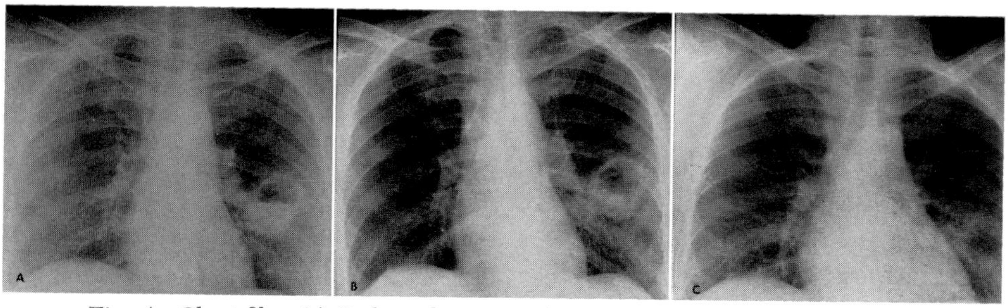

Fig. 4. Chest film. A) Prebronchoscopy. B) Immediate postbronchoscopy. C) One month postbronchoscopy.

---

* 3 mm length, 2 mm width. Olympus Corp., New Hyde Park, NY.
** Winthrop Laboratories, New York, NY.
*** The Purdue Frederick Co., Norwalk, CT.
† Emi Medical Inc., Northbrook, IL.

A chest film disclosed a cavitating lesion with an air-fluid level in the superior segment of the left lower lobe (Fig. 4A). Under multiplanar fluoroscopic control, using a fiberoptic bronchoscope,* an arterial catheter was introduced into the cavity. Approximately 50 cc of mucopurulent material was obtained, which contained on Gram stain, many polymorphonuclear leukocytes and Gram positive cocci in chains.

Following bronchoscopy, her fever immediately defervesced and a postbronchoscopy film demonstrated the absence of an air-fluid level in the cavity (Fig. 4B). Culture grew group A streptococcus. She was treated with intravenous aqueous penicillin 20 million units per day in divided doses for two weeks, followed by an additional two weeks of oral phenoxymethyl penicillin 500 mg four times per day. At the time of discharge four weeks after admission, the cavity had almost completely resolved (Fig. 4C). A chest film taken two months later showed complete resolution of the abscess.

DISCUSSION

This technique provides a useful method for employing the fiberoptic bronchoscope in the diagnosis and management of a wide spectrum of pulmonary disease. In addition, it recognizes the effect of bronchofiberscopy upon pulmonary physiology. It is flexible in that either regional or general anesthesia may be used. Careful attention to the dosages of premedication, and regional and topical anesthetics used, avoids the major complications associated with fiberoptic bronchoscopy. As surveyed by Credle *et al,* most of the major complications reported occurring with bronchofiberoscopy were related to the systemic toxic effects of these agents.[11] In many cases, this was due to tetracaine which has a significantly smaller margin of safety than lidocaine which we use.

During fiberoptic bronchoscopy, a number of investigators have found a mean decrease in arterial oxygen of 12 mm Hg (range 2-20 mm Hg), which is felt to be secondary to a loss of effective tidal volume through suctioning and bronchial lavage.[12,13] Ventilation-perfusion abnormalities due to localized atelectasis are produced by prolonged suctioning or by increased resistance to airflow into the bronchus.

These problems are minimized in the present technique by a continuous flow of inspired oxygen content through a closed system, by using intermittent suction and lavage with small aliquots of normal saline, and by the maintenance of intermittent positive end-expiratory pressure during ventilation to prevent alveolar collapse. Increased airway resistance is avoided by using a greater than 8.5 mm inside diameter endotracheal tube.[14]

The C-arm fluoroscopic control with image intensification system provides a continuous multiplanar fluoroscopic technique, facilitating intralesional placement of brushes, biopsy forceps or catheters. An image retrieval system yields additional radiographic documentation for review of the procedure and photography.

Presently, a prototype flexible fiberoptic bronchoscope is being clinically tested which solves some of the problems created by bronchofiberoscopy. Lightweight, allowing easier mobility, it contains a 2 mm suction channel controlled with an open-close lever mounted on the control section. This enables the operator to aspirate secretions simultaneously and independently of the placement of instruments. The collection port has been placed on the light carrier, away from the operator, allowing manipulation of the bronchoscope without interference.

There are several problems, however, still posed by flexible fiberoptic bronchoscopy, including the small size of the biopsy, crush artifact, and the small size of the optic image. In order to get more precise control of the instruments, the development of flexible manually-guided biopsy forceps which can be manipulated independent of the bronchofiberscope, is underway. A pediatric fiberoptic bronchoscope and the construction of specialized grasping forceps for the removal of peripherally lodged foreign bodies is also anticipated.

* Model BF-B2. Olympus Corp. of America, New Hyde Park, NY.

REFERENCES

1. Ikeda S, Yanai N, Ishikawa S: Flexible bronchofiberscope. Keio J Med 17:1-16, 1968

2. Davidson TM, Bone RC, Nahum AM: Flexible fiberoptic laryngobronchoscopy. Laryngoscope 84:1876-1882, 1974

3. Sackner MA: State of the art—bronchofiberscopy. Am Rev Respir Dis 111:62-88, 1975

4. Marsh BR, Frost JK, Erozan YS, *et al*: Flexible fiberoptic bronchoscopy: its place in the search for lung cancer. Ann Otol Rhinol Laryngol 82:757-764, 1973

5. Stoloff IL: The prognostic value of bronchoscopy in primary lung cancer. JAMA 227:299-301, 1974

6. Christensen ES, Michaelson M, Mossing N: The diagnostic value of bronchial washing in lung cancer. J Thorac Cardiovasc Surg 68:313-317, 1974

7. Fennessy JJ: Bronchial brushing. Ann Otol Rhinol Laryngol 79:924-932, 1970

8. Richardson RH, Zavala DC, Mukerjee PK: The use of fiberoptic bronchoscopy and brush biopsy in the diagnosis of suspected pulmonary malignancy. Am Rev Respir Dis 109:63-66, 1974

9. Zavala DC: Diagnostic fiberoptic bronchoscopy: techniques and results of biopsy in 600 patients. Chest 68:12-19, 1975

10. Sanderson DR, Fontana RS, Woolner LB, *et al*: Bronchoscopic localization of radiographically occult lung cancer. Chest 65:608-612, 1974

11. Credle WF, Smiddy JF, Elliot RC: Complications of fiberoptic bronchoscopy. Am Rev Respir Dis 109:67-72, 1974

12. Pierson DJ, Iseman MD, Sutton FD, *et al*: Arterial blood gas changes in fiberoptic bronchoscopy during mechanical ventilation. Chest 66:495-497, 1974

13. Lampton LM: Bronchofiberscopy: caution, Letter. JAMA 231:138, 1975

14. Tahir AH: General anesthesia for bronchofiberscopy. Anesthesiology 37:564-566, 1972

Reprints—Joseph P. Atkins, Jr., MD, Department of Otorhinolaryngology and Human Communication, University of Pennsylvania School of Medicine, 3400 Spruce Street, Philadelphia, PA 19104.

Ann Otol 85: 1976

PERCUTANEOUS JET VENTILATION

EDWARD CARDEN, FRCP(C)

GARY BECKER, MD HASSNEY HAMOOD, MD

LOS ANGELES, CALIFORNIA

SUMMARY – A method of ventilation utilizing an S-shaped cannula placed through the cricothyroid membrane and hooked up to a conventional jetting system is described. Its advantages are reduced morbidity, better ventilation, and an unobstructed view of the operating site for the surgeon. The system allows ventilation of the patient with oxygen prior to the induction, or at the end of anesthesia if necessary, and allows the surgeon to perform a tracheostomy in the usual manner if it is indicated. The system is not proposed as a routine method of ventilation during anesthesia for laryngeal surgery but is reserved for cases in which other methods would not perform adequately.

Much progress has been made over the last few years in developing jet ventilation systems for use during general anesthesia for laryngeal surgery. Jets have been placed in the trachea via the transoral,[1,2] transnasal,[3] or transtracheal[4] route and by intermittently jetting gas from the tip of these jets, positive pressure ventilation can be accomplished while the patient is anesthetized and the vocal cords are paralyzed.

The advantage of these techniques is that the vision for the surgeon is much improved over the standard endotracheal tube, allowing more precise surgical maneuvers to be performed. In some patients, large obstructing upper airway lesions make it impossible to place a Carden tube[1] or even a catheter[2,3] through the vocal cords and also, the introduction of a catheter through the vocal cords could obstruct exhalation to a significant degree. It is in these patients that a cannula placed percutaneously through the tracheal wall or cricothyroid membrane into the trachea and used as the jet to ventilate the patient assumes paramount importance. In this manner, ventilation of the patient can be accomplished without added obstruction to exhalation and assisted ventilation with 100% oxygen may be instituted prior to anesthesia being induced.

This technique, however, has unique hazards. There exists the possibility of the cannula being placed through the posterior wall of the trachea or into the subcutaneous tissues of the neck. Attempted ventilation at this point will cause emphysema which can track down into the mediastinum, into the chest, or up around the area of the vocal cords.[5] In this paper, we will show the design of a special cannula which will minimize these unique hazards while affording maximum ventilatory support during the period of surgery.

METHOD

It has been shown that the optimum position of the jetting cannula in the trachea is in the center of the lumen with the direction of flow parallel to the side walls of the trachea.[6] Adequate ventilation is possible through a 14-gauge 2¼ inch cannula utilizing pressures less than 50 pounds per square inch (the usual pipeline pressure in a hospital). It therefore became apparent that a simple way to solve the problem of optimal intratracheal position of the needle would be to make a plastic cannula which was S-shaped. Ideally, after insertion through the cricothyroid membrane

---

From the Departments of Anesthesiology and Otorhinolaryngology, UCLA School of Medicine, and the Department of Otorhinolaryngology, VA Wadsworth Medical Center, Los Angeles, California.

Presented at the meeting of the American Broncho-Esophagological Association, Palm Beach, Florida, April 27-28, 1976.

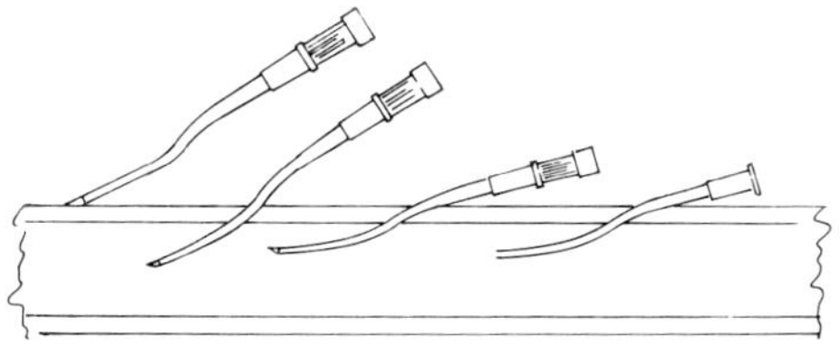

Fig. 1. The method of insertion of the S-shaped cannula into the trachea, showing from left to right; the needle entering the skin, the first part of the needle in the trachea, the hub lowered, and last, the stylet removed.

or tracheal wall the plastic cannula should retain its shape after removing the stylet. The terminal segment of the S would then be parallel to the longitudinal axis of the trachea and in the center of the trachea (the optimum position); the middle section of the S would be in the tissues of the patient's neck and the proximal portion of the S would be parallel to the skin of the neck at which point the jetting system would be attached (Fig. 1). We investigated various possibilities and looked at many different intravenous cannulas. We found that the Medicut R®* cannula could be bent into an S-shape by hand and after heating to 81.2 C the plastic cannula would retain its shape after removal of the stylet. The cannula (Fig. 2) has a hub which is integral with its shaft, making removal of the stylet simple.

CLINICAL STUDIES

Having determined that this cannula would serve our purpose in providing ventilation, yet increasing safety, we decided to carry out a clinical trial on five patients who were having laryngeal surgery. These patients were specially selected because they had upper airway obstructing lesions, making the use of jets placed into the trachea by any other method extremely difficult if not impossible. In two patients (Cases 1 and 2) the S-shaped cannulas were placed through the cricothyroid membrane under local anesthesia and ventilation assisted prior to induction of general anesthesia. A conventional balanced anesthetic technique, together with intratracheal injection of nitrous oxide oxygen mixtures from the 14-gauge cannula, was used (Fig. 3). Arterial blood samples were obtained after 10-20 minutes of surgery and analyzed for PaO_2,

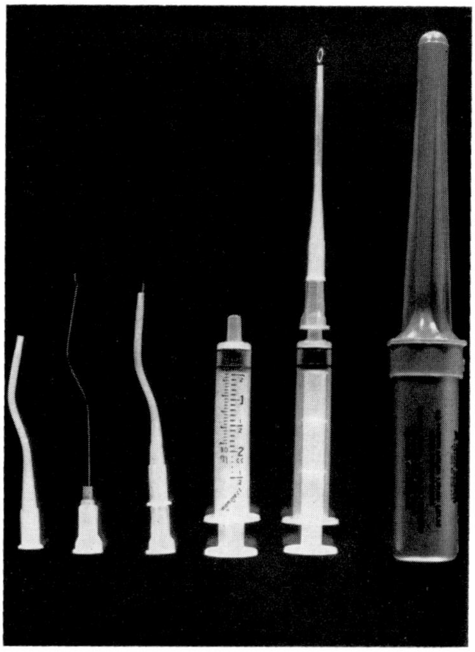

Fig. 2. Showing from top to bottom: the Medicut R® cannula in its case; the case removed; the cannula removed; the S-shaped cannula; the stylet; the cannula with stylet removed.

$PaCO_2$ and pH. These results are seen in Table I.

DISCUSSION

Results shown in Table I reveal that this technique gives adequate ventilation of these anesthetized paralyzed patients.

The shape of the cannula is such that by inserting it in the method shown in Figure 1, perforation or damage to the posterior tracheal wall becomes virtually impossible unless it is being used on a child. Its center segment surrounded by skin acts as a stabilizing factor, keeping it in position and minimizing the problem of accidental withdrawal which is prone to occur when the patient's neck is extended prior to insertion of the laryngoscope blade. In patients with very thick necks, its center section is not as efficient in doing this and a longer cannula is needed. The case reports of patients 1, 2 and 3 are

* Sherwood Medical Industries, St. Louis, MO.

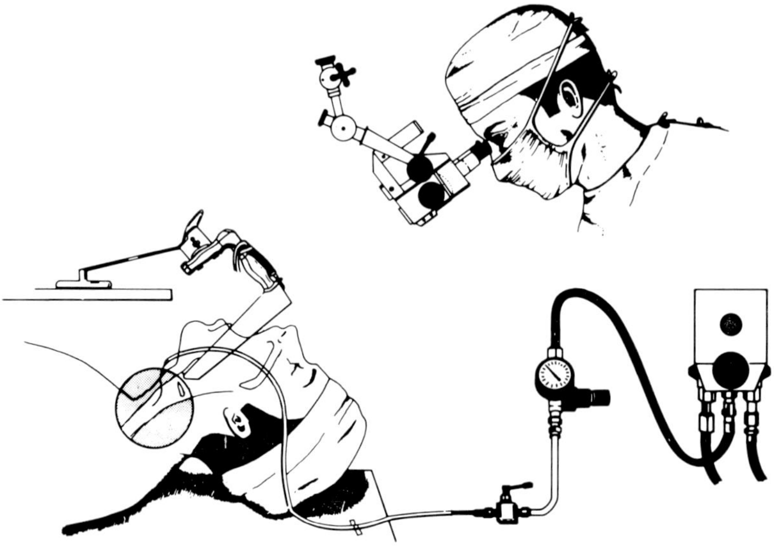

Fig. 3. A schematic representation of the complete system in use.

used to demonstrate the distinct advantages of this technique.

CASE REPORTS

Case 1. This 75-year-old male developed acute upper airway obstruction and was brought to surgery for an emergency tracheostomy. Because of his distressed condition, adequate visualization of the larynx was not possible with the patient awake. The special cannula was placed through the cricothyroid membrane after infiltrating the area with local anesthesia and his ventilation was assisted with 100% oxygen for two minutes prior to anesthesia being induced in the usual manner. Then anesthesia was maintained with intravenous narcotic (fentanyl) and 70% nitrous oxide with 30% oxygen jetted from the cannula. A succinyl choline drip (0.2%) was used to maintain paralysis. Visualization of the cords with the laryngoscope demonstrated a true vocal cord web which was dilated with the bronchoscope. No other pathology was found and the etiology of the web was unknown. A tracheostomy was not performed.

Case 2. This 99.9 kg, 74-year-old female came to surgery with acute upper airway obstruction. As before, the special cannula was placed through the

TABLE I

BLOOD GAS DATA ON PATIENTS ANESTHETIZED USING THIS TECHNIQUE

Patient No.	*%N_2O*	*PaO_2 mm Hg*	*$PaCO_2$ mm Hg*	*pH*	*Age (yr)*	*Lesion*
1	60	140	30	7.50	75	Web across the vocal cords
2	50	201	43	7.33	74	Carcinoma of larynx
3	60	202	31	7.49	70	Edema of larynx
4	60	170	31.8	7.46	63	Large right posterior cord lesion
5	60	170	34	7.4	54	Two large laryngeal polyps

cricothyroid membrane under local anesthesia and ventilation assisted for two minutes with 100% oxygen. A large carcinoma of the larynx had created a gross distortion of the anatomy, and the airway through the larynx was noted after induction of anesthesia to be circular and approximately 4 mm in diameter. This would have precluded the use of the standard endotracheal tube or the use of a catheter placed through the larynx, since the added resistance to flow caused by the catheter would have impaired exhalation. Anesthesia proceeded as with the patient in Case 1, but using a 50% nitrous oxide oxygen mixture. After the extent of the lesion was determined and biopsies obtained, an orderly tracheostomy was performed through the third and fourth tracheal rings.

Case 3. This 70-year-old man had a small degree of upper airway osbtruction due to edema of the aryepiglottic folds following radiation. After induction of anesthesia in the usual manner, he could not be intubated or ventilated by the anesthesiologist. The S-shaped cannula was placed through the cricothyroid membrane at this time and the patient ventilated with the nitrous oxide oxygen mixture while the surgeons viewed the larynx and took appropriate biopsies. At the end of this procedure the cannula was left in position to see if the patient would be able to maintain a satisfactory airway and only when the patient was fully awake and breathing well on his own was the cannula removed.

As with any technique, careful patient selection shows a successful outcome. As the complication rate from percutaneous cannula jetting techniques is high,[7] other methods should be utilized if at all possible. The design of this cannula has meant that better ventilation can be accomplished and the likelihood of emphysema is much reduced as compared to utilizing a conventional straight needle. By using this technique, ventilation can be assisted prior to beginning of anesthesia and at the end of anesthesia, and the cannula need only be withdrawn when an adequate airway in the patient is apparent. By utilizing the cricothyroid membrane as the puncture site, a tracheostomy can be performed immediately with an unobstructed surgical view.

CONCLUSION

A technique of ventilation for patients with obstructing lesions of the larynx has been presented. It maximizes visualization by avoiding an endotracheal tube, allows ventilatory support prior to and at the end of anesthesia and also allows a tracheostomy to be performed in a routine manner at the end of surgery if necessary. We reserve this technique for special cases and have found that the S-shape cannula permits adequate ventilation with a minimum of hazard.

REFERENCES

1. Carden E, Vest HR: Further advances in anesthetic techniques for microlaryngeal surgery. Anesth Analg (Cleve) 53:584-587, 1974

2. Carden E, Ferguson GB: A new technique for microlaryngeal surgery on infants. Laryngoscope 83:691-699, 1973

3. Spoerel WE, Greenway RE: Techniques of ventilation during endolaryngeal surgery under general anesthetic. Can Anaesth Soc J 20:369-377, 1973

4. Spoerel WE, Narayanan PS, Singh NP: Transtracheal ventilation. Br J Anaesth 43: 932-939, 1971

5. Carden E, Calcaterra TC: Pneumatocoel of the larynx. Anesth Analg, to be published

6. Carden E: An improved percutaneous jetting system for use during microlaryngeal surgery. Can Anaesth Soc J, to be published

7. Smith RB, Schaer WB, Pfaeffle H: Percutaneous transtracheal ventilation for anesthesia and resuscitation. Can Anaesth Soc J 22:607-612, 1975

Acknowledgments—The authors would like to thank Medical Engineering of Racine, Wisconsin for providing the jetting system, the Bird Corporation of Palm Springs, California for the nitrous oxide oxygen blender, and Sherwood Medical Industries of St. Louis, for the cannulas. We would also like to thank Sara Fulwiler for her secretarial help.

Reprints—Edward Carden, MD, Department of Anesthesiology, UCLA School of Medicine, Los Angeles, CA 90024.

Ann Otol 85: 1976

ENDOTRACHEAL INTUBATION AND VENTURI (JET) VENTILATION FOR LASER MICROSURGERY OF THE LARYNX

MARTIN LLOYD NORTON, MD

M. STUART STRONG, MD CHARLES W. VAUGHAN, MD

JOHN C. SNOW, MD BENJAMIN J. KRIPKE, MD

BOSTON, MASSACHUSETTS

SUMMARY – Meeting the exacting requirements for microsurgery of the larynx is a challenge for the anesthesiologist. To accomplish the necessary dissection, the otolaryngologist has several requirements. They are a quiet relaxed field, excellent illumination with magnification, binocular vision for depth perception, and, above all, an unobstructed field. The management of anesthesia for suspension microsurgery on the larynx presents many problems, the most vexing of which is the fact that the otolaryngologist and anesthesiologist are in competition for access to the patient's airway. In sharing this, neither has been able to perform with the degree of control that he would like due to either inadequate operating conditions or insufficient access to ventilatory mechanisms. Several anesthetic techniques have been used for inspection or operative laryngoscopy: topical anesthesia, apneic techniques, translaryngeal topical anesthesia, chest respirator,* neuroleptanalgesia, and general endotracheal anesthesia with muscle relaxants. The latter has proven most popular, particularly in children, because ventilation and surgical conditions are considered to be most controllable. However, the presence of the requisite endotracheal tube obscures the full view of the larynx and vocal cords, and the tube may itself become obstructed. Additionally, use of the laser involves the further risk of heat effects on the endotracheal tube if the beam hits the tube. This report presents our experience and development of the combined technique of endotracheal intubation and Venturi (jet) ventilation. We believe it represents the safest available approach while providing near ideal working conditions for the otolaryngologist during laser microsurgery of the larynx.

The management of anesthesia for suspension microsurgery on the larynx presents many problems because the otolaryngologist and the anesthesiologist are in competition for control of the patient's airway. In sharing this control, neither has been able to perform the quality work that he would like to perform due to inadequate operating conditions or insufficient ventilation.

Several anesthetic techniques have been used for inspection or operative laryngoscopy: 1) topical anesthesia, 2) apneic technique, 3) translaryngeal topical anesthesia, 4) chest respirator, 5) neuroleptanalgesia, and 6) general endotracheal anesthesia with muscle relaxants. The last anesthetic technique has been most popular, particularly in children, because ventilation and surgical conditions are considered to be relatively adequate. However, the presence of an endotracheal tube obscures the full view of the larynx and vocal cords. This has required the use of undersized tubes and occasionally less than adequate ventilation. In addition, during carbon dioxide laser microsurgery on the larynx and trachea, there is the risk of fire if the laser beam repeatedly hits the endotracheal tube.

* Model No. 33CRC. J. H. Emerson Co., Cambridge, MA.

From the Boston University Medical Center, University Hospital, Boston, Massachusetts.

Presented at the meeting of the American Broncho-Esophagological Association, Palm Beach, Florida, April 27-28, 1976.

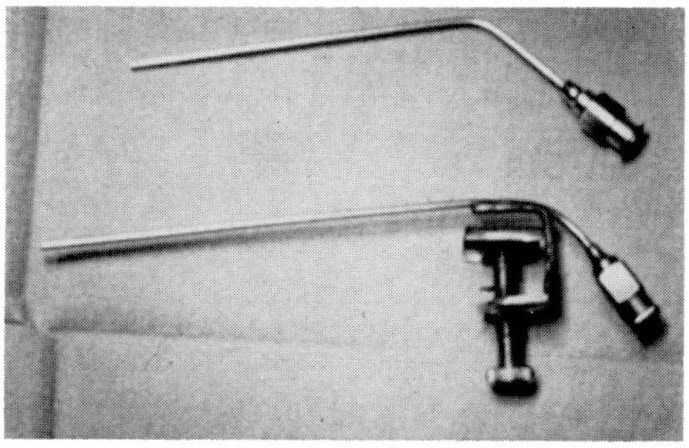

Fig. 1. Jet needle mounted on clamp.

We have approached the problem using the concepts originally presented by Sander,[1] Spoerel and Grant,[2] as modified by Rajagopalan *et al*,[3] and McGrail.[4]

Venturi or jet ventilation affords an excellent view of the vocal cords while maintaining adequate ventilation, but has significant disadvantages. The preoperative airway must not be compromised. Examination and treatment of the airway is largely limited to the vocal cords. Proper placement of the suspension system for microsurgery requires many minutes of unhurried manipulation. Fortunately, a combination of endotracheal intubation and Venturi systems may be easily and alternatively used to enjoy the advantages of the one to overcome the disadvantages of the other.

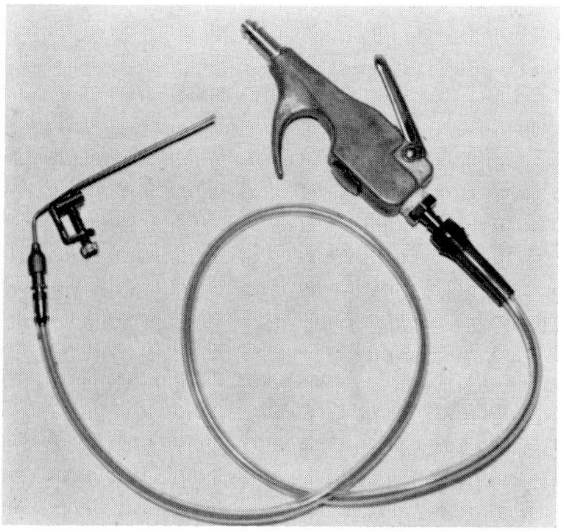

Fig. 2. Modified Speedaire® Blo-gun.

TABLE I

GENERAL STUDY GROUP DATA

Age range (yr)	3-78
Weight (kg)	13.5-104.4
Height (cm)	97.5-182.5
Male = 54	
Female = 46	
Case Studies = 100	

INSTRUMENTATION

The special equipment required for laser microsurgery anesthesia management includes aluminum foil* wrapping for the endotracheal tube. Additionally, we designed an inexpensive jet needle (16 and 14 g) mounted on a clamp (Fig.1). A two-stage reducing valve mounted on an "H" tank of medically pure oxygen with tubing leading to a modified Speedaire Blo-gun®** completes the system (Fig. 2).

The 16 g needle is used for pediatric patients and the 14 g needle for adults. Pressure gauge settings have not exceeded 13.5 kg for adults or 9 kg for children. However, using clinical movement of the chest as the primary guide for ventilatory adequacy, we use as low as 3.6 to 5.4 kg pressure in most of our pediatric cases and 9 kg in adults.

SUBSTRATE STUDY GROUP

Our study population consisted of 100 cases with an age range from 3 to 78 years (Table I). Ninety percent of our study patients were in the pediatric age grouping (2 to 12). Weights varied from 13.5 to 104.4 kg, and height varied from 97.5 to 182.5 cm. The ratio of male to female cases is 54/46. Of these patients, almost all have been studied more than once. It must be noted that the primary diagnosis was laryngotracheal papillomatosis (juvenile papillomatosis), though we did include patients with other vocal cord tumor masses. As is well known, laryngotracheal papillomatosis is presumably of viral etiology and has a very high recurrence rate.[5-7]

* Realistic, 100" metallic sensing tape. Radio Shack Corp., Fort Worth, TX.
** No. 2X492. Dayton Electric Mfc. Co., Chicago, IL.

TABLE II

PREMEDICATION SCHEDULE FOR LASER MICROSURGERY CASES WITH VENTURI VENTILATION

Age *yr*	*Weight* *kg*	*Nembutal®** *mg*	*Morphine* *mg*	*Atropine* *mg*
0.5	7.2	15	0.75	0.1
1	9.45	25	1.00	0.1
2	12.15	30	1.50	0.2
4	15.75	45	2.00	0.25
6	20.25	50	2.5	0.3
8	24.75	60	3.0	0.35
10	29.25	75	3.5	0.4
12	38.25	100	3.5	0.45

Dosage scheduled to be reduced if patient is demonstrably in respiratory distress. Morphine is to be omitted if patent is demonstrably in respiratory distress. If premedication is inadequate, use rectal thiopental (Abbott) in doses never exceeding 17.6 mg/kg.

* Abbott Laboratories, North Chicago, IL.

PREMEDICATION

It is of major importance that these patients have carefully chosen premedication. The children particularly, should be well sedated. Special care, however, must be given not to either over or under medicate those patients with massive accumulations of papillomas. Pharmacologic respiratory depression may be superposed on an already borderline mechanical airway. We found the use of rectal thiopental* in doses never exceeding 17.6 mg/kg of great help in pediatric management both for induction and the maintenance of anesthesia during the Venturi phase in lieu of intravenous barbiturates as used for adults. Generally, our premedicant schedule is as indicated in Table II. The reader will note that this is a modification of the schedule recommended by Smith.[8]

MONITORING

We routinely monitor our patients with electrocardiogram (Leads I or II), precordial stethescopes, and sphygmomanometry (Riva Rocci technique). Where specifically indicated, the Block-Aid ®** monitor has been of some use. On randomly sampled cases, we have also studied arterial blood gases (Table III). A subsequent study is in preparation reporting electrocardiographic findings and comparing various anesthetic agents during these procedures.

PROCEDURE

Induction of anesthesia in adults follows routine procedures and usually is initiated with intravenous barbiturate (thiamylal sodium). Pediatric patients are routinely induced by mask. All patients received the inhalation agents nitrous oxide, oxygen, and enfluorane in proportions of 3 liters: 2 liters, 3000-4000 cc flows. Relaxation is maintained with 0.2% succinylcholine chloride intravenous drip.

Subsequent to induction, the patient is intubated with a small diameter aluminum foil protected red rubber tube following the techniques of Snow *et al.*[9] Thus, the surgeon is not rushed in the placement of his suspension laryngoscope. Furthermore, the trapdoor effect of jet ventilation on massive polyposis is avoided. A further modification is the introduction of a gastric suction tube for gravity drainage of gases and secretions, and is accomplished in *all* pediatric cases and some adults.

Suspension laryngoscopy is then performed by the surgeon, and the microscope and CO_2 laser are utilized to treat any pathology that is not obscured by the presence of the tube. The endotracheal tube is then withdrawn, the larynx inspected and suctioned, and Venturi ventilation initiated. We place the jet needle within the lumen of the laryngoscope resting above the channel of the light carrier. This will not interfere with vision or instrumentation, does not require reduction of illumination by removal of one of the light carriers, and provides unqualified access to the posterior one-third of the vocal

* Pentothal® sodium, No. 7236, rectal suspension, Abbott Laboratories, North Chicago, IL.
** Burroughs Wellcome Co., Greenville, NC.

TABLE III

BLOOD GAS STUDIES

Study Case	*Age*	*Wt kg*		*On Endotracheal Tube*	*Pressure Kg*	*Needle g*	*On Venturi System*
21	3½	13.5	pO_2	80	3.6	16	80
			pCO_2	44			41
			O_2sat	94.0			94.1
			HCO_3	22.8			20.6
			pH	7.35			7.33
22	12	34.9	pO_2	120	5.4	16	135
			pCO_2	48			45
			O_2sat	98.5			98.7
			HCO_3	28.5			25.5
			pH	7.38			7.38
23	6	18.9	pO_2	130	5.4	16	235
			pCO_2	48			46
			O_2sat	98.5			99.3
			HCO_3	25.5			24.3
			pH	7.40			7.35
30	5	19.575	pO_2	155	4.5	16	247
			pCO_2	44			35
			O_2sat	98.5			99.3
			HCO_3	24.3			21.2
			pH	7.44			7.41
40	13	42.75	pO_2	160	5.4	16	177
			pCO_2	44			40
			O_2sat	98.8			99.3
			HCO_3	22.5			20.6
			pH	7.40			7.34
45	58	81.0	pO_2	100	13.5	14	148
			pCO_2	44			32
			O_2sat	98.5			98.9
			HCO_3	18.5			16.9
			pH	7.39			7.35
46	22	104.4	pO_2	88	13.5	14	100
			pCO_2	44			37
			O_2sat	95.5			96.8
			HCO_3	22.0			19.1
			pH	7.35			7.34
47	10		pO_2	150	9.0	16	210
			pCO_2	46			31
			O_2sat	98.6			99.3
			HCO_3	25.5			23.7
			pH	7.39			7.39
55	51	96.75	pO_2	72	13.5	14	155
			pCO_2	42			29
			O_2sat	92.9			QNS
			HCO_3	22.6			QNS
			pH	7.36			QNS
57	5	25.65	pO_2	170	5.4	16	250
			pCO_2	62			52
			O_2sat	98.9			99.3
			HCO_3	25.4			22.3
			pH	7.24			7.26
59	46	19.50	pO_2	180	13.5	14	190
			pCO_2	48			46
			O_2sat	99.3			99.3
			HCO_3	27.8			23.7
			pH	7.39			7.34

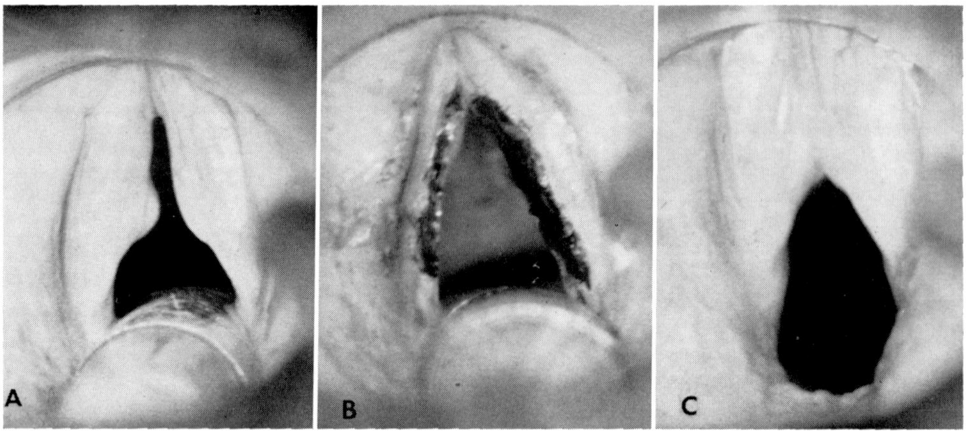

Fig. 3. A) Laryngeal orifice before surgery with endotracheal tube. B) Laryngeal orifice after surgery with endotracheal tube. C) Laryngeal orifice without endotracheal tube; Venturi ventilation system in use.

cords as well as the interarytenoid area. The surgeon must be particularly attentive to the placement of the laryngoscope. The instrument must have the tip as close to the cords as possible and the axis of the laryngoscope lumen in line with the axis of the trachea.

On completion of the surgery, an oropharyngeal airway is inserted and respiration is supported by bag and mask until the effects of the succinylcholine chloride drip wears off. It is during this time that the benefits of the gastric drainage tube are most manifest.

ADVANTAGES OF THE COMBINED SYSTEM

The primary and unparalleled advantage of Venturi ventilation techniques in laryngeal surgery is the total access to the larynx and trachea without visual and/or mechanical obstruction by an endotracheal tube (Fig. 3). While this is not a dominant factor in the anterior commissure and anterior two-thirds of the vocal cord region, it is of controlling significance in the posterior and lateral aspects of the subglottic and interarytenoid areas. Furthermore, we have kept patients on this system for a long as 40 minutes and see no limitation of time other than the surgeon's needs.

DISADVANTAGES AND REMEDIES

The problems noted herein, real and theoretic, are presented in no particular order of significance. Their importance is dominant, however, when we consider the narrow margins of safety we deal with in our particular substrate patient population.

1. *Pneumomediastinum and Pneumothorax.* This hazard presents itself in the presence of an unsealed opening in the mucosa of larynx, or trachea, or other of the fascial planes of this region. The Venturi end pressure rise enhances the risk of paratracheal fascial plane dissection. This is a particular hazard in knife surgery situations where there is no immediate seal of lacerations in contradistinction to laser, plasma vapor, or cryosurgery. This would only be true if the tip of the injection tube is at or close to the mucosal opening, since away from the injector tip, the end pressure falls off rapidly. Thus distal to this peak end pressure area there would exist a hazard no greater than with an intratracheal tube.

In this situation, we recommend the use of the least Venturi pressures, individualized for adequate ventilation. Clinical suspicion of the development of this complication requires immediate cessation of the Venturi technique, diagnostic radiologic confirmation, and requisite therapy. A postsurgery neck and chest x-ray should be done in the recovery room for proper evaluation.

2. *Gastric Distention and Regurgita-*

tion. Gastric distention with vagal effects and concomitant regurgitation presents as a significant hazard. Air insufflated into the stomach prior to intubation (during induction due to aerophagia, and/or while assisting the patient until spontaneous ventilation returns) can be quite efficiently managed with the routine introduction of a gastric drainage tube immediately after endotracheal intubation. The gastric tube should remain *in situ* until the patient is fully awake and cooperative. Adequate premedication will, similarly, reduce the degree of aerophagia and hydrochloric acid secretion by the gastric mucosae.

3. *Trap-door Obstruction.* In patients with a significant proliferation of polypoid masses, ball-valve obstruction of the airway secondary to the jet effect may take place. The technique we have stressed (initial endotracheal intubation, clearance of the airway in the anterior two-thirds of the larynx — and only *after* this — initiation of the Venturi system) will obviate this problem.

The converse of this situation should also be kept in mind. If, after following the proposed techniques and procedures, adequate ventilation is not achieved, the surgeon should seek out the hidden polypoid masses producing obstruction, *e.g.*, in the ventricles or subglottic area.

4. *Vocal Cord Motion.* Spontaneous movement of the vocal cords during surgery and jet blast can be partially averted by the use of muscle relaxants. We have found 0.2% intravenous drip of succinylcholine chloride to meet the needs of short duration, rapid reversal, and avoidance of the adverse effects of neuromuscular blocking reversal agents (atropine and Prostigmin®* or edrophonium chloride). Cord movement produced by the jet blast itself and magnified by the operating microscope can be limited by a) using the minimum oxygen delivery Venturi pressures needed for ventilation, and b) synchronizing the laser burn with the respiratory rhythm.

5. *Mucosal Dehydration.* Vocal cord dehydration is a constant problem. If the recently traumatized (laser burn) mucosae, particularly in the anterior commissure, come into apposition, edema and adhesions could occur more readily. Theoretically, an increased incidence of anterior commissure web formation might result. We have approached this problem in four ways. First, repeated humidification by hand spray (4% lidocaine); second, corticoid administration (Solu-Medrol®)** 40 mg intravenously to reduce tissue reaction; third, systemic hydration by the intravenous route; and lastly (and perhaps most important), immediate postoperative use of ultrasonic and macrosonic nebulization of water.

6. *Lower Respiratory Tract Involvement.* There is a real risk of blasting particulate matter and blood into the tracheobronchial tree. This is more of a problem with cold surgery (in contradistinction to cryosurgery). The laser usually vaporizes the affected tissue. However, particulate matter could still be introduced into the lower respiratory tract. This may be obviated by synchronization of the surgical suction with the ventilatory rhythm.

In one of our patients (vocal cord stripping using forceps), we noted blasting of the resultant blood into the tracheobronchial tree with dehydration. The potential for cast formation and obstructive phenomena are evident. Similarly, at the end of the jet blast, there is an aerodynamic back pressure which will disperse some of the blood toward the microscope and laser mirrors. This can produce significant damage to the laser system, and must be constantly kept in mind when doing knife surgery.

7. *Inadequate Ventilation.* This is obviously our primary concern. It therefore becomes the entire team's responsibility (both anesthesiologist and sur-

* Roche Laboratories, Nutley, NJ.
** The Upjohn Company, Kalamazoo, MI.

geon) to provide a) a maximally compliant chest (with muscle relaxants and other agents as indicated), b) placement of the suspension laryngoscope tip as close to the vocal cords as possible, *i.e.*, within the rima glottidis, and c) placement of the suspension laryngoscope in an axis as closely related to the tracheal axis as possible so that "baffling" of the Venturi effect is avoided. This will often require that the patient's head be placed in the classic Jackson position (neck antiflexed and chin extended).[10]

8. *Hypocarbia.* Over ventilation could theoretically occur. Certainly we have seen a significant change from the relative borderline hypercarbia during the use of less-than-adequate endotracheal tube sizes previously required for adequate ventilation with the Venturi system. We have seen no clinical evidence of adverse effects of this change despite the rapidity of effects. However, we do a) use minimum jet pressure/volume relationships required for ventilation, b) limit the duration of jet ventilation to that part of the surgical procedure actually requiring its use, and c) recognize that we are, in fact, using an oxygen enriched system. While we deliver 100% oxygen through our jet needle, it is significantly diluted by the room air entrained through the lumen of the laryngoscope barrel tube.[2] This latter is also a function of the smallest cross-sectional diameter of the tube and the aerodynamic properties produced thereby. Studies are now being developed to clearly delineate these aerodynamic characteristics.

9. *Hypercarbia.* While this is more frequently seen while using the aforementioned limited-sized endotracheal tubes, we periodically monitor clinical observation of chest movement adequacy as correlated to arterial blood gas studies.

There are several other admonitions we must present. While not problems directly related to the instrumentation, they may present as hazards to satisfactory accomplishment of the procedure. First, we suggest avoiding use of Innovar®* injection because of the "rigid chest syndrome" sometimes seen with this agent. Similarly, we do not use ketamine hydrochloride due to the "sensitization" of the laryngeal mechanism and poor relaxation produced, except in most unusual circumstances. This is of heightened importance in our study population, recognizing the inherent difficulties of intubation. Lastly, we pay particular attention to avoiding trauma to the eyes. We use 5% boric acid opthalmic ointment applications to the cornea and conjunctiva, and wet eye patches. This combination provides maximum protection from dehydration, mechanical trauma, and the theoretic reflection of the laser beam retrograde into the eyes.

SUMMARY AND CONCLUSIONS

A relatively recent development, Venturi ventilation for laryngeal surgery affords us an alternative and a valuable addition to our armamentarium. The authors present their experience in 100 cases presented for laser microsurgery of the larynx. Most of the patients are children, and many of them have previously had multiple surgical/anesthetic experiences. The techniques of anesthetic management followed the approach of Snow *et al*[9] for initial management. After the placement of the suspension laryngoscope and completion of the surgical procedure in the anterior commissure area and anterior cord area, we converted to Venturi ventilation management. Our experience indicates that a Venturi tube pressure of as low as 3.6 kg gauge using a 16 g needle is effective in children, while most adults require approximately 6.75 to 9 kg gauge using a 14 g needle.

We have developed criteria for Venturi ventilation management which suggest to the authors that case selection for this procedure assumes significant proportions. The complications, potential and real, that we have noted (dehydration effects, *etc.*), while minimal,

* McNeil Laboratories, Inc., Fort Washington, PA.

must receive due consideration though they have not previously been fully delineated. Conversely, the patients can be demonstrated to be most adequately ventilated while affording unparalleled access to the larynx for the necessary microsurgery. This is particularly important in the interarytenoid area as well as in the region of the larynx just distal to the true and false vocal cords.

In conclusion, we do not consider Venturi ventilation as a substitute for endotracheal intubation. It provides an adjunct to our armamentarium with the ultimate objective of meeting the otolaryngologist's needs for unobstructed access to his surgical field. Furthermore, we believe the routine we have evolved presents the safest approach to anesthetic management of laser microsurgery of the larynx. Still, the ultimate success of any procedure depends upon the interrelationship of surgeon, anesthesiologist, and patient.

REFERENCES

1. Sander RD: Two ventilating attachments for bronchoscopes. Del Med J 30:170-176, 1967

2. Spoerel WE, Grant PA: Ventilation during bronchoscopy. Can Anaesth Soc J 18:178-188, 1971

3. Rajagopalan R, Smith F, Ramachandran PR: Anesthesia for microlaryngoscopy and definitive surgery. Can Anaesth Soc J 19:83-86, 1972

4. McGrail JS: Suspension microlaryngoscopy. Can J Otolaryngol 1:129-134, 1972

5. Majoros M, Parkhill EM, Devine KD: Papilloma of the larynx in children. Am J Surg 108:470-475, 1965

6. Szpunar J: Laryngeal papillomatosis. Acta Otolaryngol (Stockh) 63:74-86, 1967

7. Foster GH: Papillomatosis laryngis. Ann Otol Rhinol Laryngol 42:548-551, 1933

8. Smith RM: *Anesthesia for Infants and Children.* St. Louis, C.V. Mosby 1959

9. Snow JC, Kripke BJ, Strong MS, *et al*: Anesthesia for carbon dioxide laser microsurgery on the larynx and trachea. Anesth Analg (Cleveland) 53:507-512, 1974

10. Dripps RD, Eckenhoff JE, Vadam LD: *Introduction to Anesthesia: The Principles of Safe Practice,* ed 45. Philadelphia, W.B. Saunders, 1972, chap 14, p 192

REPRINTS—Martin Lloyd Norton, MD, 48 Clark Street, Newton Centre, MA 02159.

Ann Otol 85: 1976

TRACHEAL AFFERENT NERVES

ROGER M. TRAXEL, MD

WILLIAM F. PRUDLOW, MD JOHN P. KAMPINE, MD

ROBERT L. COON, PHD EDWARD J. ZUPERKU, PHD

MILWAUKEE, WISCONSIN

SUMMARY – The individual fibers of the inferior laryngeal nerve and anastomosing branch of the superior laryngeal nerve arising from the upper five to six tracheal rings were studied. In 30 mongrel dogs using single and multifiber nerve preparations, afferent nerve activity was studied both in the intact trachea and in an isolated segment of trachea with artificial stimuli of graded pressure and flow. The adaptation rate, threshold, spontaneous firing frequency, maximum firing frequency, and rate of change in afferent discharge were recorded. Subsequently, these fibers were electrically stimulated to determine what reflex effects could be produced. Afferent nerve activity recorded from the upper trachea was found to be sensitive to tracheal pressure changes of 0.5 to 12 mm Hg. Nerve activity paralleled the frequency of pressure changes. Electrical stimulation of these fibers demonstrated reflex bradycardia, bradypnea and alteration of blood pressure. These data and that of other investigators indicate that upper airway mechano-receptors may be significant, not only in the initiation of upper airway protective reflexes, but also in the regulation of normal respiration.

Upper airway reflexes are initiated by stimulation of specialized receptors in the hypopharynx, larynx, and trachea. When stimulated during intubation, endoscopy, assisted respiration, or surgery of the head and neck, these receptors may initiate reflex alterations in respiration and circulation.[1,2] Nerve activity arising from receptors in the hypopharynx and larynx has been demonstrated in the superior laryngeal nerve.[3] Widdicombe has defined and attempted to localize rapid, slow, and intermediate adapting pulmonary stretch receptors in the tracheobronchial tree.[4] Afferent as well as efferent nerve activity has been studied in the inferior laryngeal nerve.[5]

The purpose of this study was to characterize the afferent nerve activity in paratracheal nerve fibers arising from mechano-receptors within the submucosa of the upper trachea in dogs. The fibers innervating the upper five to six tracheal rings, and also the branch of the inferior laryngeal nerve which anastomoses with the superior laryngeal nerve, were studied. During graded pressure and flow stimulation, the adaptation rate, the threshold, spontaneous firing frequency, maximum firing frequency, and change in rate of afferent nerve discharge were recorded using single and multifiber nerve preparations. In addition, afferent nerve activity during quiet, spontaneous respiration was studied. These same afferent fibers were then stimulated to determine what reflex effects could be produced.

METHODS AND MATERIALS

Thirty mongrel dogs (18-25 kg) were anesthetized with thiopental 10-15 mg/kg, followed by halothane (0.5-1.0%) in O_2.

In two dogs, changes in tracheal afferent nerve activity were recorded with an intact trachea during spontaneous respiration. In the remainder of the animals, the trachea was isolated through a vertical midline incision from the hyoid bone to the suprasternal notch. A low tracheotomy was performed, and a tracheotomy tube was connected to an Ohio Chemical Co. anesthesia machine with a calibrated vaporizer. All animals were studied

From the Departments of Otolaryngology and Anesthesiology, The Medical College of Wisconsin and the Veterans Administration Center, Wood, Wisconsin.

Presented at the meeting of the American Broncho-Esophagological Association, Palm Beach, Florida, April 27-28, 1976.

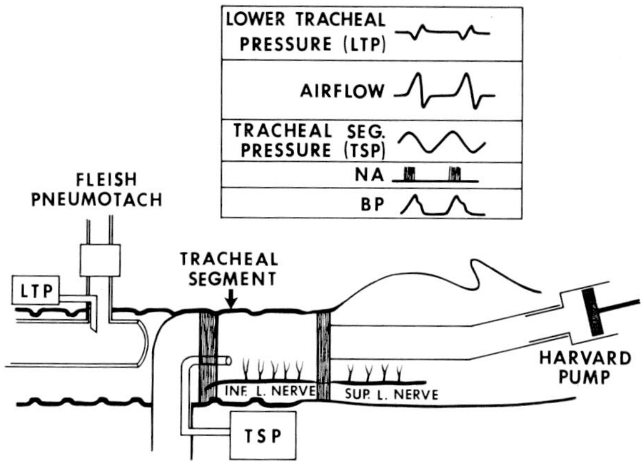

Fig. 1. Model for evaluation of tracheal afferent nerves.

during spontaneous respiration. Air flow was measured with a Fleisch pneumotactograph and differential pressure transducer* and integrated to obtain ventilation volume. Cardiac function was monitored by EKG (Lead II). Femoral arterial blood pressure was monitored with a transducer.* The upper trachea was sealed just below the cricoid cartilage by ligating in position a No. 36 Lanz endotracheal tube. The midtrachea was sealed likewise by ligating in position a No. 36 Lanz endotracheal tube. The pressure within the isolated segment (tracheal segment pressure) was then measured with a low pressure transducer* when square wave, ramp, and sinusoidal pressure changes were produced in the isolated tracheal segment (Fig. 1).

Slips of paratracheal branches of the inferior laryngeal and the anastomosing branch between the inferior and superior laryngeal nerves were dissected into fine filaments under oil using a dissecting microscope.** Single and multifiber nerve filaments were placed on a pair of fine tungsten hook electrodes held in position by a micromanipulator.*** The bipolar electrodes were connected to a high impedance preamplifier and filter system with photoelectric coupling. A Faraday cage was used to reduce 60 Hz interference. Afferent spike activity was analyzed as unit potential

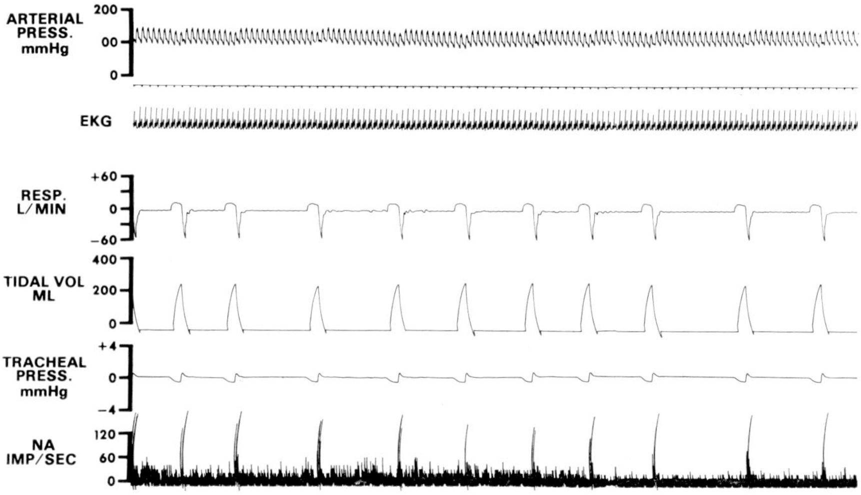

Fig. 2. Illustration of minimal tracheal pressure changes (0.5 mm Hg) during spontaneous respiration producing changes in paratracheal nerve activity.

* Statham Instruments, Inc., Oxnard, CA.
** Bausch and Lomb, Rochester, NY.
*** Eric Sobotka Co., Inc., Sarasota, FL.

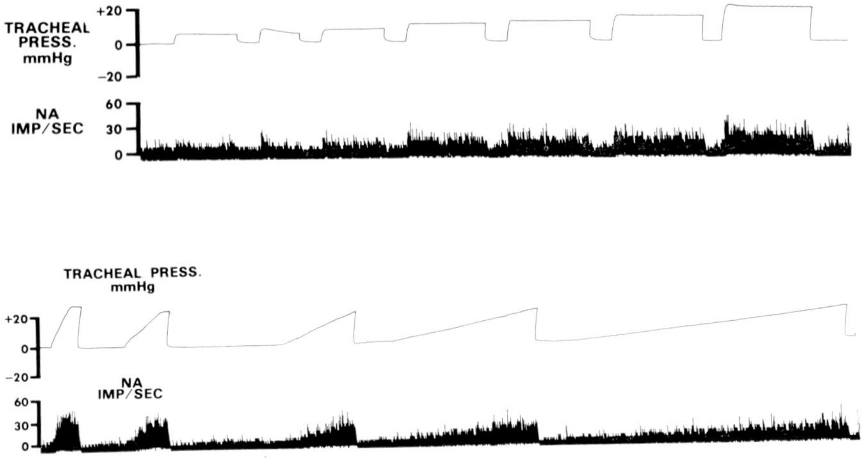

Fig. 3. Changes in tracheal afferent nerve activity in response to square wave and ramp tracheal pressure changes in an isolated tracheal segment.

in single or multifiber preparations using a window discriminator with spike frequency analyzer.

Afferent nerve activity was monitored from the upper trachea during spontaneous respiration and from the isolated tracheal segment while varying volumes of air were injected. Air was injected with a syringe to obtain a square wave stimulus. Sinusoidal positive and negative pressure changes were produced by utilizing an animal respirator* to vary tracheal segment pressure and cycle frequency. Ramp pressure changes were effected with an infusion pump.* Variations in the rate of positive pressure change were produced by changing the infusion pump speed.

Either the central end of the transected left or right inferior laryngeal nerve or the central ends of the individual upper tracheal nerves were stimulated using a constant current stimulator. Supramaximal stimulation strengths were used (1-5 ma) with 0.1-0.5 m/sec spike duration and frequencies from 1-50 Hz. Repetitive stimuli of 15, 30, and 60 sec duration were studied at varying frequencies. Generally, maximum changes in respiratory rate and heart rate occurred at stimulation frequencies of 10-15 Hz.

RESULTS

Changes in afferent nerve activity were recorded consistently with changes

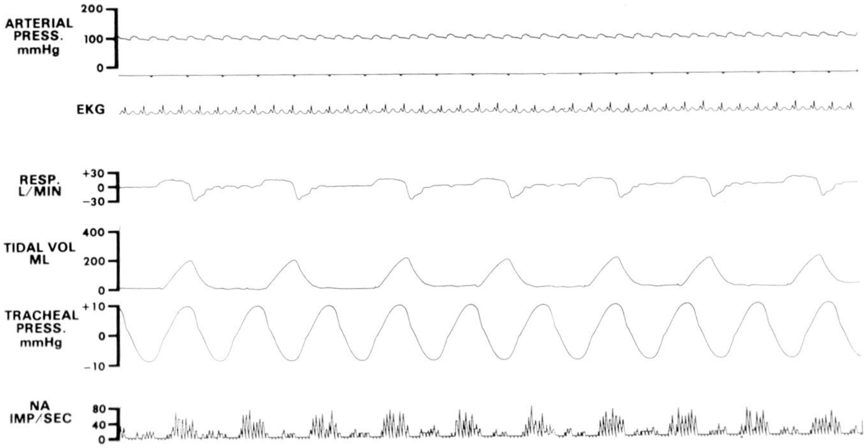

Fig. 4. Demonstration of negative intratracheal pressure changes in the range of 8-10 mm Hg required to elicit a response.

* Harvard Apparatus Co., Inc., Millis, MA.

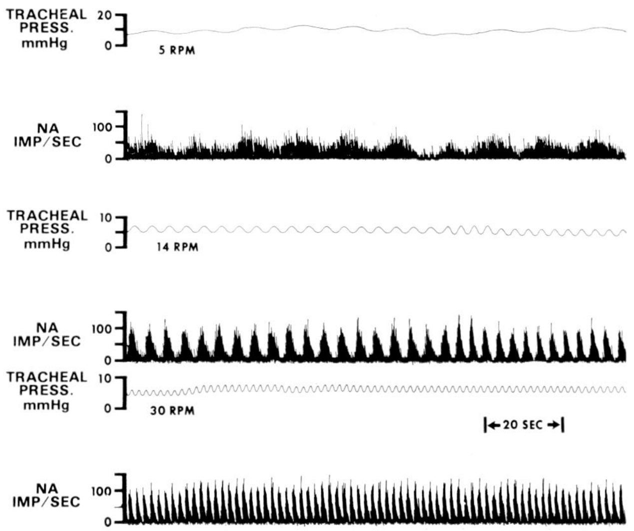

Fig. 5. Changes in afferent tracheal nerve activity in response to sinusoidal tracheal pressure changes at three different frequencies.

in intratracheal pressure. Variations of intratracheal pressure as small as 0.5 mm Hg produced changes in afferent nerve activity. Figure 2 shows changes in average nerve activity recorded from a paratracheal nerve during spontaneous respiration. As positive airway pressure occurred during expiration, there was a large increase in nerve activity. An increase in average nerve activity is recorded as a positive deflection in the averaged neurogram displayed in the bottom trace.

Stimulation by square wave and ramp changes show increased nerve activity directly in proportion to increases of tracheal pressure up to 12 mm Hg as shown in Figure 3. Higher pressures failed to produce a significant increase in nerve activity in most nerve preparations. With release of intratracheal pressure to zero, a transient off response was elicited in afferent activity.

Sinusoidal changes in intratracheal pressure from a positive to negative range demonstrates that negative intratracheal pressures in the 8-10 mm Hg range were necessary to stimulate afferent activity. Positive deflections in the pressure tracing were accompanied by sharp increases in average nerve activity. Much smaller increases in nerve activity were associated with the development of negative pressure portions of the pressure curves as indicated in Figure 4. Changes in sinusoidal frequency at the same amplitude of pressure stimulus in the isolated tracheal segment did affect afferent nerve discharge frequency. As shown in Figure 5, higher frequency pressure stimulation resulted in greater afferent nerve activity compared to lower frequency pressure stimulation. This was a consistent finding and was independent of peak developed pressure as shown in this example. The increase in maximum nerve activity at higher frequency pressure stimulation indicates some degree of rate sensitivity in these receptors.

Reflex responses to stimulation of intact and sectioned paratracheal and inferior laryngeal nerves are shown in Figure 6. Decreases in breathing frequency and heart rate were consistent findings in all of the animals studied. The decrease in breathing frequency is more obvious than bradycardia in Figure 6. In some instances the bradycardia was associated with a decrease in arterial blood pressure, and in other instances there was little or no change in arterial blood pressure.

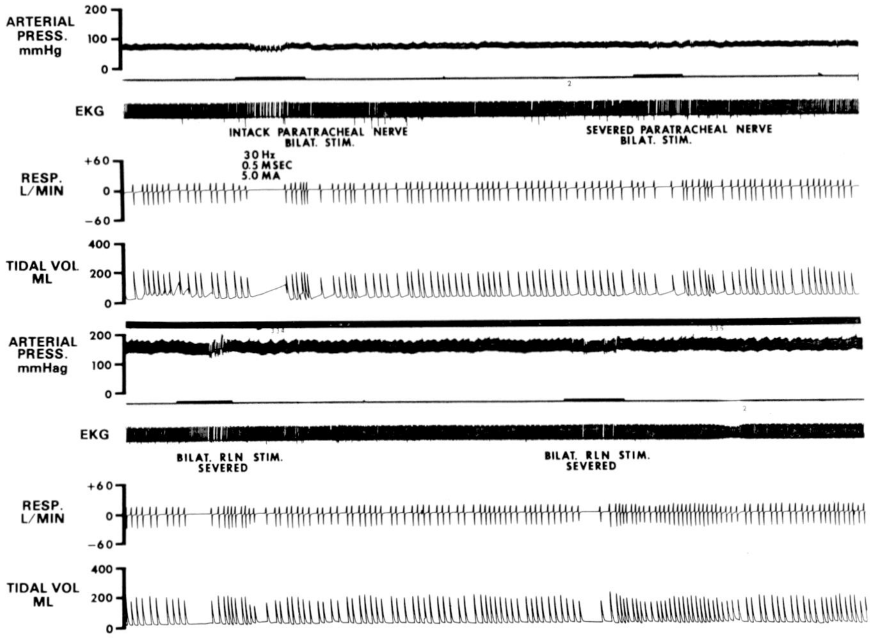

Fig. 6. Reflex responses to stimulation of intact and sectioned paratracheal and inferior laryngeal nerves demonstrating bradypnea and bradycardia. Alteration in blood pressure varied in different animals.

DISCUSSION

Laryngeal and tracheal afferent nerve activity in animals has been clearly demonstrated by several investigators and is well summarized in the work of Hirose.[5] Ogura and co-workers have likewise confirmed this afferent activity in man.[6] In this study, some of the electrophysiologic characteristics of this nerve activity are further demonstrated.

Recordings were taken directly from the peripheral (tracheal) end of sectioned tracheal branches of the inferior laryngeal nerve. Identical activity was also found in the larger branch of the inferior laryngeal nerve which anastomoses with the superior laryngeal nerve. Only slow adapting afferent nerve activity was positively identified within the tracheal segment studied. Previous investigators have also found rapid adapting nerve activity in this area.[4]

The afferent activity found was both pressure and frequency sensitive. With graded pressure increases, the nerve activity increased in direct proportion up to a maximum at approximately 12 mm Hg pressure within the airway. As frequecny of pressure stimulation increased, afferent nerve discharge frequencies likewise increased. Of particular interest is the finding that with very minimal changes in tracheal pressure (0.5 mm Hg) significant nerve activity could be demonstrated. This fine sensitivity of afferent discharge was confirmed by the identical finding in intact tracheal segments within the physiological range of normal respiration.

Reflex effects of stimulation of the proximal end of these same inferior laryngeal nerve branches were briefly studied. The findings of bradycardia, bradypnea and altered blood pressure concur with those of several previous investigators.[5]

The demonstration of afferent activity in the upper trachea together with the reflex effects which have been elicited leads to further speculation about the function of these inferior laryngeal nerve branches in the control of intrinsic laryngeal musculature during respiration and phonation. Gautier *et al*[7] demonstrated the importance of upper airway resistance determining expiration time and respiratory frequency. Suzuki and Kirchner[8] have shown that a reflex motor response can be elicited in the inferior laryngeal nerve by electrical stimulation of afferent fibers in the same nerve trunk with a reflex latency of about 25 to 40 msec. The data presented by these investigators and the results of studies reported in this paper indicate that upper airway mechano-receptors may be important not only in the initiation of upper airway protective reflexes, but also may be importantly involved in the regulation of normal respiration.

REFERENCES

1. Nadel JA, Widdicombe JG: Reflex effects of upper airway irritation on total lung resistance and blood pressure. J Appl Physiol 17:861-865, 1962
2. Widdicombe JG: Respiratory reflexes from the trachea and bronchi of the cat. J Physiol (Lond) 123:55-70, 1954
3. Andrew BL: A functional analysis of the myelinated fibers of the superior laryngeal nerve of the rat. J Physiol (Lond) 133:420-433, 1956
4. Widdicombe JG: Receptors of the trachea and bronchi of the cat. J Physiol (Lond) 123:71-104, 1954
5. Hirose H: Afferent impulses in the recurrent laryngeal nerve in the cat. Laryngoscope 71:1196-1206, 1961
6. Ogura JH, Lam RL: Anatomical and physiological correlations on stimulating the human superior laryngeal nerve. Laryngoscope 63:947-959, 1953
7. Gautier H, Remmers JE, Bartlett D Jr Control of the durations of expiration. Respir Physiol 18:205-221, 1973
8. Suzuki M, Kirchner JA: Sensory fibers in the recurrent laryngeal nerve. Ann Otol Rhinol Laryngol 78:21-31, 1969

REPRINTS—Roger M. Traxel, MD, Department of Otolaryngology, Medical College of Wisconsin and the Veterans Administration Center, Wood, WI 53193.

Ann Otol 85: 1976

TRANSBRONCHOSCOPIC CRYOSURGERY OF RESPIRATORY STRUCTURES: EXPERIMENTAL AND CLINICAL STUDIES

ARYEH GORENSTEIN, MD

H. BRYAN NEEL III, MD DAVID R. SANDERSON, MD

ROCHESTER, MINNESOTA

SUMMARY — Although resection is the only treatment proven effective for localized malignant tumors in the tracheobronchial tree, alternative methods for cure or control of unresectable or recurrent tumor should be explored. In 24 dogs, cryonecrosis of sizable portions of carina, main stem bronchi, first division bronchi, and lung parenchyma was well tolerated, and the necrosis was localized, reproducible, and followed by prompt healing of frozen tissue. The gross architecture of the bronchi was not permanently altered, and no strictures formed. Six patients with endobronchial tumors were treated transbronchoscopically with cryosurgery. All patients tolerated the procedures well, and there were no complications. Palliation was achieved in five of the six patients.

Cryosurgery has been used clinically for both cure and palliation of malignant neoplasms in several anatomic regions.[1-5] The temporal and physical factors required to produce predictable areas of cell death have been delineated.[6-9] Moreover, tumor-specific immunologic consequences of tumor necrosis *in situ* by freezing have been identified in several syngeneic murine tumor-host systems.[10]

Investigation of cryotherapy as a form of treatment for tumors arising in the trachea and tracheobronchial tree is merited, because surgical excision or radiotherapy cannot always be used, and radiation and chemotherapy, the usual alternative forms of therapy, seldom lead to cure. The present study was designed to 1) develop probes for endobronchial cryosurgery, 2) determine the feasibility of performing cryosurgery within the bronchi and the lung through a bronchoscope, and 3) assess the pathophysiologic effects of extensive cryosurgery in the bronchial tree and adjacent lung.

METHODS AND MATERIALS

A 57 cm long cryoprobe and several tips of various sizes and shapes were developed for standard liquid nitrogen cryosurgical equipment (Fig. 1A, B). Through an 8 mm rigid bronchoscope, each site was frozen three times, each time for 2 minutes, and allowed to thaw spontaneously. Probe-tip temperature was maintained at –170 C.

Twenty-four mongrel dogs weighing 10 to 15 kg were divided into four groups. Animals in each group had two or more of the following areas frozen: carina, main stem bronchi, first division bronchi, and lung (by wedging the probe into the lung parenchyma). Each dog was anesthetized with intravenously administered pentobarbital.

The entire carina was frozen using a V-shaped probe tip in 10 dogs. In 14 dogs the main stem bronchi were frozen using a tapered cylindrical probe tip (Fig. 2). The proximal portion of the right upper lobe, the right middle lobe, and the first division bronchi of the right lower lobe were frozen using the same tip in five dogs. In 13 dogs a skewed teardrop-shaped or tapered cylindrical probe tip was passed into the distal bronchus of the left lower lobe or the right lower lobe parenchyma and left *in situ* during spontaneous thaw to freeze pulmonary parenchyma transbronchoscopically (Fig. 3).

The extent of the ice ball and regional

From the Mayo Clinic and Mayo Foundation, Rochester, Minnesota. This investigation was supported in part by NIHPHS Research Contract CB-53886.

Presented at the meeting of the American Broncho-Esophagological Association, Palm Beach, Florida, April 27-28, 1976.

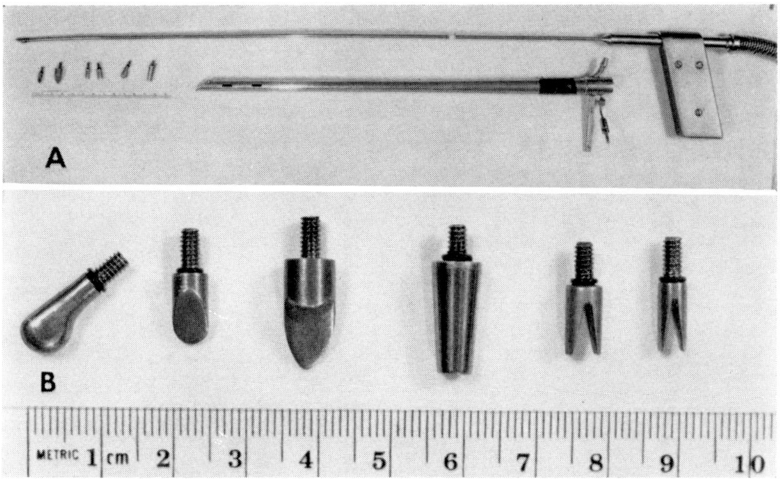

Fig. 1. A) Cryoprobe and tips. B) Cryoprobe tips.

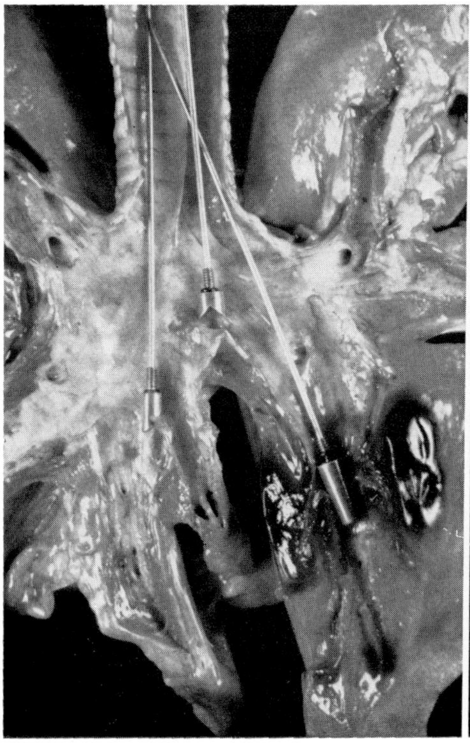

Fig. 2. Cryoprobe tips on wire carriers for illustration; V-shaped tip resting on carina (center); tapered cylindrical tip passed into distal bronchus of left lower lobe (right); beveled cylindrical tip resting on spur of divisional bronchus (left).

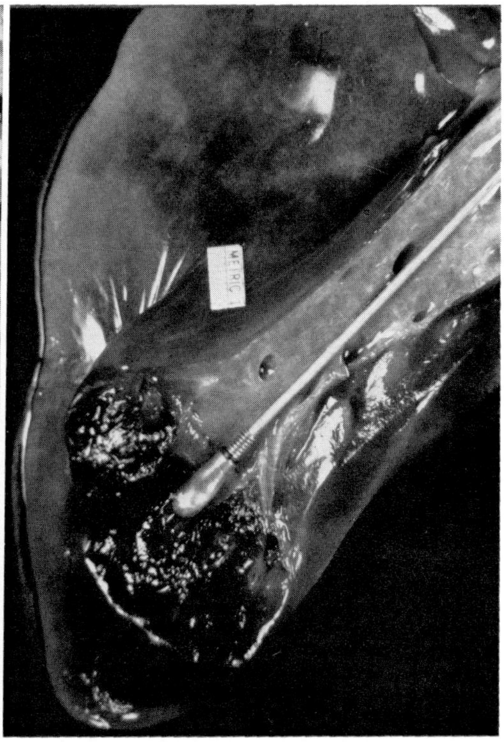

Fig. 3. Skewed teardrop-shaped probe tip wedged peripherally into lower lobe, with surrounding cryonecrosis one day postoperatively.

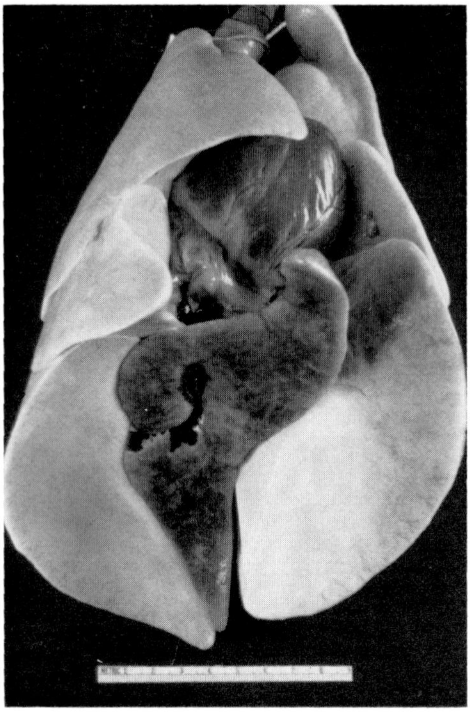

Fig. 4. Right lower lobe one day postoperatively. Central target zone shows complete infarction.

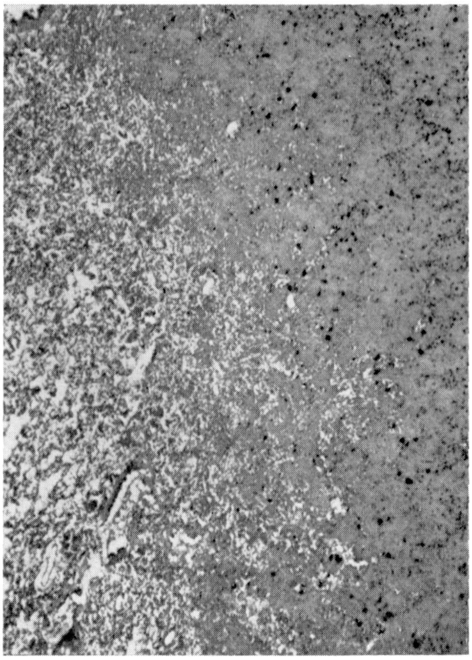

Fig. 5. Intense local hemorrhage and complete coagulation necrosis of lung in central target zone (upper right). Transitional zone (lower left) shows partial necrosis (H. & E. X64).

temperature changes around the lobar bronchus were assessed at thoracotomy during cryosurgery in two dogs. Needle thermocouples were embedded along the bronchus and in the adjacent lung to measure temperature changes directly.

After cryosurgery, each dog was returned to his cage and offered his usual diet of commercial dog chow and water. Nine of 24 dogs received 1,000,000 units of long-acting intramuscularly administered penicillin immediately after cryosurgery. One dog from each group was killed at 1, 7, 14, 21, and 180 days postoperatively, and the rest have been retained for further follow-up. After autopsy and fixation in 10% buffered formaldehyde, the trachea, bronchi, and lungs were retained for detailed gross and microscopic evaluation; sections were prepared with H. and E. stain.

RESULTS

Survival. With the exception of one death caused by an overdose of pentobarbital, all dogs survived the procedures initially and resumed normal activity within 24 hours after the operation. However, in the peripheral wedge group, there were three deaths: one attributable to the anesthetic overdose, one to pneumothorax (at 5 days postoperatively), and one to pneumonia (at 15 days). Pneumothorax was attributed to wedging of the probe tip through the visceral pleura. None of these dogs had been given penicillin. Fibrinous pleural adhesions were seen in dogs of this group at one and seven days postoperatively, but not thereafter. There were no deaths or pleural-space complications in the other groups of dogs.

Gross Findings. Ice balls extended 2.5 to 3.0 cm beyond the probe tip and into the tissues surrounding the bronchus after two minutes of freezing, and temperatures 0.5 to 1 cm from the bronchial wall were consistently below –30 C.[6-9] Two to six minutes was required for spontaneous thaw and return of target temperature to 37 C. Immediately after freezing, petechiae appeared beneath the mucosa and the target site became violaceous and edematous. Blood-tinged mucous secretions appeared within the lumen of the bronchus by 10 to 15 minutes. Hyperemia,

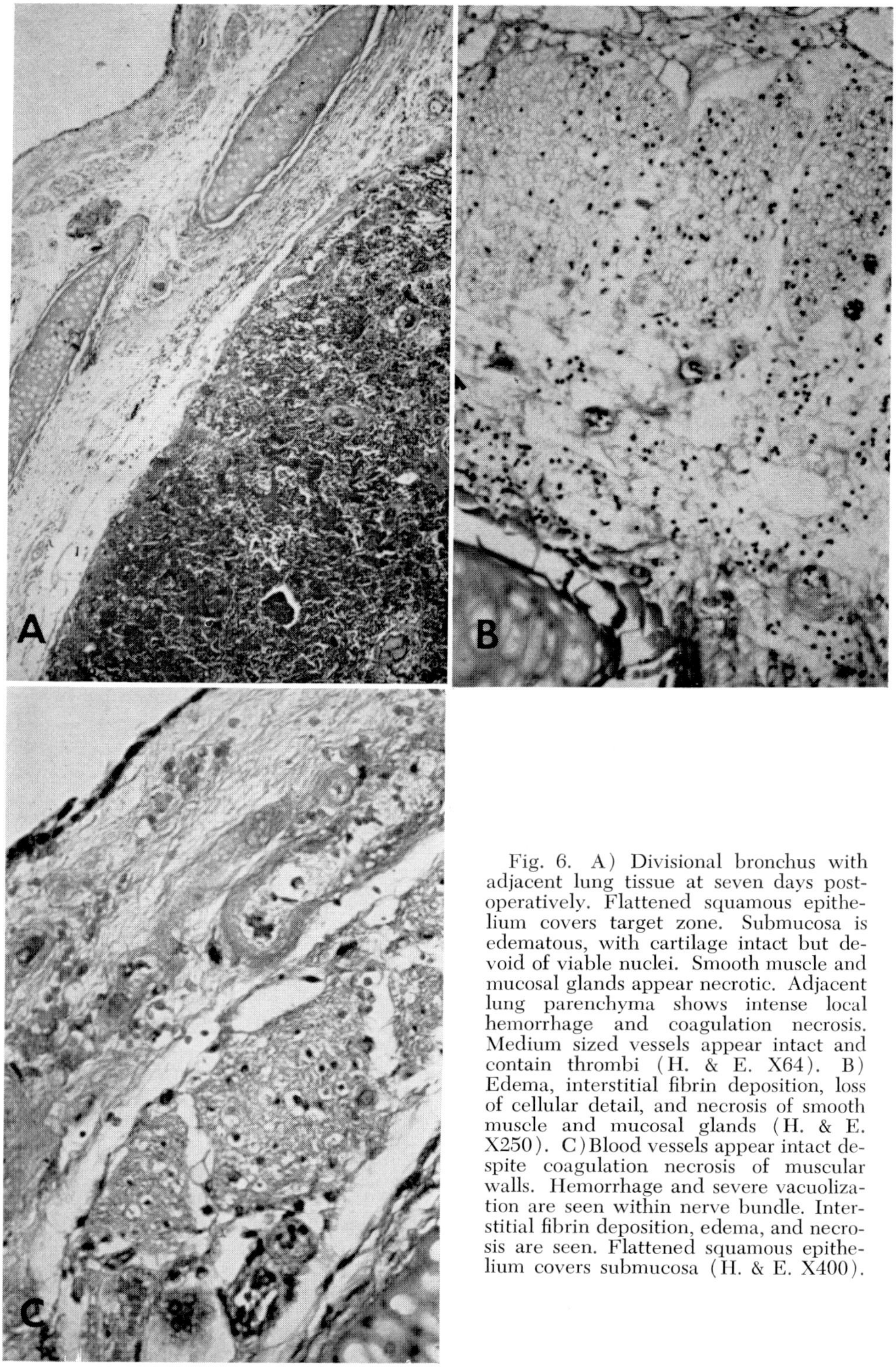

Fig. 6. A) Divisional bronchus with adjacent lung tissue at seven days postoperatively. Flattened squamous epithelium covers target zone. Submucosa is edematous, with cartilage intact but devoid of viable nuclei. Smooth muscle and mucosal glands appear necrotic. Adjacent lung parenchyma shows intense local hemorrhage and coagulation necrosis. Medium sized vessels appear intact and contain thrombi (H. & E. X64). B) Edema, interstitial fibrin deposition, loss of cellular detail, and necrosis of smooth muscle and mucosal glands (H. & E. X250). C) Blood vessels appear intact despite coagulation necrosis of muscular walls. Hemorrhage and severe vacuolization are seen within nerve bundle. Interstitial fibrin deposition, edema, and necrosis are seen. Flattened squamous epithelium covers submucosa (H. & E. X400).

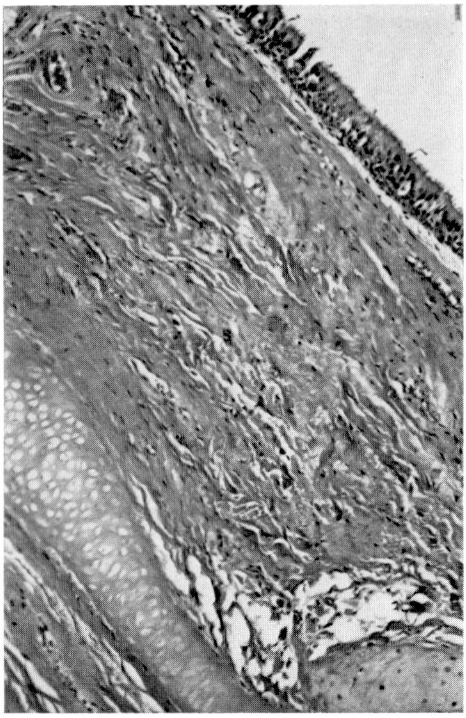

Fig. 7. Normal respiratory epithelium overlies submucosa, which contains dense fibrous tissue with no smooth muscle or mucosal glands at 180 days (H. & E. X160).

edema, necrosis, and inspissated mucus disappeared from within the frozen bronchus by the 21st day. When first division bronchi were frozen, necrosis and, later, fibrosis of adjacent lung occurred, but there was neither bronchial narrowing nor stricture formation at all observation times.

Histologic Findings. The target sites had gradations of tissue destruction, tissue necrosis being virtually complete in the center of the cryolesion. This region was bounded by a markedly congested, partially necrotic transitional zone that was sharply demarcated from adjacent healthy tissue, a finding typical of cryolesions in general.

In the peripheral wedge group, at one day, lung tissue in the center of the cryolesion had all the histologic features of an acute hemorrhagic infarct — intense local hemorrhage and complete coagulation necrosis (Figs. 4, 5). By seven days, the center of the lesion appeared the same, but interstitial edema, fibrin deposition, swollen alveolar epithelial cells, and many fibroblastic and histiocytic cells were seen in the transitional zone. By 180 days, dense fibrous scar tissue gradually replaced the central target zone; microcystic spaces and thickened interalveolar septae were seen in the transitional zone.

Main stem bronchi, first division bronchi, and carinal target sites were denuded of epithelium one day postoperatively. By seven days, edema in the submucosal region, vascular congestion, thrombosis, and a polymorphonuclear leukocyte infiltrate within the subepithelial connective tissue were evident (Fig. 6A). In addition, the cartilage in the central zone at the target site appeared intact, but smudging of smooth muscle, loss of cellular detail, and complete necrosis of mucosal glands were seen (Fig. 6B). Simple flattened squamous epithelium covered the target zone, and the cartilage was devoid of viable nuclei. Smooth muscle appeared necrotic and hemorrhagic and there were infiltrations of polymorphonuclear cells. Blood vessels in the transitional zone appeared congested and many contained thrombi. Large vessels appeared intact despite coagulation necrosis of muscular walls. Hemorrhage and severe vacuolization were seen within nerve bundles (Fig. 6C). By 14 days, flattened squamous epithelium completely covered the target zone, within which cartilage appeared to be undergoing necrosis. A prolific fibroblastic response accompanied by many mononuclear cells was seen in the transitional zone adjacent to the central necrotic area. By 21 days, necrotic glands and smooth muscle were no longer present, apparently replaced by fibrous tissue. By 180 days, there was partial transformation of flattened squamous epithelium to a normal appearing respiratory epithelium covering the luminal surface (Fig. 7). Cartilage in the target zone appeared nonviable; however, new cartilage had developed at the margins of the necrotic cartilage (Fig. 8A). Submucosally there was no evidence of

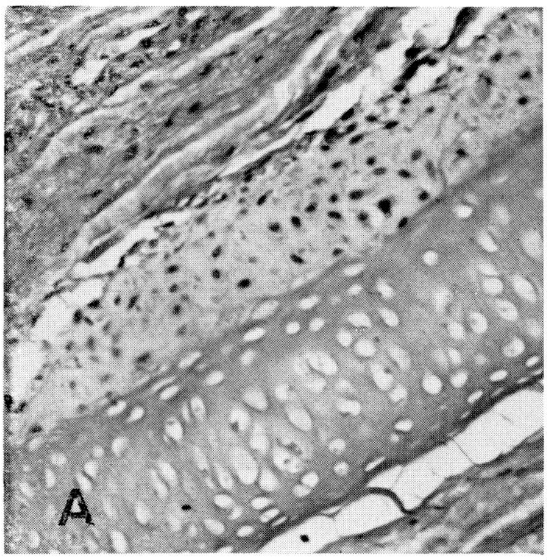

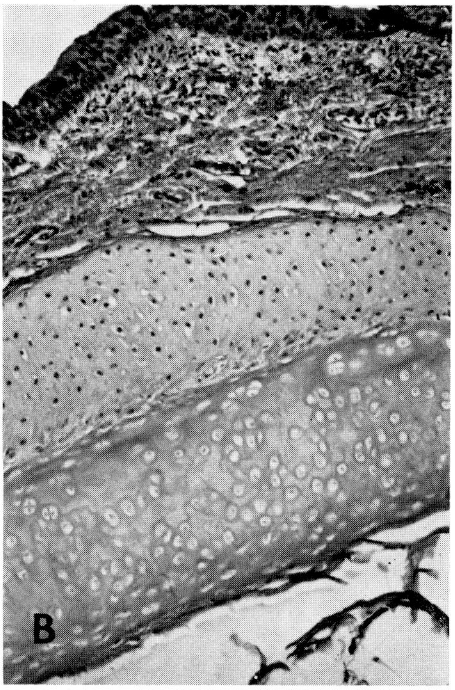

Fig. 8. At 180 days, generation of new cartilage at margins of necrotic cartilage, which served as a scaffold. A) H. & E. X250. B) H. & E. X160.

smooth muscle or mucosal gland regeneration (Fig. 8B). Blood vessels and nerve ganglia in the transitional zone appeared intact.

Presently, four dogs are under observation six to nine months after treatment and are doing well.

DISCUSSION

By using transbronchoscopic techniques and appropriate apparatus, extensive areas of carina, accessible bronchus, and portions of central lung can be frozen safely and repetitively at the same operation to induce large areas of necrosis. Predictable areas of cell death can be induced, and necrosis is localized, reproducible, and followed by prompt regeneration of mucosa. The gross architecture of the bronchopulmonary tissue is not altered extensively, and no strictures occur in the bronchi. Perhaps necrotic cartilage serves as a scaffold for generation of new cartilage, in part preventing stricture formation. Submucosal glands are destroyed and do not regenerate.

Recent investigations suggest that sputum cytology and chest roentgenography permit early detection and localization of bronchogenic carcinomas.[11] Various alternatives to standard forms of therapy are desirable, particularly when other medical problems preclude resection or when a tumor recurs. Under such circumstances, resection or radiation treatment may be poorly tolerated and endoscopic cryosurgery may be an alternative form of therapy, because the tracheobronchial tree and more distal areas can be frozen safely through the bronchoscope. Further studies may establish this approach as primary therapy in apparently localized disease, particularly if it can be proved of comparable therapeutic efficacy in instances in which classic extensive resection produces undesirable functional disability, as in those patients with marginal respiratory reserve. Cryosurgery may also be a useful surgical adjunct in patients with residual cancer after tumor resection when pulmonary function will not permit further operation or in patients in whom it is impossible to remove all tumor because

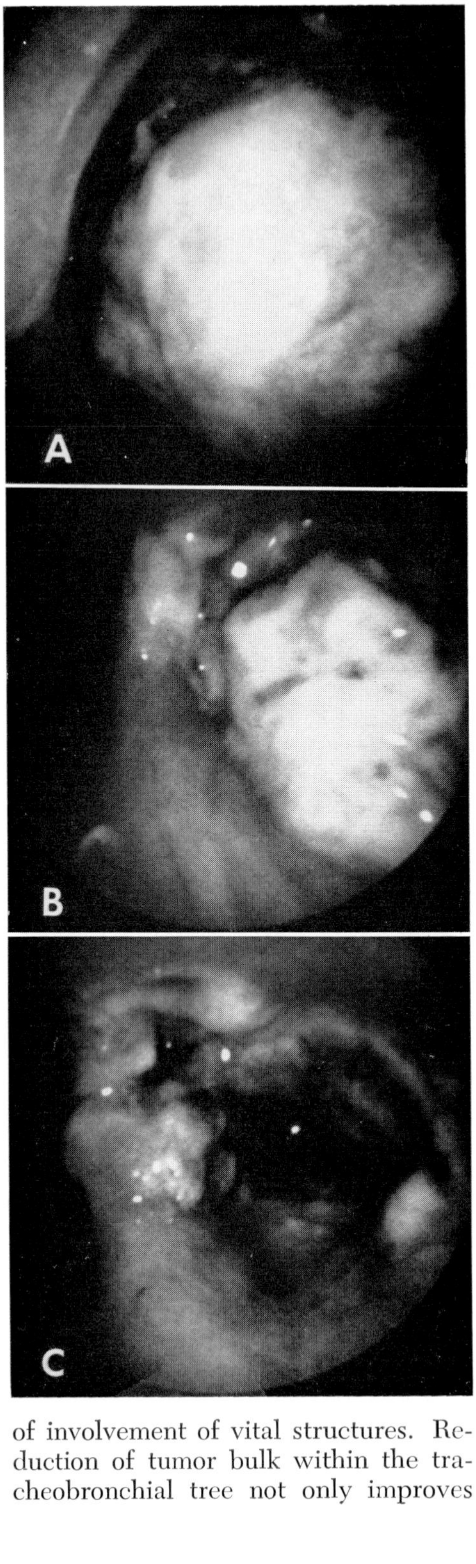

of involvement of vital structures. Reduction of tumor bulk within the tracheobronchial tree not only improves the airway, but also may allow drainage of secretions and pulmonary infection caused by obstructing tumor. Because target areas in the trachea and bronchi are accessible, they may be examined for tumor control sequentially at bronchoscopy.

In syngeneic murine tumor-host systems, destruction of tumor *in situ* by cryosurgery provides greater immunity than does excision. Apparently the immunologic effects are induced by a mechanism involving tumor kill *in situ*, prolonged absorption of tumor antigen(s), or both.[10] In view of the experimental findings, the immunotherapeutic effects of *in situ* cryogenic necrosis should be studied clinically in patients with primary or metastatic tumor.

CLINICAL EXPERIENCE

Six patients (five men and one woman) with endobronchial tumors were treated with cryosurgery by the transbronchoscopic technique developed in the animal studies. The mean age of the patients was 65 years, with a range of 51 to 77 years.

Four patients had had surgical procedures for high grade squamous cell carcinoma and subsequent radiation therapy (5,000 to 5,500 rads) for residual or recurrent tumor. One patient had had operation but no irradiation for carcinoid tumor. Tumors in all five patients were localized, involving the main stem bronchial stump, carina, or both. The one female patient presented with adenoid cystic carcinoma (cylindroma) involving the distal trachea, carina, and right main stem bronchus. Additional surgical resection was not considered possible in any of the six patients. Because distant metas-

Fig. 9. A) Entire right main stem bronchus and 90% of left main stem bronchus obstructed by tumor. B) Marked regression of tumor size and restoration of airway two weeks after biopsy and cryotherapy. C) Further regression of tumor after two cryotreatments.

tases were not evident in these patients, systemic chemotherapy was not used. Furthermore, because all the tumors were localized and accessible at bronchoscopy and for subsequent follow-up examinations, cryosurgery seemed to be acceptable therapy.

Using topical anesthesia in five patients and general anesthesia in one, we did standard open-tube bronchoscopic examinations on all patients. Inspection was facilitated by using Storz-Hopkins lens telescopes*, and color photographs were taken before and after each procedure. Under direct vision, the open tip of the bronchoscope was held against a selected part of the tumor. Supplemental oxygen was delivered through the ventilating side arm of the bronchoscope. Vital signs were observed and electrocardiograms were monitored during the procedure. The cryoprobe tip was applied to grossly visible tumor and, on contact, was cooled to a temperature of –170 C; this temperature was maintained for two minutes. On each occasion, the cryoprobe was applied to the tumor three to five times, with spontaneous thaw between freezes. Large contact surfaces between probe tip and tumor ensure rapid heat extraction. Because the open bronchoscope limits the size of the probe tip, tip-to-tumor contact is restricted, necessitating several overlapping applications to freeze large tumors.

Electrocardiograms showed no changes during cryosurgery. All patients tolerated the cryosurgical procedures well, and there were no immediate or delayed complications. Patients resumed their normal activity and were dismissed from the hospital the next day.

Local control (tumor shrinkage or disappearance, or both) was evident endoscopically in five of the six patients. The one patient with no reduction in tumor size had extensive tumor that was only superficially destroyed by cryotherapy. Two patients with severe airway obstructive symptoms (90% of lumen obstructed by tumor) (Fig. 9A-C) were successfully palliated. Although complete tumor destruction was not accomplished, adequate airways were restored. In two patients, tumor growth was controlled and no gross recurrence was seen at follow-up bronchoscopic examinations at two to seven months postoperatively. Episodic hemoptysis has been less frequent in one patient for the past ten months. A more detailed report of our clinical series is planned.

REFERENCES

1. Cahan WG: Cryosurgery of malignant and benign tumors. Fed Proc 24 Suppl 15: 241-248, 1965

2. Cooper IS: Cryogenic surgery: a new method of destruction or extirpation of benign or malignant tissues. N Engl J Med 268:743-749, 1963

3. DeSanto LW: The curative, palliative, and adjunctive uses of cryosurgery in the head and neck. Laryngoscope 82:1282-1291, 1972

4. Miller D: Cryosurgery for the treatment of neoplasms of the oral cavity. Otolaryngol Clin North Am 5:377-388, 1972

5. Bridgman AH, King FW, Dunn RC, *et al*: Experimental freezing of intrathoracic organs. J Cryosurg 1:193-196, 1968

6. Neel HB III, Ketcham AS, Hammond WG: Requisites for successful cryogenic surgery of cancer. Arch Surg 102:45-48, 1971

7. Neel HB III, DeSanto LW: Cryosurgical control of cancer: effects of freeze rates, tumor temperatures, and ischemia. Ann Otol Rhinol Laryngol 82:716-723, 1973

8. Neel HB III, Farrell KH, DeSanto LW, *et al*: Cryosurgery of respiratory structures. I. Cryonecrosis of trachea and bronchus. Laryngoscope 83:1062-1071, 1973

9. Neel HB III, Farrell KH, Payne WS, *et al*: Cryosurgery of respiratory structures. II. Cryonecrosis of the lung. Laryngoscope 84: 417-426, 1974

10. Neel HB III, Ketcham AS, Hammond WG: Experimental evaluation of *in situ* oncocide for primary tumor therapy: comparison

* Storz-Hopkins lens telescopes, Karl Storz Endoscopy-America, Inc., Los Angeles, CA.

of tumor-specific immunity after complete excision, cryonecrosis and ligation. Laryngoscope 83:376-387, 1973

11. Fontana RS, Sanderson DR, Woolner LB, *et al*: The Mayo lung project for early detection and localization of bronchogenic carcinoma: a status report. Chest 67:511-522, 1975

ACKNOWLEDGMENTS—We thank Drs. L. H. Weiland and L. B. Woolner for histopathologic interpretation, and Mrs. B. Elford, RN, for assistance at bronchoscopy.

REPRINTS—A. Gorenstein, MD, c/o Section of Publications, Mayo Clinic, 200 First Street SW, Rochester, MN 55901.

Ann Otol 85: 1976

TEST-RETEST RELIABILITY IN CLINICAL ELECTROCOCHLEOGRAPHY

L. M. Bergholtz, M.D.
Linkoping, Sweden

R. E. Hooper, M.D.
Bronx, New York

D. C. Mehta, M.D.
Bronx, New York

SUMMARY — The intratest test-retest reliability in clinical electrocochleography was studied by measuring the difference between amplitude of the test and retest and latency of the test and retest. Eighty-four comparisons were made in 40 patients with different types of hearing losses. The type of hearing loss and whether test and retest were performed in sequence or not did not affect the variability of the amplitude. The test and retest correlation between amplitudes was good. Small amplitudes mainly found near the action potential (AP) "threshold" showed less absolute variability than larger amplitudes found at higher intensities. The correlation between the intratest latencies was excellent. The latency showed less variability at higher intensities than near AP "threshold."

Electrocochleography has now become established as a physiological hearing test. Data is being used to establish thresholds[1-9] often at different frequencies[1,2,5,8-10] and also in diagnosing the nature of the hearing loss by study of waveform and other suprathreshold parameters such as the input-output functions of amplitude and latency of AP response.[1,2,8,9,11-13]

Electrocochleography is a particularly valuable test in evaluating hearing in patients who are unable to cooperate for routine behavioral audiometry because they are very young, mentally handicapped or emotionally disturbed.[1-4,6,14] Electrocochleographic suprathreshold parameters such as the study of waveforms and input-output graphs of amplitude and latency of response may be valuable tools in diagnosing the site and type of peripheral hearing loss.

However, the limitations of the method must be considered. The action potential (AP) "threshold" is usually found to be higher than the behavioral threshold.[7-9,15] The interpretation of frequency specific thresholds even using filtered clicks or tone bursts is difficult. Also, some form of general anesthesia is necessary when the transtympanic technique is used in young children.[1,2,5,6,9]

It is important to establish the reliability of any hearing test. The limitations and disadvantages must, therefore, be recognized before data is interpreted. This paper will report the investigation of intratest test-retest reliability in clinical electrocochleography.

METHODS AND MATERIALS

Forty subjects, whose ages ranged from 20 to 74 years with a mean age of 58 years, were studied. There were 25 female and 15 male subjects. Half the group had pure tone audiograms showing low and high frequency sensorineural losses with normal or near normal hearing for at least one of the speech frequencies. The other half showed either a high frequency sensorineural loss, flat sensorineural loss or a conductive loss. The pure tone average (PTA) at 500, 1000 and 2000 Hz within the whole group ranged from 10 to 55 dB with a mean of 30 dB. Only the poorer hearing ear was tested in each subject.

The subject, after being otoscopically examined, lies supine on a bed in a sound treated room. The tympanic membrane was anesthetized with 2% Xylocaine®* with 1:2000 parts epinephrine using an iontophoretic anesthetizer.**[16] If the tympanic membrane was re-

* Astra Pharmaceutical Products, Inc., Worcester, MA.
** Medicon, Portland, OR.

From the Department of Otolaryngology, Albert Einstein College of Medicine, Yeshiva University, Bronx, NY. This work was supported by the Deafness Research Foundation and the International Foundation for Children's Hearing, Education and Research, Inc.

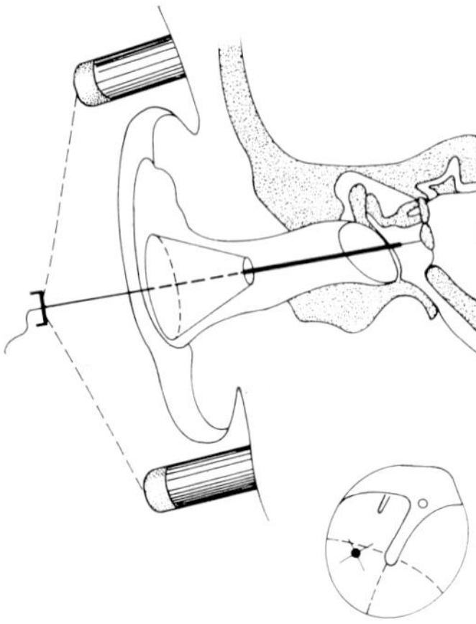

Fig. 1. Placement of the electrode.

tracted or perforated, a small piece of cotton impregnated with Xylocaine® jelly was placed on the tympanic membrane of the ear to be tested.

The ground and reference electrodes were silver cup electrodes filled with electrode jelly placed on the center of the forehead and the ear lobe of the ear to be tested. The active electrode was of stainless steel, 5 cm long, 0.4 mm in diameter and insulated to within 0.5 mm of its tip. It was placed transtympanically on the promontory of the middle ear, using a plastic aural speculum under microscopic control. The aim was to place this electrode halfway between the umbo and the annulus at approximately eight o'clock.[17] The electrode was secured with a rubber band on a "doughnut" placed circumaurally (Fig. 1). The DC resistance between all three electrodes was recorded before and after testing. The aim was to keep the resistance between the surface electrodes (*i.e.*, ground and reference electrodes less than 10,000 ohms whenever possible). The electrodes were connected to a preamplifier which led to the amplifier.* The band pass setting was set at 32 Hz to 3.2 kHz. The signal then passed to the averager.* All components are part of the electrocochleography unit* (Fig. 2). One hundred to fifteen hundred responses were averaged depending on the magnitude of the response. The averaging window was 10 msec. It was increased to 15 msec when necessary. The averager had a 200 address memory and its address time was 50 μsec (75 μsec for a sweep time of 15 msec).

The acoustic clicks were generated by a pulse generator** using a rectangular pulse of 0.5 msec duration. The rate of click stimulation was 10/sec made up of alternate rarefaction and condensation clicks. The stimulus pulses were fed via an attenuator*** and audio-power amplifier† to the sound treated room. A driver speaker†† was placed 70 cm from the ear to be tested (Fig. 2). The maximum level of the click was 95 dB peak equivalent sound pressure level measured at the entrance of the ear canal. This corresponds to 75 dB above detection threshold as measured on ten normally hearing subjects (who all reached the same threshold), *i.e.*, 75 dB hearing level (HL). The main energy of the stimulus was contained in the frequency range 0.5 - 2 kHz.

The investigation was used clinically to establish the whole nerve AP "threshold," *i.e.*, minimum averaged AP visual detection level of the cochlear division of the VIII nerve. The

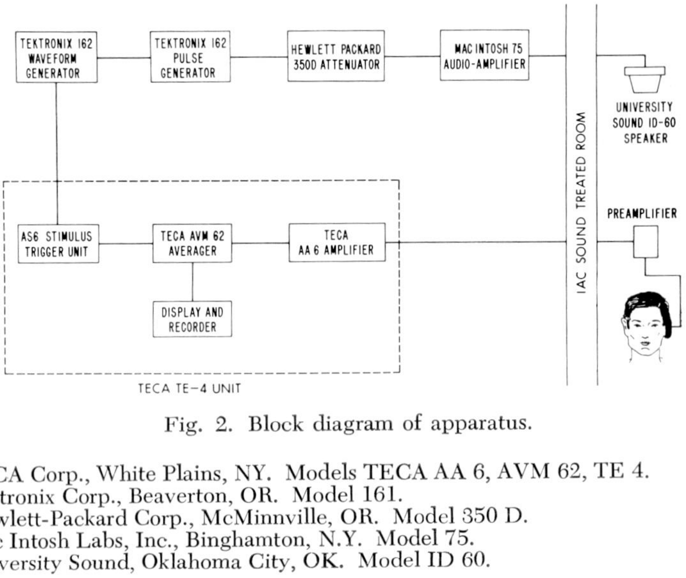

Fig. 2. Block diagram of apparatus.

---

* TECA Corp., White Plains, NY. Models TECA AA 6, AVM 62, TE 4.
** Tektronix Corp., Beaverton, OR. Model 161.
*** Hewlett-Packard Corp., McMinnville, OR. Model 350 D.
† Mac Intosh Labs, Inc., Binghamton, N.Y. Model 75.
†† University Sound, Oklahoma City, OK. Model ID 60.

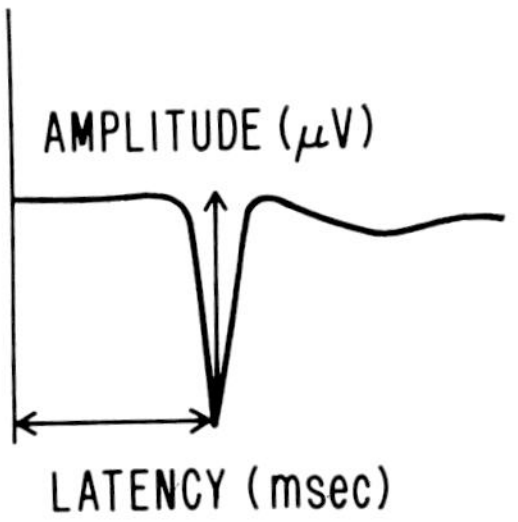

Fig. 3. Measurement of amplitude and latency.

stimuli were initially presented at maximum intensity of 75 dB HL and the resulting response averaged and recorded. This procedure was repeated at decreasing 10 dB levels until no response was visible. Five dB decrements were used when approaching the AP "threshold."

In order to analyze the intratest test-retest reliability, those tests which were repeated twice at the same intensity in the same patient were studied.

The procedure for determining the AP "threshold" as described lasted approximately one hour. Test and retest were either performed in sequence or at intervals of up to one hour. An attempt was made to keep all test conditions constant during the procedure, *i.e.*, stimulus and recording conditions remained the same and both active and reference electrodes were kept in the same position.

Latency was measured on the cathode ray display of the TE 4 when the averaging was completed. It was measured from the time of the stimulus reaching external auditory canal to the point of maximum deflection of the N_1 or N_2 when that was the only visible response (Fig. 3).

Responses were recorded on the TE 4 optic recorder. The amplitude of the response was measured after the test, from the baseline to the point of maximum deflection of the N_1 or N_2 respectively (Fig. 3).

TABLE I

DISTRIBUTION OF TYPES OF HEARING LOSSES IN THE SETS OF TESTS

Type of Hearing Loss	*No.*	*%*
Low and high frequency sensorineural loss	46	55
High frequency sensorineural loss	21	25
Flat sensorineural loss	8	9
Conductive loss	9	11
Total	84	100

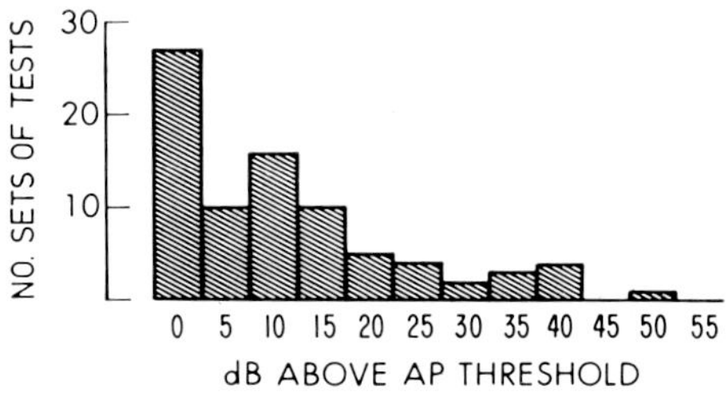

Fig. 4. Number of sets of tests at different intensities above AP "threshold."

RESULTS

Eighty-four sets of tests, each set consisting of test and retest, were performed in the 40 subjects studied. The distribution of the different kinds of hearing losses is shown in Table I. Intensities at which the tests were run ranged from the AP "threshold" to 50 dB above the AP "threshold" (Fig. 4). Seven of the 84 sets of tests had a retest in which no response was recorded. These will be considered separately and only the results of the remaining 77 sets of tests (154 tests) will now be presented.

The standard deviation of the differences between the amplitudes of test and retest for the 77 sets of tests was 1.0 μv. The scattergram of the amplitudes of test and retest are shown (Fig. 5). The correlation coefficient (r) was +0.78 ($p < .001$). The analysis of variance for the regression is shown in Table II.

The standard deviation of the differences between the latencies of test and retest was 0.24 msec. The scattergram of the latencies of test and retest are shown (Fig. 6). The correlation coefficient was +0.98 ($p < .001$). The analysis of variance for the regression is shown in Table III.

In order to make a more detailed study of the variability of the response amplitude and latency on test and retest, the effect of: 1) the N_1 amplitude; 2) stimulus intensity; 3) type of hearing loss; and 4) whether test and retest were performed in sequence or not, were evaluated.

First, the amplitude was studied. The mean of the two amplitudes in each set

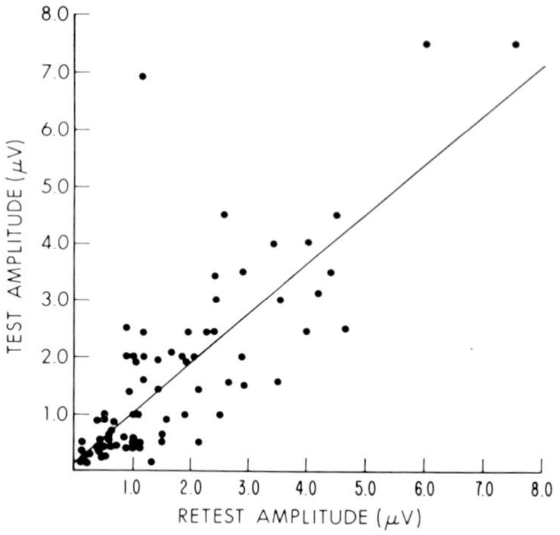

Fig. 5. Correlation between response amplitude of test and amplitude of retest.

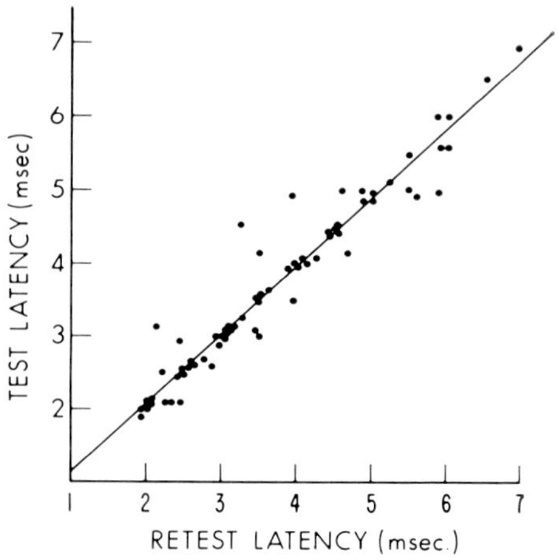

Fig. 6. Correlation between latency of test and latency of retest.

of tests was calculated and the data then was divided into three groups using a distribution of class intervals. Ten class intervals were used. The intervals were plotted against frequency of occurrence and the resulting histogram could be divided into three groups: large amplitudes (2.3-7.5 μv), medium amplitudes (0.8-2.25 μv) and small amplitudes (0.1-0.75 μv). The distribution of the different groups of amplitudes is seen in Table IV.

As would be expected, small amplitudes were found in decreasing frequency with increasing intensity of the stimulus while large amplitudes were found in increasing frequency with increasing intensity. Medium amplitudes were more evenly distributed over the intensities (Fig. 7). When amplitude was plotted against the standard deviation of the amplitude differences between test and retest, the standard deviation for large and medium amplitudes was significantly larger ($p < .05$) than for small amplitudes (Fig. 8).

When test-retest variability between the amplitudes was plotted against stimulus intensity, the standard deviation was seen to increase with increasing intensity (Fig. 9). The differences between the test-retest amplitudes were analyzed according to type of hearing loss but no significant difference was seen. Decreasing variability of the latencies occurred with increasing stimulus intensity (Fig. 10).

No significant difference was seen when the differences between the test-retest latencies were plotted against amplitudes and type of hearing loss. The standard deviation of the differences between the amplitude of test and retest done in sequence was 1.2 μv. There is

TABLE II

ANALYSIS OF VARIANCE FOR THE REGRESSION (TEST-RETEST AMPLITUDE)

Source of Variation	*Degrees of Freedom*	*Sum of Squares*	*Mean Squares*	*F Value*
Attributable to regression	1	123.28	123.28	121.11
Deviation from regression	75	76.34	1.02	
Total	76	199.62	2.63	

TABLE III

ANALYSIS OF VARIANCE FOR THE REGRESSION (TEST-RETEST LATENCY)

Source of Variation	Degrees of Freedom	Sum of Squares	Mean Squares	F Value
Attributable to regression	1	114.27	114.27	1867.79
Deviation from regression	75	4.59	.06	
Total	76	118.86	1.56	

no significant difference from the standard deviation of tests not done in sequence (0.9 μv) or among all tests including those done in sequence (1.0 μv).

DISCUSSION

Seven of the 84 sets of tests included in the study had a retest in which no response was visible. In each case a small response amplitude (0.15-0.7 μv) was recorded in the test and the stimulus intensity was either at AP "threshold" or within 10 dB above.

TABLE IV

DISTRIBUTION OF AMPLITUDES IN THE SETS OF TESTS

Amplitude		No.	%
Large	2.3-7.5 μv	22	26
Medium	0.8-2.25 μv	30	36
Small	0.1-0.75 μv	32	38
Total		84	100

The response amplitude is less consistent than the latency. Biological variability may exist and affect the amplitude more than the latency.

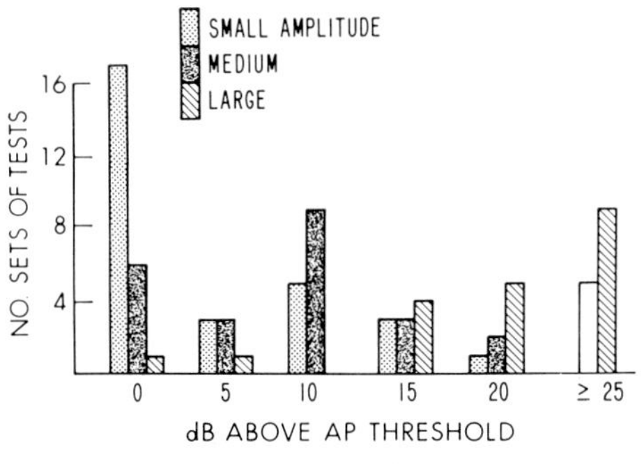

Fig. 7. Distribution of amplitudes at different stimulus intensities above AP "threshold."

That the amplitude decreases with decreasing stimulus intensity is what one would expect (Fig. 7). It is also natural that the amplitude variability of test and retest is larger for large and medium amplitudes than for small amplitudes (Fig. 8). A small amplitude cannot vary very much. It can increase but if it decreases substantially, no response will be visible.

The amplitude variability is seen to increase with increasing stimulus intensity (Fig. 9). The reason for this is probably that at higher intensities there are more larger amplitudes (Fig. 7) and larger amplitudes have larger standard deviations. There was no significant difference between the response amplitude for test and retest whether the tests are in sequence or not.

The latency variability of test and retest is larger for lower stimulus intensities than for higher intensities (Fig. 10). One explanation for this is that latencies at lower intensities are more difficult to

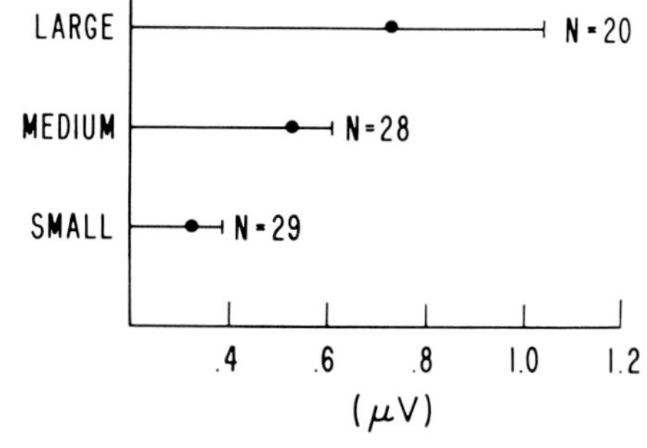

Fig. 8. Difference between amplitude of test and retest for different amplitudes showing mean difference (•) and standard deviation of difference (——|).

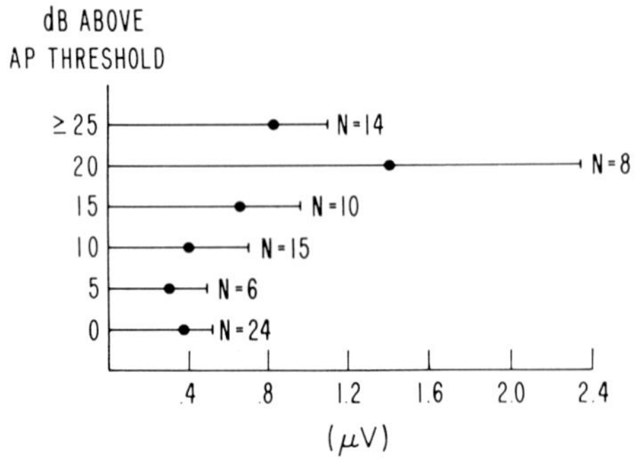

Fig. 9. Difference between amplitude of test and retest at different intensities above AP "threshold" showing mean difference (•) and standard deviation of difference (———|).

measure because of the broad response associated with small amplitudes.

The type of hearing loss does not seem to affect the test-retest reliability. There was no significant difference in amplitude or latency variability when analyzed according to type of hearing loss.

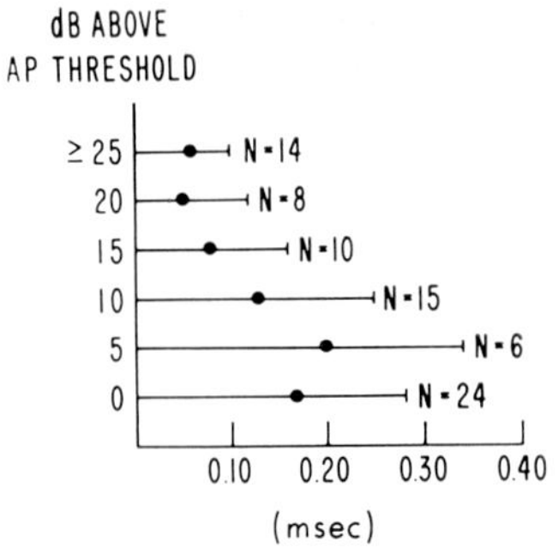

Fig. 10. Difference between latency of test and retest at different intensities above AP "threshold" showing mean difference (•) and standard deviation of difference (———|).

The seven retests in which no response was visible were all run near AP "threshold" where the averaged AP responses are small. These responses also tend to be broad because of less synchronized neuronal firing and difficult to detect in the background noise activity. The exact stimulus intensity at each test and retest was not checked. However, the acoustic system was regularly calibrated. It was also checked during the test that the patient remained in exactly the same position so there was no reason to believe that the stimulus intensity varied. During the test the position of the electrode was checked and a few times the response could be seen to improve if the electrode pressure was slightly increased. Biological variability could explain why the response could be seen at test but not at retest.

CONCLUSIONS

The intratest test-retest reliability in clinical electrocochleography has been studied. This was done by measuring the variability of amplitude and latency from test to retest. The correlation between amplitude of test and retest was good ($r = +0.78$) and even better between latency of test and retest ($r = +0.98$). However, in 7 of the 84 sets of tests there was no visible response in the retest. These were all within the range of 10 dB or less from the AP "threshold" and all had small amplitudes. It is, therefore, important that the apparent AP "threshold" be checked by repeating the test at the same intensity and also at intensities above and below in order to be sure that a reliable "threshold" response is obtained. This is important because the background noise can mask the response at "threshold" stimulus intensities.

Large response amplitudes are mainly found at higher intensities and they show the greatest variability. Small amplitudes show less variability but it is important to realize that around AP "threshold" the response may be visible in one test but not in another at the same intensity.

Changes in position of the electrode and individual biological variability may explain differences between the response amplitude of test and retest. Naturally it is also important to have the same stimulus intensity at test and retest. Occasionally this may be influenced by the patient changing position in relation to the loudspeaker.

The latency shows less variability than the amplitude. At higher intensities the difference between latency of test and retest is less than at lower intensities where the latency is more difficult to accurately measure because the response is broad when the amplitude is small.

REFERENCES

1. Portmann M, Aran JM: Electrocochleography. Laryngoscope 81:899-910, 1971

2. Portmann M, Aran JM: Electrocochleographie sur le nourrisson et le jeune enfant. Methode d'audiometrie objective. Acta Otolaryngol (Stockh) 71:253-261, 1971

3. Sohmer H, Feinmesser M, Bauberger-Tell L, *et al*: Routine use of cochlear audiometry in infants with uncertain diagnosis. Ann Otol Rhinol Laryngol 81:72-75, 1972

4. Sohmer H, Feinmesser M: Routine use of electrocochleography (cochlear audiometry) on human subjects. Audiology 12:167-173, 1973

5. Aran JM: Clinical measures of VIIIth nerve function. Adv Otorhinolaryngol 20:374-394, 1973

6. Beagley HA: Electrocochleography in clinical otology. J Laryngol Otol 87:441-448, 1973

7. Hooper RE: Electrocochleography. J Laryngol Otol 87:919-927, 1973

8. Yoshie N: Diagnostic significance of electrocochleography in clinical audiometry. Audiology 12:504-539, 1973

9. Eggermont JJ, Odenthal DW, Schmidt PH, *et al*: Electrocochleography: basic principles and clinical application. Acta Otolaryngol [Suppl] (Stockh) 316:37-74, 1974

10. Zerlin S, Naunton RF: Whole nerve response to third-octave audiometric clicks at moderate sensation level, to be published

11. Yoshie N, Ohashi T: Clinical use of cochlear nerve action potential responses in man for differential diagnosis of hearing loss. Acta Otolaryngol [Suppl] (Stockh) 252:71-87, 1969

12. Portmann M, Aran JM, Lagourgue P: Testing for "recruitment" by electrocochleography: preliminary result. Ann Otol Rhinol Laryngol 82:36-43, 1973

13. Bergholtz LM, Hooper RE, Mehta DC: Response patterns in clinical electrocochleography, to be published

14. Leiberman A, Sohmer H, Szabo G: Cochlear audiometry (electrocochleography) during the neonatal period. Dev Med Child Neurol 15:8-13, 1973

15. Hooper RE, Bergholtz LM, Mehta DC: Electrocochleography: A comparison of action potential and behavioral thresholds, to be published

16. Comeau M, Brummett R, Vernon J: Local anesthesia of the ear by iontophoresis. Arch Otolaryngol 98:114-120, 1973

17. Aran JM, Le Bert G: Les responses nerveuses cochlaires chez l'homme: image du fonctionnement de l'oreille et nouveau test d'audiometrie objective. Rev Laryngol Otol Rhinol (Bord) 89:361-378, 1968

ACKNOWLEDGMENTS—The authors would like to express their gratitude to Roy F. Sullivan, Ph.D. for his advice in the statistical interpretation of our data.

REPRINTS—L.M. Bergholtz, MD, Department of Otolaryngology, University Hospital, 5-581 85, Linkoping, Sweden.

Ann Otol 85: 1976

ANTIHISTAMINES

GUIDELINES AND IMPLICATIONS

ANTHONY S. KRAUSEN, MD

ST. LOUIS, MISSOURI

SUMMARY — Antihistamines may be used to maximum benefit for the allergic patient if the physician adheres to four guidelines. These guidelines are based upon 1) an appreciation of certain structural and pharmacologic differences among antihistamines, and 2) an understanding of their mechanism of action. Around the clock administration is advisable, the dosage should be titrated for the individual patient, substitutions to another antihistamine should be to a different class of antihistamine, and the efficacy of any single antihistamine usually will diminish with prolonged use, either on the basis of true tolerance or because of psychic factors. There is good theoretical evidence why α-adrenergic sympathomimetics, employed as decongestants in combination with antihistamines, should not be given to allergic patients. Two newer drugs, disodium cromoglycate and beclomethasone, may provide symptomatic relief for allergic rhinitis patients. They may benefit the patient who does not obtain full symptomatic relief from antihistamines.

Antihistamines have long been a cornerstone in the practice of otolaryngology and in the treatment of allergy. Nevertheless, these drugs have been consistently employed in a less than systematic fashion. There are, however, certain guidelines for antihistamine administration. These guidelines enable an otolaryngologist to make some intelligent selections with regard to his choice of drugs and dosage. Consider the patient with refractory symptoms of allergic rhinitis for whom a change in antihistamines is often prescribed. In many such instances, a simple alteration in dosage would have sufficed. On the other hand, when a substitution should be made, it is frequently done in a manner that totally disregards distinct pharmacologic differences among antihistamines. Thus, certain guidelines should be kept in mind in hopes of minimizing patient discomfort and maximizing therapeutic efficacy.

Historically, the use of antihistamines in the treatment of allergic rhinitis is based upon the work of Bartosch[1] and Dragstedt[2] in 1932. They demonstrated that histamine was released during antigen-antibody reactions following which allergic phenomena ensued.

ALLERGIC RHINITIS

Recent immunologic research has shown that histamine production and release is a complex event centering around tissue-bound mast cells. In the face of stimulation by an antigen, previously sensitized lymphocytes in an allergic individual will release IgE immunoglobulin. This IgE binds to mast cells in "target organs," such as the nasal mucosa. Subsequent exposure to the same antigen results in the bridging of two IgE molecules on the surface of these mast cells. The interaction of the antigen and the IgE molecules effects intracellular alterations within the mast cells. Granules in which histamine had been stored undergo degenerative changes leading to histamine release into adjacent tissues.[3,4] Histamine in turn induces smooth muscle contraction and increased vascular permeability. Other mediators are released during granule breakdown, in particular eosinophile chemotaxic factor of asthma (ECF-A). This substance leads to the

From the Department of Otolaryngology, Washington University School of Medicine, St. Louis, Missouri. This work supported in part by NIH-NINDS Grant No. 5 T01 NS05190-17.

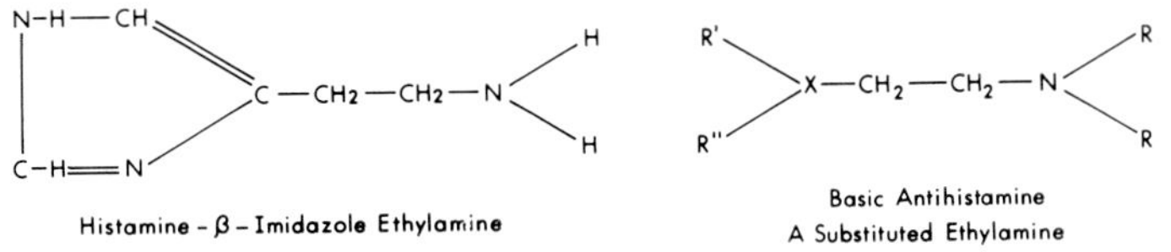

Fig. 1. Similarity in the structures of histamine and antihistamine molecules enabling antihistamines to compete for histamine binding sites. (Modified from RE Wilhelm, *Medical Clinics of North America* 45:888, 1961. Permission of S. B. Saunders and Co.

attraction of eosinophils to the target organs.[5]

Recent asthma research also suggests that slow-reacting substance of anaphylaxis (SRS-A) may be released from basophils (the circulating counterparts of mast cells) during antigen stimulation. This substance produces slow contraction of tracheobronchial smooth muscle. Extrapolating, it is possible that such a substance is also released by mast cells or basophils in the nasal mucosa.

ROLE OF ANTIHISTAMINES

Antihistamines, by counteracting only the effects of histamine, block most of the untoward events of an allergic response. Antihistamines in no way affect antibody production, antigen-antibody interaction, or histamine release.[6] They play no role in inhibiting SRS-A or ECF-A activity.

Antihistamines do act by occupying the same cellular receptor site on target organs as does histamine. Antihistamines can do this by virtue of a similarity in their molecular configuration to the configuration of the histamine molecule. Histamine is β-imidazole ethylamine, whereas the basic antihistamine structure is a substituted ethylamine (Fig. 1).[7] Substitutions are made

TABLE I

FIVE CLASSES OF ANTIHISTAMINES

Class of Antihistamine	*Generic Name*	*Trade Name*	*Dose (mg)*	*Drowsiness*
I. Ethylene diamines	Tripelennamine	Pyribenzamine®	25-50	+
	Pyrilamine	NeoAntergan (Triaminic®)	25-50	
	Thonzylamine	Anahist®	25-50	
II. Ethanolamines	Diphenhydramine	Benadryl®	25-50	++
	Phenyltoloxamine	Histionex® (Naldecon®, Sinubid®)	88	
	Dimenhydrinate	Dramamine®	50	
III. Propylamines	Chlorpheniramine	Chlor-Trimeton® (Teldrin®, Ornade®, Histaspan®, Naldecon®)	4	+
	Brompheniramine	Dimetane® (Dimetapp®)	4	
	Brompheniramine (d-isomer)	Disomer® (Drixoral®)	2	
	Pyrrobutamine	Pyronil® (Co-Pyronil®)	15-30	
	Triprolidine	Actidil® (Actifed®)	2-5	
IV. Phenothiazines	Promethazine	Phenegran®	12.5-25	++
	Trimeprazine	Temaril®	2.5	
V. Miscellaneous	Cyproheptadine	Periactin®	4	+
	Phenindamine	Theophorin®	25	

* Adapted from Goodman and Gilman, ed 3. Drugs in parentheses are common combination drugs containing the antihistamine plus decongestant.

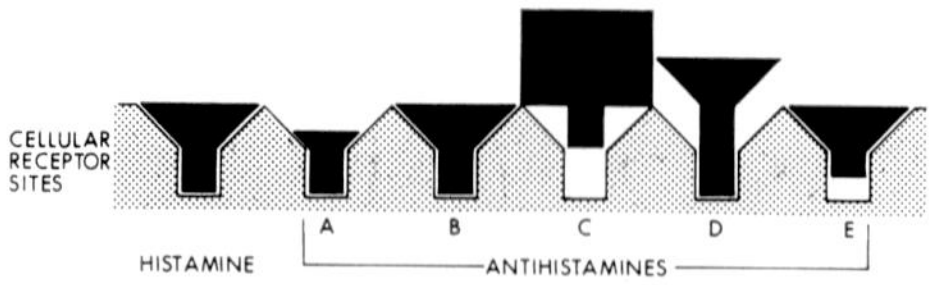

Fig. 2. Optimal structures of antihistamines. A – Aromatic radical too small, side chain adequate; B – Aromatic radical adequate, side chain adequate; C – Aromatic radical too large, side chain adequate; D – Aromatic radical adequate, side chain too long; E – Aromatic radical adequate, side chain too short. (RE Wilhelm, *Medical Clinics of North America* 45:888, 1961. Permission of S.B. Saunders and Co.)

on the ethylamine chain, -C-C-N. The R′ and R″ radicals are both aromatic moieties while R respresents a straight side chain. Based upon the aromatic substitution, five distinct classes of antihistamines can be delineated (Table I).[8] These will be discussed later.

The schematic representation in Figure 2 shows how an antihistamine molecule with an adequate side chain and adequate aromatic radicals, as in case B, can successfully occupy the same cellular receptor sites as does histamine. In this way histamine is prevented from acting upon a target cell.[7]

A dynamic relationship of competing for, and of blocking receptor sites is thus established. Such a relationship is known as competitive inhibition. This means that the concentration of the antihistamine molecule must be considerably greater than the concentration of the histamine molecule in order for most receptor sites to be blocked. Only then will inhibition of histamine activity be clinically evident.[3]

Histamine causes marked capillary dilatation and increased capillary permeability. By blocking histamine from receptor sites, antihistamines prevent such events from occurring. Thus, turbinate swelling and nasal congestion with mucosal edema, all secondary to increased capillary permeability, are prevented.[7]

Secondary Pharmacologic Properties. Secondary pharmacologic properties of antihistamines provide additional uses as well as drawbacks. Most important among such adjunctive effects are the central nervous system actions. All antihistamines exert a depressive effect centrally. The degree of sedation and drowsiness produced varies with the class of the preparation and with the individual patient. It is this side effect of drowsiness which causes the bulk of patient dissatisfaction with antihistamine therapy.[6,8,9]

All antihistamines also have atropinic or anticholinergic effects. This results in decreased production of tears and airway secretions.[10] Patients thus may complain of dry eyes, dry mouth, and viscid sputum. Additionally, blurred vision and constipation may also be problems. Some antihistamines, such as promethazine and diphenhydramine, are also local anesthetics when injected.

Lastly, antihistamines may evoke contraction of vascular smooth muscle by direct action, *i.e.*, by dipolarization of the smooth muscle cell membrane coupled with a release of bound calcium ions.[11]

Class Structure of Antihistamines. It is most helpful to consider the antihistamines as being separable into five classes based upon structural differences, with each class having distinct pharmacologic properties.[8]

Class I, the ethylenediamines, includes tripelennamine. These exhibit a low incidence of drowsiness. Their duration of action is short, usually three to six hours, during which time they have been transformed and metabolized by the liver as are all the other antihistamines.[12]

Class II, the ethanolamines, represented by diphenhydramine, causes marked sedation in over 50% of patients. Atropine-like side effects are also prominent during their three to six hours' duration of action.[8,9]

Class III, the propylamines, includes chlorpheniramine and brompheniramine. These produce drowsiness in only 10-30% of patients. The duration of action for the simple tablet is again three to six hours. This class is often used in sustained release capsules and tablets, in which case, the duration of action is 8 to 12 hours.[13]

Class IV, the phenothiazines, includes promethazine. They are often employed as tranquilizers or antiemetic agents, and not surprisingly, produce a high incidence of drowsiness. Most members of this group have a long duration of antihistamine action, up to 12 to 24 hours, due to slow liver metabolism.[14]

Class V, designated miscellaneous, includes cyproheptadine and phenindamine. These have a low incidence of drowsiness and a three to six hours' duration of action.[8]

Palliation Therapy. In the management of nasal allergy, palliation is the keyword with regard to antihistamine therapy. Avoidance of the offending allergen by diet and environmental manipulation or hyposensitization injection therapy can provide more definitive protection against nasal allergy.[15] Antihistamines, however, only palliate the clinical complex of sneezing, nasal obstruction, nonpurulent rhinorrhea, excessive lacrimation, and ocular pruritus. These drugs exert a "favorable influence" on such symptoms for an estimated 60-80% of patients.[10]

Therapy Guidelines. For maximal palliation, four guidelines should be considered.

First, around-the-clock administration is advisable. Antihistamines are rapidly absorbed when taken orally with some clinical effect observable in 15-30 minutes. Peak effect is reached in one to two hours. Often real clinical usefulness has passed within four hours.[8] Acting as competitive inhibitors, antihistamine molecules must be present in high concentration for the drug to be effective. Thus, most antihistamines should be given four times a day, around-the-clock, for maximal benefit.

Second, the choice of dosage is important. The average clinical dose of a given antihistamine may provide only partial relief in a particular patient. However, a slight increase in dosage may produce a more complete palliation of symptoms by placing an adequate concentration of antihistamines into circulation. For example, 6 mg of chlorpheniramine given every six hours might provide marked relief whereas 4 mg every six hours might have no favorable effect. The dosage is *titrated* for the individual patient, with the therapeutic dose being slightly less than that causing troublesome drowsiness.[16] In patients with liver damage, dosage must, of course, be reduced to coincide with decreased metabolism.

Third, occasional inadequate palliative response or excessive drowsiness is encountered with a particular drug despite dosage adjustment. Substituting another antihistamine in a systematic fashion may lead to a favorable result. This necessitates substitution to a different class of antihistamine.[8]

Fourth, the efficacy of any single antihistamine preparation will usually diminish with prolonged use. Whether this is due to a true tolerance or due to psychic factors is not certain. It is possible that once the novelty of partial relief has worn off, the patient concentrates his attention on the unrelieved portion of his symptoms.[10] Nevertheless, a change in regimen, in accordance with previous guidelines, should center around substitution to a different antihistamine class.

ORAL DECONGESTANTS

Among the myriad of preparations prescribed for allergic rhinitis, many contain a decongestant in combination with an antihistamine. The decongestants most commonly employed are pseudoephedrine, phenylpropanolamine, and phenylephine. Each acts predominantly as a α-adrenergic sympathomimetic in the dosage administered. As such, each provides vasoconstrictive action on arterioles which might counteract histamine-induced vasodilatation at the capillary level. These sympathomimetics are also psychomotor stimulants. Acting upon the central nervous system, they overcome some of the drowsiness produced by antihistamines.

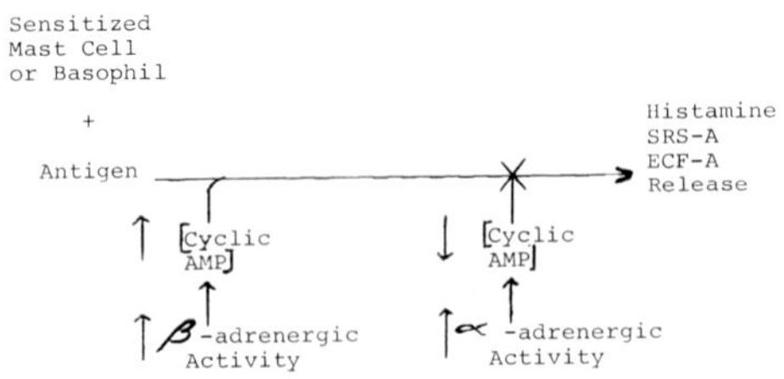

Fig. 3. Schematic representation of the pharmacologic controls of the immunologic release of chemical mediators. Cyclic AMP modulates histamine, SRS-A, and ECF-A release. The concentration of cyclic AMP varies inversely with the amount of mediator released. Increased concentration of cyclic AMP inhibits mediator release while decreased cyclic AMP allows mediators to be released.

However, recent asthma research provides some theoretical questions as to the advisability of employing decongestants to treat allergic rhinitis. Figure 3, based upon human lung fragment studies, illustrates that cyclic adenosine 3′5′ monophosphate (cyclic AMP) suppresses the histamine released, which follows IgE and antigen interaction. On the other hand, α-adrenergic drugs depress cyclic AMP levels resulting in a loosening of the constraints on histamine release.[6] The implications of such an action with regard to allergic rhinitis are evident. By giving α-adrenergic decongestants, one may be increasing the histamine load against which antihistamines must compete.[16] Recently, Kaliner *et al*[17] showed that in tissue from human polyps, incubation with cyclic AMP inhibited histamine, SRS-A, and ECF-A release in a dose-dependent fashion. Also, α-adrenergic stimulation was shown to increase histamine and SRS-A release.

Pharmacologic studies of oral decongestants employing rhinomanometric techniques reveal interesting findings. McLaurin *et al*[18] in 1961 tested ephedrine, phenylephrine, pseudoephedrine, and phenylpropanolamine alone, and not in combination with antihistamines. Testing 88 individuals with nasal congestion due to a variety of causes, including allergic rhinitis, they found that only ephedrine produced significant nasal mucosa shrinkage.* Ephedrine is one of the few drugs which, like epinephrine, directly increases the AMP levels, thereby diminishing histamine release. A later McLaurin study of Actifed,®** a combination of pseudoephedrine and the antihistamine tripolidine, showed that this drug had decongestant properties.[19] This suggested that adrenergic agents may act synergistically with antihistamines. The 74 patients studied were not separated as to allergic or other etiologies for nasal congestion, thus making it difficult to ascertain the rationale for using this drug in strictly allergic rhinitis.

In short, the theoretical reason for withholding α-adrenergic decongestants other than ephedrine in the treatment of allergic rhinitis still remains. Unfortunately, ephedrine produces cardiac irritability and excessive psychomotor stimulation in so many patients that its usefulness may be limited.

As with any combination of drugs, knowledge of the side effects and hazards of all the components is important. Most of the sympathomimetics, particularly ephedrine, cause nervousness and irritability. Furthermore, patients with glaucoma, hypertension, and diabetes mellitus all have their conditions exacerbated by the α-adrenergics. There is a distinct risk of precipitating a hypertensive crisis by giving these oral decongestants to patients taking monamine oxidase inhibtors (Eutonyl®***, Parnate®****) or tricyclics (Elavil®†, Triavil®†).[6] So, not only may decongestants be inappropriate in treating allergic rhinitis, additionally, their use may be ill considered in numerous patients.

ADDITIONS TO THE ARMAMENTARIUM

Two new drugs have recently been

---

* Farr. Personal oral communication, 1974.
** Burroughs Wellcome Co., Research Triangle Park, NC.
*** Abbott Laboratories, North Chicago, IL.
**** Smith Kline & French Laboratories, Philadelphia, PA.
† Merck Sharp & Dohme, West Point, PA.

added to the armamentarium for the symptomatic treatment of allergic rhinitis. The first, disodium cromoglycate, has been used for some time in the treatment of asthma. Administered by inhalation in a powder form, this drug stabilizes mast cells and basophils, thereby preventing degranulation and mediator release. The drug is awaiting FDA approval for intranasal use. According to Toogood in Canada[20] disodium cromoglycate, administered as a nasal inhalant, significantly suppresses clinical hay fever symptoms.

The second new drug is a topically administered steroid with little, if any, systemic absorption. Steroids, by virtue of their antiinflammatory properties, act directly on cells to inhibit capillary dilatation and edema formation seen in allergic responses. The controlled studies of Smith *et al*[21] show that beclomethasone dipropionate aerosol, in allergic rhinitis patients, produces a significant improvement in nasal forced expiratory volume.

Whether these two newer drugs will supplant antihistamines completely is impossible to say. Certainly, since each drugs acts in a pharmacologically different way, the combined use of the three should find application in the difficult allergic patient.

REFERENCES

1. Bartosch R, Feldberg M, Nagel E: Das Freiwerden eines Histaminähnlichen Stoffes bei der Anaphylaxie des Meerschweinchens. Pfluegers Arch 230:120-153, 1932

2. Dragstedt CA, Gebauer-Fuelneigg E: Studies in Anaphylaxis I: the appearance of a physiologically active substance during anaphylactic shock. Am J Physiol 102:512-519, 1932

3. Wells JA: General discussion I. Ann NY Acad Sci 50:1202-1206, 1948-50

4. Kelly JF, Patterson R: Anaphylaxis—course, mechanisms and treatment. JAMA 227:1431-1436, 1974

5. Austen KF: A review of immunologic, biochemical and pharmacological factors in the release of chemical mediators from human lung, in Austen KF, Lichtenstein LM (eds): *Asthma-Physiology, Immunopharmacology, and Treatment.* New York, Academic Press, 1973, chap 8

6. Hartman MM: Capabilities and limitations of major drug groups in allergy: their role within current theories. Ann Allergy 27:164-181, 1969

7. Wilhelm RE: The newer anti-allergenic agents. Med Clin North Am 45:887-906, 1961

8. Douglas WW: Histamine and antihistamines, in Goodman LS, Gilman A (eds): *The Pharmacologic Basis of Therapeutics,* ed 3. New York, Macmillan Co, 1966, pp 615-643

9. Aviado DM (ed): *Krantz and Carr's Pharmacologic Principles of Medical Practice,* ed 8. Baltimore, Williams and Wilkins Co, 1972, pp 382-394, 797-826

10. Feinberg SM: Antihistamine therapy, experimental and clinical correlation. Ann NY Acad Sci 50:1186-1199, 1948-50

11. Altura BM, Altura BT: Contractile actions of antihistamines on isolated arterial smooth muscle. J Pharmacol Exp Ther 191:262-267, 1974

12. Mayer RL: The activity of pyribenzamine and related compounds with special reference to their mode of action. Ann NY Acad Sci 50:1127-1114, 1948-50

13. Aaronson AL, Ehrlich NJ, Frankel DB, *et al*: Effective oral nasal decongestion: a double-blind crossover analysis. Ann Allergy 26:145-150, 1966

14. Wood CD, Graybiel A, Kennedy RS: Human centrifuge studies on the relative effectiveness of some antimotion sickness drugs. Aerosp Med 37:187-190, 1966

15. Willoughby JW: Serial dilution titration skin tests in inhalant allergy. A clinical quantitative assessment of biologic skin reactivity to allergenic extracts. Otolaryngol Clin North Am 7:579-615, 1974

16. Pincus WB: Current status of allergic immunotherapy. Trans Am Acad Ophthalmol Otolaryngol 80:356-361, 1975

17. Kaliner M, Wasserman SI, Austen KF: Immunologic release of chemical mediators from human nasal polyps. N Engl J Med 289:277-281, 1973

18. McLaurin JW, Shipman WF, Rosedale R Jr: Oral decongestants: a double-blind comparison study of the effectiveness of four sympathomimetic drugs: objective and subjective. Laryngoscope 71:57-67, 1961

19. McLaurin JW, Graves TA, Komet H: Efficacy of Actifed as a decongestant. Laryngoscope 76:1612-1614, 1966

20. Toogood JH: Disodium cromoglycate for allergic rhinitis. J Allergy Clin Immunol 50:188, 1972

21. Smith JM, Clegy RT, Cook N, *et al*: Intranasal beclomethasone dipropionate in allergic rhinitis. Br Med J 2:255, 1975

REPRINTS—Anthony S. Krausen, MD, 517 S Euclid Avenue, St. Louis, MO 63110.

X-RAY OF THE MONTH

AMELOBLASTOMA

Alfred L. Weber, MD
Walter Guralnick, DMD
Boston, Massachusetts

PATIENT

Following treatment of an upper respiratory tract infection, a swelling of the right cheek and hard palate, together with loose teeth, were noted in a 7-year-old boy.

RADIOGRAPHS

The Water's projection (A) revealed an expansile mass (arrows) in the region of the right antrum with inferior displacement of the molar teeth (T). AP polytome sections (B and C) revealed a homogeneous density, displacing the intact nasoantral wall medially (B) and a thinned alveolar ridge and hard palate displaced inferiorly (C). D) A lateral tomogram demonstrating the superior displacement of the orbital floor by the mass. O - Inferior orbital rim.

DIAGNOSIS

The patient was explored surgically and a well encapsulated mass was found in the right alveolar ridge of the maxilla, extending into the antrum with no invasion of the orbit. The interface between the well encapsulated mass and the mucoperiosteum was well defined. The tumor was freely lifted off the adjacent bone and completely removed. The histological diagnosis was ameloblastoma.

DISCUSSION

This benign cystic tumor is composed of ameloblasts which are derived from ectodermal epithelium of the enamel organ, follicle and periodontal membrane.[1,2] If incompletely excised, this neoplasm has a high recurrence rate and metastases have been reported rarely. More than half of the tumors are found between the ages of 20 and 40 but may occur at any age. About 80% of ameloblastomas originate in the mandible and the majority of these occur in the molar tooth area. The remaining 20% are found in the maxilla, usually in the molar area and if large enough, extend into the antrum and adjacent nasal cavity. The radiological picture is characterized by unilocular or multilocular[3] cystic areas separated by distinct septae of various thickness. Coalescence of the smaller cysts into a large unilocular cyst may occur with expansion of the tumor. This pattern of slow growth also produces a sharply defined margin of expanded cortical bone which allows differentiation from the destruction of a malignant neoplasm. There is often displacement of teeth or resorption of the roots of the teeth. If teeth are incorporated, the lesion may simulate a dentigerous cyst. The radiological differential diagnosis includes ossifying fibroma, mucocele of the antrum and other benign tumors.

From the Department of Radiology, Massachusetts Eye & Ear Infirmary, Massachusetts General Hospital, Boston, Massachusetts.

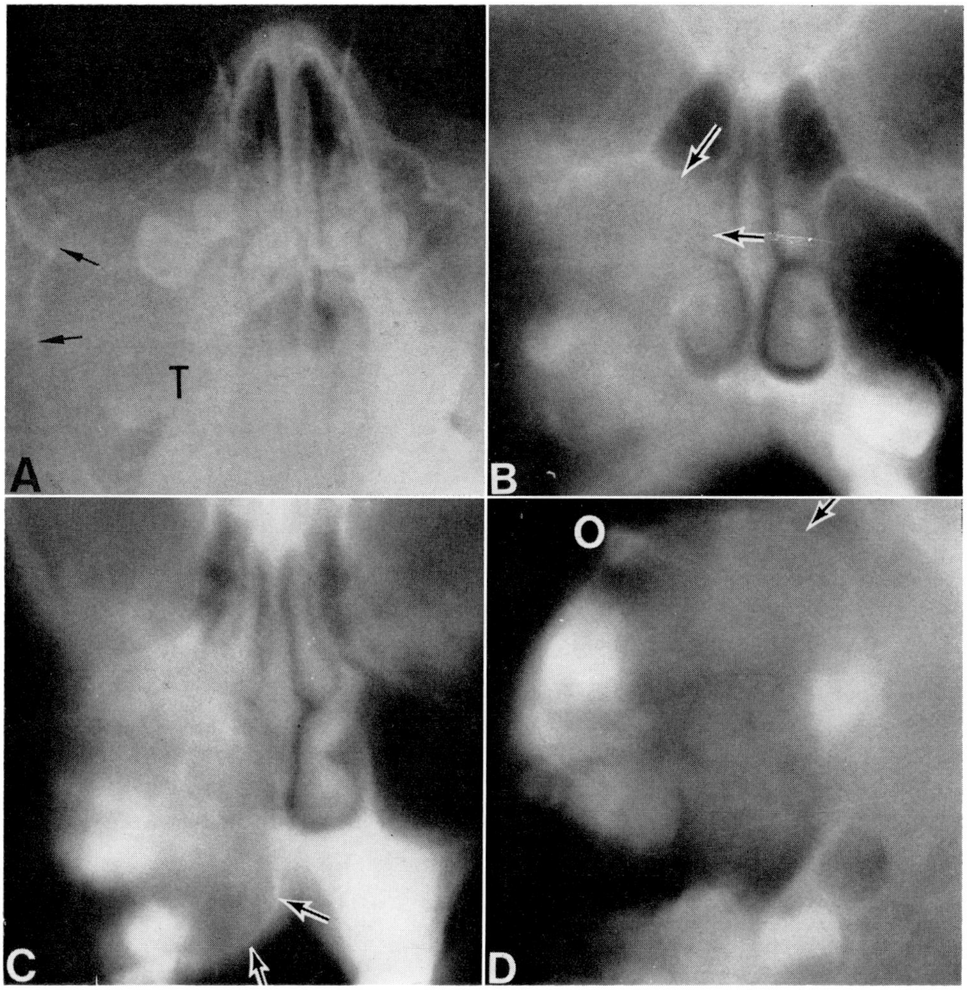

REFERENCES

1. Stafne EC, Gibilisco JA: *Oral Roentgenographic Diagnosis. Philadelphia,* WB Saunders Co, 1975

2. Small IA, Waldron CA: Ameloblastomas of jaws. Oral Surg 8:281-297, 1955

3. Sherman RS, Caumartin H: The roentgen appearance of adamantinoma of the mandible. Radiology 65:361-366, 1955

BOOK REVIEWS

Handbook of Auditory and Vestibular Research Methods

By *Catherine A. Smith* and *Jack A. Vernon* (eds). Hard cover, black and white illustrations, referenced, indexed by subject and author, 600 pp, 1975. Charles C. Thomas, Springfield, Illinois. Price $43.75

I must confess that when I began this review, I did it with some degree of prejudice against the work. After all, one cannot teach research methods from a book, so why bother writing or editing one? I still do not believe that research can be learned outside the laboratory, but the legitimacy of this book is no longer doubtful. In it there is a storehouse of interesting information, often offering fascinating details, about a wide variety of subjects. The information on any given subject is more useful, I suspect, to the interested bystander than to the practitioner of the art. Thus, material on biochemical techniques was of more interest to me than that on, say, physiology or experimental audiology, simply because the former material was less familiar. A biochemist undoubtedly would have found the opposite. The book will assist those who are reading in the broad spectrum of hearing science to acquire a taste in areas other than their specialty for best methodology, preferred techniques, and possible pitfalls. It is recommended for that use.

The topics are intelligently chosen and much of the material is very competently written. Included are sections on anatomical methods (microdissection, surface preparation, temporal bone preparation, transmission and scanning electron microscopy, and tissue culture methods), electrophysiological methods (inner ear and central pathways, unit and gross recording techniques, computer processing and sound measurement methods), biochemical methods, behavioral methods (animal conditioning techniques and experimental audiology). There is very little to quarrel with in the chosen array of topics or the content of any individual section. There might be minor disagreement about the lack of uniformity of detail from contributor to contributor. In a handbook more detail would have been expected on some topics. For example, in the material pertaining to the electrophysiology of the central pathways, there is no information on anesthesia, surgical techniques, and physiological monitoring of the state of the animal. Other minor editorial problems, admittedly hairsplitting on my part, are the following: in one chapter a great deal is made of the inadequacy of coupler-calibration of the sound field in animal research, whereas, in another, coupler-calibration methods for human work are described in detail. Of course these are two traditional methods resulting from different needs; however, it would be good to tie the two together. The editors should have clipped without mercy all photos of racks of equipment, unplugged cords, *etc*; these contain no information whatsoever. They should have also made sure that such anachronisms as the English system of units are not used in a scientific text.

The one major shortcoming of the book, probably a casualty of the customarily endless production time of handbooks and compendia, is the noninclusion of electrocochleography (ECochG) and brain stem evoked response (BER) audiometry. While neither of these methods is new, they both came into their own within the past two to three years, hence the possible cause for not including them. Compared to these two extremely promising and significant procedures, the averaged response audiometry dealing with long latency responses (a chapter is included on these) is chiefly of historical interest today.

All-in-all, this is a good book and a useful reference. I am pleased to recommend it.

PETER DALLOS, MD

Review of Speech Therapy

By *P. Pialoux, M. Valtat, G. Freyss and F. Legent*. Masson and Cie, Editeurs. 129 Boulevard Saint Germain, Paris-VIe, 1975. In French.

In this text the different aspects related to speech and hearing are outlined.

The work is divided in four parts: The first section is an introduction which describes the anatomy and physiology of the organs involved in speech and hearing. The second section exposes the different methods of evaluating hearing, speech, articulation and language. The third section describes the different problems associated with these two functions. In the fourth and last section, the different methods of treatment are outlined as they relate to specific problems.

SAMIR BISHARA, DDS

Carcinomas of the Floor of the Oral Cavity

By *Pierre Cerneo*, Ed. Masson and Cie, Eds. 120 Boulevard Saint-Germain, Paris-VIe, 1975. In French.

In this volume, carcinomas involving the floor of the oral cavity are discussed in detail. The general characteristics of these malignancies and the clinical signs are described. Separate chapters on the treatment of epitheliomas, epidermoid carcinomas, adenocarcinomas and intraepithelial lesions are included. The indications and contraindications of different treatment philosophies as they relate to a particular lesion are outlined. These include surgery, electrosurgery, curie-puncture, chemotherapy and irradiation.

The last four chapters address different complications which result from these various therapeutic procedures.

SAMIR BISHARA, DDS

PHYSIOLOGICAL BASIS OF COCHLEAR TRANSDUCTION AND SENSITIVITY

VICENTE HONRUBIA, MD

DAVID STRELIOFF, PHD STEPHAN T. SITKO, PHD

LOS ANGELES, CALIFORNIA

SUMMARY – Experiments were conducted in the guinea pig cochlea and the *Xenopus laevis* lateral line organ to obtain information about the electrical impedance properties of the cochlea, the sources and characteristics of the cochlear potentials, and to determine if hair cells are electrically excitable. The significance of the resting and evoked cochlear potentials in the transduction process leading to excitation of the acoustic nerve fibers was evaluated by comparing the results of electrophysiological experiments with the prediction of a model of the cochlea designed after the mechanoelectric theory of hair cell function. The results of these experiments 1) were compatible with the prediction of the mechoelectric theory of cochlear function; 2) made it possible to estimate and compare the energy dissipated in generating and maintaining the cochlear potentials with the stores of biochemical energy available in the cochlea; and 3) showed that the hair cells are electrically excitable, from which it was concluded that interaction between the hair cells is feasible.

The mechanism of excitation in most sensory organs involves the production of a receptor potential by the receptor cells.[1,2] The significance of this intermediate step in the transduction process leading to the excitation of the afferent neuron of the acoustic nerve is a long-debated and unresolved issue.

Information basic to the understanding of this problem is being derived from studies in different hair cell systems, the lateral line organs, the cochlea and vestibular receptors, all of which point toward a common physiological process. In lateral line organs it has been shown that water displacements, not hydrostatic pressure changes, in the vicinity of the hair cells constitute the effective stimulus for the excitation of the afferent nerve fibers.[3] Furthermore, excitation in the semicircular canal preparation occurs when the displacement of the cilia is in the direction toward the kinocilium.[4,5] In the mudpuppy lateral line and the basilar papilla of the lizard, stimulation of the hair cells results in modulation of the membrane potential at the frequency of the stimulus.[6,7] It has also been shown that the firing of action potentials in the afferent nerve is also modulated at the stimulus frequency.[8-11] However, the precise relationship between hair cell membrane potential changes and the neural activity is not yet known. It has been suggested that afferent transmission at the hair cell-neuron synapse is a neurochemical process and that transmitter release is modulated by the currents associated with hair cell membrane potential changes during physiological stimulation.[12,13] Recently Sand *et al*[14] were able to modulate the neural activity of afferent dendrites in the mudpuppy lateral line by injecting current into the hair cell.

The hair cell membrane has the characteristic of being nonuniform with the peculiarity that its morphological appearance at the top is different from the

From the Department of Surgery, Head and Neck Division (Otolaryngology), University of California, Los Angeles, CA. This work was supported by grants from the U.S. Public Health Service (NS 08193, NS 09823), the Deafness Research Foundation, and the Castera Estate Fund.

Presented at the meeting of the American Otological Society, Inc., Palm Beach, Florida, April 25-26, 1976.

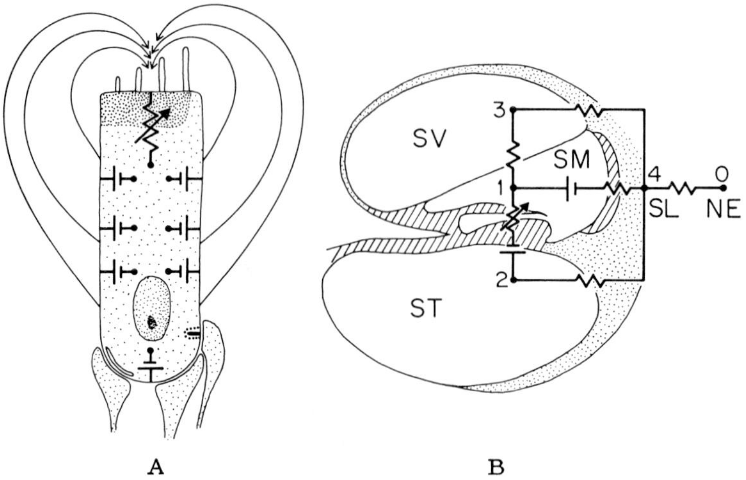

Fig. 1. A) Hair cell model with nonuniform membrane properties. Apical (hair-bearing) end is assumed to be a purely passive (ohmic) resistance whose value, as indicated by the schematic variable resistor, is modulated during mechanical displacement of the sensory hairs. The remainder of the cell membrane is assumed to exhibit active ion transport and maintain a transmember potential as indicated by the schematic batteries. The nonuniformity of the membrane's electrical properties results in local currents through the hair cells as indicated by the arrows. B) Network model of the cochlea incorporating the concepts of the hair cell model of Figure 1A. The network branches represent the lumped-equivalent electrical resistances between the scala media (SM), scala vestibuli (SV), scala tympani (ST) and the neck muscles (NE). The schematic batteries represent the biochemical sources of electromotive force in the stria vascularis and organ of Corti.

rest of the cell (Fig. 1A). It has been postulated that this section of the cell membrane also has different physiological properties: that it is nonelectrogenic and that its ohmic resistance changes during acoustic stimulation.[15] The nonuniformity of the membrane results in local currents between other areas of the membrane and the top and gives rise to a negative extracellular potential above the cilia relative to the scala tympani or the neck of the animal. The magnitude of the current is modulated by resistance changes at the top of this section of the membrane produced by mechanical displacements of the cilia during acoustic stimulation. The changing current, in turn, affects the synaptic transmission at the afferent synapse. The voltage produced by the changing current is recorded as the well known microphonic potential.

Experimental testing of these postulates, collectively referred to as the mechanoelectric theory of hair cell function, presents great difficulties. Through the evolutionary process many elaborate features have been incorporated in the auditory receptor organ which have greatly increased the complexity of its anatomical and physiological properties. They include the mechanical travelling waves in the basilar membrane,[16] differential features of innervation and anatomical configuration of the inner and outer hair cells,[17-19] and a positive resting potential, endocochlear potential (EP), in the cochlear duct generated in the stria vascularis.[16,20,21]

In the cochlea the hair cells are situated between two fluid compartments: the scala media, filled with endolymph and maintained at +80 mV with respect to plasma, and the spaces inside the organ of Corti filled with perilymph and believed to be equipotential with the scala tympani (+5 mV with respect to plasma). The +80 mV EP of the scala media together with the –70 to –80 mV intracellular membrane potential results in a net 150-160 mV potential gradient across the variable-resistance section at

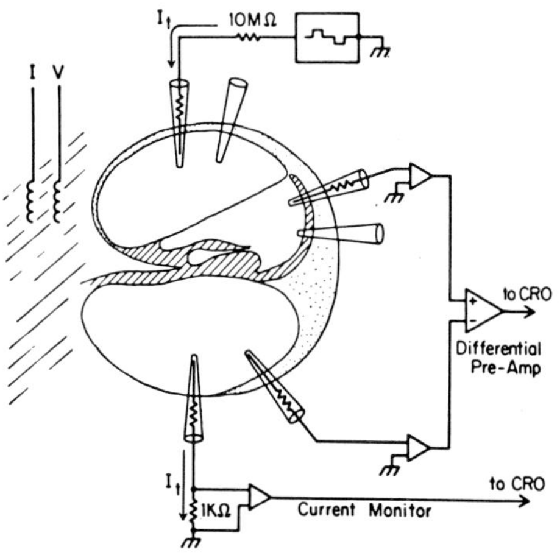

Fig. 2. Schematic drawing outlining the procedure used for determining the electrical resistances between the SM, the ST, the SV and the body. Pairs of glass capillary microelectrodes were inserted into each of the three scalae and a pair of chlorided wire electrodes was placed subcutaneously in the neck. Constant test currents (I_t) were applied between two points and the induced voltage was measured using all six possible differential recording configurations. This procedure allowed 36 total resistance measurements to be made in a single cochlear turn of which six are independent.

the top of the sensory hair cell surface. The action of the hair cells by the gating control they have in this potential gradient is thought to be that of transducing and amplifying the mechanical acoustic energy into bioelectric energy.[16]

Insights into the role of the hair cells and determination of the magnitude and distribution of the currents through the cochlear partition require precise information about the electrical impedances of the cochlear membranes and fluids. This paper summarizes the results of work conducted in the cochlea of the guinea pig and in the lateral line organ of the toad *Xenopus laevis*, designed to obtain specific information about the amplifier action of the cochlea and quantitative information about the magnitudes of the electric currents associated with the excitation of hair cells. To this end the following physiological questions were investigated:

1. What are the electrical impedance properties of the cochlea? This information is necessary to adequately interpret the resting and evoked cochlear potentials, to compute the magnitudes of electric current associated with their production, and to estimate the energy requirements of the cochlea.

2. What are the sources and characteristics of the cochlear resting potentials and microphonics?

3. Are hair cell systems sensitive to electrical stimulation? Is the electric current associated with the microphonics essential for synaptic transmission?

METHODS AND MATERIALS

Healthy young guinea pigs weighing 250-350 gm were anesthetized with Nembutal®* (35 mg/kg) and fixed in a rigid head holder. Following a tracheotomy the animal was immobilized with Flaxedil®** and placed on artificial respiration. Small holes were drilled in the otic capsule for the insertion of glass microelectrodes into the cochlear scalae to pass extrinsic currents and measure potential changes. Microelectrodes for insertion into the scala media and the perilymphatic scalae were pulled from glass capillary tubing to tip diameters of 2μ and 50μ, respectively. The scala media electrodes were filled 0.11 M KCl; the scala vestibuli and scala tympani electrodes were filled with a gel of Ringer-agar solution. Reference electrodes placed on the exposed muscles of the neck were large Ag-AgCl wires covered with cotton soaked in Ringer's. The potential inside the organ of Corti was measured using ultrafine pipettes (.5μ tip diameter) filled with 3M KCl. Following removal of the round window membrane the pipette was advanced with a motorized hydraulic microdrive at a constant rate of 2-3μ/second through the basilar membrane-organ of Corti (BM-OC) into the scala media.

Acoustic stimuli were generated in a closed system using a condenser microphone cartridge as the driving source. The stimuli were monitored within 1 mm of the tympanic membrane using a calibrated probe microphone. In cochlear experiments involving ethacrynic acid the drug was administered as the sodium salt in dextrose Ringer's solution in a standard dose of 50 mg/kg by infusion into the external carotid artery. Perfusion of the perilymphatic space was accomplished using a 50μ diameter pipette connected to a column of the perfusate by flexible tubing. The perfusate was introduced into the scala vestibuli or scala tympani

* Abbott Laboratories, North Chicago, IL.
** Davis and Geck, div. of American Cyanamid Co., Pearl River, NY.

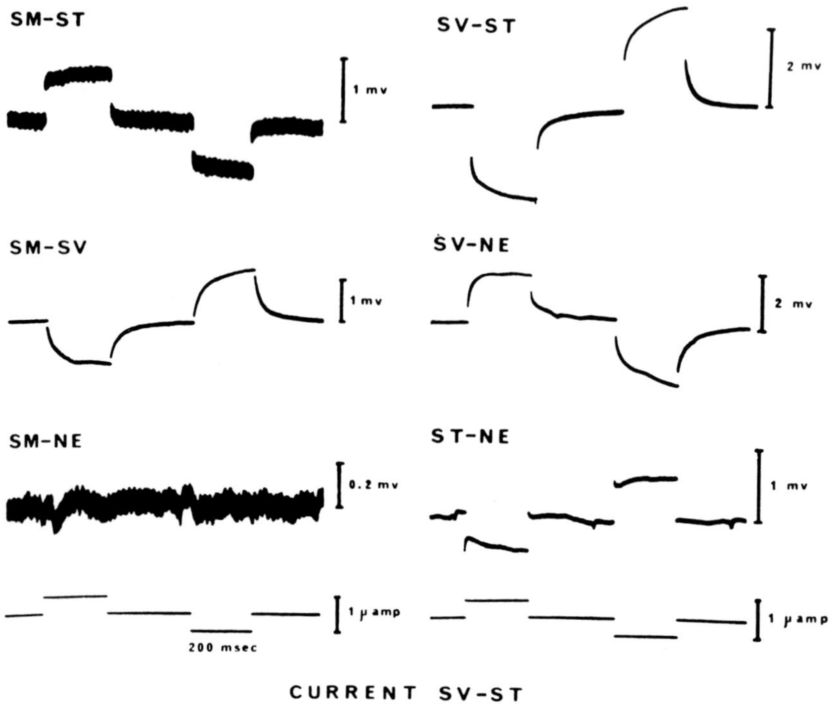

Fig. 3. Photographic records of the six differential voltages observed between the four measurement points in a typical preparation during application of the test current between the SV and the ST in turn I. The recording configuration associated with each record is given at the upper left and the amplitude scale is given to the right. The bottom traces represent the output of the current monitor.

through a fenestra in the otic capsule in the basal turn and escaped via a hole in the apex, where it was removed from the bulla by aspiration. These techniques are described in detail in earlier publications.[22-24]

The *in vitro* preparation of the lateral line organ of the African clawed toad *Xenopus laevis* consisted of a segment of skin including the lateral line organ with its attached nerve. The preparation was mounted in a chamber separating two fluid-filled compartments. The end organ with its cupula projected into oxygenated water which was moved by electromagnetic drivers to provide the physiological (mechanical) stimulus. The inside surface of the skin was covered with a thin layer of Ringer's solution. A short segment of the nerve was attached to a pair of recording electrodes and manipulated so that activity from one or two fibers from a single stitch was recorded. The signals from the electrodes were amplified by a differential ac preamplifier. The remainder of the upper chamber was filled with mineral oil and sealed. To stimulate the preparation electrically, current was passed between a chlorided silver disk in the water chamber and a chlorided silver wire ring attached to the inside of the upper chamber. The voltage across the skin was monitored with chlorided silver wire electrodes. Data processing consisted of the determination of the mean firing rates, PST or cycle histograms, interspite interval histograms as well as analog-to-digital conversion of the stimulus signals. Detailed descriptions of the experimental techniques have been presented in two previous publications.[3,25]

RESULTS

DC Electrical Network Properties of the Guinea Pig Cochlea. The electrical impedances of the walls of the cochlea in 20 guinea pigs were determined using a four-electrode technique in which current was applied between one pair of electrodes and the resulting voltage was measured with another pair. Three pairs of electrodes were introduced into the cochlear fluid spaces of one turn as outlined in Figure 2 and a fourth pair was placed in the subcutaneous space of the neck of the animal. This arrangement made possible 36 different resistance measurements in a given cochlear turn. An example of six recordings made dur-

TABLE I

COMPARISON OF EXPERIMENTAL AND MODEL DRIVING-POINT RESISTANCES BETWEEN DIFFERENT POINTS IN THE COCHLEA

	Experimental	*Model*
SM-ST	9.77 ± 1.19 kΩ	9.76 kΩ
SM-SV	10.85 ± 2.62	10.62
SM-NE	11.43 ± 1.12	12.04
SV-ST	2.72 ± 1.03	2.51
SV-NE	4.06 ± 1.30	4.19
ST-NE	3.22 ± 0.25	3.14

ing application of the test current between the scala vestibuli (SV) and the scala tympani (ST) in the first turn is shown in Figure 3. The measurement of these voltages produced by known amounts of current was used to derive the values of the resistances separating the fluid compartments of the cochlear partition.

The electrical model of the cochlea shown in Figure 1 was found to provide the best quantitative description of the experimental results. The values of the model resistors were determined with the aid of an iterating computer program designed to converge on a best-fit solution for the model resistance values. Table I compares the values of the experimental data (mean ± standard deviation) of the driving point resistance obtained in 20 animals between each of the measuring points in the preparation and the model values selected for the first turn of the cochlea. Since the characteristic length (λ) of the scala media was found to average 3.2 mm, these figures refer essentially to the whole length of the basal cochlear turn. Of significance are the impedances between the scala media (SM) and the rest of the preparation (SM-ST, SM-neck [NE], SM-SV), indicative of the degree of electrical insulation of the endolymph from the perilymph. The model resistance values giving the best fit to the experimental data are listed in Table II. Also tabulated are the voltages and currents in the model after incorporating batteries simulating the biological electromotive sources in the stria vascularis and organ of Corti. To maintain a +80 mV potential in the cochlear duct, the model stria vascularis battery required a value of 304 mV. The estimated energy dissipation associated with the current through the membranes (except that inside the stria vascularis) is approximately 0.19μ watts per millimeter length of the cochlea in the first turn.

TABLE II

VOLTAGE, CURRENT AND RESISTANCE IN THE COCHLEAR NETWORK MODEL

Model Branches	*R (kΩ)*	*V (mV)*	*I (μamp)*
1-2	23.0	74.9	6.74
1-3	42.5	76.7	1.80
1-4	26.0	80.0	3.07
2-4	.75	5.05	6.74
3-4	1.85	3.34	1.80
4-0	2.40	0	0

Resting Cochlear Potentials. According to the model of the cochlea described in Figure 1, there are two sources of current which produce the resting potentials of the cochlea. The major one, highly sensitive to oxygen supply, is located in the stria vascularis.[20] We postulated that the second one is located in the organ of Corti.[26,27] As described in Figure 1A and due to the anatomical and functional asymmetries in the hair cells, there is a constant flow of current from the side of the cells towards their apical surface. This current, by Ohm's law, is proportional to the value of the resting potential in the hair cell and inversely proportional to the resistance in the current loop. The present model predicts that if the current source in the stria vascularis in inhibted, the SM will retain a resting potential due to the currents produced by the hair cells and will become negative relative to the ST or neck by as much as 30 mV. Such a situation has been postulated to occur during anoxia where the potential of the organ of Corti seems to have a survival half-time of 20-30 minutes, much longer than that of the stria vascularis.[22,28] An alternative hypothesis for the negative EP has been that Reissner's membrane is selectively permeable to K^+ ions and,

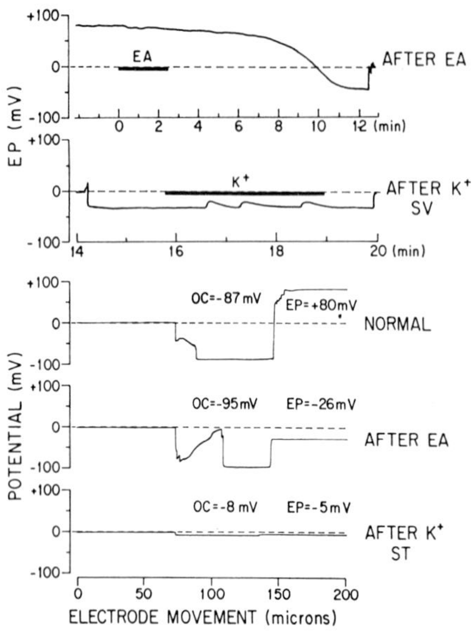

Fig. 4. Effect of ethacrynic acid (EA) administration and K^+ perfusion of the perilymphatic spaces on the cochlear resting potentials. From top to bottom: The first record shows the time course of the decline of the EP following EA administration from +80 to −40 mV. The second record shows the change of the −EP in the scala media during perfusion of the scala vestibuli with .11 M KCl. The third record shows the voltage profile recorded during advancement of a microelectrode from the scala tympani through the basilar membrane and organ of Corti into the scala media in a normal preparation. The fourth record shows a subsequent profile obtained after the EP had been made negative by EA administration. The last record shows the voltage profile recorded subsequent to perfusion of the scala tympani with .11 M KCl.

due to the different concentration of potassium in the endolymph and perilymph, there is a K^+ diffusion potential across the membrane, which becomes evident when the much larger, positive stria vascularis potential is abolished.[29]

Previous attempts to test these two alternatives gave conflicting results because in the anoxic animal perfusion of the scala vestibuli produces a restoration of the EP independently of the ionic composition of the perfusate for different Na^+ or K^+ concentrations. Apparently this is due to the pervasiveness of oxygen in the perfusate fluid.[30,31] The possibility of solving this dilemma was presented after the effect of ethacrynic acid (EA) in the cochlea was demonstrated.[32-34] This drug produces a negative potential in the scala media by interfering with oxidative metabolism, inhibiting the utilization of ATP in spite of the availability of oxygen. Therefore, it was thought that changes in the scala media potential following perfusion of the scala vestibuli with fluid of different ionic compositions would be independent of the oxygen content of the perfusate and would reflect only the effect of differences in the ionic species. Such experiments were conducted in 12 animals. Following the administration of EA the potentials in the scala media and organ of Corti were monitored during perfusion of the scala vestibuli and scala tympani with potassium solutions. A typical example of the changes in the resting potentials produced by EA is shown in Figure 4, top. Within 12 minutes after drug administration the value of the endocochlear potential declined from +80 mV to −40 mV. The change in the magnitude of the EP was similar to that observed during anoxia.[35] In a first series of experiments, replacement of the perilymph in the scala vestibuli with KCl having a K^+ concentration similar to that of the endolymph failed to alter the negative value of the EP except for transient fluctuations due to hydrostatic pressure changes (Fig. 4, top). Perfusion of the scala vestibuli with KCl in normal animals also failed to change the EP. Since the negative EP, if due to a diffusion potential across Reissner's membrane, would have been immediately abolished when the K^+ concentration of the perilymph was made equal to that of the endolymph, it is clear that a K^+ diffusion process cannot be the origin of this potential.

In another series of experiments the perilymph in the scala tympani was replaced by a 0.1 M K^+ solution, also after EA administration. As shown in Figure 4, bottom, the organ of Corti potential remained highly negative while the EP changed from +80 to −26 mV. Following perfusion of the scala

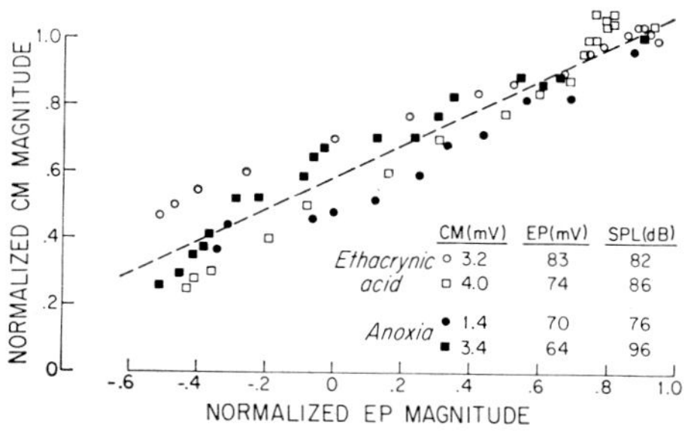

Fig. 5. Plot of peak-to-peak CM magnitude to constant-intensity tone pips vs EP magnitude during EP changes produced by anoxia and administration of ethacrynic acid. The dashed least-square regression line fitting the pooled data has a slope of 0.49 and a correlation coefficient of 0.98.

tympani with K^+, the organ of Corti and the negative endocochlear potentials were greatly reduced. These results are consistent with the hypothesis that the organ of Corti is the source of the negative EP.

Dependence of the Cochlear Microphonics (CM) on the Value of the EP. Three sets of experiments were conducted to test the prediction of the mechanoelectric theory that the magnitude of the CM is proportional to the potential gradient across the top of hair cells. This was accomplished by measuring the CM while the value of the EP was modified by administration of EA, the induction of asphyxic anoxia, and electrical polarization of the scala media in normal and anoxic animals. The changes in the CM concomitant with the change in the EP produced by anoxia and EA in four representative animals are summarized in Figure 5. The amplitude of the CM can be accurately described by a linear function of the EP; the regression line fitted to the data has a slope of 0.49 and a correlation coefficient of 0.98.

A similar linear dependence of the CM amplitude upon the EP magnitude was observed during electrical polarization of the SM in normal animals. Results of experiments in anoxic animals are exemplified in Figure 6, which shows the measurements of the CM and EP obtained from an animal made anoxic half an hour previously. The magnitude of the 300 Hz acoustic stimulus was kept constant while the peak magnitude of the 3 Hz polarizing current was doubled in each of the successive records. In the first record there is approximately 100% modulation of the CM amplitude where the increase in the CM corresponds to an increase in the EP. For large decreases of the EP the initial decrease in the CM is followed by an increase in its magnitude, indicating greater than 100% modulation. The scatter plot on the right shows the relationship between the CM and the EP for the 0 dB record, and the scatter plot on the left shows the variation of CM at different times during the electrical stimulus cycle. When the EP increases there is a linear relationship between the CM and EP. However, when the EP decreases the CM decreases linearly until it reaches a zero value, and further decrease in the EP results in a subsequent increase of the CM but with the phase of the CM changed by 180°. This finding is the strongest experimental evidence obtained to date in support of the mechanoelectric theory of cochlear function. The phase reversal of the CM is due to the change in direction of the current through the variable resistor of the hair cells. A detailed description of these experiments has been published in earlier papers.[22,26]

Electrical Excitability of Hair Cells. The following sequence of events pictorially described in Figure 7, left, is believed to take place in the cochlea during acoustic stimulation: Movement of the stapes towards the vestibule results in a displacement of the basilar membrane towards the ST, whereas an outward movement of the stapes results in a displacement of the basilar membrane towards the SV. During the latter there is a decrease in the resistance of the hair cells, the potential in the SM diminishes, and more current flows through the hair cells. This in turn results in an increase of the frequency of action potentials in the acoustic nerve.

In Figure 7, right, are shown the

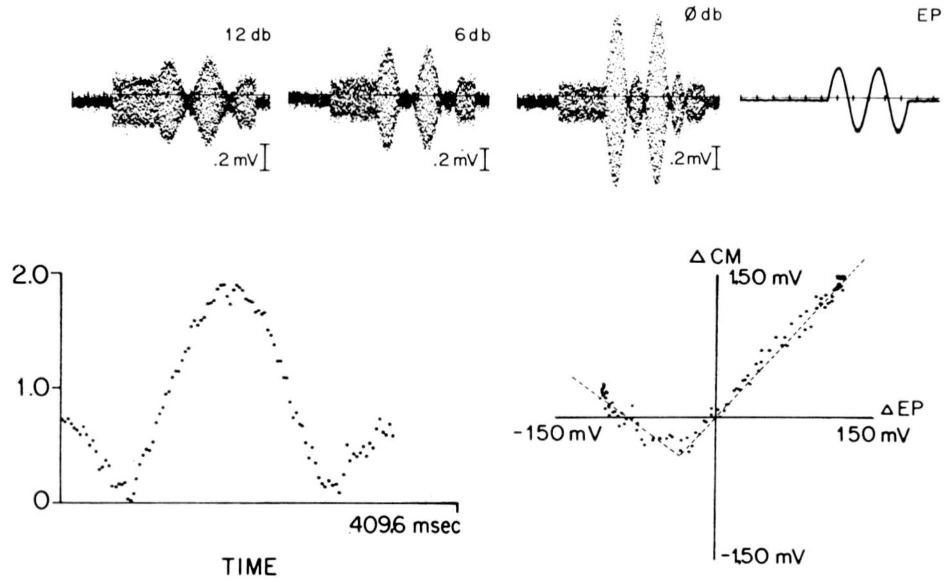

Fig. 6. Modulation of the CM response inside the scala media to 300 Hz acoustic stimuli by 3 Hz extrinsic currents. The upper three left records illustrate the degree of modulation achieved at three different test current magnitudes. The record to the upper right shows the variation of the EP during polarization. The bottom left record shows the variation of the CM amplitude over one cycle of the polarizing current; in this example the current amplitude corresponds to 0 dB of the upper records. The bottom right figure is a plot of peak-to-peak CM amplitude vs the magnitude of the EP during polarization at the 0 dB level of extrinsic current. The inflection of the curve is due to the phase reversal of the CM as the EP swings through −20 mV.

changes that should occur during electrical polarization of the SM with extrinsic currents. If the hair cells are electrically excitable in the absence of basilar membrane motion, an increase of the SM potential would increase the current through the hair cells and the firing of action potentials in the afferent fibers. It is significant that during acoustic stimulation the increase in neural activity should take place during decrease of the EP, whereas during electrical stimulation the increase should be concomitant with the increase of the EP.

To obtain experimental evidence that the hair cell systems are sensitive to changes in electrical potential in their vicinity, measurements were made of the change in firing rate of the two afferent nerve fibers innervating one stitch of the lateral line of the *Xenopus laevis* during mechanical stimulation and during the application of voltage across the hair cells. This preparation was selected because it is easily accessible for well controlled electrical and mechanical stimulation.[25]

In Figure 8, left, are shown the responses of the fibers (A and B) to a 16 Hz, 158mμ peak-to-peak water movement past the cupula of the stitch. On the right are shown the responses of the same fibers to a 16 Hz, 43 mV peak-to-peak electrical potential applied across the skin near the stitch. Whereas the two fibers responded approximately 180° out of phase when stimulated mechanically, suggesting that they innervate groups of hair cells having different morphological polarization, they responded in phase when stimulated electrically. This result is predicted by the mechanoelectric hypothesis and also demonstrates that the electrical stimulus does not produce suprathreshold mechanical movements. The electrical threshold for a 16 Hz sinusoidal electrical stimulus in six fibers ranged from 0.23 to 0.93 mV with a mean value of

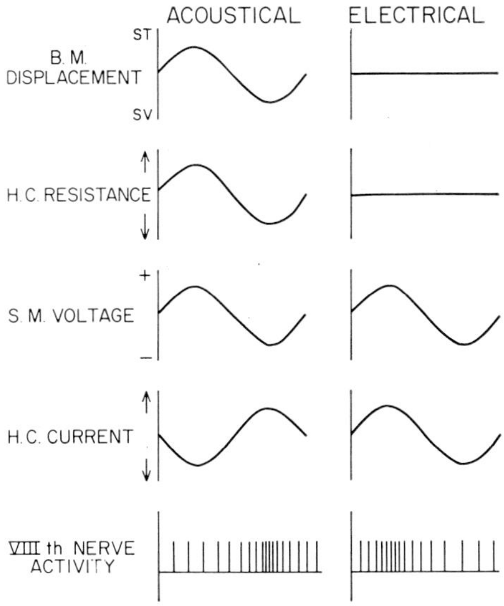

Fig. 7. Summary of the theory of changes taking place in the peripheral auditory system at different stages in the sequence of events culminating in modulation of the impulse activity in the VIII nerve fibers. The left column depicts the changes occurring during acoustic stimulation while the right column depicts the changes occurring during stimulation with extrinsic currents applied across the organ of Corti. It is important to note that for acoustic stimuli the theory predicts an increase in hair cell current and increased neural activity during the decrease of the EP, whereas during polarization with extrinsic currents, increased hair cell current and increased neural activity is associated with the increase of the EP.

0.59 mV. The slopes of the regression lines (on log-log plots) describing the relationship between the amplitudes of the neural responses and the electrical and mechanical stimuli were not significantly different, having slopes of 0.822 ± 0.031 and 0.738 ± 0.115, respectively, and exhibiting a dynamic range of 40 dB. Thus, at any point within the fiber's dynamic range an equal change in the firing rate occurs when the amplitude of the stimulus is changed by a given amount in decibels, be it mechanical or electrical.

The wide dynamic range and the low threshold of the response to electrical stimuli support the hypothesis that the extrinsic electric potentials act upon the hair cells rather than on the myelinated nerve fibers directly. During anoxia the spontaneous and evoked response activity to physiological and electrical stimuli were abolished while the nerve fibers remained excitable and able to propagate nerve impulses antidromically towards the epithelial layers of the stitch. This suggests that the lack of oxygen initially affects transmission at the hair cell-neuron synapse but not the excitability of the myelinated axons.

It was also demonstrated (Fig. 9) that the neural response to a high-frequency (32 Hz) mechanical stimulus is modulated by low-frequency (2 Hz) electrical stimuli. At any instant during the electrical stimulus cycle the magnitude of the neural response evoked by the mechanical stimulus was directly proportional to the magnitude of the applied voltage. That the response is proportional to the product rather than to the sum of the two stimuli is a significant finding which should be incorporated in any model of the transduction process of hair cell systems and is also consistent with the postulates of the mechanoelectric theory.

DISCUSSION

Two important aspects of the physiological properties of the peripheral auditory system have recently been pointed out by quantitative biochemical studies in the inner ear and measurements of the neural responses of single auditory nerve fibers: 1) there is a high rate of energy consumption in the cochlea,[34] and 2) the frequency selectivity of the auditory fibers is greater than can be accounted for by the mechanical filter properties of the basilar membrane.[36,37]

The results of the present experiments are significant in relation to the above observations. They corroborate the conclusions of biochemical investigations, showing that the production of the cochlear potentials requires a high rate of energy expenditure. The information obtained from electrical measurements regarding the energy expenditure in the cochlea provides an opportunity for gaining insight into the

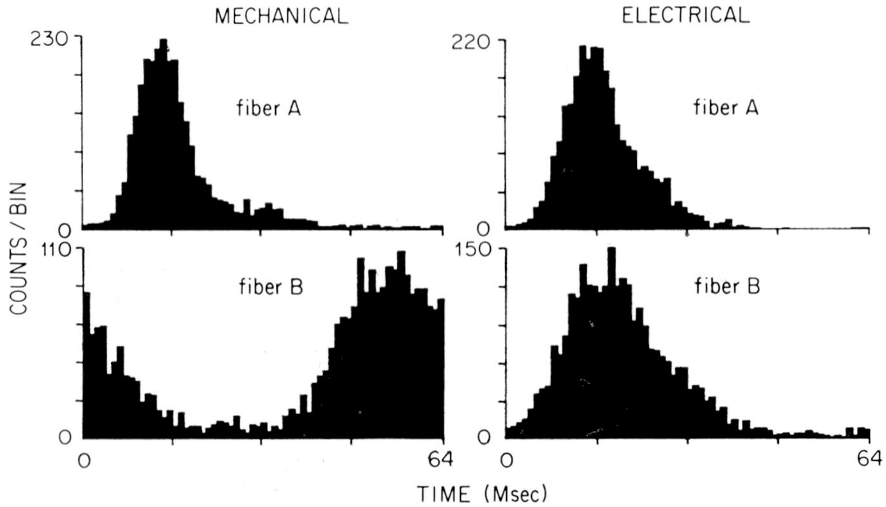

Fig. 8. Cycle histograms of the evoked neural responses recorded simultaneously in the two afferent nerve fibers (A and B) innervating a single stitch in the lateral line organ of *Xenopus laevis.* The left column shows the responses in the two fibers during mechanical stimulation of the cupula by 16 Hz sinusoidal water movements. The right column shows the responses recorded in the same two fibers during application of a 16 Hz sinusoidal extrinsic current across the skin near the stitch.

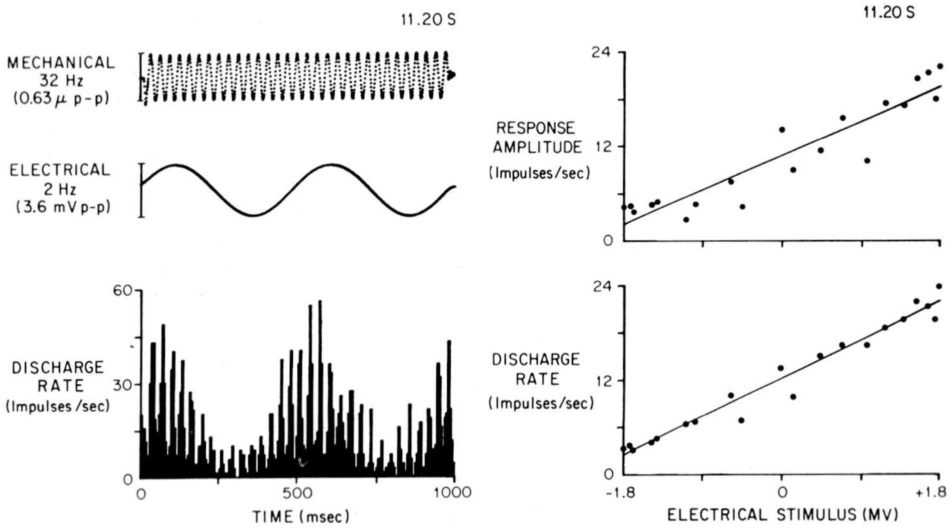

Fig. 9. Neural response of a fiber innervating the *Xenopus laevis* lateral line organ (bottom left) in response to the combination of mechanical (top left) and electrical (middle left) stimuli. Peak-to-peak amplitude of the neural response to the mechanical stimulus (top right) and average discharge rate (bottom right) as functions of the value of the electrical stimulus.

relationship between the bioelectric and biochemical events taking place in the peripheral auditory transduction process. The finding that hair cell systems are electrically excitable suggests that the microphonics are not an epiphenomenon but play an important role in the excitatory process in the cochlea and that electrical interactions (at the hair cell level) may contribute to enhance the frequency selectivity of the cochlea.

Biochemical investigations have revealed two major energy stores in the cochlea which could serve as the necessary sources of electromotive force for generating and maintaining the cochlear potentials. In the stria vascularis the "total energy reserve"* amounts to 245 mmoles of ~P/KDW. A minimum estimate of the rate of consumption of this energy is 65-80 mmoles of ~P/KDW/minute, equivalent to a dissipation of approximately 125μcal/hour/mm of stria vascularis or 0.15μwatts/mm. The second major pool of energy is in the organ of Corti. The "total energy reserve" of average organ of Corti amounts to 500-530 mmoles of ~P/KDW, and the estimated rate of consumption of this energy is 15-21 mmoles/KDW/minute, equivalent to 31μcal/hour/mm or 0 036μwatt/mm**. The amount of energy dissipated in the cochlea by the constant flow of electric current according to our estimates is 0.19μwatt/mm, not including the stria vascularis resistance of Figure 1B. Of this energy 0.16μwatt/mm or 84% is dissipated at the site of transduction in the hair cells.

A strong parallelism exists between the rate of expenditure of biochemical energy in the stria vascularis and organ of Corti and the sources of electromotive force required in the network model of Figure 1B to generate and maintain the cochlear resting potentials. In the model, for example, the organ of Corti battery contributes about 2μamp or 30% of the total 6.7μamp current through the hair cells. On the basis of the biochemical data the consumption of energy in the organ of Corti appears to amount to 20% of the total energy consumed in the organ of Corti and stria vascularis combined. Considering the vastly different approaches used to arrive at these two figures the agreement is quite remarkable. Another interesting parallelism exists between the decline of ATP in the organ of Corti and the decline of its resting potential with a half-time for both of approximately 20-30 minutes.[34] Evidently, due to efficient anaerobic energy generation and because of a relatively low rate of energy utilization, the resting potential of the organ of Corti can be maintained during anoxia for prolonged periods. By contrast, ATP levels in the stria vascularis cannot be maintained for any length of time in the absence of oxygen, presumably due to its extremely high rate of energy utilization. This estimate is supported by the experimental finding that the half-time of the positive component of the EP following anoxemia is approximately one minute.[35]

In the cochlear network model the change in the hair cell resistance required to produce a microphonic having an amplitude similar to that recorded in the guinea pig[24,39] is consistent with the impedance change of the cochlear partition observed during acoustic stimulation.[23,40]

In the guinea pig first turn the amplitude of the microphonics elicited by a 200 Hz acoustic stimulus at 60 dB SPL is about 0.2 mV peak-to-peak. According to the present model such a microphonic is generated by hair cell resistance changes amounting to 34 ohms peak-to-peak. This impedance change results in a change in the power dissipation by 5.6×10^{-14} watts. When compared with the power of the acoustic input (2.5×10^{-14} watts) a ratio of 2.2 is obtained for the energy gain of a 6.4 mm length of the cochlea. However,

---

* The "total energy reserve" represents the sum of high energy phosphate (~P) in mmoles/kg dry weight (KDW) available from preformed ATP and P-creatine and potentially available from glycolytic breakdown of glucose and glycogen to lactate.[38]

** Thalmann R: Personal communication

over the whole length of the cochlea the power dissipated in the hair cell resistances over the length of the travelling wave is conservatively estimated to be 7.4 x 10^{-12} watts which gives a total power gain of 296. Thus, the quiescent current through the hair cells makes possible the amplification of acoustic energy in the sequence of events leading to excitation of the VIII nerve fibers. It should be noted that the mechanical energy losses in the middle ear and basilar membrane were not taken into account in these computations and that the actual effective power gain may be many times greater than the amount given.

The magnitude of the changes in the endocochlear potential during acoustic stimulation due to the production of the microphonic and summating potentials is significantly greater than the voltages required to evoke neural responses in the *Xenopus* lateral line. Interactions between inner and outer hair cells are therefore quite plausible, and if the effective mechanical stimuli upon each group of cells or their responses are different, as has been suggested,[16,41,42] frequency selectivity could be enhanced.

Recent experimental evidence suggests that interactions do exist between inner and outer hair cells[41,43-45] and that the electrical properties of the cochlea influence the characteristics of neural responses.[37,46] Theoretical studies on the model to investigate this possibility indicate that the magnitude of the current changes in the inner hair cells during simulated acoustic stimulation of the outer hair cells may be only 6 dB smaller than in the outer hair cells themselves,[47] with the characteristic that the direction of current flow is opposite in each group of hair cells as depicted in Figure 7. Consequently, if the extracellular potentials measured in the cochlea do in fact reflect the relative magnitudes of the inner and outer hair cell currents accurately, a rather complicated interaction can be produced if the amplitude ratios and phase differences of the currents vary nonlinearly with frequency and sound pressure level. Such an interaction could play an important role in determining the frequency selectivity of the auditory nerve fibers.

REFERENCES

1. Davis H: Some principles of sensory receptor action. Physiol Rev 41:391-416, 1961
2. Fuortes MGF: Generation of responses in a receptor, in Lowenstein WR (ed): *Handbook of Sensory Physiology: I.* New York, Springer-Verlag, 1971, pp 243-268
3. Bauknight RS, Strelioff D, Honrubia V: Effective stimulus for the *Xenopus laevis* lateral line hair cell system. Laryngoscope, to be published
4. Lowenstein O, Wersäll J: A functional interpretation of the electron microscopic structure of the sensory hairs in the cristae of the elasmobranch *Raja clavata* in terms of directional sensitivity. Nature (Lond) 184:1807-1810, 1959
5. Goldberg JM, Fernández C: Physiology of peripheral neurons innervating semicircular canals of the squirrel monkey. I. Resting discharge and response to constant angular accelerations. J Neurophysiol 34:635-660, 1971
6. Harris GG, Frishkopf FS, Flock Å: Receptor potentials from hair cells of the lateral line. Science 167:76-79, 1970
7. Weiss TF, Mulroy MJ, Altmann DW: Intracellular responses to acoustic clicks in the inner ear of the alligator lizard. J Acoust Soc Am 55:606-619, 1974
8. Davis H, Derbyshire AJ, Lurie MH, *et al*: The electric response of the cochlea. Am J Physiol 107:311-332, 1934
9. Tasaki I: Nerve impulses in individual nerve fibers of guinea pig. J Neurophysiol 17: 97-122, 1954
10. Kiang NYS, Watanabe T, Thomas EC, *et al*: *Discharge Patterns of Single Fibers in the Cat's Auditory Nerve.* Res Monograph 35, Cambridge, MIT Press, 1965
11. Rose JE, Brugge JF, Anderson DJ, *et al*: Phase-locked response to low-frequency tones in single auditory nerve fibers of the squirrel monkey. J Neurophysiol 30:769-793, 1967
12. Furukawa T, Ishii Y: Neurophysiological studies on hearing in gold fish. J Neurophysiol 30:1377-1403, 1967
13. Flock Å: Sensory transduction in hair cells, in Lowenstein WR (ed): *Handbook of Sensory Physiology: I.* New York, Springer-Verlag, 1971, pp 396-441
14. Sand O, Ozawa S, Hagiwara S: Electrical and mechanical stimulation of hair cells

in the mudpuppy. J Comp Physiol Psychol 102:13-26, 1975

15. Davis H: A model for transducer action in the cochlea. Cold Spring Harbor Symp Quant Biol 30:181-190, 1965

16. von Békésy G: *Experiments in Hearing.* New York, McGraw-Hill, 1960

17. Lorente de Nó R: The sensory endings in the cochlea. Laryngoscope 47:373-377, 1937

18. Kimura RS: The ultrastructure of the organ of Corti. Int Rev Cytol 42:173-222, 1975

19. Spoendlin H: The innervation of the cochlear receptor, in Møller A (ed): *Basic Mechanisms in Hearing.* New York, Academic Press, 1973, pp 185-234

20. Tasaki I, Spyropoulos CS: Stria vascularis as source of endocochlear potential. J Neurophysiol 22:149-155, 1959

21. Davis H, Deatherage BH, Rosenblut B, *et al*: Modification of cochlear potentials produced by streptomycin poisoning and by extensive venous obstruction. Laryngoscope 68: 596-627, 1958

22. Honrubia V, Ward PH: Dependence of the cochlear microphonics and summating potential on the endocochlear potential. J Acoust Soc Am 46:338-392, 1969

23. Strelioff D, Haas G, Honrubia S: Sound-induced electrical impedance changes in the guinea pig cochlea. J Acoust Soc Am 51:617-620, 1972

24. Honrubia V, Strelioff D, Ward PH: A quantitative study of cochlear potentials along the scala media of the guinea pig. J Acoust Soc Am 54:600-609, 1973

25. Strelioff D, Honrubia V, Bauknight RS: Stimulus control for the study of the *Xeopus laevis* lateral line hair cell system. J Electrophysiol Tech 5:35-43, 1976

26. Honrubia V, Ward PH: Mechanism of production of cochlear microphonics. J Acoust Soc Am 47:498-503, 1970

27. Strelioff D: A computer simulation of the generation and distribution of cochlear potentials. J Acoust Soc Am 54:620-628, 1973

28. Butler RA: Some experimental observations on the dc resting potentials in the guinea pig cochlea. J Acoust Soc Am 37:429-433, 1965

29. Kuijpers W, Bonting SL: The cochlear potentials: II. The nature of the cochlear resting potentials. Pfluegers Arch 320:359-372, 1970

30. Honrubia V, Johnstone BM, Butler RA: Maintenance of cochlear potentials during asphyxia. Acta Otolaryngol (Stockh) 60:105-112, 1965

31. Johnstone BM: Genesis of the cochlear endolymphatic potential, in Sanadi DR (ed): *Current Topics in Bioenergetics.* New York, Academic Press, 1967, pp 335-352

32. Prazma J, Thomas WG, Fisher ND, *et al*: Ototoxicity of ethacrynic acid. Arch Otolaryngol 95:448-456, 1972

33. Bosher SK, Smith C, Warren RL: The effects of ethacrynic acid upon the cochlear endolymph and stria vascularis. Acta Otolaryngol 75:184-191, 1973

34. Thalmann R, Kusakari J, Miyoshi T: Dysfunction of energy releasing and consuming processes of the cochlea. Laryngoscope 83:1690-1712, 1973

35. Konishi T, Kelsey E, Singleton GT: Negative potentials in scala media during early stages of anoxia. Acta Otolaryngol (Stockh) 64:107-118, 1967

36. Geisler CD, Rhode WS, Kennedy DT: Responses to tonal stimuli of single auditory nerve fibers and their relationship to basilar membrane motion in the squirrel monkey. J Neurophysiol 37:1156-1172, 1974

37. Robertson D: Cochlear neurons: frequency selectivity altered by perilymph removal. Science 186:153-155, 1974

38. Lowry OH, Passonneau JV, Hasselberger FX, *et al*: Effect of ischemia on known substrates and cofactors of the glycolytic pathway in the brain. J Biol Chem 239:18-20, 1964

39. Honrubia V, Strelioff D, Sitko ST: Electroanatomy of the cochlea: Its role in cochlear potential measurements, in Ruben RJ, Elberling C, Salamon G, (eds): *Electrocochleography.* Baltimore, University Park Press, to be published

40. Geisler CD, Adrian HO, Mountain DC, *et al*: Electrical impedance changes in the guinea pig cochlea recorded during tonal stimuli. J Acoust Soc Am 58, Suppl No. 1:S31, 1975

41. Karlan MS, Tonndorf J, Khanna SM: Dual origin of the cochlear microphonics, inner and outer hair cells. Ann Otol Rhinol Laryngol 81:696-704, 1972

42. Dallos P: Cochlear potentials and cochlear mechanics, in Møller A, (ed): *Basic Mechanisms of Hearing.* New York, Academic Press, 1973, pp 335-372

43. Kiang NYS, Moxon EC, Levine RA: Auditory-nerve activity in cats with normal and abnormal cochleas, in Wolstenholme GEW, Knight J, (eds): *Sensorineural Hearing Loss.* London, Churchill, 1970, pp 241-268

44. Ryan A, Dallos P: Effect of absence of cochlear outer hair cells on behavioural auditory threshold. Nature 253:44-46, 1975

45. Zwislocki JJ, Sokolich WG: Neuro-mechanical frequency analysis in the cochlea, in Zwicker E, Terhardt E, (eds): *Facts and Models in Hearing.* New York, Springer- Verlag, 1974, pp 107-177

46. Johnstone JR, Johnstone BM, Yates GK: Cochlear neurons: frequency selectivity altered by conductance change in scala tympani. J Acoust Soc Am 57:1210-1211, 1975

47. Strelioff D, Sitko ST, Honrubia V: Role of inner and outer hair cells in neural excitation. Trans Am Acad Ophthalmol Otolaryngol, to be published

-----

ACKNOWLEDGMENTS—We wish to acknowledge the cooperation of Doctors D. McPherson, G. Haas, and T. Dodson, Mr. J. Shallit and Mr. R. Metson, who participated in the performance of different experiments. We thank Dr. Ruediger Thalmann for his critical reading of our manuscript and helpful suggestions. Thanks are due to Ms. M. Oreck for her editorial help.

REPRINTS—Vicente Honrubia, MD, Division of Head and Neck Surgery (Otolaryngology), University of California, Los Angeles, CA 90024.

PSYCHOSOCIAL CARE OF THE DYING PATIENT

A postgraduate course in Psychosocial Care of the Dying Patient will be presented June 3-4, 1977 by the Cancer Research Institute and Extended Programs in Medical Education, University of California School of Medicine, San Francisco, CA.

ESSAY CONTEST

The American Cleft Palate Education Foundation, Inc. announces its annual essay contest for high school students, lay persons, graduate students and novice professionals. Winners will receive cash and a plaque. For information contact: Dr. Curtis Weiss, Essay Contest Committee Chairman, University of Nevada, Department of Speech Pathology and Audiology, Reno 89557, telephone (702) 784-4887.

Ann Otol 85: 1976

SAFE LEVEL FOR NOISE EXPOSURE?

Barbara A. Bohne, PhD
St. Louis, Missouri

SUMMARY – The safety of long, continuous exposure to several different levels of noise was determined. Chinchillas were exposed for two or nine days to an octave band of noise with a center frequency of .5 kHz or 4 kHz. By examining the inner ear for evidence of acute cellular degeneration, exposures which produced minimal permanent damage could be identified easily. Differences were found between the two bands of noise in the level required to produce injury, and the type, location and extent of damage which occurred as the level was increased. The findings help explain why exposure to industrial noise, which is generally low frequency, first produces measurable auditory changes for high frequency tones.

A number of studies have shown that both man[1-4] and animals[5-8] sustain temporary hearing losses following some exposures to noise. The losses are termed "temporary" because pure-tone auditory thresholds return to preexposure levels after the subjects are removed from the noise field. In this situation, use of the word temporary may be misleading since the ability to detect slight permanent damage in the ear is dependent on the technique used to assess the condition of the auditory system. Minimal damage to the organ of Corti cannot be detected if only pure-tone thresholds are determined at discrete frequencies. Examination of the inner ear shortly after exposure to noise for evidence of recent cellular degeneration is the best technique for determining whether or not the exposure produced any permanent injury. The safety of exposure to noise at several different levels was assessed using this anatomical technique. The findings in this study are the subject of the present report.

Carder and Miller[5,6] were first to describe the production of stable or asymptotic temporary threshold shifts in chinchillas following prolonged exposure to noise. They found that the pure-tone thresholds of chinchillas exposed to an octave band of noise with a center frequency of .5 kHz continued to worsen for 24 hours after the start of the exposure. At this time, the thresholds reached an asymptote and continued exposure for up to nine days resulted in no additional loss of sensitivity. The amount of shift at asymptote (in dB) increased regularly with increasing sound pressure level (SPL) of the exposing band. Following removal from the noise field, the animals' thresholds returned to preexposure levels within three to seven days. These results were later duplicated using an octave band of noise centered at 4 kHz.[7,8]

Preliminary anatomical study of ears which had recovered completely from asymptotic threshold shifts (ATS) of 50 dB revealed that all ears were missing small to moderate numbers of outer hair cells.[9] The finding of hair cell loss after recovery from an ATS was later confirmed by Lim and Melnick.[10] This unexpected finding prompted the question, "Are any long, continuous exposures to noise safe?" The present study concerning the condition of the organ of Corti shortly after exposure to noise was designed to give at least partial answers to this question.

From the Department of Otolaryngology, Washington University School of Medicine, St. Louis, Missouri. This work was supported by NINCDS with NIH grants NS-01791 and NS-11417 to the Department of Otolaryngology, Washington University School of Medicine, and grant NS-03856 to the Central Institute for the Deaf, St. Louis, Missouri.
Presented at the meeting of the American Otological Society, Inc., Palm Beach, Florida, April 25-26, 1976.

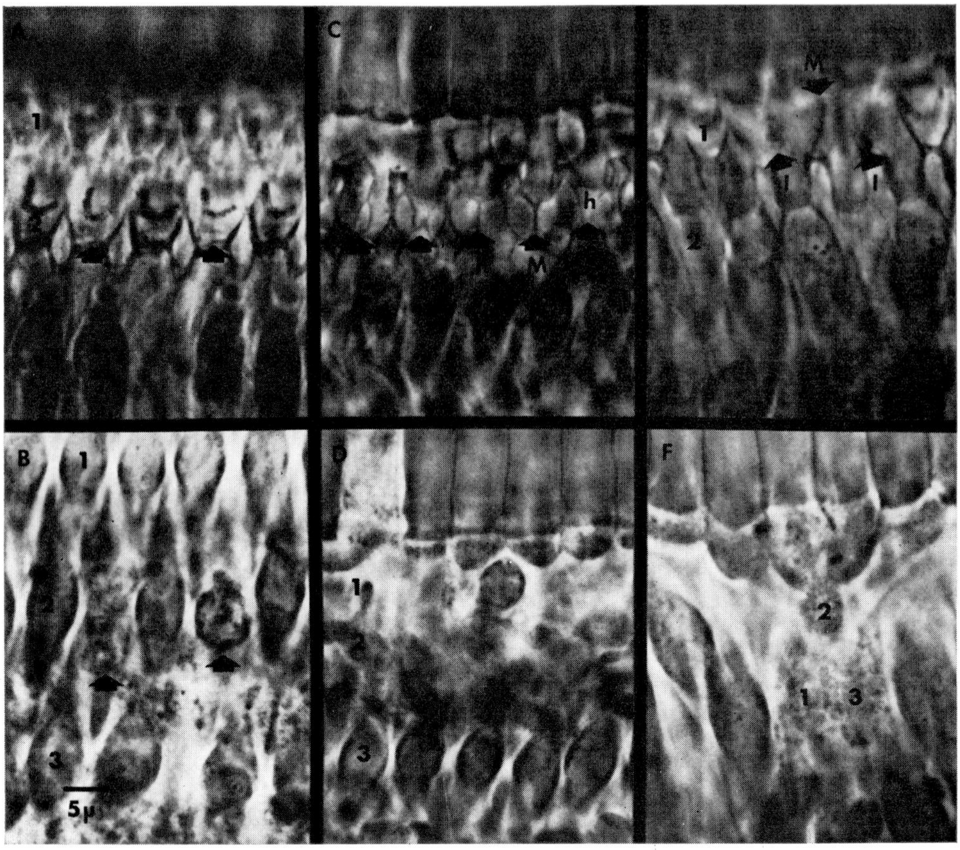

Fig. 1. Phase contrast photomicrographs illustrating acute acoustical injury in outer hair cells. All specimens were perfused less than one hour after termination of noise exposure. A) Two cells in second row (arrows) seem paler than normal and have fewer stereocilia. B) Below reticular lamina in "A." Cells with pale apices are in process of degenerating since cellular debris (arrows) is all that remains. C) All cells in second row have degenerated. Phalangeal scars are in process of forming so small holes (h) (arrows) remain in reticular lamina. One immature scar, characterized by a faint central line (I), is also present. This stage follows complete closure of the hole in the reticular lamina and is reached when phalangeal processes first come together. Mature scar differs from immature scar by having a dense central line (M) between phalangeal processes. D) Below reticular lamina in "C." One cell body is present in first row and none in second. E) Three cells are missing in first row. Scar in center has dense central line (M) and hence must be considered mature. Scars on either side have pale central junctions (I) and are therefore immature. F) Below reticular lamina in "E." Cellular debris is found beneath each missing cell (1, 2, 3). Thus, the cell replaced by the mature scar in "E" had only recently degenerated.

METHODS AND MATERIALS

For this experiment, 27 chinchillas* averaging 13.4 months of age (range 8-28 months) without a history of noise or ototoxic drug exposure were used. All were housed in sound-shielded animal quarters until the time of their exposure. They were removed from their quarters and exposed to noise in the unanesthetized state in the chamber described by Carder and Miller.[5,6] The chinchillas were exposed for two or nine days to an octave band noise (OBN) with a center frequency of either .5 kHz or 4 kHz. For the .5-kHz OBN, the sound pressure level of the exposure was 65, 75, 85, 95 or 108 dB (re .0002 μbar). For the 4-kHz OBN, the sound pressure level was 57, 65, 72, 80 or 86 dB (re .0002 μbar).

* There were 49 ears available for study. In five animals, one ear had been sectioned before the method for determining acute cell loss had been developed.

Thus, the experimental animals were exposed for two or nine days to one of two different octave bands of noise at one of five different sound levels. The rationale behind the use of multiple exposure levels was to have ears with asymptotic threshold shifts which varied from approximately 10 dB, the minimum detectable, to greater than 50 dB, the level already shown to produce sensory cell loss. Some of the levels used for these exposures (.5-kHz OBN at 75, 85 and 95 dB SPL; 4-kHz OBN at 57, 65, 72 and 80 dB SPL) were the same as those used in the earlier behavioral studies.[5-8] Other animals were exposed to the .5-kHz OBN at 65 dB SPL. This level was chosen because straight-line extrapolation of the ATS data[5,6] suggested that no threshold shift would result from this exposure. Finally, additional chinchillas were exposed at levels known or suspected to produce permanent threshold shifts (.5-kHz OBN at 108 dB SPL; 4-kHz OBN at 86 dB SPL). Animals were exposed at the different levels for two or nine days in order to determine whether or not the ear reaches an "asymptote" as far as sensory cell loss is concerned.

Following termination of their exposures, the chinchillas were anesthetized, their bullae surgically exposed and the cochleae perfused with a buffered solution of 1% osmium tetroxide (pH 7.4) at 4 C. The cochleae of all animals were perfused less than one hour following termination of the noise exposure. After fixation, the specimens were dehydrated, infiltrated with plastic and prepared for phase contrast microscopic examination as embedded whole mounts.[11]

In cochleae preserved shortly after the termination of a noise exposure, the damaged cells in the organ of Corti will be in various stages of degeneration and the reticular lamina will still be in the process of healing.[12,13] For this reason, it is possible to differentiate between cells which degenerated prior to exposure and those which degenerated as a result of it. As an outer hair cell begins to degenerate, that portion of its plasma membrane which borders on the Nuel spaces is first to disintegrate. When this occurs, cytoplasmic and nuclear debris can be found beneath the intact apical membrane of the hair cell (Figs. 1A, B). Once the apical membrane disappears, a hole the exact size of the missing cell is left in the reticular lamina. The phalangeal processes which surround the degenerated sensory cell soon begin to enlarge so that smaller holes of variable sizes and shapes are found in the reticular lamina (Figs. 1C, D). When the phalangeal processes first come together, a faint central line of union between the processes is visible (Fig. 1C). Later, with deposition of electron-dense material adjacent to the cell membranes, the central line appears much darker (Fig. 1C). These phalangeal scars are designated "immature" and "mature" respectively.[12,13] If the mature scar has only recently formed, cellular debris can still be seen beneath the scar (Figs. 1E, F).

Mature phalangeal scars require approximately 48 hours to form.[13] Thus, one would not expect to find a large number of mature scars* in the cochleae of animals exposed to noise for two days. In chinchillas exposed for nine days, more mature scars may be present because some immature scars could have matured during the exposure. Nevertheless, there should still be evidence of acute injury (cellular debris, *etc.*) in ears exposed for nine days. If an ear perfused shortly after exposure has numerous mature phalangeal scars and little or no cellular debris, one can postulate that the majority of missing cells could not have degenerated very recently. In this case, it would be impossible to determine how many cells would have been damaged by the exposure since so many were missing prior to the exposure.

When counting missing sensory cells in ears exposed for two days, only those cells which were in the process of degenerating, or replaced by open holes or immature scars were included in the totals. All missing cells were included in the totals in ears exposed for nine days since some scars may have matured during the exposure. After tabulating the number of missing sensory cells, the percentage loss** was calculated for each segment of the organ of Corti.

In addition to calculating the percentage of missing sensory cells, the extent (from base to apex) of the lesions was determined. A given segment of the organ of Corti was considered to be involved in the injury if there were ten or more recently-degenerated sensory cells in any single row or if there was one recently-degenerated cell in at least two rows. Thus, areas having mature scars only were not included. Very rarely one finds a cell in the process of degenerating in nonexposed ears. By setting the above criteria, areas with small "spontaneous" cell losses were presumably eliminated.

RESULTS

Of the original group, two experimental animals were judged to have

* Nonexposed chinchilla ears have an average of 39 mature phalangeal scars replacing missing outer hair cells. These scars are scattered throughout the organ of Corti and never amount to more than 1.5% in any segment, excluding the apical half-turn of the organ of Corti.[14]

** In a series of 18 normal ears, it has been found that the chinchilla organ of Corti averages 18.37 mm in length and has 405 OHC and 102 IHC/mm. To determine percentage missing, the number missing (based on actual counts) was divided by the calculated total (based on above averages) in the segment.

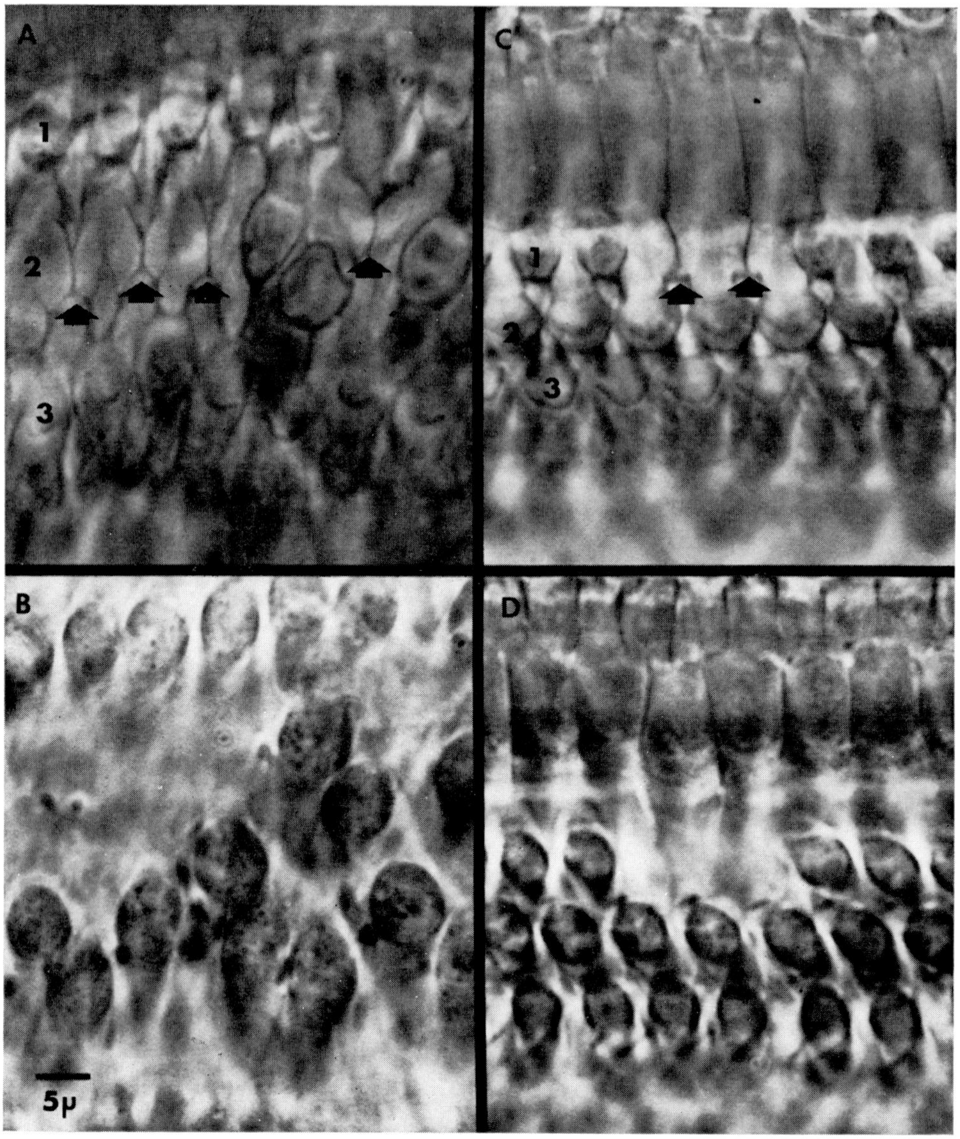

Fig. 2. Phase contrast photomicrographs of noise-exposed cochleae which were judged to have had large cellular losses prior to exposure. A) Third turn of ear exposed for nine days to .5-kHz OBN at 75 dB SPL. Four mature phalangeal scars (arrows) are visible in reticular lamina. B) Below reticular lamina in "A." No cellular debris is present beneath scars. Thus, it is unlikely that these cells degenerated very recently. C) First turn of ear exposed for nine days to 4-kHz OBN at 57 dB SPL. Two mature scars (arrows) are present in first row. D) Below reticular lamina in "C." No cellular debris is present.

had large cellular losses prior to their noise exposures. One had been exposed for nine days to the .5-kHz OBN at 75 dB SPL and the other for nine days to the 4-kHz OBN at 57 dB SPL. Both ears of each animal had a large number of mature phalangeal scars and little cellular debris (Fig. 2). The percentage loss of sensory cells in these ears was far in excess of that in other ears exposed at higher levels. Therefore, these animals were dropped from the study

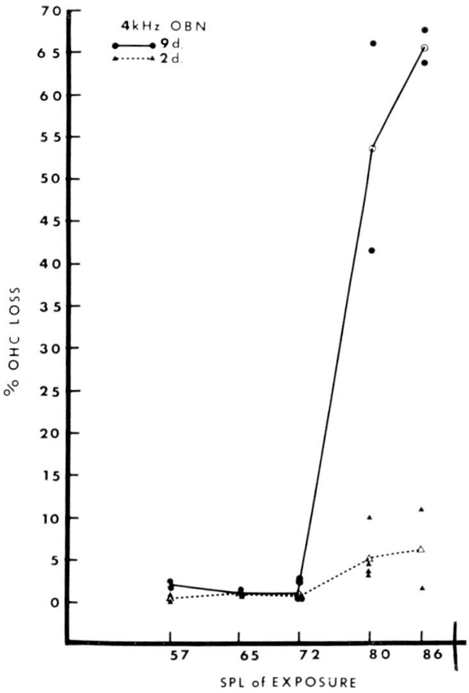

Fig. 3. Graph showing average percentage missing OHC in segment with worst injury in lower first turn of ears exposed for two or nine days to 4-kHz OBN at 57, 65, 72, 80 or 86 dB SPL. Solid data points show percentages from individual ears. There were at least two ears at each exposure level.

and replaced by two other animals with comparable ages and histories.

Although the percentage loss of sensory cells was calculated for each segment of the organ of Corti from every cochlea, presentation of all values would make this report unnecessarily long. Therefore, in order to condense the data, the "severity of injury" in each ear was determined by locating the segment having the greatest percentage loss of sensory cells. The only restriction was that the segment be between 10% and 40% of the distance from the apex for ears exposed to the .5-kHz OBN and between 70% and 90% for ears exposed to the 4-kHz OBN. These are the regions thought to be stimulated maximally by the respective exposures, according to the traveling wave theory. At the higher intensity levels, exposure to the .5-kHz OBN produced damage over a large extent of the basilar membrane. In some of these cases, the percentage loss of hair cells in the base exceeded that in the upper turns. Nevertheless, data on "severity of injury" in ears exposed to the .5-kHz OBN was taken from the lower third to upper second turns only.

Severity of Injury: 4-kHz OBN

Two-Day Exposure. Ears exposed for two days to the 4-kHz OBN at 57, 65 or 72 dB SPL had no more than five acutely-injured outer hair cells in the lower first turn of the cochlea. The percentage of missing outer hair cells never exceeded 1% in any segment (Fig. 3). Four of the six ears exposed at these levels had lost at least one outer pillar in the same area. When the level was increased to 80 or 86 dB SPL, the severity of injury increased to 5.2% and 6.4% respectively (Fig. 3). All ears exposed at the two higher levels had lost some outer pillars. The ears with the greatest loss of outer hair cells were missing the largest number of outer pillars.

Nine-Day Exposure. Ears exposed for nine days to the 4-kHz OBN at 57 or 65 dB SPL had fewer acutely-injured outer hair cells than those exposed for two days. However, the percentage of missing cells in the nine-day ears increased slightly (2.1% and 1.2% respectively) because counts of mature scars were included in the totals (Fig. 3). None of these ears was missing any pillar cells. Exposure at 72 dB SPL produced variable damage in the individual ears. Two ears had no acute cell losses at all, whereas two other ears averaged 13 acutely-injured outer hair cells in the lower first turn. Of the latter two ears, one was missing two inner and one outer pillar while the other was missing five outer pillars in the region of injury. The amount of damage in these ears was still minimal (Fig. 3).

There was a dramatic increase in damage in the ears exposed at 80 dB SPL over those exposed at 72 dB. In the 80-dB ears, outer hair cell loss averaged 54% (Fig. 3). In addition, a large number of inner and outer pillars

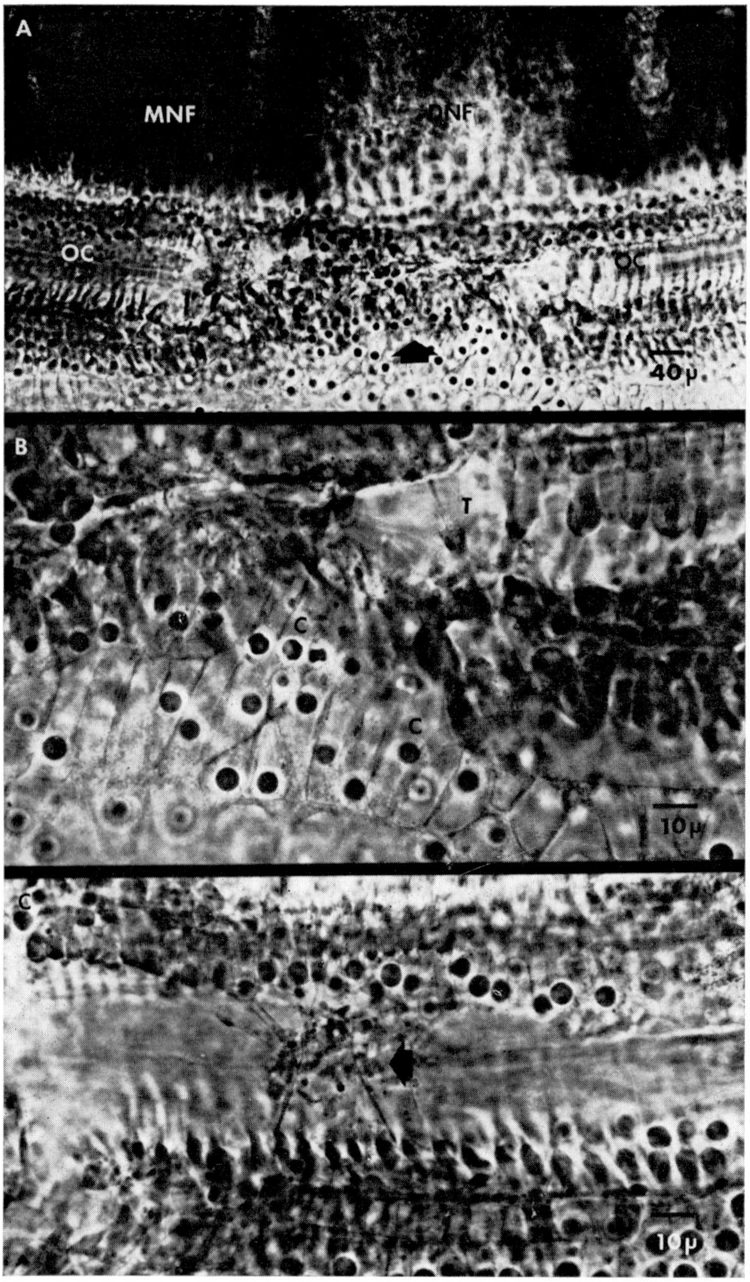

Fig. 4. Phase contrast photomicrographs of first turn of ear exposed for nine days to 4-kHz OBN at 80 dB SPL. A) At low power, area of complete destruction (arrow) of organ of Corti (OC) can be seen. Myelinated nerve fibers (MNF) in osseous spiral lamina adjacent to damaged organ of Corti have already begun to degenerate (DNF). B) Higher power of destroyed area shows Claudius' cells (C) have begun to seal off open ends of tunnel (T). C) Focused on tunnel space (T) in area adjacent to destroyed region in "A." Many radial tunnel fibers have ruptured and extruded axoplasm (arrow) into tunnel space.

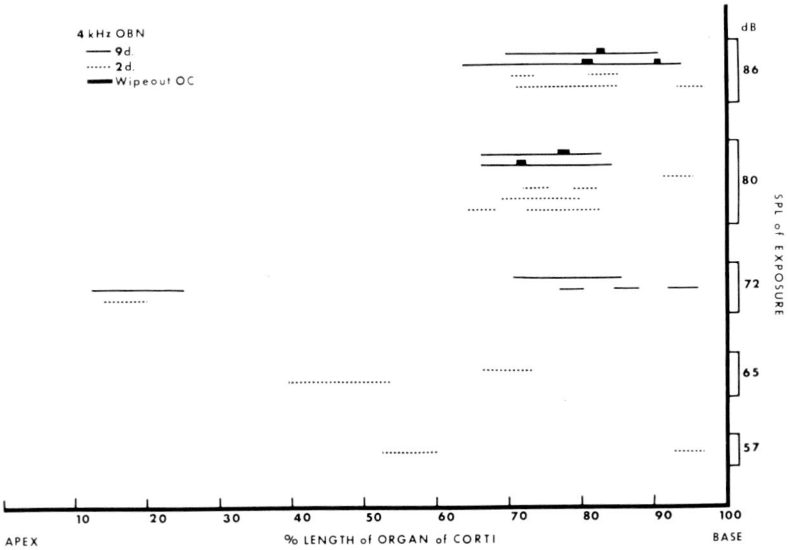

Fig. 5. Graph showing extent and location of acute OHC damage (see text) in individual ears exposed for two or nine days to 4-kHz OBN at 57, 65, 72, 80 at 86 dB SPL. Some ears are not shown because exposure at lower levels did not injure enough cells to meet criterion for identifying areas of acute injury. Wide black bar indicates area in which entire organ of Corti (all sensory and supporting cells) had degenerated.

had degenerated (41 and 43 respectively). In regions where all inner and outer pillars were gone, all inner hair cells were missing too. Exposure at 86 dB SPL produced outer hair cell loss which averaged 66% (Fig. 3). Inner and outer pillar loss had increased to 49 and 62 respectively. All inner hair cells were gone in areas where the inner and outer pillars had degenerated.

Figure 4 illustrates the appearance of the area of maximal injury in an ear exposed for nine days to the 4-kHz OBN at 80 dB SPL. A .27 mm long portion of the organ of Corti has degenerated and nerve fibers to that area are already in an advanced state of degeneration (Fig. 4A). Evidently the missing portion of the organ of Corti had degenerated within a few days after the start of the exposure. Evidence of sealing of the open ends of the tunnel space and reepithelialization of the bare portion of the basilar membrane by the Claudius' cells was clearly visible at the end of the nine-day exposure (Fig. 4B). In areas of the organ of Corti adjacent to the degenerated region, radial tunnel fibers showed signs of severe damage including clumping of axoplasm and extrusion of it into the tunnel space (Fig. 4C).

Extent of Injury: 4-kHz OBN

As indicated above, the area of maximal injury in the organ of Corti following exposure to the 4-kHz OBN was located in the lower first turn. Occasionally (4 ears), a few degenerating outer hair cells (<7) were seen in the second or third turns (Fig. 5). However, this cell loss never amounted to more than 2% in any segment and averaged only 1.2%.

The extent of the acute injury in the lower first turn was slightly greater in ears exposed for nine days at 86 dB SPL than ears exposed at the lower levels (Fig. 5). The only ears in which an entire segment of the organ of Corti had degenerated were those which had been exposed for nine days at 80 or 86 dB SPL (Fig. 5). In these ears, all the degenerated portions of the organ of Corti had appearances quite similar to that illustrated in Figure 4.

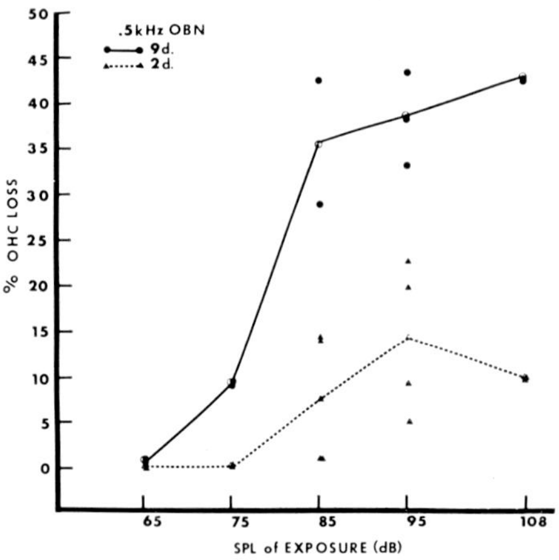

Fig. 6. Graph showing average percentage missing OHC in region with worst damage in lower third turn of ears exposed for two or nine days to .5-kHz OBN at 65, 75, 85, 95 or 108 dB SPL. Solid data points show percentages from individual ears. There were at least two ears at each exposure level.

Severity of Injury: .5-kHz OBN

Two-Day Exposure. Figure 6 summarizes data on the percentage loss of outer hair cells in the lower third to upper second turns as a function of exposure level. Ears exposed for two days at 65 or 75 dB SPL had no more than six acutely-injured outer hair cells in that region. The percentage of missing outer hair cells averaged .3% and .2%, respectively. None of these ears was missing any pillar cells. Exposure at 85 dB SPL produced variable results in the individual ears. Two ears averaged 11 acutely-injured outer hair cells and no pillar loss, whereas two other ears averaged 170 missing outer hair cells (14%). In the area of damage, one of the latter two ears was missing three outer and one inner pillar. Increase of the level of the exposure to 95 or 108 dB SPL resulted in outer hair cell losses which averaged 14.2% and 9.7% respectively. There were no degenerated pillar cells in the third turn in any of these ears.

Nine-Day Exposure. Exposure for nine days to the .5-kHz OBN at 65 dB SPL did not produce any increase in the number of acutely-injured outer hair cells over that seen in the two-day ears. Ears exposed at 75 dB SPL averaged 76 acutely-injured outer hair cells which amounted to 9.3% loss in the third turn (Fig. 6). In the same area, one of the 75-dB ears was missing three outer and four inner pillars while the other had lost only one inner pillar.

Outer hair cell loss averaged 35.7% in the third turn in ears exposed at 85 dB SPL (Fig. 6). In the same region, one ear had lost 12 outer pillars while the other was missing seven outer and three inner pillars. Exposure at 95 dB SPL produced outer hair cell losses averaging 38.2% (Fig. 6). Two of the three 95-dB ears had lost two outer pillars in this area. Average outer hair cell loss in the third turn of ears exposed at 108 dB SPL was 42.9% (Fig. 6). One of these ears was missing 17 outer and 15 inner pillars while the other was missing 48 outer and 44 inner pillars.

All seven of the ears exposed for nine days at 85, 95 or 108 dB SPL had one or more regions in the third turn where a number of adjacent outer hair cells had degenerated (Figs. 7A, B). In only one case (one of the 108-dB ears) was there an associated large loss of inner and outer pillars. In these same ears, myelinated nerve fibers in the osseous spiral lamina showed no signs of damage. There was some indication of injury to the radial tunnel fibers as evidenced by slight axoplasmic clumping (Fig. 7C).

Extent of Injury: .5-kHz OBN

Exposure for two days to the .5-kHz OBN at 75 dB SPL produced minimal hair cell damage which was restricted to the lower third turn of the cochlea (Fig. 8). Exposure for nine days at 75 dB SPL did not increase cell loss in any segment. However, damage was found to extend both apically and basally from the lower third turn. In addition, one of the latter ears had an area of acute cell loss in the lower first turn. Increasing the level of the exposure produced damage that spread over a larger extent of the basilar membrane in the third and second turns and the lesion

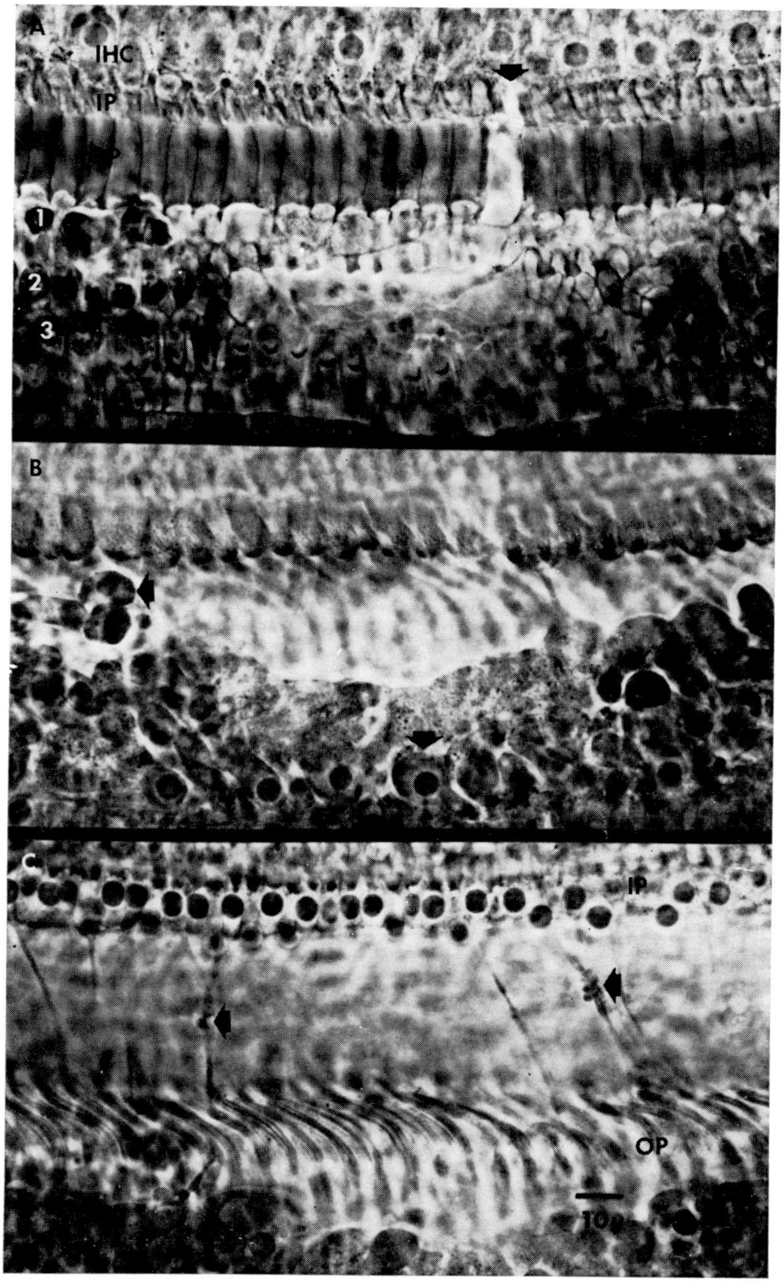

Fig. 7. Phase contrast photomicrographs of third turn of ear exposed for nine days to .5-kHz OBN at 108 dB SPL. A) Reticular lamina (partly out-of-focus) shows large number of missing cells in first (1) and second (2) rows. One outer pillar (OP) and one inner pillar (IP) have degenerated (arrow). Most inner hair cells (IHC) are present. B) Below reticular lamina in "A." The few OHC bodies that remain are swollen and/or distorted (arrows). C) Focused on tunnel space (T) in "A." Minimal damage, as evidenced by clumping of axoplasm (arrows) in radial tunnel fibers, can be seen. IP - inner pillar bases; OP - outer pillar bodies.

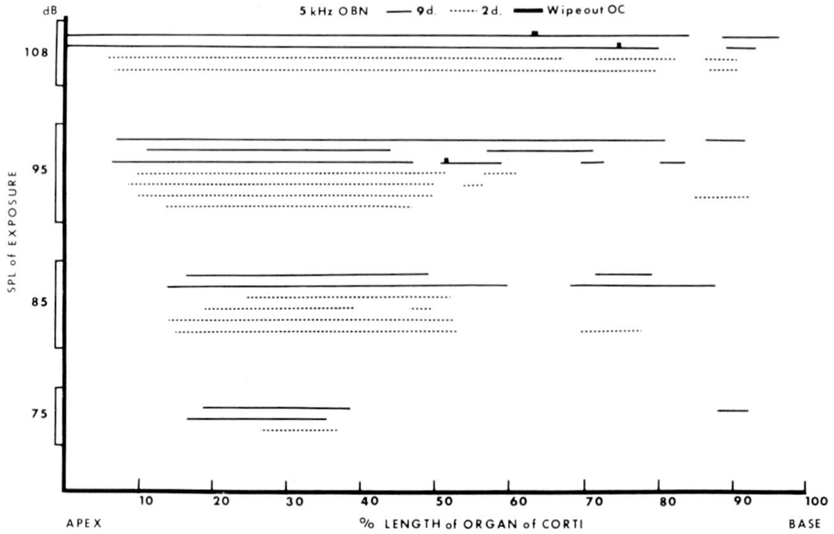

Fig. 8. Graph showing extent and location of acute OHC damage (see text) in individual ears exposed for two or nine days to .5-kHz OBN at 75, 85, 95 or 108 dB SPL. Some ears are not shown because exposure at lower levels did not injure enough cells to meet criterion for identifying areas of acute injury. Wide black bar indicates area in which entire organ of Corti (all sensory and supporting cells) had degenerated.

in the lower first turn appeared more frequently. The basal turn lesion was present in all ears exposed for nine days at 85, 95 or 108 dB SPL and became progressively worse as the level increased. In general, the lesion in the base was located between 70% and 90% of the distance from the apex. In one of the three ears exposed for nine days at 95 dB SPL and three of the four ears exposed at 108 dB SPL, the lesion in the upper turns extended far enough basally to merge with the lesion in the base.

In one of the three ears exposed for nine days at 95 dB SPL and both exposed for nine days at 108 dB SPL, there was a small area in which the entire organ of Corti had degenerated. The location of the region of degeneration was not consistent. It was found in the upper first turn in one ear, the middle first turn in the second ear, and the lower first turn in the third ear (Fig. 8).

Figure 9 illustrates the appearance of the degenerated portion of the organ of Corti in the upper first turn of the ear exposed at 95 dB SPL. Only the most peripheral parts of the nerve fibers in the osseous spiral lamina were beginning to disintegrate and demyelinate (Fig. 9A). This is indicative of the recent loss of the organ of Corti. It must have degenerated quite late during the nine-day exposure period as there is little evidence of sealing of the open ends of the tunnel space (Fig. 9B). In areas of the organ of Corti adjacent to the degenerated region, the radial tunnel fibers appeared moderately damaged with clumping of axoplasm and some extrusion of it into the tunnel (Fig. 9C). The degenerated portions of the organ of Corti in the ears exposed at 108 dB SPL had appearances very similar to that illustrated in Figure 9.

Summary of Pillar Damage

All ears (14) exposed to the 4-kHz OBN having losses of outer hair cells in the first turn of .7% or greater were missing some pillar cells. The more hair cells that had been lost, the greater was the loss of pillars. In contrast, 14 out of 17 ears exposed to the .5-kHz OBN which sustained losses of outer hair cells in the lower third turn ranging from .5% to 38% had no pillar damage in

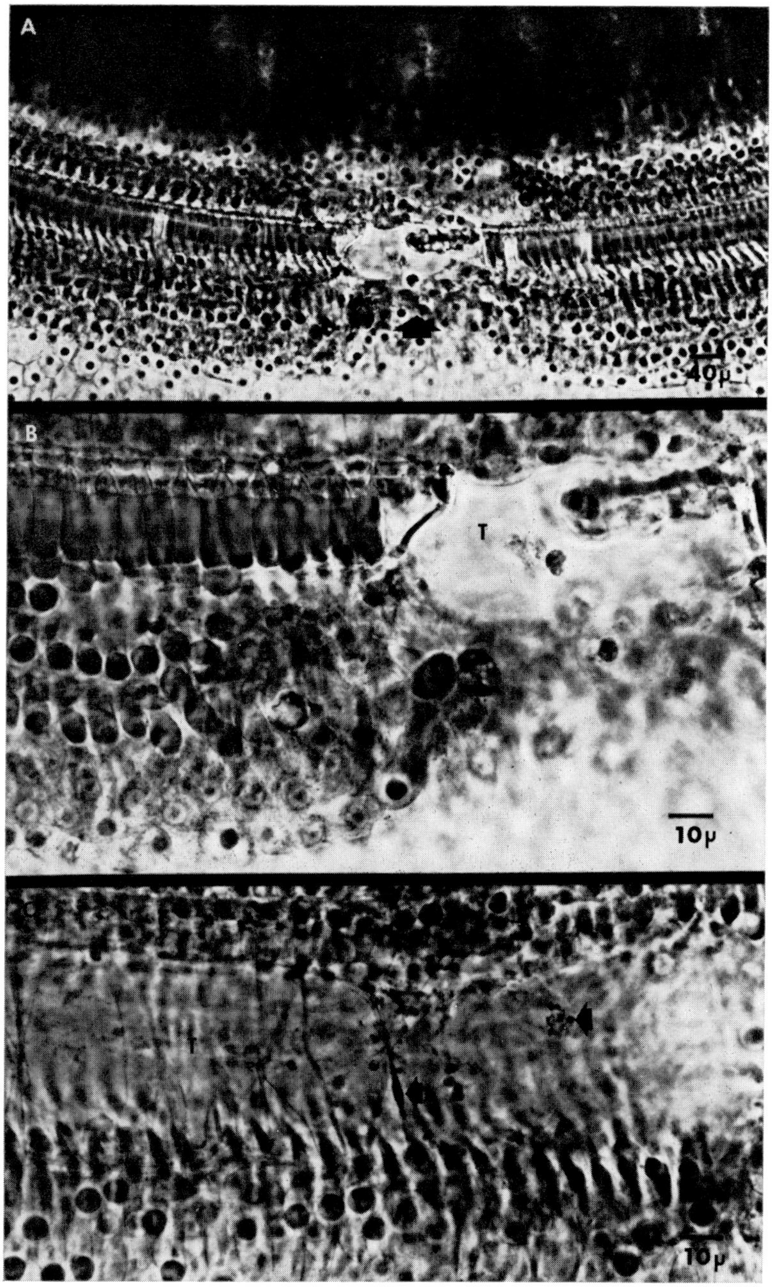

Fig. 9. Phase contrast photomicrographs of first turn of ear exposed for nine days to .5-kHz OBN at 95 dB SPL. A) Low power showing region in which all OHC and OP have degenerated (arrow) as have most IP and IHC. Myelinated nerve fibers to area show minimal damage. B) Higher power of region adjacent to severely-damaged area in "A." Healing of region has not yet begun so tunnel space (T) still communicates with scala media. C) Focused on tunnel space (T) in organ of Corti adjacent to severely-damaged area in "A." Radial tunnel fibers are beginning to show signs of axoplasmic clumping and extrusion (arrows).

the same area. The other three ears had small pillar losses, the largest of which was seven outer and three inner pillars. Only in one of the two ears exposed for nine days at 108 dB SPL did pillar losses become significant in the lower third turn. In the first turn of ears exposed to the .5-kHz OBN, pillar loss was present in one half of the ears (4 out of 8) with outer hair cell losses between .5% and 13% and in all ears (5) with losses greater than 16%.

DISCUSSION

The anatomical technique used to prepare the cochleae for microscopic examination permitted detailed study of the entire organ of Corti at 1250X magnification. All portions of the organ of Corti were available for study since there were no dissection errors. Also, since the organ of Corti was divided into segments by thin pieces of razor blade, there was no loss of material at the cut edges. By examining 100% of each organ of Corti, the possibility of overlooking minimal damage was eliminated.

Fixation of the inner ear shortly after termination of a noise exposure enables one to distinguish between recent and old injuries in the organ of Corti. This is important for two reasons. First, ears which have large lesions which are not related to the exposure can be identified and discarded. Secondly, exposures which produce no acute injury in the ear can be deemed safe, at least for the durations they were presented. In addition, one can be fairly certain that, when present, small cellular losses in the organ of Corti are the direct result of the exposure.

Hair Cell Losses in Relation to ATS

Behavioral studies[7,8] have shown that chinchillas exposed to the 4-kHz OBN sustain asymptotic threshold shifts after 24 hours of continuous exposure. When the octave band values were 57, 65, 72 and 80 dB SPL, the shifts in threshold for a 5.7-kHz tone were 17, 30, 42 and 50 dB, respectively. Once at asymptote, the animals' thresholds remained unchanged until the end of the nine-day exposure. Generally, thresholds returned to preexposure values three to six days after cessation of the exposure. Results of the present study have shown that exposure for two or nine days to the 4-kHz OBN at 57, 65 or 72 dB SPL produces minimal sensory cell degeneration in the organ of Corti. Thus, chinchillas can be exposed to a 4-kHz OBN at 72 dB SPL, the level which results in an ATS of approximately 42 dB, without incurring any significant permanent damage in their inner ears.

Exposure to the 4-kHz OBN for two days at 80 dB SPL, the level which results in a threshold shift of approximately 50 dB[7,8] produces some sensory and supporting cell loss in the lower first turn of the cochlea. Although exposures for up to nine days at this level produced no additional change in threshold, in this study sensory and supporting cell losses continue to increase. Exposure for two or nine days at 86 dB SPL resulted in a threshold shift of 64.6 dB.[8] Sensory and supporting cell losses are always present in ears exposed at this level and are greater in ears exposed for nine days than those exposed for two days. Thus, chinchillas exposed for more than two days to a 4-kHz OBN at a level greater than 72 dB SPL will always have permanent inner ear damage.

Chinchillas exposed to the .5-kHz OBN at 75, 85 or 95 dB SPL sustained asymptotic threshold shifts for a 715-Hz tone of 17, 31 and 49 dB, respectively.[5,6] The magnitude of the shifts remained unchanged for exposures lasting from two to nine days. Thresholds returned to preexposure levels three to seven days after termination of the exposure. Results of the present study have shown that ears exposed for two days at 75 dB SPL have no significant sensory cell loss. However, exposure at this level for nine days does produce outer hair cell losses averaging 10% in the lower third turn of the cochlea. Cell losses were always present in ears exposed at 85 or 95 dB SPL. Ears exposed for nine days at these levels had significantly more damage than those exposed for two days.

Chinchillas exposed for nine days at 65 dB SPL had no more acutely-injured outer hair cells than those exposed for two days. However, straight-line extrapolation of the asymptotic threshold shift data of Carder and Miller[5,6] suggested that no threshold shift would result from this exposure. Since no level has been tested between 65 and 75 dB SPL, the true threshold for injury lies somewhere between the level which is thought to produce no ATS and that which produces an ATS of 17 dB.

Not enough data has been collected to determine if the presence of damage after an ATS exposure follows more closely the level of the exposure or the magnitude of the shift. It is noteworthy that permanent inner ear damage is associated with a .5-kHz OBN exposure producing an ATS of as little as 17 dB. The possibility cannot be rejected that the presence of any ATS after exposure to the .5-kHz OBN indicates that the ear has been permanently damaged. This contrasts with the apparent safety of exposure to the 4-kHz OBN at a level which produces an ATS of 42 dB.

Hair Cell Losses in Relation to Pillar Losses

In cochleae damaged by the 4-kHz OBN, loss of pillars began in the first turn when outer hair cell losses were quite small (.7%) and continued to increase as more and more hair cells degenerated. This contrasts with the situation in ears exposed to the .5 kHz OBN where pillar losses were insignificant in the third turn until outer hair cell loss reached 38%. In the first turn of ears exposed to the .5-kHz OBN, pillar losses were present in some cases when outer hair cell losses were small and in all cases when the hair cell losses were greater than 16%. Thus, it appears that pillars have different susceptibilities to noise exposure depending on their location within the organ of Corti. In the base, pillars are only slightly less susceptible to noise than outer hair cells, whereas in the apex, the pillars are much more resistant than the outer hair cells. These differences in pillar loss may explain the differences in the loss of inner hair cells. Once several adjacent inner and outer pillars had been lost, inner hair cells began to degenerate. Therefore, lesions in the basal turn always included loss of inner hair cells. In the third turn, however, inner hair cell loss was insignificant except in the one ear exposed for nine days at 108 dB SPL which had large pillar losses.

Nerve Fiber Damage in Relation to Sensory and Supporting Cell Loss

The nonmyelinated nerve fibers in the organ of Corti did not show signs of damage until several pillar cells in a restricted region had degenerated. Thus, nerve fiber damage was frequently associated with lesions in the first turn but rarely associated with lesions in the third turn. These findings support the hypothesis that nerve fibers are not damaged during the noise exposure but are injured subsequently by entrance of endolymph into the fluid spaces of the organ of Corti through holes in the reticular lamina.[15,16] Demyelination and degeneration of nerve fibers in the osseous spiral lamina closely followed loss of supporting and inner hair cells.

CONCLUSIONS

1. The method for determining acute cellular degeneration enables one to distinguish between recent and old injuries and therefore to identify clearly noise exposures which produce minimal damage in the organ of Corti.

2. Some long exposures to noise are safe. For the 4-kHz OBN, no significant inner ear damage was seen following an exposure which produced a fairly large ATS (42 dB). In contrast, for the .5-kHz OBN, permanent damage was associated with an exposure which produced a small ATS (17 dB).

3. In the first turn, pillars are nearly as susceptible to noise exposure as outer hair cells. This is not true for pillars in the third turn. These findings help explain why inner hair cells are lost more

readily in the first turn and also why nerve fiber degeneration is generally associated with lesions in the first turn but rarely associated with those in the third turn. These results may explain why exposure to industrial noise, which is usually low frequency, first produces measurable auditory changes for high frequency tones.

4. At the levels of exposure which caused damage, ears exposed for nine days always had more damage than those exposed for two days. The levels used were one which had been shown to produce asymptotic threshold shifts. Although more data is needed (*i.e.*, ears exposed for longer durations), it appears that there is no "asymptote" as far as sensory cell loss is concerned.

5. Because ears exposed for nine days at the lower levels had fewer acutely-injured cells than those exposed for two days, it is hypothesized that these levels would be safe for any duration of exposure. The few acutely-injured cells which were found in these ears probably belong to a small, finite population of cells which are extremely sensitive to noise and are lost quite early during an exposure.

REFERENCES

1. Mills JH, Gengel RW, Watson CS, *et al*: Temporary changes of the auditory system due to exposure to noise for one or two days. J Acoust Soc Am 48:524-530, 1970

2. Mosko JD, Fletcher JL, Luz GA: Growth and recovery of temporary threshold shifts following extended exposure to high-level, continuous noise: report No. 911. Exp Psych Div, US Army Med Res Lab, Ft Knox, Kentucky, 1970

3. Melnick W: Human temporary threshold shift from 16-hour noise exposures. Arch Otolaryngol 100:180-189, 1974

4. Ward WD: Temporary threshold shift and damage-risk criteria for intermittent noise exposures. J Acoust Soc Am 48:461-574, 1970

5. Carder HM, Miller JD: Temporary threshold shifts produced by noise-exposure of long duration. Trans Am Acad Ophthalmol Otolaryngol 75:1346-1354, 1971

6. Carder HM, Miller JD: Temporary threshold shifts from prolonged exposure to noise. J Speech Hear Res 15:603-623, 1972

7. Mills JH, Talo SA: Temporary threshold shifts produced by exposure to high-frequency noise. J Speech Hear Res 15:624-631, 1972

8. Mills JH: Temporary and permanent threshold shifts produced by nine-day exposures to noise. J Speech Hear Res 16:426-438, 1973

9. Eldredge DH, Mills JH, Bohne BA: Anatomical, behavioral and electro-physiological observations on chinchillas after long exposures to noise. Adv Oto-Rhino-Laryng Otophysiology 20:64-81, 1973

10. Lim DJ, Melnick W: Morphological correlates of asymptotic temporary threshold shifts in chinchillas. J Acoust Soc Am 53:292, 1973

11. Bohne BA: Location of small cochlear lesions by phase contrast microscopy prior to thin sectioning. Laryngoscope 82:1-16, 1972

12. Bohne BA, Ward PH, Fernández C: Irreversible inner ear damage from rock music. Trans Am Acad Ophthalmol Otolaryngol 82: 50-59, 1976

13. Bohne BA: Healing of the noise-damaged inner ear, in Hirsh SK, Eldredge DH. Hirsh IJ, *et al* (eds): *Hearing and Davis: Essays Honoring Hallowell Davis.* St. Louis, Washington University Press, 1976, pp 85-96

14. Bohne BA, Eldredge DH, Mills JH: Cochlear potentials and electron microscopy applied to the study of small cochlear lesions. Ann Otol Rhinol Laryngol 82:595-608, 1973

15. Bohne BA: Mechanism for continuing degeneration in the organ of Corti. J Acoust Soc Am 55:S77-S78, 1974

16. Bohne BA: Mechanisms of noise damage in the inner ear, in Henderson D, Hamernik R, Dosanjh DS, *et al* (eds): *The Effects of Noise on Hearing.* New York, Raven Press, 1976, pp 41-68

Acknowledgments—Excellent technical assistance was provided by Rosie Saito and Virginia Schnettgoecke.

Reprints—Barbara A. Bohne, PhD, 517 So. Euclid, St. Louis, MO 63110.

DEGENERATION PATTERNS IN HUMAN EARS EXPOSED TO NOISE

LARS-GÖRAN JOHNSSON, MD
JOSEPH E. HAWKINS, JR., PHD
ANN ARBOR, MICHIGAN

SUMMARY – Various forms of sensorineural degeneration patterns related to noise exposure are illustrated in six pairs of temporal bones selected from a group of 33 male patients with histories of noise exposure. For the entire group the commonest form of lesion, associated with a 4-kHz dip in the audiogram, was a relatively diffuse degeneration in the second quadrant of the basal turn, in the 9-13 mm area. An advanced form of this lesion had a wide gap of more or less complete sensorineural degeneration affecting the entire second quadrant and displaying various degrees of extension toward the apex and base. The pattern associated with an "abrupt high-tone loss," with more or less complete hair cell and nerve degeneration in both the second and first quadrants and extending to the basal end of the cochlea, was rare. In one case this pattern appeared to have evolved from the first type of lesion as the remaining nerve fibers in the first quadrant had degenerated. The protective effect of the acoustic shadow of the head for the right ear, in shooting from the right shoulder, is demonstrated for the higher frequencies. Two almost identical cases of sharply-circumscribed single areas of degeneration in the first quadrant and one case with two such areas represent the third type of lesion. In one of these cases there was a history of firearm usage. It is postulated that this type of lesion is caused by impulse noise. In most of the material the degeneration pattern differed markedly from the diffuse degeneration seen with presbycusis. Degeneration patterns with knife-sharp transitions between completely degenerated and apparently undamaged areas appear to be characteristic of noise-induced injuries.

In the course of our study of human temporal bones by the technique of microdissection,[1,2] we have found a number of specimens displaying distinctive patterns of sensorineural degeneration, obtained at autopsy from patients with a history of noise exposure. The method used enjoys a major advantage over the conventional histological technique employing serial sections, in that it affords an overall view of the organ of Corti and its innervation as well as a detailed view of the pattern of degeneration. Six representative pairs of ears from a total of 33 patients known to have been exposed to noise will be described here. We hope to encourage others to look for similar sensorineural lesions, which may be characteristic of various forms of noise exposure and may be associated with hearing losses having specific audiometric configurations.

In recent years numerous descriptions of noise damage in laboratory animals have been published, while only two reports, involving only a few cases, are available on noise damage in man.[3,4] The more recent of these, that by Bredberg, is also based on microdissection. Both reports confirm the presence of maximum damage in the 5 to 15-mm area of the basal turn, corresponding to the well known noise-induced audiometric "dip" in the 4-6 kHz region. Early reports of cochlear pathology due to noise published by Habermann,[5,6] Brühl,[7] and Zange[8] simply describe se-

From the Kresge Hearing Research Institute and Department of Otorhinolaryngology, University of Michigan Medical School, Ann Arbor Michigan. This investigation was supported by grants from the Research Fund of the American Otological Society, Inc., and from the John A. Hartford Foundation, and by USPHS Research Grants NS 12706, NS 05065, and Program Project Grant NS 05785.

Presented at the meeting of the American Otological Society, Inc., Palm Beach, Florida, April 25-26, 1976.

vere degeneration in the basal turn without specifying the location more precisely.

The recent investigations of the effects of noise exposure on other primate cochleas[9-11] are more instructive for the otopathologist than the studies of laboratory rodents, because of the similarity in cochlear structure and susceptibility to noise between man and monkey, which permits direct comparison of degeneration patterns in human and nonhuman primate specimens. In our laboratory we have studied the effects of octave-band noise on the macaque cochlea.[9,11] In addition to the expected tonotopical damage we found a juxtafenestral lesion[9,12] in the form of complete hair cell loss and severe nerve degeneration at the extreme basal end of the cochlea. Jordan *et al*[10] exposed their monkeys to impulse noise, but some of the degeneration patterns in their animals were similar to ours; in addition to a severe damage in the 10-mm area, they observed degeneration at the basal end corresponding to our juxtafenestral lesion. Their area of degeneration, however, was about twice as extensive as ours.

It is of interest to compare the audiometric patterns recorded in surveys of noise-exposed individuals with temporal bone findings. Audiometric data of Gallo and Glorig[13] indicate that for long-term exposure to fairly steady-state industrial noise, most hearing level changes occur at 3, 4, and 6 kHz in the initial 15 years while at 0.5, 1, and 2 kHz the hearing loss is approximately linear with exposure time. Those authors also found more severe hearing loss in males than in females, although they emphasized that this was due, at least in part, to differences in exposure. There were also great individual differences as to the degree of loss in both sexes. High-tone audiometry has shown that noise also has a deleterious effect on the frequencies above 8000 Hz, and that the characteristic "dips" are not as deep as one would predict from conventional audiograms.[14]

It has often been suggested that impulse noise causes a rather specific type of cochlear damage[15,16] and an audiometric pattern different from that found as a consequence of steady-state noise. In this view, impulse noise would be characterized by abrupt losses or "dips,"[17] and steady-state exposure by more gently sloping losses. This notion is strongly opposed by Ward *et al*,[18] who found no differences in the slopes and patterns of audiograms when hearing losses caused by steady-state noise were compared with those caused by gunfire.

In any case, noise-induced hearing loss is initially most pronounced at 4 kHz, followed by loss at 6, 3, 2, 1, and 0.5 kHz.[13] Several hypotheses attempting to explain the origin of the 4-6 kHz dip have been offered,[15,16] but the exact cause of its occurrence at these frequencies remains obscure.

METHODS AND MATERIALS

The temporal bones were prepared according to our standard technique,[1,2] except that the length of staining time for human material was reduced from ten minutes as previously recommended[1] to five minutes. After perilymphatic perfusion and staining, the otic capsule was removed with burrs and middle ear instruments. After the spiral ligament, Reissner's membrane, and the tectorial membrane were dissected out, the specimens were photographed under a dissecting microscope* while immersed in 70% alcohol and transilluminated by four A-O Model 651 lights. The entire length of the organ of Corti was then removed and mounted as surface preparations.[2] In selected cases all remaining hair cells were counted and plotted as the percentage of the number normally present.[9,11,19] The percentage of cells remaining was calculated on the basis of a regular arrangement of three rows of outer hair cells.[20] However, the pattern of hair cells in man is irregular, especially in the middle and apical turns, where an incomplete fourth and sometimes a fifth row of outer hair cells are present.[2] Such hair cell counts are, therefore, not entirely satisfactory, but they give a fairly reliable picture of the extent of sensory cell loss. The apparent reduction in the number of outer hair cells present and seen in the apical turn beyond the 30-mm point in all cytocochleograms, should probably be regarded as normal, although in some cases it may reflect an apical hair cell loss.[21]

The cases to be reported were selected from our collection of more than 200 pairs of human

---

* Model M-5, Wild Heerbrugg Instruments Inc., Farmingdale, NY.

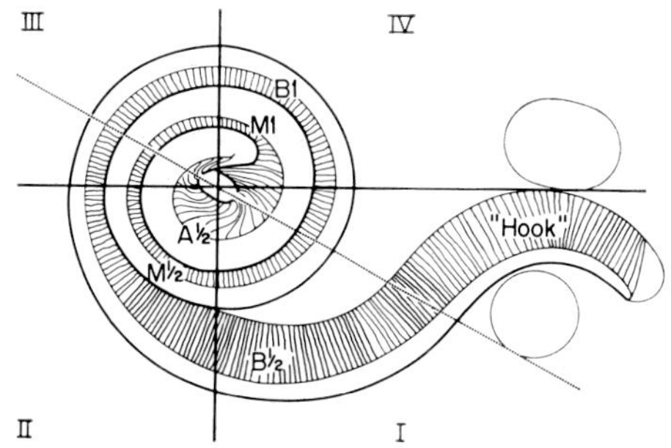

Fig. 1. Division of the basal turn of the human cochlea into four quadrants by axes passing through the helicotrema, as described in the text. The upper turns could be subdivided in the same way. In addition to the imaginary axes (solid), the "Nabeya line" (broken) is indicated, together with the subdivisions of the cochlear turns referred to in our previous publications.[1,2] B½ and B1 are segments of the basal turn, M½ and M1 of the middle turn, and A½ the apical turn. A1, at the extreme apex, is shown but not labeled. It is often small or absent.

temporal bones, most of which were obtained at autopsy in the University of Michigan Hospital, the Ann Arbor Veterans Administration Hospital, or other associated institutions. In response to a questionnaire routinely sent to the next of kin, information indicating a history of vocational and/or recreational noise exposure was obtained in 33 cases. In 20 pairs of bones from this group of patients the pattern of circumscribed degeneration in the basal turn of the cochlea was easily recognized. Cochleas from eight other patients with characteristic dips in their audiograms and a history of noise exposure did not differ markedly from specimens obtained from patients in the same age group who had no such history. Another five pairs of bones were classified as representing patients who had probably been exposed to noise because they showed the characteristic pattern of sensorineural degeneration, even though we were unsuccessful in eliciting information about their owners' histories. For ten of the cases, good clinical audiograms were available, taken one to three years before death.

It should be noted that all of these 33 pairs of bones were obtained from male patients. In the left ear from one female patient we found circumscribed complete loss of hair cells and nerve fibers similar to the lesion in Figure 7b, but there was no history of noise exposure. Many of the patients had worked in the automotive or other noisy industries in the Detroit area, and a number of them had also done game and target shooting.

Six of the cases will be considered in greater detail here.

OBSERVATIONS

For describing and locating cochlear lesions and degeneration patterns we have found it helpful to divide the basal turn into four quadrants by means of imaginary axes passing through the helicotrema (Fig. 1). Since the right and left cochleas are mirror images of each other, the numbering of the quadrants cannot follow the convention of analytical geometry. Instead, the quadrants of the right cochlea are numbered counter-clockwise from the base, and those of the left cochlea clockwise. The first and largest quadrant includes the "hook" and the lower portion of the segment we have referred to elsewhere as B½. The second quadrant includes most of the upper portion of B½, and the third and fourth quadrants most of the upper portion of the basal turn (B1). The middle turn, M½ and M1, and the apical turn A½, could be subdivided in the same way. A1, shown in the diagram but not labeled, is often of negligible size.

I. Lesions of the Second Quadrant

This quadrant is the site of the lesion associated with the 4-kHz dip and is the most common site of maximum damage in our 33 cases.

Case 1. The temporal bones were obtained from a male of 24 years. He had worked for six months in noisy surroundings as a press operator, and had served in the US Army for more than five years as a tank driver on Okinawa and in Vietnam. The audiogram taken at the bedside shows a typical 4-kHz dip of 70 dB in both ears.

Three distinct, small areas of complete absence of the organ of Corti with corresponding areas of nerve degeneration in the osseous spiral lamina are seen in the second quadrant of the basal turn of the left cochlea (Fig. 2), giving the appearance of patchy degeneration similar to that described by Crowe *et al.*[20] The lesion appears to be relatively recent, since the areas of nerve degeneration are not sharply defined, and because there is no visible nerve degeneration associated with a

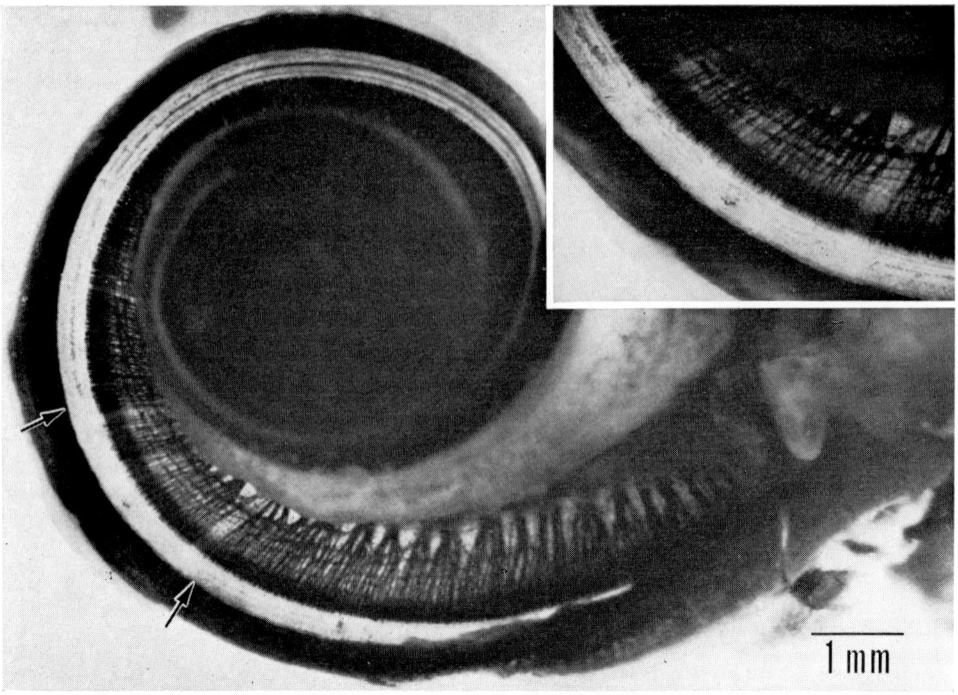

Fig. 2. The left cochlea from Case 1. Note the lesion in the second quadrant between the arrows (insert) with three small sectors of nerve degeneration corresponding to three areas of complete absence of organ of Corti. (OsO_4).

fourth small, bare area of the basilar membrane, halfway between the main lesion and the round window area (not clearly seen in the photomicrograph). The right ear does not display any obvious nerve degeneration, except for the usual changes seen at the basal end.[21]

The type of degeneration pattern observed in this patient is the most frequent in our material, and similar patterns or variations are seen in specimens from seven other patients.

Case 2. The patient, 72-years-old, had not been exposed to industrial noise, but was described as an enthusiastic hunter. The asymmetry of the degeneration seen in his left and right ears (Figs. 3, 4) gives a striking illustration of the protective effect of the acoustic shadow of the head for the right ear of a person shooting right-handed, *i.e.*, from the right shoulder.[22,23] The left ear shows an almost complete absence of the organ of Corti and nerve fibers in the second quadrant. In the first quadrant the pattern of degeneration is more diffuse, and the presence of scattered nerve fibers is well correlated with the survival of supporting elements of Corti's organ. At the beginning of the third quadrant there is a small island of supporting cells, also with a few remaining nerve fibers.

It is important to note that the areas of the osseous spiral lamina which appear light on the photomicrographs and are described as displaying "complete" nerve degeneration are not totally devoid of nerve fibers. When they are scrutinized by phase- contrast or bright-field microscopy a few scattered myelinated nerve fibers are usually found.

In the shadow-protected right ear the injury is much less (Fig. 4). Only one small area of complete absence of sensory and neural elements is seen at the beginning of the third quadrant. There appears to be some thinning out of the nerve pattern in the upper portion of the first quadrant.

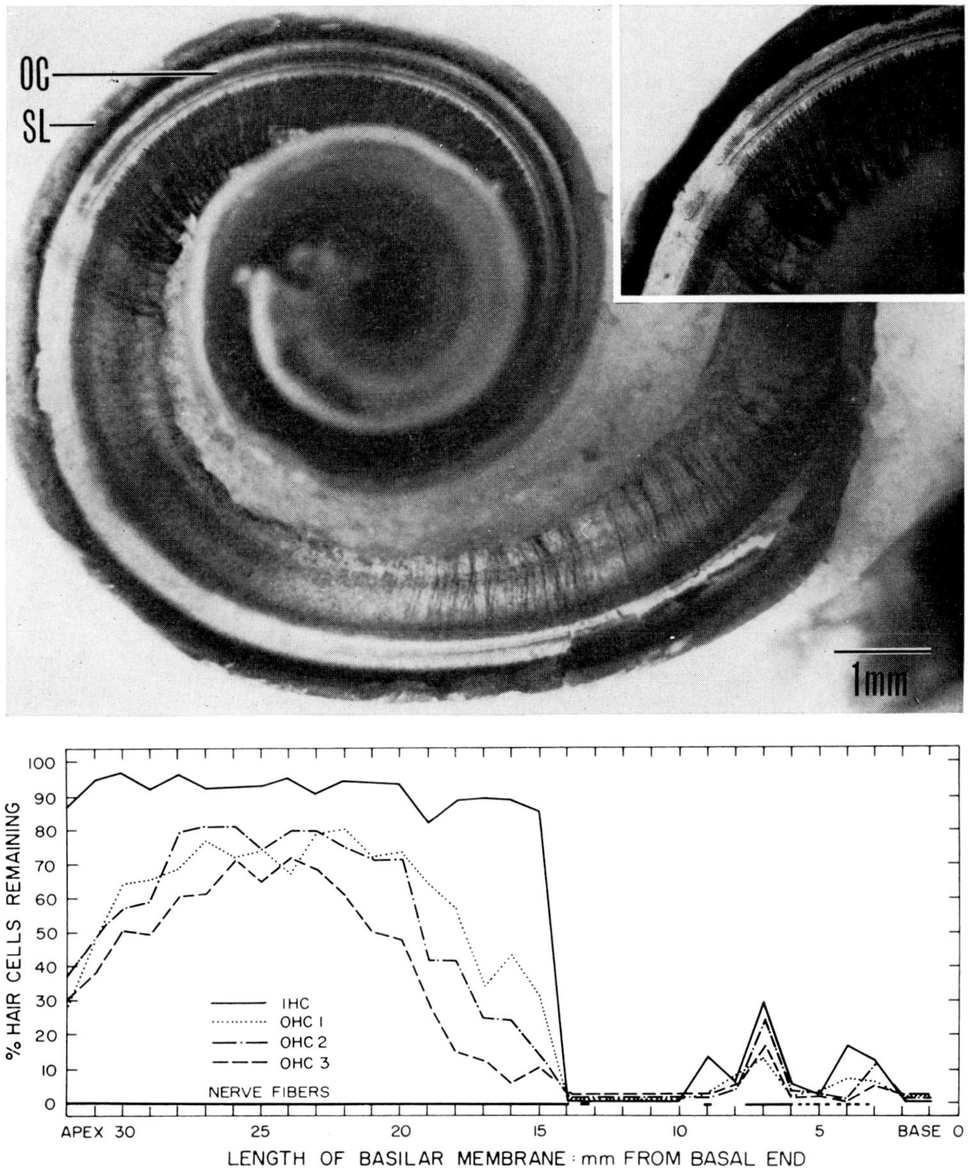

Fig. 3. The left cochlea from Case 2. Organ of Corti (OC), is seen as one wide and one narrow dark stripe, corresponding to outer and inner hair cells. There is a wide gap in the second quadrant with complete loss of organ of Corti and nerve fibers. Note at the upper border of the lesion a small island of supporting cells (insert) with a few nerve fibers. Compare Figure 4, right ear. (OsO_4) SL - Spiral ligament. The cytocochleogram is shown below. The black horizontal bar indicates presence of nerve fibers in the osseous spiral lamina, see text. The apparent hair cell loss at the apex represents the normal irregularity of pattern in the apical turn; see Methods. IHC - Inner hair cells, OHC - Outer hair cells.

Cytocochleograms for these two ears are shown in Figures 3 and 4. The difference in the extent and severity of the lesions in the basal turn is striking. Hair cells are largely absent from the first 14 mm of the left cochlea, but only from the first 3 mm of the right. There is a second area of severe loss of outer

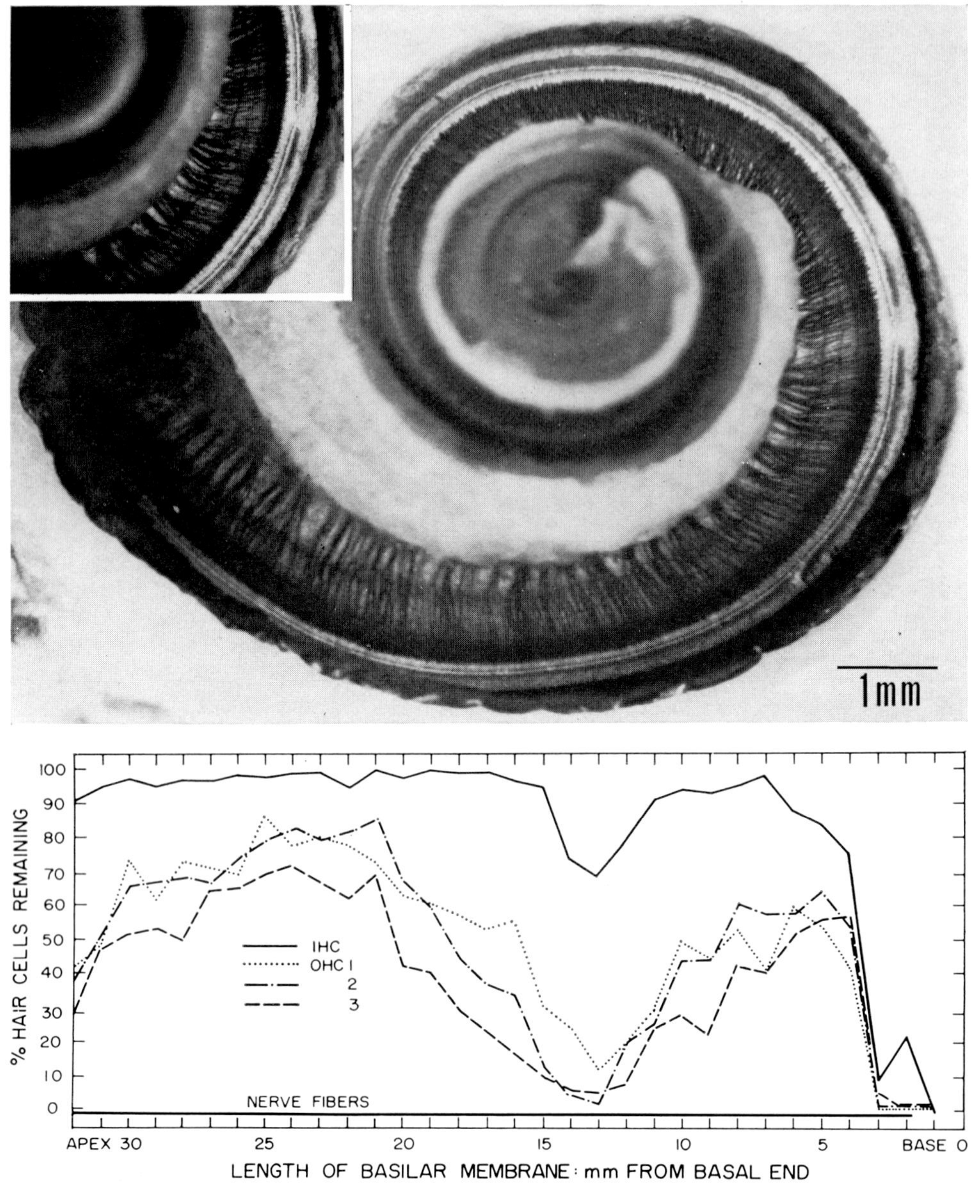

Fig. 4. The right cochlea from Case 2. There is a comparatively mild sensorineural degeneration (See Fig. 3), because of the acoustic shadow of the head. Note a small area with absence of Corti's organ and corresponding nerve degeneration (insert). The cytocochleogram is shown below. Above the 15-mm point the pattern of hair cell loss is almost identical with that in Figure 3, indicating that the head shadow was effective only for the higher frequencies.

hair cells from the right cochlea between 10 and 14 mm. Above the 15-mm point the patterns of hair cell loss in the two ears are almost identical, indicating that the head shadow was effective only for the higher frequencies.[22] To judge by the right cochlea, there appears to be surprisingly little hair cell loss, *viz* that in the basal 3 mm alone, which can be attributed to pres-

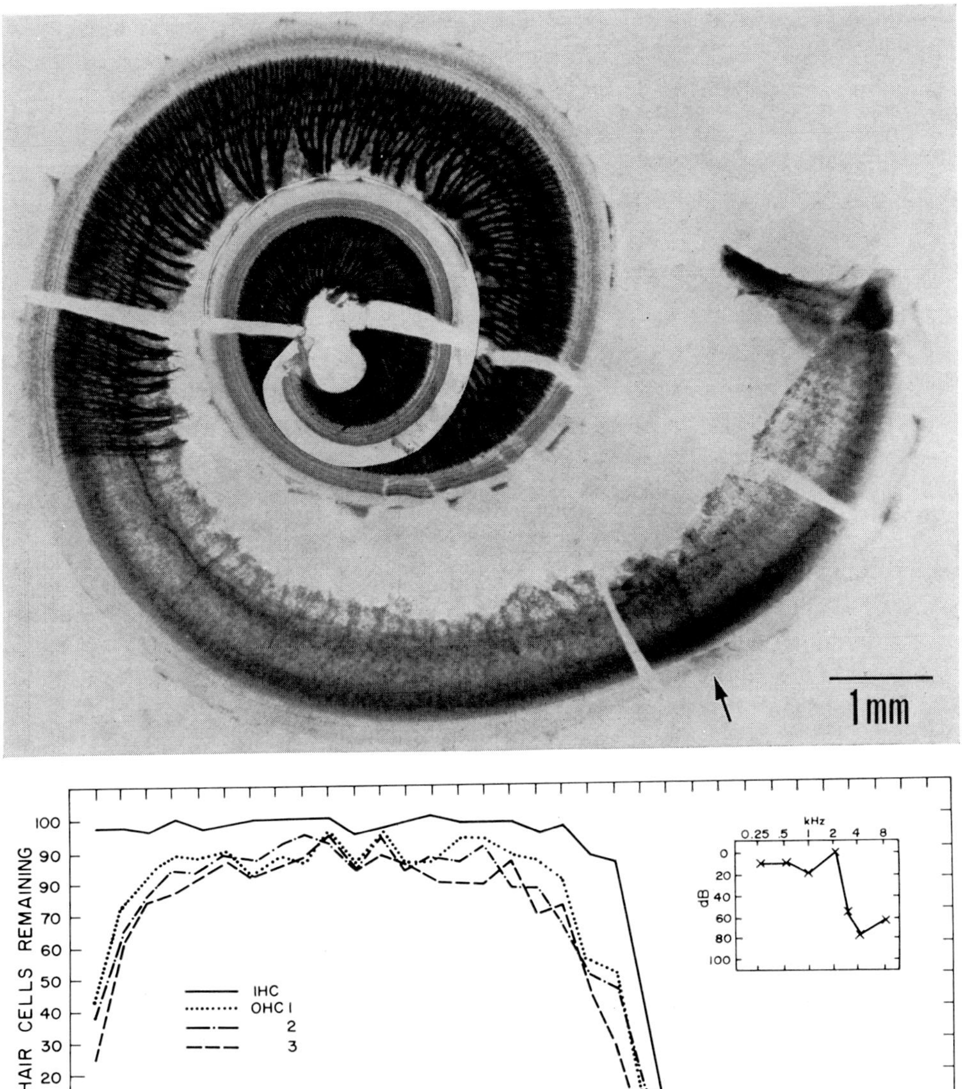

Fig. 5. Osseous spiral lamina with basilar membrane dissected out from the left cochlea of Case 3. There is a knife-sharp transition between the normal-appearing organ of Corti with dense nerve network and an area of complete absence of both. The opposite ear had an identical lesion; see Figure 6. Note a small island of Corti's organ with a few nerve fibers (arrow), implying previous presence of sensory cells in the first quadrant as in Figure 3. Cytocochleogram and audiogram are shown below.

bycusic changes, in spite of the patient's 72 years.

The degeneration pattern in the left cochlea of this case is the second most common type and is seen in the specimens from another four patients. It is worth noting that the little island of supporting elements with nerve fibers seen in the third quadrant in Figure 3 is not an isolated observation. Narrow

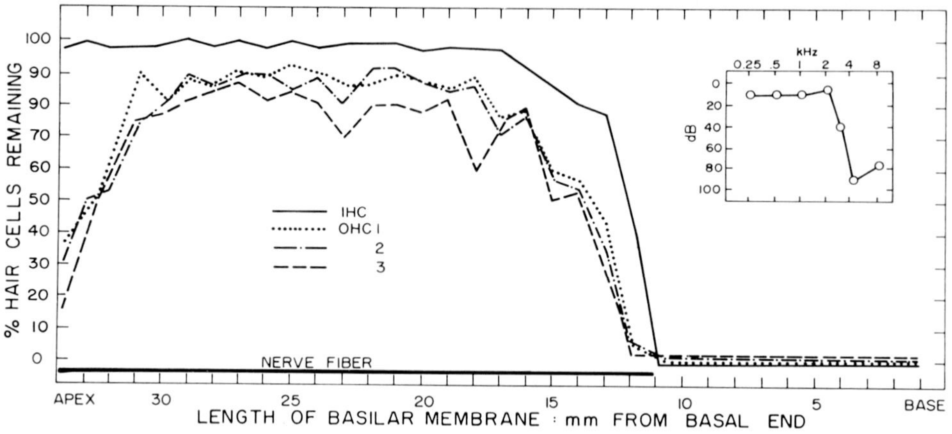

Fig. 6. Cytocochleogram and audiogram for the right ear from the same patient as in Figure 5. Note the marked symmetry of hair-cell and hearing losses.

patches, similar in size and location, are seen in at least three other specimens and have also been reported by Crowe *et al*[20] and Bredberg.[4]

II. Lesions Involving the First Quadrant As Well As the Second

The lesions of this type apparently represent extension of the second-quadrant lesion, as seen in Case 1, basalward to the first quadrant.

Case 3. The patient was 50 years old when he died. He had not been in military service, but he had worked on and off for five or six years in the press room of a factory making automobile bodies, and he liked hunting. Both ears show an almost complete loss of sensory and neural elements throughout the lower half of the basal turn (Figs. 5, 6). A knife-sharp transition occurs at 12 mm between the areas where neither nerve fibers nor organ of Corti can be seen and where both are present. Cytocochleograms for the two ears are remarkably symmetrical. An audiogram taken about a year before the patient's death indicates an abrupt hearing loss for frequencies above 2 kHz, with a maximum shift at 4 kHz of 80 and 90 dB in the respective ears. The slight upturn at 8 kHz may have been the contribution of the tiny island of surviving organ of Corti and nerve fibers at 4 mm, although by the time of the patient's death no hair cells were present there.

This type of degeneration, so common in material of Crowe *et al*,[20] is rare in our study. Only one similar pair of bones was obtained from a 78-year-old sheet metal worker with a 20-year history of noise exposure. However, the zone of transition is not as sharp and is located lower in the second quadrant.

III. Lesions of the First Quadrant

The following three cases are of special interest, differing markedly from the first two cases described above. The loss of hair cells and nerve fibers is confined almost entirely to the first 8 mm of the basal turn.

Case 4. The patient, aged 31, had worked eight years on the assembly line but was not reported to have been a hunter. The left ear shows a single, sharply-delimited lesion in the lower basal turn, 1.84 mm long, with its lower border 3.24 mm and its upper border 5.08 mm from the basal end of the basilar membrane (Fig. 7a). There is a similar 0.12-mm lesion in the right ear, located 3.75 mm from the base.

Case 5. A 62-year-old male had worked in what was described as a "very noisy paper mill" for 36 years. He hunted irregularly with a shotgun, and was right-handed. There is a 1.08-mm lesion in the right cochlea (Fig. 7b), although not so sharply defined as in the previous case. The distances of the lower and upper border from the basal

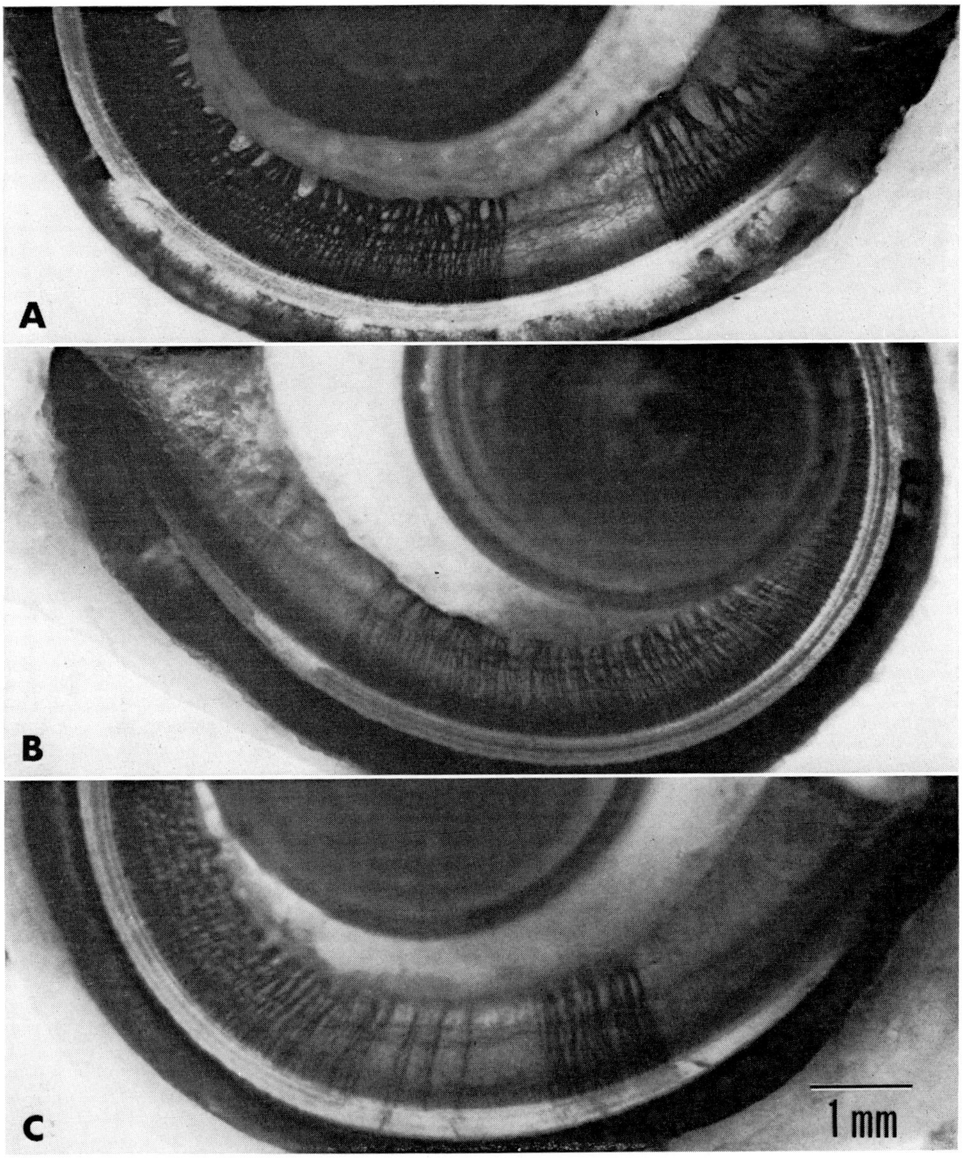

Fig. 7. Lower half of basal turn (first and second quadrants) from a) Case 4; b) Case 5; c) Case 6. Note the striking similarity in appearance and location between the 1.08-mm lesion in b) and the 1.84-mm lesion in a) where a few intralaminar spiral fibers are seen traversing the gap. In c) the lesion to the left extends for 1.88 mm and encloses three small bundles of nerve fibers, two of which supply small islands of Corti's organ. A second area of degeneration begins to the right at 5.14 mm from the base. This transition is located at almost the same distance, *i.e.,* 5 mm, from the basal end as the upper borders of the lesions in a) and b). It is postulated that the lesion in c) and possibly those in a) and b) are characteristic of impulse noise.

end are 4.11 mm and 5.07 mm respectively. There is also a complete loss of outer hair cells in the area below the lesion, and considerable hair cell loss above the lesion, especially in the same area of the second quadrant as in Case 1 (Fig. 2).

Case 6. This male was 25 years of

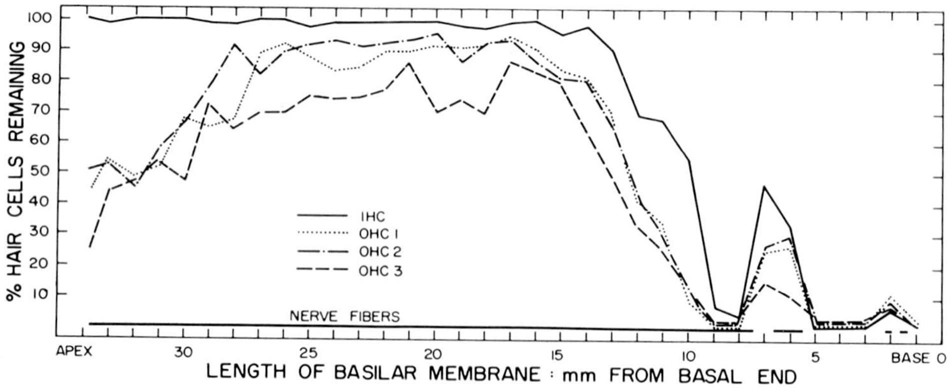

Fig. 8. The cytocochleogram of the specimen in Figure 7c.

age and had not been exposed to industrial noise, but was reported to have used guns regularly, both 16-gauge shotgun and .22-caliber rifle, shooting right-handed (Fig. 7c). The gap in the left organ of Corti is 1.88 mm wide with the lower border 6.4 mm and the upper border 8.29 mm from the basal end. Within the lesion there are three tiny fascicles of nerve fibers, two of which supply minute islands of Corti's organ, of which only the one to the left contains sensory cells — more precisely, three inner hair cells and one first-row outer hair cell. Below this lesion a second area of degeneration begins abruptly at 5.14 mm and extends down to the basal end, leaving a small block of Corti's organ with a dense nerve network between the two areas of degeneration. There is a tiny patch of supporting cells with a few nerve fibers remaining in the cecum vestibulare, but it is not visible in Figure 7c. The right ear, with the exception of the extreme basal portion, displays a normal, dense nerve network, again probably due to the effect of the head shadow.[22,23] The cytocochleogram for the left ear is shown in Figure 8.

The left ear from Case 4 and the right ear from Case 5 are almost identical so far as the locations and dimensions of their lesions are concerned (Fig. 7a, b), despite the fact that they represent different age groups and types of exposure. They also show similarities with the last case. The major difference is that Cases 4 and 5 have more or less the usual amount of hair cells and nerve fibers present below the gap, while Case 6, despite the youthful age of the patient, displays an almost complete nerve degeneration in the basal end. It should be noted that the transition of this 5.14 mm stretch of degeneration is located almost at the same distance from the basal end as the upper borders of the lesions in Cases 4 and 5, (5.08 and 5.07 mm, respectively).

Single, circumscribed lesions, like those in Figure 7a, b, were observed in two ears from different patients, in the first and second quadrant respectively. Multiple lesions resembling Figure 7c, but less sharply outlined, were seen in three patients, two of whom used shotguns and rifles fairly regularly.

DISCUSSION

The question whether a given cochlear injury has been caused by industrial or recreational noise, by gunfire, or by skull trauma,[3,16] aging,[21] or hereditary factors[24,25] is often difficult to answer because histories tend to be incomplete. In our material it was impossible to determine in some of the cases whether the damage was due primarily to occupational noise, to gunfire, or to both. Judging from our patients' histories, the pathology we have described is in all likelihood related to noise exposure in one form or another and is not just a coincidental finding. The industrial noise usually involved metal work and included strong elements of impulse noise. The nearly steady-state type of noise found in textile mills[26] was not represented.

The diffuse sensorineural degeneration associated with presbycusis[21] differs markedly from most of the degeneration patterns seen in this study. Yet, as stated earlier, some of the cochleas examined do not differ from our presbycusis material. Until a larger body of material with complete histories and reliable audiograms has been obtained, we cannot be sure whether noise exposure in certain cases might perhaps cause a type of sensory and neural degeneration similar to, or indistinguishable from that of presbycusis.

The left ears from Cases 1 and 2 and both ears from Case 3 probably represent successive stages of noise damage. Initially there appears to be a small second-quadrant lesion corresponding to an audiometric 4-kHz dip (Fig. 2). The lesion then slowly expands (Fig. 3), involving a greater length of the organ of Corti and additional frequencies (although audiometric documentation is missing for this case). Finally, further noise exposure and/or aging destroys the remaining sensory and neural elements in the first quadrant. The upper limb of the audiogram "breaks away"[27] and the 4-kHz dip becomes the abrupt high tone loss of Crowe *et al*[20] (Fig. 5). We do not mean that this is a rigidly-determined progression, but it appears to be the logical sequence of events. This is also in agreement with the conclusions of Gallo and Glorig[13] mentioned earlier. The ears in Figures 3 and 5 certainly seem to have passed the initial 15-year stage of the maximal hearing loss above 2 kHz that these authors describe, and would presumably have shown, if further exposed, a hearing loss at and below 2 kHz progressing more slowly and "linear with time."

The minute island of supporting elements and nerve fibers in the first quadrant of Case 3 (Fig. 5) implies that there had been a longer survival of sensory cells in this area, which was perhaps reflected by the upturn at 8 kHz in the patient's audiogram taken one year earlier. A similar small island, seen in the third quadrant in the left ear from Case 2 (Fig. 3), is probably also the remnant of a larger patch of sensory cells and could hypothetically have been responsible for a "divided dip" such as that described in the 2-3 kHz region in audiograms of military personnel.[17]

The right ear of Case 2 (Fig. 4) shows the protective effect of the head shadow, at least at the higher frequencies, when shooting from the right shoulder.[22,23] Nevertheless, there is considerable loss of outer hair cells in the 10-15 mm region. The nerve degeneration is slight, because inner hair cells and supporting elements are still present.[28] A similar asymmetry between the two cochleas is seen in Case 6 and to a lesser extent in Case 1.

The degeneration patterns seen in Figures 2 and 3 are similar to those described by Igarashi *et al*[3] and by Bredberg[4] and can be considered common. Figure 5, showing the ear with abrupt loss above 2 kHz, represents a form of pathology which appears to be relatively uncommon in recent investigations. The great number of these cases in the Johns Hopkins study[20] is something of a mystery, unless the ears were from patients with service in World War I or other exposure to the noise of gunfire. However, there was no statement to that effect.

The conspicuous types of degeneration patterns of the first quadrant of Cases 4, 5 and 6 have not been described earlier. The similar dimensions of the lesions and the almost identical distance from the base of three sharp transitional areas in the specimens, all from different individuals, could imply that the pattern and location of the damage are related to the geometry of the lower basal turn and the position of the windows. The damage in Figure 7c was caused by gunfire, and this type of degeneration with multiple, sharply-circumscribed lesions in the first quadrant may be characteristic of certain types of impulse noise. So are perhaps the patterns of Figure 7a and b, but they could only be related to industrial noise of a relatively steady-state character. It is of interest to note that the forms of degeneration in Figure 7 show similarities with patterns of both hair cell and nerve degeneration seen in some of the monkeys exposed to impulse noise.[10] In experimental animals the area of maximal damage spreads toward the basal end with increased intensity.[29] The sharp wave-fronts of impulse noise might be expected to set up waves of high amplitude which travel for only a short distance and injure Corti's organ in its first few millimeters.[12]

It is unfortunate that no audiograms were available for any of these ears with lesions of the first quadrant. Conventional audiometry, however, might not have revealed measurable hearing loss, since the lesions are restricted to the area which, according to Crowe *et al*,[20] should respond only to frequencies above 8 kHz.

Varying degrees of nerve degeneration are found at the basal end of the cochlea in adult human subjects, regardless of the type of material studied. Therefore, the role of noise in producing lesions in this region is difficult to evaluate. However, a clear-cut juxtafenestral lesion[9,12] is seen only in Case 6 (Fig. 7c), corresponding to that found in our noise-exposed monkeys and in those of Jordan *et al.*[10]

In discussion of diplacusis[30] and recruitment, the presence of localized damage to hair cells is often suggested as a possible cause for these phenomena. Figure 7 amply demonstrates such lesions. One may readily infer that a low-intensity stimulation of the damaged areas in Figure 7 would not elicit any sensation of sound, while a more intense stimulation would involve the areas surounding the gap, causing the displacement of pitch characteristic of diplacusis as well as the rapid growth of loudness characteristic of recruitment. A high-pitched tinnitus could also have been associated with these lesions initially when the hair cells were in process of degeneration. However, none of the cases shown in Figure 7 had complained of tinnitus, according to their next of kin.

A question of both theoretical and medico-legal importance is whether some of the degeneration patterns, notably the symmetrical lesions associated with abrupt high-tone loss, could have been caused by hereditary factors.[24,25,,31] We believe that such sharp transitions, symmetrical or otherwise, are simply the result of nerve degeneration, sharply localized and secondary to noise-induced hair cell loss. These presumably reflect the orderly spatial arrangement of nerve fibers in the osseous spiral lamina and their dependence on Corti's organ. The arrangement of ganglion cells in the modiolus is probably not precise enough to permit a primarily ganglionic lesion to cause a loss of dendrites as clearly defined as those in Figures 5 and 7. We have seen relatively abrupt transitions in the organ of Corti in various forms of cochlear pathology, including congenital deafness and ototoxicity,[19] but the neural lesions have always lacked the crisp demarcation demonstrated here. However, both the clinician and the otopathologist should bear in mind that a number of factors, unrelated to noise and skull trauma,[3,16] can cause audiometric changes more or less closely mimicking the classical 4-kHz dip and the abrupt high-tone loss. Among the possible etiologies are the following: 1) hereditary hearing loss.[24,25,31] 2) ototoxicity[19,32] 3) sudden hearing loss, idiopathic[33,34] or secondary to acoustic neurinoma;[35] 4) sensorineural hearing loss secondary to barotrauma in diving;[36] and 5) various forms of systemic toxicity.[37] Hereditary deafness is the most common cause, at least in males.[24] To what extent the degeneration pattern in such cases may resemble the noise-induced injuries described here remains for the most part to be determined.

It should be noted that with one small exception there is an excellent correlation between the existence of hair cells and/or supporting cells and the presence of nerve fibers (Fig. 3). This is in agreement with our previous statement that secondary nerve degeneration occurs in the osseous spiral lamina when the supporting elements, notably the pillar cells, have degenerated.[28] Only in one single specimen was there a short stretch of a nerve network of almost normal density in the osseous spiral lamina, corresponding to a bare area of the basilar membrane. Early nerve degeneration, possibly simultaneous with hair cell damage, has been described in guinea pigs exposed to noise.[38,39] One isolated instance of limited nerve degeneration without comparable hair cell and supporting cell loss has also been observed in a monkey.[10] Such findings imply primary neural damage. In none of our cases could we see evidence of such independent nerve degeneration. Neither did we observe any of the sporadic regeneration of nerve fibers we have described earlier in animals.[40]

The myelinated spiral fibers of the human cochlea comprise the spiral bundle of the modiolus and the intralaminar spiral fibers of the osseous spiral lamina.[21] Only the latter fibers are visible in our illustrations (Figs. 2, 7a and c). In our earlier discussion we stated our belief that such fibers are afferent in nature. They are seen crossing the relatively narrow gap in the first quadrant in Figure 7a. It is not clear why they are absent in the much wider gap in Figure 3, or why only a single, relatively short fascicle is to be seen below the zone of transition in Figure 5, in view of the limited loss of hair cells which they would innervate above these lesions, and the presence there of a full complement of supporting cells.

Strial atrophy was not more pronounced in the noise-damaged cochleas than in the rest of our material. It appears that noise-induced strial injury, which occurs in laboratory rodents,[40,41] is rare in man and monkey.[9] It should also be mentioned that we did not observe any obvious pathology of the tectorial membrane. Even in areas where Corti's organ was completely absent and where the tectorial membrane was lying against the flat epithelium covering the basilar membrane, it appeared normal by phase-contrast microscopy.

Hair cell degeneration produced in human cochleas by noise is probably caused by biological changes in the sensory cells which, when prolonged or aggravated, lead to cell death and permanent hearing loss. It appears unlikely that a purely mechanical type of cochlear damage occurs in everyday life, except perhaps in some cases of skull trauma or acoustic trauma due to blast or to exposure to intense impulse noise. In addition to sensorineural degeneration, endolymphatic hypoxia,[42] decreased turnover of perilymph,[43] alteration of the composition of the cochlear fluids,[44] disturbed microcirculation,[45,46] and increased permeability of Corti's organ[47] have been demonstrated in guinea pigs exposed to noise. Such factors may play important roles in the causation of sensory cell damage, at least in laboratory rodents. Yet the sharply circumscribed lesions which we[9,11] and others[10] have demonstrated in man and experimental animals suggest that the hair cells and their supporting cells still constitute the primary target, and that the cause of their death may be metabolic exhaustion, closely related to the vibration patterns of the basilar membrane in response to intense stimulation.

Audiometric surveys have revealed a high proportion of 4-kHz dips as well as more extensive high-frequency hearing losses which appear to have been caused by noise exposure. The peculiar tendency for the left ear to show more hearing loss than the right, reported in the 1954 Wisconsin State Fair Hearing Survey,[48] appears to find a natural explanation in our material, which included several firearm users. In view of the widespread interest in the mechanisms of noise-induced hearing impairment and its prevention, the scarcity of reports of cochlear pathology in such cases is surprising. We are convinced that further studies of temporal bones from patients with histories of noise exposure, accompanied by reliable audiometric data, can make valuable contributions toward the solution of these problems which cannot be gained from laboratory investigations, even in nonhuman primates.

REFERENCES

1. Hawkins JE Jr, Johnsson LG: Microdissection and surface preparations of the inner ear, in Smith CA, Vernon JA (eds): *Handbook of Auditory and Vestibular Research Methods.* Springfield, Illinois, Charles C Thomas, 1975, pp 5-52

2. Johnsson LG, Hawkins JE Jr: A direct approach to cochlear anatomy and pathology in man. Arch Otolaryngol 85:599-613, 1967

3. Igarashi M, Schuknecht HF, Myers EN: Cochlear pathology in humans with stimulation deafness. J Laryngol Otol 78:115-123. 1964

4. Bredberg G: Cellular pattern and nerve supply of the human organ of Corti. Acta Otolaryngol [Suppl] (Stockh) 236, 1968

5. Habermann J: Ueber die Schwerhörigkeit der Kesselschmiede. Arch Ohrenheilkunde 30:1-25, 1887

6. Habermann J: Beitrag zur Lehre von der professionellen Schwerhörigkeit. Arch Ohrenheilkunde 69:106-130, 1906

7. Brühl G: Beiträge zur pathologischen Anatomie des Gehörorgans. Z Ohrenheilk 52: 232-246, 1906

8. Zange J: Beitrag zur Pathologie der professionellen Schwerhörigkeit. Arch Ohrenheilkunde 86:167-174, 1911

9. Hawkins JE Jr, Johnsson LG, Stebbins WC, *et al*: Hearing loss and cochlear pathology in monkeys after noise exposure. Acta Otolaryngol (Stockh) 81:337-343, 1976

10. Jordan VM, Pinheiro ML, Chiba K, *et al*: Cochlear pathology in monkeys exposed to impulse noise. Acta Otolaryngol [Suppl] (Stockh) 312, 1973

11. Moody DB, Stebbins WC, Johnsson LG, *et al*: Noise-induced hearing loss in nonhuman primates, in Henderson D, Hamernik RP, *et al* (eds): *The Effects of Noise on Hearing–Critical Issues.* New York, Raven Press, 1976

12. Hawkins JE Jr, Johnsson LG: Patterns of sensorineural degeneration in human ears exposed to noise, in Henderson D, Hamernik RP, *et al* (eds): *The Effects of Noise on Hearing–Critical Issues.* New York, Raven Press, 1976

13. Gallo R, Glorig A: Permanent threshold shift changes produced by noise exposure and aging. Am Ind Hyg Assoc J 25:237-245, 1964

14. Sataloff J, Vassallo L, Menduke H: Occupational hearing loss and high frequency thresholds. Arch Environ Health 14:832-836, 1967

15. Schuknecht HF, Tonndorf J: Acoustic trauma of the cochlea from ear surgery. Laryngoscope 70:479-505, 1960

16. Schuknecht HF: *Pathology of the Ear.* Cambridge, Mass, Harvard University Press, 1974, pp 295-297, 300-308

17. Salmivalli A: Acoustic trauma in regular army personnel. Clinical audiologic study. Acta Otolaryngol [Suppl] (Stockh) 222, 1967

18. Ward WD, Fleer RE, Glorig A: Characteristics of hearing losses produced by gunfire and by steady noise. J Aud Res 1:325-356, 1961

19. Stebbins WC, Miller JM, Johnsson LG, *et al*: Ototoxic hearing loss and cochlear pathology in the monkey. Ann Otol Rhinol Laryngol 78:1007-1025, 1969

20. Crowe SJ, Guild SR, Polvogt LM: Observations on the pathology of high-tone deafness. Bull Johns Hopkins Hosp 54:315-380, 1934

21. Johnsson LG, Hawkins JE Jr: Sensory and neural degeneration with aging, as seen in microdissections of the human inner ear. Ann Otol Rhinol Laryngol 81:179-193, 1972

22. Keim RJ: Sensorineural hearing loss associated with firearms. Arch Otolaryngol 90: 581-584, 1969

23. Taylor GD, Williams E: Acoustic trauma in the sports hunter. Laryngoscope 76: 863-879, 1966

24. Anderson H, Wedenberg E: Genetic aspects of hearing impairments in children. Acta Otolaryngol (Stockh) 69:77-88, 1970

25. Fisch L: The aetiology of congenital deafness and audiometric patterns. J Laryngol Otol 69:479-493, 1955

26. Taylor W, Pearson J, Mair A, *et al*: Study of noise and hearing in jute weaving. J Acoust Soc Am 38:113-120, 1965

27. Hinchcliffe R: Occupational noise-induced hearing loss. Proc R Soc Med 60:1111-1117, 1967

28. Johnsson LG: Sequence of degeneration of Corti's organ and its first-order neurons. Ann Otol Rhinol Laryngol 83:294-303, 1974

29. Covell WP: Histologic changes in the organ of Corti with intense sound. J Comp Neurol 99:43-59, 1953

30. Davis H, Morgan CT, Hawkins JE Jr, *et al*: Temporary deafness following exposure to loud tones and noise. Acta Otolaryngol [Suppl] (Stockh) 88, 1950

31. Huizing EH, Van Bolhuis AH, Odenthal DW: Studies on progressive hereditary perceptive deafness in a family of 335 members. Acta Otolaryngol (Stockh) 61:34-41; 161-167, 1966

32. Dayal VS, Whitehead GL, Smith EL: Gentamicin–progressive cochlear toxicity. Can

J Otolaryngol 4:348-351, 1975

33. Hallberg OE: Sudden deafness and its relation to atherosclerosis. JAMA 165:1649-1652, 1957

34. Lindsay JR, Zuidema JJ: Inner ear deafness of sudden onset. Laryngoscope 60:238-265, 1950

35. Higgs WA: Sudden deafness as the presenting symptom of acoustic neurinoma. Arch Otolaryngol 98:73-76, 1973

36. Soss SL: Sensorineural hearing loss with diving. Arch Otolaryngol 93:501-504, 1971

37. van Dishoeck HAE: Akustisches Trauma, in Berendes J, Link R, Zöllner F (eds): *Hals-Nasen-Ohren-Heilkunde Band III*. Stuttgart, Georg Thieme, 1966, pp 1764-1799

38. Spoendlin H: Primary structural changes in the organ of Corti after acoustic overstimulation. Acta Otolaryngol (Stockh) 71: 166-176, 1971

39. Wright CG: Neural damage in the guinea pig cochlea after noise exposure. A light microscopic study. Acta Otolaryngol (Stockh) 82:82-95, 1976

40. Johnsson LG, Hawkins JE Jr: Strial atrophy in clinical and experimental deafness. Laryngoscope 82:1105-1125, 1972

41. Ward WD, Duvall AJ III: Behavioral and ultrastructural correlates of acoustic trauma. Ann Otol Rhinol Laryngol 80:881-896, 1971

42. Misrahy GA, Arnold JE, Mundie JR, *et al*: Genesis of endolymphatic hypoxia following acoustic trauma. J Acoust Soc Am 30: 1082-1088, 1958

43. Schnieder EA: A contribution to the physiology of the perilymph. Part III: On the origin of noise-induced hearing loss. Ann Otol Rhinol Laryngol 83:406-412, 1974

44. Nakashima T, Meiring NL, Snow JB: Cations in the endolymph with noise-induced deafness. Arch Otolaryngol 94:109-113, 1971

45. Hawkins JE Jr: The role of vasoconstriction in noise-induced hearing loss. Ann Otol Rhinol Laryngol 80:903-913, 1971

46. Kellerhals B: Acoustic trauma and cochlear microcirculation. An experimental and clinical study on pathogenesis and treatment of inner ear lesions after acute noise exposure. Adv Otorhinolaryngol 18:91-168, 1972

47. Goldstein AJ: Permeability of the organ of Corti. Ann Otol Rhinol Laryngol 82: 166-174, 1973

48. Glorig A, Wheeler D, Quiggle R, *et al*: 1954 Wisconsin State Fair Hearing Survey. Am Acad Ophthalmol Otolaryngol, Los Angeles, 1957

REPRINTS—Lars-G. Johnsson, MD, Kresge Hearing Research Institute and Department of Otorhinolaryngology, University of Michigan Medical School, Ann Arbor, MI 48109.

INTERNATIONAL CONGRESS ON THE EDUCATION OF THE DEAF

The International Congress on the Education of the Deaf voted in August 1975 to establish an International Congress Committee on the Education of the Deaf with the aim of creating a mechanism to insure a more orderly continuity in the congresses. For information write to Dr. S. Richard Silverman, Chairman, International Congress Committee on the Education of the Deaf, 818 South Euclid Avenue, St. Louis, MO 63110, U.S.A.

Ann Otol 85: 1976

ULTRASTRUCTURAL COCHLEAR CHANGES FOLLOWING ACOUSTIC HYPERSTIMULATION AND OTOTOXICITY

DAVID J. LIM, MD

COLUMBUS, OHIO

SUMMARY – Using guinea pigs and chinchillas as experimental animals, modes and patterns of sensory cell damage by acoustic hyperstimulation and kanamycin intoxication were compared. In general, outer hair cells were more vulnerable to both acoustic trauma and ototoxicity (particularly in the basal turn) than inner hair cells. However, in kanamycin ototoxicity, the inner hair cells were more vulnerable in the apical coil. Nerve endings and nerve fibers generally were resistant to both acoustic trauma and kanamycin intoxication, and their degeneration appears to be secondary to the sensory cell degeneration. A large number of unmyelinated nerve fibers were seen in both the organ of Corti and the osseous spiral lamina even three months after the organ of Corti had been completely degenerated by ototoxicity. The total number of unmyelinated and myelinated nerve fibers in the osseous spiral lamina far exceeded the scanty surviving ganglion cells in Rosenthal's canal, indicating the possibility of regeneration of these fibers following kanamycin intoxication. The remaining few ganglion cells were mainly type II or type III cells, and a majority of the type I ganglion cells appeared to be degenerated. Signs of strial damage were observed in both acoustic trauma and ototoxicity, but their pattern did not correlate well with that of sensory cell degeneration.

Cochlear pathologies following acoustic trauma and ototoxicity have been investigated for the last 25 years,[1] and it has been established that the sensory cell and subsequent neural degeneration are the main histologic findings.[2-9] Although the mode of insult is different between acoustic trauma and antibiotic ototoxicity, the end result is commonly sensory cell degeneration and subsequent sensorineural hearing loss. The purpose of this paper is to compare cochlear pathologies caused by these two agents, to elucidate the mechanism by which the sensory cell degenerates, and to examine the fate of nerve fibers and ganglion cells following complete degeneration of sensory cells. The latter information may be useful in the theoretical consideration of cochlear implants.

METHODS AND MATERIALS*

A total of 25 guinea pigs was used for the kanamycin ototoxicity study. Nine animals which were received from Dr. Peter Dallos' laboratory are also included in this report. The animals received kanamycin** (400 mg/kg body weight daily) until Preyer's reflex disappeared. One group was sacrificed immediately after the first sign of loss of Preyer's reflex, and the other group was sacrificed after two to three months following the loss of Preyer's reflex.

A total of 30 chinchillas was used for the acoustic trauma study.*** One group was exposed to 85 dB for 48 to 92 hours at 200 to 300 Hz octave band noise. Another group was exposed to 120 to 130 dB at 1 or 2 kHz for 30 to 60 minutes. A third group served as control.

The specimens were either fixed directly in 1.22% *s*-collidine-buffered osmic acid or prefixed in cacodylate-buffered 3% glutaraldehyde and postfixed in *s*-collidine buffered 1.33% osmic acid. Following fixation, the

---

* The experiments reported herein were conducted according to the "Guide for the Care and Use of Laboratory Animals," Institute of Laboratory Animal Resources, National Research Council.

** Kantrex® was partly provided by Bristol Laboratories, Syracuse, NY.

*** Part of a study conducted jointly with Dr. William Melnick, Audiological Research Laboratory, Ohio State University.

From the Otological Research Laboratories, Ohio State University College of Medicine, Columbus, Ohio. Supported in part by the Deafness Research Foundation and by the USAF research contract (F33615-74-C-4049) awarded through the 6570th Aerospace Research Laboratory, Aerospace Medical Division, Air Force Systems Command, Wright-Patterson AFB, Ohio. This article is identified as AMRL-TR-76-56 by the Air Force.

Presented at the meeting of the American Otological Society, Inc., Palm Beach, Florida, April 25-26, 1976.

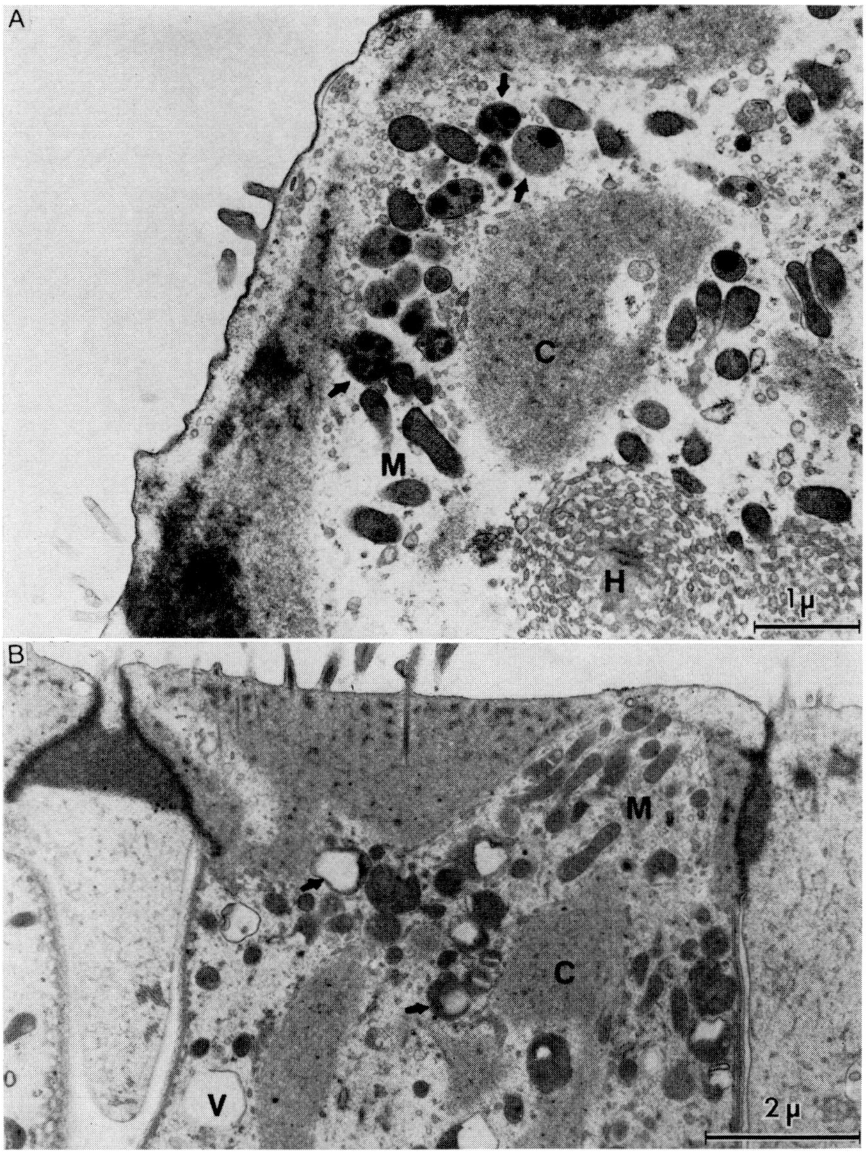

Fig. 1. A) Top portion of outer hair cell from a guinea pig exposed to noise (117 dB, 300-600 Hz, for six hours and ten days' recovery) shows lysosome-like structures (arrows) which resemble some of mitochondria (M), cuticle-like structures (C), and proliferated Hensen's body (H). Observe heavy accumulation of vesicles in the cuticle-free area of the hair cell. B) Top portion of outer hair cell of kanamycin-treated guinea pig shows vacuoles (V), lysosomal granules, vacuole formation of degenerating mitochondria (arrow), normal mitochondria (M), and cuticle-like structure (C).

specimens were washed in buffer and then dehydrated in graded ethanol and embedded in epoxy resin. Sections 1μ thick were made for light microscopy, and thin sections were made for transmission electron microscopy,*

For scanning electron microscopy, some specimens were prefixed in cacodylate-buffered 3% glutaraldehyde and then incubated in a tannin-osmic acid mixture to enhance the conductivity of the specimen, as described by

* Philips 300. Philips Electronic Instruments, Inc., Mount Vernon, NY.

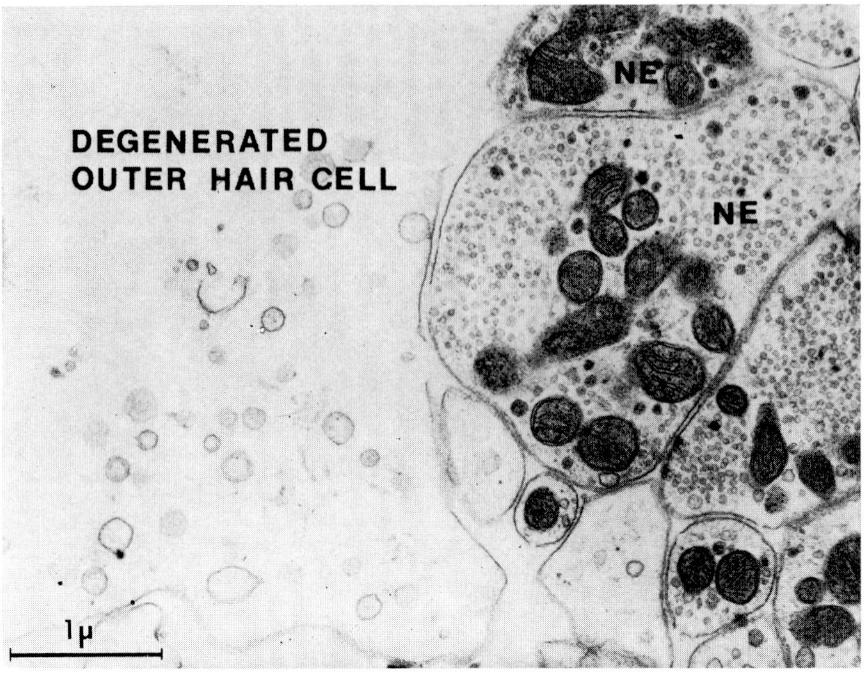

Fig. 2. Basal portion of completely degenerated outer hair cell due to kanamycin ototoxicity shows cell debris and seemingly intact nerve endings (NE).

Murakami.[10] The specimens were then washed in buffer and dehydrated using graded ethanol and critical point dried using CO_2. Dried specimens were gold coated for scanning electron microscopy.*

RESULTS

Evidence of mechanical stress on the organ of Corti can be found in the ear exposed to excessive noise. These are separation of Deiters'-Hensen's cell junction, rupture of Reissner's membrane, and detachment of the organ of Corti from the basilar membrane. These types of lesions are well described by other investigators[11,12] and will not be discussed in detail here.

More subtle pathologies in acoustic trauma which may be attributed to the metabolic stress and resultant damage were compared to those pathologies observed in the kanamycin-intoxicated ear. Similarities were noted in the modification of the cuticular plate and sensory hairs in both the kanamycin-intoxicated ears and the acoustically traumatized ears. These were the fusion of sensory hairs, softening of cuticular plates, and excessive cuticle formation (Fig. 1). Vesiculation of the smooth endoplasmic reticular (ER) system and eventual cell rupture were also noted in both groups. The vesiculation of afferent nerve endings noted in the acoustic trauma group was not found in the kanamycin-intoxicated group. The orderly proliferation of the ER system, including Hensen's body, that was noted in acoustic trauma was not observed in the kanamycin-treated ears.

Dark granules were accumulated in the top portions of cells in both groups. They are interpreted as lipofuscin granules or lysosomes. In the kanamycin-treated group, some of the lamellar bodies apparently derived from degenerated mitochondria (Fig. 1).

Sensory cells may have disintegrated, but nerve endings seemed intact in the kanamycin-treated animals (Fig. 2). As in the acoustic trauma cases, the cell debris in Nuel's space was phagocytized

* Cambridge Stereoscan Mark IIa. Cambridge Instrument Co., Inc., Ossining, NY.

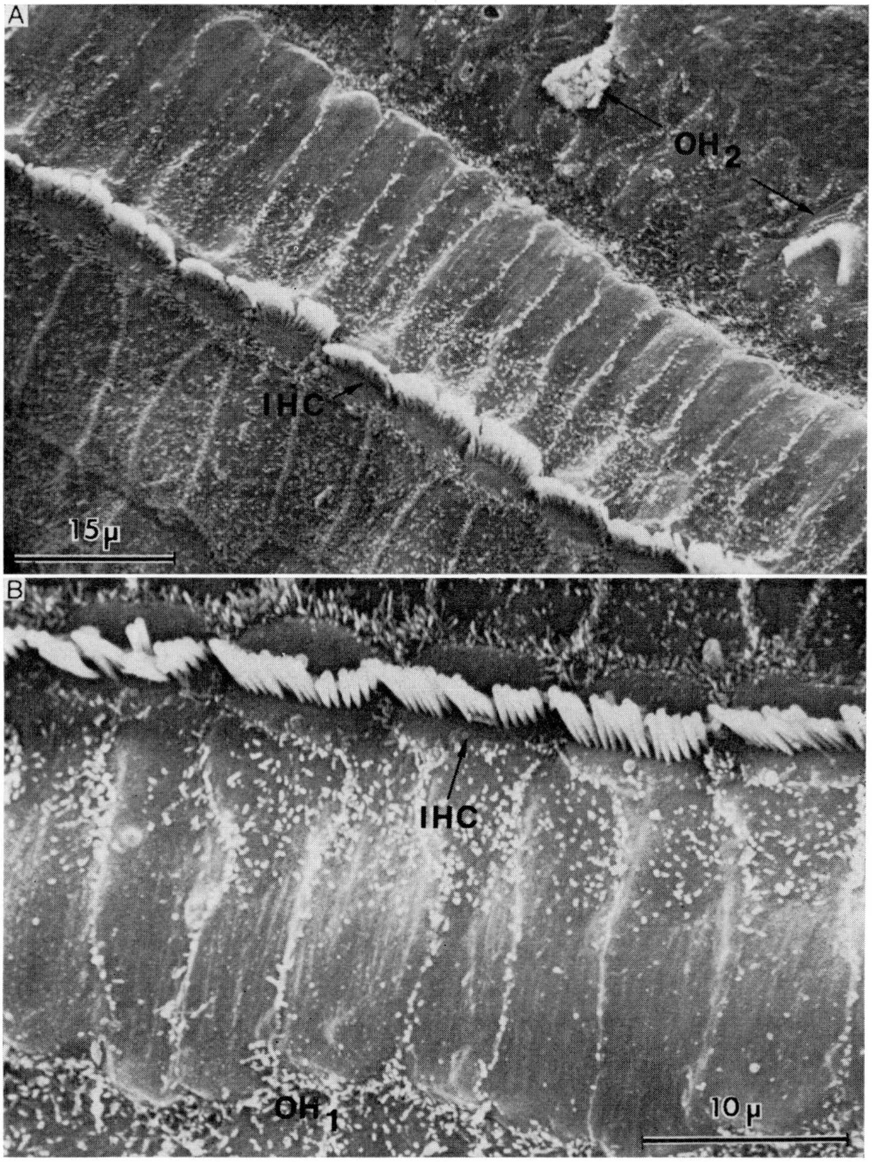

Fig. 3. A) A basal turn of cochlea of kanamycin-treated guinea pig shows nearly complete degeneration of outer hair cells. One outer hair cell in the second row is still identifiable (OH_2). Observe intact inner hair cells (IHC). B) Another example of normal inner hair cells (IHC) despite complete degeneration of outer hair cells (OH_1) at the basal turn of kanamycin-treated guinea pig. Most of the area where outer hair cells were located is not shown.

by wandering macrophages in kanamycin-intoxicated ears.

A sharp contrast between these two groups was noted in the pattern of sensory cell degeneration. Sensory cell degeneration in acoustic trauma was frequently observed in the outer hair cells and less in the inner hair cells, regardless of the cochlear turns. This general statement can also be made about the kanamycin-treated ears, at least in the basal turn (Fig. 3). However, in the

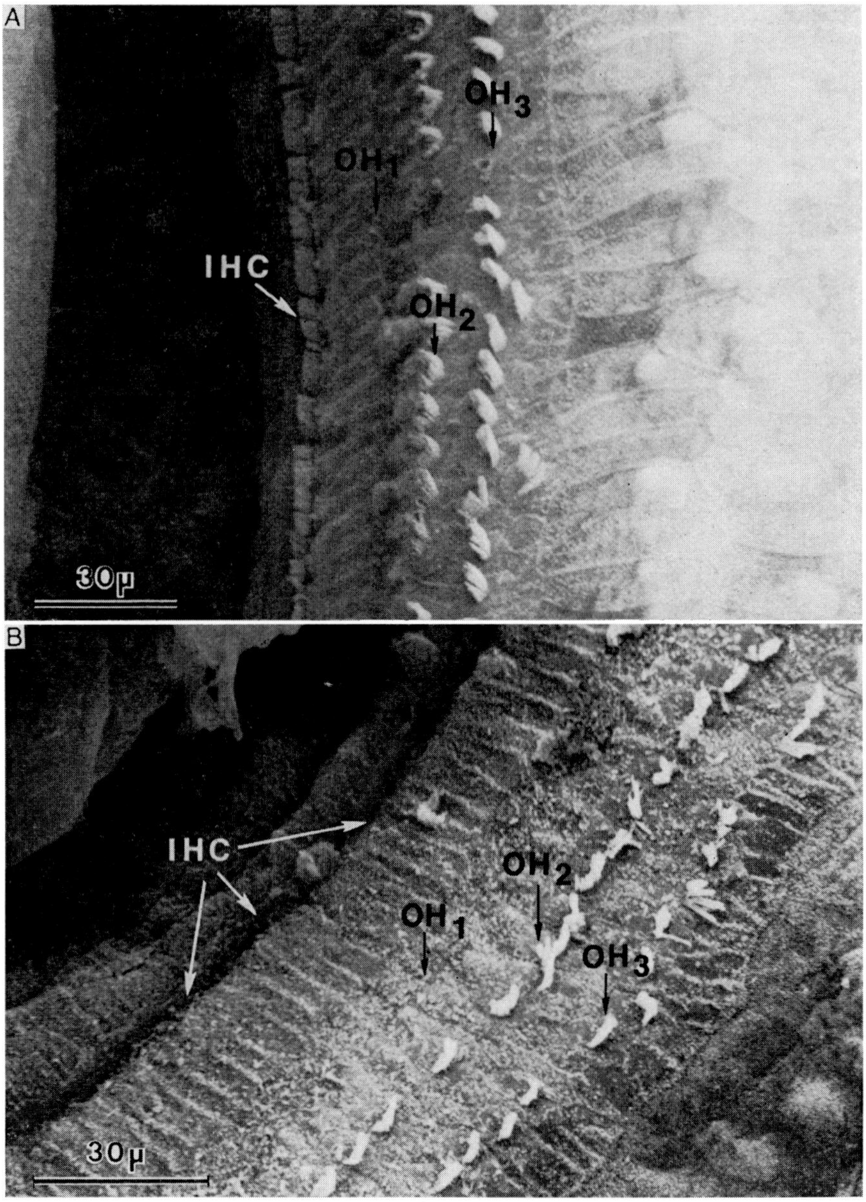

Fig. 4. A) Midturn of kanamycin-intoxicated cochlea (same animal as Fig. 3B) shows total destruction of first row of outer hair cells (OH_1) and normal inner hair cells (IHC). Some cells are missing in second and third rows of outer hair cells (OH_2, OH_3). B) Same animal as A but in the apical turn, which shows complete destruction of inner hair cells (IHC) and first row of outer hair cells (OH_1). Outer hair cells in general are intact in second and third rows.

apical turn of kanamycin-intoxicated ears, the damage was most frequently observed mainly in the inner hair cells (Fig. 4A). In the middle turn, however, the first row of the outer hair cells was the most vulnerable (Fig. 4B). This peculiar sensory cell degeneration pattern was not observed in acoustic trauma, where the lesions were either sharply delineated or broadly affected,

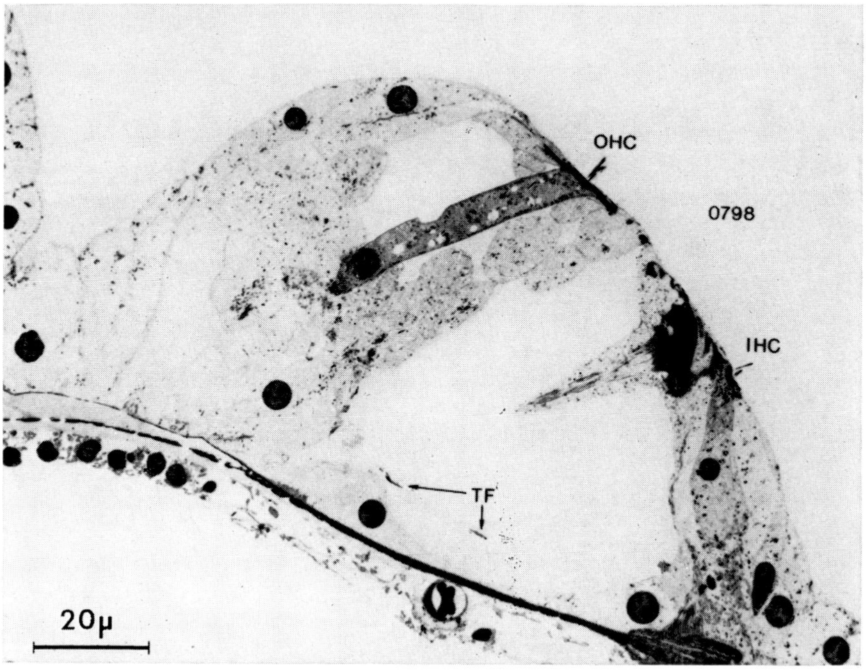

Fig. 5. A middle turn of the cochlea of kanamycin-treated guinea pig shows missing first and second outer hair cells but intact inner hair cells (IHC). Surviving third row hair cell (OHC) shows extensive vesiculation in the cytoplasm. Tunnel fibers (TF) can also be seen.

depending on the nature and characteristics of the sound stimuli.

When neighboring sensory cells had completely degenerated, some sensory cells survived with minimum injury to the outer as well as inner hair cells of both groups (Fig. 5).

Only a few reticular holes created by degenerated sensory cells in acoustic trauma[13] were observed in cases of acoustic trauma and kanamycin treatment (Fig. 6). These holes were observed in acute cases within six days following the experiments and were not observed in animals that were kept alive more than a week. A majority of the neighboring sensory cells around the holes appear grossly normal on scanning electron microscopic photographs (Fig. 6).

Strial pathology was occasionally prominent in the acoustically traumatized ears. The cell injury appeared to be exclusively in the intermediate cells. These cells reappeared in the recovered ear. As in sensory cell death, the cell debris derived from degenerated strial cells was largely taken up by the macrophages. In kanamycin-treated ears, the strial pathology observed in the present experiment was not nearly as remarkable as in the cases of acoustic trauma examined, although some swelling of the root cells of the limbus spiralis and intermediate cells of the stria was noted.

When the organ of Corti was completely destroyed by kanamycin intoxication, the bare nerve fibers were readily found in the intercellular spaces of the cuboidal cells that replaced the organ of Corti cells (Fig. 7A). The nerve fibers were more abundant in ears where some supporting structures of the organ of Corti remained (Fig. 7B). The scanty unmyelinated nerve fibers that survived in the collapsed organ of Corti devoid of sensory cells three months after the kanamycin treatment resemble tunnel basilar fibers.

In the osseous spiral lamina of the

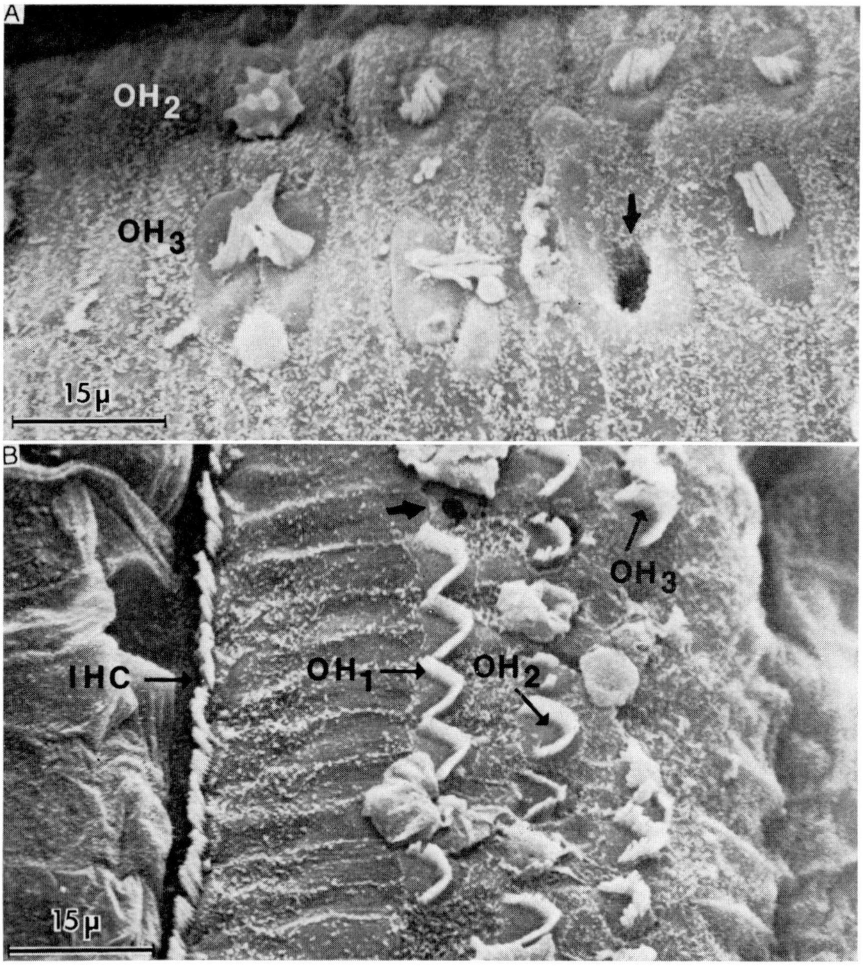

Fig. 6. A) A noise-exposed (1 kHz, 130 dB, for 30 min.) chinchilla cochlea in midturn shows degenerating outer hair cells in second and third rows (OH_2, OH_3). An arrow indicates a reticular hole created by sensory cell degeneration. This animal was sacrificed six days after the noise exposure. B) A portion of basal turn of guinea pig cochlea two days after kanamycin treatment shows intact inner hair cells (IHC) and numerous degenerating outer hair cells in first, second and third rows (OH_1, OH_2, OH_3). An arrow indicates a reticular hole.

cases where the organ of Corti had disappeared, some myelinated fibers survived after three months of kanamycin intoxication. In these specimens numerous unmyelinated fibers also could be seen in the osseous spiral lamina (Fig. 8). Most of the intraganglionic efferent spiral fibers remained intact, while a majority of the ganglion cells degenerated. Although a few type I cells were seen, the remaining ganglion cells were mainly type II or type III cells (Fig. 8A). The latter cells have thin myelin sheets. There are many more myelinated and unmyelinated nerve fibers in the osseous spiral lamina than the total number of ganglionic cells. With our present sound exposure methods, none of our ears showed complete degeneration of the organ of Corti; therefore, it is not possible to compare them with the pathology obtained by kanamycin.

DISCUSSION

It is well established that excessive

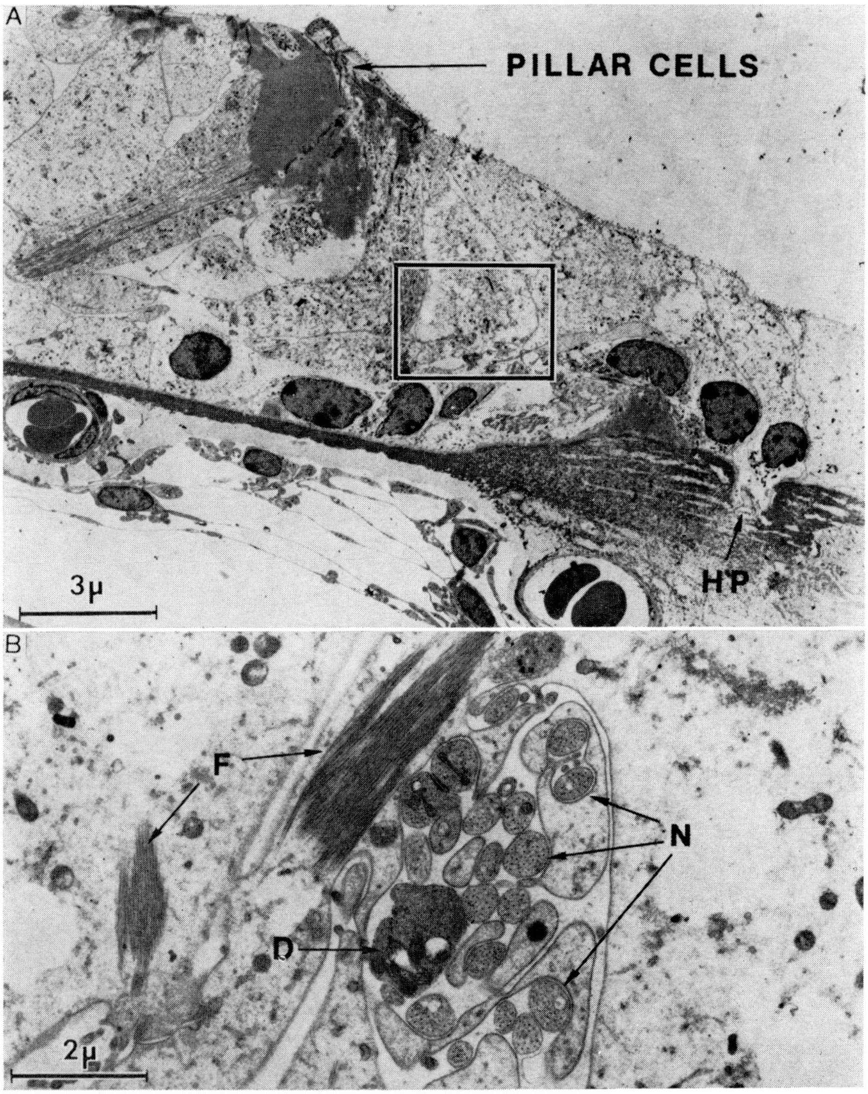

Fig. 7. A) Partially collapsed organ of Corti due to kanamycin intoxication (three months' survival) possesses some remaining inner spiral bundles shown in square. Some unmyelinated nerve fibers are also seen in habenula perforata (HP). B) Similar area as A of same animal shows numerous inner spiral fibers (N). One granulated nerve fiber shows signs of degeneration (D). F - Fibrils of collapsed supporting cells.

noise can cause direct mechanical damage to the organ of Corti.[11,14] Besides the mechanical mode of damage mentioned, there is supportive evidence to suggest that sensory cell degeneration is brought about by metabolic stress[12,14,15] and is presumably due to poor circulation in the sensory regions.[6,16] The other mode of sensory cell degeneration can be secondary to the intermixing of fluids in the cochlear partition. Bohne[17] noted holes in the reticular lamina created by the degenerated sensory cells following noise exposure, and the present finding also supports the notion that intermixing of fluids may occur in acute lesions. The extent to which this type of lesion causes further sensory cell damage can-

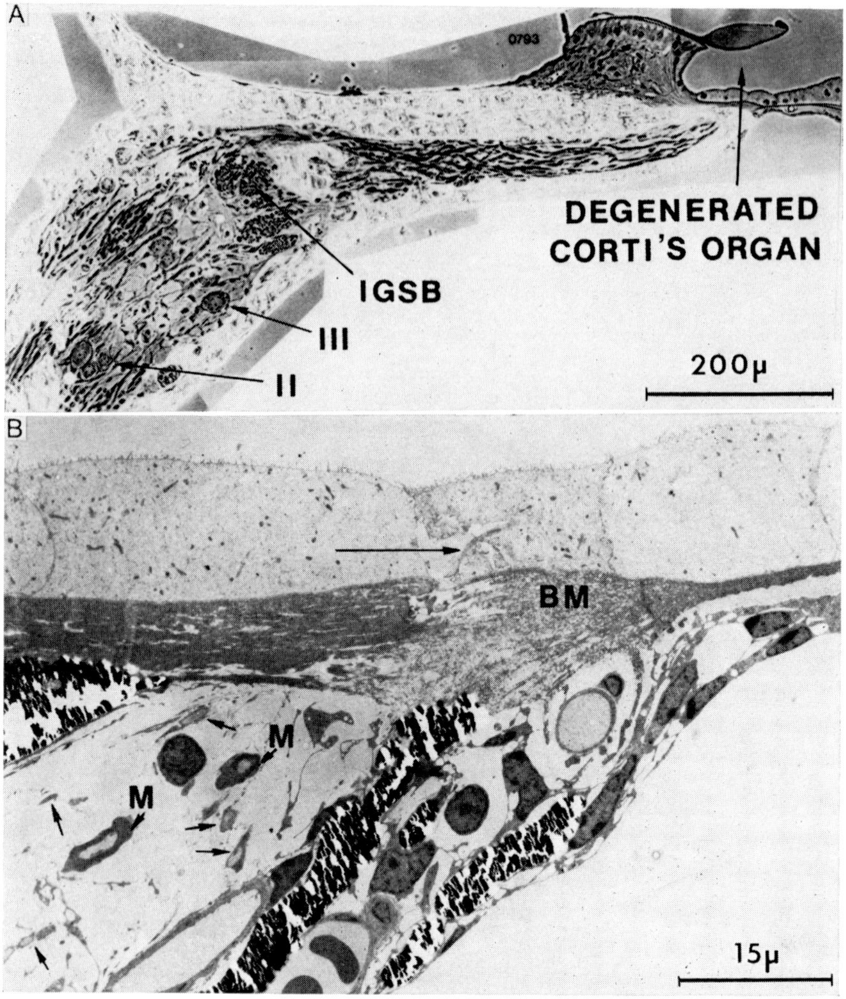

Fig. 8. A) A phase contrast light micrograph of basal turn of cochlea intoxicated with kanamycin examined 100 days after the last injection shows total degeneration of organ of Corti, heavy loss of ganglion cells, and intact intraganglionic efferent spiral bundle fibers (IGSB). Surviving ganglion cells are either small (II) or large (III). Numerous myelinated fibers are seen in osseous spiral lamina. B) Electron micrograph of same specimen as A shows a few unmyelinated nerve fibers (long arrow) above the habenula perforata of the basilar membrane (BM), numerous unmyelinated fibers (small arrows), and a few myelinated fibers (M).

not be determined.

Sensory hair fusions are also considered a sign of hair cell degeneration in acoustic trauma,[8,12,18] in ototoxicity,[19] and in the waltzing guinea pig.[5,20] However, how sensory hairs fuse together is not wholly understood. Wersäll *et al*[19] postulated that perhaps there is direct incorporation of the antibiotics into the surface membrane, which in turn may change the properties of the membrane. On the other hand, it could change the metabolism of the cell with a secondary defect in the plasma membrane or change a membrane-attached substance which stabilized the cell surface. While it is possible that ototoxic antibiotics (aminoglycosides) are incorporated into the surface membrane to cause the fusion it is also possible that any insult which alters the protein-lipid metabolism of the membrane[21] may result in sensory hair fusions, regardless of their stimulus, in view of the fact that similar sensory hair fusions in acoustic stimulation and in genetic sensory cell degeneration have identical pathologies.

Softening and modification of cuticular plates are also observed in acoustically stimulated, aminoglycoside-intoxicated, or genetically degenerating cochlear sensory cells.[5,8,12] Again, this commonality of the pathology caused by diverse factors suggests that protein-lipid metabolism in the sensory cells is altered by the insults. The normal chemical composition of the dense substance forming the cuticular plates and the amorphous ground substance is known to show a filamentous appearance when certain fixatives were used.[22] Whether these substances are indeed chemically altered in damaged sensory cells may be suspected but cannot be confirmed with certainty in the absence of biochemical proof.

Degeneration patterns of sensory cells in both acoustic trauma and ototoxicity have been observed by many investigators. No single hypothesis can explain these patterns satisfactorily. Why the outer hair cells are more vulnerable than the inner cells, and even among outer hair cells how some cells degenerate while neighboring cells are relatively intact in acoustic trauma, is not wholly understood. It has been suggested that the outer hair cells are metabolically more active than the inner hair cells, and cells that are active will suffer proportionally more.[12] It also may be that the outer hair cells are more physically exposed to the fluid motion generated by sound than the inner hair cells.

The degeneration pattern of kanamycin-intoxicated ears is more puzzling. Some ears showed a typical pattern described by Kohonen[4] and Engström *et al.*[23] In the basal turn, the damage occurs preferentially in the outer hair cells from the third to the first rows, in the order of sensitivity to ototoxicity. In the middle turn, the ototoxicity occurs mostly in the first row of the outer hair cells; the second and third rows and inner hair cells are the last to go. On the other hand, in the apical coil the inner hair cells were the first to degenerate and the outer hair cells last. This peculiar characteristic of sensory cell degeneration patterns caused by ototoxicity cannot be explained by the cell's metabolic activity alone. Engström and Kohonen[3] suggested that the cells with large efferent nerve endings are more susceptible to ototoxic damage, and the sensory cell degeneration pattern observed in the ototoxic experiments coincides well with the number of efferent nerve endings present. The present investigation supports the peculiar pattern of sensory cell degeneration by kanamycin similar to that of other aminoglycosides; however, whether the efferent system promotes sensory cell degeneration cannot be determined.

Resistance of nerve endings to kanamycin intoxication and also to acoustic trauma is also puzzling. Ototoxic drugs apparently are less toxic to nerve fibers than to the sensory cells. Neural degeneration appears to be secondary to sensory cell degeneration. Kimura[24] also observed the durability of the nerve endings in the inner ear following arterial blockage.

Pathology involving the stria vascularis has been reported in acoustic trauma[6,12,13] and in ototoxicity.[6,25,26] It is generally believed that the intermediate cells are the primary target of the insults.[26] Hawkins[6] suggested that these cellular changes, including the swelling of the root cells, are secondary to capillary injuries in these regions. The present investigation supports his observation. In agreement with the findings of Bohne *et al*,[13] however, the strial pathology correlates poorly with the patterns of sensory cell degeneration.

It is well established that when sensory cells degenerate by VIII nerve section,[27] acoustic trauma,[27-29] or ototoxic drug,[30] the majority of cochlear ganglion cells and myelinated nerve fibers also degenerate in time following these insults. Although it is generally assumed that the ganglion cell degeneration in acoustic trauma is secondary to sensory cell degeneration, it is also possible that ganglion cell degeneration is the primary process in ototoxicity.

Spoendlin[28] further observed that following nerve section and acoustic trauma the surviving ganglion cells are mainly type II cells, which innervate outer hair cells primarily, and some type III cells. Our present data on kanamycin-intoxicated ears also confirmed his observation in that when all sensory cells in the organ of Corti have completely degenerated, most type I cells are also degenerated, leaving mainly type II and a few type I and III cells. The unmyelinated fibers in the osseous spiral lamina have increased in number compared to normal, as in the case of VIII nerve sectioning.[31] Even if the sensory cells have disappeared, a few unmyelinated fibers are found in the organ of Corti that are replaced by cuboidal cells. Since the neurons of type II ganglion cells are unmyelinated,[32,33] it is possible that some of the unmyelinated fibers belong to type II ganglion cells. On the other hand, the number of unmyelinated fibers far exceeds the ganglion cell population, as in the case of myelinated fibers. Spoendlin and Suter[31] observed regeneration of both myelinated and unmyelinated nerve fibers in cats that were examined one year or more following the VIII nerve sectioning. The present study appears to suggest that even in the ototoxic ear similar, if not identical, neural regeneration occurs. Since the present study covers only three months following kanamycin treatment, it is not possible to predict how long the unmyelinated fibers will survive in the absence of sensory cells. Further study is needed to clarify the regenerative ability of the cochlear nerve and the nature of the unmyelinated nerve fibers to learn whether they are afferent, efferent, or autonomic.

REFERENCES

1. Hawkins JE Jr, Lurie MH: The ototoxicity of streptomycin. Ann Otol Rhinol Laryngol 61:789-806, 1952

2. Hawkins JE Jr, Engström H: Effects of kanamycin on cochlear cytoarchitecture. Acta Otolaryngol [Suppl] (Stockh) 188, 1963

3. Engström H, Kohonen A: Cochlear damage from ototoxic antibiotics. Acta Otolaryngol (Stockh) 59:173-178, 1965

4. Kohonen A: Effect of some ototoxic drugs upon the pattern and innervation of cochlear sensory cells in the guinea pig. Acta Otolaryngol [Suppl] (Stockh) 208, 1965

5. Wersäll J: Problems and pitfalls in studies of cochlear hair cell pathology, in Møller AR (ed): *The Auditory Periphery.* New York, Academic Press, 1973, pp 235-256

6. Hawkins JE Jr: Comparative otopathology: Aging, noise, and ototoxic drugs. Adv Otorhinolaryngol 20:125-141, 1973

7. Bredberg G, Hunter-Duvar IM: Behavioral tests of hearing and inner ear damage, in Autrum H, Jung R, Lowenstein WR, *et al* (eds): *Handbook of Sensory Physiology.* Berlin, Springer-Verlag, 1975, pp 261-306

8. Spoendlin H: Primary structural changes in the organ of Corti after acoustic overstimulation. Acta Otolaryngol (Stockh) 71:166-176, 1971

9. Lundquist P-G, Wersäll J: Kanamycin induced changes in cochlear hair cells of the guinea pig. Z Zellforsch Abt Histochem 72: 543-561, 1966

10. Murakami T: A revised tannin-osmium method for non-coated scanning electron microscope specimens. Arch Histol Jap 36:189-193, 1974

11. Beagley HA: Acoustic trauma in the guinea pig: II. Electron microscopy including the morphology of cell junctions in the organ of Corti. Acta Otolaryngol (Stockh) 60:479-495, 1965

12. Lim DJ, Melnick W: Acoustic damage of the cochlea: A scanning and transmission electron microscopic observation. Arch Otolaryngol 94:294-305, 1971

13. Bohne BA, Ward PH, Fernández C: Irreversible inner ear damage from rock music. Trans Am Acad Ophthalmol Otolaryngol 82: 50-59, 1976

14. Lim DJ, Melnick W: Mode of cochlear damage by excessive noise – an overview. AGARD Conference Proc No 171, AGARD, Washington, DC, 1975

15. Vinnikov YA, Titova LK: *The Organ of Corti: Its Histophysiology and Histochemistry.* Consultants Bureau, New York, 1964

16. Kellerhals B: Pathogenesis of inner ear lesions in acute acoustic trauma. Acta Otolaryngol (Stockh) 73:249-253, 1972

17. Bohne BA: Locations of small cochlear lesions by phase contrast microscopy prior to

thin sectioning. Laryngoscope 82:1-16, 1972

18. Bredberg G, Lindeman HH, Ades HW, *et al*: Scanning electron microscopy of the organ of Corti. Science 170:861-863, 1970

19. Wersäll J, Björkroth B, Flock Å, *et al*: Experiments on ototoxic effects of antibiotics. Adv Otorhinolaryngol 20:14-41, 1973

20. Ernstson S: Cochlear morphology in a strain of the waltzing guinea pig. Acta Otolaryngol (Stockh) 71:469-482, 1971

21. Schacht J: Interaction of neomycin with phosphoinositide metabolism in guinea pig inner ear and brain tissues. Ann Otol Rhinol Laryngol 83:613-618, 1974

22. Angelborg C, Engström H: The normal organ of Corti, in Møller AR (ed): *Basic Mechanisms of Hearing*. New York, Academic Press, 1973, pp 125-183

23. Engström H, Ades HW, Andersson A: *Structural Pattern of the Organ of Corti*. Baltimore, The Williams & Watkins Company, 1966

24. Kimura RS: Cochlear vascular lesions, in de Lorenzo AJD (ed): *Vascular Disorders and Hearing Defects*. Baltimore, University Park Press, 1973, pp 205-218

25. Ostyn F, Tyberghein J: Influence of some streptomyces antibiotics on the inner ear of the guinea pig. Acta Otolaryngol [Suppl] (Stockh) 234, 1968

26. Quick CA, Duvall AJ: Early changes in the cochlear duct from ethacrynic acid: An electronmicroscopic evaluation. Laryngoscope 80:954-965, 1970

27. Spoendlin H: Degeneration behavior of the cochlear nerve. Arch Klin Exp Ohren Nasen Kehlkopfheilkd 200:275-291, 1971

28. Spoendlin H: The innervation of the cochlear receptor, in Møller AR (ed): *The Auditory Periphery*. New York, Academic Press, 1973, pp 185-234

29. Rossi G, Robecchi MG, Penna M: Effects of acoustic trauma on Corti's ganglion. Acta Otolarnygol (Stockh) 81:270-277, 1976

30. Ward PH, Fernández C: The ototoxicity of kanamycin in guinea pigs. Ann Otol Rhinol Laryngol 70:132-142, 1961

31. Spoendlin H, Suter R: Regeneration in the VIII nerve. Acta Otolaryngol (Stockh) 81: 228-236, 1976

32. Spoendlin H: Innervation patterns in the organ of Corti of the cat. Acta Otolaryngol (Stockh) 67:239-254, 1969

33. Kellerhals B, Engström H, Ades HW: Die morphologie des Ganglion spirale Cochleae. Acta Otolaryngol [Suppl] (Stockh) 226, 1967

ACKNOWLEDGMENT—The author acknowledges the invaluable assistance of Ilija Karanfilov, David Stutes, Jonathan Darby, Nancy Sally, and Katherine Adamson.

REPRINTS—David J. Lim, MD, Otological Research Laboratories, The Ohio State University Hospitals, 410 West 10th Ave., Columbus, OH 43210.

XV INTERNATIONAL CONGRESS OF BRONCHOESOPHAGOLOGY

The XV International Congress of Bronchoesophagology will be held in Sao Paulo, Brazil, March 24-26, 1977, following the II World Congress of Otolaryngology in Buenos Aires. For information write: Dr. Plinio de Mattos Barretto, President of the Congress, Rua Cons. Torres Homem, 371, 01432, Sao Paulo, Brazil.

Ann Otol 85: 1976

AUDITORY-NERVE ACTIVITY IN CATS EXPOSED TO OTOTOXIC DRUGS AND HIGH-INTENSITY SOUNDS

NELSON Y. S. KIANG, PHD

M. CHARLES LIBERMAN, PHD   ROBERT A. LEVINE, MD

BOSTON, MASSACHUSETTS

SUMMARY – The response characteristics of auditory-nerve fibers in normal cats are compared with those in cats exposed to kanamycin and high-intensity sounds. The pathophysiology is characterized by an elevation of the tuning-curve "tips," which is sometimes associated with hypersensitivity of the "tails." Plots of unit thresholds are correlated with patterns of sensory-cell losses in the cochlea. There can be significant shifts in unit threshold without significant loss of hair cells; however, significant hair cell loss is always accompanied by highly abnormal unit thresholds. The presence of inner hair cells seems to be essential for the long-term survival of spiral ganglion cells. An incidental observation is that in the "normal" animal there is almost always a prominent "notch" at 3-4 kHz in the plots of threshold at characteristic frequency, which may have been produced by environmental noise.

The treatment of sensorineural hearing disorders is a major clinical problem. Damage to sensory end organs must modify the activity of primary neurons in order to create sensorineural disorders; thus, it is somewhat surprising that there have been few reports on the activity of single auditory-nerve fibers after injury to the cochlea. Two of the more easily-controllable agents of permanent cochlear damage are ototoxic drugs and high-intensity sounds.[1-5] Both are being used by us in studies designed to elucidate the mechanisms within the cochlea that generate auditory-nerve activity. The present paper is an attempt to select a few of these results that might have special significance for otologists. The intention is to describe the kinds of abnormal neural activity that can result from damage to the end organ; little attempt will be made to present systematically the parameters that influence the nature and extent of the damage.

METHODS

Healthy young cats were chosen for this study. Most of the animals were under 2 kg in weight at the time of recording. Kanamycin was administered as described previously.[6] To produce acoustic trauma, the animals were first anesthetized with Nembutal® (48 mg/kg body weight). The head was then clamped firmly so that the left tragus was 1-2 cm from an acoustic driver. The electric input to the driver was the amplified output of a noise generator. For narrow-band stimuli the output of a noise generator was fed through a tracking filter before amplification. A ¼" condenser microphone was placed between the driver and the entrance to the ear canal so that the sound pressure level (dB rms) could be monitored throughout the exposure. Sample spectra for narrow- and broad-band traumatizing stimuli, as measured at the ¼" microphone, are shown in Figure 1.

The animals were kept for variable lengths of time after treatment before recordings were made from the auditory nerve. The surgical exposures, the methods of recording from single fibers, the presentation of acoustic stimuli, and the processing of neural responses were as described earlier.[6] The stimuli used in searching for single units were 10/sec, moderate-level, acoustic clicks in cats MCL14, MCL48 to 66, and MCL75 to 85. Electric

----

From the Eaton-Peabody Laboratory of Auditory Physiology, Massachusetts Eye and Ear Infirmary; the Research Laboratory of Electronics, Massachusetts Institute of Technology; and the Neurology Service, Massachusetts General Hospital, Boston, Massachusetts. This work was supported by U. S. Public Health Service Grants 5 R01 NS01344, 5 R01 NS11000, and 5 T01 MH07084.

Presented at the meeting of the American Otological Society, Inc., Palm Beach, Florida, April 25-26, 1976.

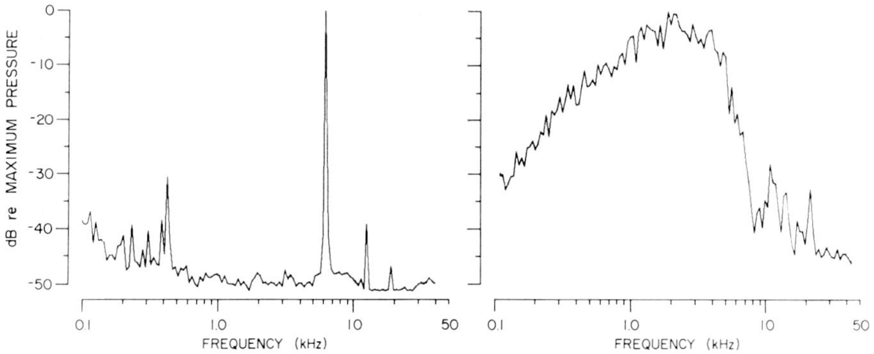

Fig. 1. Spectral magnitudes of typical narrow- (left) and broad-band (right) stimuli used to produce cochlear lesions. Analysis was performed by passing the output of the ¼" microphone (positioned at the tragus) through a tunable filter with a bandwidth of 5 Hz (Spectral Dynamics Corporation Model SD-131 Tracking Filter). The levels of the particular narrow- and broad-band stimuli shown here were 102 and 115 dB SPL (rms), respectively.

stimulation was used as a search stimulus in MCL71 to 74, MCL36, and RAL25. The 10/sec shocks were delivered either through the recording microelectrode or between two wires placed on the bony capsule of the cochlea. The shocks were most useful in finding units that did not respond to sound and had low rates of spontaneous discharge. Round-window potentials were recorded in each animal.

In all experiments, several microelectrode passes were made through the auditory nerve. The usual procedure was to note the position

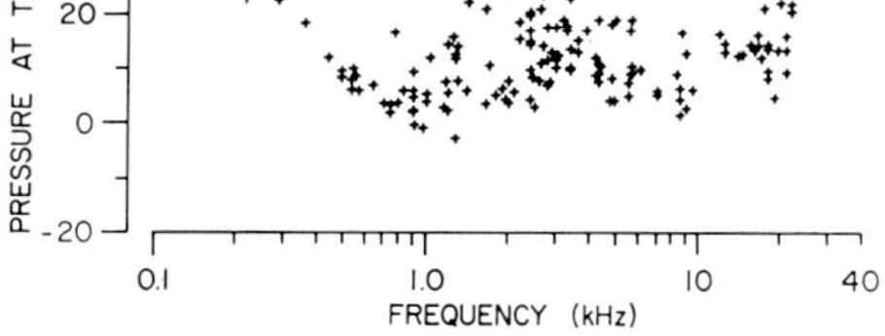

Fig. 2. Threshold at the characteristic frequency (CF) for 176 units in a normal cat. Thresholds were based on tuning curves obtained by the procedure described[6] and are repeatable within a few dB for the same unit. Since one of the objectives of this experiment was to determine the spread in threshold among units with similar CF, the distribution of thresholds is somewhat biased in favor of units with high thresholds.

of each penetration on a calibrated drawing of the nerve bundle. The angle of the microelectrode with respect to the cat's head was constant from pass to pass and from animal to animal. Each time a unit was encountered, its position in the pass was recorded. With this procedure, the tonotopic organization of the auditory nerve in normal animals was reconstructed by analyzing the distribution of unit characteristic frequency (CF) as a function of position within the nerve. The repeatability of this organization was exploited when searching for units of a given CF in abnormal animals and in estimating grossly the original CF of fibers which had lost their responsiveness to sound.

At the end of most of the auditory-nerve experiments the animal was sacrificed by intra-aortal perfusion with Heidenhein-Susa solution. For RAL25 a surface preparation of the temporal bone was made as described previously.[6] All the acoustically-traumatized and the rest of the kanamycin-treated cochleas were decalcified, dehydrated, embedded in celloidin, and cut in 20μm sections in the horizontal plane. Routinely, every fifth section was stained with H. and E. before mounting on slides. Whenever examination showed that the cochlear lesion was small, a second set of sections (each one between two successive sections of the first set) was stained and mounted. For cats MCL36 and MCL48, every section in the vicinity of the lesion was evaluated.

The organs of Corti were reconstructed as described by Schuknecht.[7] The histograms depicting cell population (hair cells and supporting cells) as a function of distance along the cochlea were constructed by computing the percentage of cells of each type remaining in each section (through the cochlear duct) and then averaging the percentages across all sections in each 1% increment of cochlear

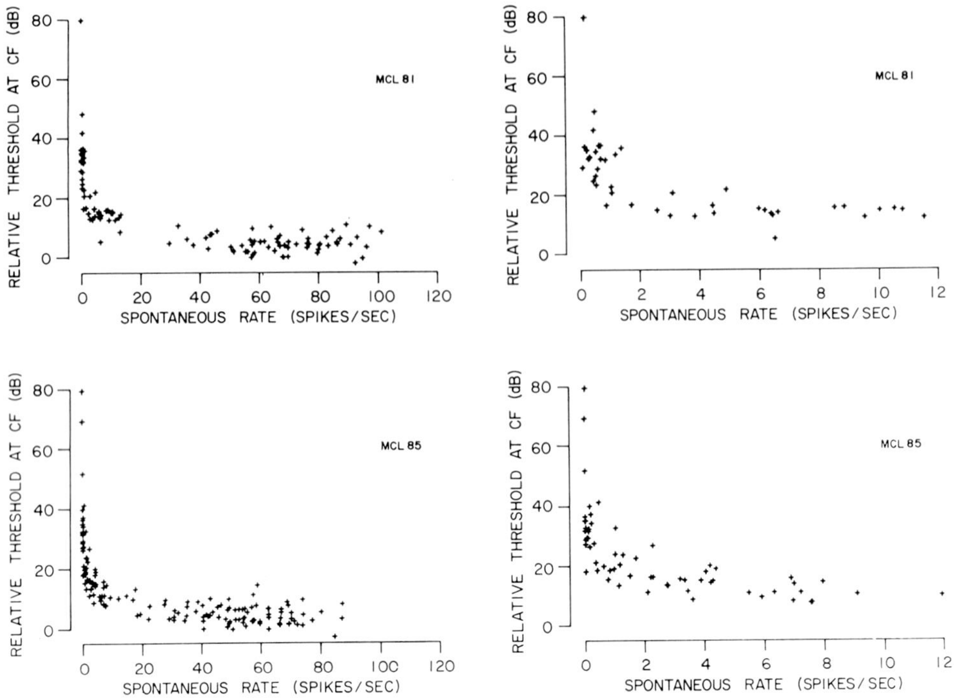

Fig. 3. Spontaneous discharge rates (Spont) for units from two normal cats plotted against their relative thresholds at CF. Relative threshold is defined as the difference between a unit's threshold and the threshold of the most sensitive units with similar CF for that animal. Only units with CF between 1 and 10 kHz are included, because at other frequencies the thresholds change with CF too rapidly to permit accuracy in determining the relative threshold. The data from each cat are shown on the left with coarse resolution in rate and on the right with fine resolution for units with Spont below 12/sec.

length. When every fifth section is evaluated, the condition of cochlear structures can be sampled at 140 positions along the length of the basilar membrane; but, because of the spiral shape, the sampling density is higher in the midmodiolar regions than in regions where the cochlea is cut tangentially. All anatomical data describing cell population vs location along the cochlea are plotted in terms of percent distance from the base. The logarithmic frequency scale along which the physiological data are plotted is aligned with the anatomical scale so that 52 kHz corresponds to the most basal point and 0.18 kHz to the most apical point. This method of display is equivalent to Schuknecht's map correlating frequency with cochlear location for all frequencies above 1 kHz.

Loss of nerve fibers in the habenula region was estimated by visual inspection. For every cross section through the cochlear duct the fiber density was rated as 100, 75, 50, 25, 12, or 0 percent of normal. Histograms were then computed in the same way as for the hair cells and supporting cells.

Loss of spiral ganglion cells was measured by determining the density of cells in a given 20μm section through the ganglion (number of cells/total area of section through Rosenthal's canal) and comparing it to the densities obtained from several normal animals at the corresponding location along the spiral ganglion. The density in abnormal animals was examined qualitatively in every fifth section but quantitatively at 30 positions along the course of the ganglion. The distance along the ganglion was related to distance along the organ of Corti in the following way: the number of spiral ganglion cells in an increment of ganglion length can be estimated from the counts on normal animals; the density of innervation as a function of distance along the organ of Corti has been reported by Spoendlin;[8] these two functions can be combined to estimate the length of organ of Corti innervated by each increment of the ganglion.

RESULTS

Responses in "Normal" Animals. There are many parameters of auditory-nerve responses that can be studied when comparing recordings from normal and

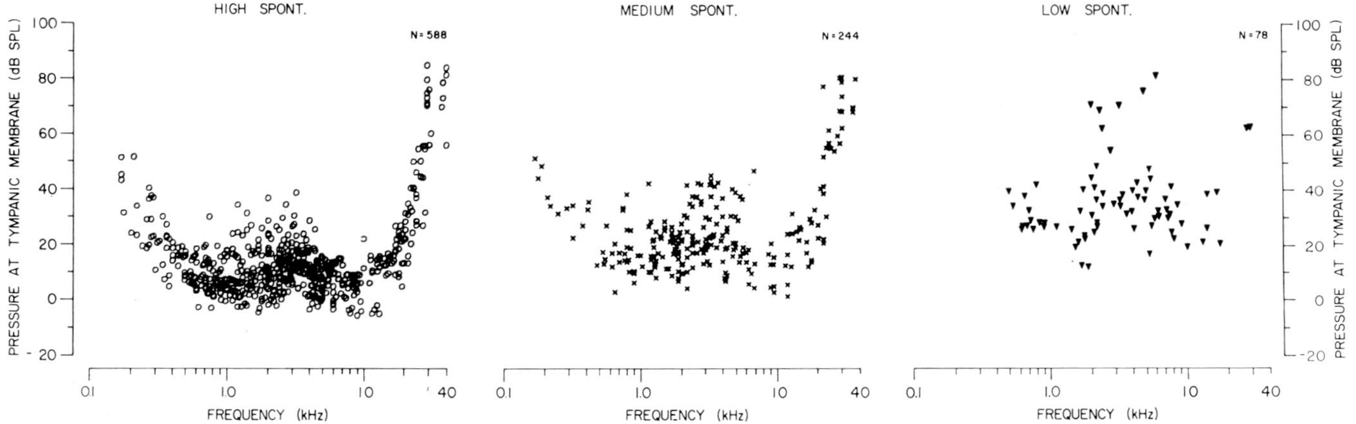

Fig. 4. Threshold at CF for 910 units from 11 normal cats segregated according to Spont. The high-Spont group contains units with rate higher than (or equal to) 18 spikes/sec. The low-Spont group consists of units with rates lower than 0.5 spikes/sec. The medium-Spont group includes units with intermediate rates. Subsequent figures will use the same symbols to designate the three Spont groups.

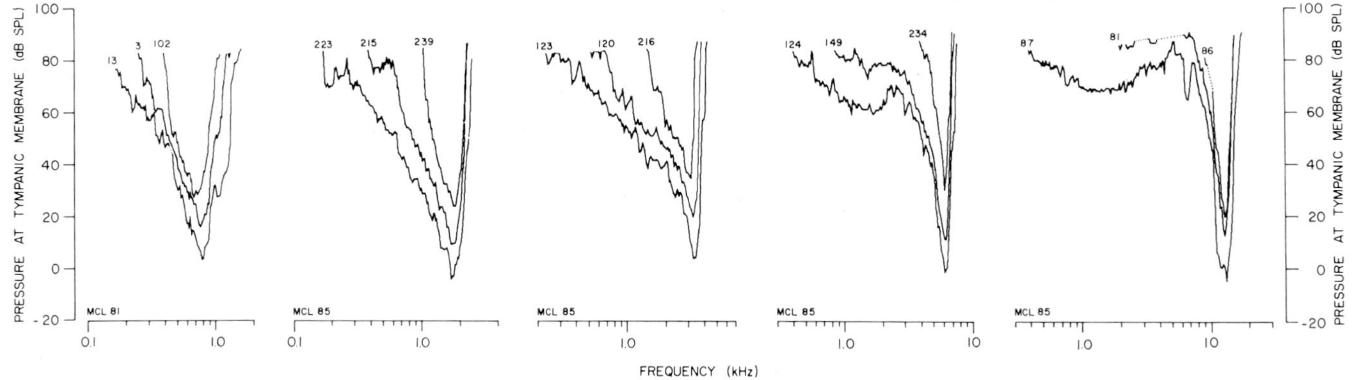

Fig. 5. Tuning curves of units with high, medium, and low Spont from normal cats. One typical unit of each Spont group was selected for five different ranges of CF. The Spont for units 13, 223, 123, 124, and 87 were 59.2, 40.6, 53.7, 62.6, and 105.0 spikes/sec. The Spont for units 3, 215, 120, 149, and 81 were 2.1, 1.13, 4.03, 2.2, and 1.83 spikes/sec. The Spont for units 102, 239, 216, 234, and 86 were 0.17, 0.03, 0.13, 0, and 0.17. The approximate CF are, from left to right, 0.8, 1.8, 3.2, 6, and 13 kHz. The tuning curve for unit 87 has a sharp dip at 6.5 kHz which is a response to a second-harmonic distortion component in the acoustic stimulus.

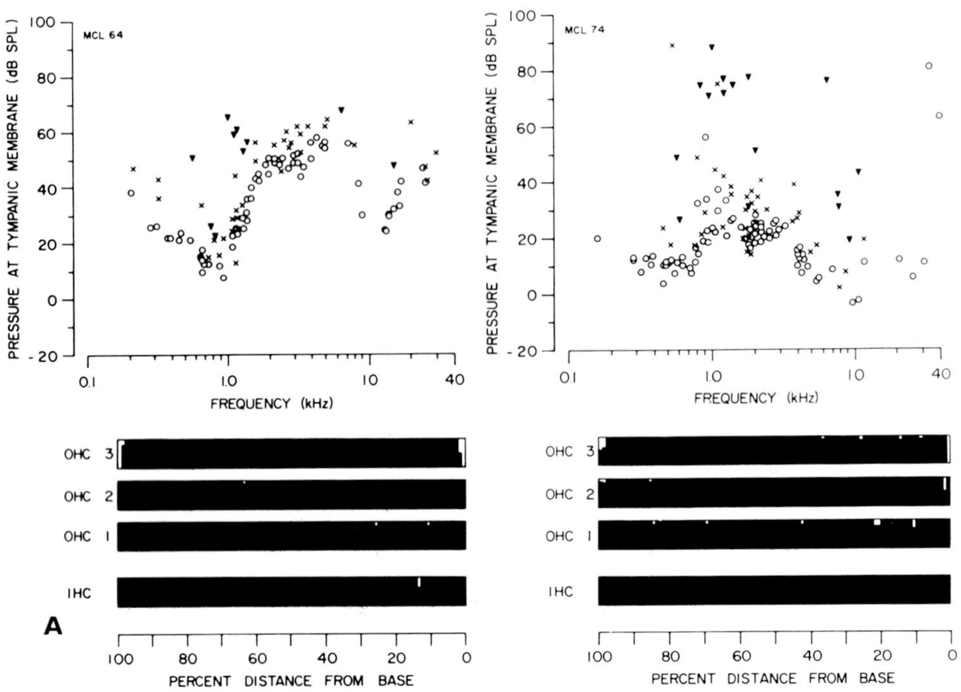

Fig. 6. A) Plots of unit thresholds for two acoustically-traumatized cats with minimal loss of hair cells. Each of the plots on the top shows the thresholds at CF for all units obtained in one ear. The box graphs below comprise the cytocochleogram for that ear. The percentage of hair cells which remains in each of the four rows is plotted (in black) as a function of percentage distance along the cochlea. The traumatic stimulus for both animals was 1.5 kHz, narrow-band (50 Hz) noise at 110 dB SPL for two hours. The survival times between traumatization and experimentation were 28 and 37 days for MCL64 and MCL74, respectively. The cochlear lengths were 23.3 mm for MCL64 and 24 mm for MCL74. Acoustic clicks were used as search stimuli in MCL64 as the microelectrode was advanced through the nerve; electric shocks were used as search stimuli in MCL74.

abnormal cats. The focus of the present paper will be on plots of threshold for single units as a function of stimulus frequency (threshold tuning curves). For each unit in a normal animal, the characteristic frequency (CF) is defined as that frequency to which the unit is maximally sensitive. There is considerable spread in the threshold at CF for units with similar CF (Fig. 2), even when the tuning curves are obtained by automated procedures. Throughout most of the frequency range the spread of thresholds at CF is approximately 30-40 dB. However, for units tuned near 3 kHz, there is a larger spread of thresholds as well as a higher average threshold, even when there is virtually no hair cell loss.

Previous studies have suggested that auditory-nerve units with low spontaneous discharge rates (Spont) tend to have higher thresholds than high-Spont units with similar CF.[6,9] The relationship between Spont and threshold is demonstrated in Figure 3. Units with the highest relative thresholds tend to have Spont lower than 0.5 spikes/sec; units with the lowest thresholds tend to have Spont higher than 18 spikes/sec; and units with intermediate thresholds tend to have intermediate Spont. In experiments performed without conscious bias in unit selection, 10% of the units have Spont less than 0.5/sec.

Differences in thresholds for units with high, medium, and low Spont can be seen in data pooled from many ani-

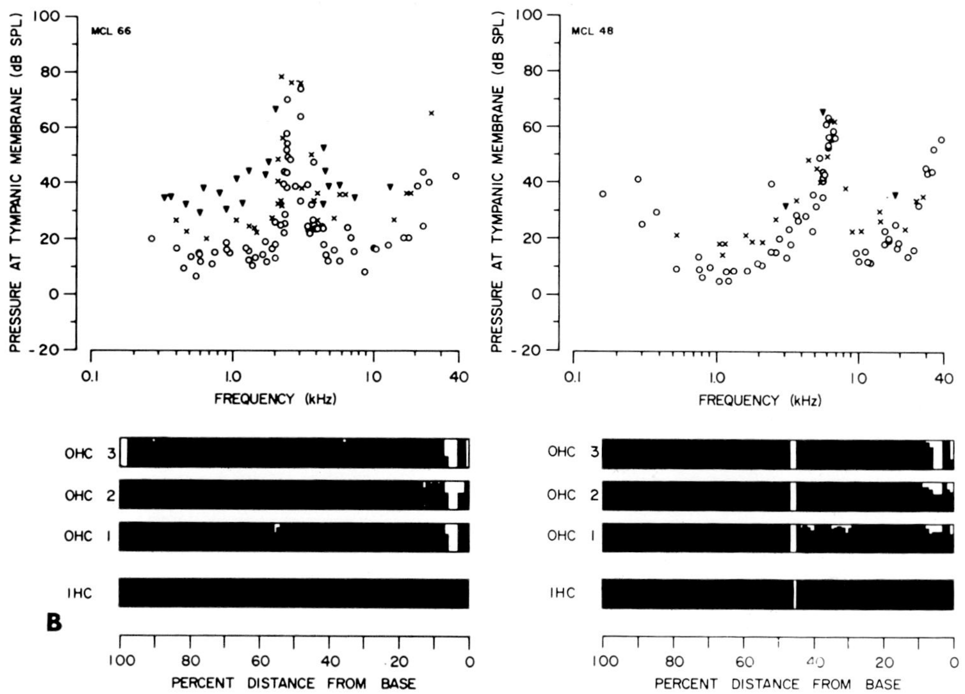

Fig. 6. B) Plots of unit thresholds for two acoustically-traumatized ears with minimal loss of hair cells. Conventions of display are as described in Figure 6A. The traumatic stimuli and survival times were as follows: MCL66 was exposed to 3 kHz, narrow-band (50 Hz) noise at 108 dB SPL for two hours and had a survival time of 57 days; MCL48 was exposed to 6 kHz, narrow-band (100 Hz) noise at 102 dB SPL for two hours and had a survival time of 54 days. The cochlear lengths were 23.1 and 22.5 mm for MCL66 and MCL48, respectively. Acoustic clicks were used as search stimuli in these ears. The absence of hair cells in the extreme base is unilateral.

mals (Fig. 4). Note that for each Spont group the units with CF near 3-4 kHz tend to have higher thresholds than units with neighboring CF. This relationship is especially evident for low-Spont units.

Tuning curves for units of similar CF with high, medium, and low Spont are displayed in Figure 5. Note that the low-Spont units tend to be more sharply tuned than high-Spont units. The differences in tuning-curve shapes argue against the idea that the high thresholds of the low-Spont units merely reflect the normal scatter of thresholds within a single population of units.

Responses in Acoustically-Traumatized Animals. Exposure to high-intensity sounds can create different patterns of damage to cochlear structures depending on the acoustic parameters. The effects of exposure to narrow-band noise on thresholds at CF are shown in Figure 6A, B for four different animals.

The two examples in Figure 6A were both exposed to 1.5 kHz, narrow-band noise. Although neither animal shows significant loss of hair cells, both show deviations from normal in unit-threshold plots (plots of threshold at CF vs CF). In MCL74 there is a threshold shift of approximately 20 dB for all of the high-Spont units with CF between 1 and 4 kHz. In MCL64, the threshold shifts extend to units with higher CF and are as great as 50 dB in some frequency regions. Apparently, extensive physiological abnormalities can be found in the absence of significant hair cell loss. Since the survival time after exposure was more than four weeks in each case, the physiological changes

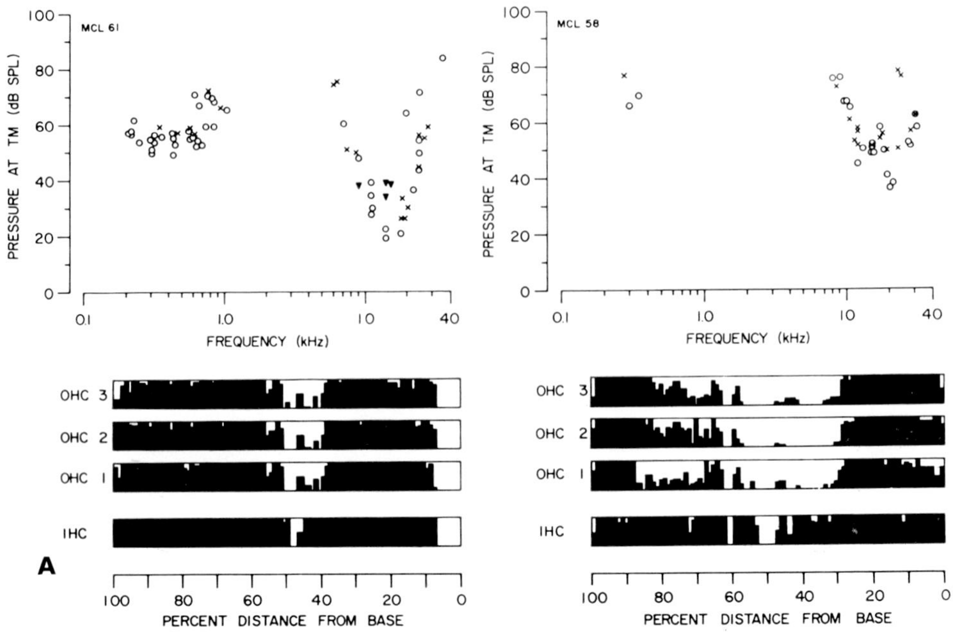

Fig. 7. A) Plots of unit thresholds for two acoustically-traumatized ears with extensive hair cell losses. The traumatic stimuli and survival times were as follows: MCL61 was exposed to low-pass (5 kHz cutoff) noise at 115 dB SPL for four hours and had a survival time of 49 days; MCL58 was exposed to low-pass (5 kHz cutoff) noise at 120 dB SPL for two hours and had a survival time of 28 days. The cochlear lengths were 23.9 and 23.2 mm for MCL61 and MCL58, respectively. Acoustic clicks were used as search stimuli for the auditory-nerve experiments in these ears.

are probably permanent.

The two cats in Figure 6B, MCL66 and MCL48, were exposed to narrow-band noise centered at 3 and 6 kHz, respectively. In each case, it is the units with CF near the center-frequency of the traumatizing stimulus that show the greatest elevation in threshold (approximately 60-70 dB). The elevation of thresholds is restricted to narrow CF regions, and normal tuning curves can be found for units with CF above and below the traumatizing frequency. The locations of hair-cell loss in these two animals do not correlate well with the usual map that is based on a simple linear-distance-to-log-frequency relation. The frequency assigned by such a map is apparently too low, at least in this particular region of the cochlea.

Data from four traumatized animals in which greater losses of hair cells were found are shown in Figure 7A, B. For each of these animals there is an extensive gap in the unit-threshold plot. Passes through regions of the nerve where the "missing" CFs would normally be found revealed many units with either no response to sound or with tuning curves so broad that no CF could be assigned. Many of the unresponsive units had no spontaneous activity; of the unresponsive units with spontaneous activity, many showed highly abnormal time-patterns of discharge. CF gaps were always found in animals with substantial regions of outer-hair cell loss. A more detailed analysis of the correlation between structural change and functional abnormality will depend upon having a more accurate cochlear frequency map upon which damage more subtle than the absence of hair cells can be plotted.

Figure 8 shows sample tuning curves from one animal with a restricted coch-

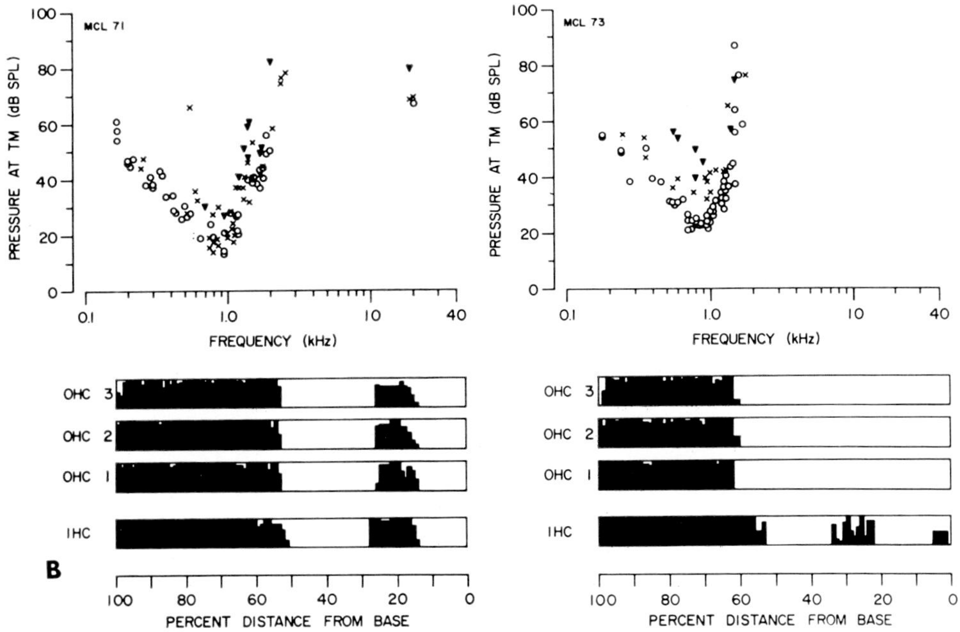

Fig. 7. B) Plots of unit thresholds for two acoustically-traumatized ears with extensive hair cell losses. The traumatic stimuli and survival times were as follows: MCL71 was exposed to 6 kHz, narrow-band (200 Hz) noise at 110 dB SPL for two hours and had a survival time of 273 days; MCL73 was exposed to 6 kHz, narrow-band (200 Hz) noise at 116 dB SPL for two hours and had a survival time of 30 days. The cochlear lengths were 23.0 and 21.9 mm for MCL71 and MCL73, respectively. Electric shocks were used as search stimuli for the auditory-nerve experiments in these ears.

lear lesion. The CF gap is well delimited because several passes were made through the regions of the nerve where 5-9 kHz units should be found. Tuning curves with CF just above and below the gap have raised thresholds at the tip. In this animal, the broadly-tuned tails seem to be relatively normal, but in other traumatized animals there are examples of tuning curves with comparable threshold shifts of both tip and tail. The tuning curves in panel E illustrate that, when the tips are elevated, prominent " clefts" can appear between the tip and the tail. This type of tuning curve has been obtained in almost all CF regions and on both the low- and high-frequency sides of the lesion. The units whose tuning curves are shown in panel F responded to frequencies from 5-9 kHz at intensities near 70 dB SPL. Of all units encountered in this animal, these four had the lowest thresholds in this frequency range, despite the fact that their CF were in the 13 kHz range.

It is often the case in acoustically-traumatized animals that the lowest thresholds to a particular frequency are found for units with CF in a much higher frequency range. A particularly striking example is shown in Figure 9. The thresholds at CF for this animal are shown in Figure 7A (left). The units whose tuning curves showed the highest thresholds were not assigned CFs since there were no regions of sharp tuning. However, based on where these three units were found in the nerve, they probably had CF between 1 and 8 kHz before the exposure to high-intensity sounds. Although their thresholds are high, these units represent the most sensitive of all the broadly-tuned units whose CFs might have fallen between those of the two stippled regions before the acoustic trauma. These stippled region delineate the response areas of two sharply-tuned units with CF just at the borders of the CF gap. Of all the units studied in this animal, the lowest

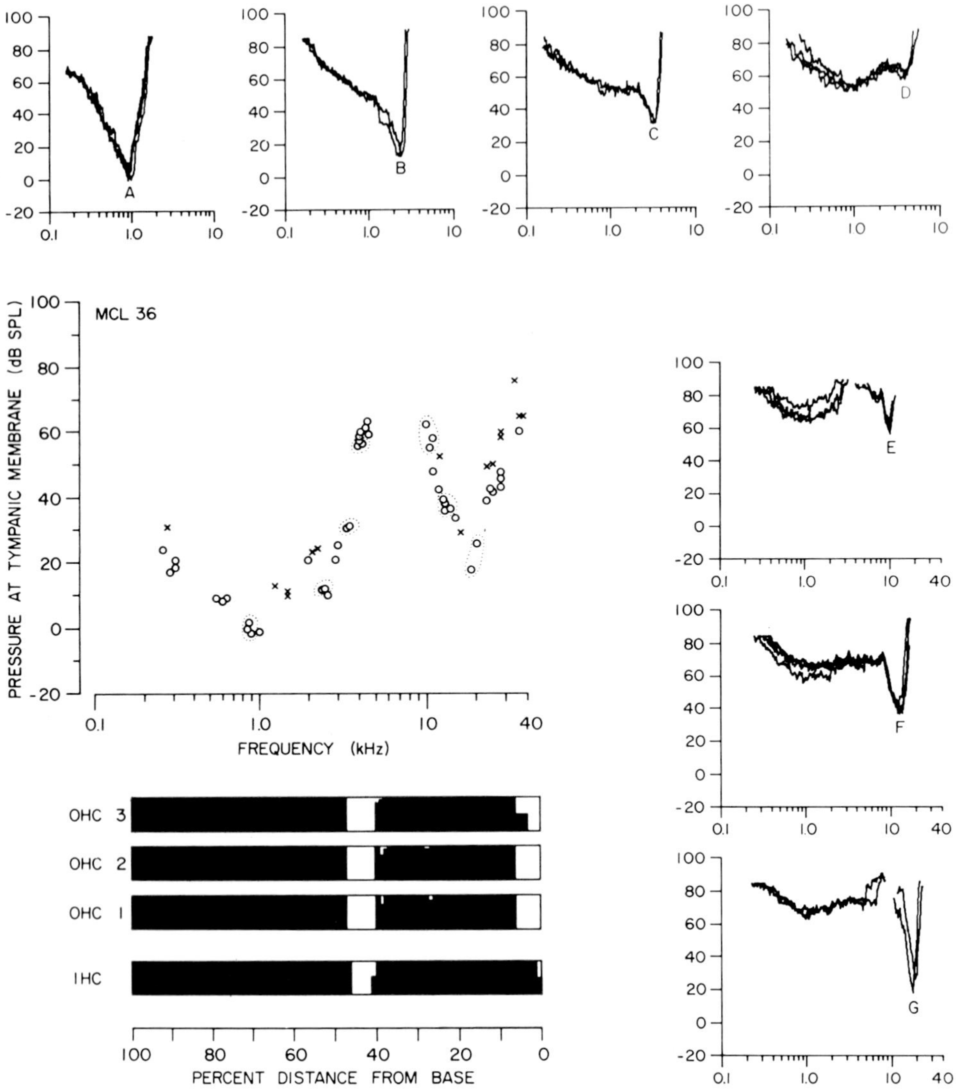

Fig. 8. Histopathology and pathophysiology in an acoustically-traumatized cat. The cat was exposed to narrow-band (200 Hz) noise centered around 6 kHz, at 105 dB SPL. The duration of exposure was two hours, and the physiological recordings were made 37 days after traumatization. Thresholds at CF of units with high and medium Spont are plotted in the middle of the figure. The seven clusters of points enclosed by the dotted circles correspond to the tips of the seven groups of tuning curves arranged in CF order along the top and the right side of the figure. Breaks in the tuning curves occur because the input to the earphones was limited in level at each frequency. The Spont of all the units whose tuning curves are shown lie between 19 and 85 spikes/sec. The cochleogram at the bottom of the figure shows the percentage of hair cells present (in black) as a function of distance along the cochlea. The total length of the basilar membrane was 25 mm. The absence of hair cells in the extreme base is unilateral.

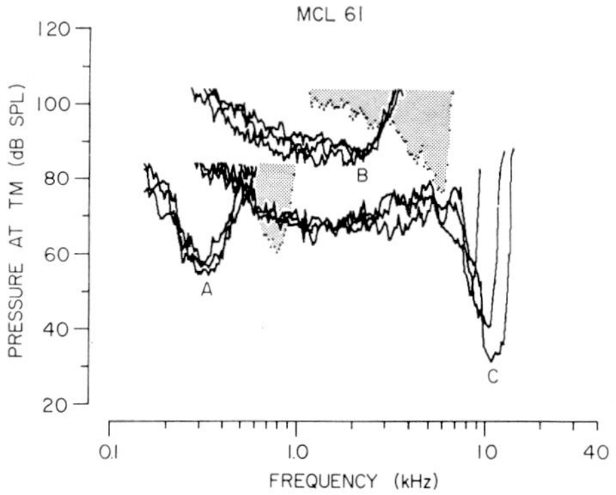

Fig. 9. Selected tuning curves from one acoustically-traumatized cat. The thresholds at CF for this animal are shown in Figure 7A. For exposure information, see the caption for Figure 7A. The Spont for these units ranged between 21.8 and 82.7 spikes/sec with the exception of the 6 kHz (stippled) unit which had a Spont of 15.2 spikes/sec. See text for further explanation.

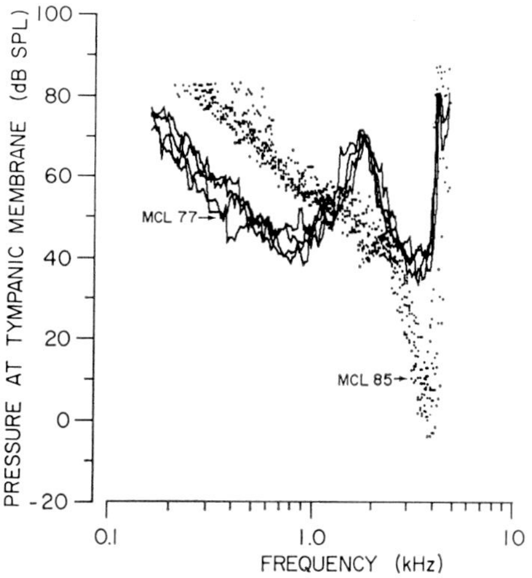

Fig. 10. Tuning curves with hyposensitive tails compared with normal tuning curves for units in the same CF range (3.5 - 4.0 kHz). The four solid curves are from MCL77, which was exposed to narrow-band (50 Hz) noise, centered at 3 kHz, for two hours at 110 dB SPL, 58 days before the auditory-nerve experiment. The eight dotted curves are from one of the most sensitive normal animals, MCL85. All units had high Spont.

thresholds for frequencies between 1 and 10 kHz were found among the high-Spont units with CF near 10 kHz (C).

The description of unit activity in acoustically-traumatized animals is further complicated by the phenomenon shown in Figure 10. When the thresholds near CF are elevated, the units can be hypersensitive at other frequencies. It appears that the effects of cochlear damage need not be limited to loss of responsiveness in the nerve; abnormal units can also respond actively to stimuli that were subthreshold before the injury.

Kanamycin-Treated Animals. Unit-threshold plots, tuning curves, and cochleograms in kanamycin-treated cats have been described previously.[6] The data from one such animal (RAL25) are shown in Figure 11 for comparison with the data from acoustically-traumatized cats. The kanamycin-induced lesion differs from the lesion in MCL36 in two ways: there is a sizeable region where outer hair cells are lost without concomitant loss of inner hair cells, and there are no hair cells left in the basal turn.

Most of the abnormal tuning curves from RAL25 resemble those seen in MCL36 for CF regions below the gap. Other tuning curves from RAL25 are so broad that no CF can be assigned (curves E and F); such units were not seen in MCL36. Although it is tempting to suggest that these broad tuning curves belong to fibers that innervate inner hair cells in regions where outer hair cells are missing, the lack of a more precise cochlear frequency map precludes such a specific conclusion.

In kanamycin-treated animals, the regions of the nerve where high-CF units are normally found are occupied by units that are unresponsive to sound but responsive to electric stimulation. The density of such units seems to be within the normal range when the survival time is on the order of several months. However, with surface preparations it is difficult to obtain quantitative measures of the presence or absence of spiral ganglion cells. Therefore, several kanamycin-intoxicated cats were prepared for serial sectioning, including some animals with survival times of more than four years.

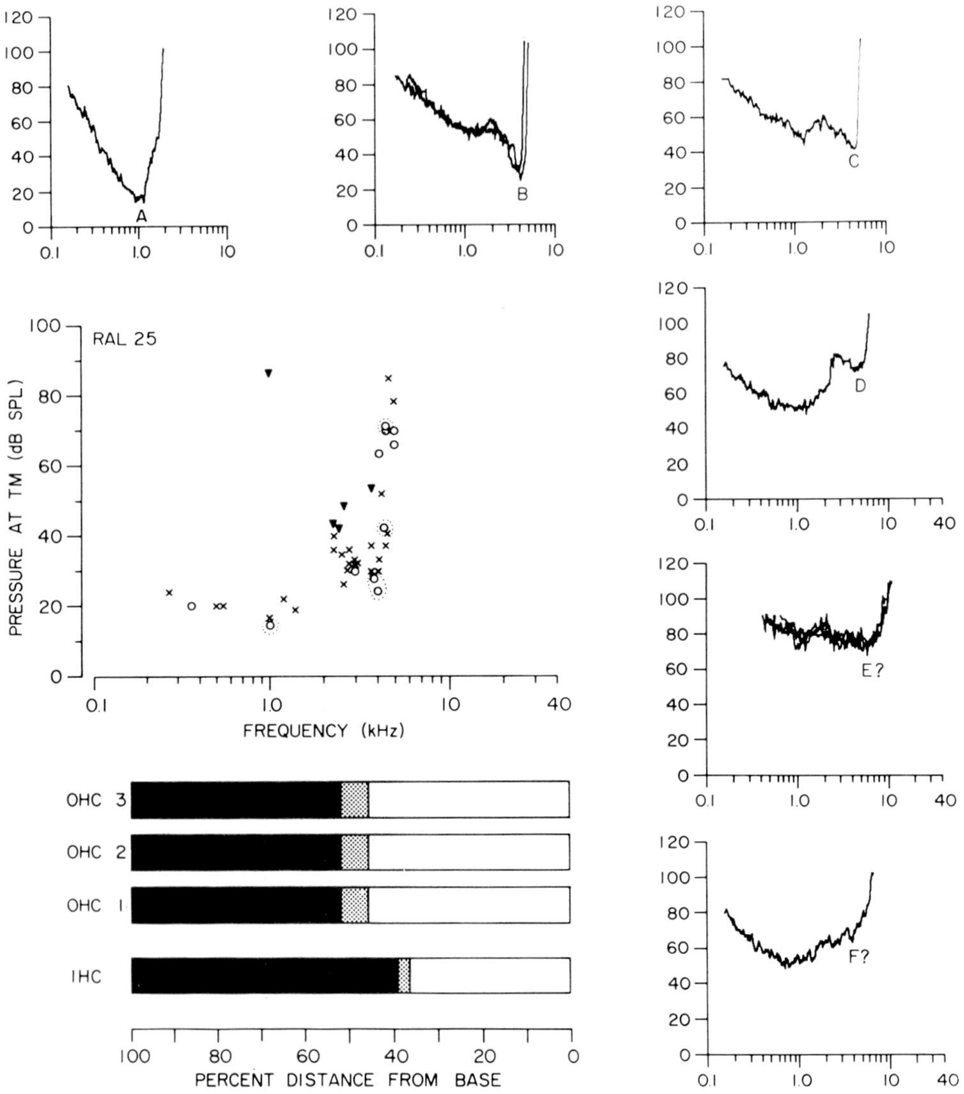

Fig. 11. Histopathology and pathophysiology of a cat treated with kanamycin (200 mg/kg for eight days). One hundred and forty-eight days after the last injection, physiological recordings were made and the animal was perfused. Surface-preparation techniques were used to examine the cochleas. The thresholds at CF for single units in the auditory nerve are plotted in the center panel. The tuning curves of the units surrounded by dots are shown in panels A, B, C, and D. The units whose tuning curves are shown in panels E and F were not assigned CFs because none showed clear signs of sharp tuning. The cochleogram, constructed from the surface preparations, is shown with black representing 90% or more present and white representing 90% or more absent; regions where 10-90% of the hair cells remain are shown with stippling. The length of the basilar membrane was 22.5 mm.

After long-term survival from kanamycin poisoning there is clear evidence, both histological and physiological, that significant loss of neural elements occurs. The pattern of destruction of sensory cells, supporting cells, and nerve fibers in one animal, sacrificed four years after treatment, is shown in Figure 12. Note that the loss of nerve fibers (as evaluated in the habenular region)

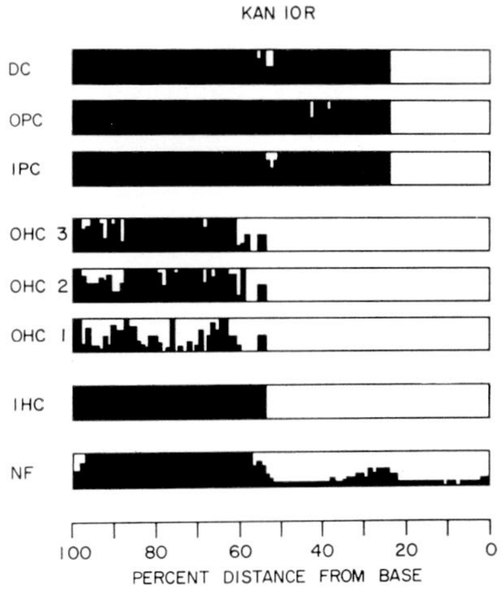

Fig. 12. Cochlear pathology in a cat four years after kanamycin intoxication. The dosage was 200 mg/kg for nine successive days. The histograms show, in black, the percentage of cells remaining. From the top down, the elements are: Deiters' cells, outer pillar cells, inner pillar cells, the three rows of outer hair cells, inner hair cells, and nerve fibers (as seen in the region of the habenula perforata).

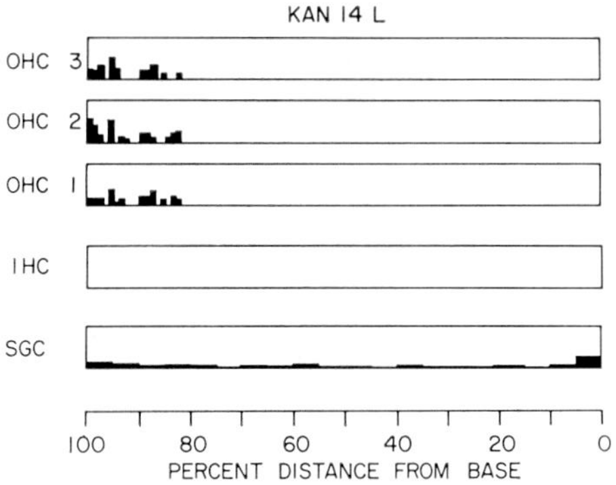

Fig. 13. Depopulation of spiral ganglion cells compared to pattern of hair cell loss in a cat 5½ years after kanamycin intoxication (200 mg/kg/day for nine successive days). Histograms show, in black, the percentage of cells remaining. In this animal no gross or unit response was found to acoustic stimuli.

correlates more closely with the pattern of inner-hair cell loss than with loss of either outer hair cells or supporting cells. However, nerve-fiber loss is not complete in regions where no inner hair cells remain; it is not even complete where the entire organ of Corti is missing. There was massive depopulation in the spiral ganglion of this animal with a pattern resembling that of inner-hair cell loss.

In another of the long-term animals, the destruction of inner hair cells was complete (Figure 13). The depopulation of the spiral ganglion was nearly complete in all regions of the cochlea. In recording from this animal, no units that responded to sound could be found, and only a few units responded to electric stimulation. There were no gross responses of the cochlea or nerve. Thus, the idea that a normal complement of viable nerve fibers might survive indefinitely after ototoxic destruction of the sensory cells seems not to have been justified. On the other hand, a few cells do remain, and they may well be electrically excitable.

For comparison, in acoustically-traumatized animals, loss of nerve fibers in the habenula perforata can be seen in regions radial to areas of inner-hair cell loss as early as two weeks after the exposure. Significant loss of spiral ganglion cells has not been seen for survival times of less than two months. In one animal with a survival time of about a year, there was extensive ganglion-cell loss following the pattern of the inner-hair cell loss. The final pattern of spiral ganglion cell losses may be similar for both the kanamycin-treated and the acoustically-traumatized cats, but the time course of degeneration need not necessarily be the same.

DISCUSSION

The results described in this paper bear upon several topics of current interest to otologists.

Cochlear Implants. The advisability of using cochlear implants to bypass a malfunctioning cochlea depends, at least in part, on the availability of excitable auditory-nerve elements. Total deafness associated with a normal complement of auditory-nerve fibers is apparently rare, but previous studies indicate that such a situation might arise among patients treated with ototoxic drugs.[6,10,11] Our present results indicate that many years after kanamycin-induced loss of inner and outer hair cells only a small proportion of spiral ganglion cells will remain. It is conceivable that chronic, electric stimulation of the neurons would prevent their degeneration unless there is some essential trophic influence exerted by elements of the sensory epithelium.

These results are of practical importance in considering whether electric stimulation could restore usable hearing in ears where only a small proportion of neural elements remains in any region of the cochlea. We do know that single- channel devices implanted in the ears of ototoxically-deafened patients are not effective in restoring normal speech discrimination.[12,13] Even if multichannel devices should prove to be more successful than single-channel devices for cases where the nerve is largely intact, it remains to be seen whether they could be effective in human ears with neural degeneration as drastic as in KAN14 (Fig. 13).

It should be noted that monitoring behavioral thresholds for electric stimuli might not reveal progressive degeneration in the nerve. Because the electrical tuning curves of auditory-nerve fibers are broad,[14] the presence of only a few fibers could be sufficient for the detection of such stimuli.

Environmental Noise. Standards for "normal" human hearing are based on averages over many individuals and probably include hearing losses due to environmental noise even when the sample is restricted to healthy young subjects.[15] The existence of a 3-4 kHz notch in the unit-threshold plots for all of the "normal" cats in this study suggests that in the present environment it may be difficult to find cats with undamaged hearing. If it could be established that the notch reflects a sensorineural loss due to acoustic trauma, as seems to be the case with the well-known 4 kHz notch in human threshold functions,[16] then the cat might be a useful animal model in which to study this phenomenon. Since there is no increase in threshold near 3-4 kHz in the tails of tuning curves of high-CF units, the notch is probably not the result of a conductive loss.

There are signs that a 3 kHz notch may exist in behavioral threshold curves of cats.[17] However, caution should be exercised in comparing such results with our physiological results because several conductive stages of the system are strongly frequency-selective in the 3-4 kHz range.[18,19] In our physiological experiments the external auditory meatus and the middle-ear septum were surgically removed; this was not the case in the behavioral studies.

Interpretation of Hearing Tests. In a normal animal, it seems reasonable to assume that a threshold audiogram would correspond to the envelope of the unit-threshold plot, since the lowest thresholds for each stimulus frequency are obtained in units with CF at that frequency. This correspondence may break down in abnormal animals, where for certain stimulus frequencies the most sensitive units can be those with CF at other frequencies (Fig. 9). It could be difficult to determine, on the basis of behavioral audiograms alone, which region of the cochlea is mediating the response to a given frequency. In an animal like MCL61, a behavioral audiogram might show a flat, 60-70 dB loss for all frequencies between 700 and 7000 Hz although there is a region in the middle of the cochlea where all hair cells are missing. More sophisticated measures such as psychophysical tuning curves based on masking function[20-22] might also be difficult to interpret in the light of these considerations.

The presence of high-threshold, broadly-tuned units in kanamycin-treated cats led to a general formulation for the physiological basis of loudness recruitment.[6] It was proposed that selective damage to the sensitive tips of the tuning curves could eliminate all responses in the nerve to low-intensity stimuli but would not affect the total amount of auditory-nerve activity in response to a stimulus level higher than the thresholds of the broadly-tuned tails. In view of the fact that noise-induced hearing loss is also characterized by the recruitment of loudness,[23] it is significant that selective damage to the tuning-curve tips is also routinely seen in acoustically-traumatized ears.

If perceptions of complex sounds are based on patterns of activity in the total array of auditory-nerve fibers,[24] alterations in patterns associated with hypo- and hypersensitivity (Fig. 10) would distort the normal cues for speech discrimination. One could imagine that, under some circumstances, the presence of abnormal responses might be more detrimental than a complete absence of responses from the same region.

Correlation of Pathophysiology with Histopathology. Any correlation of auditory-nerve physiology with cochlear histology is based on the premise that the CF dimension in the auditory nerve maps in some continuous way onto the longitudinal dimension in the cochlea. If an accurate, quantitative expression for this relationship were derived, many facts could be given meaningful interpretation. The most commonly used cochlear frequency map for cats is based on Schuknecht's study of behavioral audiograms of cats with lesions in the cochlea.[25] Using this map, the frequencies assigned to punctate regions of hair cell loss do not correlate with the frequency range of the CF gaps (MCL48 in Fig. 6B, MCL36 in Fig. 8). This discrepancy is not surprising given the relatively coarse frequency resolution of the behavioral audiograms and the relatively dispersed nature of the lesions in Schuknecht's animals. The results of a more recent study correlating lesions with behavioral threshold shifts in cats[26] seem to support the idea that Schuknecht's map needs some revision.

Even without an accurate cochlear frequency map, certain relationships between abnormal responses and cochlear lesions can be found in our data:

1. If there is a region in the cochlea which is devoid of outer hair cells, there will be a gap in the range of assignable CF.

2. If there are tuning curves with assignable CF at all frequencies, there will not be extensive regions of outer-hair cell loss.

3. Significant increases in threshold of tuning-curve tips can be seen with virtually no loss of hair cells, but significant hair cell loss is always associated with drastic threshold shifts.

Physiological Bases for Tuning Curves of Auditory-Nerve Units. In previous papers,[6,27] the point has been made that the sharply-tuned, low-threshold tips of the tuning curves are elevated relative to the more broadly-tuned, high-threshold tails by certain types of background noise, high-intensity sounds, ototoxic drugs, and stimulation of the crossed olivocochlear bundle. It has also been observed that the threshold of the tips can be raised by anoxia, removal of perilymph from scala tympani, and certain drugs.[28,29] These observations have led some workers to propose the existence of a physiologically-vulnerable "second filter" that sharpens the supposedly broad tuning curves for the mechanical vibrations of the basilar membrane.[30,31] Actually, the term *second* filter is inappropriate because the tuning curves of auditory-nerve fibers result from the superposition and interaction of a great many components of the outer, middle, and inner ear. Even if the term is taken only to mean some mechanism by which sharp tuning is introduced after the basilar membrane response, it must first be established that the basilar membrane motion is not as sharply tuned as the nerve fibers. Some of the currently available studies on the basilar membrane suggest that its tuning is significantly broader than that of auditory-nerve fibers.[32,33] Others are less clear on this issue.[34,35] Given the technical difficulties in measuring such small motions in physiologically intact cochleas, it is not surprising that the validity of these measurements has not been fully established. It is somewhat disquieting that most of the uncontrolled biases in the methods would tend to make the measured mechanical tuning curves broader than they really are. There is, however, one study on the cat that reports mechanical tuning curves that are comparable in sharpness to the neural.[36] If these results are accurate, it may not be necessary to invoke the concept of a second filter as a sharpening mechanism. However, the final shapes of the neural tuning curves might still be infiuenced by factors other than the tuning of the basilar membrane. Indeed it would be surprising if the complex of cells that lies on the membrane did not contribute to the frequency-selectivity of the auditory-nerve fibers.

There has been much recent speculation on the roles of inner and outer hair cells in generating neural activity. The evidence for assigning specific functional characteristics to outer or inner hair cells is based largely on data from pathological ears in which one type of hair cell is missing.[37,38] Although there have been rapid advances in the techniques for assessing the status of damaged sensory cells at the ultrastructural level,[39-46] these methods have not yet been fully applied to work of this nature.

One method to investigate the roles of the inner and outer hair cells, without causing structural damage to either, is to electrically stimulate the crossed olivocochlear bundle. It has been reported that the crossed olivocochlear bundle innervates, almost exclusively, the outer hair cells.[47] Stimulating the crossed bundle selectively elevates the tips of tuning curves.[6,48] Since the innervation of the outer hair cells constitutes approximately 5% of the afferent fibers,[49] the fact that virtually all units encountered in the auditory nerve are affected by crossed-bundle stimulation poses a problem. Presumably, at least some of the radial fibers, which innervate inner hair cells, are also influenced by crossed-bundle activity. Such a picture would require that inner and outer hair cells interact in some as yet unknown way to generate the entire tuning curve in normal fibers.

REFERENCES

1. Lurie MH, Davis H, Hawkins JE Jr: Acoustic trauma of the organ of Corti in the guinea pig. Laryngoscope 54:375-386, 1944

2. Hawkins JE Jr: The ototoxicity of kanamycin. Ann Otol Rhinol Laryngol 68:698-715, 1959

3. Hawkins JE Jr: Comparative otopathology: aging, noise and ototoxic drugs. Adv Otorhinolaryngol 20:125-141, 1973

4. Kellerhals B: Acoustic trauma and cochlear microcirculation. Adv Otorhinolaryngol 18:91-168, 1972

5. Matz GJ: Toxic cochlear and vestibular disorders, in Tower DB (ed): *The Nervous System, Vol 3: Human Comunication and Its Disorders.* New York, Raven Press, 1975, pp 333-349

6. Kiang NYS, Moxon EC, Levine RA: Auditory-nerve activity in cats with normal and abnormal cochleas, in Wolstenholme GEW, Knight J (eds): *Sensorineural Hearing Loss.* London, J & A Churchill, 1970, pp 241-268

7. Schuknecht HF: Techniques for study of cochlear function and pathology in experimental animals. Arch Otolaryngol 58:377-397, 1953

8. Spoendlin H: Innervation densities of the cochlea. Acta Otolaryngol (Stockh) 73: 235-248, 1972

9. Kiang NYS, Watanabe T, Thomas EC, *et al*: *Discharge Patterns of Single Fibers in the Cat's Auditory Nerve.* Research Monograph No. 35, Cambridge, Mass., M.I.T. Press, 1965

10. Lindsay JR, Proctor LR, Work WP: Histopathologic inner ear changes in deafness due to neomycin in the human. Laryngoscope 70:382-392, 1960

11. Kerr A, Schuknecht HF: The spiral ganglion in profound deafness. Acta Otolaryngol (Stockh) 65:586-598, 1968

12. House WF, Urban J: Long term results of electrode implantation and electronic stimulation of the cochlea in man. Ann Otol Rhinol Laryngol 82:504-510, 1973

13. Merzenich MM, Michelson RP, Schindler RA, *et al*: Neural encoding of sound sensation evoked by electrical stimulation of the acoustic nerve. Ann Otol Rhinol Laryngol 82: 486-503, 1973

14. Kiang NYS, Moxon EC: Physiological considerations in artificial stimulation of the inner ear. Ann Otol Rhinol Laryngol 81:714-730, 1972

15. Ward WD: Acoustic trauma and noise-induced hearing loss, in Tower DB (ed): *The Nervous System, Vol 3: Human Communication and Its Disorders.* New York, Raven Press, 1975, pp 221-229

16. Taylor W, Pearson J, Mair A, *et al*: Study of noise and hearing in jute weaving.

J Acoust Soc Am 38:113-120, 1965

17. Miller JD, Watson CS, Covell WP: Deafening effects of noise on the cat. Acta Otolaryngol [Suppl] (Stockh) 176, 1963

18. Weiner FM, Pfeiffer RR, Backus ASN: On the sound pressure transformation by the head and auditory meatus of the cat. Acta Otolaryngol (Stockh) 61:255-269, 1965

19. Guinan JJ, Peake WT: Middle-ear characteristics of anesthetized cats. J Acoust Soc Am 41:1237-1261, 1967

20. Zwicker E: On a psychoacoustical equivalent of tuning curves, in Zwicker E, Terhardt E (eds): *Facts and Models in Hearing.* New York, Springer-Verlag, 1974, pp 132-141

21. Houtgast T: *Lateral Suppression in Hearing, doctoral dissertation.* Institute for Perception TNO, University of Amsterdam, 1974

22. Vogten LLM: Pure-tone masking; a new result from a new method, in Zwicker E, Terhardt E (eds): *Facts and Models in Hearing.* New York, Springer-Verlag, 1974, pp 142-155

23. Salmivalli A: Acoustic trauma in regular army personnel. Acta Otolaryngol (Stockh) Suppl 222, 1967

24. Kiang NYS: Stimulus representation in the discharge patterns of auditory neurons, in Tower DB (ed): *The Nervous System, Vol 3: Human Communication and Its Disorders.* New York, Raven Press, 1975, pp 81-96

25. Schuknecht HF: Neuroanatomical correlates of auditory sensitivity and pitch discrimination in the cat, in Rasmussen GL, Windle WF (eds): *Neural Mechanisms of the Auditory and Vestibular Systems.* Springfield, Illinois, Charles C. Thomas, 1960, pp 76-90

26. Dolan TR, Ades HW, Bredberg G, *et al*: Inner ear damage and hearing loss after exposure to tones of high intensity. Acta Otolaryngol (Stockh) 80:343-352, 1975

27. Kiang NYS, Moxon EC: Tails of tuning curves of auditory-nerve fibers. J Acoust Soc Am 55:620-630, 1974

28. Robertson D: Cochlear neurons: frequency selectivity altered by perilymph removal. Science 186:153-155, 1974

29. Evans EF: Auditory frequency selectivity and the cochlear nerve, in Zwicker E, Terhardt E (eds): *Facts and Models in Hearing.* New York, Springer-Verlag, 1974, pp 118-129

30. Evans EF, Wilson JP: The frequency selectivity of the cochlea, in Møller AR (ed): *Basic Mechanisms in Hearing.* New York, Academic Press, 1973, pp 519-551

31. Evans EF, Wilson JP: Cochlear tuning properties: concurrent basilar membrane and single nerve fiber measurements. Science 190: 1218-1221, 1975

32. Kohllöffel LUE: A study of basilar membrane vibrations III. The basilar membrane frequency response curve in the living guinea pig. Acustica 27:82-89, 1972

33. Wilson JP, Johnstone JR: Basilar membrane and middle-ear vibration in guinea pig measured by capacitive probe. J Acoust Soc Am 57:705-723, 1975

34. Rhode WS: Observations of the vibration of the basilar membrane in squirrel monkeys using the Mössbauer technique. J Acoust Soc Am 49:1218-1231, 1971

35. Johnstone BM, Yates GK: Basilar membrane tuning curves in the guinea pig. J Acoust Soc Am 55:584-587, 1974

36. Helfenstein WM: *Beitrag zur messung der akustisch bedingten bewegungen und identifikation des mechanischen teils des innenohrs der katze,* doctoral dissertation. Eidgenoessischen Technischen Hochschule Zurich, Institut für Automatik und Industrielle Elektronik, 1973

37. Ryan A, Dallos P: Effect of absence of cochlear outer hair cells on behavioural auditory threshold. Nature 253:44-46, 1975

38: Zwislocki JJ, Sokolich WG: Neuromechanical frequency analysis in the cochlea. in Zwicker E, Terhardt E (eds): *Facts and Models in Hearing.* New York, Springer-Verlag, 1974, pp 107-117

39. Beagley HA: Acoustic trauma in the guinea pig II. Acta Otolaryngol (Stockh) 60: 480-495, 1965

40. Spoendlin H: Auditory, vestibular, olfactory and gustatory organs, in Bischoff A (ed): *Ultrastructure of the Peripheral Nervous System and Sense Organs.* St. Louis, CV Mosby Co., 1970, pp 173-337

41. Engström H, Ades HW, Bredberg G: Normal structure of the organ of Corti and the effect of noise-induced cochlear damage, in Wolstenholme GEW, Knight J (eds): *Sensorineural Hearing Loss.* London, J & A Churchill, 1970, pp 127-152

42. Lim DJ, Melnick W: Acoustic damage of the cochlea. Arch Otolaryngol 94:294-305, 1971

43. Lindeman HH, Bredberg G: Scanning electron microscopy of the organ of Corti after intense auditory stimulation: effects on stereocilia and cuticular surface of hair cells. Arch Klin Exp Ohren Nasen Kehlkopfheilkd 203: 1-15, 1972

44. Bohne BA, Eldredge DH, Mills JH: Cochlear potentials and electron microscopy applied to the study of small cochlear lesions. Ann Otol Rhinol Laryngol 82:595-608, 1973

45. Spoendlin H, Brun JP: Relation of structural damage to exposure time and intensity in acoustic trauma. Acta Otolaryngol (Stockh) 75:220-226, 1973

46. Wërsall J: Problems and pitfalls in studies of cochlear hair cell pathology, in Møller AR (ed): *Basic Mechanisms in Hearing.* New York, Academic Press, 1973, pp 235-256

47. Iurato S: Fibre efferenti dirette e cro-

ciate alle cellule acustiche dell 'organo del Corti. Monitore Zoologico Italiano Suppl 72: 62-63, 1964

48. Wiederhold ML: Variations in the effects of electric stimulation of the crossed olivocochlear bundle on cat single auditory-nerve-fiber responses to tone bursts. J Acoust Soc Am 48:966-977, 1970

49. Spoendlin H: Neuroanatomy of the cochlea, in Zwicker E, Terhardt E (eds): *Facts and Models in Hearing.* New York, Springer-Verlag, 1974, pp 18-32

ACKNOWLEDGMENTS—We are pleased to acknowledge the assistance of A. R. Kahn, S. M. Liberman, E. M. Marr, J. B. Miller, A. Morino, E. C. Moxon, and G. S. Roberts. Special thanks are due C. C. Northrop, whose assistance in temporal bone histology was a major factor in this study. Grateful appreciation is extended to Dr. Moses H. Lurie, whose early work and generous support have been of great help.

REPRINTS—Nelson Y. S. Kiang, PhD, Eaton-Peabody Laboratory of Auditory Physiology, Massachusetts Eye and Ear Infirmary, 243 Charles St., Boston, MA 02114.

FIRST OTOPEDIATRIC CONGRESS

The First Otopediatric Congress will be held in Sirmione on the Lake of Garda, April 26-May 1, 1977. For further information write: Otopediatric Congress, PO Box 30, Brescia 25100, Italy.

ALLERGY AND IMMUNOLOGY SELF-ASSESSMENT PROGRAM

The Allergy and Immunology Self-Assessment Program 1977, sponsored by the American Academy of Allergy, the American Association for Certified Allergists, the American Association for Clinical Immunology and Allergy, the American Board of Allergy and Immunology — A Conjoint Board of the American Board of Internal Medicine and the American Board of Pediatrics, and the American College of Allergists, will be available in January, 1977. The National Board of Medical Examiners is assisting in the project.

Subscription details may be obtained by writing to AISAP, 3930 Chestnut Street, Philadelphia, PA 19104.

Ann Otol 85: 1976

SODIUM LOADING OF INNER EAR FLUIDS

HERBERT SILVERSTEIN, MD

SARASOTA, FLORIDA

TIERO TAKEDA, MD

KYOTO, JAPAN

SUMMARY – A slow intracarotid infusion of hypertonic sodium chloride solution, 350 mEq/L, and potassium chloride, 5 mEq/L, was used to increase serum sodium chloride over a 90-minute period in 85 cats. A slow, steady rise in serum sodium occurred, which reached almost 208 mEq/L at the end of 90 minutes. A concomitant rise in sodium occurred in the cerebrospinal fluid and perilymph. In contrast, the sodium showed only a transient slight increase in the cochlear and vestibular endolymph. Endolymph potassium appeared to rise in order to balance out the increase in sodium concentration of the surrounding and extracellular fluids. The ratio of sodium to potassium ions in both the endolymph and perilymph compartment remained relatively constant before and after the infusion with hypertonic NaCl. After infusion, the total concentration of ions in endolymph was similar to that of perilymph. These experiments indicate that the endolymph compartment has a built-in mechanism for maintaining a low-sodium concentration while keeping ionic balance with the surrounding perilymph and serum.

There is still a controversy concerning whether the ingestion of excessive quantities of sodium chloride will affect the clinical course of Ménière's disease. One theory has been that ingested sodium chloride becomes incorporated into the endolymph, thus increasing osmotic pressure and causing endolymphatic hydrops with an exacerbation of Ménière's attacks. Furstenberg[1] first proposed a low-salt diet as part of the treatment for patients with Ménière's disease. In order to evaluate this form of treatment, Perlman[2] admitted patients with Ménière's disease to the hospital, "loaded" them with excessive salt, and found there was no increase in the incidence of vertiginous episodes.

This study was undertaken to determine whether artificially increasing the sodium content of the serum in cats produces alterations of the sodium and potassium in inner ear fluids.

METHODS AND MATERIALS

Inner ear fluids, cerebrospinal fluid (CSF) and serum were collected from 85 normal healthy cats before and after intracarotid infusion of hypertonic sodium chloride solution.

Cats weighing 1.5-3.0 kg, unfed for 20 hours prior to the experiment, were anesthetized by intraperitoneal injection of sodium pentobarbital (35 mg/kg). Using a Jelco intravenous catheter, Cathlon IV Teflon® needle, 20 g, 2.5-3.8 cm, and Venoset – 198 cm long (approximately 15 drops = 1 ml), hypertonic sodium chloride solution, which included 350 mEq/L of sodium as NaCL and 5 mEq/L of potassium as KCl, was infused into the left common carotid artery at a rate of 260 ml/hour. Samples of inner ear fluid were obtained from the scala tympani, scala vestibuli, scala media and utricle by techniques described in earlier publications.[3,4] Samples from 67 ears were taken just prior to the beginning of the infusion. After the onset of infusion, fluid samples were taken from 147 ears during a 90-minute period. Samples of CSF from the cisterna magna and serum from the femoral vein were obtained prior to and after the onset of the infusion, and also at the time of inner ear collection. These blood samples were centrifuged immediately after the collection and the serum separated.

After a tracheotomy and wide exposure of the left common carotid artery, a midline scalp incision was made; then the auditory bulla and dura overlying the cisterna magna were exposed. To minimize the flow of CSF through the cochlear aqueduct, a polyethylene tube (No. 190) was inserted through the dura mater into the cisterna magna for continuous drainage of CSF. The auditory bulla was then

Presented at the meeting of the American Otological Society, Inc., Palm Beach, Florida, April 25-26, 1976.

TABLE I

CHANGE OF SODIUM CONCENTRATION (mEq/L) IN VARIOUS FLUIDS DURING INTRACAROTID INFUSION OF HYPERTONIC SODIUM CHLORIDE SOLUTION

(Data are expressed as a mean ± standard error)

	Before Infusion	*During Infusion (Minutes)* 5	10	20	30	40	60	90
Serum	163.69 ± 1.78 (N=33)	166.85 ± 0.77 (N=13)	177.46*** ± 1.59 (N=14)	182.35*** ± 2.69 (N=10)	188.65*** ± 2.06 (N=10)	194.25*** ± 2.19 (N=14)	197.06*** ± 3.38 (N=24)	207.96** ± 3.74 (N=22)
CSF	159.71 ± 2.33 (N=33)	166.65 ± 2.21 (N=13)	163.43 ± 1.89 (N=14)	168.07* ± 1.82 (N=14)	174.90** ± 1.58 (N=10)	177.25*** ± 2.09 (N=14)	181.62*** ± 2.71 (N=17)	192.35** ± 2.06 (N=17)
Perilymph of scala tympani	164.14 ± 0.99 (N=56)	173.42*** ± 1.19 (N=13)	166.30 ± 1.05 (N=20)	182.94*** ± 1.87 (N=16)	181.05*** ± 1.18 (N=20)	175.90*** ± 2.05 (N=10)	185.20*** ± 0.74 (N=10)	191.79** ± 1.98 (N=12)
Perilymph of scala vestibuli	157.08 ± 1.03 (N=65)	158.06 ± 1.92 (N=14)	165.42** ± 1.75 (N=12)	175.08*** ± 1.76 (N=12)	183.50*** ± 1.75 (N=15)	168.86*** ± 1.45 (N=25)	160.10 ± 3.32 (N=10)	172.91** ± 2.34 (N=11)
Cochlear endolymph	6.97 ± 0.29 (N=35)	11.25*** ± 1.37 (N=10)	13.62*** ± 1.02 (N=13)	17.33*** ± 1.26 (N=18)	4.63*** ± 0.36 (N=19)	6.62 ± 0.73 (N=13)	10.57*** ± 0.78 (N=22)	10.38** ± 0.80 (N=16)
Utricular endolymph	18.28 ± 1.09 (N=18)	22.75* ± 2.41 (N=8)	31.50*** ± 2.29 (N=9)	22.30* ± 1.50 (N=10)	23.96** ± 1.53 (N=11)	24.00** ± 2.05 (N=18)	20.92 ± 1.39 (N=26)	19.02 ± 1.39 (N=27)

*Significantly different ($P<0.05$) from "before infusion" value
**Significantly different ($P<0.01$) from "before infusion" value
***Significantly different ($P<0.001$) from "before infusion" value

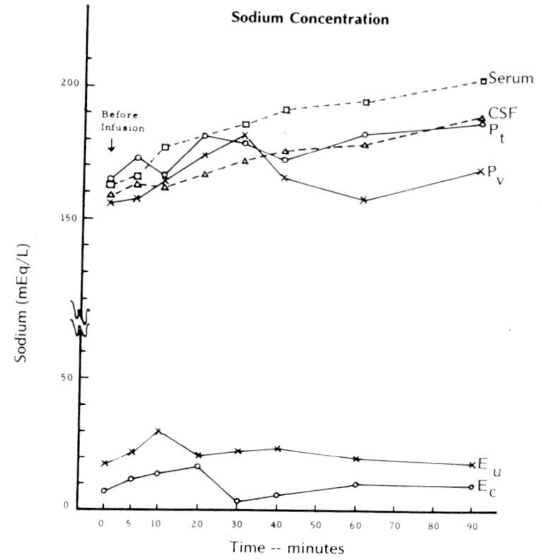

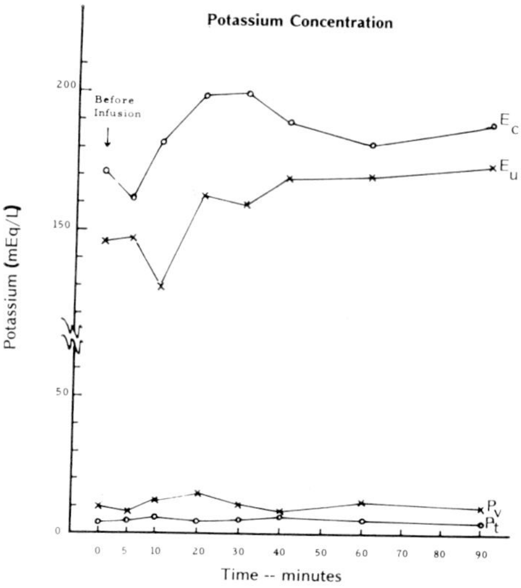

Fig. 1. Graph showing the changes of the sodium concentrations in perilymph, endolymph, CSF and serum during infusion of hypertonic sodium chloride solution. P_v - Perilymph of scala vestibuli; P_t - Perilymph of scala tympani; E_c - Cochlear endolymph; E_v - Vestibular endolymph. Note that there is a linear sodium increase in serum, CSF, and perilymph sodium.

Fig. 2. Graph showing the changes of the potassium concentration in the inner ear fluids during the hypertonic sodium chloride solution infusion. Note that there is a progressive increase in the endolymph potassium concentration.

opened and the middle ear exposed. With the aid of an operating microscope, a sample of the scala vestibuli perilymph was obtained by introducing the tip of a glass capillary through the stapes footplate into the vestibular cistern. The sample from the scala tympani was collected by inserting the glass capillary through the round window membrane into the scala tympani. Using a fine pick, a second hole was made in the footplate and in the round window membrane to allow air to enter as the sample was aspirated from each scala. Usually 3-4μl of perilymph were collected from each area.

Before collecting cochlear endolymph, the round window membrane was removed and the basilar membrane dried with Gelfoam®*. One to three microliters of endolymph were collected by capillary action after directing the tip (20-25μ) of the glass pipette through the basilar membrane into the scala media. Utricular endolymph was obtained from the crus commune after removing the bony wall between the oval and round windows. In most of the cats, it was possible to collect 1-4μl of utricular endolymph.

The ends of the glass capillary were sealed with mineral oil and the samples were centrifuged and examined for blood contamination. Samples contaminated with blood were discarded.

Each inner ear fluid sample from one ear, and each CSF and serum sample from one animal represented one sample in chemical analysis.

A digital flame photometer** was used for sodium and potassium determinations. In principle, this flame photometer measures concentration of sodium and potassium against a lithium standard and requires a sample volume of one-half to one microliter for analysis. The sample is diluted in 200μl of lithium blank before analysis. (The details of this method have been described earlier.[3])

RESULTS

The changes in sodium concentration in serum, CSF and inner ear fluids during infusion of hypertonic sodium chloride solution are shown in Table I and Figure 1. The serum sodium concentration slowly rose over a period of 90 minutes at which time the concentration was 207.9 mEq/L or a 44 mEq increase. Sodium concentration in CSF appeared to mirror the increase in serum sodium concentration. At the end of 90 minutes, the concentration was 192 mEq/L or a 33 mEq increase. Perilymph, likewise, showed an increase in sodium concen-

* The Upjohn Company, Kalamazoo, MI.

** Model 143. Instrumentation Laboratory Inc., Lexington, MA.

TABLE II

CHANGE OF POTASSIUM (mEq/L) CONCENTRATION IN VARIOUS FLUIDS DURING THE INTRACAROTID INFUSION OF HYPERTONIC SODIUM CHLORIDE SOLUTION

(Data are expressed as a mean ± standard error)

	Before Infusion	*During Infusion (Minutes)* 5	10	20	30	40	60	90
Serum	4.59 ± 0.12 (N=33)	4.50 ± 0.18 (N=13)	4.36 ± 0.14 (N=14)	4.70 ± 0.19 (N=10)	4.55 ± 0.20 (N=10)	4.82 ± 0.09 (N=14)	4.42 ± 0.12 (N=24)	4.58 ± 0.15 (N=22)
CSF	3.49 ± 0.15 (N=33)	3.62 ± 0.29 (N=13)	3.69 ± 0.14 (N=14)	3.54 ± 0.21 (N=14)	3.60 ± 0.18 (N=10)	3.54 ± 0.25 (N=14)	3.88 ± 0.42 (N=17)	4.06* ± 0.14 (N=17)
Perilymph of scala tympani	4.41 ± 0.16 (N=56)	4.69 ± 0.32 (N=13)	5.48** ± 0.43 (N=20)	4.81 ± 0.25 (N=16)	4.93 ± 0.29 (N=20)	6.00** ± 0.71 (N=10)	5.25* ± 0.43 (N=10)	4.83 ± 0.32 (N=12)
Perilymph of scala vestibuli	10.83 ± 0.27 (N=65)	9.68 ± 0.64 (N=14)	12.63* ± 1.06 (N=12)	14.25*** ± 0.94 (N=12)	10.24 ± 0.67 (N=15)	7.78*** ± 0.34 (N=25)	11.40 ± 0.92 (N=10)	11.18 ± 0.91 (N=11)
Cochlear endolymph	171.89 ± 1.57 (N=35)	162.70* ± 4.09 (N=10)	183.69*** ± 2.98 (N=13)	200.44*** ± 3.15 (N=18)	201.74*** ± 4.06 (N=19)	192.96*** ± 1.72 (N=13)	184.05*** ± 2.36 (N=22)	192.28*** ± 2.02 (N=16)
Utricular endolymph	147.33 ± 1.76 (N=18)	148.38 ± 3.04 (N=8)	130.89*** ± 3.92 (N=9)	163.20*** ± 3.20 (N=10)	161.41*** ± 1.95 (N=11)	170.94*** ± 1.83 (N=18)	171.44*** ± 2.00 (N=26)	177.13*** ± 1.88 (N=27)

*Significantly different (P 0.05) from "before infusion" value
**Significantly different (P 0.01) from "before infusion" value
***Significantly different (P 0.001) from "before infusion" value

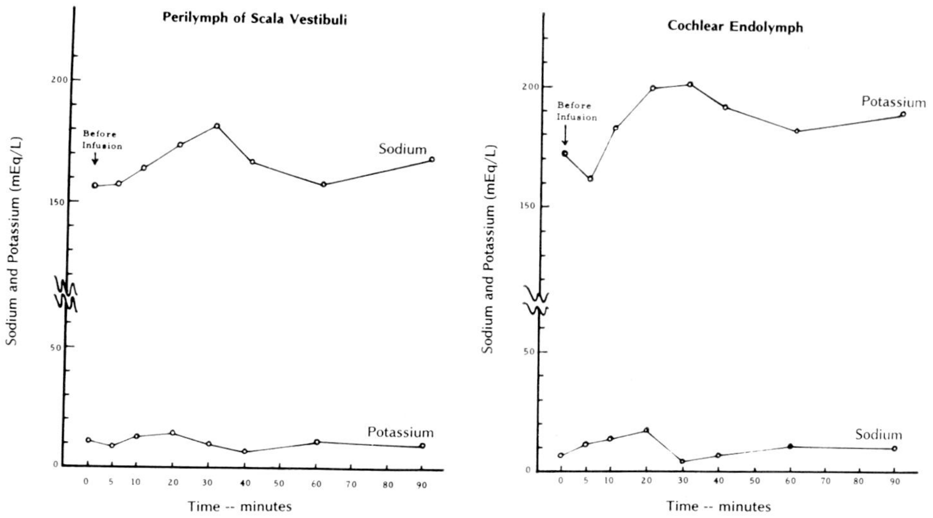

Fig. 3. Graph showing the changes of sodium and potassium concentration in A) scala vestibuli perilymph and B) cochlear endolymph during the hypertonic sodium chloride solution infusion. Note that the elevation of perilymph sodium concentration causes an increase of potassium concentration in cochlear endolymph.

tration during the infusion of hypertonic sodium chloride solution. Perilymph of the scala tympani appeared to run very close to the curve of CSF. At the end of 90 minutes, the sodium concentration in perilymph of the scala tympani was 191.7 mEq/L or a 27 mEq increase. Sodium concentration in the perilymph of the scala vestibuli increased during the first 30 minutes as rapidly as the CSF and perilymph of the scala tympani. However, after this time, the curve appeared to change. At the end of 90 minutes, the concentration was 172.9 mEq/L or a 15 mEq increase. The sodium concentration in cochlear and vestibular endolymph during the first 10 to 20 minutes, showed a transient increase. Cochlear endolymph increased from 6.9 to 17 mEq/L. The utricular endolymph increased from 18 to 31.5 mEq/L. After this time, the sodium concentration decreased, so that at the end of 90 minutes, the sodium concentration returned to normal levels.

Table II and Figure 2 show changes in potassium concentration in the serum, CSF and inner ear fluids during infusion of hypertonic sodium chloride solution. There was no significant increase in serum, CSF or perilymph concentration of potassium. In contrast, there was an increase in endolymph potassium over the 90-minute period. Greatest changes were seen at 30 minutes after the infusion. Potassium concentration in cochlear endolymph reached 201 mEq/L and utricular endolymph, 161.4 mEq/L. At the end of 90 minutes, there was approximately a 20 mEq increase in potassium concentration as compared to the values before infusion. The increase in potassium concentration in the endolymph appeared to balance the increase in sodium content in the perilymph space. This can be seen in Figures 3 and 4, which show the comparison of sodium and potassium in both perilymph and endolymph.

The ratio of sodium to potassium in the perilymph and endolymph compartment were similar before and at the end of the 90-minute sodium chloride infusion.

DISCUSSION

The present study shows that during infusion of hypertonic sodium chloride solution, a significant increase in sodium concentration occurs in serum, CSF and perilymph compartments. There is also a transient rise in sodium concentration

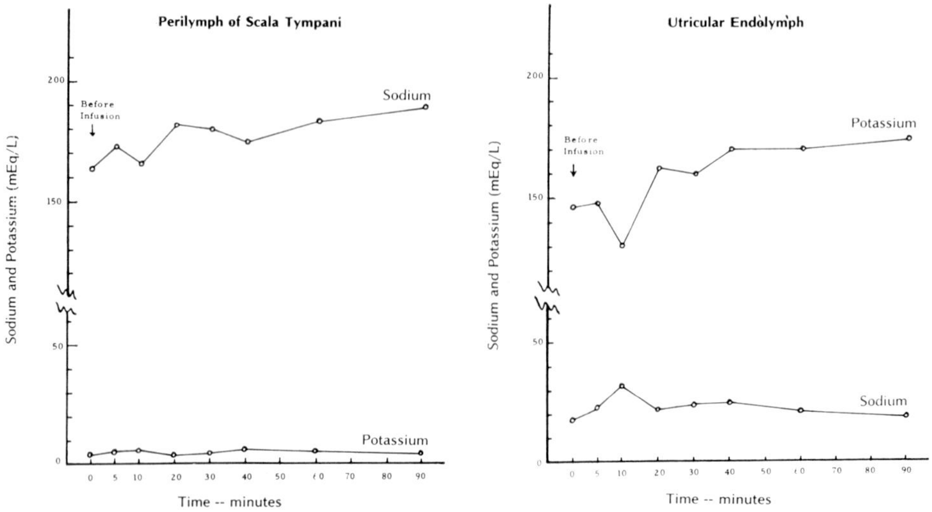

Fig. 4. Graph showing the changes of sodium and potassium concentration in A) scala tympani perilymph and B) utricular endolymph during the hypertonic sodium chloride infusion. Note changes are similar to cochlear endolymph of Figure 3B.

in the endolymph compartments, but this is not sustained and the endolymph sodium returns to normal by the end of 40 minutes. The greatest increase in sodium concentration occurred in the serum. Less increase occurred in CSF with a smaller increase found in the perilymph. It appeared that the dynamic increase in perilymph sodium produced a concomitant increase in endolymph potassium. The total concentration of sodium and potassium ions on either side of Reissner's or the vestibular membranes appeared to remain constant. Thus, it does not appear that more water would be drawn only into the endolymph space. Infusion of large quantities of sodium into the body is distributed to most extracellular spaces while the endolymph compartment appears to regulate its own metabolism to counteract or balance this increase.

From this data, it appears that the regulation of the near-normal sodium concentration in the endolymph space is controlled by the stria vascularis. Sodium and potassium concentrations in the endolymph compartment are probably regulated by the (Na, K) — ATPase and other enzyme groups which participate in the transport of sodium and potassium.[5-7] The activity of these enzyme groups are governed by the amount of sodium and potassium concentration in the surrounding fluids.[8,9]

Lawrence and McCabe[10] postulated that the attack of vertigo in Ménière's disease is caused by an increase in potassium concentration in the perilymphatic cavity which is due to repeated rupture and healing of the saccule. Schuknecht *et al*[11] also suggested that the rupture of the labyrinthine membrane is the histopathologic finding most reasonably explaining the episodic nature of Ménière's disease.

From these studies, it does not appear that an increase in osmotic pressure in endolymph can be caused by ingestion of large quantities of sodium chloride. It is apparent that in the normal ear, the endolymph compartment has a built-in, powerful mechanism for maintaining low-sodium concentration while keeping ionic balance with the surrounding perilymph and serum. Correlating this work with clinical studies showing no increase in vertiginous episodes during ingestion of sodium chloride, one could assume, in Ménière's disease, that the inner ear may still have the ability to maintain ionic balance during periods of excessive salt ingestion. There does not appear to be any rationale in subjecting patients to a very low-salt diet in order to prevent the attacks of Ménière's disease.

REFERENCES

1. Furstenberg AC: Ménière's syndrome complex, medical treatment. Trans Am Otol 24:126-136, 1934

2. Perlman H: Electrolyte studies in Ménière's disease. Laryngoscope 63:640-651, 1953

3. Silverstein H: The biochemistry of the inner ear fluids in the cat. Ann Otol Rhinol Laryngol 75:48-64, 1966

4. Makimoto K, Silverstein H: Sodium and potassium concentrations in the endolymph and perilymph of the cat. Ann Otol Rhinol Laryngol 83:174-179, 1974

5. Whittam R: The asymmetrical stimulation of a membrane adenosine triphosphatase in relation to active cation transport. Biochem J 84:110-118, 1962

6. Rendi R, Uhr ML: Sodium, potassium — requiring adenosine triphosphatase activity. I. Purification and properties. Biochem Biophys Acta 89:520-531, 1964

7. Skou JC: Enzymatic basis for active transport of Na^+ and K^+ across cell membrane. Physiol Rev 45:596-617, 1965

8. Hoffman JF: The red cell membrane and the transport of sodium and potassium. Am J Med 41:666-680, 1966

9. Hodgkin AL, Keynes RD: Active transport of cations in giant axons from sepia and loligo. J Physiol 128:28-60, 1955

10. Lawrence M, McCabe B: Inner ear mechanics and deafness. JAMA 171:1927-1932, 1959

11. Schuknecht HF, Benitez JT, Beekhuis J: Further observation on the pathology of Ménière's disease. Ann Otol Rhinol Laryngol 71: 1039-1053, 1962

REPRINTS—Herbert Silverstein, MD, 1849A Hawthorne Street, Sarasota, FL 33579.

THIRD DANIEL C. BAKER JR. LECTURESHIP

The American Laryngological Association is pleased to announce that the Third Daniel C. Baker, Jr. Lectureship in Laryngology will be presented by Dr. Lewis Thomas, President of the Sloan Kettering Institute, New York City. The lecture will be given at the time of the annual meeting of the American Laryngological Association on May 8, 1977 at the Sheraton Boston Hotel, Boston, Mass.

Dr. Thomas is the author of the best seller "The Lives of a Cell" and also a series of articles which appeared in the New England Journal of Medicine called "The Biology Watcher."

Ann Otol 85: 1976

HEARING LOSS IN PATIENTS WITH DIALYSIS AND RENAL TRANSPLANTS

CEDRIC A. QUICK, MD

MINNEAPOLIS, MINNESOTA

SUMMARY — Hearing loss in renal dialysis and renal transplant patients occurs quite frequently. An assessment of the likely etiological factors is nearly impossible in a retrospective analysis of any one patient because many factors exist simultaneously. In a prospective study of a large series of patients an identification of factors contributing to the hearing loss was possible in the majority of patients. During the study it became increasingly apparent that what was observed at any one time was the combined effect of many factors. Although one factor seemed to precipitate the hearing loss it was inadvisable to attribute total responsibility to that agent or circumstance. Further, this combined effect was not a simple addition of effects but potentiation. The serious implications of this phenomenon are discussed.

In the United States today about eight million people suffer from some form of kidney disease, and every year 70 to 80 thousand deaths are attributable to kidney disease. Patients with end-stage renal disease are either maintained on chronic dialysis or receive a kidney transplant. Both groups of patients have abnormal life expectancies. Dialysis patients are more susceptible to cardiovascular disease and premature arteriosclerosis, whereas transplant patients are susceptible to complications from immunosuppression and steroid treatment, particularly infections. Improved methods of dialysis, newer agents for immunosuppression, and more reliable methods of tissue typing have resulted in a marked increase in survival of these patients. Longer survival has permitted the emergence of changes in many organ systems.[1] It was noted quite early in renal transplantation that the ears, nose and throat had not escaped complications.[2,3] One of the most perplexing problems facing an otolaryngologist in consultation is the evaluation of hearing loss in renal and transplant patients. It is frequently noted that many factors in the patient's medical history contribute to the cause of the hearing loss. Consequently, assessment of the effects of individual factors is nearly impossible in a retrospective analysis. A prospective analysis was initiated at the University of Minnesota to determine which factors were responsible for the hearing loss, with the ultimate hope that modification of the management of these patients would prevent the onset of hearing loss or reduce its magnitude.

METHODS AND MATERIALS

A prospective transplant recipient in end-stage renal disease entering the Unversity of Minnesota transplant program would undergo a series of routine procedures for evaluation of the renal and other organ systems. After an initial stabilizing period on dialysis the patient would undergo bilateral nephrectomy and splenectomy. A renal transplant from a living related donor would take place within two weeks of this procedure. Transplant recipients with no available donor usually were transferred to other hemodialysis units from which they were recalled when a cadaver kidney became available. As part of the initial assessment, the prospective transplant recipient underwent an ENT interview, examination and full audiological evaluation. If the interval between the initial evaluation and transplantation was unduly long the ENT and audiological evaluation was repeated prior to trans-

---

From the Department of Otolaryngology, University of Minnesota, Minneapolis, Minnesota.
Supported in part by NIH Grant 2P02-AM-13083-05 and NS Grant 12125-01.
Presented at the meeting of the American Otological Society, Inc., Palm Beach, Florida, April 25-26, 1976.

TABLE I

TYPES OF RENAL DISEASE IN PATIENTS WITH HEARING LOSS

Nephrotic syndrome	6
Nephrosclerosis	1
Chronic pyelonephritis	17
Hypertension	2
Glomerular nephritis	21
Diabetes	22
Polycystic, medullary, cystic	12
Goodpasture's syndrome	4
Alport's syndrome	9
Hydronephrosis	1
Hypoplastic	1
Fabry's disease	3
Renal dwarfism	1
Acute	2
Unknown	5
Total	107

plantation. Repeated ENT examinations were performed following transplantation and at the onset of any symptoms referable to an otologic disorder.

Data concerning the hearing status and probable causes of hearing loss were recorded in the patient's chart. In addition to the hospital charts, extensive flow charts were routinely kept on each patient. These flow charts recorded clinical chemical data, urine production and other factors related to the kidney disorder. Analysis of patients with a hearing loss, as defined by our criteria, would include an otological history, otological examination, audiological examination, and analysis of therapy charts and of clinical flow charts. Hearing loss on initial testing was defined as a hearing threshold with two readings greater than 15 dB or one reading greater than 25 dB between 250 Hz and 8000 Hz. The incidence of sensorineural hearing loss attributable to noise-induced hearing loss for the adult male population caused modification of our criteria to exclude single readings of 25 dB or greater hearing loss at 4000 Hz. In addition, any patient demonstrating deterioration in hearing threshold of any measurable amount was categorized as having hearing loss.

Temporal bones were obtained whenever possible and histopathological investigation carried out by the temporal bone laboratory of the Department of Otolaryngology under the direction of Dr. M. M. Paparella. Animal laboratory studies were needed to explain certain aspects uncovered by this clinical investigation. Materials and methods utilized in these studies are described in prior publications.

TABLE II

MAIN FACTORS IMPLICATED IN HEARING LOSS IN RENAL PATIENTS

Multiple transplant	1
Idiopathic sudden hearing loss	6
Congenital (nonhereditary)	2
Congenital and hereditary (Alport's, *etc*)	9
Diuretics	14
Aminoglycosides	3
Drug potentiation (diuretic + aminoglycoside)	8
Dialysis	5
Metabolic disorders (diabetes, Fabry's, *etc*)	7
Otologic (conductive, infective, *etc*)	9
Noise induced hearing loss	9
Unknown: occurring before transplant	26
Unknown: occurring after transplant	8
Total	107

RESULTS

In a prospective study of hearing in dialysis and transplant patients at the University of Minnesota between July 1968 and December 1975, a total of 602 patients were screened, 363 males and 239 females. A total of 676 transplants were performed, comprising 278 cadaver kidney transplants and 398 kidney transplants from living related donors. According to our criteria, 107 patients had identifiable hearing loss upon initial evaluation or developed it later. No single type of renal disease appeared dominant in patients with hearing loss. The distribution of diseases is shown in Table I and closely approximates the overall distribution of kidney disease in the transplant program.

A likely precipitating cause for the hearing loss was identified in 71 patients. Hearing loss of unidentifiable cause was present in 26 patients before they entered the transplant program, and in eight patients who developed hearing loss while being monitored after transplantation (Table II). The single most frequent factor identified as responsible for hearing loss was the

TABLE III

ASSOCIATED FACTORS IMPLICATED IN HEARING LOSS OF RENAL PATIENTS

Congenital and hereditary (Alport's)	2
Diuretics	6
Aminoglycosides	2
Drug potentiation (diuretics + aminoglycosides)	5
Dialysis	10
Metabolic (diabetes, Fabry's, *etc*)	7
Otologic (conductive, infective, *etc*)	3
Noise induced hearing loss	2
Multiple transplant	4
Minimal hearing loss	7
Unknown before transplant	1
Improvement following transplant	3
Total	52

use of ototoxic diuretics and antibiotics. The diuretics considered to be ototoxic were furosemide and ethacrynic acid. The antibiotics most frequently incriminated in ototoxicity were kanamycin and gentamicin, although hearing loss caused by streptomycin was seen in one patient. As yet no cases of tobramycin hearing loss have been seen. In the past two years, greater control of ototoxic antibiotics and ototoxic diuretics has been implemented, however, hearing loss has now occurred when both diuretics and aminoglycoside antibiotics were used simultaneously in doses that would not be expected to cause ototoxicity if either were used alone. A potentiation of drug effects was clearly seen in eight patients and may have contributed to the hearing loss in another five patients. Otological disorders such as otosclerosis, acute otitis media, chronic otitis media and temporal bone trauma accounted for hearing loss in nine patients and may have contributed to the hearing loss in another three patients. In some patients it was evident that more than one factor contributed to the hearing loss (Table III).

In several patients a reversible hearing loss was seen following the use of some ototoxic drugs, and in three patients an improvement in the hearing thresholds followed a successful transplant.

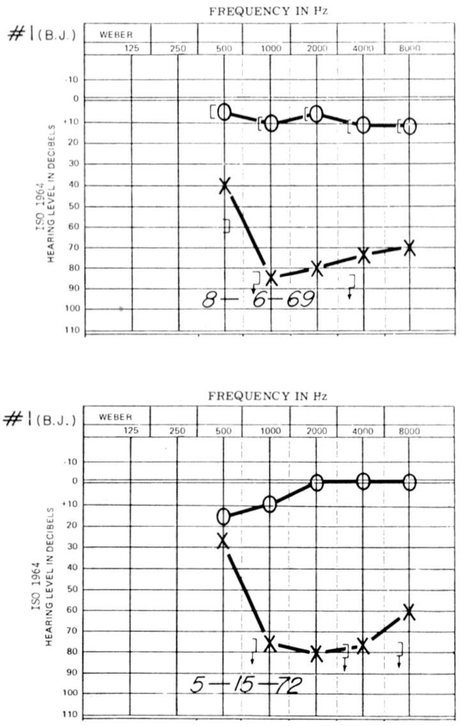

Fig. 1. Pure tone audiogram for Case 1 showing a sensorineural hearing loss.

CASE REPORTS

It is inappropriate and impractical to recount in this paper cases histories of all patients in this study. The following case reports represent hearing losses which are unusual or illustrate points for discussion.

Case 1. A 29-year-old female with juvenile onset of diabetes mellitus had slowly progressive uremia for five years, during which time she had a progressive retinopathy which was treated by pituitary ablation but eventually progressed to total blindness. The patient was admitted to hospital on July 13, 1969 for investigation and treatment of peripheral edema and a low serum sodium value of 116 mEq/liter. At this time uremia was controlled by a Giovanetti diet with sodium and fluid intake restrictions. On July 18, 1969, sodium intake was increased and serum sodium rose progressively to normal levels. On July 21, 1969, the patient stated that upon waking she noticed a hearing loss in her left ear. This was not accompanied by vertigo or tinnitus. Prior to this she had excellent hearing. An

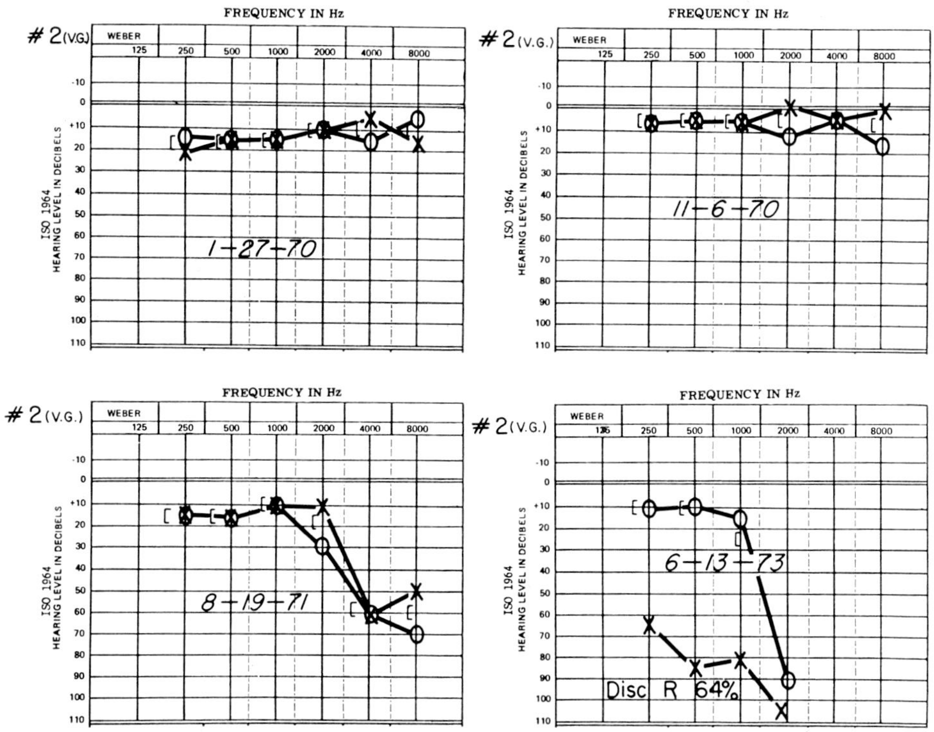

Fig. 2. Pure tone audiogram for Case 2 showing a sensorineural hearing loss.

audiogram on August 6, 1969, was within normal limits for the right ear but showed a moderate-severe hearing loss in the left ear (Fig. 1). At the time of the hearing loss the patient's medication consisted of insulin, alpha-methyl-dopa, chloral hydrate, secobarbital, allopurinol, amphogel and diazepam. On the day of the loss of hearing, electrolytes were within normal limits, her BUN was 100 mg/100 ml and serum creatine approximately 20 mg/100 ml. The hearing thresholds remained unchanged following this loss and no explanation could be given for her idiopathic sudden hearing loss.

Case 2. A 29-year-old female, weighing 31 kg, with end-stage renal failure due to juvenile onset diabetes mellitus, entered the transplant program in November 1970. At that time she was also noted to have peripheral neuropathy, retinopathy and hypertension. Bilateral nephrectomy and splenectomy took place in December 1970, and a cadaver kidney transplant was performed on January 4, 1971. An audiogram performed six months prior to transplant was normal and her hearing had not changed since then (Fig. 2). No ototoxic antibiotics or diuretics were administered prior to transplant. From the ninth postoperative day the patient exhibited spiking fevers which ultimately were shown to be caused by an infected urinary fistula. Surgical exploration of the fistula tract was performed on January 22, 1971. Gentamicin therapy was commenced on January 22, 1971, with a starting dose of 40 mg IV followed by 40 mg IM q. 8 hours. This dose was continued until January 30, 1971, when the patient was given gentamicin 30 mg q. 12 hours until February 8, 1971. At this time the gentamicin dose was adjusted to 35 mg IM, postdialysis, three times weekly. Peak serum levels of gentamicin obtained at intervals were not above 5.9 μg/ml.

Furosemide therapy was commenced during surgery on January 22, 1971, with intravenous doses of 50 mg, 50 mg and 30 mg. This was followed by a postoperative intravenous infusion of 200 mg with mannitol. This was followed by 40 mg intramuscularly q. 8 hours until February 3, 1971, when transplant nephrectomy was performed for rejection. Mild tinnitus was reported following this two-week period. A repeat audiogram performed at the time of the second successful uncomplicated cadaver transplant six months later showed a bilateral high frequency hearing loss (Fig. 2). Potentiation of furosemide and gentamicin was thought to be responsible for this audiological picture.

The patient's health remained good for almost two years and there was no reported decrease in hearing levels. In May 1973, the

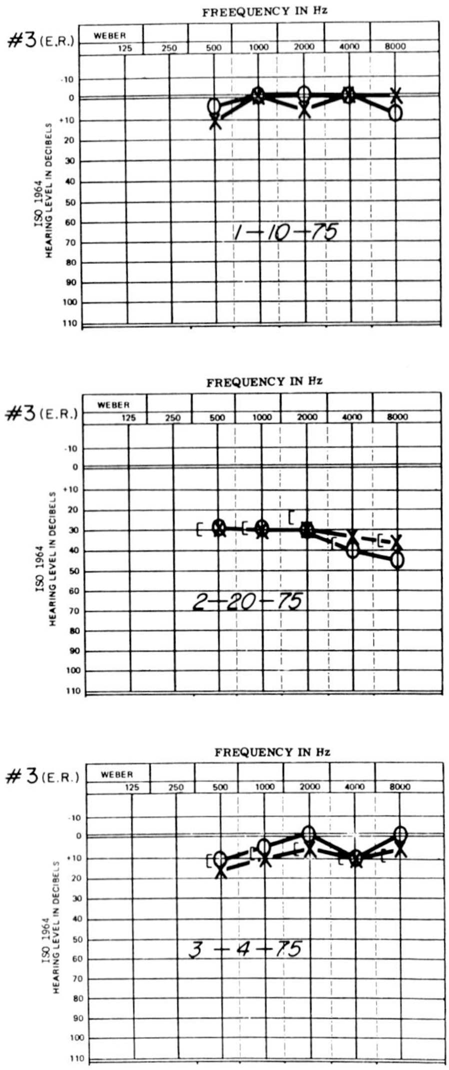

Fig. 3. Pure tone audiogram for Case 3 showing a sensorineural hearing loss

patient was readmitted with a painful abdominal mass. A diagnosis of mycotic aortic aneurysm was made and surgical resection of the aorta with axillary femoral bypass was performed on May 12, 1973. One day prior to surgery the patient was given prophylactic gentamicin 60 mg IV, q. 12 hours and oral neomycin 1 gram q. 1 hour for four hours then 1 gram q. 6 hours for two doses as a bowel preparation. Infusion of furosemide in mannitol was commenced preoperatively at a rate of 4 mg/hour. The postoperative course was extremely difficult and gentamicin was continued in doses of 60 mg q. 12 hours. Regular serum levels were obtained and were between 2.0 μg/ml and 11.5 μg/ml. The total dose of furosemide given during the operation was 200 mg, and in the first 12 hours postoperatively a further 260 mg was given IV. Thereafter occasional small doses of intravenous furosemide were given in addition to a regular administration of 40 mg p.o. twice daily. On May 24, 1973, the patient noticed a decrease in hearing. This progressed markedly over the next few days and an audiogram on June 13, 1974, showed essentially no hearing in the left ear and a severe sensorineural hearing loss in the right ear. The patient's condition continued to deteriorate and she died one month later. Potentiation was again thought to be the cause of the second and more serious hearing loss, since ototoxic levels of gentamicin never reached the critical level of 16 μg/ml. The oral administration of neomycin may also have contributed to the hearing loss but was felt unlikely since the onset of the hearing loss occurred 12 days after its administration.

Case 3. This 31-year-old female with juvenile onset diabetes mellitus was admitted on January 5, 1975 with deteriorating renal function and pneumonia. At the time of admission she was also noted to have nephropathy, retinopathy, neuropathy and premature arteriosclerosis which had resulted in a previous myocardial infarction. Admission chemistries were: creatine 5.9 mg/100 ml, BUN 73 mg/100 ml, sodium 127 mEq/liter, and potassium 4.2 mEq/liter. The patient's medications were: furosemide 40 mg p.o. daily, digoxin, alpha-methyl-dopa and insulin. A sudden deterioration in renal function necessitated IV furosemide 80 mg and 160 mg on January 10 and January 11, 1975, respectively. Gentamicin 200 mg daily was given in divided doses from January 26 to February 3, 1975. An audiogram performed early in this admission showed normal hearing (Fig. 3). Bilateral nephrectomy and splenectomy was performed on February 11, 1975 and the patient commenced on dialysis. A kidney transplant from a related donor was performed on February 24, 1975. Prior to transplant an audiogram showed a sensorineural hearing loss of 30 to 45 dB bilaterally. During surgery the patient received IV furosemide 150 mg and 60 mg, followed by 40 mg p.o. q.i.d. until March 7, 1975. Gentamicin prophylaxis was given at the time of surgery and postoperatively in doses of 60 mg IM daily until March 11, 1975. A repeat audiogram performed following transplant on March 4, 1975, showed essentially normal hearing, which confirmed the patient's observations of improved hearing (Fig. 3). This improvement in hearing following transplantation was even more remarkable in view of the simultaneous use of furosemide and gentamicin.

Case 4. This 27-year-old female with juvenile onset diabetes mellitus entered the transplant service on October 4, 1975 for evaluation of terminal renal failure. On admission she had gross anasarca and congestive heart fail-

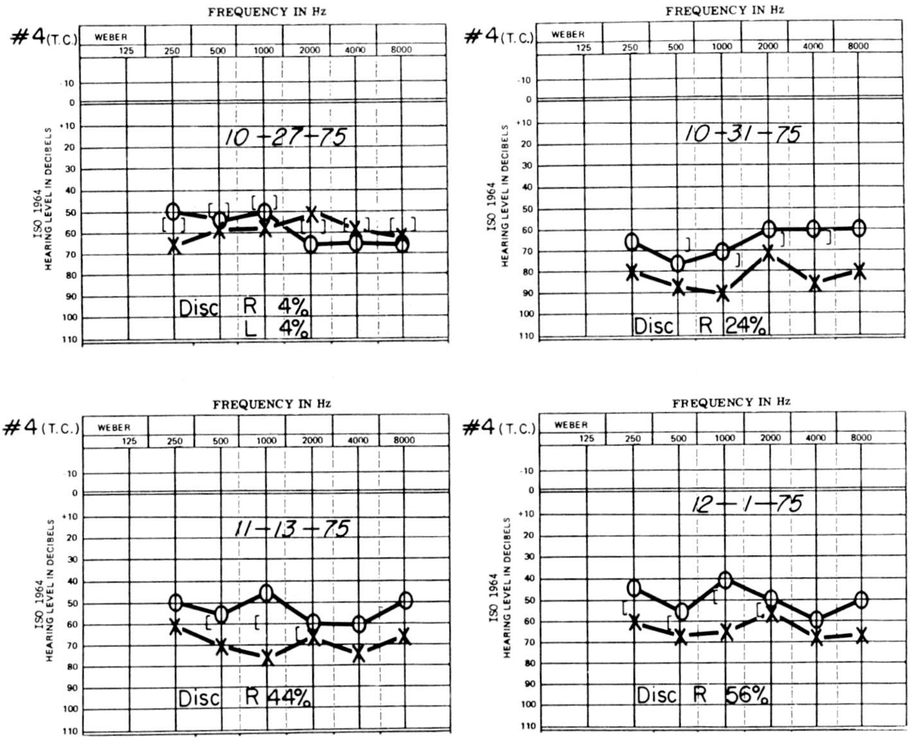

Fig. 4. Pure tone audiogram for Case 4 showing a sensorineural hearing loss.

ure. The BUN was 200 mg/100 ml and creatine 18.8 mg/100 ml. The edema had not responded to massive doses of oral furosemide prior to admission. Hemodialysis was begun on an emergency basis on October 17, 1975 via Shaldon catheters. For four consecutive days large amounts of fluid were removed and occasionally the patient was noted to have "disequilibrium syndrome" during dialysis, which was easily controlled by mannitol infusion. Unfortunately, an audiogram was not performed due to the patient's critical condition but the hearing was normal to clinical testing. On October 24, 1975 a Buselmeier shunt was inserted into the right arm and the fifth dialysis was performed via this shunt on the same day. During the fifth dialysis the patient complained of a rapid deterioration of hearing. This coincided with a fall in blood pressure from 130/60 to 100/50. An audiogram performed two days later showed a sensorineural hearing loss and very poor discrimination scores (Fig. 4). During this dialysis run electrolytes were normal, glucose was normal and coagulation studies were within acceptable limits for this dialysis. The rate of dialysis was 3 ml/min/kg of BUN which is the average rate for this dialysis center and not in the range of ultrafiltration. No further hearing loss occurred on successive dialyses. The discrimination scores gradually improved over the next two weeks and the pure tone audiogram also improved slightly. A transplantation of a kidney from a living related donor was performed on November 24, 1975. A further improvement in pure tone thresholds and discrimination was seen following the transplant period.

The hearing loss in this patient occurred during hemodialysis and corresponded to a time when hypotension was observed. A slight improvement occurred subsequently, but with renal transplantation a more significant increase in hearing was observed by the patient and the ward staff and confirmed audiometrically.

DISCUSSION

Renal failure is a severe systemic disorder which not only causes disturbances of fluid and electrolyte balances of the body, but also affects many other organs of the body directly or indirectly. Merrill and Hampers studied chronic kidney disease patients to determine if there were specific toxins of uremia.[4,5] They reported disorders in neurological, ophthalmological, gastrointestinal, cardiovascular, hemopoietic, mineral metabolic, lipid and protein metabolic systems. Organ transplantation with its accompanying altered immune mechanisms has also been shown to produce changes in organ systems not anatomically or physiologically related to the transplant organ. Over a decade ago it was recognized that otolaryngological disorders were caused by or accompanied the uremic state.[2,3]

Great advances have been made in the management of patients on chronic dialysis and those undergoing transplantation, so that the life expectancy of these patients has been increased dramatically. With increased patient survival and control of renal disease, the problems in other systems have become more prominent. Directors of large transplant units therefore have gathered teams of medical and surgical specialists to act as consultants. This is the case at the University of Minnesota, which has the distinction of being the largest transplant program in existence, performing over 100 kidney transplants each year.

In the early 1960s the advent of chemical agents of immunosuppression permitted the beginning of successful transplantation. New techniques of tissue typing and the use of antilymphocytic sera and other techniques of immunological enhancement have permitted increased survival of transplants. At the present time, the six-year survival of nondiabetic transplant patients independent of age is approximately 90% for related donor kidney grafts and 68% for cadaver grafts. The survival for diabetics is less; about 70% of patients receiving related donor grafts and 60% receiving cadaver grafts survive.[6] Renal transplantation is an established procedure for the treatment of end-stage renal disease, and with a few exceptions, is probably the treatment of choice.

Despite encouraging results, both dialysis and transplantation are not without serious risks or complications. Fifty percent of all deaths in transplantation are directly or indirectly caused by infections.[7] Fifty percent of the deaths in chronic hemodialysis are caused by cardiovascular accidents.[8] Cardiovascular premature aging may be an important survival limiting factor in chronic dialysis programs.[9] Many of the factors which influence the morbidity or mortality of the kidney patient may potentially affect the integrity and performance of the otologic system. In addition, as survival increases there is evidence that the transplanted kidney may start to show signs of the original renal disease. This is particularly evident in those diseases which have an immunological basis such as membrano-proliferative glomerulo-nephritis and Goodpasture's syndrome. The otological implications of these immunological factors will be alluded to later.

In our study, about one in six patients had some form of hearing disorder. Most of the hearing losses encountered were markedly greater than the arbitrary levels set for this study. Only seven patients exhibited borderline or minimal losses (Table III). As might be expected, the majority of hearing losses could be attributed to ototoxic agents used either alone or in combination. In very few cases could one factor alone be incriminated in the hearing loss. At best, single factors could be isolated that had precipitated the hearing loss. In order to understand the role of certain factors in the production of hearing loss, it was necessary to conduct laboratory experiments where the environment of the experimental animals could be controlled. Several of these ancillary investigations have been reported previously.[10-12] The patients entering our study were in terminal renal failure and most had suffered kidney disease for many years. Some patients had a life-long illness, such as juvenile onset diabetes mellitus. Previous medical records and drug charts frequently were not available for perusal, so that in 26 patients there was lack of evidence to determine the cause of hearing loss that was present when the patient entered the transplant program.

It became increasingly apparent that what we observed at any one instance during the study was the combination of the effects of many factors and that it was inadvisable to apportion total responsibility to any single agent or clinical circumstance. Bearing in mind this important concept, the factors which contributed in varying degrees to the hearing loss of our patients can be conveniently described in the following categories.

Otological Disorders. In any large group of patients it is expected that some will have or have had otological disorder. In our series, otologic disorders contributed to the hearing loss in 21 instances. Acute and chronic otitis media occurred most frequently, but one patient with Alport's syndrome suffered a basilar skull fracture, resulting in bilateral moderate sensorineural loss. In the upper Midwest, where the majority of our kidney patients originate, firearms, tractors, and other noisy farm machinery play an important role in the lives of many young men. It is not surprising that a positive history of noise exposure was observed in many of the male patients. Allowance for this was necessary in establishing the threshold criteria. In addition, it seemed that those patients with previous noise induced hearing loss were more susceptible to other damage. There is experimental evidence to lend support to this clinical observation.[13] Following transplant, immunosuppressed patients are more susceptible to infections, and the clinical presentation of such infections is markedly altered. In one patient with a diagnosis of acute otitis media there was only a mild otalgia, a temperature of 37.2 C and the tympanic membrane appeared only moderately erythematous. When the diagnosis of unilateral acute otitis media was made, appropriate antibiotics were started. The otitis media took three weeks to subside and resulted in a moderate sensorineural hearing loss in that ear. In retrospect it was evident that not only did this patient have otitis media, but he also had a labyrinthitis resulting in a hearing loss.[14] A serious result of an apparent mild infection has been the rule rather than the exception in otolaryngological disorders such as sinusitis, laryngitis, and tracheitis that we have encountered. The classical clinical signs may be absent or minimal in the immunosuppressed patient and may lead the unwary observer to give routine treatment. All infections in transplant patients must be treated vigorously as soon as the disease is suspected.

Excluding dialysis and other known or suspected causes of rapid hearing loss, six patients exhibited idiopathic sudden hearing loss, as illustrated in Case 1. A hypercoagulative state was evident in one patient when the hearing loss followed bilateral nephrectomy and splenectomy. However, the syndrome of sudden hearing loss was without explanation in the remainder of the cases.

Renal Disease. The similarities between physiological roles of the kidney and the cochlea have led to speculation that uremia may be associated with hearing loss. Electrolyte imbalance has been suggested as a possible cause for hearing loss in these patients.[15] Despite documented fluctuations in electrolytes in our study, no cases of hearing loss could be attributed to these occurrences, and in those cases where hearing loss did occur the electrolytes were usually within acceptable limits. Occasionally there were abnormalities of a single electrolyte in patients with hearing loss, but this was not consistently associated with any particular electrolyte.

Uremia has been shown to cause disturbances in many organ systems, but the relationship between hearing and urea levels has not clearly been established.[4,5] Patients in whom the blood urea or creatinine is markedly raised are very sick, lethargic, and have difficulty in performing audiological procedures. We have not been able to show convincingly that uremia itself causes impairment of hearing.

The concomitant diseases that occur in the kidney and ears, such as Alport's

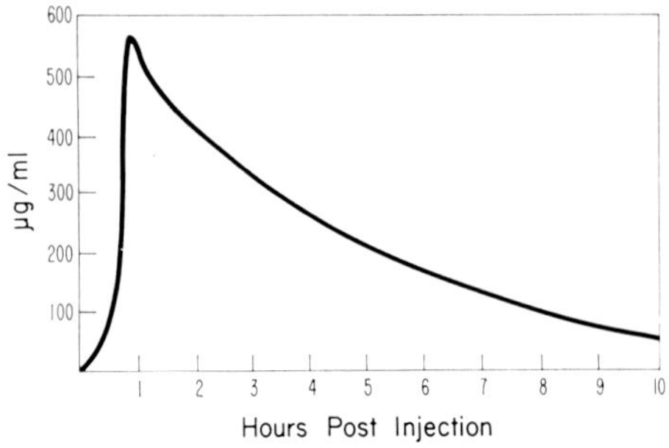

Fig. 5. Serum level of kanacycin following a single I.P. injection of 300 mg/kg in healthy guinea pig. Averaged readings of multiple estimations are shown.

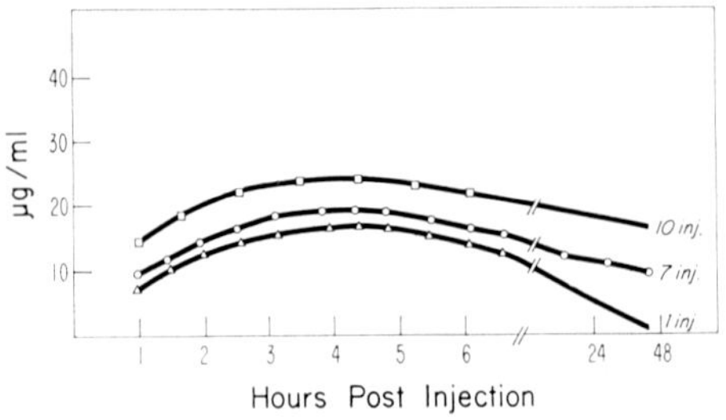

Fig. 6. Levels of kanamycin in inner ear fluids of guinea pigs following I.P. injections of 300 mg/kg daily. Averaged readings of multiple estimations are shown.

syndrome, occasionally can be very difficult to categorize. As yet there is no characteristic renal histopathology for these diseases and no serological or biochemical tests exist that can identify these syndromes. It is possible, therefore, that congenital hearing disorders may be present in patients with kidney disease which are not able to be classified into set syndromes, such as Alport's, Weil's, or Alstrom's disease. In our studies, 11 patients had hearing loss and hereditary nephropathy, and two patients had a congenital hearing loss but no history of hereditary nephropathy. Confusing patterns occur when the onset of hearing loss occurs after the onset of renal failure, as is sometimes the case in these disorders.

Uremia is known to cause neuropathy, the exact mechanism of which is uncertain.[16] This neuropathy has never been reported to be associated with hearing loss. In fact, it affects the peripheral nerves, sparing the cranial nerves, as illustrated in Case 2.

Ototoxicity. The ENT literature is replete with discussions of the temporal bone changes, ultrastructural effects, biochemical changes and histochemical patterns caused by the ototoxic antibiotics of the aminoglycoside group. There is no shortage of evidence that distinct changes occur in the cochleo-vestibular system with toxic levels of these antibiotics. Similarly, with undaunted repetition, in the general medical literature articles appear extolling the virtues of mathematic equations which help determine the exact dosage and frequency of administration of the aminoglycoside antibiotics to prevent toxic blood levels in patients with impaired renal function. Despite the endeavors of researchers, and the care and precautions taken by clinicians, ototoxic damage still occurs. It is therefore imperative that some of the factors responsible for this paradoxical situation be reviewed.

It is well known that a high level of antibiotic in the blood is necessary to produce toxic effect. This level is the resultant of the quantity and rate at which the drug is given and the rate of its excretion or degradation. However, it is not the blood level per se that is damaging, but it is thought that only in this circumstance will the drug be able to enter the cochlea. Stupp and his coworkers suggested that an active secretion of the drug into the cochlear fluids occurs, resulting in accumulation.[17] Experiments performed on normal guinea pigs in our laboratory showed that a peak kanamycin level in serum was reached after 30 to 60 minutes following an intraperitoneal injection. Excretion of the drug was usually complete within eight hours. Cochlear fluids, however, showed presence of this drug for much longer periods. Repeated daily intraperitoneal injections caused higher levels of the drug in the cochlear fluids even though the curve of the serum levels was exactly the same after the last daily injection (Figs. 5, 6). It seems, therefore,

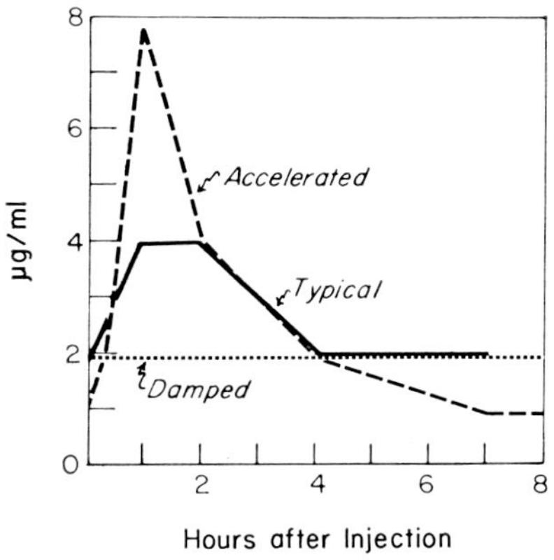

Fig. 7. Responses to gentamycin dosage of 3 mg/kg/day in patients with normal renal function. (After Riff and Jackson.[18])

that only above a certain level in the serum will the drug enter the ear, but can remain there for long periods, allowing further injections to cause an accumulation of the drug. A simple method of preventing ototoxicity would be to prevent the peak level of the antibiotic from reaching threshold that is necessary for entrance into the inner ear. These toxic levels have been estimated in humans as being 16 μg/ml for gentamicin and kanamycin, and 10μg/ml for streptomycin. To achieve adequate therapeutic blood levels, dosages are usually calculated according to body weight or surface area. This does not take into consideration the variation of individual susceptibility to drugs. It has been pointed out that response to dosages of gentamicin in patients with normal renal function falls into three categories: "typical" response, "accelerated" response, or "dampened" response (Fig. 7).[18] Prescription of aminoglycoside antibiotics on a milligram per kilogram body weight basis will result in variable plasma concentrations even in patients with normal renal function. One cannot overemphasize the importance of individualizing treatment regimens of aminoglycoside antibiotics according to the patient's own pharmacokinetics.

Microbiological and immunochemical procedures are now available that permit accurate and rapid assay of antibiotic levels of the aminoglycosides. This allows calculation of the size and interval of the doses that should avoid toxicity. Sawchuk and Zaske, using a radioimmune assay of serum antibiotic levels following a test dose, are able to calculate the half-life and distribution of the drug.[19] With the aid of computers they are then able to predict with incredible accuracy the rate at which the drug must be given and the interval between doses, which is individualized to the patient and irrespective of the renal status. This exciting work has great potential in the effort to avoid ototoxic damage because it is designed to avert some of the toxic peak levels that exist 30 to 60 minutes after administration of these drugs.

Ethacrynic acid was the first of the potent diuretics shown to cause hearing loss. Since this drug is excreted exclusively by the kidney, impaired renal function would be expected to increase the ototoxicity of this drug by maintaining a high blood level for longer periods. This fact has been substantiated experimentally.[20] Following some irreversible hearing loss in our renal patients and as a result of animal experiments demonstrating the ototoxic effect of ethacrynic acid, this drug has rarely been used at the University of Minnesota dialysis and transplant service since 1970.[10] The second potent toxic diuretic, furosemide, however, has been increasingly used. At first it was thought that only reversible hearing loss occurred with this drug. Animal experiments, however, showed that the mode of action in the ear was similar to that of ethacrynic acid, and gradually cases of irreversible hearing loss have been reported.[12,21,22] Furosemide is unlike ethacrynic acid in that it is not excreted exclusively by the kidneys, thus its action is independent of renal function. In our series the hearing loss occurred during rapid and repeated administration of the drug. The policy of "intravenous push" has now been abandoned and the drug is given by slow infusion. The recommended rate of infusion for adults is not to exceed 4 mg of furosemide per minute per kilogram of body weight.

As illustrated in Case 2, we have become increasingly aware of the existence of the potentiation of ototoxicity of potent diuretics and aminoglycoside antibiotics. The circumstances for potentiation of the ototoxicity of these drugs are pharmacologically ideal. Two sites of primary action exist, the stria vascularis and the organ of Corti. Second, there is probably a direct dependence of the hair cells on the stria vascularis and third, damage to the stria vascularis may permit increased entry of the antibiotic into the cochlear fluids. Potentiation of hearing loss by diuretics and aminoglycoside antibiotics has been conclusively shown.[23,24] In our clinical survey, eight patients were thought to have suffered hearing loss as a direct result of potentiation of these two types of drugs and in five other patients drug potentiation contributed significantly to the hearing loss.

Utmost caution must be exercised in giving ototoxic diuretics and aminoglycoside antibiotics together or closely following each other. The rules mentioned above regarding the serum antibiotic levels and rate of administration of drugs and even the newer half-life, blood distribution studies are not applicable in potentiation.

A new concept of ototoxicity must also be considered. In addition to the potentiation of known ototoxic drugs, it is possible that drugs which have not hitherto been regarded as ototoxic may become so when used in combination with other drugs. Much more experimental work in this area is needed.

Diabetes and Other Metabolic Disorders. Diabetes mellitus, Fabry's disease and partial lypodystrophy were thought to be directly responsible for the gradual loss of hearing in seven patients and contributed significantly to the hearing loss in seven others. In one patient, a sudden decrease in hearing accompanied a rather prolonged hypoglycemic episode, however, there was no overall correlation in these few patients between control of the diabetes and the onset of hearing loss. Most of our cases developing hearing loss had been diabetic for many years, and the possibility of premature arteriosclerosis causing decreased cochlear blood flow must be considered. There has been an increasing number of reports regarding hearing in diabetics. It seems to be universally held that, in general, diabetics have poorer hearing than comparable groups of nondiabetics, particularly when the diabetes is of long standing.[25] In histopathological studies of the temporal bones of diabetic patients, positive PAS staining is seen in the stria vascularis with thickening of the capillary walls and arteriosclerotic changes in the vessels of the ear.[26,27] This histological picture has been reported by others in relation to chronic renal disease and will be referred to later. It is possible that some of the 22 diabetics developing hearing loss may belong to the familial syndrome of juvenile diabetes, optic atrophy, and neurogenic deafness.[28] No attempt was made to distinguish these from other forms of diabetes and it is possible that this syndrome may account for some of the unknown causes of hearing loss in Table I. In Fabry's disease, the hearing loss seems to be quite variable and no definite correlation can be made at the present time as to what proportion of patients with Fabry's disease do have a hearing loss.

Dialysis. Before embarking on the present prospective study, a retrospective evaluation of hearing in chronic dialysis patients at our institution was performed. In this pilot study it seemed that patients on chronic dialysis all had high-tone sensorineural hearing loss, however, too many variables existed to draw any scientific conclusions. Therefore, this prospective study was initiated. With increased awareness of certain specific causes of hearing loss it became apparent that hemodialysis could be responsible for hearing loss in a variety of ways. Other investigators have also reported hearing loss in dialysis patients.[29,30]

It has been stated previously that long term dialysis results in premature arteriosclerosis, a condition similar to that occurring in long-standing diabetes mellitus. When compared with established standards of hearing for the general population, our dialysis patients who had been on long-term dialysis before kidney transplant had a high-frequency hearing loss similar to that of diabetics and similar to the pattern seen in presbyacusis. Temporal bone studies performed at the University of Minnesota have revealed the presence of blue concretions in the stria vascularis of patients who had undergone multiple dialyses.[31] Bergstrom and her co-workers, in another excellent clinical pathological study of renal patients, independently identified similar deposits.[32] Temporal bone studies of diabetics have shown similar changes in the stria vascularis.[26] It is tempting to assume that these findings can be explained on the basis of degenerative vascular changes. However, several other factors merit consideration.

Acute mononeuritis multiplex has been reported in connection with the rapid ultrafiltration form of hemodialysis.[33,34] It has been postulated that the rapid decrease in blood and extracellular fluid volume leads to neuronal ischemia. Veverbrants and coauthors point out the role of ultrafiltration, $2M^2$/hour dialysis, in the etiology of cochleovestibular disturbances in their series of five patients.[29] As illustrated in Case 4, the rapid loss of hearing occurring during dialysis was consistently associated with hypotension. It must, however, be pointed out that ultrafiltration was not used in this patient and the rate of dialysis was fairly typical for this center. One other patient, not summarized here, had a repeated drop of blood pressure on each dialysis run and complained that during dialysis her hearing was always markedly decreased but returned at the end of the run. It is unlikely that hypotension itself is responsible for the hearing loss since one would have expected greater incidence of hearing loss in such clinical conditions as myocardial infarction where hypotension is a common feature. It is conjectural that subtle movements of body fluids or changes in osmolality which result in hypotension during dialysis may also cause changes in the fluid compartments of the inner ear.

During rapid dialysis the well recognized "disequilibrium syndrome" occurs. The exact nature of this syndrome is unclear, but neurovestibular signs and symptoms have been well documented.[35] A condition may therefore exist that bears some similarity to endolymphatic hydrops and, like this condition, may result in sensorineural hearing loss.

Finally, although hypotension is unlikely to be a major cause of hearing loss, hypoxia has recently been shown to cause decreased cochlear action potentials.[36] The effect of hypoxia due to hypotension, together with other factors mentioned above, must be considered. Furthermore, it has been suggested that the ototoxicity of tobramycin in experimental animals was more likely to be the result of hypotension caused by the drug than the direct chemical poisoning effect.[37] The full answer on these factors has obviously not yet been discovered.

Transplantation. Occasional hearing loss has occurred during kidney transplantation and furosemide used to encourage renal blood flow and glomerular filtration during the operation, as well as in the immediate postoperative period, may have been a factor in some of our cases. The practice of neomycin solution irrigation of the wound and peritoneal cavity prior to closure was evaluated as a potential ototoxic hazard. Blood neomycin levels were drawn prior to the operation, immediately after the irrigation and one hour later. Measurable serum levels were found only occasionally, the highest level being 12 μg/ml. In the patient with the highest serum level of neomycin, the postoperative hearing evaluation showed normal hearing. Serum neomycin levels of 6.7 μg/ml have been reportedly associated with hearing impairment but these levels were maintained for longer periods.[38] The practice of irrigation with neomycin solution does pose a potential ototoxic risk, particularly in the presence of other ototoxic agents. Because neomycin is nephrotoxic it would similarly impose a risk on the newly acquired kidney. This technique therefore, needs close scrutiny and reassessment. In two patients who received four kidney transplantations the hearing loss observed was not easily accounted for by other factors. The possibility of immunological factors was considered and a laboratory experiment was designed to investigate possible antigenic similarities between the cochlea and the kidney.[11] The results of this study suggest that an antigenic relationship might indeed exist between the kidney and the cochlea. Although no direct clinical correlation can be extrapolated from this experimental study, immunological factors cannot be ignored either in the effect on the ear or in the kidney disease. It has been observed that in patients with renal failure due to immunologic kidney disease a return of the original disorder sometimes does occur following transplantation.[6]

In four patients in our series hearing improved following transplantation. A typical case is illustrated in Case 3. This curious phenomenon has also been reported by Mitschke and co-workers, who thought that successful transplantation removed the uremic toxin.[39] It seemed to us more plausible that the restoration of a physiological renal system would remove the exogenous ototoxic influences of repeated dialysis, diuretics, or other ototoxic agents necessary for the control of chronic renal failure.

There is insufficient clinical and experimental evidence as yet to formulate definite conclusions with respect to kidney transplantation or immunological factors in the cause or relief of hearing impairment. This is an exciting concept, however, and one that is well worth keeping in mind in clinical observations and worth pursuing in ancillary laboratory experiments.

CONCLUSIONS

A prospective study of hearing in patients of the dialysis and transplant program has been presented. Since this program is the largest in existence and attracts patients from all over the world, the magnitude of the task was enormous. In addition, monitoring the hearing of these patients was not easy. Hearing evaluations understandably are not of primary importance when the patient is fighting for life or in a comatose state from an overwhelming infection. Patients receiving cadaver transplants are recalled to the hospital when donor kidneys are available. This means that scheduling of admissions is impossible and they frequently occur outside the normal working day. As a result, these patients may not receive an audiological evaluation until after the immediate postoperative period, which can be quite stormy and beset with ototoxic hazards. Despite the difficulties, it was possible to identify the factors contributing to hearing loss in the majority of patients. Many of these factors were previously known and in these instances suggestions have been made for either management or avoidance of the problem. It was rewarding to observe a decrease of the overall incidence of hearing loss resulting from the instigation of corrective measures indicated by this study. The main purpose of every clinical study is that it will directly benefit the patient. Several new theories were brought to light by this study, which in some instances necessitated laboratory and experimental studies to assist in the evaluation of these concepts. A satisfactory explanation of some of these issues is still wanting, but may be forthcoming with further clinical and laboratory investigations. Application of experience gained by these issues may in the future increase our knowledge of the fundamental mechanisms associated with sensorineural hearing loss in general.

The most striking result of this work has been the realization that hearing loss is rarely due to one cause but stems from the interaction of many factors. Further, this interaction is not a simple addition of effects but may be the result of potentiation. Potentiation of effects means that physical, clinical or immunological factors not previously ototoxic may become ototoxic in the presence of other agents. This survey provided the rare opportunity of combining a clinical study for the direct benefit of patients, with basic investigations of fundamental issues of hearing and hearing loss.

REFERENCES

1. Bricker NS, Bourgoignie J, Weber H, *et al*: Pathogenesis of the uremic state; A new perspective, in Hamburger J, Crosnier J, Maxwell MH (eds): *Advances in Nephrology*. Chicago, Yearbook Medical Publishers, 1972, vol 2, chap 13
2. Beaney GP: Otolaryngeal problems arising during the management of severe renal failure. J Laryngol Otol 78:506-515, 1964
3. Yassin A, Safwat F, Fatt-Hi A: Ear, nose and throat manifestations in cases of renal failure treated by dialysis, hemodialysis and peritoneal dialysis. Ann Otol Rhinol Laryngol 75:192-201, 1966
4. Merrill JP, Hampers CL: Uremia. N Engl J Med 282:953-961, 1970
5. Merrill JP, Hampers CL: Uremia II. N Engl J Med 282:1014-1021, 1970
6. Kjellstrand CM, Simmons RL, Buselmeier TJ, *et al*: Renal transplantation at the University of Minnesota. Minn Med 57:886-891, 1974
7. U.S. Kidney Transplant Fact Book. DHEW Publication No. (NIH) 73-335, Bethesda, 1973
8. Guland HJ, Brunner FP, Dehn H, *et al*: Combined report on regular dialysis and transplantation in Europe, 111, 1972. Proc European Dialysis Transplant Association 10:LVII, 1973
9. Lindner A, Charra B, Sherrard DJ, *et al*: Accelerated atherosclerosis in prolonged maintenance hemodialysis. N Engl J Med 290:697-701, 1974
10. Quick CA, Duvall AJ: Early changes in the cochlear duct from ethacrynic acid: An electronmicroscopic evaluation. Laryngoscope 80:954-965, 1970
11. Quick CA, Fish A, Brown C: The relationship between cochlea and kidney. Laryngoscope 83:1469-1482, 1973
12. Quick CA, Hoppe W: Permanent deafness associated with furosemide administration. Ann Otol Rhinol Laryngol 84:94-101, 1974
13. Falk SA: Combined effects of noise and ototoxic drugs. Environ Health Perspect 2: 5-22, 1972
14. Paparella MM, Oda M, Hiraide F, *et al*: Pathology of sensorineural hearing loss in otitis media. Ann Otol Rhinol Laryngol 81:632-647, 1972
15. Yassin A, Badry A, and Fatt-Hi A: The relationship between electrolyte balance and cochlear disturbances in cases of renal failure. J Laryngol Otol 84:429-435, 1970
16. Kjellstrand CM, Peterson RJ, Evans RL, *et al*: Considerations of the middle molecule hypothesis. II: Neuropathy in nephrectomized patients. Trans Amer Soc Artif Int Organs 19:325-336, 1973
17. Stupp H, Rauch S, Sous H, *et al*: Dee Vrsache der spezifischen ototoxizitat der basischen Streptomyces - Antibiotika-ein Permeabilitatsproblem. Med Hyg (Geneve) 23:706, 988, 1965
18. Riff LJ, Jackson GG: Pharmacology of gentamicin in man. J Infect Dis (Suppl) 124: 98-105, 1971
19. Sawchuk RJ, Zaske DE: Pharmacokinetics of dosing regimens which utilize multiple intravenous infusions: gentamicin in burn patients. J Pharmacokinet Biopharm 4:183-195, 1976
20. McCurdy JA, McCormick JG, Harrill JA: Ototoxicity of ethacrynic acid in the anuric guinea pig. Arch Otolaryngol 100:143-147, 1974
21. Wigand ME, Heidland A: Ototoxic side-effects of high doses of furosemide in patients with uremia. Postgrad Med J (Suppl) 47:54-56, 1971
22. Vargish T, Benjamin R, Sherkman L: Deafness from furosemide administration. Ann Otol Rhinol Laryngol 84:94-101, 1974
23. West BA, Brummett RE, Himes DL: Interaction of kanamycin and ethacrynic acid. Arch Otolaryngol 98:32-37, 1973
24. Prazma J, Browder JP, Fischer ND: Ethacrynic acid ototoxicity potentiation by kanamycin. Ann Otol Rhinol Laryngol 83:111-118, 1974
25. Chochinov RH, Ullyot GL, Moorhouse JA: Sensory perception thresholds in patients with juvenile diabetes and their close relatives. N Engl J Med 286:1233-1237, 1972
26. Jorgenson MG: Changes in aging in the inner ear and the inner ear in diabetes mellitus. Histologic studies. Acta Otolaryngol [Suppl] (Stockh) 188:125-128, 1963
27. Makishima K, Tanaka K: Pathological changes of the inner ear and central auditory pathway in diabetics. Ann Otol Rhinol Laryngol 80:218-228, 1971
28. Stevens PR, Macfadyean WA: Familial incidence of juvenile diabetes mellitus pro-

gressive optic atrophy and neurogenic deafness. Br J Ophthalmol 56:496-500, 1972

29. Veverbrandts E, Lowry K, Rainer D, *et al*: Hearing loss associated with double-gambro dialysis. Proc Dial Transpl Forum 3: 252-257, 1973

30. Johnson DW, Mathod RH: Hearing function and chronic renal failure. Ann Otol Rhinol Laryngol 85:43-49, 1976

31. Oda M, Preciado MC, Quick CA, *et al*: Labyrinthine pathology of chronic renal failure patients treated with hemodialysis and kidney transplantation. Laryngoscope 84:1489-1506, 1974

32. Bergstrom L, Jenkins P, Sardo I, *et al*: Hearing loss in renal disease: Clinical and pathological studies. Ann Otol Rhinol Laryngol 82:555-576, 1973

33. Meyrier A, Fardeau M, Richet G: Acute asymmetrical neuritis associated with rapid ultrafiltration dialysis. Br Med J 2:252-254, 1972

34. Bosl R, Shideman JR, Meyer RM, *et al*: Effects and complications of high efficiency dialysis. Nephron 15(2):151-160, 1975

35. Rosen JA, Nicotera J: Nystagmus during dialysis. Trans Am Neurol Assoc 92:283, 1967

36. Lawrence M, Nuttali AL, Burgio PA: Cochlear potentials and oxygen associated with hypoxia. Ann Otol Rhinol Laryngol 84:499-512, 1975

37. Brummett RE, Brown RT: Tobramycin ototoxicity: A second look. Arch Otolaryngol 101:540-543, 1975

38. Sugarbaker PH, Sabath LD, Morgan AP: Neomycin toxicity from porcine skin xenografts. Ann Surg 179:183-185, 1974

39. Mitschke H, Schmidt P, Kopsa H, *et al*: Reversible uremic deafness after successful renal transplantation. N Engl J Med 292(20): 1062-1063, 1975

ACKNOWLEDGMENT—The contribution of Dr. W. Hoppe, D. Colburn and P. McKeon in the painstaking analysis of the data is gratefully acknowledged. The author is indebted to Dr. C. Kjellstrand, Director of the Dialysis Unit, and Drs. J. Najarian and R. Simmons of the Transplant Service for the stimulating intellectual experience of working with them and for the opportunity of reviewing and reporting their cases.

REPRINTS—Cedric A. Quick, MD, 412 Union St. S.E., Minneapolis, MN 55455.

CURRENT THERAPY FOR MALIGNANCY OF THE ORAL CAVITY

The Department of Otolaryngology, National Naval Medical Center, is sponsoring a symposium on Current Therapy for Malignancy of the Oral Cavity and Related Structures, June 2-4, 1977 in Bethesda, Maryland. For further information, contact Alan D. Kornblut CDR MC USNR, Department of Otolaryngology, National Naval Medical Center, Bethesda, MD 20014.

Ann Otol 85: 1976

ELECTRON MICROSCOPIC COCHLEAR OBSERVATIONS IN BILATERAL MÉNIÈRE'S DISEASE

ROBERT S. KIMURA, BA CAROL Y. OTA, BA
HAROLD F. SCHUKNECHT, MD TADAHIKO TAKAHASHI, MD
BOSTON, MASSACHUSETTS

SUMMARY – Electron microscopic study of the cochleas of an individual with bilateral Ménière's disease revealed the presence of many abnormal sensory cells in the apical regions of the cochleas. The pathological alterations were greater in the left ear with the greater hearing loss. There were some giant cilia, fusion of cilia, and loss of cilia. The outer hair cells contained diffuse cuticular bodies near or basal to the nuclei. Many outer hair cells were retracted away from the reticular membrane. The population of the nerve endings appeared normal. The inner hair cells of the apical turns appeared essentially normal. The spiral ganglia were normal in number and morphology at the apical turns, and a majority of their cell bodies were of the unmyelinated or partly myelinated types. The stria vascularis showed atrophy; however, the magnitude of this change was consistent with that known to occur in the aging ear. In the distended areas Reissner's membrane showed areas devoid of mesothelial cells, as well as atrophic epithelial cells. The blood vessels were no different from other human cochlear vessels. These abnormalities seen in the stereocilia, the outer hair cells, and Reissner's membrane are a matter of fact. We must admit, however, that not enough electron microscopic studies have been performed on ears from aging individuals or ears with other pathologies to state that these changes are unique to Ménière's disease. Furthermore, there is currently insufficient knowledge to predict whether these changes affect auditory function.

The light microscopic observations on temporal bones from individuals with Ménière's disease have been thoroughly studied by numerous investigators. By this technique the cochleas have uniformly shown enormous distention of Reissner's membrane and normal or near normal populations of sensory cells.[1,2] The existence of an apparently normal organ of Corti in association with severely impaired hearing has puzzled these investigators. It is obvious that other, more penetrating methods of investigation of these structures is needed. We obtained the temporal bones from an individual with the clinical manifestations of Ménière's disease and processed them for study by electron microscopy. Our objective was to define the ultrastructural features of the organ of Corti, spiral ganglia, Reissner's membrane and stria vascularis in a search for possible explanations for the hearing loss.

METHODS AND MATERIALS

Otologic History. A Caucasian male traveling salesman (T.M.), first experienced recurring episodes of severe vertigo, nausea, and vomiting, and progressive left hearing loss at the age of 25. After several years, the vertigo subsided but the hearing loss persisted. At the age of 40, he again reported having had several episodes of vertigo. At the age of 52, audiometric studies showed a severe sensorineural hearing loss in the left ear with zero speech discrimination score and a mild loss in the right with 100% speech discrimination score. At age 57, he again experienced acute recurring vertiginous episodes with nausea and vomiting. Audiograms showed a further progression of the hearing loss in the left ear and a moderate sensorineural hearing loss in the right ear. Discrimination scores were 4% in the left and 80% in the right ear. The SISI test was negative on the right and 100% on the left. The tone decay test was negative bilaterally, and the Rinne test was positive

From the Department of Otolaryngology at the Massachusetts Eye and Ear Infirmary and Harvard Medical School, Boston, Massachusetts. This work was supported by US Public Health Grant 5 RO1 NSO3932-14.

Presented at the meeting of the American Otological Society, Inc., Palm Beach, Florida, April 25-26, 1976.

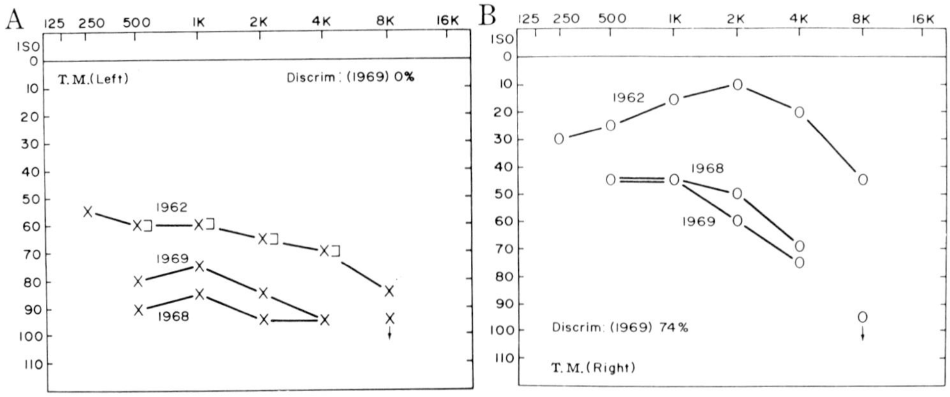

Fig. 1. Audiograms. Caucasian male, age 59. A) Left ear. Ménière's disease for 34 years. B) Right ear. Ménière's disease for seven years.

bilaterally. Cold caloric tests were reported to be normal in the right. There was no response to 20 cc of ice water in the left. At the age of 58, he continued to complain of vertiginous episodes and stated that his hearing seemed improved at times, although this was not confirmed by audiometric tests. The discrimination scores were 0% on the left and 74% on the right (Fig. 1). Radiologic studies of the temporal bones, including laminograms, at ages 57 and 58 were normal. At age 59 he experienced severe acute chest pain and died 17 days later. Autopsy revealed recent acute myocardial infarction.

One and one-half hours after death, both temporal bones were fixed by perfusion of 1% phosphate buffered osmium. The specimens were trimmed to reduce their size, the apices of the cochleas were opened, and the vestibular labyrinths were dissected out. After each whole cochlea was imbedded in Epon®*, it was bisected through the midmodiolar region. Then each half was further subdivided, and each cochlear turn was separated out. The location of each piece was plotted on the cochlear spiralgraph. These pieces were examined from the base to the apex at about 1 to 2 mm intervals. Some pieces were serially sectioned from the reticular lamina of the organ of Corti to the nerve endings. The sections were examined and photographed** at magnifications of 1,000 to 40,000 X. Many composite photographs of the entire cochlear ducts were made to provide panoramic views of the cytoarchitectural features of these cochleas.

RESULTS

Structural alterations in the organ of Corti of the left ear were more severe and extensive than the right ear. Hydrops was very extensive throughout the left cochlea while the distention was noted at the apical and second turns in the right cochlea. The stria vascularis was severely atrophic in the left, and to a lesser degree in the right ear.

Left Ear. From the basal end to the 8 to 9 mm area, there was severe atrophy of both outer hair cells (OHC) and inner hair cells (IHC); the OHC were missing more frequently than the IHC. Abnormal or degenerated OHC were not attached to the reticular lamina and appeared pushed down toward the basilar membrane (Fig. 2). In the area where the OHC were totally missing, some unmyelinated nerve fibers were discernible between the Deiters' cells. As the organ of Corti was followed apicalward, the hair cell populations became normal or near normal. Some of the OHC showed loss of stereocilia, fusion of cilia or giant cilia. The apical cytoplasm showed an accumulation of lipofuscin granules, and the middle or basal part of the cells showed a decrease in the number of subsurface cisternae. Usually there were 2 to 3 nerve endings per hair cell (15 mm area). One of these nerve endings was large, but only a few vesicles were shown inside. In general, the nerve endings remained attached to the hair cells even though the cells were clearly

---

* Shell Chemical Co., N.Y., NY.

** Elmiskop 1. Siemens Corp., Iselin, NJ.

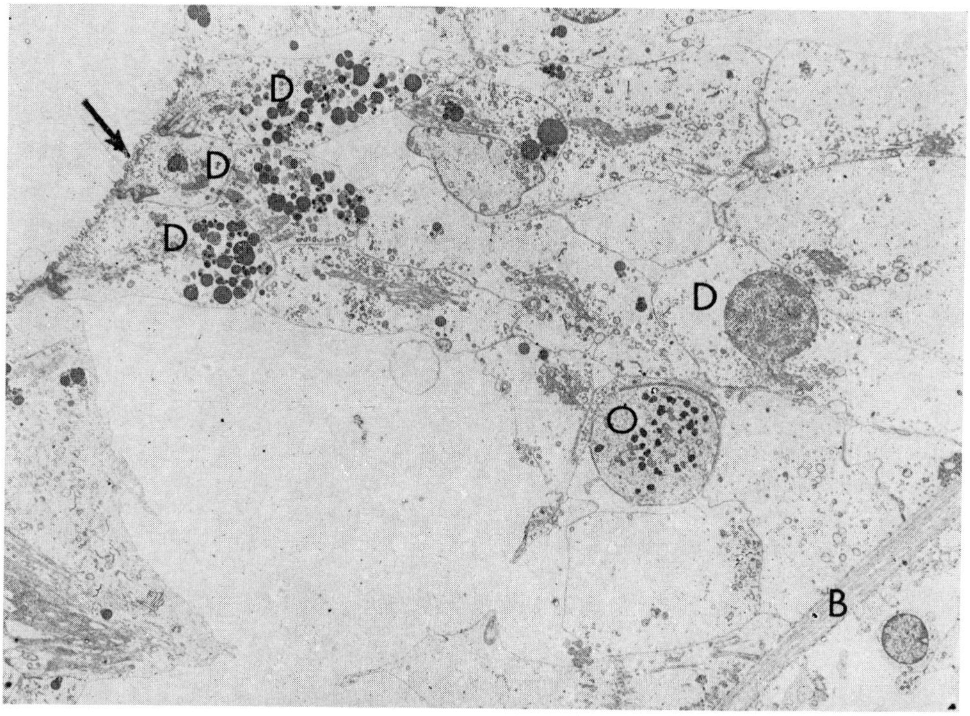

Fig. 2. Degenerated organ of Corti from the basal turn of the left cochlea. Note the reticular lamina (arrow) without OHC; however, detached hair cell (O) with dense granules is shown closer to the basilar membrane (B) than the usual position. D - Deiters' cell.

atrophied. A few hair cells were devoid of nerve endings.

As the serial sections cut parallel to the reticular lamina were followed toward the basilar membrane, more OHC began to emerge adjacent to the existing ones (Fig. 3). Evidently, these cells were not connected to the reticular lamina. In one specimen, in the 2 kHz area (about 15 mm from the basal end), we counted 83 OHC just below the reticular lamina, but 105 OHC were present nearer the nerve endings (20% increase). The cytoplasmic and nuclear morphology of the disconnected cells was similar to those which were connected to the reticular lamina; however, they often contained a homogeneous diffuse body intermixed with dense substances near or at the infranuclear zone. The disconnected cells retained well-developed subsurface cisternae and abutting nerve endings or nerve fibers. A pair of these disconnected or unattached hair cells showed cell junctions (reticular lamina type) among themselves at their nuclear levels (Fig. 4A).

Fine morphological changes in the IHC were difficult to detect. These cells were often displaced by swollen nerve endings and nerve fibers. In some cells the number of coated vesicles was increased. Synaptic bodies, which are so common in animal ears, were infrequently found adjacent to the nerve endings; however, thickenings of opposing plasma membranes were often found on the hair cell and nerve endings. The stereocilia were of giant size in some cells (Fig. 5). There was no obvious loss of nerve endings below normal appearing hair cells; however, a decrease was noted below the abnormal hair cells. When the hair cells were completely missing, the entire area was filled by the inner supporting cells and border cells with only a few scattered nerve fibers clearly evident.

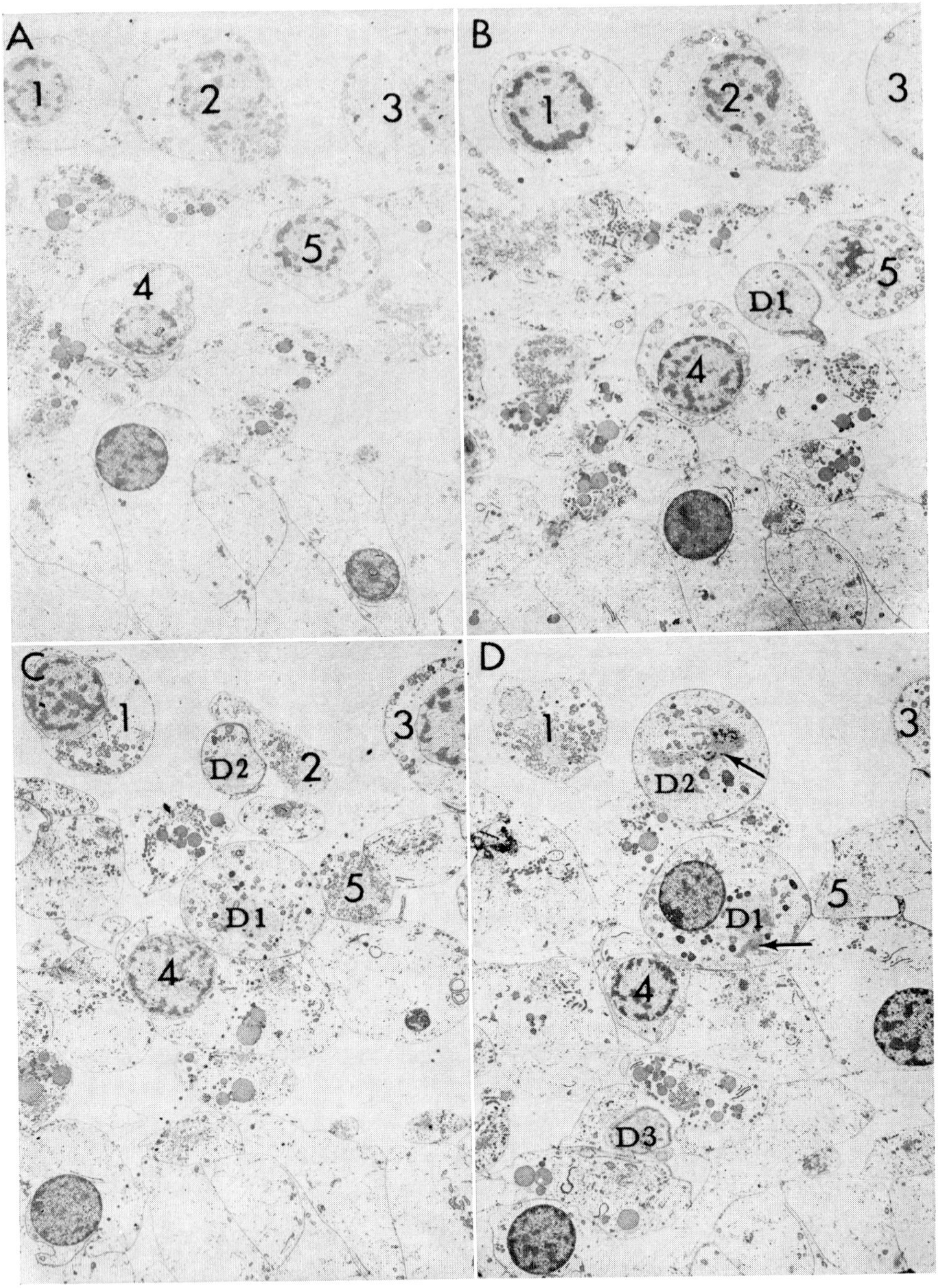

Fig. 3. Serial sections of the OHC followed from the top of the organ of Corti to the nerve ending areas (15 mm area). A) Five OHC are shown. B) Another OHC (D1) appears. C) A second hair cell (D2) appears. D) A third hair cell (D3) emerges. These three cells are not attached to the reticular lamina. The arrows point to the diffuse cuticular bodies in the detached hair cells.

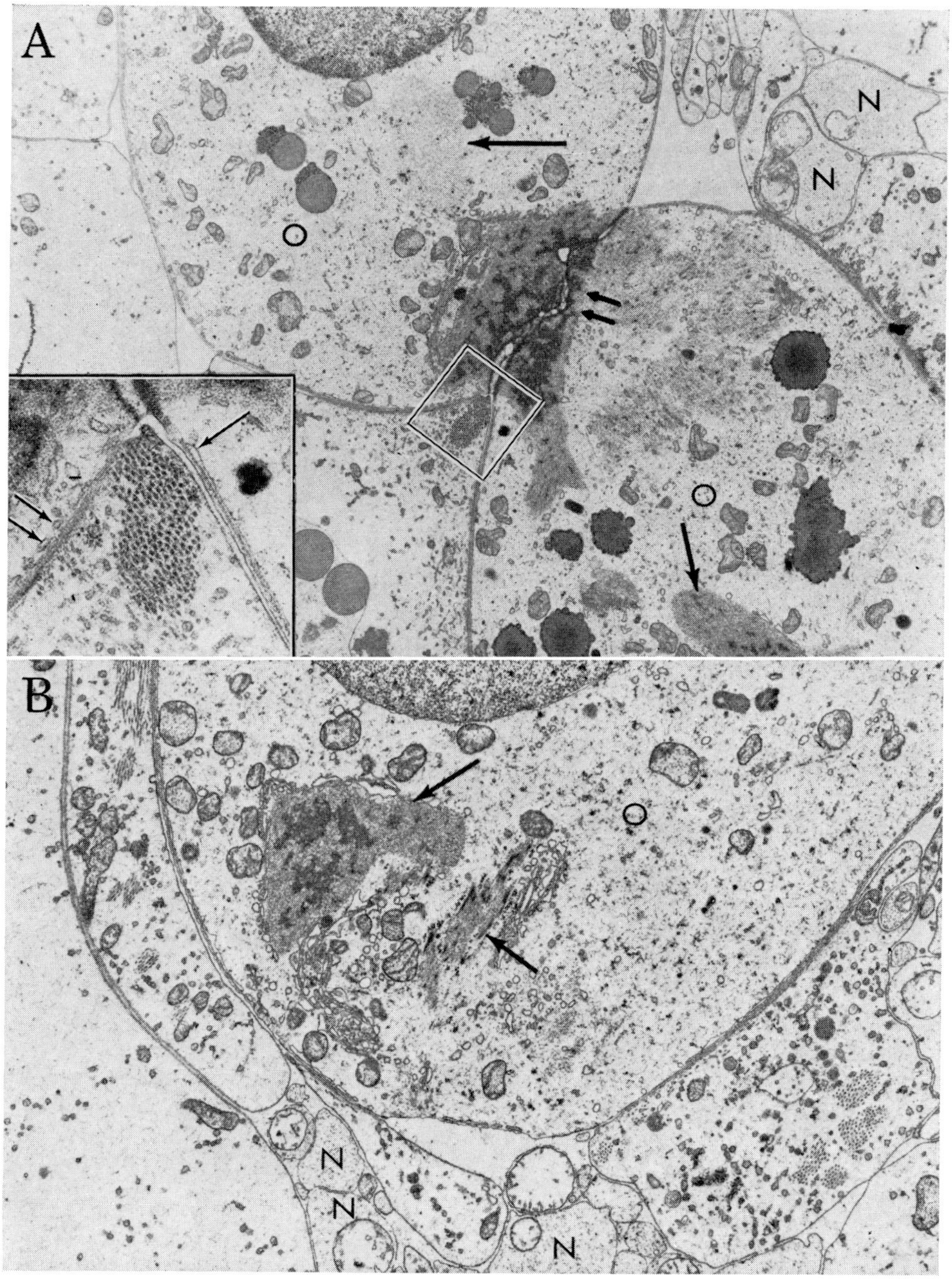

Fig. 4. The diffuse cuticular bodies in the OHC which were unattached to the reticular lamina. A) Two outer hair cells (O) establish cell junctions at the nuclear level (two arrows). Note the presence of diffuse bodies in these cells (long arrows). The bracketed area is shown at higher magnification in the lower left corner. Arrows point to the subsurface cisternae of the two abutting hair cells. N - Nerve fibers of the outer spiral bundle. Left cochlea. B) A high magnification of the diffuse cuticular bodies (arrows) in the infranuclear zone of the OHC (O). N - Nerve fibers of the outer spiral bundle. 21 mm area of the right cochlea.

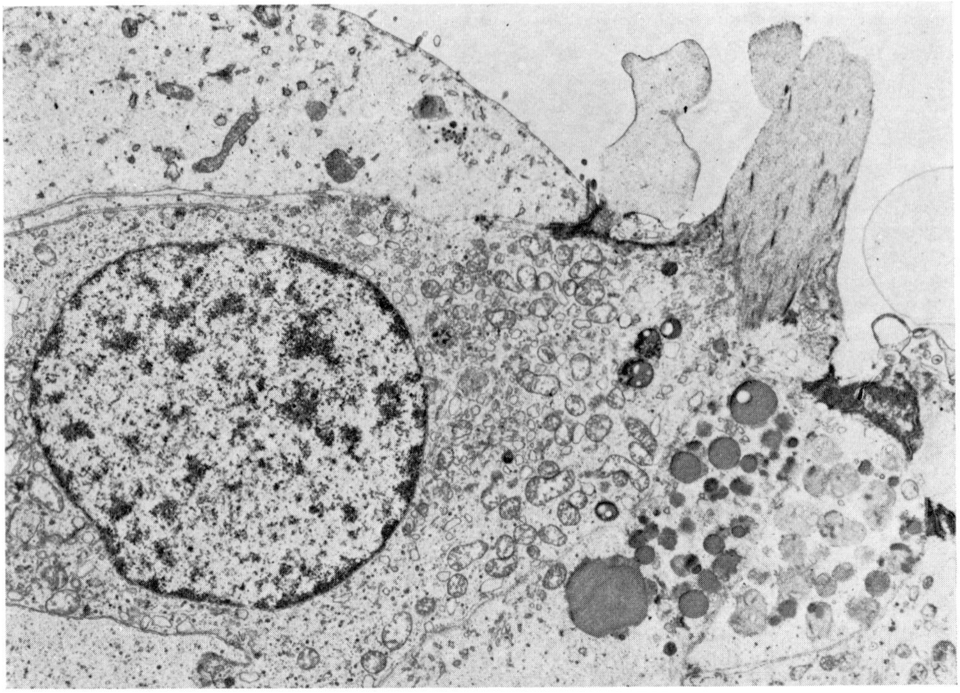

Fig. 5. The IHC demonstrates a giant or fused cilia. The cell body is essentially normal. In the adjacent area the OHC were missing. 8 mm area of the left cochlea.

The nerve fibers of the tunnel spiral bundles and outer spiral bundles appeared to exist in normal populations in the apical region. There were no unusual structural alterations in these fibers. A desmosomal type of thickening of the neurilemma was occasionally found, though some were of the synapse type. Synaptic vesicles were absent or few, possibly as the result of postmortem changes. There were numerous bundles of unmyelinated nerve fibers running in the spiral direction at the tympanic lip of the limbus spiralis. Unlike those of the tunnel and outer spiral bundles of the organ of Corti, these fibers were surrounded by Schwann cell cytoplasm. Some of these fibers contained vesicles with dense cores.

The spiral ganglia were examined in all cochlear turns. Almost all these ganglion cells were the unmyelinated or scantily myelinated type (Fig. 6). The heavily or compactly myelinated type, which is common in animal ears, was rarely seen. Some ganglion cells were atrophic, showing dense cytoplasm at the basal turns. Many unmyelinated fibers were found among the spiral ganglion cells.

The pillar cells, Hensen's cells, Claudius' cells, spiral prominence cells and outer sulcus cells appeared normal. Their cell apices usually contained lipofuscin granules, a common occurrence at this age. In the apical region, the Deiters' cells were large and filled in the spaces between the OHC.

Atrophy of the margins of the stria vascularis was common in the basal turn. Adjacent to the areas of atrophy, the stria vascularis appeared hypertrophied. In these areas, the marginal cells were compactly arranged, and their nuclei appeared to exist in clusters. The marginal cells contained many dense oval granules. A large mass containing aggregates of ribosomes surrounded by a capsule or by a cytoplasmic cup was found in the wide fluid space within a marginal cell. Areas of mild atrophy showed marginal cells with decreased cytoplasmic infoldings.

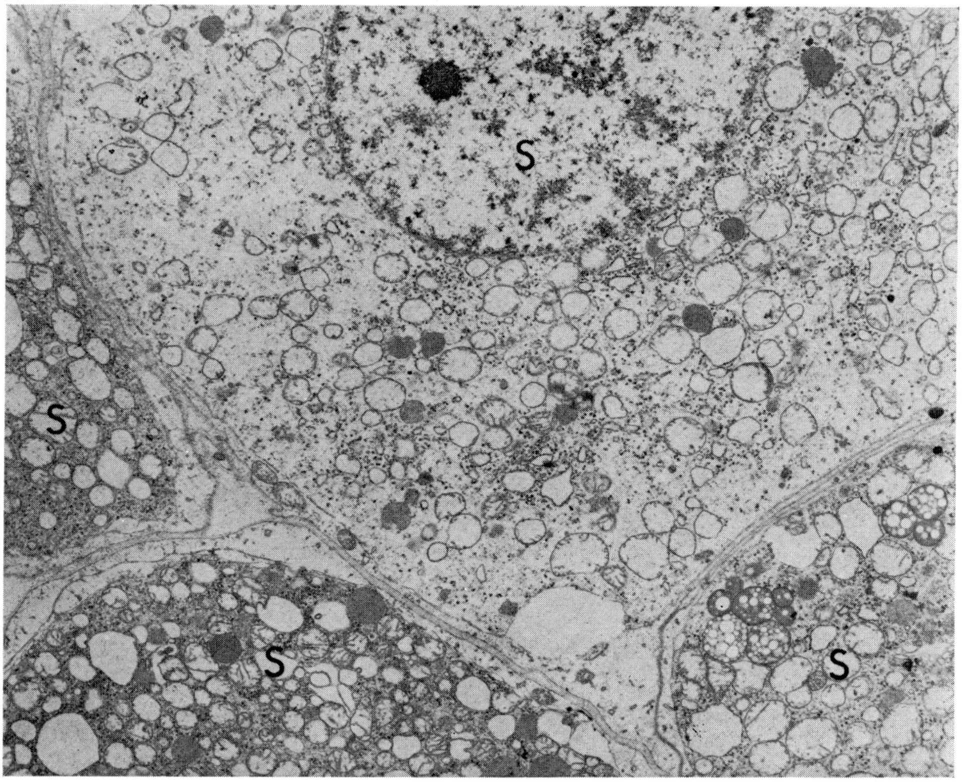

Fig. 6. Spiral ganglion cells (S) of the unmyelinated type which are in the majority. Heavily myelinated neurons are few in number and are not shown in this photograph.

Their pinocytotic activities were decreased, and mitochondria and ribosomes were decreased in number. A large portion of the cytoplasm was occupied by masses of filaments. The number of intermediate cells was decreased. In the severely atrophic areas, the marginal cells were very flat and were abutted by the basal cells. The basal lamina was thickened in some of the strial vessels. However, in general, the strial vessels were no different from those of other non-Ménière's disease specimens.

The distended Reissner's membrane was flat, and the mesothelial cells often showed wide gaps between their cells or were missing entirely (Fig. 7A). The epithelial cells often had dense cytoplasm presumed to be an atrophic change. At the apex of the cochlea, Reissner's membrane had herniated through the helicotrema and extended into the scala tympani. Thus, the surface of the basilar membrane facing the scala tympani was lined by the endolymphatic epithelium and mesothelial cells of Reissner's membrane.

Right Ear. At the basal end of the cochlea, the OHC showed severe atrophic changes; however, the remainder of the cochlea showed only small scattered changes. In some outer hair cells, stereocilia were missing. Just as in the left cochlea, diffuse bodies interspersed with dense substances were found occasionally in the outer hair cells (Fig. 4B). It was also obvious that some hair cells were not attached to the reticular lamina, although a cell count was not made. The subsurface cisternae were decreased in number. The cytoplasm became more electron dense and the entire cell body tilted toward the basilar membrane. Usually two to four nerve endings were found at

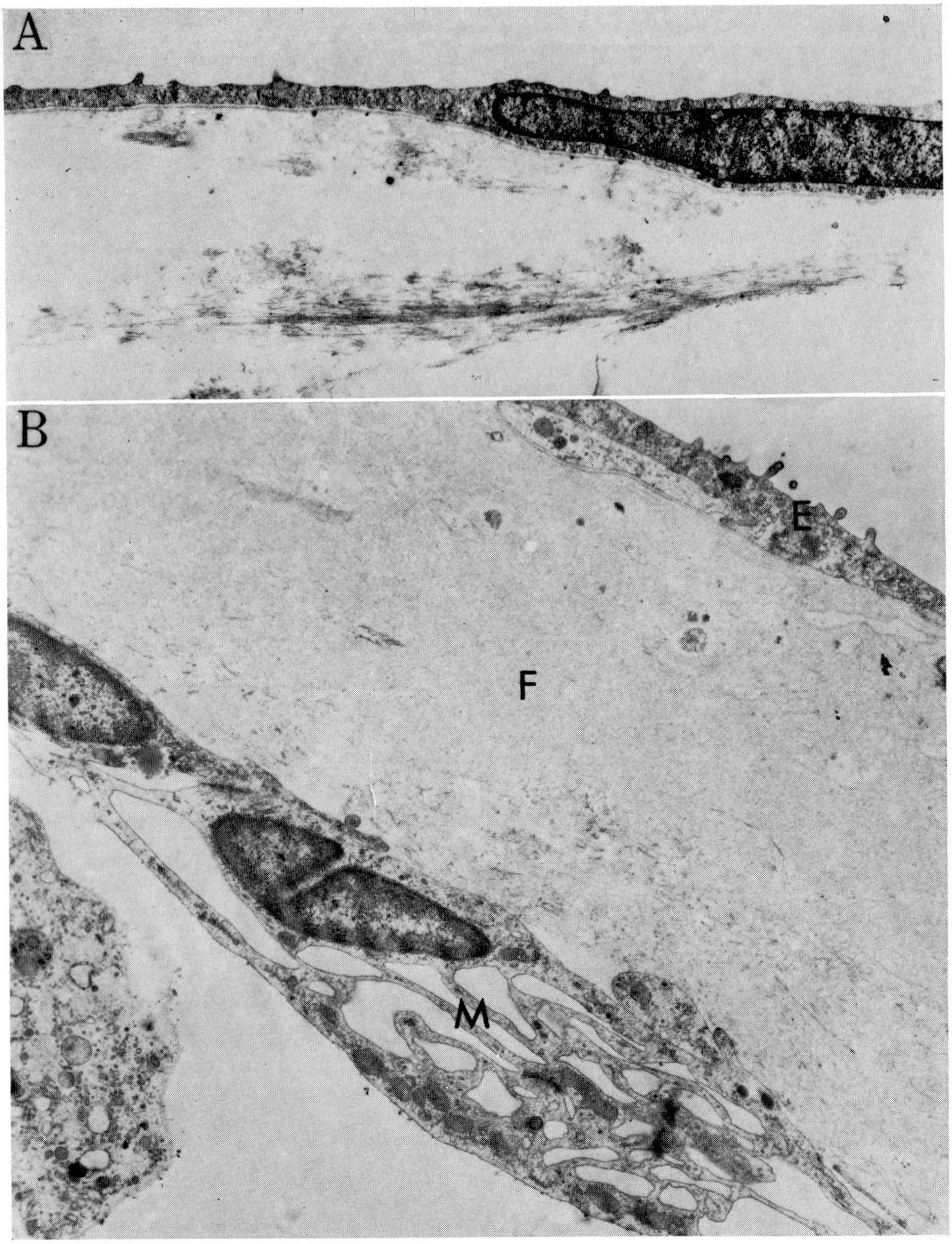

Fig. 7. A) Distended Reissner's membrane showing a single layer of endolymphatic epithelial cells. The mesothelial cells are totally missing. B) Thick Reissner's membrane with a wide filamentous (F) or homogeneous zone between the epithelial layer (E) and mesothelial layer (M). The mesothelial cells show unusual plasma membrane infoldings. Taken from the basal end of the right cochlea where the distention was minimal.

the base of each OHC, although as many as six were seen (11 and 23 mm areas). In some areas the nerve endings were detached from the outer hair cells. Occasionally nerve fibers of the outer spiral bundle touched the basal sides of the OHC. The populations of nerve fibers of the outer spiral bundles and tunnel spiral bundles were normal.

Structural alterations within the IHC were too minimal to be significant. The stereocilia of some cells were enlarged. The nerve endings were swollen in a vacuolar honeycomb arrangement, and no decrease in their number was observed. A count of nerve fibers at the tympanic lip (20 mm area) revealed that about 10% of the fibers crossed the tunnel toward the OHC. The nerve fiber count at the tympanic lip appeared similar to that of normal ears; however, the tunnel fiber population was at the lower limit of normal.[3] Thus, a majority of nerve fibers (90%) appeared to terminate below or at the IHC areas. The synaptic bodies so common in animal inner hair cells were rarely evident.

The nerve fibers of the tympanic spiral bundle at the limbus were numerous, as in the left cochlea. The spiral ganglia of the basal and apical turns showed a majority of unmyelinated or partly myelinated neurons with the heavily myelinated neurons appearing infrequently.

Some Deiters' cells contained numerous granules of varying size with dense cores near the basilar membrane. The dense cores were surrounded by clear zones which were delimited by a membrane. The other supporting cells showed cytological characteristics similar to the left ear. No obvious abnormalities could be detected in the basilar or tectorial membranes. Structural changes in the stria vascularis were similar to those described in the left ear.

In the less distended area Reissner's membrane was thickened by a wide filamentous and homogeneous layer which was located between the endolymphatic epithelial and mesothelial cells (Fig. 7B). Another finding was deep penetrations of the basal surface of the epithelial cells toward the mesothelial layer. Here, a microorganism was found lying on the mesothelial cell surface. As Reissner's membrane was followed apicalward, distention increased, and the thickness of the membrane decreased. There was a reduction in filamentous materials, and both cell types became flat and wide gaps began to appear between the mesothelial cells.

DISCUSSION

Our study of the organ of Corti focused especially on three areas: the stereocilia, the hair cell bodies, and the nerve endings. Although we found that stereocilia were missing, or had fused together, or were projecting as giant cilia above the cuticular plates, the extent of these alterations appears to be too minimal to account for the severe hearing loss. Similar changes can be seen in human cochleas without hearing loss.[4]

The OHC in the apical region showed a nearly normal population, yet many of these cells were not connected to the reticular lamina. It seems improbable that this change was caused by postmortem degeneration, because our controlled studies in animals have shown that in postmortem autolysis the hair cell cytoplasm is blanched out, the cell is detached from Deiters' cup, becomes round, and is displaced closer to the reticular lamina. We have frequently observed in other human ears showing postmortem autolysis that the OHC become detached from the Deiters' cups. In the present Ménière's specimens, the OHC appeared to sink deeper into the Deiters' cells. Another factor which supports the hypothesis that the detachment of these cells was not due to postmortem changes are that these cells appear morphologically similar to adjacent normal hair cells. Also near the nucleus or basal to it, they often contain diffuse bodies which resemble the cuticular plate. Such bodies were not observed in the postmortem study on animal ears. In our experimental hydrops study, we noted the cuticular substance with hair rootlets was often found sagging toward the nucleus in abnormal hair cells.[5] In an experiment on acoustic trauma, Lim and Melnick[6] reported extention of a similar substance deep into the cytoplasm of the hair cell. The significance of the diffuse cuticular body is not clear, though it implies an abnormality affecting cell function.

It seems probable that this subtle change, retraction of the OHC from the cuticular plate, would not be detected by light microscopy. Although we admit a high level of enthusiasm for the concept, we are not certain that this change is sufficient to cause the severe hearing loss.

The third major area of possible dysfunction in these cochleas is the nerve endings. Synaptic bodies and vesicles are rarely observed, but this may have been caused by postmortem change. The functional significance of synaptic bodies is not yet clear, for some studies have shown them to be absent in the OHC of the cat.[7,8] In postmortem specimens such as these, no definite statement can be made about the synaptic gap since the hair cells tend to be detached from Deiters' cups. As far as the population of nerve endings is concerned, it appears to be normal in the upper cochlear turns when compared with normal ears. In general, the number of nerve endings below the OHC is surprisingly small in comparison to that of small animals. Also, it is difficult to identify efferent nerve endings, though there are numerous tunnel spiral bundles which are considered to consist mainly of efferent fibers. These observations hold for both Ménière's and non-Ménière's specimens.

The IHC areas were difficult to evaluate because of the extensive swelling of nerve endings. Again, synaptic bodies in the hair cells, which are so common in experimental animals, are rarely shown. However, nerve endings appear in great number. With the population of the IHC so good in the apical region, it is not clear why the hearing for low tones is so poor. According to Spoendlin,[9] in the cat almost 95% of the afferent fibers go to the IHC. Anatomical and pathological observations on the IHC do not correlate with the hearing loss.

The presence of numerous unmyelinated or partly myelinated spiral ganglia is surprising. In small animals the compactly myelinated type is in the majority.[9,10] Our own observations on the spiral ganglia of the bat, guinea pig, squirrel monkey and Rhesus monkey indicate that the compactly myelinated type is numerous. Our postmortem studies on the squirrel monkey showed that the myelin sheath of the spiral ganglia remains nearly intact at three hours postmortem, though some unraveling was noted. We examined ten human specimens (not Ménière's disease) ranging from 9 months to 92 years of age with an even age distribution and found that about 92% of a total 540 spiral ganglion cells examined were of the unmyelinated or partly myelinated type. There tended to be more unmyelinated neurons (99%) under age 40, but a variation was noted above this age; for example, the lowest tally was 72% at age 75. In the Ménière's specimens 97% of a total 181 spiral ganglion cells were unmyelinated or partly myelinated. It seems that these numerous unmyelinated neurons were not the result of postmortem change, nor is the high incidence of unmyelinated neurons specific to Ménière's disease.

Fine morphological alterations of the stria vascularis of Ménière's disease was reported earlier by us.[11] At that time we concluded that the atrophic changes could not be differentiated from those caused by aging. The findings in these two ears is again consistent with that opinion.

It is not clear why Reissner's membrane is so thick in the less distended area (basal turn). We have sometimes observed a thick membrane in the basal turns of other human ears.

In the distended area, Reissner's membrane showed wide gaps between mesothelial cells, thus leaving a thinly stretched epithelial layer. The same conditions were noted in experimentally induced hydrops in animals.[5] Tonndorf[12] suggested that such distention would interfere with the motion mechanics of the cochlear partition. The extent to which this distention affects hearing is not clearly established.

Morphological changes found in the

sensory cells, stria vascularis, and Reissner's membrane in the cochleas of the present case may be considered either too subtle or too similar to the changes of postmortem autolysis or aging to be conclusively ascribed as the cause of hearing loss. Other possible explanations are changes in the chemical composition of endolymph or perilymph. Schuknecht[13] proposed potassium intoxication associated with ruptures of the endolymphatic system as a possible cause for the acute cochlear and vestibular symptoms.

REFERENCES

1. Lindsay JR: Histopathology of Ménière's disease as observed by light microscopy. Otolaryngol Clin North Am 1:319-329, 1968

2. Schuknecht HF: Ménière's disease: A correlation of symptomatology and pathology. Laryngoscope 73:651-665, 1963

3. Kimura RS: The ultrastructure of the organ of Corti. Int Rev Cytol 42:173-222, 1975

4. Kimura RS, Schuknecht HF, Sando I: Fine morphology of the sensory cells in the organ of Corti of man. Acta Otolaryngol (Stockh) 58:390-408, 1964

5. Kimura RS: Experimental production of endolymphatic hydrops. Otolaryngol Clin North Am 1:457-471, 1968

6. Lim DJ, Melnick W: Acoustic damage of the cochlea. A scanning and transmission electron microscopic observation. Arch Otolaryngol 94:294-305, 1971

7. Spoendlin H: *The Organization of the Cochlear Receptor.* New York, Karger, 1966

8. Dunn RA, Morest DK: Receptor synapses without synaptic ribbons in the cochlea of the cat. In press

9. Spoendlin H: Degeneration behavior of the cochlear nerve. Arch Klin Exp Ohren Nasen Kehlkopfheilkd 200:275-291, 1971

10. Kellerhals B, Engström H, Ades HW: Die Morphologie des Ganglion spirale cochleae. Acta Otolaryngol (Stockh) 226:1-78, 1967

11. Kimura RS, Schuknecht HF: The ultrastructure of the human stria vascularis. Part II. Acta Otolaryngol (Stockh) 70:301-318, 1970

12. Tonndorf J: Pathophysiology of the hearing loss in Ménière's disease. Otolaryngol Clin North Am 1:375-388, 1968

13. Schuknecht HF: Pathophysiology of Ménière's disease. Otolaryngol Clin North Am 8:507-514, 1975

REPRINTS—Robert S. Kimura, Department of Otolaryngology, Massachusetts Eye and Ear Infirmary, 243 Charles St., Boston, MA 02114.

OTOLARYNGIC PATHOLOGY TRAINING PROGRAM

A training program on otolaryngic pathology, presented by the Armed Forces Institute of Pathology (AFIP) in conjunction with the Committee on Otolaryngic Pathology, AAOO, is currently being offered at the Department of Otolaryngic Pathology, AFIP. The course covers both temporal bone pathology as well as surgical pathology of the head and neck area.

Requirements are flexible but preference is given to residents and practitioners in Otolaryngology and Pathology, both military and civilian, who wish to expand their knowledge of ENT pathology. The course, for which there is no charge, is designed to be given quarterly, beginning in January, April, July and October; however, consideration will be given to those seeking shorter training periods.

Requests for course applications should be directed to: The Director, Armed Forces Institute of Pathology, ATTN: AFIP-EDZ, Washington, DC 20306.

Ann Otol 85: 1976

HISTOPATHOLOGIC AND EXPERIMENTAL MODELS FOR SENSORY AND NEURAL DEAFNESS

GERSHON J. SPECTOR, MD

ST. LOUIS, MISSOURI

SUMMARY – Six selected cases with neonatal and fetal cochlear pathology are presented. Those denoting cochlear sepsis are: *H. influenza* purulent labyrinthitis, cytomegalovirus endolabyrinthitis, and aseptic meningitis and labyrinthitis. Those denoting cochlear neural aplasia are Goldenhar's syndrome, left-sided cardiac hypoplasia with partial basal turn neural aplasia, and cerebral cortical and ventricular hemorrhage with modiolar extension. These findings are compared to the fluorocitrate ototoxicity model for neural deafness in the guinea pig. This study suggests hypotheses for viral trophism in the inner ear and neural degeneration of the cochlea as mechanisms for sensorineural deafness.

Heredity and the environment often interact strongly and only in extreme cases is it possible to differentiate the etiologic factors of deafness on a histopathologic basis.[1] Thus, the clinical manifestations and the underlying pathology may be identical in certain widely divergent disorders of hearing.[2]

Classifications based on genetics,[3,4] clinical picture,[5] pathology[6-11] or a combination of factors[2] provide a toxonomy or a nomenclature. However, a real understanding of pathophysiology is still lacking in many areas. For example, cochlear neural degeneration or dystrophy may pathologically be indistinguishable, whether it is due to mumps, measles, toxic neuropathies, dominant or recessive heredity nerve deafness, or a myriad of other disorders which affect neural tissues. Other examples of diseases which can give a similar histopathologic picture are the numerous causes for endolymphatic hydrops or the extensive list of disorders which can produce serous labyrinthitis.[2]

We can infer that the inner ear has a predictable and perhaps a limited response to different pathologic insults. It, therefore, behooves us to understand the underlying pathophysiology.

It is important, therefore, to compare the temporal bone histopathology with experimental studies in animals where conditions are more readily controlled and studied.[12] In addition, it is imperative that we develop new experimental models which simulate the pathologic picture.

The purpose of this report is to evaluate a series of fetal and neonatal temporal bones which demonstrate sensory and neural cochlear pathology. The findings are compared to a biochemical model for cochlear neural degeneration which can selectively damage different nerve populations.

METHODS AND MATERIALS

Temporal Bone Studies. Forty-seven consecutive pairs of temporal bones were obtained from fetuses and neonates who died of various medical disorders over a period of three years. Complete autopsies were performed in all instances. The duration of time from death to fixation ranged from 3 to 17 hours.

The fixative was prepared just prior to use and consisted of 4% glutaraldehyde in sodium phosphate buffer (pH 7.4, 0.1 M). Sucrose was added to raise the osmolarity to 280 milliosmoles.*

From the Department of Otolaryngology, Washington University School of Medicine, St. Louis, Missouri. This work supported by a grant from the Deafness Research Foundation.

* Osmette A digital osmometer, Precision Instrument, Danbury, MA.

Presented at the meeting of the American Otological Society, Inc., Palm Beach, Florida, April 25-26, 1976.

The temporal bones were injected with the fixative by the transtympanic route and then were removed with a Stryker saw. After overnight fixation in 4% glutaraldehyde, the bones were decalcified with RDO,* dehydrated in graded alcohols and embedded in celloidin. The temporal bones were sectioned in the horizontal plane at 10 micra. Every tenth section was mounted and stained with H. and E.

RESULTS

Temporal Bone Studies

Six selected temporal bones illustrate congenital as well as acquired fetal and neonatal inner ear disorders which would result in deafness. These are subdivided into infections, hemorrhagic diathesis, and congenital disorders.

Infections

Cytomegalovirus Endolabyrinthitis.[13] The first case demonstrates a congenital hearing loss which is due to intrauterine cytomegalovirus infection. A premature infant who died at 22 days after birth with hyaline membrane disease was found to have diffuse cytomegalovirus (CMV) inclusion disease at autopsy.

The pathology of both bones showed a similar histopathologic picture of CMV infection. The CMV inclusions were found only in the endolymphatic compartments of the inner ear; including scala media (Fig. 1A), utricle, saccule and semicircular canals. The viral inclusions were most prominent on the stria vascularis (Fig. 1B), the vascular prominence (Fig. 1B), Reissner's membrane (Fig. 1C), and in the planum semilunatum at the bases of the ampullae (Fig. 2). Almost all nonneural and nonsensory epithelial surfaces were involved. The sensory cells of the organ of Corti, maculae of the utricle and saccule, and the three canal ampullae were free of viral inclusions. The neural tissues of the cochlear and the vestibular nerves were also free of viral inclusions. The spiral ligament was normal and there was no strial atrophy. The bony labyrinth was free of infection. The cochlear aqueduct and duct, and the endolymphatic duct and sac had no evidence of viral inclusions. The internal auditory canals were normal.

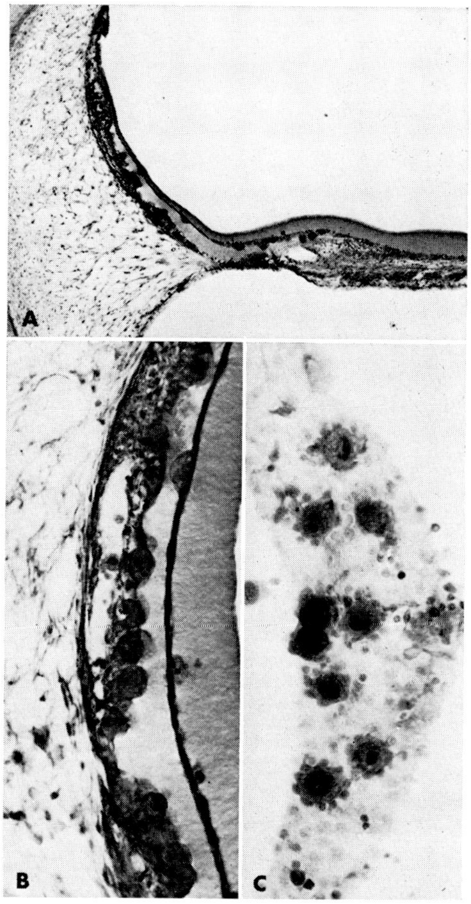

Fig. 1. A) CMV inclusions in cells lining the stria vascularis, vascular prominence and Reissner's membrane. Organ of Corti is collapsed. Eosinophilic material in collapsed cochlear duct and scala tympani (H & E X90). B) CMV infection in the stria vascularis and vascular prominence (H & E X300). C) CMV infection of tangentially cut Reissner's membrane (H & E X300).

There was no evidence of viral infection in the nerves, vessels, bone and immediately adjacent meninges. The infected cells were evenly distributed throughout all cochlear turns. There was an associated serous endolabyrinthitis with mild inflammatory cell exudate. The organ of Corti in many areas was collapsed. The canal of Corti was free of eosinophilic deposits. There was no evidence of teratogeny of maldevelopment.

---

* DuPage Kinetic Laboratories, Inc., Downers Grove, IL.

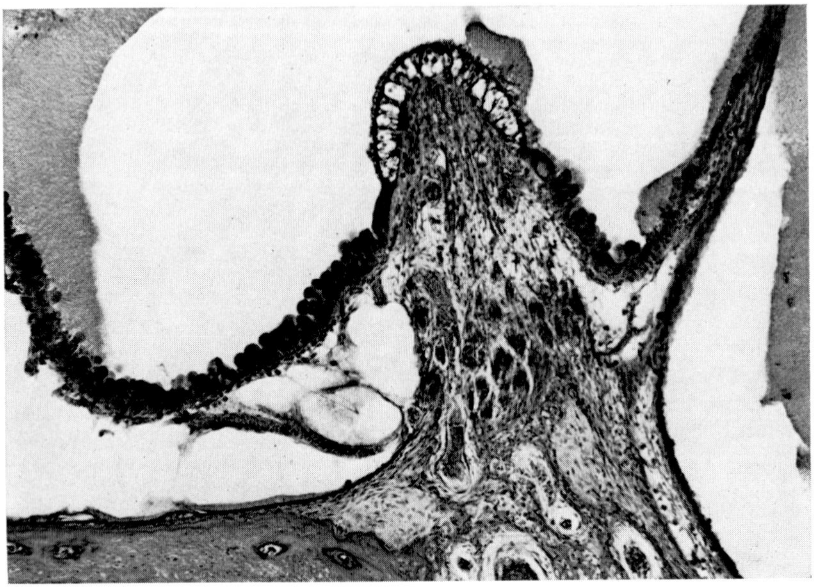

Fig. 2. CMV infects the epithelial cells at the base of the crista ampularis of the semicircular canal. The sensory epithelium and the vestibular nerve are not infected (H & E X175).

Hemophilus Influenza, Otitic Meningitis. A female infant was the 1.2 kg product of an uncomplicated gestation and premature delivery. The child, having respiratory distress, was thought to have mild hyaline membrane disease which required one day of oxygen therapy. On four occasions between November 6, 1973 and November 27, 1973, minimal pulmonary infiltrates were seen on chest x-rays. The question of aspiration pneumonia was raised.

On November 29, 1973 the child became pale and tachypneic and was admitted to the hospital. A lumbar puncture revealed cloudy spinal fluid. Examination of right ear showed acute otitis media. Counter-immunoelectrophoresis of right middle ear and spinal fluid was positive against *H. influenza* antigen. The infant became bradycardic and sustained a cardiorespiratory arrest for which resuscitation was successful. Following treatment with kanamycin, ampicillin, and hydrocortisone, the child continued to have bradycardia with inability to maintain blood pressure despite the use of pressors. A second cardiorespiratory arrest occurred from which she was unable to be resuscitated. Terminally the child began oozing from puncture sites, and postmortem blood exhibited a clotting time of 30 minutes. It is of interest to note that this patient had a sibling who expired from *H. influenza* meningitis 13 months previously.

Autopsy findings confirmed the presence of acute meningitis. *Hemophilus* sp was grown postmortem from the right middle ear and cerebrospinal fluid. The pulmonary findings were of interest in that peripheral alveoli exhibited numerous alveolar macrophages and foreign body giant cells consistent with aspiration pneumonia.

The clinical picture of shock and *H. influenza* sepsis was correlated with the observation of bilateral adrenal hemorrhages. Secondary to the state of sepsis was the clinical picture of disseminated intravascular coagulation which was confirmed histologically by the finding of fibrin thrombi in pulmonary and renal vessels.

The right temporal bones showed a chronic subacute otitis media of at least one week duration. The middle ear was filled with proliferative granula-

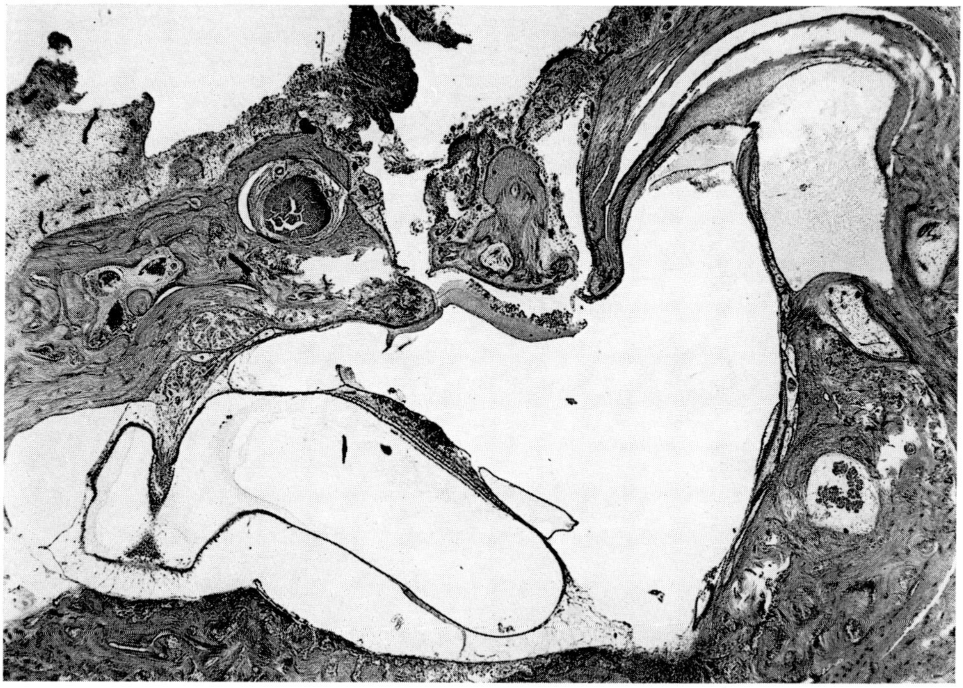

Fig. 3. *H. influenza* otitis meningitis. Note proliferative middle ear granulation with extension around the oval window into the vestibule. The utricle has a mild eosinophilic precipitate. The caecum cochleae has a purulent debris which extends into the cochlear aqueduct (H & E X20).

tion, organized thrombi in microvessels, and new blood vessel formation. Pus surrounded the stapes footplate and invaded the vestibule through the oval window (Fig. 3). Leukocytes were present in all perilymphatic spaces. Leukocytes were noted in the patent cochlear aqueduct, the adjacent meninges, and dura of the posterior cranial fossa. The internal auditory canal was filled with a leukocytic infiltrate. The organ of Corti was degenerated throughout, but the neural tissues were grossly and microscopically normal.

Prenatal Hepatitis, Meningitis, and Labyrinthitis. This full-term baby was a frank breech delivery following premature rupture of the membranes. The baby was heavily meconium-stained and never able to breathe on its own. There was also hypotension, oliguria and hypoglycemia and it died on the fourth day of life. The maternal history, including VDRL testing, was negative. The baby had no evidence of hemolytic anemia.

Autopsy disclosed a full-term baby with marked cyanosis. There was congestion and incomplete expansion of the lungs. In addition, there were focal alveolar hemorrhages in the lungs, pleural petechiae, subcutaneous generalized edema and interstitial fibrosis of the pancreas. Microscopically there was a large amount of meconium aspiration.

The meninges were darkly stained and there were bilateral cerebral ventricle hemorrhages. The brain was severely macerated and demonstrated tertiary convolutions. An unexpected finding in the liver was numerous fibrotic bands and a nonspecific inflammatory infiltrate with a few giant cells. Possible causes of a neonatal hepatitis such as cytomegalovirus and extrahepatic biliary atresia were not evident in the autopsy. There was no history of rubella. The mother was subsequently

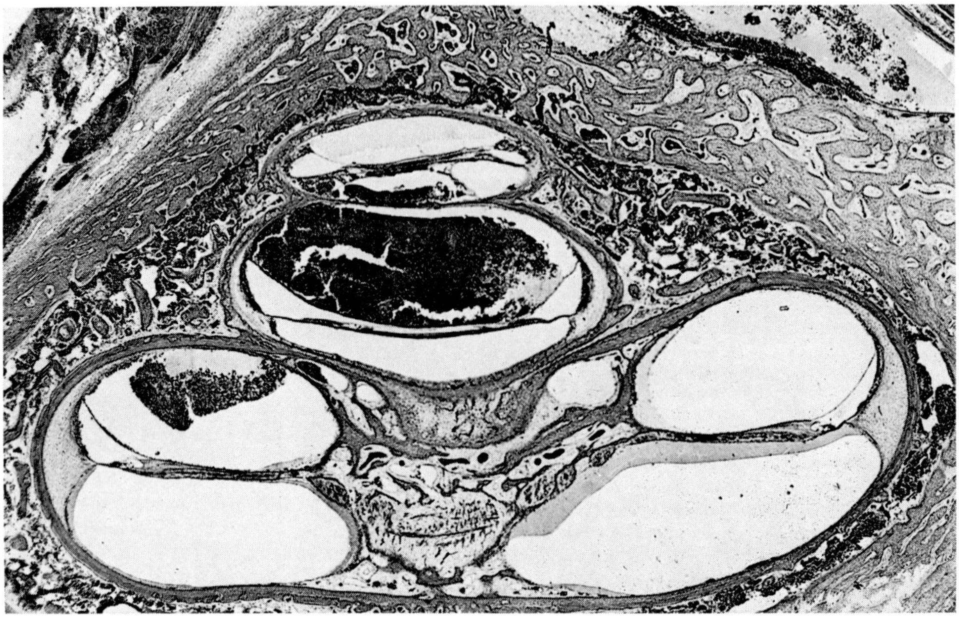

Fig. 4. Purulent labyrinthitis secondary to aseptic meningitis. Note the inflammatory reaction in the scala tympani and vestibuli in the two apical turns (H & E X20).

found to be negative for hepatitis associated antigen. With our inability to assign a specific etiology, this was classified as a case of nonspecific prenatal hepatitis. The amount of liver fibrosis would suggest a process that had been active for more than two weeks.

Both temporal bones demonstrated a similar pathologic picture. The middle ear showed no evidence of sepsis. There was a long-standing organized purulent accumulation in the scala vestibuli and tympani (Fig. 4). There were leukocytes in the modiolus and cochlear aqueduct. The organ of Corti was degenerated but the neural structures appeared grossly normal.

Cerebral Hemorrhage with Extension to the Modiolus

This 7-day-old baby boy was a product of a normal gestation and delivery. Two days later he developed profuse hemorrhagic diarrhea, nausea, and vomiting. A diagnosis of necrotizing enterocolitis with Gram negative septicemia was made. On the following day the ileum of the child had perforated. This area was resected. However, the extensive peritonitis was associated with progressive disseminated intravascular coagulation syndrome. The patient became progressively obtunded and comatose. After the onset of bradycardia and hypotension, repeated cardiorespiratory resuscitations were unsuccessful and he died.

The autopsy demonstrated blood over the cerebellar tonsils which was indicative of intraventricular hemorrhage. On cut sections this hemorrhage was noted to have originated from the periventricular cortex. It extended interventricularly and finally into the subarachnoid space.

Both temporal bones demonstrated massive hemorrhage in the internal auditory canals with extension into the modiolus and Rosenthal's canal (Fig. 5). There was involvement of the spiral ganglia and bleeding into the scala vestibuli and tympani basal cochlear turn. The cochlear aqueduct was free of blood.

Congenital Cochlear Nerve Dysplasia

Goldenhar's Syndrome.[14-19] This 2-day-old female presented with multiple

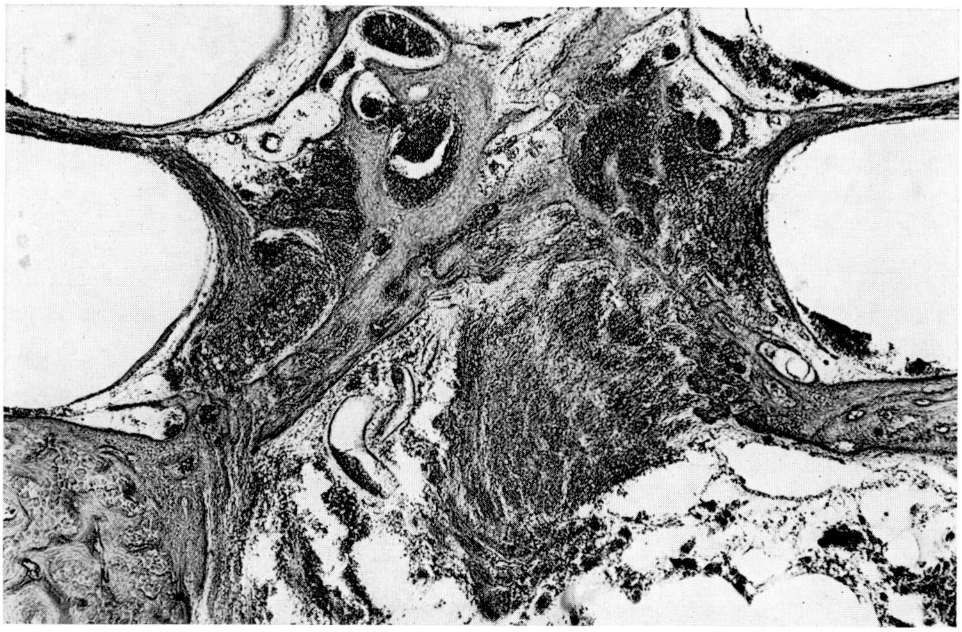

Fig. 5. Subarachnoid hemorrhage with extension into the modiolus. Note extension of blood along the nerves to involve the spiral ganglia (H & E X40).

congenital anomalies which were oculo-auriculo-vertebral dysplasias. She had bilateral epibulbar dermoids, cleft palate, bilateral auricular appendices with a hypoplastic left external ear, blind-ended pretragal fistulas and multiple congenital skeletal anomalies (on x-rays) which included vertebral anomalies. In addition, there was complete transposition of the great vessels with pulmonary atresia, high ventricular septal defect, patent ductus arteriorosus and cardiomegaly with right ventricular hypertrophy. Other findings included accessory spleen and bi-lobed right lung. The second and third toes of both feet were syndactile.

At autopsy the brain was grossly normal except that a thin fibrous band represented the cochlear nerve on the left side and the internal auditory canal was very small. The temporal bone studies demonstrated a normal inner ear on the right. The left temporal bone demonstrated no cochlear nerve or spiral ganglia. The internal auditory canal and the porus acousticus were small. The falciform crest and the vestibulo-facial bar were thick (Fig. 6). Only the efferent nerves of the olivocochlear bundle were present in the internal auditory canal and as interganglionic fibers in the modiolus (Fig. 6). The organ of Corti was missing throughout all turns. The bony and membranous labyrinth otherwise appeared normal.

Hypoplasia of the Left Heart and Spiral Ganglia in the Basal Cochlear Turn. This patient, a product of a normal gestation and delivery, developed progressive congestive heart failure in his third day of life which was fatal 14 hours later. The heart failure was characterized radiographically by diffuse cardiomegaly, electrocardiographically by right ventricular hypertrophy and p-pulmonale, and cardioangiographically by hypoplasia of the left cardiac chambers. Pathologically, this progressive terminal heart failure resulted from a classic example of congenital aortic atresia, *i.e.*, left ventricular outflow complex hypoplasia.[20,21]

At autopsy there was hypoplasia of the left ventricle and atrium with hypertrophy and dilatation of the right ventricle and atrium. There was a widely patent ductus arteriosus and

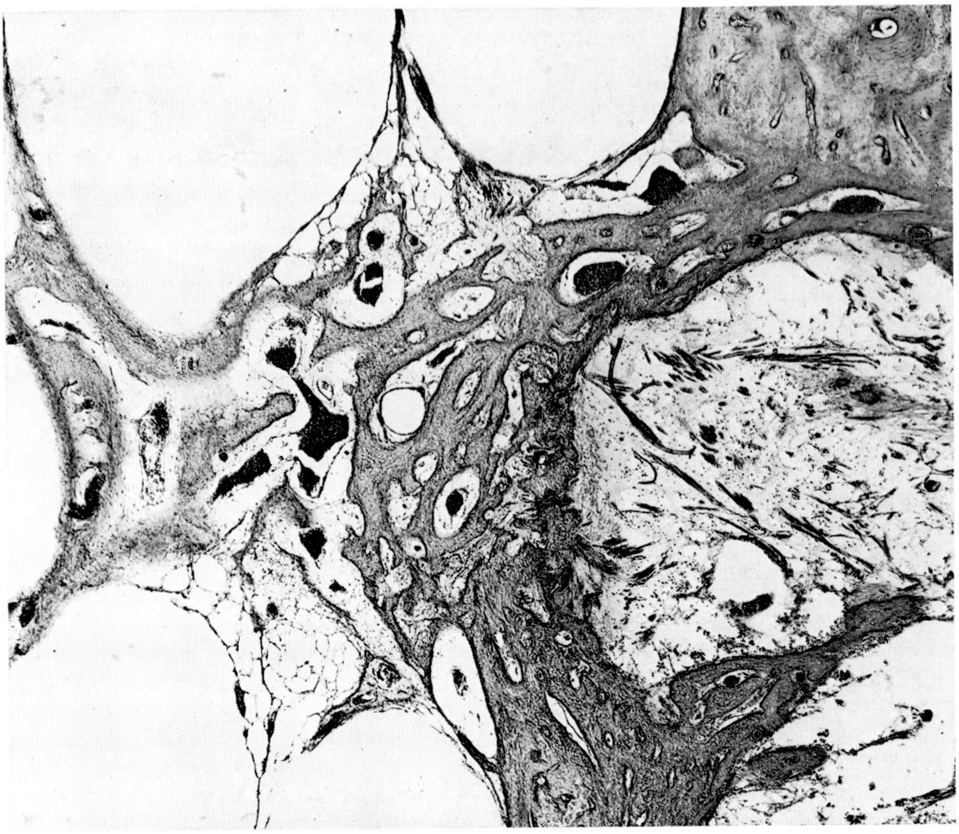

Fig. 6. Goldenhar's syndrome. Note missing afferent nerve in internal auditory canal, as well as missing spiral ganglia. The efferent nerves appear to be present (H & E X40).

foramen ovale. There was passive congestion and hemorrhages of the lung, pleura, liver, colon and abdominal structures, spleen, adrenals, and kidneys. The lungs showed emphysema and focal centroacinar emphysema. In addition, there was a left temporal lobe hemorrhage with extension into the subarachnoid space.

Both temporal bones showed blood in the internal auditory canal and mild serous perilabyrinthitis. There was a marked diminution of sensory cells in the spiral ganglia of both basal cochlear turns and a diminution of afferent nerve fibers (Fig. 7). The organ of Corti was collapsed in the basal cochlear turns.

DISCUSSION

Temporal Bone Studies

Fetal and neonatal sepsis of the inner ear can occur in a variety of ways: extension from the middle ear via the oval window *(H. influenza)*; vascular spread (CMV); retrograde invasion from the central nervous system via the cochlear aqueduct (aseptic meningitis and labyrinthitis), or the modiolus (cochlear hemorrhage). In this respect, since CMV is readily visible and can be used as its own marker, a careful study of CMV endolabyrinthitis may be of interest to further explore the exact pathophysiology of specific cochlear sepsis.

Meyers and Stool[22] and Davis[23] have previously demonstrated CMV endolabyrinthitis in newborn infants. Clinical studies by McCracken *et al*[24] of patients with congenital cytomegalic

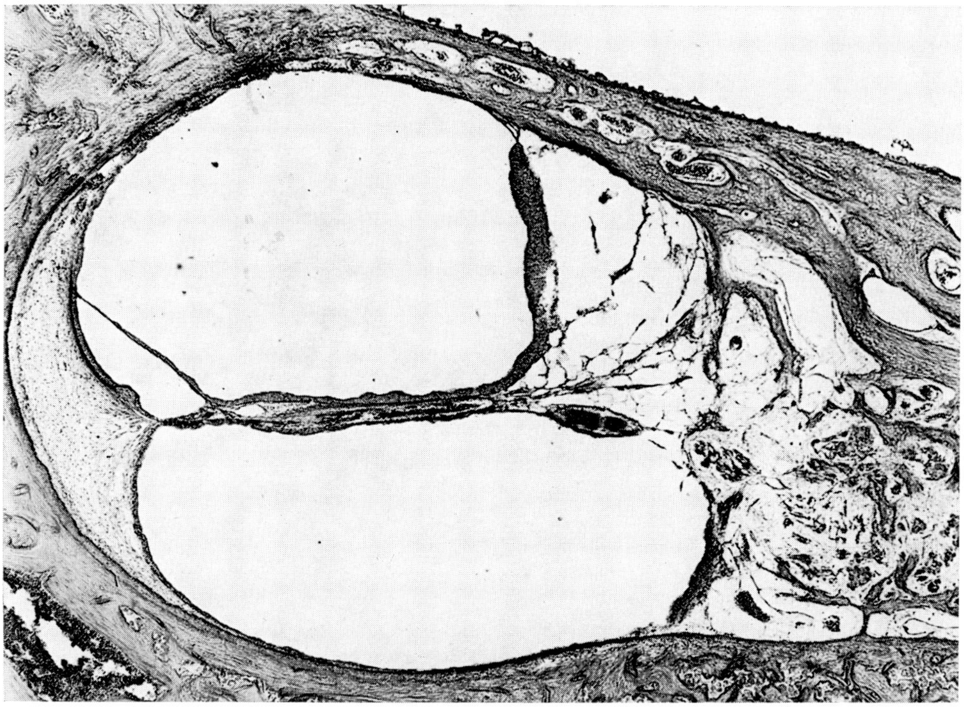

Fig. 7. Partial aplasia of basal cochlear turn spiral ganglia. Note the paucity of cells in spiral ganglion of basal turn (H & E X40).

inclusion disease (CID) and with inapparent (nonclinical) congenital CMV infection[25,26] indicated a higher incidence of hearing losses in this population. The correlation of these studies suggested that CMV could be a significant cause of congenital deafness.

Histologic examination of the temporal bone with CID confirms that CMV causes an endolymphatic labyrinthitis without direct involvement of the nerves, sensory cells or perilymphatic spaces even in the presence of CMV meningoencephalitis. These findings support hematogenous spread (viremia) and secretion (or release) directly into the endolabyrinth via the stria vascularis and vascular prominence.

CMV may infect an infant by the hematogenous route, transplacentally, by direct contact during passage through an infected birth canal, cervical gland infection, or by ingestion of infected mother's milk.[27] A fourth means of infection is secondary to blood transfusion.[28,29]

Davis and Strauss[30] infected the inner ear of mice by direct intracranial inoculation. Secondary extension of the meningoencephalitis through the cochlear aqueduct caused perilymphatic CMV labyrinthitis. This pattern of mouse CMV infection is similar to that seen in varicella-zoster in humans.[31]

Davis *et al*[32] directly inoculated hamster inner ears with hamster adapted strains of influenza, mumps, and measles virus. They showed three different immunohistologic patterns of infection: influenza was essentially perilymphatic; mumps infected the organ of Corti, stria vascularis and Reissner's membrane; and rubella infected the crista of the semicircular canal. Similar retrospective, immunohistologic studies may document the varying patterns of viral trophism in the human ear.

The importance of a patent cochlear aqueduct as a conduit for fetal and neonatal sepsis is well documented.[11,30] The *H. influenza* case demonstrates a fatal meningitis which was secondary to a necrotizing otitis media which had invaded the vestibule via the oval window niche and extended to the meninges via the cochlear aqueduct. However, the case of prenatal aseptic meningitis demonstrates the reverse pattern, with the disease process entering the cochlear aqueduct and destroying the inner ear. These disorders would presumably affect the sensory structures primarily, at least in the initial phase.

On the other hand, in the case of the cerebral hemorrhage with extension into the spiral ganglia, there is damage to neural tissues first, with the sensory structures being spared initially. The clinical implications of such injuries are at present not known. Furthermore, the cochlear nerve congenital aplasia demonstrates another model of neural damage.[33] In the Goldenhar's syndrome, one ear demonstrated total absence of spiral ganglia and afferent nerve fibers. Only the efferent nerves and some interganglionic fibers were present. The organ of Corti was missing throughout. The case of hypoplasia of the left heart outflow tract and partial basal turn cochlear afferent nerve aplasia demonstrates limited neural damage. Nevertheless, the efferent nerve fibers are still present in the basal cochlear turns.

The question arises, Why do nerve tissues degenerate and why are the efferent fibers present in the modiolus when the afferent nerves are missing? It is my contention that the major injury occurs in the perikaryon of the primary sensory neurons. The pathophysiology is that of a biochemical block which prevents the cochlear neuron from utilizing organic fuel molecules efficiently. This leads to a direct or indirect inhibition of oxydative phosphorylation and respiration in the nerve cells. In addition, because of the spatial separation of the cell bodies of the afferent nerves (located in Rosenthal's canals of the modiolus) and the efferent nerves (located near the superior olivary nucleus of the pons) pathologic insults selectively damaged isolated neural populations of cells. The experimental animal model of the fluorocitrate induced cochlear nerve dystrophy substantiates this conclusion.

The evidence for the importance of aerobic metabolic energy for the cochlea[34] and the function of the electron transport system in the cochlear hair cell of the guinea pig have been described.[35] Recently, I have demonstrated the reaction of the cochlear neural tissues to fluorocitrate toxicity.[36] However, on careful evaluation, a differential neural dystrophy in the cochlear nerves was noted, *i.e.*, the afferent nerves were damaged earlier than the efferent nerves.

In a previous report,[12] it was demonstrated that fluorocitrate is a metabolic inhibitor of the aconitase reaction in the Krebs' cycle [E.C. 4.2.1.3][37,38] and succinic dehydrogenase in the cochlear nerves.[39] Both enzymes are located in the mitochondria and the latter one is located on the cristate membrane.[40] On the other hand, fluorocitrate does not inhibit the respiratory chain enzymes *per se*, *i.e.*, $NADH_2$-dehydrogenase and cytochrome oxidase via cytochrome c (cytochrome c, a, and a_3). Since $NADH_2$-D and succinic dehydrogenase are the main sources of input to the electron transport system, the net effect is that of an indirect reduction of respiratory activity, *e.g.*, a decrease in the rate of oxidative phosphorylation ($ADP + P_1 \rightarrow ATP$).

The swelling of perikaryon mitochondria and the early destruction of the mitochondrial inner membrane are the initiating events for subsequent extrusion of cytoplasmic organelles into the axons. There is a diminution of cell bodies of the afferent nerves in the spiral ganglia of the modiolus.[41] The preferential, earlier destruction of the afferent nerves could be due to two reasons. One, the afferent nerves may be more dependent than the efferent nerves, on respiration for generation of energy in order to fulfill their metabolic requirements. However, a second reason appears more plausible. Fluorocitrate acts on nerve cell bodies and not directly on axons.[42] The afferent nerves are affected first because, having their cell bodies in the spiral ganglion, they are in the immediate zone of perfusion. The efferent nerves, their cell bodies near the superior olivary nucleus of the pons, were not in the immediate zone of perfusion; consequently, their axons would be unaffected initially. Presumably, some fluorocitrate would diffuse into the nearby CNS structures after a time and would then act directly on the efferent nerve cell bodies to produce the delayed dystrophic lesions.

Therefore, these cytochemical and morphological models achieve three goals. One, it demonstrates that neural degeneration does occur when biochemical reactions are dissociated and the aerobic metabolism is directly or indirectly damaged. Two, the morphologic picture is indistinguishable from neural and axonal dystrophy which occurs in the spinal cord and the brain.[12,42] Three, it demonstrates that toxic agents can affect selectively, spatially separated neural populations of cells.

At the present time there is no evidence that, metabolically, the cochlear nerves behave any differently from neural tissue in general. Substantial evidence indicates that mitochondria from different organs are indistinguishable with respect to their oxido-reductive properties.[35] Therefore, we must assume the validity of these observations.

In conclusion, these correlations of temporal bone histopathology and experimental animal models put forward two major hypotheses:

1. Despite the route of infection into the inner ear, there is evidence to suggest that viruses have a specific trophism (proclivity to infect specific cells) for structures in the inner ear.

2. Neural degenerations, dysplasias or dystrophies in the cochlear nerve, are due to separation of biochemical processes which interfere with aerobic metabolism of the perikaryon mitochondria. The main injury occurs in the *primary sensory nerve cell body.* A corollary to this hypothesis is that the peculiar spatial orientation of the perikarya allows selective damage to specific populations of nerves.

REFERENCES

1. McConnell E, Ward PH: *Deafness in Childhood.* Vanderbilt University Press, 1962, pp 69-169

2. Proctor CA, Proctor B: Understanding hereditary nerve deafness. Arch Otolaryngol 85:23-40, 1967

3. Martensson B: Dominant hereditary nerve deafness. Acta Otolaryngol (Stockh) 52:270-274, 1960

4. Konigsmark BW: Hereditary deafness in man. N Engl J Med 281:713-720; 774-778; 827-832, 1969

5. Kinney CE: Pathology of hereditary deafness. Ann Otol Rhinol Laryngol 59:1117-1122, 1950

6. Ormerod FC: Pathology of congenital deafness. J Laryngol Otol 74:919-950, 1960

7. Lindsay JR: Profound childhood deafness: Inner ear pathology. Ann Otol Rhinol Laryngol 82:(Suppl 5), 1973

8. Gacek R: The pathology of hereditary sensorineural hearing loss. Ann Otol Rhinol Laryngol 80:289-298, 1971

9. Schuknecht HF: Pathology of sensorineural deafness of genetic origin, in McConnell E, Ward PH (eds): *Deafness in Childhood.* Vanderbilt University Press, 1962, chap 7

10. Schuknecht HF, Igarashi M, Gacek RR: The pathological types of cochleo-saccular degeneration. Acta Otolaryngol 59:154, 1968

11. Schuknecht HF: *Pathology of the Ear.* Cambridge, MA, Harvard University Press, 1974, pp 388-403

12. Spector GJ, Carr CD: Fluorocitrate ototoxicity: a morphologic and cytochemical model for primary neural degeneration in the guinea pig cochlea. Ann Otol Rhinol Laryngol 85:185-198, 1976

13. Davis G, Spector GJ, Strauss M: Cytomegalovirus endolabyrinthitis. Arch Pathol, to be published

14. Gorlin RJ, Jue KL, Localsen U, *et al*: Occuloauriculo vertebral dysplasia. J Pediatr 63:991-999, 1963

15. Aubrey M, Morand: The epibulbar dermoid auricular appendix-preauricular fistula triad or Franchescetti-Goldenhar's syndrome. Ann Otolaryngol Chir Cervicofac 81:69-71, 1964.

16. Goldenhar M: Associations malforma-

tives de l'oeil et l'oreille, en particulier le syndrome dermoide epibulbaire-appendices auriculaires-fistula auris congenita et ses relations aves la depostose mandibulofaciale. J Genet Humaine 1:243-283, 1952

17. Neimann N, Cordier J, Manciaux M, *et al*: Franchescetti's syndrome associated with Goldenhar's syndrome and with vertebral abnormalities. Ann Pediatr (Paris) 7:460, 1960

18. Smithills RW: Oculo-auriculo-vertebral syndrome (Goldenhar's syndrome). Dev Med Child Neural 6:406, 1964

19. Budden SS, Robinson GC: Oculoauricular vertebral dysplasia. Its association with sensorineural deafness and other abnormalities. Am J Dis Child 125:431-433, 1973

20. Anderson WAD: *Pathology*. St. Louis, C. V. Mosby, 1971, pp 725-726

21. Keith JD: *Heart Diseases in Infancy and Childhood.* New York, McMillan Co., 1967, pp 466-474

22. Meyers EN, Stool S: Cytomegalic inclusion diseases of the inner ear. Laryngoscope 78:1904-1915, 1968

23. Davis GL: Cytomegalovirus in the inner ear. Case report and electron microscopic study. Ann Otol Rhinol Laryngol 78:1179-1189, 1969

24. McCracken GH Jr, Shinefield HR, Cobb K, *et al*: Congenital cytomegalic inclusion disease. A longitudinal study of 20 patients. Am J Dis Child 117:522-529, 1969

25. Reynolds DW, Stagno S, Stubbs G, *et al*: Inapparent congenital cytomegalovirus infection with elevated cord IgM levels. Casual relationship with auditory and mental deficiency. N Engl J Med 290:291-296, 1974

26. Dahle AJ, McCollister FP, Hammer BA, *et al*: Subclinical and congenital cytomegalovirus infection and hearing impairment. J Speech Hear Disord 39:320-329, 1974

27. Reynolds DW, Stagno S, Hosty JS, *et al*: Maternal cytomegalovirus excretion and perinatal infection. N Engl J Med 289:1-5, 1973

28. Kane RC, Rousseau WE, Noble GR, *et al*: Cytomegalovirus infection in a volunteer blood donor population. Infect Immun 11: 719-723, 1975

29. Yeager AS: Transfusion-acquired cytomegalovirus infection in newborn infants. Am J Dis Child 128:478-483, 1974

30. Davis GL, Strauss M: Viral disease of a labyrinth. II. Ann Otol Rhinol Laryngol 82: 584-593, 1973

31. Friedmann I: Cochlear pathology in viral disease. Adv Otorhinolaryngol 20:155-177, 1973

32. Davis LE, Shurin S, Johnson RT: Experimental viral labyrinthitis. Nature 254:339-340, 1975

33. Ward PH, Kinney CE, Lindsay JR: Inner ear pathology in congenital deafness. Laryngoscope 72:435-455, 1962

34. Spector GJ, Lucente FE: Aerobic metabolism of the inner ear. Results of a critical evaluation. Laryngoscope 84:1663-1672, 1974

35. Spector GJ: The ultrastructural cytochemistry of lactic dehydrogenase, succinic dehydrogenase, dihydronicotinamide adenine dinucleotide diaphorase and cytochrome oxidase activities in hair cell mitochondria of the guinea pig cochlea. J Histochem Cytochem 23:216-234, 1975

36. Spector GJ, Carr CD, Arenberg IK, *et al*: Fluorocitrate neural dystrophy of the guinea pig cochlea. Proceedings 33rd Annual Proc Electron Microscopy Soc Amer, Las Vegas, Nevada, 1975. G. W. Bailey (ed)

37. Peters RA: Mechanism of the toxicity of the active constituent of Dichapetalum cymosum and related compounds. Adv Enzymol 18:113-159, 1957

38. Carrell HL, Glusker JP, Villafranca JJ, *et al*: Fluorocitrate inhibition of aconitase: Relative configuration of inhibiting isomer by x-ray crystallography. Science 170:1412-1414, 1970

39. Spector GJ, Carr CD, Arenberg IK: Fluorocitrate induced neural dystrophy in the guinea pig cochlea: An ultrastructural and cytochemical study. J Cell Biol 67:413a, 1975

40. Spector GJ, Carr CD: The electron transport system in the cochlear hair cell: The ultrastructural cytochemistry of respiratory enzymes in hair cell mitochondria of the guinea pig. Laryngoscope 84:1673-1706, 1974

41. Spector GJ: Fluorocitrate neurotoxicity of guinea pig cochlea: An ultrastructural cytochemical model of neural deafness. J Histochem Cytochem, to be published

42. Koenig H: Acute axonal dystrophy caused by fluorocitrate: The role of mitochondrial swelling. Science 164:310-312, 1969

REPRINTS—Gershon J. Spector, MD, Department of Otolaryngology, Washington University School of Medicine, 517 S. Euclid Ave., St. Louis, MO 63110.

Ann Otol 85: 1976

THE COMBINED CORRELATED AUDIOHISTOGRAM

INCORPORATION OF THE SUPERIOR VENTRAL COCHLEAR NUCLEUS

WILLIAM B. DUBLIN, MD

MARTINEZ, CALIFORNIA

SUMMARY – The state of the spheroid cells of the superior ventral cochlear nucleus (SVCN) must be accounted for along with that of stria vascularis, hair cells, and spiral ganglion neurons in the development of the combined correlated audiohistogram in cases of sensorineural hearing loss. For the stated evaluation, transverse sections through SVCN are marked off into ventrodorsally progressive zones corresponding to the frequency levels of the audiometric chart, and the loss of spheroid cells in each level is estimated on a percentage basis. The resultant "best fit" of pattern of cell injury with audiometric curve suggests that the anatomic frequency scale of SVCN parallels the logarithmic frequency scale of the standard audiometric chart.

In an earlier publication,[1] the cellular architecture of the cochlear nucleus (CN) was described. Of six nerve cell types found in CN, spheroid (large spherical) cells appeared to constitute the main second-order neurons of the principal afferent pathway. Their injury was considered to be the pathologic basis of sensorineural hearing impairment of central type. The state of the spheroid cells observed in the superior ventral cochlear nucleus (SVCN) was compared with the expected audiometric curve, positioned in keeping with the low-frequency-ventral to high-frequency-dorsal tonotopic gradient of SVCN, and the result was termed the cochlear nucleogram.[1]

In the past, the state of stria vascularis, hair cells, and spiral ganglion neurons has been employed in the production of the cochleogram, and has been charted parallel with the audiometric curve.[2] This plan of procedure can now be extended by the addition of the aforementioned cochlear nuclear information, with the production of a combined correlated audiohistogram (for brevity, audiohistogram). Such a plan of procedure serves as part of the whole-auditory-pathway study of cases of sensorineural deafness. The histopathologic data obtained offers the best means of properly determining the anatomic frequency gradient, and any other similarly accessible functional characteristics, of the ventral cochlear nucleus (VCN) in the human. Conclusions reached to date are but tentative, and broad in scope; it is hoped, however, that a basis has been established from which further investigative efforts can proceed.

In the study appropriate to this presentation of VCN, standard histologic technique is employed, including fixation of brains in formaldehyde solution, embedding in paraffin, and staining with the usual methods, such as H.&E., cresyl violet, protargol, and/or luxol fast blue. A tissue block transverse to the brain stem that includes the auditory nerves with a 2 to 3 mm margin on each side, is needed. The block is sectioned at step levels. While passing through the auditory nerve(s), a series of sections (for the different stains) is made at intervals of roughly 100μ. This provides some six to eight sections of SVCN, including one at the point of greatest dorsoventral expansion of the nucleus (Fig. 1). The anatomic relations of CN subdivisions were shown previously.[1]

SVCN as seen in greatest dimension

From the Laboratory of Auditory Pathology, Veterans Administration Hospital, Martinez, California.

Presented at the meeting of the American Otological Society, Inc., Palm Beach, Florida, April 25-26, 1976.

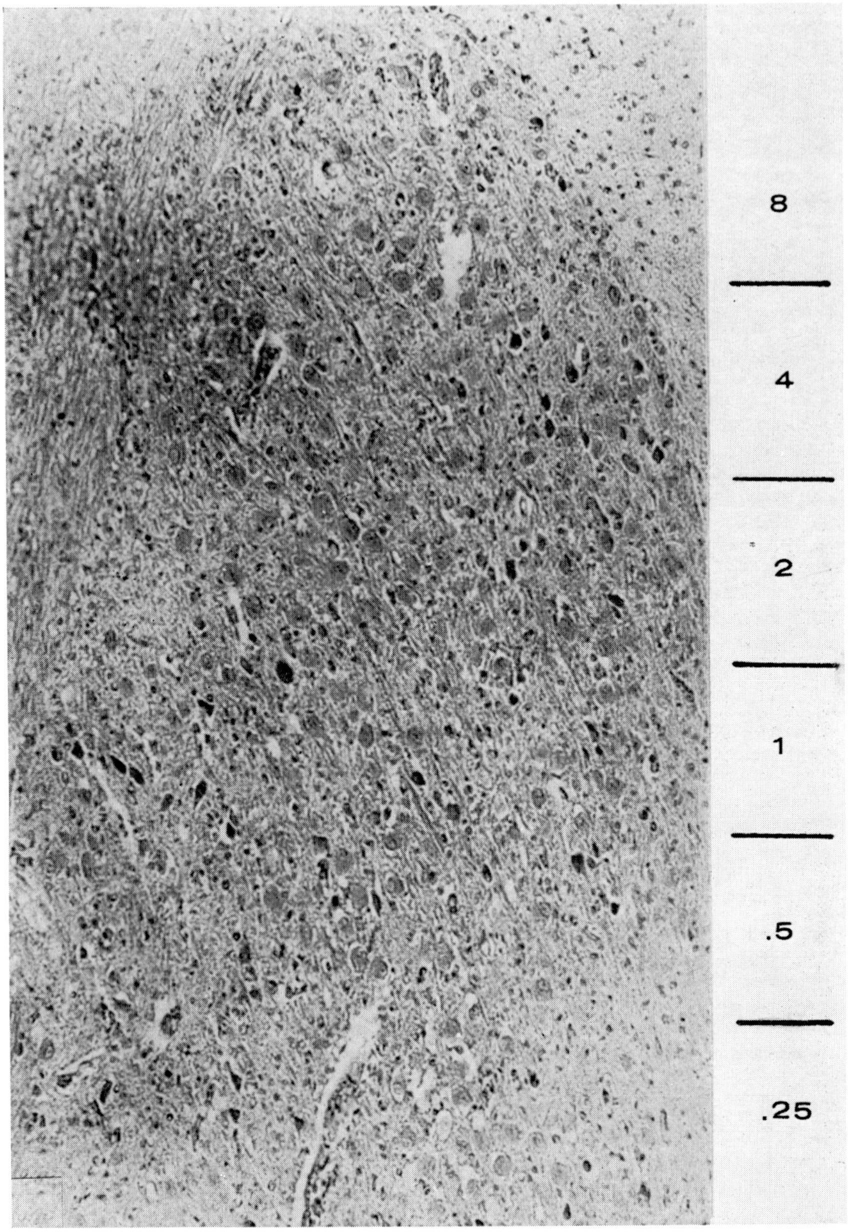

Fig. 1. Transverse section through greatest dimension of normal SVCN; frequency levels are indicated in kHz.

section is marked off in ventrodorsally progressive zones of frequency, using a microphotograph, or by simply marking the coverslip with ink, and based on the frequency intervals of a standard audiometric chart (Fig. 1). In so doing, one must begin with an assumption regarding the anatomic frequency scale, to be tested by ensuing "best fit" of audiometric curve with pattern of spheroid cell injury. The zone for 250 Hz is positioned fairly near the ventral margin of SVCN, allowing some space (approximately 10% of the nucleus) for still

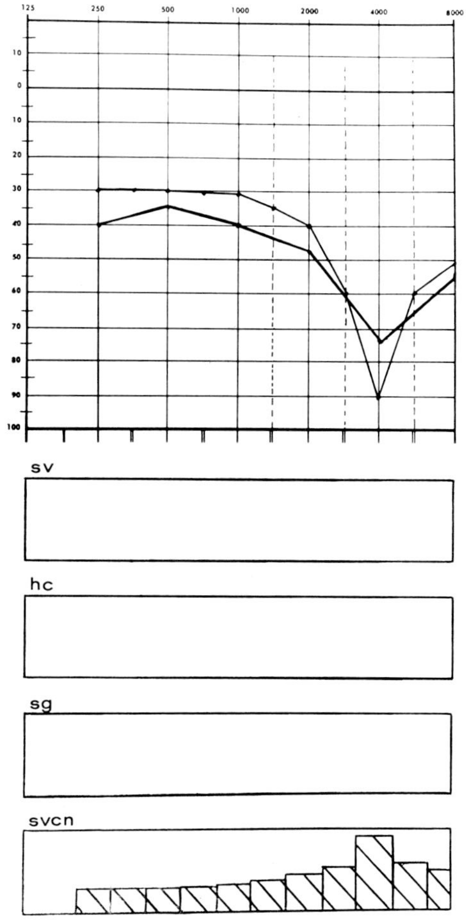

Fig. 2. Same case as in Figure 4. Audiohistogram. An audiogram was not available. The lighter line results from using the ordinate values as percent of spheroid cell loss. The heavier line is an audiogram found characteristically in postanoxic deafness.[3-6] sv - Stria vascularis. hc - Hair cells. sg - Spiral ganglion nerve cells. svcn - Spheroid cells of SVCN. Estimated percentage of injury in the different frequency zones is represented by height of crosshatched columns.

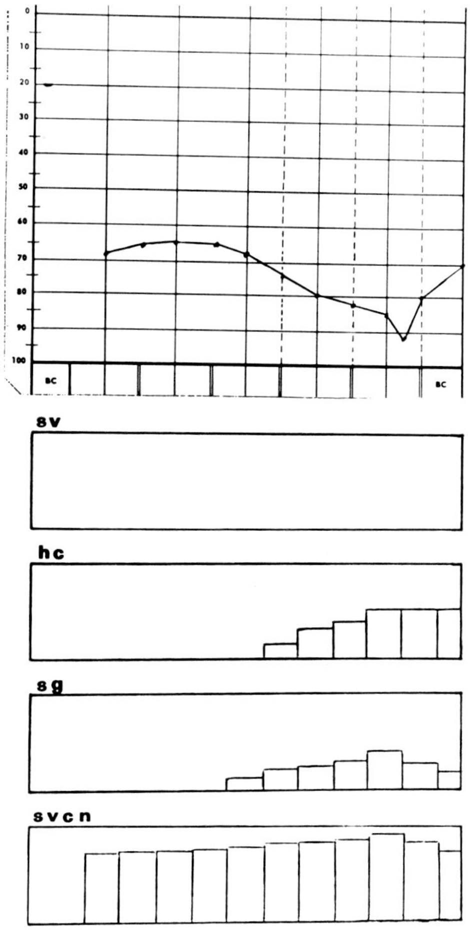

Fig. 3. Same case as in Figure 5. Audiohistogram. Audiometric curve is that for bone conduction (BC). The symbols have the same meaning as in Figure 2. In the present case, spheroid cell loss in SVCN is relatively marked; in various cases, it may range from little or no alteration to virtually complete destruction. In the audiohistogram, the graph for spheroid cell loss in SVCN, the frequency zones being delineated according to the logarithmic scale of the audiometric chart, parallels the audiometric curve as well as the graph for loss of spiral ganglion nerve cells.

lower frequencies; 8,000 Hz being placed, correspondingly, fairly near the dorsal margin (leaving approximately 15% of the nucleus dorsally). The portion of the nucleus between the two points is divided evenly according to the frequency intervals provided in the audiometric chart. The degree of spheroid cell injury is estimated on a percent basis for each frequency zone, somewhat as the percent of injury of spiral ganglion nerve cells has been estimated for various positions along the cochlea. The estimated injury of spheroid cells observed in sections other than that at the greatest dimension of SVCN is prorated as to weight accord-

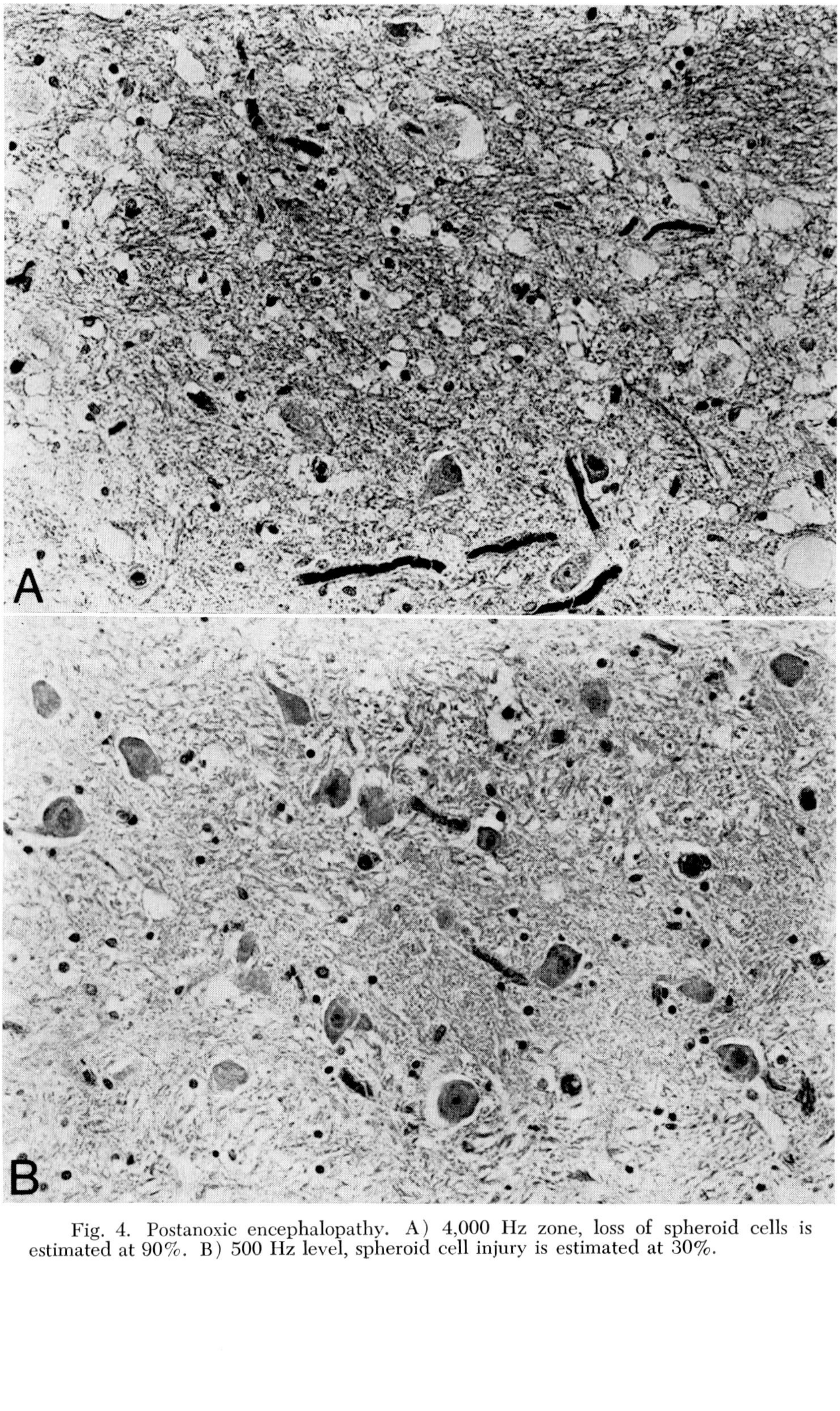

Fig. 4. Postanoxic encephalopathy. A) 4,000 Hz zone, loss of spheroid cells is estimated at 90%. B) 500 Hz level, spheroid cell injury is estimated at 30%.

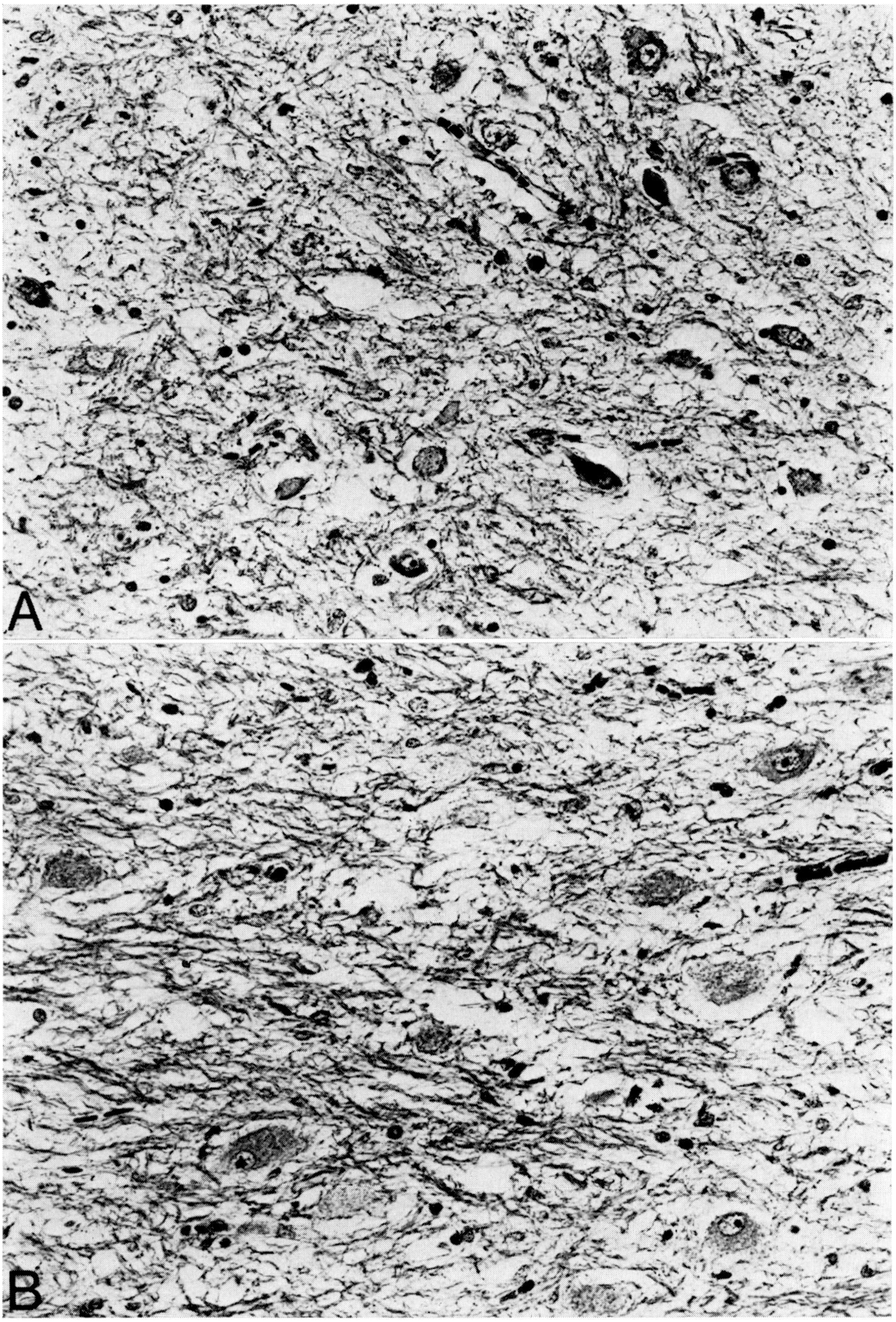

Fig. 5. Presbycusis. Microphotographs of SVCN. A) 4,000 Hz level, loss of spheroid cells is estimated at 90 - 95%. B) 500 Hz level, loss of spheroid cells is estimated at 65%.

ing to estimate of original population before injury, considering the curved outline of the nucleus. The percent values (which are not absolute, but only relative) of cell injury thus obtained for the different frequency levels are recorded by height of columns in the construction of an audiohistogram (Figs. 2, 3). To date, the pattern of injury has extended essentially at a comparable level craniocaudally through SVCN, so that the largest dimension section has served, for practical purposes, in the formulation of the graph, without employment of the other transverse (craniocaudally progressive) section levels. Indeed, especially in view of the approximate nature of the values involved, if the individual worker is among those who do not habitually construct a cochleogram, but prefer simply to position estimates(s) of injury of cochlear elements in general terms, as in (a) certain portion(s) of one or other of the cochlear turns, it will be found that the distribution and severity of spheroid cell injury in SVCN can, comparably, be estimated by simple inspection. Considerable flexibility is possible in plan of reporting the finding of importance relative to the present discussion — the condition of the spheroid cell population of SVCN.

The orientation of the sections frequency-wise is facilitated by perforating the tissue block with a needle fairly close to CN; this is enhanced by the deposit of India ink along the track as the needle is withdrawn. The marking of frequency zones is maintained at a constant scale space-wise through the sections.

By means of the described procedure, the "best fit" of pattern of spheroid cell injury with that of the cochlear elements and with the audiometric curve is determined, and appropriate conclusion, such as may be possible, is made regarding the anatomic frequency scale of SVCN in the human.

Owing to variation encountered in normal distribution and population density of spheroid cells, the employment of estimates remains practical for individual cases. If a statistically significant number of cases of a given clinical condition should be available, the investigative problem becomes quite different. Surviving spheroid cells could be counted and totalled for each frequency level throughout the series of cases, the sections having been made at a constantly spaced interval (for example, at every 100μ); the mean values for numbers of spheroid cells found in the different frequency levels could be compared with those of spheroid cell population of appropriate controls (whose procurement may be difficult). The means of cell losses can thus be determined, and can be compared with losses suffered by the cochlear elements and with the mean of audiometric curves.

The application of the method is illustrated with cases of anoxia and presbycusis. The former category offers particular value in the study of CN, inasmuch as it appears to be essentially uncomplicated by histopathologic changes of the cochlear elements. Unfortunately, audiograms tend not to be available; auditory pathway tissues from a case of anoxic hearing loss provided with audiometric curve has not as yet been studied by the author. Presbycusis involves the appearance of peripheral and central alterations in varying proportions. The contribution of findings in SVCN to the determination of the anatomic frequency scale of the stated nucleus is correspondingly less pointed, but the inclusion of SVCN still provides a more complete accounting of the structural basis of the hearing deficit than would otherwise be possible, and the "best fit" of the pattern of spheroid cell injury with that of the cochlear elements and with the audiometric curve, can be observed.

The case of anoxia is that of a man, aged 47 years, who died after nine years of mental deficiency and athetosis, resulting from severe carbon monoxide anoxia (Figs. 2, 4). The case of presbycusis is that of a man expiring at age 83, who showed progressive high frequency hearing deficit over a number of years (Figs. 3, 5).

It appears that increasing experience with the whole auditory pathway study of cases of sensorineural deafness has yielded a useable method of procedure for the evaluation of CN. The "best fit" of the pattern of spheroid cell injury with that of the audiometric curve is in keeping with the tentative impression that the anatomic frequency scale of VCN is in general parallel with the logarithmic frequency scale of the standard audiometric chart. This is on a basis of the study of cases of high-frequency deafness; to date, injury of spheroid cells especially marked in lower frequency zones, thus providing point for establishing "best fit" in that frequency range, has not been observed. The performance of cell counts in the different frequency levels of SVCN in a statistically significant number of cases of postanoxic deafness in which audiograms are available, and the comparison of the results with the audiometric curves, appears to offer the best opportunity of developing the anatomic frequency scale in SVCN of the human. A broad pattern trend could thus be established; however, owing to the variation in pattern and population density of distribution of spheroid cells, the scale might not necessarily apply in exact detail in individual cases.

REFERENCES

1. Dublin WB: Cytoarchitecture of the cochlear nuclei. Arch Otolaryngol 100:355-359, 1974

2. Schuknecht HF: *Pathology of the Ear.* Cambridge, Harvard University Press, 1974

3. Crabtree N, Gerrard J: Perceptive deafness associated with severe neonatal jaundice. J Laryngol Otol 69:482-506, 1950

4. Matkin ND, Carhart R: Auditory profiles associated with Rh incompatibility. Arch Otolaryngol 84:502-513, 1966

5. Buch NH, Tygstrup I, Jörgensen MB: Erythroblastosis fetalis and the hearing organ. Acta Otolaryngol (Stockh) 61:387-397, 1966

6. Flottorp G, Morley DE, Skatvedt M: The localization of hearing impairment in athetoids. Acta Otolaryngol (Stockh) 48:404-414, 1957

REPRINTS—William B. Dublin, MD, Laboratory of Auditory Pathology, Veterans Administration Hospital, Martinez, CA 94553.

Ann Otol 85: 1976

MASKING LEVEL DIFFERENCES FOR COCHLEAR AND BRAIN STEM LESIONS

WAYNE O. OLSEN, PhD

ROCHESTER, MINNESOTA

DOUGLAS NOFFSINGER, PhD

CHICAGO, ILLINOIS

SUMMARY – Masking level differences (MLD) for 500 Hz pure tones and for spondees were obtained from 48 subjects. Twelve were without otologic or neurologic complaints (normal), 12 had high frequency, noise-induced hearing losses, 12 were diagnosed otologically as having Ménière's disorder, and 12 had neurologically diagnosed central nervous system (CNS) disorders. Results indicated that high frequency, noise-induced hearing losses do not affect MLD for 500 Hz stimuli, but do diminish the size of MLD for speech. Masking level differences for both 500 Hz and spondees were decreased for the Ménière's disorder group. The group of patients having CNS disorders attributed to multiple sclerosis, to inflammatory lesion of the pons, to degenerative processes of the cerebellum and adjacent nervous tissue, or to brain stem cerebrovascular accident had normal hearing according to conventional pure tone and speech testing, but attained smaller than normal MLD for 500 Hz and spondees. These findings agree closely with results obtained in an earlier study and continue to suggest that, given normal peripheral auditory function, MLD tests may have unique value in detection of subtle lesions of the central auditory nervous system.

The fact that a normal auditory system can make advantageous use of subtle differences in simultaneous acoustic events at the two ears is well known. A number of laboratories have devoted much time and effort to determine to what extent the auditory system can utilize differences in various auditory stimuli delivered to both ears simultaneously or almost simultaneously.

One such phenomenon which has been investigated extensively is known as binaural release from masking, or more commonly, masking level differences (MLD). The phenomenon involved concerns the ability of the auditory system to take advantage of phase differences in a masking noise or in a signal delivered to the two ears simultaneously.

Figure 1 depicts some of the more common experimental conditions used for investigating binaural release from masking. The lettering on the forehead of each caricature gives the designation for the different listening conditions. The large letters "S" and "N" represent signal and noise respectively. The small letters reveal whether the signal or noise are presented monaurally, "m," or the phase relationship between ears of the signal or the noise when presented binaurally. The small "o" represents no phase difference between ears for the signal or the noise, while "π" indicates a phase reversal, *i.e.*, 180° phase difference between the signal or the noise at the two ears.

The top left drawing reveals delivery of the signal and the noise monaurally (SmNm), a difficult condition for the listener. If, however, the signal is main-

From the Department of Otorhinolaryngology, Mayo Clinic, Rochester, Minnesota, and the Auditory Research Laboratory, Northwestern University Medical School, Chicago, Illinois. This work was supported by the Mayo Foundation and by grant NSO 7791 to Northwestern University by NINCDS.

Presented at the meeting of the American Otological Society, Inc., Palm Beach, Florida, April 25-26, 1976.

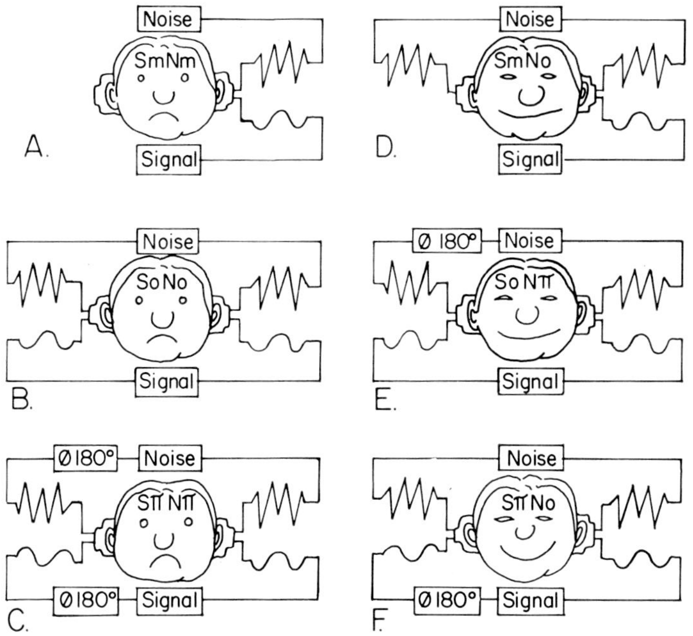

Fig. 1. Stimulus conditions for MLD tests. S - Signal, N - Noise, m - Monaural, o - In phase at two ears, π - 180° out of phase at two ears.

tained in the noise at a just-audible level for monaural hearing, the addition of an identical noise at the opposite ear results in easier detection of the signal. This condition is labelled SmNo. When identical signals and noises are presented bilaterally (SoNo), the listening situation reverts to a difficult one. Signal detection under this condition is similar to that experienced when the signal and noise are presented monaurally. However, putting the noise 180° out of phase between ears ($N\pi$), while the signal remains in phase between ears (So) eases the listening situation. If both the signal and noise are 180° out of phase with themselves ($S\pi N\pi$), the listening task is difficult and similar to that encountered in the SmNm and SoNo conditions. The best listening condition occurs when the signal is out of phase by 180° at the two ears while the noise is maintained in phase bilaterally, $S\pi No$. In this condition, a low frequency tone or speech can be heard at levels less intense than required for hearing in the more difficult SmNm, SoNo and $S\pi N\pi$ conditions. A similar but smaller advantage occurs for the SmNo and $SoN\pi$ conditions.

The fact that masked thresholds improve for normal hearers in the noted conditions has been known since the reports of Licklider[1] and of Hirsh[2] in 1948. Since then, these observations have been confirmed in a variety of experiments. Further, since MLD phenomena obviously involve more than separate processing of information from each ear, it has been theorized that some form of correlational processes within the central auditory nervous system (CANS) are responsible.[3]

Until recently, MLD tests have not been administered to persons having known hearing losses, or to persons with medically diagnosed lesions of the CNS. Three separate investigations have established that smaller than normal MLD are obtained from persons having hearing impairments attributed to Ménière's disorder.[4-6] One study has found normal MLD for 500 Hz, but decreased binaural release from masking for speech in persons having high frequency, noise-induced hearing losses.[6]

The observation of MLD of normal

size for persons having temporal lobe lesions or even hemispherectomies is of considerable interest.[6,7] Such findings indicate that unqualified participation by both cortical hemispheres is not necessary to attain binaural release from masking. It would appear that MLD are mediated in the CANS at some level or levels below the auditory cortex. In this context, our earlier observations of small MLD for patients having multiple sclerosis (MS)[6,8] take on added interest, particularly since the brain stem and midbrain seem to be sites of predilection for MS plaques. The critical point here is that both the MS subjects and the cortical lesion subjects typically have normal hearing for pure tones and speech. Since the MS group yields small MLD and the cortical lesion group normal MLD, an obvious speculative conclusion is that MLD may have unique value in detection of brain stem and/or midbrain lesions. The recent report of Noffsinger *et al*[9] showing reduced MLD for a patient having a lateromedial inferior pontine syndrome lends further credence to such a supposition.

SUBJECTS AND PROCEDURES

For further evaluation of MLD behavior for patients having otologic or neurologic abnormalities, four groups of subjects were tested. The same test procedures and materials employed in our previous work[6,8] were utilized. Briefly, masked thresholds for 500 Hz pure tone stimuli and for spondees were determined. As in most other studies of MLD the SoNo condition served as the reference condition. Our interest was in the masked threshold improvement observed when either the signal ($S\pi No$) or the noise ($SoN\pi$) was 180° out of phase with itself at the two ears. Thresholds for a pulsed 500 Hz tone were determined via Békésy audiometry. A continuous narrow band noise centered at 500 Hz was maintained at 80 dB SPL at both earphones throughout the three pure tone test conditions. White noise set at 80 dB SPL served as the masker in the same listening conditions when spondees were the stimuli. Speech reception thresholds were determined via a descending approach.[10]

Twelve normal hearing subjects (pure tone thresholds at 250-8000 Hz and speech reception thresholds no poorer than 25 dB HL bilaterally re ANSI 1969[11]) having no otologic or neurologic complaints were tested to serve as a control group. This group was tested to assure that the equipment utilized at a new test site would yield results similar to those obtained earlier with other apparatus.

Additional groups of 12 patients having unilateral Ménière's disorder and of 12 individuals with noise-induced sensorineural hearing loss were also tested for comparison to our earlier findings with larger samples having the same otologic diagnoses. All hearing impaired patients had unmasked thresholds no poorer than 50 dB HL at 500 Hz and speech reception thresholds no poorer than 40 dB HL bilaterally. These criteria assured that each patient would experience at least 10 dB threshold shift in the SoNo reference condition.

Finally, a group of 12 patients having neurologically diagnosed CNS disorders was tested. The disease process was ongoing in ten; two others had suffered brain stem insults earlier, but had essentially recovered at the time of testing. Nine patients had a diagnosis of MS. Of the others, one had an idiopathic inflammatory lesion of the pons, one was afflicted with progressive degeneration of the cerebellum and adjacent nervous tissue, and one had suffered a brain stem cerebrovascular accident involving the medial longitudinal fasciculus between the III and VI cranial nerve nuclei. At the time of testing the latter had recovered to the point of having minimal neurologic symptomatology. Each of the 12 subjects in this group had 25 dB HL or better 250-4000 Hz and speech reception thresholds bilaterally. Seven ears revealed mild hearing losses at 6000 or 8000 Hz.

RESULTS

The averaged data for each group are given in Table I. The values in the columns headed $S\pi No$ and $SoN\pi$ reveal

TABLE I

MEAN MLD IN dB OBTAINED FOR FOUR GROUPS OF SUBJECTS ($N = 12$ IN EACH GROUP)

	500 Hz		*Spondees*	
Group	$S\pi No$	$SoN\pi$	$S\pi No$	$SoN\pi$
Normal	11.7	9.3	7.3	6.9
Noise-induced loss	11.6	8.4	5.1	4.9
Ménière's disorder	4.8	2.9	3.0	2.9
CNS	9.8	7.3	5.0	3.8

the dB improvement in masked thresholds for these conditions relative to the SoNo reference.

Masking level differences for 500 Hz stimuli were about the same size for the normal subjects and for the patients with noise-induced hearing losses. These values are virtually identical to those obtained in earlier studies with larger samples ($N = 50$).[6] Hence, these results support our earlier observations that MLD at 500 Hz are not affected by high frequency, noise-induced hearing losses.

Binaural release from masking was reduced considerably for the group of patients having unilateral Ménière's disorder. These results are also in agreement with other reports on MLD for such patients.[4-6] It is apparent that low frequency sensorineural hearing loss such as associated with unilateral Ménière's disorder does alter the input from one side sufficiently to diminish binaural release from masking.

The 500 Hz MLD for the MS and brain stem lesion group are about 2 dB smaller than those of the normal group. This difference is not large, but given the similarity of the results for the normal and noise-induced loss groups who also had normal hearing at 500 Hz, the fact that there was a difference at all is of interest. The average 500 Hz MLD observed for this CNS group was about 2 dB larger than that observed for a group of 100 MS patients in an earlier study.[6]

Mean speech MLD for the control group (Table I) were virtually identical to those obtained in an earlier study.[6]

The results for the noise-induced hearing loss group are of particular interest for two reasons. First, mean MLD for the noise-induced hearing loss group are smaller than those observed for the normal group in spite of the fact that both had normal speech reception thresholds bilaterally. Second, these results closely match those obtained previously. Thus it appears that high frequency hearing losses such as those produced by excess noise exposure can influence binaural release from masking. Persons having noise-induced, high frequency sensorineural hearing losses frequently complain of difficulty in understanding conversational speech against speech or noise backgrounds in spite of normal speech reception thresholds and excellent speech discrimination in quiet and in noise.[12] Further research is needed to explore this aspect of their difficulty.

Masking level differences for speech attained by the Ménière's disorder patients were small as were their 500 Hz MLD. The data reported here are within 0.2 dB of the average we observed earlier for a group of 20 such subjects. Apparently the disturbance in end organ function accompanying this pathological condition disrupts the quality of transduction necessary for normal MLD.

Binaural release from masking for spondees on the order of 5 dB for the $S\pi No$ condition, and 4 dB for the $SoN\pi$ condition was obtained for the MS and brain stem lesion patients. These results almost exactly replicate those obtained earlier from 100 MS patients, being within 0.1 dB and 0.6 dB for the $S\pi No$ and $SoN\pi$ conditions respectively. The reduction in MLD size for these patients cannot be attributed to hearing loss since their speech reception thresholds and 250-4000 Hz thresholds were normal; in only a few instances were there mild losses at 6000 and 8000 Hz. Therefore, reduced MLD for these patients is more logically tied to some

TABLE II

NUMBER OF SUBJECTS ACHIEVING MLD SMALLER THAN INDICATED VALUES

Group	*500 Hz* <8 dB $S\pi No$ and/or <5 dB $SoN\pi$	*Spondees* <6 dB $S\pi No$ and/or <4 dB $SoN\pi$
Normal	0	0
Noise-induced loss	0	7
Ménière's disorder	8	12
CNS	1	7

disruption in the CANS integration of binaural input than to peripheral auditory damage.

Another way of comparing these data to our earlier work is to consider the incidence of "abnormally small" MLD. In the earlier data, only 2 (4%) of our 50 normal subjects attained 500 Hz MLD smaller than 8 dB for the $S\pi No$ condition or smaller than 5 dB for the $SoN\pi$ condition. Only 3 (6%) of the 50 normals achieved MLD for speech smaller than 6 dB and 4 dB for the $S\pi No$ and $SoN\pi$ conditions respectively. On this basis, MLD at 500 Hz smaller than 8 dB ($S\pi No$) and 5 dB ($SoN\pi$), or smaller than 6 dB ($S\pi No$) or 4 dB ($SoN\pi$) for speech were considered to be "reduced."[6]

If these criteria are applied in the present instance as shown in Table II, none of the 12 normal subjects attained MLD for either 500 Hz or spondees smaller than the lower limits of normal. The same was true for 500 Hz MLD for the high frequency, noise-induced hearing loss subjects. However, seven of the noise-induced hearing loss cases experienced reduced MLD for speech. In the Ménière's disorder group, 8 of 12 failed to achieve MLD at or above the indicated levels for 500 Hz; all attained binaural release from masking less than the indicated cutoff levels for speech.

Of the CNS patients, only the patient with an inflammatory lesion of the pons attained reduced MLD for 500 Hz. This patient, four of the nine MS patients, and the patient with ongoing degeneration of the cerebellum and adjacent nervous tissue also obtained reduced MLD for speech. The incidence of reduced MLD for speech observed for the MS patients is similar to that observed in our earlier sample of 100 such patients. It is also imporatnt that of the three other CNS lesion patients in the present sample, those with active pathology at the time of testing demonstrated reduced MLD, at least for speech. The other patient who had reassumed nearly normal neurological status at the time of testing, attained 8 dB of binaural release from masking for speech for the $S\pi No$ condition and 5 dB for the $SoN\pi$ condition.

CONCLUSION

From the preceding review of data, it is clear that binaural release from masking is influenced by disturbances in cochlear function. Noise induced-hearing losses do not affect MLD for 500 Hz, but do diminish binaural release from masking for spondees. The alteration in cochlear transduction associated with unilateral Ménière's disorder disrupts processing to the extent that binaural release from masking is sharply reduced.

Given normal peripheral function, however, it appears that MLD are frequently affected by lesions of the CNS associated with MS, or other pathologies in the brain stem and/or midbrain region.

The data presented here indicate that MLD tests utilizing speech are more sensitive to subtle CANS dysfunctions than are tests utilizing 500 Hz pure tone stimuli. This observation is in accord with other attempts directed at detecting auditory lesion beyond the cochlea and VIII nerve. That is, complex tasks utilizing complex stimuli such as speech are necessary for detection of dysfunction in the CANS.

REFERENCES

1. Licklider JCR: The influence of interaural phase relations upon the masking of speech by white noise. J Acoust Soc Am 20:150-159, 1948

2. Hirsh IJ: The influence of interaural phase on interaural summation and inhibition. J Acoust Soc Am 20:536-544, 1948

3. Jeffress LA: Binaural signal detection: vector theory, in Tobias, TV (ed): *Foundations of Modern Auditory Theory.* New York, Academic Press, 1972, vol 2, pp 351-368

4. Shoeny ZG, Carhart R: Effects of unilateral Ménière's disease on masking level differences. J Acoust Soc Am 50:1143-1150, 1971

5. Quaranto A, Cervellera G: Masking level differences in normal and pathological ears. Audiology 13:428-431, 1974

6. Olsen WO, Noffsinger D, Carhart R: Masking level differences encountered in clinical populations. Audiology 15:287-301, 1976

7. Cullen JK Jr, Thompson CL: Masking release for speech in subjects with temporal lobe resections. Arch Otolaryngol 100:113-116, 1974

8. Noffsinger D, Olsen WO, Carhart R, *et al*: Auditory and vestibular aberrations in multiple sclerosis. Acta Otolaryngol [Suppl] (Stockh) 303, 1972

9. Noffsinger D, Kurdziel S, Applebaum EL: Value of special auditory tests in the latero-medial inferior pontine syndrome. Ann Otol Rhinol Laryngol 84:384-390, 1975

10. Tillman T, Olsen WO: Speech audiometry, in Jerger, J (ed): *Modern Developments in Audiology,* ed 2. New York, Academic Press, 1973, pp 37-74

11. American National Standards Institute: *American National Standard Specifications for Audiometers ANSI S3.6 1969.* New York, American National Standards Institute, 1969

12. Olsen WO, Noffsinger D, Kurdziel S: Speech discrimination in quiet and in white noise by patients with peripheral and central lesions. Acta Otolaryngol 80:375-382, 1975

REPRINTS—Wayne O. Olsen, PhD, Department of Otorhinolaryngology, Mayo Clinic, Rochester, MN 55901.

Ann Otol 85: 1976

HEARING LOSS OF A CENTRAL TYPE SECONDARY TO ANOXIC ANOXIA

KAZUMI MAKISHIMA, MD

FUKUOKA, JAPAN

ROGER B. KATZ, MD JAMES B. SNOW, JR., MD

PHILADELPHIA, PENNSYLVANIA

SUMMARY – The effect of anoxic anoxia on the threshold sensitivity and amplitude of the responses from the auditory cortex, inferior colliculus and cochlea to acoustic stimuli in guinea pigs was studied. Decay of the amplitude of the responses from the auditory cortex and the inferior colliculus occurs faster and is more severe than that of the cochlea. Recovery of the amplitude of the responses is slower at the auditory cortex and the inferior colliculus than at the cochlea. Loss of auditory threshold sensitivity in anoxic anoxia is most prominent at the auditory cortex. The loss of sensitivity at the inferior colliculus is the next most severe. The loss of sensitivity at the cochlea is negligible. The relative vulnerability of the central auditory pathway to anoxic anoxia as compared to the end organ is demonstrated.

Oxygen deprivation due to cardiovascular collapse or respiratory arrest causes neurologic deficits. These deficits may include hearing loss. The susceptibility of the AC cochlear potentials, the compound action potential of the VIII nerve and the DC cochlear resting potential to oxygen deprivation has been demonstrated by many investigators.[1-3] The oxygen uptake of the central nervous system is 30 times greater than that of the peripheral nerves. It would be expected that damage to the auditory system due to oxygen deprivation would occur earlier and be more severe in the central pathways than in the periphery. The loss of function due to oxygen deprivation as manifested by otoneurological symptoms and signs would appear sooner and be more severe in the central auditory pathways than in the cochlea.

The purpose of this experiment was to study the relative vulnerability of the central auditory pathways and the end organ to varying degrees of anoxic anoxia.

METHODS AND MATERIALS

Adult guinea pigs weighing 200 to 250 g were anesthetized with sodium pentobarbital (Nembutal®*) 35 mg/kg given intramuscularly. Atropine at a dosage of 0.01 mg/kg was given intramuscularly. Tracheotomy was performed, and the tracheal cannula was connected to a small animal respirator. The respirator delivered air with a tidal volume of 1.5 ml at a rate of 80 strokes/min.

The soft tissue was elevated from the skull to expose the greater part of the calvarium. The dura over the auditory cortex and the inferior colliculus was exposed with care to avoid abrading or penetrating it. Access to the round window membrane was obtained. The superior part of the right external auditory canal was incised about 3 mm lateral to the tympanic ring for insertion of a sound-probe tube which was sealed to the ear canal.

Acoustic stimuli were presented through the closed tube system to the right ear, and the responses were measured from the left cortex and the right round window. A silver bipolar electrode was used to monitor the signals from the dura overlying the auditory cortex, and a small silver ball electrode was used on the round window membrane. The signals were amplified and displayed on an oscilloscope, the sweep of which was synchronized with the tone bursts. Thresholds for the responses from

----

* Abbott Laboratories, North Chicago, IL.

From the Department of Otorhinolaryngology and Human Communication, University of Pennsylvania School of Medicine, Philadelphia, Pennsylvania.

Presented at the meeting of the American Otological Society, Inc., Palm Beach, Florida, April 25-26, 1976.

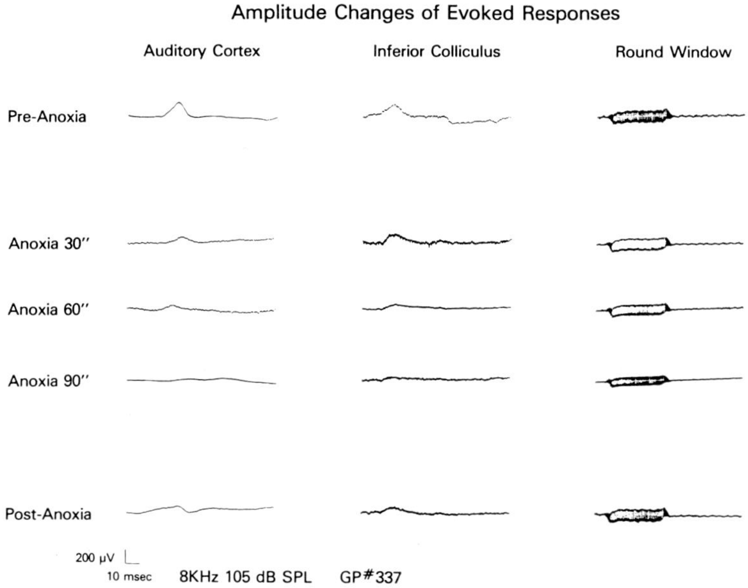

Fig. 1. Typical amplitude changes of the evoked responses from the auditory cortex, the inferior colliculus and the round window of the cochlea of a guinea pig for an 8.0 kHz tone burst with an intensity of 105 dB SPL, following anoxic anoxia, are shown. After 90 seconds of anoxia, the cortical responses disappear and the amplitude of the inferior colliculus responses decrease severely in the presence of a lesser effect on the AC cochlear potentials.

the auditory cortex were determined by visual detection on the oscilloscope.[4] The AC cochlear potentials were measured with a frequency sensitive voltmeter. Thresholds for the responses from the cortex and cochlea were obtained at 17 frequencies in successive one-third octave steps between 0.5 and 20.0 kHz.

The sound-probe tube was repositioned to the left external auditory canal, and the thresholds for the responses from the right inferior colliculus were measured as were the thresholds for right cortical responses. The thresholds for the AC cochlear potentials from the left round window were also measured. A stainless steel coaxial electrode was used to monitor the responses from the inferior colliculus. The techniques for measuring thresholds for responses from the inferior colliculus and the auditory cortex have been described.[4,5]

After collecting control thresholds for the responses from the auditory cortex, the inferior colliculus and the round window, the animal was deprived of oxygen by clamping the tracheal cannula and turning off the respirator. The initial period of the oxygen deprivation was five minutes. Subsequent periods of oxygen deprivation were four minutes with an interval to allow the animal to recover from the anoxia. The guinea pigs were divided into three groups according to the total length of the periods of oxygen deprivation, namely; mild (5 minutes of oxygen deprivation), moderate (9 to 17 minutes) and severe (more than 21 minutes). Following the periods of oxygen deprivation, the animals were given a 30-minute period for stabilization, and the thresholds for the responses from the auditory cortex, the inferior colliculus and the round window were again determined. In some animals, changes in the amplitudes of the responses from the auditory cortex, the inferior colliculus and the round window secondary to anoxia were compared to each other in successive and increasing intervals of anoxia. In others, the amplitude of the responses from the inferior colliculus and the round window following repetitive oxygen deprivation was monitored to determine decay and recovery patterns. Another group of animals were studied to determine the effects of duration of oxygen deprivation on the recovery pattern of the inferior colliculus responses. After the measurements, fixation by arterial perfusion and histological processing of the heads were carried out.

RESULTS

Typical changes in the amplitude of the responses from the auditory cortex, the inferior colliculus and the cochlea following oxygen deprivation are shown in Figure 1 for an 8.0 kHz tone burst with an intensity of 105 dB SPL. At

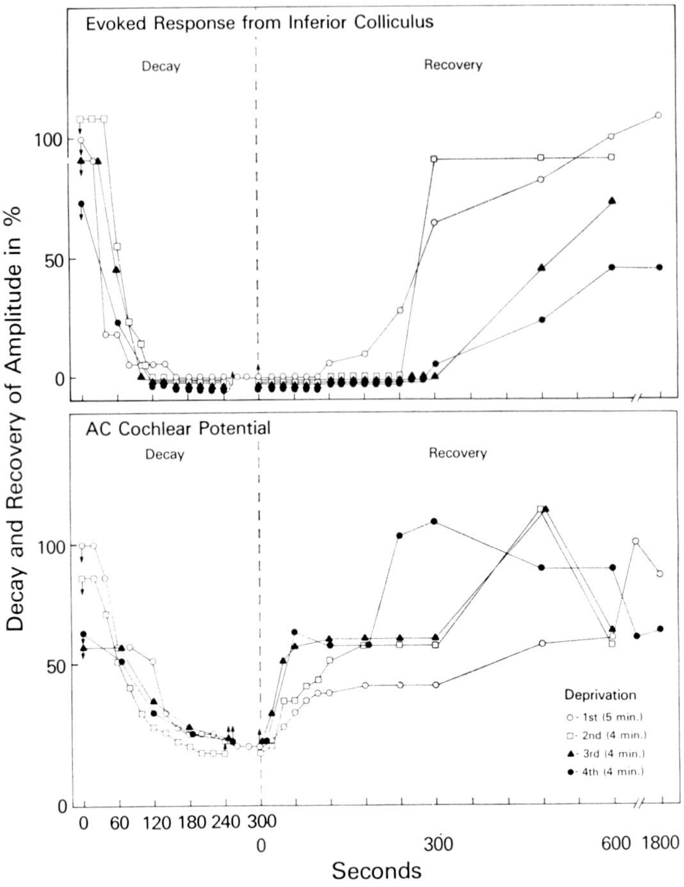

Fig. 2. Comparison of the decay and recovery patterns of the amplitude of responses from the inferior colliculus (upper segment) to that of the AC cochlear potentials, lower segment) of a typical guinea pig. The amplitude of the responses from the inferior colliculus decay faster and recover slower than those from the cochlea.

approximately 90 seconds, the cortical responses disappear, and the amplitude of the responses from the inferior colliculus decrease profoundly. On the other hand, the amplitude of the AC cochlear potentials are less affected. The recovery of the amplitude of the responses for the AC cochlear potentials is almost complete at 300 seconds after reventilation, but recovery is incomplete and slower for the responses from the cortex and the inferior colliculus. The decay and recovery times of the responses vary from animal to animal.

Decay and recovery of the amplitude of the responses from the inferior colliculus are compared to the decay and recovery of the amplitude of the AC cochlear potentials in a typical animal in Figure 2. The animal was deprived of oxygen for an initial period of five minutes and for three subsequent periods of four minutes each. The rapid decay of the amplitude of the response from the inferior colliculus occurred at approximately 60 seconds, and the response disappeared at approximately 120 seconds in each trial. At the initial oxygen deprivation, the first sign of recovery of the responses occurred at approximately 120 seconds after reventilation. The time to recovery was longer with each repetition of oxygen deprivation, and the depression of the recovered amplitude of the responses became more profound with repetition

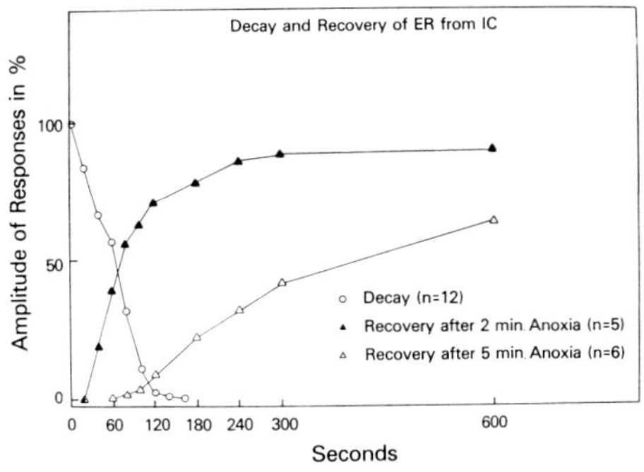

Fig. 3. Decay and recovery pattern of the responses from the inferior colliculus following two or five minutes of anoxia. Decay of the amplitude of the responses reaches approximately 0% at about 120 seconds. Recovery of the amplitude begins later and is slower in the five minutes of anoxia group than in the two minutes of anoxia group.

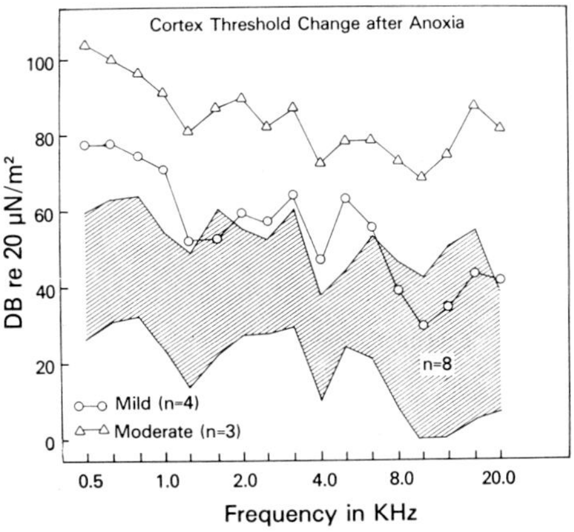

Fig. 4. Mean threshold curves of the responses from the auditory cortex for the mild and the moderate anoxia groups are illustrated. The shaded area represents one standard deviation from the mean threshold curve for the control group. The mean threshold curve for the moderate group shows a marked elevation of the thresholds throughout the entire frequency range tested.

of oxygen deprivation. Following the fourth oxygen deprivation, approximately 50% recovery of the control amplitude occurred after a 30-minute period of stabilization. On the other hand, the decay of the amplitude of the AC cochlear potentials was slower, and the amplitude remained at approximately 20% of the control level even after four or five minutes of oxygen deprivation. The recovery of the AC cochlear potentials began earlier and reached 50% of the control amplitude sooner than the recovery of the responses from the inferior colliculus. The recovering amplitude of the AC cochlear potentials often exceeded the control level. With repetition of anoxic periods, the amplitude of the AC cochlear potentials decreased more; however, a slowly progressive recovery continued for several hours. In summary, the amplitude of the responses from the inferior colliculus decays faster and recovers slower than that from the cochlea.

Decay and recovery of the responses from the inferior colliculus were studied further in a group of guinea pigs which were deprived of oxygen for two or five minutes. In the guinea pigs deprived of oxygen for two or five minutes, the mean curve of the amplitude of the responses declined rapidly to approximately 0% in 120 seconds as illustrated in Figure 3.

Recovery of the amplitude in the animals deprived of oxygen for two minutes began within 20 seconds after reventilation and reached about 90% of the control amplitude within 300 seconds. In the animals deprived of oxygen for five minutes, the recovery of the amplitude began at 60 seconds after reventilation and attained less than 50% of the control amplitude in 300 seconds. The recovery continued at a slow rate.

The changes in the thresholds of the responses to acoustic stimuli from the auditory cortex, the inferior colliculus and the cochlea following mild, moderate or severe oxygen deprivation were measured.

Auditory Cortex. The mean threshold curves of the responses from the auditory cortex for the mild and moderate groups are illustrated in Figure 4. The mean curve in the mild group showed a slight elevation of threshold, especially in the low frequencies tested. The mean curve in the moderate group showed a marked elevation of threshold throughout the entire frequency range tested.

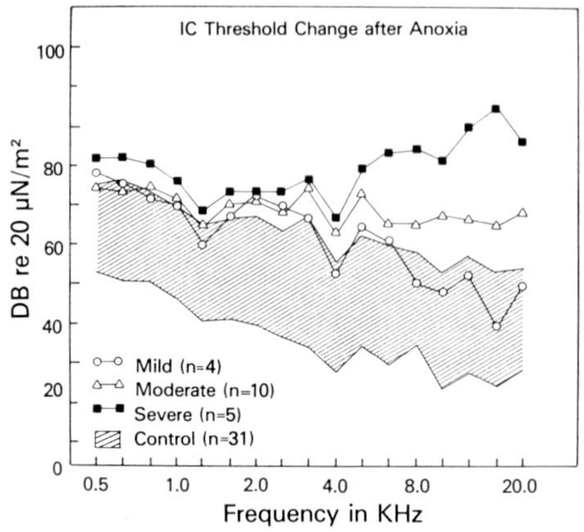

Fig. 5. Mean threshold curves of the responses from the inferior colliculus for the mild, moderate and severe anoxia groups. The shaded area represents one standard deviation from the mean threshold curve for the control group. Marked elevation of the thresholds in the higher frequency range is seen in the severe anoxia group.

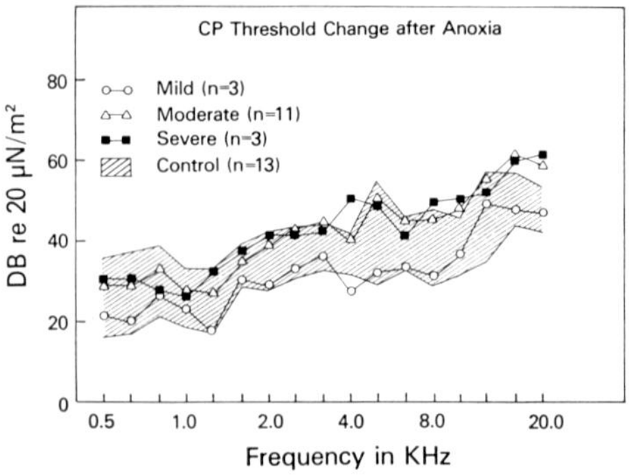

Fig. 6. Mean threshold curves for the AC cochlear potentials from the round window for the mild, moderate and severe groups. The shaded area represents one standard deviation from the mean threshold curve for the control group. Threshold curves for the three anoxia groups do not differ significantly from the control threshold curve.

Inferior Colliculus. The mean threshold curve of the responses from the inferior colliculus for the control condition is shown in Figure 5. The mean curve for the mild group was not significantly different from the control condition except that there was a slight loss of sensitivity in the middle frequencies. The mean threshold curve in the moderate group is elevated in most of the frequencies tested, especially in the higher frequencies. Elevation of the mean threshold curve is much more prominent in the severe group with slight loss of sensitivity in the low and middle frequencies and marked loss in the higher frequencies tested.

AC Cochlear Potential. The mean threshold curves for the responses from the round window of the mild, moderate and severe groups are illustrated in Figure 6. Although there was a slight elevation of the threshold in the higher frequencies in the moderate and severe groups, the thresholds of the mild, moderate and severe groups in general did not differ significantly from the control condition.

In summary, the elevation of threshold secondary to oxygen deprivation was prominent in the auditory cortex with a loss of sensitivity throughout the entire frequency range tested. The loss of sensitivity at the inferior colliculus was severe in the higher frequencies. The loss of sensitivity at the cochlea was negligible.

DISCUSSION

The animals in this study were deprived of oxygen by turning off the respirator and clamping the tracheal cannula. To describe the condition that resulted from almost complete interruption of the supply of oxygen, the term anoxic anoxia was chosen in preference to hypoxia or asphyxia. The distinction between anoxic anoxia in which only oxygen is absent from the circulating blood and ischemic anoxia in which the blood and all of the substances carried in the blood, including oxygen, are prevented from reaching the tissue, is an important one. From a histopathological point of view, the two conditions are essentially identical.

The effects of anoxia on tissues and organs are complex. Anoxia has a direct damaging effect on neurons that may be reversible or irreversible. Another prominent effect is dilatation of or stasis in small blood vessels. The vasodilatation, of course, may be in part due to the associated hypercarbia.

The susceptibility of the cochlear potentials to oxygen deprivation has been studied extensively by many workers. Recently, Lawrence *et al* demonstrated a decline in oxygen concentration in the cochlear tunnel prior to a decline in oxygen concentration in the endolymph of the scala media following interruption of ventilation. Considerably later the DC cochlear resting potential began to decline and was followed later by the decline of the AC cochlear potentials. With reventilation, the DC cochlear resting potential and the AC cochlear potentials recovered together prior to the return of oxygen concentration in the endolymph of the scala media to normal levels. Since the AC cochlear potentials were the last to decline, Lawrence *et al* suggest that the AC cochlear potentials are at least partially dependent on the DC cochlear resting potential and that there is a "storehouse" of oxygen to support the generation and maintenance of the DC cochlear resting potential and the AC cochlear potentials.[3]

Our data are in good agreement with these previous findings in demonstrating the relative survival in anoxia and recovery from anoxia of the AC cochlear potentials. Although the generators of the AC cochlear potentials exhibit increased susceptibility to damage with repetition of anoxia, there is a persistent pattern of progressive recovery of the amplitude of the AC cochlear potentials. Moreover, the threshold of the AC cochlear potentials remained unchanged after a period of stablization even in the severe anoxia group which were deprived of oxygen repeatedly.

Study of the cochleae with light microscopy demonstrated no damage in the experimental animals after acute and prolonged oxygen deprivation. This lack of morphological change suggests that the depression of the AC cochlear potentials observed in the animal is a reversible phenomenon based on undetermined biochemical derangements.[2,6]

Significant elevation of the thresholds of the responses from the inferior colliculus and the auditory cortex were observed in the presence of normal thresholds of the AC cochlear potentials. The data demonstrate the relative vulnerability of the central auditory pathway to anoxic anoxia as compared to the end organ.

Labile constituents in central nervous tissue may undergo biochemical and morphological changes during anoxia. Sugar and Gerard proposed that the requirement for oxygen is higher in the phylogenetically newer portions of the central nervous system after demonstrating shorter survival times for neurons in the cerebral cortex than for neurons in the medulla oblongata during anoxia.[7] Gildea and Cobb also indicated that periods of almost complete cessation of blood flow for not more than ten minutes resulted in permanent damage to the cortical neurons and less damage to neurons of the medulla oblongata.[8] Furthermore, a number of investigators have shown that cerebral arterial occlusion is followed by expansion and coalescence of cortical pallor and vasoconstriction in the ischemic areas.[9] This no-reflow phenomenon following cerebral ischemia might be explained by vasoconstriction, endothelial swelling and stasis and suggests that cerebral neurons might be relatively more resistant to ischemia than blood vessels.[10] The implication is that very prompt reperfusion after ischemia might prevent neural damage. Several investigators reported evidence of repair of brain damage and signs of recovery of neuronal function even following total ischemia for a one hour period.[11] Levy *et al*, however, found that light microscopic neuronal abnormalities were evident after five to ten minutes of hypoxia-ischemia, and motor behavioral abnormalities were present after 10 to 20 minutes.[12] There were no associated histological vascular changes or regional no-reflow. Furthermore, Meyer reported permanent damage in cats when the duration of respiratory or cardiac arrest lasted longer than five minutes, and severe and widespread lesions in a patient after cardiac arrest of only one minute.[13] Although some studies have been concerned with ischemic anoxia produced by occluding arteries and others with anoxic anoxia, the histopathological changes are essentially identical. The usual pathological sequelae of anoxia or profound hypoxia in the brain consists of widespread damage to cortical neuronal populations and various subcortical structures.

Widespread pathological changes in the cerebrum and the rhombencephalon including the central auditory pathway cause elevation of the auditory thresholds over a wide frequency range. Good examples of these conditions are severe edema,[14,15] widspread hemorrhage,[14] tumor invasion[15] and encephalomalacia.[16] Makishima examined the brains and temporal bones of aged patients whose hearing had been measured during life, and proposed that diffuse senile cytopathological changes in the brain played a significant role in the development of hearing loss throughout the frequency range.[16]

From our data and this discussion, we may conclude that elevation of the thresholds of the responses from the auditory cortex and the inferior colliculus in the presence of normal thresholds from the cochlea demonstrate the relative vulnerability of the central auditory pathway to anoxic anoxia as compared to the end organ. Furthermore, the loss of auditory sensitivity throughout the entire frequency range tested at the cortical level is probably caused by widespread, reversible and irreversible, acute, biochemical and morphological changes of anoxia.

REFERENCES

1. von Békésy G: D-C potentials and energy balance of the cochlear partition. J Acoust Soc Am 23:576-582, 1951
2. Fernández C, Alzate R: Modification of cochlear responses by oxygen deprivation. Arch Otolaryngol 69:82-94, 1959
3. Lawrence M, Nuttall AL, Burgio PA: Cochlear potentials and oxygen associated with hypoxia. Ann Otol Rhinol Laryngol 84:499-512, 1975
4. Makishima K, Keane WM, Katz RB, *et al*: A method for determining cortical auditory thresholds in guinea pigs. Submitted for publication
5. Makishima K, Saunders JC, Snow JB: Evoked responses from inferior colliculus as an index of hearing thresholds in guinea pigs. Acta Otolaryngol (Stockh) 80:238-244, 1975
6. Falbe-Hansen J, Christensen E, Gisselsson L *et al*: Effect of acute and prolonged oxygen deprivation on the organ of Corti in guinea pigs and cats. Arch Otolaryngol 67: 71-77, 1958
7. Sugar O, Gerard RW: Anoxia and brain potential. J Neurophysiol 1:558-572, 1938
8. Gildea EF, Cobb S: The effects of anemia on the cerebral cortex of the cat. Arch Neurol Psychiatry 23:876-903, 1930
9. Denny-Brown D, Meyer JS: The cerebral collateral circulation: 2. Production of cerebral infarction by ischemic anoxia and its reversibility in early stages. Neurology (Minneap) 7:567-579, 1957
10. Ames A, Wright RL, Kowada M, *et al*: Cerebral ischemia: II. The no-reflow phenomenon. Am J Pathol 52:437-453, 1968
11. Kleihues P, Hossmann KA, Pegg AE, *et al*: Resusitation of the monkey brain after one hour complete ischemia. III. Indications of metabolic recovery. Brain Res 95:61-73, 1975
12. Levy DE, Brierley JB, Silverman DG, *et al*: Brief hypoxia-ischemia initially damages cerebral neurons. Arch Neurol 32:450-456, 1975
13. Meyer A: Intoxication, in Blackwood W, Mc Menemey WH, Meyer A, *et al* (eds): *Greenfields Neuropathology*. Baltimore, Williams & Wilkins, 1963, pp 235-287
14. Makishima K, Snow JB: Electrophysiological responses from the cochlea and inferior colliculus in guinea pigs after head injury. Laryngoscope 85:1947-1956, 1975
15. Makishima K, Ogata J: Brain stem tumor and otoneurologic manifestations: Report of a case with autopsy. Ann Otol Rhinol Laryngol 84:391-400, 1975
16. Makishima K: Clinicopathological studies in presbycusis. Otol Fukuoka 13:Suppl 3, 333-364, 1967

Reprints—Kazumi Makishima, MD, Department of Otorhinolaryngology, Kyushu University School of Medicine, Fukuoka 812, Japan.

NEW DEVELOPMENTS IN EVALUATING CENTRAL AUDITORY MECHANISMS

CHARLES I. BERLIN, PHD

NEW ORLEANS, LOUISIANA

SUMMARY – Five tests are reviewed for their ability to assist in the evaluation of the central auditory mechanism. These are: 1) the Masking Level Difference (MLD); 2) ipsilaterally and contralaterally evoked stapedius muscle reflex; 3) electrocochleography; 4) early brain stem responses; and 5) dichotic listening. A summary chart outlining the tests most commonly in use and their areas of special productivity is also presented.

It has recently become possible for the hearing diagnostician to get new and clear insights into auditory mechanisms central to the VIII nerve. Because of anatomical constraints, lesions of the floor of the IV ventricle and lesions of the upper brain stem rarely produce either abnormalities in the pure tone audiogram or clinical complaints of hearing loss. However, neurootologic diagnosis with vestibular tests and some of the procedures to be described in this paper allow diagnosticians new techniques for the evaluation of the central auditory system in the absence of peripheral hearing loss. Figure 1 lists a set of procedures which can be used to assess various portions of the auditory nervous system. An "X" sign represents a high likelihood of positive results for lesions in the listed areas. In the interest of brevity, this paper will focus on only five of the most promising procedures available to clarify central auditory mechanisms. These procedures are:

1. the masking level difference (MLD);
2. stapedial reflex recordings (both ipsilaterally and contralaterally elicited);
3. electrocochleography;
4. brain stem potentials (1 to 12 msec);
5. dichotic listening.

CONDITIONS UNDER WHICH CENTRAL AUDITORY TESTING IS MOST USEFUL

Some of the tests to be described are most productive when the patients to be tested have voluntarily produced normal or virtually normal pure tone audiograms. For example, in the MLD test and in the dichotic listening tasks, normal hearing is almost a prerequisite to adequate interpretation and use of the tests. In the stapedial reflex test, it is important to have accompanying tympanometry, and audiometry in order to interpret the data effectively. However, the stapedial reflexes can sometimes be combined with electrocochleography (ECochG) to give important information about central auditory mechanisms without a voluntary audiogram being acquired. A sample case will be presented later. Two of these procedures, masking level difference and dichotic listening, require patient cooperation and skills roughly equivalent to those necessary to take a pure tone audiogram and a discrimination test. The other three tests (stapedial reflexes, ECochG, and brain stem potentials) are physiologic tests and require only that the subject be still enough for the examiner to acquire the

----

From the Kresge Hearing Research Laboratory of the South, Department of Otorhinolaryngology, Louisiana State University Medical Center, New Orleans, Louisiana. This investigation was supported by The Deafness Research Foundation and the National Institutes of Health, USPHS Program Project Grant No. NS-11647.

Presented at the meeting of the American Otological Society, Inc., Palm Beach, Florida, April 25-26, 1976.

POSSIBLE LOCUS OF LESION			Tone and Click Tests															Speech Tests													
	Pure tone A C	TDT	Békésy	SBMPL	MLD	Tonal Integ.	DL Intensity	DL Frequency	DL Duration	SISI (high INT.)	Reflexes (Contra)	Reflexes (Ipsi)	ABLB	Early Evoked Potentials	1-12 msec	12-50 msec	Electrocochleography	SRT	Discrim (Q)	Discrim (N)	MLD Speech	SSI	SSW	FILTERED SP.	Speeded Speech	Competing Messages	Interrupted Speech	Dichotic Simultan.	Dichotic, Time St.	Dichotic Digits	PI-PB
	1	2	3	4	5	6	7	8	9	10	11	12	13	14	15	16	17	18	19	20	21	22	23	24	25	26	27	28	29	30	31
Eighth Nerve	X	X	X	X	X	X	X	X	X	X	X	X	X		X	X	X	X	X	X	X			X			X				X
Cochlear Nuclei	X	X	X	X	X	X	X	X	X	X	X	X	X		X	X	X	X	X	X	X			X			X				X
Trapezoid Bodies					X				X		X	X			X						X						X				
Olivary Bodies					X				X		X	X			X						X						X				
Inferior Colliculi					?				X		?	?			X						?						?				
Medical Geniculate															X													X	X		
Temporal Lobe						X	X		X						X	X				X		X	X	X	X	X		X	X	X	X
Corpus Callosum															X	X												X	X	X	

Fig. 1. Summary of auditory procedures for central evaluation.

data. In children, the use of sedation or even general anesthesia has no effect on the ECochG but may have some slight effect on both reflexes and brain stem potentials, depending upon the sedatives and/or anesthetics used.

Masking Level Difference

The Phenomenon. If a target tone is presented to one ear, and then covered with noise in the same ear, the noise will mask out the tone if the proper intensity relationships exist. If the noise and tone are then left in this fixed relationship in the first ear, and an additional noise is presented to the other ear, which is 180° out-of-phase with the noise already being used to mask the target tone, the target tone will become more audible. It appears as if some form of neural cancellation of the out-of-phase noises has taken place.[1,2] What is generally seen is approximately 11 to 15 dB improvement in threshold detection of the target signal. This threshold detection difference is called a "masking level difference." This effect, incidentally, has also been found in the cat,[3] permitting new dimensions of comparative research on this phenomenon. This phenomenon of "release from masking" by the introduction of out-of-phase noise can also be seen if the *target* is introduced out-of-phase, or if the target is speech. It has been shown that this release from masking does not depend on auditory association cortex[4] but probably depends upon brain stem structures related to the trapezoid bodies and the olivary bodies.

In normal-listening subjects there is approximately an 11 to 15 dB release from masking. In patients with cortical lesions there is approximately the same level of release.[4] However, in patients with multiple sclerosis, in which diffuse lesions are seen throughout the brain stem, there is a reduction of MLD.[5] This reduction is such that one would predict a reduced MLD in patients with lesions of the IV ventricle and areas related to the trapezoid and olivary bodies in the two-ear interaction system.

STAPEDIAL REFLEXES (IPSILATERAL AND CONTRALATERAL)

In order to see a middle ear muscle reflex with currently available impedance bridges, three prerequisites must be observed.

1. The middle ear must be normal (usually evidenced by a Type A tympanogram).

2. The stimulating signal, either ipsilateral or contralateral, must be "loud enough" to elicit a reflex.

3. The reflex arc must be intact.

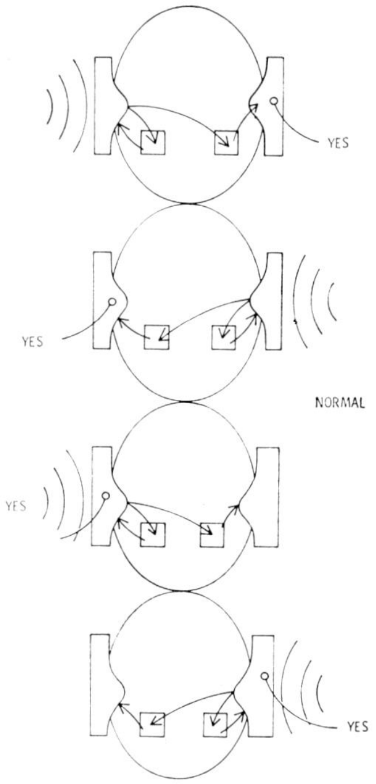

Fig. 2. Schematic of contralateral vs ipsilateral reflex testing. Dark probe is reflex measuring device; repetitive wave is reflex eliciting tone. Top two figures show tone in one ear, probe in the other. Bottom two figures show tone and probe in same ear.

The reflex arc for the stapedius muscle has only been recently found to include the medial superior olive (but not the lateral superior olive) and the nucleus of the trapezoid body.[6,7] For a review of the physical basis of impedance, see Berlin and Cullen[8] and for the application of reflexes to the study of central auditory dysfunction, see Jerger.[9]

Figure 2 shows what would happen if one presented the test tone in one ear and the probe searching for the reflex in either the opposite ear or in the same ear. The tone designed to elicit the reflex is represented as a repetitive wave, and the section of the bridge used to measure the presence of the reflex is marked as the dark probe. In a patient with a normal middle ear and normal brain stem, whether the reflex is elicited by a contralateral tone or by an ipsilateral tone, we see virtually the

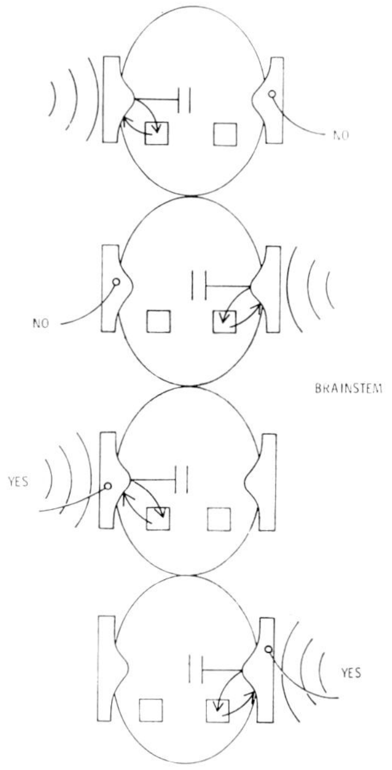

Fig. 3. Failure of a patient with a brain stem lesion to show contralateral reflexes despite normal ipsilateral reflexes.

same responses. In contrast, when a patient has a lesion of the central structures near the IV ventricle no reflex can be elicited by contralateral tones, but virtually normal reflexes are seen by ipsilateral recording of the reflex from the same ear in which stimulation is taking place (Fig. 3). We recommend, and are currently implementing, both ipsilateral and contralateral reflex recordings in appropriate patients.

ELECTROCOCHLEOGRAPHY

ECochG records the synchronous discharge of VIII nerve units from individual cochleae. It is extremely reliable and precise, as is shown in a test-retest run on a normal subject with a five-month interval (Fig. 4). In the presence of an VIII nerve tumor, for example, despite a normal pure tone audiogram, asynchronous discharge can be revealed.[10] In patients with tumors but no hearing, peripheral cochlear response can sometimes be uncovered;[11] however, in this application we are using it as an aid in the diagnosis of more central auditory dysfunction. De-

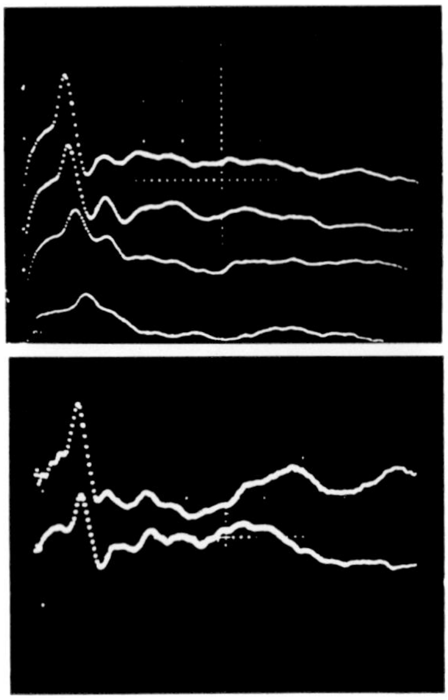

Fig. 4. Five-month test-retest of extratympanic electrocochleography.

tails of the technique of how we acquired ECochG data can be found elsewhere.[10,12] I would like to present a case here to show how ECochG helped alert us to a possible diagnosis of central auditory imperception in a very young child.

Patient K.R., a Caucasian female, was born in November 1970. She had a history of maternal rubella and when she was seen at age two for general medical and pediatric evaluation, the following observations were made: "She could sit alone, but could not walk. She had good function of her upper and lower extremities, had calconeo valgocavus feet bilaterally with marked pronation. She had a searching type nystagmus, was highly myopic, and had profound bilateral atrophy, worse in the right eye." When seen at age four she still had no speech and language, was not bladder or bowel trained, and, on the Vineland Social Maturity Scale, achieved a social age score of 1 year 3 months. She was severely retarded in virtually all intellectual and behavioral skills attempted with her, including the Callier-Azusa Scale and the Bzoch-League Receptive-Expressive Emergent Language Scale. The Slosson Intelligence Test for children placed this child at a 1 year 4-month-old level, but since many of the testing avenues require adequate visual and auditory capacities, it was premature to label her generally retarded.

ECochG showed an exceptionally sensitive extratympanic ECochG response confirming quite normal peripheral nerve activity in this child despite her apparent behavioral deafness. Conspicuously absent were stapedius muscle reflexes at 120 dB HTL at any frequency. At the time the child was tested, ipsilateral reflex testing was not available to us, and we have not been able to call her back for further testing since. However, in view of her behavioral deafness, with normal cochlear function, only a number of options remain open to us. One is, of course, that she has very poor hearing in the speech frequencies, but a normal basal turn of her cochlea gives us spuriously good ECochG responses to click stimuli. However, in a case such as that, we would expect middle ear muscle reflexes would be present at some frequencies. On subsequent testing we will perform toneburst ECochG and ipsilateral reflex testing to clarify the missing gaps in this analysis. With respect to the absent middle ear muscle reflexes, we could not elicit the reflex even by nonauditory means and she may have some developmental anomaly not uncommon in rubella children, which prevents us from seeing middle ear muscle reflexes, despite Type A tympanograms. Also at the time we tested this patient we were not able to do brain stem evoked potentials. Here, however, ECochG combined with reflex studies suggest a central auditory problem. Another patient with similar auditory behavior was studied with both ECochG *and* brain stem potentials, and in the next section, we will discuss our findings in that patient.

BRAIN STEM POTENTIALS (1-12 MSEC)

Patient C.B., born in November 1973, was referred to us for failure to develop verbal language. Her mother reported

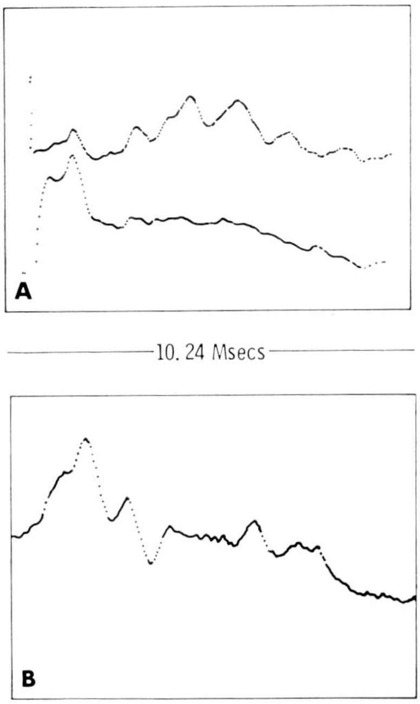

Fig. 5. A) Shows brain stem responses and extratympanic electrocochleogram from normal adult. B) Shows aberrant brain stem responses from patient CB. Stimuli were 10/sec clicks, 86 dB peak sound pressure, repeated 2048 times. Note normal N_1 (VIIIth N AP) in all traces.

that pregnancy was full-term and uncomplicated with no natal or neonatal problems reported. Aside from speech, developmental milestones appeared normal. The child seemed to have normal vision, was easily disciplined, and was cared for by the maternal grandparents in the mother's absence. At age two she showed a Vineland Social Maturity Scale social age equivalent near the 1½ year level. Extratympanic ECochG by air conduction revealed responses in both ears down to 20 dB HL for the clicks used. Bone-conduction ECochG showed normal bone-conduction responses in both ears and early evoked potential data were then taken on this child by moving the extra-tympanic electrode from the ear canal under the scalp at the vertex. Figure 5A shows an ECochG and brain stem response from a normal-hearing adult, while Figure 5B shows the responses taken from patient CB. There is an aberrant waveform at approximately 5 msec which was repeated consistently throughout the test procedure and suggests some form of interruption to the central auditory pathways being reflected in this early evoked potential data.

BACKGROUND FOR EARLY EVOKED POTENTIAL RECORDINGS

Jewett and Williston,[13] among others, have reported on the accessibility of the major nuclei of the auditory system by "far-field recording." The technique is as follows:

A recording electrode is placed at the vertex and subject receives repetitive clicks at a rate of approximately 10/sec. Broad band-pass filters (above 1,000 cycles) and high amplification (10^5 or 10^6 times preamplification) are requisites to obtaining valid data from the brain stem. Workers have acquired data which strongly suggest that the individual waves obtained can be traced to major sites in the auditory nervous system as follows:

*Wave No.**	*Presumed Locus*
1.	cochlear nerve
2.	cochlear nuclei
3.	olivary and trapezoid body nuclei
4. & 5.	interaction of the olivary, lemniscal, and collicular nuclei
6.	medial geniculate

* See Figure 5A for example.

A further review of salient features of brain stem audiometry may be found in Sohmer and Feinmesser,[14] Hecox and Galambos,[15] and Davis.[16]

The fifth wave, probably from the inferior colliculus, is most responsive to low-level stimulation and therefore ideally suited for "audiometric purposes."[17]

The important point here is that if laboratory work is accurate, each of these waves should represent a synchronous discharge of a major nucleus in the auditory system and therefore

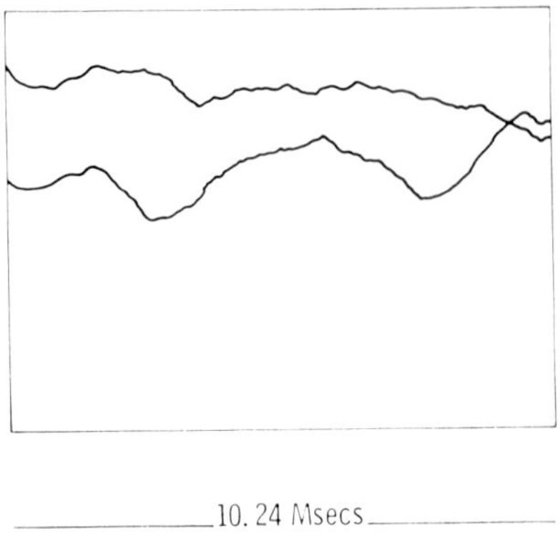

Fig. 6. Abnormal brain stem responses from patient with occlusion of the left vertebral artery. Right-ear stimulation at 111 dB peak sound pressure (approximately 90 dB hearing level).

give neuro-otologic diagnosticians insight into the integrity of these nuclei.

The following patient is a good example. A 56-year-old black male was admitted to the hospital with symptoms of severe vertigo, nausea and vomiting, right-sided headache, and claimed total hearing loss in one ear following complaints of "clicking noises." The patient's blood pressure was 150/100 and, after three-vessel angiography, he was found to have a complete occlusion of the left vertebral artery.

At the time of initial audiologic assessment, he was unable to take a pure tone audiogram, but showed no stapedius reflexes to transcranial stimulation.

He subsequently showed return of pure tone auditory function in a manner remarkably similar to a case reported by Noffsinger *et al*[18] and Applebaum and Ferguson.[19] We did not have the equipment at the time to acquire ipsilateral reflex measurements, but were able to acquire normal ECochG from both ear canals. Figure 6 shows the dysynchrony of brain stem responses in this patient with a superficially normal audiogram but persistent complaints of speech discrimination problems.

Noffsinger *et al*[18] also report their patients had a severely reduced MLD, a test our patient was unable to complete.

The patient remains with a minimal right facial weakness and a left-sided hemiplegia with hyperactive reflexes on the left. He shows that, despite normal pure tone audiometry, physiologic measures can reveal central deficits.

DICHOTIC LISTENING

When two different words are presented, one to each ear simultaneously, the normal nervous system generally perceives the right-ear message more accurately than the left-ear message. Thus, the presentation of two simultaneous signals can be expected to be correlated with the dominance of the left hemisphere for speech and language perception. Figure 7 shows development of the right-ear advantage in boys and girls 7 through 13 years old.[20] Each bar represents the performance of left and right ears, respectively, listening to simultaneous syllables. Analyses published previously show that what is really changing over age is not the differences between right and left ears, but the ability of the normal central nervous system in young children to process increasingly more accurately both members of the pair. This increase in double-correct score seems to be a reflection of central nervous system integrity. We do not see it in patients with known brain lesions, nor do we see it in children with learning disabilities or so-called auditory-processing disabilities.[21] Many people view this right-ear advantage as an index of language dominance of one hemisphere over the other. However, this is not strictly a correct interpretation.

The dichotic CV test is a much more powerful tool in revealing the presence of lesions in either of the temporal lobes, the corpus callosum, and/or the auditory areas of the thalamus. Test results on patients with confirmed lesions of the temporal lobe are, in fact, more dependable and reproducible than test results on patients with normal brains. For example, Figure 8 shows the dichotic listening scores of a right temporal

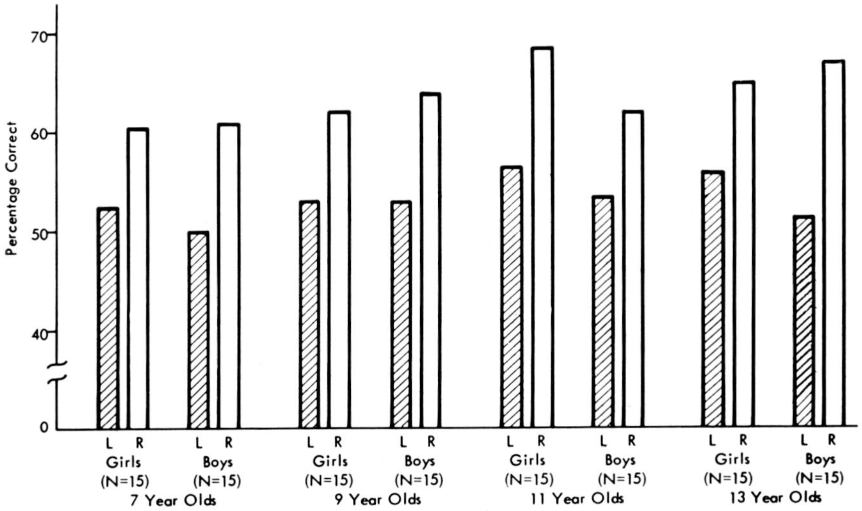

Fig. 7. Dichotic right-ear advantage for children 7 to 13 years of age. Stimuli were 60 pairs of nonsense syllables given simultaneously in both ears. (Adapted from Berlin *et al*[20])

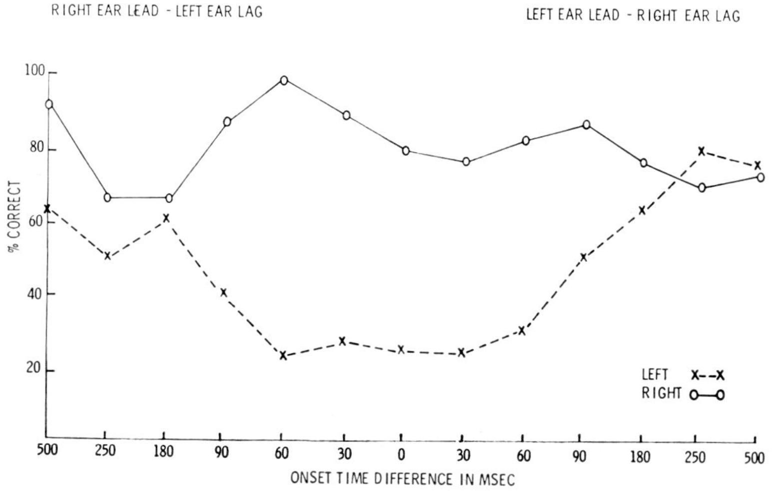

Fig. 8. Percent correct of dichotically-presented simultaneous and time-separated nonsense syllables in a patient with a right temporal lobectomy.

lobectomee at simultaneity and with time separations between the competing syllables. These data have remained stable over 3½ years. Here we see one of the salient features of dichotic listening in the presence of a temporal lobe lesion: there is no "lag effect" in which the second message normally out-performs the initial message.[22,23]

Figure 9 shows the consistency of performance of a left temporal lobectomee on dichotic listening tasks given over 16 months. The effect of his temporal lobe lesion has been to essentially suppress information coming from the right ear and actually allow his left ear to perform better than a normal subject's left ear under comparable dichotic

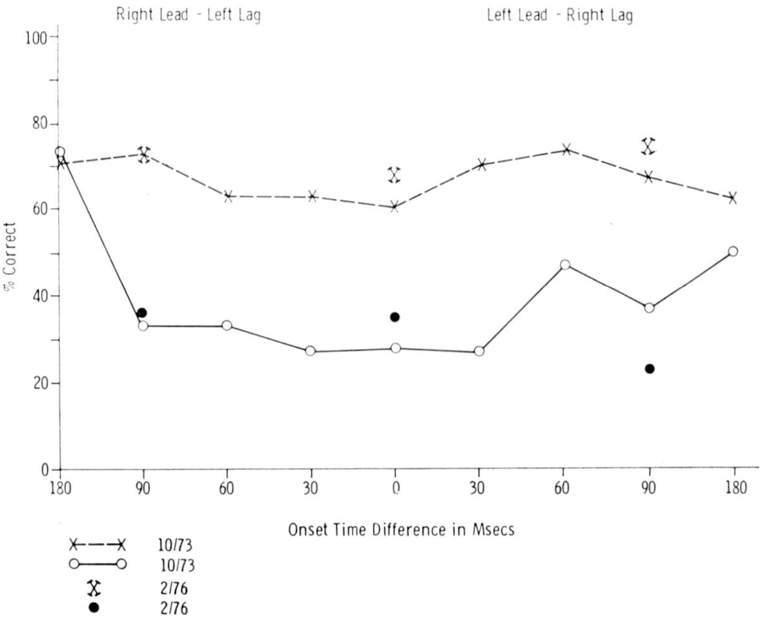

Fig. 9. Percent correct of dichotic simultaneous and time-staggered nonsense syllables presented to a patient (J.Y.) with a left temporal lobectomy. Data presented for test-retest over a 16-month period.

listening circumstances. Most provocative, but of unclear significance, is the repeated observation that the weak (contralateral) ear of these patients seems to surpass the strong ear performance at 180 msec of time separation. We do not see this paradoxical reversal in hemispherectomees or patients with corpus callosum lesions disconnecting the hemispheres.

Dichotic listening tasks have also proven useful in patients with multiple sclerosis who, on some occasions, show lesions of the corpus callosum and hence apparent disconnection between right and left temporal lobes.

SUMMARY

The outline in Figure 1 is meant to summarize the utility of most of the available tests for central auditory dysfunction. Three physiologic tests (ECochG, early brain stem potentials, and middle ear muscle reflexes) and two behavioral tests — MLD and dichotic listening — are discussed in some detail. We commend these five procedures to you as important new tools in the evaluation of central auditory mechanisms.

REFERENCES

1. Hirsh IJ: The influences of interaural phase on interaural summation and inhibition. J Acoust Soc Am 20:536-544, 1948

2. Licklider JCR: The influence of interaural phase relations upon masking of speech by white noise. J Acoust Soc Am 20:150-159, 1948

3. Cranford JL: Auditory masking-level differences in the cat. J Comp Physiol Psychol 89(3):219-223, 1975

4. Cullen JK Jr, Thompson CL: Masking release for speech in subjects with temporal lobe resections. Arch Otolaryngol 100(2):113-116, 1974

5. Olsen WO, Noffsinger D, Carhart R: Masking level differences encountered in clinical populations. Audiology 15(4):287-301, 1976

6. Borg E: On the neuronal organization of the acoustic middle ear reflex. A physiological and anatomical study. Brain Res 49:101-123, 1973

7. Browner RH, Webster DB: Projections of the trapezoid body and the superior olivary

complex of the kangaroo rat *(Dipodomys merriami)*. Brain Behav Evol 11:322-354, 1975

8. Berlin CI, Cullen JK Jr: The physical basis of impedance, in Jerger J (ed): *Handbook of Impedance Measurements.* Dobbs Ferry, New York, American Electromedics Corp., 1975, pp 1-20

9. Jerger J: Diagnostic use of impedance measures, in Jerger J (ed): *Handbook of Clinical Impedance Audiometry.* Dobbs Ferry, New York, American Electromedics Corp., 1975, pp 149-174

10. Berlin CI, Cullen JK Jr, Ellis MS, *et al*: Clinical application of recording human VIII nerve action potentials from the tympanic membrane. Trans Am Acad Ophthalmol Otolaryngol 78:401-410, 1974

11. Aran J-M: The electro-cochleogram: Recent results in children and in some pathological cases. Arch Klin Exp Ohren Nasen Kehlkopfheilkd 198:128-141, 1971

12. Cullen JK Jr, Ellis MS, Berlin CI, *et al*: Human acoustic nerve action potential recordings from the tympanic membrane without anesthesia. Acta Otolaryngol (Stockh) 74: 15-22, 1972

13. Jewett DL, Williston JS: Auditory-evoked far fields averaged from the scalp of humans. Brain 94:681-696, 1971

14. Sohmer H, Feinmesser M: Electrocochleography in clinical-audiological diagnosis. Arch Otolaryngol 206:91-102, 1974

15. Hecox K, Galambos R: Brain stem auditory evoked responses in human infants and adults. Arch Otolaryngol 99:30-33, 1974

16. Davis H: Brain stem and other responses in electric response audiometry. Ann Otol Rhinol Laryngol 85:3-14, 1976

17. Lev A, Sohmer H: Sources of averaged neural responses recorded in animal and human subjects during cochlear audiometry (electrocochleogram). Arch Klin Exp Ohren Nasen Kehlkopfheilkd 201:79-90, 1972

18. Noffsinger D, Kurdziel S, Applebaum EL: Value of special auditory tests in the latero-medial inferior pontine syndrome. Ann Otol Rhinol Laryngol 84:379-383, 1975

19. Applebaum EL, Ferguson RJL: The latero-medial inferior pontine syndrome. Ann Otol Rhinol Laryngol 84(3):379, 1975

20. Berlin CI, Hughes LF, Lowe-Bell SS, *et al*: Dichotic right ear advantage in children 5 to 13. Cortex 9(4):393-401, 1973a

21. Tobey EA, Cullen JK Jr, Rampp DL: Performance of children with auditory-processing disorders on a dichotic, stop-vowel identification task. Paper delivered at the Fourth Annual Meeting of the International Neuropsychology Society, Toronto, Ontario, Canada, February 1976

22. Berlin CI, Lowe-Bell SS, Janetta PJ, *et al*: Central auditory deficits after temporal lobectomy. Arch Otolaryngol 96:4-10, 1972

23. Berlin CI, Lowe-Bell SS, Cullen JK Jr, *et al*: Dichotic speech perception: An interpretation of right-ear advantage and temporal offset effects. J Acoust Soc Am 53:699-709, 1973b

Acknowledgments—We wish to thank Drs. M. Burton, Michael Wilensky, and Barbara Grayson of the Veterans Administration Hospital, Dr. D. G. Fourrier, Maria Gondra, Dr. D. F. Mouney, the Special Education Center of the University of New Orleans, Pamela Weaver, and Gae Decker for their assistance.

Reprints—Charles I. Berlin, PhD, Kresge Hearing Research Laboratory of the South, Dept. of Otorhinolaryngology, Louisiana State University Medical Center, New Orleans, LA 70122.

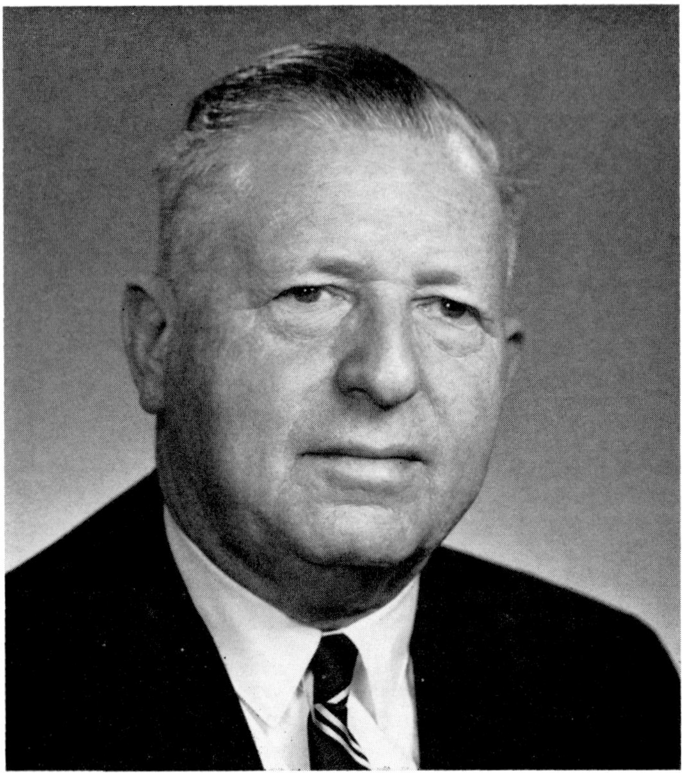

DEAN M. LIERLE, MD

1895 - 1976

DEAN M. LIERLE, MD

Dean McAllister Lierle died August 8, 1976 of natural causes at age 81. He was Professor Emeritus of Otolaryngology and Maxillofacial Surgery of The University of Iowa.

What does one say about a man who was so well known to his specialty as to defy description? He was a world renowned physician and educator. His accomplishments in his specialty were of such proportions that he bore the name "Mr. Otolaryngology" for three decades. At a time when many thought antibiotics had rung the death knell for otolaryngology, he became the acknowledged leader in bringing "ENT" resurgent into modern medicine by fostering diversification and basic research. His greatest satisfaction was in seeing almost all of our training programs respond by becoming basically head and neck surgery programs. Dean Lierle was in great measure responsible for this through his boundless energy and influence in American medicine, his prescience, and his views of the health needs of people which were far ahead of their time.

There are numerous examples of his farsightedness. He was building a training program staff when other programs consisted of essentially little more than preceptorships. He established the first cleft palate team in the United States. At a time when general surgery decried our performing radical cancer surgery and tried everywhere to interdict it on the basis of poor training, he almost single-handedly convinced the American Board of Otolaryngology to lengthen training programs by adding basic surgical training to board requirements. He developed America's first clinical audiologist, Scott N. Reger, PhD.

Dean was a prodigious organizer. As a young man and a brand new board member, he had the audacity to criticize the examination to its then Secretary-Treasurer, Dr. Harris P. Mosher. He was rewarded by being elected his successor after being obviously hand-picked by him. He then vigorously and wisely guided the board for over 20 years. He helped organize the American Board of Plastic Surgery and was a founding member of that Board. He reorganized and ran for years the Home Study Course of The Academy.

In recognition of his vast contribution to otolaryngology, he received virtually every honor his specialty could bestow. Besides being Secretary-Treasurer of the Board, Head of his department, and a Regent of the American College of Surgeons simultaneously, he was elected to the presidency of each of our major specialty societies. This has not been accomplished before or since.

He leaves a significant gap in American medicine.

Brian F. McCabe, MD

SUMMARY REPORTS ON
NATIONAL - INTERNATIONAL CONFERENCES

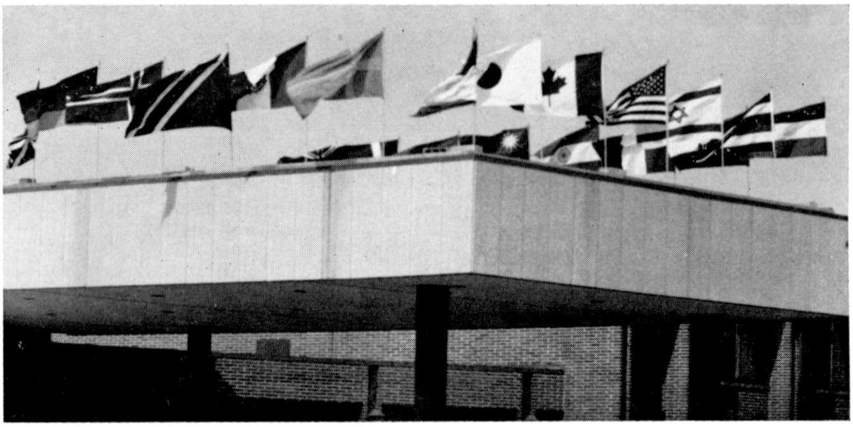

First International Conference on Cholesteatoma

May 25-29, 1976

This conference was held in Iowa City under the auspices of the Department of Otolaryngology and Maxillofacial Surgery of the University of Iowa and attended by speakers and registrants from 25 different countries.

The emphasis was principally in two areas. First, a discussion of recent developments in the biology and pathophysiology of the cells and tissues involved in the cholesteatoma problem, and secondly, a critical look at the success/failure rate of the various surgical techniques in present day use in dealing with the disease. Clinical scientists prepared reviews covering assignments given them one year previously.

The conference began with a definition of cholesteatoma in biological as well as clinical terms. Cholesteatoma was described not simply as skin in the wrong place, but as a three dimensional epidermoid structure exhibiting independent growth, replacing middle ear mucosa, resorbing underlying bone, and tending to recur after removal. The biological definition of cholesteatoma permitted a more abstract discussion so that the biological models used by the scientists in the panel applied to the understanding of the disease. We considered growth control as related to control of mitosis in skin, differentiation of cells under various influences as related to metaplasia, competition in the interphase between different epithelia in terms of cell surface properties, wound healing as a model for cell movement, epithelial mesenchymal interactions, and other factors influencing patterns of cell migration, to name some of the subjects covered.

There appeared to be a definite relationship between the inability for self-cleansing in a cholesteatoma as compared to canal skin, with the promotion of a subepithelium inflammatory reaction. The inflammatory connective tissue promotes bone resorption through decalcification, followed by sequential enzymatic breakdown of bone matrix. While osteoclasts are capable of resorbing bone under normal conditions, evidence was presented that localized bone resorption can occur from inflammatory connective tissue, the action of cells "turned on" by inflammation. This inflammatory connective tissue, while always present under the epithelium of cholesteatoma, is also present in chronic otitis media without cholesteatoma. No evidence was evinced that stratified squamous epithelium of itself had any destructive or noxious properties.

Ten experienced otologic surgeons presented their longest term results available on different operative techniques, especially including "closed cavity" techniques. This series of presentations entitled "Tell Me About Your Failures!" was followed by a panel discussion among them which engendered a considerable difference of opinion, indicating that we are far from the final word. Indeed, there appeared evidence we may be in some state of regression from the enthusiastic acceptance of the "canal up" mastoidectomy of the past decade. At the same time, in presentations on rates of complication, it was evident that not only have complications from cholesteatomatous disease in itself dropped dramatically from earlier years, but "canal up" procedures do not seem to have been attendant with any reversal of this trend. Circumscribed mastoiditis (positive fistula test) is by far the most common complication today, excluding progressive conductive deafness. The two most noteworthy features of this part of the conference were, 1) there is a definite need for longer followup in these newer operations for adequate evaluation, and 2) at least a few surgeons voiced willingness to give them up.

Epidemiologic studies pointed out that ethnic groups with a high rate of central perforations) Eskimos, Indians, Australian aborigines) did not have a disproportionately high cholesteatoma rate, whereas groups with a high rate of Eustachian tube "insufficiency" (cleft palate patients) did. Moreover, cholesteatoma patients had a higher rate of Eustachian tube "insufficiency" than noncholesteatoma patients, it appears from exisiting work, admitting the comparatively primative state of the art. Other studies seemed to establish at least a frequent *genetically* established mastoid hypocellularity, a feature of this disease chronically underestimated in terms of middle ear aerodynamics.

The three theories of genesis of cholesteatoma, *viz,* acquired, congenital, and metaplastic, were presented and discussed in detail.

While it became evident that most otologists today view cholesteatoma as a purely surgical disease, it was evident that selected patients are best served by office management. Further, a new form of medical management was introduced (without, to date, suitable controls or long term follow-up) which could be revolutionary in cholesteatoma management: topical vitamin A therapy (New Zealand). Plans were laid for the evaluation of this modality multinationally.

Finally, although an auspicious beginning was made in understanding the pathophysiology and treatment of this disease involving many of our best basic and clinical scientists, it was evident that many more questions were raised than were answered. Perhaps the greatest yield of the conference was in bringing the expertise and interest of our colleagues in basic science to bear on our problem. Future such conferences, we hope, will extend this, and through mutual effort result in the eradication of this disease.

Full proceedings of the conference including discussions, questions and answers, will be available from Aesculapius Publishing Company, Birmingham, Alabama, in four to five months.

Brian F. McCabe, MD
Jacob Sadé, MD
Maxwell Abramson, MD
Cochairmen

COMMUNICATIONS

Dear Editor:

Dr. Titche's recent communication about tetracaine reflects the enormous and gratifying experience one man has had with the use of this drug.[1] The question however, is not really whether we should use cocaine or tetracaine, but rather providing for the safe use of either.

We attempted to show that cocaine is an *unexcelled* topical anesthetic because no other compound presently available can provide cocaine's duration of topical anesthesia, margin of safety, membrane shrinkage and vasoconstriction.[2] Tetracaine requires the addition of epinephrine to provide the last two properties, and is certainly not superior in the first two.

Dr. Titche states that there have been no reports of tetracaine reactions since 1951. To account for this we may reasonably assume that a tetracaine reaction is no longer a reportable event, or that physician education in the use of this drug has precluded further disaster. Let us examine briefly the pre-1951 tetracaine morbidity.

In a study of 1000 cases, Weisel and Tella reported 19 reactions, 12 minor, 7 severe with the topical use of tetracaine.[3] In contrast to Titche's 0.5% solution, they utilized a 2% solution but claimed that the total dose was held below 30 to 40 mg. (The accepted clinical limit today is similar.) Himalstein[4] quotes Ireland's statistics showing tetracaine reactions occur twice as often as cocaine reactions. Adriani and Campbell[5] (in *1956*, incidentally) noted ten fatalities following the topical application of tetracaine for endoscopy in a 15-year period at Charity Hospital. They felt conclusively that the hospital records indicated an obvious overdosage in each case. But even more perturbing is the lack of *prodrome* with tetracaine. "The major distinction between reactions due to tetracaine and those of other topical anesthetics has been the absence of convulsions and the abrupt onset of syncope. The interval between the onset of symptoms and the moment of fatal termination was brief. The train of events occurred so quickly, and in such rapid succession, that there was little time for evaluation of symptoms, differential diagnosis, and antidotal therapy."[5] This statement implies that at least with other topical anesthetics the physician has a chance to step in.

And finally, Titche fails to mention Rubin's study[6] demonstrating tetracaine to be six times as toxic to animals as cocaine. Clinically this may be inconsequential though, as a 1% tetracaine solution would have the same toxicity as a 6% cocaine solution.

The important fact to reap from Dr. Titche's experience and the foregoing comments is that both cocaine and tetracaine are safe drugs *only* when used by experienced operators who abide by the two prime rules of limited dosage and extended time of application.

Sincerely,

Nicholas L. Schenck, MD

1281 South Hickory St.
Melbourne, FL 32901

REFERENCES

1. Titche LL: Communication to the Editor, Ann Otol Rhinol Laryngol 85:149, 1976

2. Schenck NL: Local anesthesia in otolaryngology. A Reevaluation. Ann Otol Rhinol Laryngol 84: 65-72, 1975

3. Weisel W, Tella RA: Reaction to tetracaine (pontocaine) used as topical anesthetic in bronchoscopy. JAMA 147:218-222, 1951

4. Himalstein MR: The problem in endoscopic topical anesthesia. Arch Otolaryngol 63:60-66, 1956

5. Adriani J, Campbell D: Fatalities following topical application of anesthesia to mucous membranes. JAMA 162:1527-1530, 1956

6. Rubin HJ: Toxicity of certain topical anesthetics used in otolaryngology: an experimental study. Arch Otolaryngol 53:411-420, 1951

Dear Editor:

Dr. J. Sadé, in a paper entitled "Facial Nerve Reconstruction and Its Prognosis,"[1] presented some very essential data in terms of 1) long-term evaluation; 2) electrical transmission through the nerve; and 3) effect of procaine. However, I think it appropriate to point out additional features of disorders of the facial nerve which have bearing upon some of the data he presented and therefore its interpretation.

1. With total anatomical division of the facial nerve, there is not paralysis of the upper lid. The widened palpebral fissure is due to paralysis of the lower lid and its "sagging" and to restriction of movement of the upper lid (see No. 2).

2. The degree of movement of the upper lid in permanent transection anatomically of the facial nerve is dependent upon the position of gaze, namely the eyeballs. 1) If such a patient is asked to look upward and then close his eyes – the upper lid will descend to the level of a line connecting the internal and external canthus. 2) If the same patient is asked to look straight ahead and then close his eyes, the upper lid will descend again to this line. There will be incomplete closure due to failure of elevation of the lower lid. 3) If the patient is asked to look down and then close his eyes – in fact, the descended upper lid will elevate to the meridian indicated above.

3. Tone returns to facial musculature after denervation and renervation first and for some weeks before any movement or any type is detected. Very often this increase in tone produces elevation of the lower lid so indeed the palpebral fissure is smaller in that side. This is shown in Dr. Sadé's pictures.

4. Similarly when attempt is made to close both eyes, as in one picture, part of the mass

movement on the affected side raises the lower lid, excessively closing the palpebral fissure. The closure is in no way the same or similar to that on a normal side.

5. Many types of associated movements, such as opening the jaw, *etc.*, may initiate a mass movement on the implicated side.

6. These precise movement patterns are seen in patients in whom there is recovery from nonanatomically transected nerves – so-called Bell's palsy. Here where the sheaths of involved axons allegedly are intact, that recovery, if it is due to regrowth of axons, should not be dependent upon finding proper passageway. Specifically structural sheath anatomy presumably has not been changed, only something which has happened in the axon or indeed in its conduction mechanism. Specifically, some of the so-called inflammatory lesions of facial nerve may simply be focal conductive defects without axonal loss. Similarly, even compressive lesion of the facial nerve may represent focal conduction defects as occur elsewhere with segmental demyelination. Here there should be no problem of axons finding their correct path back to appropriate structures.

7. It is of importance that electrical conductivity was demonstrated in five patients and that procaine block did not abolish upper eye lid movement. The reason for this is explained above. It shouldn't.

8. The same type of restoration of function of the face is seen after hypoglossal facial anastomosis, namely, there is return of tone. There is movement of the face – mass movement associated with movement of the tongue.

9. Indeed in nonanatomical interruption of facial nerve function, restoration of voluntary control of isolated facial movement may occur. This however, is rare and minimal in the facial nerve in which there has been anatomical interruption no matter what the anastomosis. On occasion, I think I have observed after long periods, very minimal focal voluntary contraction of muscles at angle of mouth on affected side after hypoglossal focal anastomosis – but this is unusual and it is hard to dissociate from tongue movement.

10. It is also important to note that frontalis function very often does not participate in mass action even if it involves the remainder of the face.

The significance of these points resides in specifically what Dr. Sadé has indicated regarding anastomosis of the facial nerve. In some patients when anastomosis is done early, there may be some return of real facial volitional movement, but the chances are, this will not be great. On the other side of the coin, as he mentions, in partial lesions and directly by partial section of part of the nerve, as in hemifacial spasm, there can be amazing voluntary function of the total face after some weeks. This has been my experience also in section of the facial nerve in hemifacial spasm.

In recovery from all peripheral nerve lesions, anatomically complete and resutured, the most focal skilled fine movements are the last to recover, if at all in most instances. There is a big difference between recovery of gross movements produced by radial nerve and those fine movements subserved by the ulnar nerve.

There is a basic principle involved but I am not sure it can be explained by peripheral events. Axonal sprouting has been invoked in many areas to explain restoration of function. This may indeed assume some role, but the character of recovery is another item. The return of normal precise voluntary control of movement in any area is probably dependent upon mechanisms which are not simply peripheral. Similarly, the lack of recovery of such movement also perhaps cannot be explained by hypothesis which involves only potential peripheral mechanisms. The organization of movement as "posture patterns" employs the peripheral anatomical units; peripheral nerve, plexi roots, *etc.* However, the manner in which they are employed (each unit) to produce the symphony or movement characteristic of normal voluntary function is dependent upon central mechanisms. Why if the peripheral mechanisms are intact, but there is misdirection of growth of fibers should there not be some facial, although inappropriate response to the will, emotion, *etc*? Characteristically, facial movements are engaged to express emotion by contraction of certain muscles and relaxation of others. If the problem was simply misdirection of fibers, certain emotions should indeed produce inappropriate facial contractions and inhibition – not mass movement. Although I do not propose to know the answer to these problems, I think Dr. Sadé's point is well taken regarding proper evaluation of facial movements and what can be expected from repair. Indeed, under some circumstances, a similar functional result would be just as good without operation, particularly in partial lesions.

Yours truly,
ALBERT W. COOK, MD

State University of New York
Downstate Medical Center
450 Clarkson Ave.
Brooklyn, NY 11203

REFERENCES

1. Sadé J: Facial nerve reconstruction and its prognosis. Ann Otol Rhinol Laryngol 84:695-703, 1975

BOOK REVIEWS

Early Identification of Hearing Loss

Edited by *George T. Mencher.* Soft cover, illustrated, referenced, 207 pp. (Proceedings of the Nova Scotia Conference, Halifax, Nova Scotia, September 1974) S. Karger, PO Box 352, White Plains, NY 10602. Price $20.00

This volume reports the proceedings of the Nova Scotia Conference on Early Identification of Hearing Loss held in Halifax in June 1974. There a dedicated group of over 25 participants from Canada, USA, Sweden, Israel, Poland, and Italy reported their research studies of methods of neonatal and childhood screening and auditory testing, and actual trials of the effectiveness of the high risk register as a means of increasing the efficiency of identification procedures. The volume represents an authoritative overview of the state of the art and practical procedures. The recommendations that were adopted center around the high risk register and repeated testing of the infants at risk. An earlier statement, dated July 1970, had discouraged routine neonatal hearing testing, and defined the register as follows:

> "The Committee recommends that, since no satisfactory technique is yet established that will permit hearing screening of all newborns, infants *at risk* for hearing impairment should be identified by means of history and physical examination. The criterion for identifying a newborn as *at risk* for hearing impairment is the presence of one or more of the following:
>
> A. History of hereditary childhood hearing impairment.
>
> B. Rubella or other nonbacterial intrauterine fetal infection (*e.g.*, cytomegalovirus infections, herpes infection).
>
> C. Defects of ear, nose, or throat. Malformed, low-set or absent pinnae; cleft lip or palate (including submucous cleft); any residual abnormality of the otorhinolaryngeal system.
>
> D. Birthweight less than 1500 grams.
>
> E. Bilirubin level greater than 20 mg/100 ml serum."

An important new study (Feinmesser and Tell, Israel) recommends adding to the criteria for high risk, F) apnea and cyanosis (apgar score 1-4), and G) severe neonatal infection. The most promising neonatal test seems to be the crib-o-gram (F.B. Simmons, Stanford, Calif.) which is an automated hearing screening test for newborns. The method is now well-developed. The data are carefully analyzed but are not yet sufficient for a final assessment.

The last sentence of the editor's introduction is very pertinent: "Clearly, controversy must now shift to 'how' early identification programs can be implemented as quickly as possible, and not 'which' program to use."

HALLOWELL DAVIS, MD

Patient Care and Rehabilitation of Communication-Impaired Adults

By *Ralph R. Leutenegger,* PhD. Hard cover, indexed and referenced, 178 pp, 1975. Charles C. Thomas, Springfield, IL 62717. Price $12.50

This book was written to inform those in contact with adult patients with communication problems about the extent and nature of communication problems and the role these problems present to total rehabilitation. A brief cursory treatment of specific disorders, particularly laryngectomy, and certain aspects of clinical emphasis, particularly rehabilitative audiology, eliminate it as a choice as a basic text in a speech pathology sequence. However, the book presents a good deal of information which should be helpful in understanding the role of these professionals in rehabilitative programs or home substitute settings.

A major contribution of this book is the attempt to facilitate the development of a team approach by describing the training and roles in rehabilitation of the four disciplines with which the book is most directly involved: physical therapy, occupational therapy, speech rehabilitation, and nursing. The author stresses the desirability of including patient and family as members of the team.

In addition to a valuable chapter on changes which occur with aging, special attention is directed to the hard of hearing and poststroke patients, laryngectomees, and patients with multiple sclerosis and Parkinson's disease. The book provides extensive bibliographies.

LINDA S. JORDAN, PHD

The Nervous System, Volume 3: Human Communication and Its Disorders

Editor-in-Chief, *Donald B. Tower, MD;* Volume Editor, *Eldon L. Eagles, MD.* Hard cover, black and white illustrations, indexed and referenced, 576 pp, 1976. Raven Press, 1140 Avenue of the Americas, New York, NY 10036. Price $25.00

"Human Communication and Its Disorders" is the third of a three-volume work celebrating the 25th anniversary of the National Institute of Neurological and Communicative Disorders and Stroke. It is a well-edited collection of more than 50 chapters. Each contributor was asked to describe recent research work in a defined area. They were remarkably successful in achieving a consistent standard of excellence. The compilation covers the field comprehensively. Raven Press shares the credit with the contributors for the up-to-date nature of the material because it published the volume unusually quickly.

From the first chapter, about the fine structure of the inner ear, to the last, about electrical stimulation of the cochlear nerve, the reader is exposed to the latest published work from each of the major laboratories concerned with this field in the United States.

Clinical research is included as well as basic. There is a progress report on laryngeal surgery, a description of how to manage children with communicative disorders, and a chapter on surgical management of hearing loss. Basic subjects include biochemistry and several chapters on physiology of audition. Many of the chapters have the virtue of combining basic techniques with clinical problems: *e.g.*, computer summation as used for recording evoked responses. As a group, they define the field of "human communication and its disorders."

The index seems rather sketchy and was inadequate for searching a few topics chosen at random. However, in many other instances, the index served its purpose well.

The book should serve to stimulate new research because it provides a clear picture of "where we are" in many different areas. A reader can scarcely avoid getting ideas for projects that would offer new ways to look at some of the old problems. It will certainly be helpful to investigators as a place to get started when searching the literature.

A particularly impressive feature of the book is its lack of repetition. The editorial committee is deserving of considerable credit for doing a fine job in choosing topics that avoided overlap and in assembling the contributions intelligently.

DAVID A. HILDING, MD

Self Assessment of Current Knowledge in Allergy

By *Claude A. Frazier, MD.* Soft cover, 169 pp, 1976. Medical Examination Publishing Co., Inc., 65-36 Fresh Meadow Land, Flushing, NY 11365. Price $10.00

This is a collection of 860 multiple choice questions with referenced answers. The booklet is divided into 16 sections, each compiled by a different author or authors.

A proliferation of such lists in various specialties has been occasioned by the threat or reality of recertification. One absolute requirement for a self-assessment test is that it be authoritative. The questions *and answers* must bear close resemblance to those which might be encountered in a certifying examination. Unfortunately, such is not always the case here. The book is poorly edited and uneven. Parts of it are well done and suited for the purpose intended, whereas other parts are woefully inadequate and misleading. The preparation of a test of this sort requires much time and considerable experience before suitable questions are distilled from many, including ambiguous, trivial, controversial, erroneous and otherwise unsuitable questions.

An example of a controversial area waded into carelessly is in the section on "management of CSOM" (chronic serous otitis media). The answers indicate erroneously that CSOM is usually caused by allergy, that foods play an important role as allergens in CSOM and that "low dose-Hansel - more otology related" school has delivered more benefit to patients with CSOM than the "high dose-conventional allergist related." In Section VI (Insect Sting Allergy) one learns that the principal *peptide* from honeybee venom is melittin, but in Section IX (Allergic Reactions and Immunology) we find that the major *antigen* in bee venom is phospholipase A. The latter has recently been found to be an oversimplification and the two questions taken together are confusing.

Trivial questions abound. Under Section X Aerobiology, we are asked when hayfever occurs in Tehran, Iran, and find that it occurs during the tree, grass and weed seasons!

One may profitably use this book as a casual and somewhat irregular review of allergy, provided he knows what areas are controversial and which of the references cited are authoritative and dependable. More suitable for the allergist or otolaryngologist preparing for a certifying examination and desiring such a quiz are self-assessment tests prepared by the American Board of Internal Medicine and its subspecialties. The American Board of Allergy and Immunology, in preparation for recertification, is planning a self-assessment test which should be more helpful and certainly more authoritative than the booklet reviewed here.

HAL B. RICHERSON, MD

AUTHOR INDEX

ABRAMSON, A. L., 394
Allansmith, M. R., 391
Allard, L. F., 310
Andréasson, L., 198
Andrews, A. H., Jr., 625
Antoine, J. E., 408
Arena, S., 404
Atkins, J. P., Jr., 646

BABIN, R. W., 387
Bailey, B. J., 472
Bailey, L. L., 625
Balkany, T. J., 368
Baloh, R. W., 111
Barton, R. P. E., 74
Becker, G., 652
Benjamin, B., 565
Benjamin, S. P., 387
Bergholtz, L. M., 679
Berlin, C. I., 833
Bicknell, P. G., 105
Birck, H., 50
Bloustine, S., 406
Bobbin, R. P., 247
Bohne, B. A., 711
Bone, R. C., 417
Brodnitz, F. S., 210
Bryce, D. P., 538
Burns, H. P., 538
Butcher, J., 101

CALCATERRA, T. C., 71
Carden, E., 652
Carr, C. D., 185
Clemente, M. A. C. P., 508
Coates, H. L., 504
Cohen, S. R., 484, 582
Coon, R. L., 664
Cooperband, S. R., 508

D'AMATO, R. F., 394
Davidson, T. M., 417
Davis, H., 3, Suppl. No. 28
Dedo, H. H., 451
Deeb, Z. E., 86
Devine, K. D., 504
Dropkin, L. R., 399
Drucker, I., 327
Dublin, W. B., 813
Duvall, A. J., III, 234

EDMONDS, C., 61
Everett, R., 472

FERNANDEZ, M. G., 86
Fitch, N., 268
Floyd, W. N., 147
Føns, M., 359
Frost, E. A. M., 618

GACEK, R. R., 90, 139, 215, 305, 460
Giordano, A., 631
Gondra, M. I., 247
Gorenstein, R., 670
Gould, W. J., 377
Griffiths, C. M., 472
Guralnick, W., 692
Gussen, R., 94

HAJDU, S. I., 498
Hall, C. M., 255
Hallberg, O., 286
Hamood, H., 652
Hardy, J. M., 523
Hawkins, J. E., Jr., 725
Healy, G. B., 508
Hellqvist, H., 286
Herzon, F., 408
Hirano, M., 25
Hirose, H., 334
Hirschhorn, K., 281
Holinger, L. D., 368, 428, 591
Holinger, P. C., 428
Holinger, P. H., 428, 591
Holsclaw, D. S., 631
Honrubia, V., 111, 697
Hooper, R. E., 679
House, J., 71
House, W. F., Suppl. No. 27
Hukee, M. J., 234

ISAACS, H., Jr., 484
Isenberg, H. D., 394

JACKSON, R. T., 65, 83
Jafek, B. W., 646
Janowak, M. C., 600
Johnson, D. W., 43
Johnsson, L-G., 310, 725
Jung, A. L., 573

KAMPINE, J. P., 664
Katz, R. B., 826
Khan, K. M., Suppl. No. 32
Kiang, N. Y. S., 752
Kiessling, P. J., 417
Kimura, R. S., 791
Kitajima, K., 377
Konrad, H. R., 111
Krausen, A. S., 686
Kripke, B. J., 656
Kumley, W. E., 111
Kutnick, S. L., 591

LANDING, B. H., 582
Langston, L., 406
Lawson, L. J., 613
Levine, R. A., 752
Lewis, J. S., 498
Lewy, R. B., 440
Liberman, M. C., 752
Lim, D. J., 50, 750
Lindeman, R. C., 609
Lindsay, J. R., 15, 169, 268, 343

Lingeman, R. E., 613
Liu, Y. S., 50
Lorente de Nó, R., Suppl. No. 34
Lyon, M. J., 460

MAEDA, S., Suppl. No. 31
Magnusson, P., 286
Maisel, R. H., 517
Makishima, K., 826
Marlowe, F. I., 101
Marovitz, W. F., 225, Suppl. No. 32
Martinelli, D. L., 600
Mathog, R. H., 43
McDonald, T. J., 504
McGill, T., 120
McKenzie, B., 61
Mehta, D. C., 679
Mendlowitz, J. C., 281
Mercke, U., 32
Merifield, D. O., 255
Merrell, H. B., 255
Miller, T., 406
Mogi, G., Suppl. No. 31
Montgomery, W. W., 491, 523
Moore, G. P., 553

NAFTALIN, L., 38
Nager, G. T., 204
Nathanson, S. E., 83
Neel, B., III, 670
Noffsinger, D., 820
Norton, M. L., 656

OGURA, J. H., 425, 517
Oh, M., Suppl. No. 31
Olsen, W. O., 820
Olson, N. R., 533
O'Reilly, B., 565
Ota, C. Y., 791

PAGE, R., 86
Palva, T., 410
Parker, S. W., 127
Parkin, J. L., 573
Peacor, D., 310
Pennington, C. L., 437
Pluznik, N., 276
Prudlow, W. F., 664
Pryor, W. H., Jr., 394

QUICK, C. A., 776

RAUCHBACH, E., 136
Rayl, J. E., 627
Riiber, H., 286
Roberson, G., 415
Ross, M. D., 310
Rowe, L. D., 646
Rubinstein, M., 276

SADÉ, J., 327
Sakata, E., 261
Sanderson, D. R., 670
Sando, I., 368
Sasaki, C. T., 382
Schild, J. A., 591
Schuknecht, H. F., 791
Senturia, B. H., 1, 2
Shapiro, R. S., 101
Shugar, J. M. A., 225, Suppl. No. 32
Silberman, H. D., 640
Sills, A. W., 111
Silverstein, H., 769
Sitko, S. T., 697
Sklansky, B. D., 544
Smith, S. A., 491
Snow, J. B., Jr., 826
Snow, J. C., 656
Solis, O., 415
Soudijn, E. R., Suppl. No. 29
Spector, G. J., 185, 802
Spiro, R. H., 498
Srolovitz, H., 268
Stead, J., Suppl. No. 30
Stephens, R. W., 613
Stevens, M. H., 573
Strelioff, D., 697
Strong, E. W., 498
Strong, M. S., 508, 656
Stroud, M. H., 136
Suga, F., 15, 169, 343
Sutton, D., 609
Suzuki, M., 382
Szpunar, J., 291

TAKAHASHI, T., 791
Takeda, T., 769
Tang, C. K., 399
Taylor, P. H., 105
Titche, L. L., 149
Toohill, R. J., 600
Toremalm, N. G., 32
Torok, N., 131
Traxel, R. M., 664
Trible, W. M., 86
Tucker, G. F., Jr., Suppl. No. 30
Tucker, J. A., 640, Suppl. No. 30

UMEDA, Y., 261

VANDERVEEN, T. S., 204
Van De Water, T. R., Suppl. No. 33
van Nostrand, A. W. P., 538
Vaughan, C. W., 508, 656
Vidic, B., Suppl. No. 30

WEBER, A. L., 147, 415, 544, 692
Weiland, L. H., 504
Weisman, Z., 327
Weiss, A. D., 127
Widström, A., 286
Wilf, H., 640
Williams, J. R., 399
Wilson, W. R., 391
Wood, R. P., II, 368
Woodman, D., 437

YARINGTON, C. T., JR., 609

ZUPERKU, E. J., 664

SUBJECT INDEX

ABDUCTOR Paralysis, Bilateral, 30 Years' Experience with Arytenoidectomy. D. Woodman, C. L. Pennington, 437.

Abductor Vocal Cord Paralysis, Bilateral, Etiology of. L. D. Holinger, P. C. Holinger, P. H. Holinger, 428.

Acoustic Hyperstimulation and Ototoxicity, Ultrastructural Cochlear Changes Following. D. J. Lim, 740.

Acoustic Neurinoma, Inner Ear Degeneration in. F. Suga, J. R. Lindsay, 343.

Acoustic Trauma, Effect of Anesthesia on Susceptibility to. M. Rubinstein, N. Pluznik, 276.

Acquired and Congenital Subglottic Stenosis in Infant. J. L. Parkin, M. H. Stevens, A. L. Jung, 573.

Acute Epiglottitis in Infants and Children. B. Benjamin, B. O'Reilly, 565.

Adenocarcinoma Originating in the Thyroglossal Duct. A. Widstrom, P. Magnusson, O. Hallberg, H. Hellqvist, H. Riiber, 286.

Adenoids, Human Adult, and Middle Ear Mucosa, Tissue Culture of. L. Drucker, Z. Weisman, J. Sadé, 327.

Afferent Nerves, Tracheal. R. M. Traxel, W. F. Prudlow, J. P. Kampine, R. L. Coon, E. J. Zuperku, 664.

Air Humidity and Mucociliary Activity. U. Mercke, N. G. Toremalm, 32.

Ameloblastoma, X-Ray of Month: A. L. Weber, W. Guralnick, 692.

Anesthesia, Effect on Susceptibility to Acoustic Trauma. M. Rubinstein, N. Pluznik, 276.

Anesthesia, Local for Suspension Microlaryngoscopy. T. C. Calcaterra, J. House, 71.

Angiofibroma, Juvenile Nasopharyngeal: X-Ray of Month. O. Solis, G. Roberson, A. L. Weber, 415.

Anoxic Anoxia, Hearing Loss of Central Type Secondary to. K. Makishima, R. B. Katz, J. B. Snow, Jr., 826.

Antihistamines: Guidelines and Implications. A. S. Krausen, 686.

Arnold's (Ear-Cough) Reflex. S. Bloustine, L. Langston, T. Miller, 406.

Arthrogryposis Multiplex Congenita, Otolaryngological Manifestations of. S. R. Cohen, H. Isaacs, Jr., 484.

Arytenoidectomy, 30 Years' Experience with, in Bilateral Abductor Paralysis. D. Woodman, C. L. Pennington, 437.

Aspiration, Intractable, Clinical Experience with Tracheoesophageal Anastomosis for. C. Lindeman, C. T. Yarington, Jr., D. Sutton, 609.

Audiohistogram, Combined Correlated, Incorporation of the Superior Ventral Cochlear Nucleus. W. B. Dublin, 813.

Audiometry, Electric Response, Brain Stem and Other Responses in. H. Davis, 3.

Audiometry, Electric Response, Principles of. H. Davis, Supplement No. 28.

Auditory and Vestibular Manifestations in Carcinomatous Encephalomyelitis. T. McGill, 120.

Auditory Imperception. D. O. Merifield, C. M. Hall, H. B. Merrell, 255.

Auditory Mechanisms, Central, New Developments in Evaluating. C. I. Berlin, 833.

Auditory-Nerve Activity in Cats Exposed to Ototoxic Drugs and High-Intensity Sounds. N. Y. S. Kiang, M. C. Liberman, R. A. Levine, 752.

BAROTRAUMA, Sinus in Divers. P. Fagan, B. McKenzie, C. Edmonds, 61.

Bilateral Abductor Paralysis, 30 Years' Experience with Arytenoidectomy. D. Woodman, C. L. Pennington, 437.

Brain Stem and Cochlear Lesions, Masking Level Differences for. W. O. Olsen, D. Noffsinger, 820.

Brain Stem and Other Responses in Electric Response Audiometry. H. Davis, 3.

Bronchial Abnormalities and Tracheostenosis Associated with Pulmonary Artery Sling. S. R. Cohen, B. H. Landing, 582.

Bronchoscopy, Fiberoptic, Newer Techniques in. J. P. Atkins, Jr., L. D. Rowe, B. W. Jafek, 646.

CALORIC and Optokinetic Nystagmus in Cerebellar Patients. M. H. Stroud, E. Rauchbach, 136.

Caloric Eye-Tracking Pattern Test: I. Visual Suppression and Possibility of Simplified Differential Diagnosis between Peripheral and Central Vertigo. E. Sakata, Y. Umeda, 261.

Carcinoma, Epidermoid, Arising from Within an Epidermoid Inclusion Cyst. T. M. Davidson, R. C. Bone, P. J. Kiessling, 417.

Carcinoma, Verrucous of Larynx: Management by Radiotherapy and Surgery. H. P. Burns, A. W. P. van Nostrand, D. P. Bryce, 538.

Carcinomatous Encephalomyelitis with Auditory and Vestibular Manifestations. T. McGill, 120.

Cardiopulmonary-Nasal Reflexes: Role of Larynx. R. T. Jackson, 65.

Central Auditory Mechanisms, New Developments in Evaluating. C. I. Berlin, 833.

Central Nervous System Disease, Electronystagmographic Manifestations of. S. W. Parker, A. D. Weiss, 127.

Central Nervous System Disease, Vestibular Decruitment in. Torok, 131.

Central Type Hearing Loss Secondary to Anoxic Anoxia. K. Makishima, R. B. Katz, J. B. Snow, Jr., 826.

Cerebellar Patients, Caloric and Optokinetic Nystagmus in. M. H. Stroud, E. Rauchbach, 136.

Cervical Fistula, Preauricular Pit, Hearing Loss Syndrome, Temporal Bone in. N. Fitch, J. R. Lindsay, H. Srolovitz, 268.

Cholesteatoma, First International Conference on, 844.

Cholesterol Granuloma Involving the Temporal Bone. G. T. Nager, T. S. Vanderveen, 204.

Clinical Experience with Tracheoesophageal Anastomosis for Intractable Aspiration. R. C. Lindeman, C. T. Yarington, Jr., D. Sutton, 609.

Clinical Manifestations of Leprous Rhinitis. R. P. E. Barton, 74.

CO_2 Laser Management of Recurrent Respiratory Papillomatosis. M. S. Strong, C. W. Vaughan, S. R. Cooperband, G. B. Healy, M. A. C. P. Clemente, 508.

Cochlear and Brain Stem Lesions, Masking Level Differences for. W. O. Olsen, D. Noffsinger, 820.

Cochlear Changes, Ultrastructural, Following Acoustic Hyperstimulation and Ototoxicity. D. J. Lim, 740.

Cochlear Duct, Rodent, Single Mitotic Center for. W. F. Marovitz, J. M. A. Shugar, 225.

Cochlear Findings in Bilateral Ménière's Disease, Electron Microscopic Observations. R. S. Kimura, C. Y. Ota, H. F. Schuknecht, T. Takahashi, 791.

Cochlear Function and Noise-Induced Hair Cell Loss, Effect of Nicotine on. R. P. Bobbin, M. I. Gondra, 247.

Cochlear Glycogen, Delineation of by Electron Microscopy. A. J. Duvall III, M. J. Hukee, 234.

Cochlear Implants. W. F. House, Suppl. No. 27.

Cochlear Nerve, Some Unresolved Problems Concerning. R. Lorente de Nó, Suppl. No. 34.

Cochlear Nucleus, Superior Ventral, Incorporation of; Combined Correlated Audiohistogram. W. B. Dublin, 813.

Cochlear Transduction and Sensitivity, Physiological Basis of. V. Honrubia, D. Strelioff, S. T. Sitko, 697.

Cohn, Mrs. Irene, Tribute to a Great Lady. B. H. Senturia, 2.

Combined Correlated Audiohistogram, Incorporation of the Superior Ventral Cochlear Nucleus. W. B. Dublin, 813.

Congenital Laryngeal Defects in Adult. W. W. Montgomery, S. A. Smith, 491.

Congenital Tracheoesophageal Fistulas in Adults. R. W. Stephens, R. E. Lingeman, L. J. Lawson, 613.

Correlation of Tubal Function and Volume of Mastoid and Middle Ear Space as Related to Otitis Media. L. Andréasson, 198.

Corti Organ Development, Spiral Migration Theory of. W. F. Marovitz, J. M. A. Shugar, K. M. Khan, Suppl. No. 32.

Cricoarytenoid, Posterior, as a Speech Muscle. H. Hirose, 334.

Cryosurgery, Transbronchoscopic of Respiratory Structures: Experimental and Clinical Studies. A. Gorenstein, H. B. Neel III, D. R. Sanderson, 670.

DEAFNESS, Sensory and Neural, Histopathologic and Experimental Models for. G. J. Spector, 802.

Deafness, Sudden, of Vascular Origin: Human Temporal Bone Study. R. Gussen, 94.

Decruitment, Vestibular, in Central Nervous System Disease. N. Torok, 131.

Degeneration Patterns in Human Ears Exposed to Noise. L-G. Johnsson, J. E. Hawkins, Jr., 725.

Delineation of Cochlear Glycogen by Electron Microscopy. A. J. Duvall III, M. J. Hukee, 234.

Dialysis and Renal Transplants, Hearing Loss in Patients with. C. A. Quick, 776.

Dinitrochlorobenzene Skin Sensitization and Peripheral Lymphocyte Count: Predictors of Survival in Head and Neck Cancer. R. H. Maisel, J. H. Ogura, 517.

Divers, Sinus Barotrauma in. P. Fagan, B. McKenzie, C. Edmonds, 61.

Drugs, Ototoxic and High Intensity Sounds, Auditory-Nerve Activity in Cats Exposed to. N. Y. S. Kiang, M. C. Liberman, R. A. Levine, 752.

Dysphonia, Spastic. F. S. Brodnitz, 210.

Dysphonia, Spastic, Recurrent Laryngeal Nerve Section for. H. H. Dedo, 451.

EAR-Cough (Arnold's) Reflex. S. Bloustine, L. Langston, T. Miller, 406.

Ears, Human, Exposed to Noise, Degeneration Patterns in. L-G. Johnsson, J. E. Hawkins, Jr., 725.

Editorial. B. H. Senturia, 1.

Educational Training in Endoscopy. J. E. Rayl, 627.

Effect of Anesthesia on Susceptibility to Acoustic Trauma. M. Rubinstein, N. Pluznik, 276.

Effect of Nicotine on Cochlear Function and Noise-Induced Hair Cell Loss. R. P. Bobbin, M. Gondra, 247.

Effects of Removal of Statoacoustic Ganglion Complex upon Growing Otocyst. T. R. Van De Water, Suppl. No. 33.

Effusions, Middle Ear, Recent Advances in. Suppl. No. 25.

Electric Response Audiometry, Brain Stem and Other Responses in. H. Davis, 3.

Electric Response Audiometry, Principles of. H. Davis, Suppl. No. 28.

Electrically Evoked Taste Threshold. M. Føns, 359.

Electrocochleography, Clinical, Test-Retest Reliability in. L. M. Bergholtz, R. E. Hooper, D. C. Mehta, 679.

Electron Microscopic Cochlear Observations in Bilateral Ménière's Disease. R. S. Kimura, C. Y. Ota, H. F. Schuknecht, T. Takahashi, 791.

Electron Microscopic Study, Scanning, of Organ of Corti in Normal and Sound-Damaged Guinea Pigs. E. R. Soudijn. Suppl. No. 29.

Electron Microscopy, Delineation of Cochlear Glycogen by. A. J. Duvall III, M. J. Hukee, 234.

Electronystagmographic Manifestations of Central Nervous System Disease. S. W. Parker, A. D. Weiss, 127.

Encephalomyelitis, Carcinomatous with Auditory and Vestibular Manifestations. T. McGill, 120.

Endolymphatic Hydrops, Unilateral, and Associated Abnormalities. I. Sando, L. D. Holinger, T. J. Balkany, R. P. Wood, 368.

Endoscpoy, Educational Training in. J. E. Rayl, 627.

Endotracheal Intubation and Venturi (Jet) Ventilation for Laser Microsurgery of the Larynx. M. L. Norton, M. S. Strong, C. W. Vaughan, J. C. Snow, B. J. Kripke, 656.

Epidermoid Carcinoma Arising from Within an Epidermoid Inclusion Cyst. T. M. Davidson, R. C. Bone, P. J. Kiessling, 417.

Epidermoid Inclusion Cyst, Epidermoid Carcinoma Arising from Within. T. M. Davidson, R. C. Bone, P. J. Kiessling, 417.

Epiglottic Flap and Laryngeal Suspension in Laryngopharyngeal Trauma. N. R. Olson, 533.

Epiglottitis, Acute, in Infants and Children. B. Benjamin, B. O'Reilly, 565.

Esophagus, Large Leiomyoma of, Unusual Presentation. S. Arena, 404.

Etiology of Bilateral Abductor Vocal Cord Paralysis. L. D. Holinger, P. C. Holinger, P. H. Holinger, 428.

Eustachian Tube and Vidian Nerve. S. E. Nathanson, R. T. Jackson, 83.

Experience with Vocal Cord Injection. R. B. Lewy, 440.

Eye Movement, Smooth Pursuit, Quantitative Measurement of. R. W. Baloh, W. E. Kumley, A. Sills, V. Honrubia, H. R. Konrad, 111.

Eye-Tracking Pattern Test, Caloric: I. Visual Suppression and Possibility of Simplified Differential Diagnosis between Peripheral and Central Vertigo. E. Sakata, Y. Umeda, 261.

FALSE Cord, Unilateral Lesions of: Grand Rounds. T. Palva, 410.

Fiber Components of Recurrent Laryngeal Nerve in Cat. R. R. Gacek, M. J. Lyon, 460.

Fiberoptic Bronchoscopy, Newer Techniques in. J. P. Atkins, Jr., L. D. Rowe, B. W. Jafek, 646.

Fiberoptic, Flexible Nasopharyngolaryngoscope. H. D. Silberman, H. Wilf, J. A. Tucker, 640.

Fine Structures of Normal Mucosa in Developing Rat Middle Ear. S. Maeda, G. Mogi, M. Oh, Suppl. No. 31.

First International Conference on Cholesteatoma, 844.

Fistula, Labyrinthine, and Tympanoplasty. J. Szpunar, 291.

Fistulas, Tracheoesophageal, Congenital in Adults. R. W. Stephens, R. E. Lingeman, L. J. Lawson, 613.

Flexible Fiberoptic Nasopharyngolaryngoscope. H. D. Silberman, H. Wilf, J. A. Tucker, 640.

Flourocitrate Ototoxicity: Morphologic and Cytochemical Model for Primary Neural Degeneration in Guinea Pig Cochlea. J. Spector, C. D. Carr, 185.

Frontal Sinus, Mucopyocele of: X-Ray of Month. A. L. Weber, B. D. Sklansky, 544.

Frontal Sinusotomy, Osteoplastic: Analysis of. J. M. Hardy, W. W. Montgomery, 523.

GANGLION Complex, Statoacoustic, Effects of Removal upon Growing Otocyst. T. R. Van De Water, Suppl. No. 33.

Glottic Closure Reflex, Initiation of. M. Suzuki, C. T. Sasaki, 382.

Glottic Reconstruction, Technique for, Following Vertical Partial Laryngectomy: A Preliminary Report. M. Hirano, 25.

Grand Rounds, Massachusetts Eye and Ear Infirmary Tumor Clinic. R. R. Gacek, 139.

Grand Rounds: Unilateral Lesions of False Cord. T. Palva, 410.

Granular Cell Tumors of Larynx. H. L. Coates, K. D. Devine, T. J. McDonald, L. H. Weiland, 504.

Granuloma, Cholesterol Involving the Temporal Bone. G. T. Nager, T. S. Vanderveen, 204.

HAIR Cell Loss, Noise-Induced, and Cochlear Function, Effect of Nicotine on. R. P. Bobbin, M. I. Gondra, 247.

Head and Neck Cancer, Predictors of Survival in: Dinitrochlorobenzene Skin Sensitization and Peripheral Lymphocyte Count. R. H. Maisel, J. H. Ogura, 517.

Head and Neck Surgery, Progress of Otolaryngology in. J. H. Ogura, 425.

Hearing Function and Chronic Renal Failure. D. W. Johnson, R. H. Mathog, 43.

Hearing Loss in Patients with Dialysis and Renal Transplants. C. A. Quick, 776.

Hearing Loss of Central Type Secondary to Anoxic Anoxia. K. Makishima, R. B. Katz, J. B. Snow, Jr., 826.

Hearing Mechanism, Peripheral. A Biochemical and Biological Approach. L. Naftalin, 38.

Hereditary Abductor Vocal Cord Paralysis. R. R. Gacek, 90.

High-Intensity Sounds and Ototoxic Drugs, Auditory-Nerve Activity in Cats Exposed to. N. Y. S. Kiang, M. C. Liberman, R. A. Levine, 752.

Histopathologic and Experimental Models for Sensory and Neural Deafness. G. J. Spector, 802.

Histopathological Observations of Presbycusis. F. Suga, J. R. Lindsay, 169.

Histopathology, Temporal Bone, of Osteopetrosis. F. Suga, J. R. Lindsay, 15.

Humidity, Air, and Mucociliary Activity. U. Mercke, N. G. Toremalm, 32.

Hydrops, Unilateral, Endolymphatic, and Associated Abnormalities. I. Sando, L. D. Holinger, T. J. Balkany, R. P. Wood, 368.

IMMUNOCYTOCHEMICAL Localization of Secretory Lysozyme in Human Middle Ear Mucosa. D. J. Lim, Y. S. Liu, H. Birck, 50.

Imperception, Auditory. D. O. Merifield, C. M. Hall, H. B. Merrell, 255.

Implanted Electronic Laryngeal Prosthesis. B. J. Bailey, C. M. Griffiths, R. Everett, 472.

Implants, Cochlear. W. F. House. Suppl. No. 27.

Initiation of Reflex Glottic Closure. M. Suzuki, C. T. Sasaki, 382.

Inner Ear Degeneration in Acoustic Neurinoma. F. Suga, J. R. Lindsay, 343.

Inner Ear Fluids, Sodium Loading of. H. Silverstein, T. Takeda, 769.

JET Ventilation, Percutaneous. E. Carden, G. Becker, H. Hamood, 652.

Jugular Foramen, Schwannoma of. R. R. Gacek, 215.

Juvenile Laryngeal Papillomatosis, Nonirradiated, Malignant Degeneration of. R. S. Shapiro, F. I. Marlowe, J. Butcher, 101.

Juvenile Nasopharyngeal Angiofibroma: X-Ray of Month. O. Solis, G. Roberson, A. L. Weber, 415.

LABYRINTHINE Fistula and Tympanoplasty. J. Szpunar, 291.

Laryngeal Behavior, Voice, and Laryngeal Disease, Observations on. G. P. Moore, 553.

Laryngeal Defects, Congenital in Adult. W. W. Montgomery, S. A. Smith, 491.

Laryngeal Disease, Laryngeal Behavior, and Voice, Observations on. G. P. Moore, 553.

Laryngeal Epithelium, Survey of Development of. J. A. Tucker, B. Vidic, G. F. Tucker, Jr., J. Stead, Suppl. No. 30.

Laryngeal Granular Cell Tumors. H. L. Coates, K. D. Devine, T. J. McDonald, L. H. Weiland, 504.

Laryngeal Laser Microsurgery, Endotracheal Intubation and Venturi (Jet) Ventilation for. M. L. Norton, M. S. Strong, C. W. Vaughan, J. C. Snow, B. J. Kripke, 656.

Laryngeal Nerve in Cat, Recurrent, Fiber Components of. R. R. Gacek, M. J. Lyon, 460.

Laryngeal Nerve, Recurrent, Section for Spastic Dysphonia. H. H. Dedo, 451.

Laryngeal Papillomatosis, Juvenile, Nonirradiated, Malignant Degeneration of. R. S. Shapiro, F. I. Marlowe, J. Butcher, 101.

Laryngeal Prosthesis, Electronic, Implanted. B. J. Bailey, C. M. Griffiths, R. Everett, 472.

Laryngeal Stenosis Repair with Nasal Septal Grafts. R. J. Toohill, D. L. Martinelli, M. C. Janowak, 600.

Laryngeal Suspension and Epiglottic Flap in Laryngopharyngeal Trauma. N. R. Olson, 533.

Laryngeal Tuberculosis Masquerading as Carcinoma. S. Naraqi, M. W. Raiser, N. M. Richards, B. R. Andersen, 547.

Laryngeal Verrucous Carcinoma: Management by Radiotherapy and Surgery. H. P. Burns, A. W. P. van Nostrand, D. P. Bryce, 538.

Laryngectomy, Vertical Partial, Technique for Glottic Reconstruction Following: A Preliminary Report. M. Hirano, 25.

Laryngopharyngeal Trauma, Laryngeal Suspension and Epiglottic Flap in. N. R. Olson, 533.

Larynx and Laryngopharynx, Mucus Gland Tumors of. R. H. Spiro, J. S. Lewis, S. I. Hajdu, E. W. Strong, 498.

Larynx, Role of in Nasal-Cardiopulmonary Reflexes. R. T. Jackson, 65.

Laser Adapter for Tracheoscopy. A. H. Andrews, Jr., L. L. Bailey, 625.

Laser Microsurgery of Larynx, Endotracheal Intubation and Venturi (Jet) Ventilation for. M. L. Norton, M. S. Strong, C. W. Vaughan, J. C. Snow, B. J. Kripke, 656.

Leiomyoma, Large, of Esophagus, Unusual Presentation of. S. Arena, 404.

Leiomyosarcoma of Nasal Cavity and Paranasal Sinuses. L. R. Dropkin, C. K. Tang, J. R. Williams, 399.

Leprous Rhinitis, Clinical Manifestations of. R. P. E. Barton, 74.

Loading of Sodium of Inner Ear Fluids. H. Silverstein, T. Takeda, 769.

Local Anesthesia for Suspension Microlaryngoscopy. T. C. Calcaterra, J. House, 71.

Lymphocyte Count, Peripheral, and Dinitrochlorobenzene Skin Sensitization: Predictors of Survival in Head and Neck Cancer. R. H. Maisel, J. H. Ogura, 517.

Lysozyme, Secretory, of Human Middle Ear Mucosa: Immunocytochemical Localization. D. J. Lim, Y. S. Liu, H. Birck, 50.

MALIGNANT Degeneration of Nonirradiated Juvenile Laryngeal Papillomatosis. R. S. Shapiro, F. I. Marlowe, J. Butcher, 101.

Manpower Resources and Needs in Otolaryngology. Suppl. No. 24.

Masking Level Differences for Cochlear and Brain Stem Lesions. W. O. Olsen, D. Noffsinger, 820.

Mastoid and Middle Ear Cavity Obliteration for Control of Otitis Media. R. R. Gacek, 305.

Maxillary Sinus (Mega-Antrum). F. Herzon, J. E. Antoine, 408.

Mega-Antrum. F. Herzon, J. E. Antoine, 408.

Ménière's Disease, Bilateral, Electron Microscopic Cochlear Observations in. R. S. Kimura, C. Y. Ota, H. F. Schuknecht, T. Takahashi, 791.

Microbiology of Canine Nasal Cavities. A. L. Abramson, R. F. D'Amato, H. D. Isenberg, W. H. Pryor, Jr., 394.

Microlaryngoscopy, Suspension, Local Anesthesia for. T. C. Calcaterra, J. House, 71.

Middle Ear Cavity and Mastoid Obliteration for Control of Otitis Media. R. R. Gacek, 305.

Middle Ear Effusions, Recent Advances in. Suppl. No. 25.

Middle Ear Effusions, Report of Research Conference on. Suppl. No. 26.

Middle Ear, Fine Structures of Normal Mucosa in Developing Rat. S. Maeda, G. Mogi, M. Oh, Suppl. No. 31.

Middle Ear Mucosa and Human Adult Adenoids, Tissue Culture of. L. Drucker, Z. Weisman, J. Sadé, 327.

Middle Ear Mucosa, Human Secretory Lysozyme: Immunocytochemical Localization. D. J. Lim, Y. S. Liu, H. Birck, 50.

Middle Ear, Pigmented Lesion of, Report of a Case. R. W. Babin, S. P. Benjamin, 387.

Middle Ear Space and Mastoid, Volume of as Related to Otitis Media. Correlation of Tubal Function. L. Andréasson, 198.

Mitotic Center, Single, for Rodent Cochlear Duct. W. F. Marovitz, J. M. A. Shugar, 225.

Models, Histopathologic and Experimental for Sensory and Neural Deafness. G. J. Spector, 813.

Mucociliary Activity and Air Humidity. U. Mercke, N. G. Toremalm, 32.

Mucociliary Clearance and Tracheal Resection. A. Giordano, D. S. Holsclaw, 631.

Mucopyocele of Frontal Sinus: X-Ray of Month. A. L. Weber, B. D. Sklansky, 544.

Mucosa, Middle Ear, and Human Adult Adenoids, Tissue Culture of. L. Drucker, Z. Weisman, J. Sadé, 327.

Mucosa, Normal, Fine Structures of in Developing Rat Middle Ear. S. Maeda, G. Mogi, M. Oh, Suppl. No. 31.

Mucus Gland Tumors of Larynx and Laryngopharynx. R. H. Spiro, J. S. Lewis, S. I. Hajdu, E. W. Strong, 498.

Mucus, Nasal, Rapid, Atraumatic Method for Obtaining Samples. W. R. Wilson, M. R. Allansmith, 391.

NASAL-Cardiopulmonary Reflexes: Role of the Larynx. R. T. Jackson, 65.

Nasal Cavities, Canine, Microbiology of. A. L. Abramson, R. F. D'Amato, H. D. Isenberg, W. H. Pryor, Jr., 394.

Nasal Cavity and Paranasal Sinuses, Leiomyosarcoma of. L. R. Dropkin, C. K. Tang, J. R. Williams, 399.

Nasal Mucus Samples; Rapid, Atraumatic Method for Obtaining. W. R. Wilson, M. R. Allansmith, 391.

Nasal Septal Grafts, Use of in Repair of Laryngeal Stenosis. R. J. Toohill, D. L. Martinelli, M. C. Janowak, 600.

Nasopharyngeal Angiofibroma, Juvenile: X-Ray of Month. O. Solis, G. Roberson, A. L. Weber, 415.

Nasopharyngolaryngoscope, Flexible, Fiberoptic. H. D. Silberman, H. Wilf, J. A. Tucker, 640.

Neural Degeneration, Primary, in Guinea Pig Cochlea, Morphologic and Cytochemical Model for: Flourocitrate Ototoxicity. G. J. Spector, C. D. Carr, 185.

Neurinoma, Acoustic, Inner Ear Degeneration in. F. Suga, J. R. Lindsay, 343.

Neurinomas, Acoustic, Bilateral: X-Ray of the Month. W. N. Floyd, A. L. Weber, 147.

New Developments in Evaluating Central Auditory Mechanisms. C. I. Berlin, 833.

Newer Techniques in Fiberoptic Bronchoscopy. J. P. Atkins, Jr., L. D. Rowe, B. W. Jafek, 646.

Nicotine, Effect on Cochlear Function and Noise-Induced Hair Cell Loss. R. P. Bobbin, M. I. Gondra, 247.

Noise Exposure of Human Ears, Degeneration Patterns in. L-G. Johnsson, J. E. Hawkins, Jr., 725.

Noise Exposure, Safe Level for? B. A. Bohne, 711.

Noise-Induced Hair Cell Loss and Cochlear Function, Effect of Nicotine on. R. P. Bobbin, M. I. Gondra, 247.

Nystagmus, Caloric and Optokinetic in Cerebellar Patients. M. H. Stroud, E. Rauchbach, 136.

OBITUARY, D. M. Lierle, 842.

Obituary, R. Carhart, 546.

Observations on Laryngeal Disease, Laryngeal Behavior, and Voice. G. P. Moore, 553.

Observations on Normal and Degenerating Human Otoconia. M. D. Ross, L-G Johnsson, D. Peacor, L. F. Allard, 310.

Optokinetic and Caloric Nystagmus in Cerebellar Patients. M. H. Stroud, E. Rauchbach, 136.

Organ of Corti Development, Spiral Migration Theory of. W. F. Marovitz, J. M. A. Shugar, K. M. Khan, Suppl. No. 32.

Organ of Corti, Scanning Electron Microscopic Study in Normal and Sound-Damaged Guinea Pigs. E. R. Soudijn. Suppl. No. 29.

Osteopetrosis, Temporal Bone Histopathology of. F. Suga, J. R. Lindsay, 15.

Osteoplastic Frontal Sinusotomy: Analysis of 250 Operations. J. M. Hardy, W. W. Montgomery, 523.

Otitis Media, Control of by Mastoid and Middle Ear Cavity Obliteration. R. R. Gacek, 305.

Otitis Media, Correlation of Tubal Function and Volume of Mastoid and Middle Ear Space as Related to. L. Andréasson, 198.

Otoconia, Normal and Degenerating Human, Observations on. M. D. Ross, L-G Johnsson, D. Peacor, L. F. Allard, 310.

Otocyst, Growing, Effects of Removal of Statoacoustic Ganglion Complex upon. T. R. Van De Water, Suppl. No. 33.

Otolaryngological Manifestations of Arthrogryposis Multiplex Congenita. S. R. Cohen, H. Isaacs, Jr., 484.

Otolaryngology, Progress of in Head and Neck Surgery. J. H. Ogura, 425.

Otosclerosis, Polygenic Inheritance of. J. C. Mendlowitz, K. Hirschhorn, 281.

Ototoxic Drugs and High-Intensity Sounds, Auditory-Nerve Activity in Cats Exposed to. N. Y. S. Kiang, M. C. Liberman, R. A. Levine, 752.

Ototoxicity and Acoustic Hyperstimulation, Ultrastructural Cochlear Changes Following. D. J. Lim, 740.

Ototoxicity, Flourocitrate: Morphologic and Cytochemical Model for Primary Neural Degeneration in Guinea Pig Cochlea. G. J. Spector, C. D. Carr, 185.

PAPILLOMATOSIS, Juvenile Laryngeal, Nonirradiated, Malignant Degeneration of. R. S. Shapiro, F. I. Marlowe, J. Butcher, 101.

Papillomatosis, Recurrent Respiratory, Management with CO_2 Laser. M. S. Strong, C. W. Vaughan, S. R. Cooperband, G. B. Healy, M. A. C. P. Clemente, 508.

Parathyroid Tumors as Lateral Pharyngeal Masses: Report of a Case. Z. E. Deeb, W. M. Trible, R. Page, M. G. Fernandez, 86.

Percutaneous Jet Ventilation. E. Carden, G. Becker, H. Hamood, 652.

Peripheral Hearing Mechanism: A Biochemical and Biological Approach. L. Naftalin, 38.

Pharyngeal Masses, Lateral, Parathyroid Tumors as: Report of a Case. Z. E. Deeb, W. M. Trible, R. Page, M. G. Fernandez, 86.

Phonation, Sustained, Vocal Shimmer in Normal and Pathologic Voice. K. Kitajima, W. J. Gould, 377.

Physiological Basis of Cochlear Transduction and Sensitivity. V. Honrubia, D. Strelioff, S. T. Sitko, 697.

Pigmented Lesion of Middle Ear, Report of a Case. R. W. Babin, S. P. Benjamin, 387.

Polygenic Inheritance of Otosclerosis. J. C. Mendlowitz, K. Hirschhorn, 281.

Posterior Cricoarytenoid as a Speech Muscle. H. Hirose, 334.

Preauricular Pit, Cervical Fistula and Hearing Loss Syndrome, Temporal Bone in. N. Fitch, J. R. Lindsay, H. Srolovitz, 268.

Presbycusis, Histopathological Observations of. F. Suga, J. R. Lindsay, 169.

Principles of Electric Response Audiometry. H. Davis, Suppl. No. 28.

Progress of Otolaryngology in Head and Neck Surgery. J. H. Ogura, 425.

Pulmonary Artery Sling Associated with Tracheostenosis and Bronchial Abnormalities. S. R. Cohen, B. H. Landing, 582.

QUANTITATIVE Measurement of Smooth Pursuit Eye Movement. R. W. Baloh, W. E. Kumley, A. Sills, V. Honrubia, H. R. Konrad, 111.

RAPID, Atraumatic Method for Obtaining Nasal Mucus Samples. W. R. Wilson, M. R. Allansmith, 391.

Recent Advances in Middle Ear Effusions. Suppl. No. 25.

Recurrent Laryngeal Nerve in Cat, Fiber Components of. R. R. Gacek, M. J. Lyon, 460.

Recurrent Laryngeal Nerve Section for Spastic Dysphonia. H. H. Dedo, 451.

Recurrent Respiratory Papillomatosis, Management with CO_2 Laser. M. S. Strong, C. W. Vaughan, S. R. Cooperband, G. B. Healy, M. A. C. P. Clemente, 508.

Reflex Glottic Closure, Initiation of. M. Suzuki, C. T. Sasaki, 382.

Renal Failure, Chronic and Hearing Function. D. W. Johnson, R. H. Mathog, 43.

Renal Transplants and Dialysis, Hearing Loss in Patients with. C. A. Quick, 776.

Repair of Laryngeal Stenosis with Nasal Septal Grafts. R. J. Toohill, D. L. Martinelli, M. C. Janowak, 600.

Report of Research Conference on Middle Ear Effusions. Suppl. No. 26.

Respiratory Structures, Transbronchoscopic Cryosurgery of: Experimental and Clinical Studies. A. Gorenstein, H. B. Neel III, D. R. Sanderson, 670.

Rhinitis, Leprous, Clinical Manifestations of. R. P. E. Barton, 74.

Round Window Membrane, Rupture of. P. H. Taylor, P. G. Bicknell, 105.

Rupture of Round Window Membrane. P. H. Taylor, P. G. Bicknell, 105.

SAFE Level for Noise Exposure? B. A. Bohne, 711.

Scanning Electron Microscopic Study of Organ of Corti in Normal and Sound-Damaged Guinea Pigs. E. R. Soudijn. Suppl. No. 29.

Schwannoma of Jugular Foramen. R. R. Gacek, 215.

Secretory Lysozyme of Human Middle Ear Mucosa: Immunocytochemical Localization. D. J. Lim, Y. S. Liu, H. Birck, 50.

Single Mitotic Center for Rodent Cochlear Duct. W. F. Marovitz, J. M. A. Shugar, 225.

Sinus Barotrauma in Divers. P. Fagan, B. McKenzie, C. Edmonds, 61.

Sinus, Frontal, Mucopyocele of: X-Ray of Month. A. L. Weber, B. D. Sklansky, 544.

Sinuses, Paranasal, and Nasal Cavity, Leiomyosarcoma of. L. R. Dropkin, C. K. Tang, J. R. Williams, 399.

Sinusotomy, Osteoplastic Frontal: Analysis of. J. M. Hardy, W. W. Montgomery, 523.

Smooth Pursuit Eye Movement, Quantitative Measurement of. R. W. Baloh, W. E. Kumley, A. Sills, V. Honrubia, H. R. Konrad, 111.

Sodium Loading of Inner Ear Fluids. H. Silverstein, T. Takeda, 769.

Some Unresolved Problems Concerning the Cochlear Nerve. R. Lorente de Nó, Suppl. No. 34.

Sound Damaged and Normal Guinea Pigs, Scanning Electron Microscopic Study of Organ of Corti. E. R. Soudijn. Suppl. No. 29.

Spastic Dysphonia. F. S. Brodnitz, 210.

Spastic Dysphonia, Recurrent Laryngeal Nerve Section for. H. H. Dedo, 451.

Speech Muscle, Posterior Cricoarytenoid as. H. Hirose, 334.

Spiral Migration Theory of Organ of Corti Development. W. F. Marovitz, J. M. A. Shugar, K. M. Khan, Suppl. No. 32.

Statoacoustic Ganglion Complex, Effects of Removal upon Growing Otocyst. T. R. Van De Water, Suppl. No. 33.

Stenosis, Laryngeal, Repair of with Nasal Grafts. R. J. Toohill, D. L. Martinelli, M. C. Janowak, 600.

Stenosis, Subglottic, Acquired and Congenital in the Infant. J. L. Parkin, M. H. Stevens, A. L. Jung, 573.

Stenosis, Subglottic, in Infants and Children. P. H. Holinger, S. L. Kutnick, J. A. Schild, L. D. Holinger, 591.

Subglottic Stenosis, Acquired and Congenital, in the Infant. J. L. Parkin, M. H. Stevens, A. L. Jung, 573.

Subglottic Stenosis in Infants and Children. P. H. Holinger, S. L. Kutnick, J. A. Schild, L. D. Holinger, 591.

Sudden Deafness of Vascular Origin: Human Temporal Bone Study. R. Gussen, 94.

Survey of Development of Laryngeal Epithelium. J. A. Tucker, B. Vidic, G. F. Tucker, Jr., J. Stead, Suppl. No. 30.

TASTE Threshold, Electrically Evoked. M. Føns, 359.

Technique for Glottic Reconstruction Following Vertical Partial Laryngectomy: A Preliminary Report. M. Hirano, 25.

Temporal Bone, Cholesterol Granuloma Involving. G. T. Nager, T. S. Vanderveen, 204.

Temporal Bone Histopathology of Osteopetrosis. F. Suga, J. R. Lindsay, 15.

Temporal Bone in Preauricular Pit, Cervical Fistula, Hearing Loss Syndrome. N. Fitch, J. R. Lindsay, H. Srolovitz, 268.

Temporal Bone Study, Human: Sudden Deafness of Vascular Origin. R. Gussen, 94.

Test-Retest Reliability in Clinical Electrocochleography. L. M. Bergholtz, R. E. Hooper, D. C. Mehta, 679.

Thyroglossal Duct, Adenocarcinoma Originating in. A. Widstrom, P. Magnusson, O. Hallberg, H. Hellqvist, H. Riiber, 286.

Tissue Culture of Human Adult Adenoids and of Middle Ear Mucosa. L. Drucker, Z. Weisman, J. Sadé, 327.

Tracheal Afferent Nerves. R. M. Traxel, W. F. Prudlow, J. P. Kampine, R. L. Coon, E. J. Zuperku, 664.

Tracheal Resection and Mucociliary Clearance. A. Giordano, D. S. Holsclaw, 631.

Tracheoscopy, Laser Adapter for. A. H. Andrews, Jr., L. L. Bailey, 625.

Tracheoesophageal Anastomosis, Clinical Experience with, for Intractable Aspiration. R. C. Lindeman, C. T. Yarington, Jr., D. Sutton, 609.

Tracheoesophageal Fistulas, Congenital in Adults. R. W. Stephens, R. E. Lingeman, L. J. Lawson, 613.

Tracheostenosis and Bronchial Abnormalities Associated with Pulmonary Artery Sling. S. R. Cohen, B. H. Landing, 582.

Tracheostomy, Tracing of. E. A. M. Frost, 618.

Tracing the Tracheostomy. E. A. M. Frost, 618.

Transbronchoscopic Cryosurgery of Respiratory Structures: Experimental and Clinical Studies. A. Gorenstein, H. B. Neel III, D. R. Sanderson, 670.

Tribute to a Great Lady. B. H. Senturia, 2.

Tubal Function, Correlation of, and Volume of Mastoid and Middle Ear Space as Related to Otitis Media. L. Andréasson, 198.

Tuberculosis of Larynx Masquerading as Carcinoma. S. Naraqi, M. W. Raiser, N. M. Richards, B. R. Andersen, 547.

Tumors, Granular Cell of Larynx. H. L. Coates, K. D. Devine, T. J. McDonald, L. H. Weiland, 504.

Tumors, Mucus Gland of Larynx and Laryngopharynx. R. H. Spiro, J. S. Lewis, S. I. Hajdu, E. W. Strong, 498.

Tumors, Parathyroid, as Lateral Pharyngeal Masses: Report of a Case. Z. E. Deeb, W. M. Trible, R. Page, M. G. Fernandez, 86.

Tympanoplasty and Labyrinthine Fistula. J. Szpunar, 291.

ULTRASTRUCTURAL Cochlear Changes Following Acoustic Hyperstimulation and Ototoxicity. D. J. Lim, 740.

Unilateral Endolymphatic Hydrops and Associated Abnormalities. I. Sando, L. D. Holinger, T. J. Balkany, R. P. Wood, 368.

Unusual Presentation of a Large Leiomyoma of Esophagus. S. Arena, 404.

VENTURI (Jet) Ventilation and Endotracheal Intubation for Laser Microsurgery of Larynx. M. L. Norton, M. S. Strong, C. W. Vaughan, J. C. Snow, B. J. Kripke, 656.

Verrucous Carcinoma of Larynx: Management by Radiotherapy and Surgery. H. P. Burns, A. W. P. van Nostrand, D. P. Bryce, 538.

Vertigo, Possibility of Simplified Differential Diagnosis between Peripheral and Central; Visual Suppression; Caloric Eye-Tracking Pattern Test. E. Sakata, Y. Umeda, 261.

Vestibular and Auditory Manifestations in Carcinomatous Encephalomyelitis. T. McGill, 120.

Vestibular Decruitment in Central Nervous System Disease. N. Torok, 131.

Vidian Nerve and Eustachian Tube. S. E. Nathanson, R. T. Jackson, 83.

Visual Suppression and Possibility of Simplified Differential Diagnosis between Peripheral and Central Vertigo: Caloric Eye-Tracking Pattern Test. E. Sakata, Y. Umeda, 261.

Vocal Cord Injection, Experience with. R. B. Lewy, 440.

Vocal Cord Paralysis, Abductor, Hereditary. R. R. Gacek, 90.

Vocal Cord Paralysis, Bilateral Abductor, Etiology of. L. D. Holinger, P. C. Holinger, P. H. Holinger, 428.

Vocal Shimmer In Sustained Phonation of Normal and Pathologic Voice. K. Kitajima, W. J. Gould, 377.

Voice, Laryngeal Behavior, and Laryngeal Disease, Observations on. G. P. Moore, 553.

Voice, Normal and Pathologic, Vocal Shimmer in Sustained Phonation of. K. Kitajima, W. J. Gould, 377.

X-RAY of Month: Ameloblastoma. A. L. Weber, W. Guralnick, 692.

X-Ray of the Month: Bilateral Acoustic Neurinomas. W. N. Floyd, A. L. Weber, 147.

X-Ray of the Month: Juvenile Nasopharyngeal Angiofibroma. O. Solis, G. Roberson, A. L. Weber, 415.

X-Ray of Month: Mucopyocele of Frontal Sinus. A. L. Weber, B. D. Sklansky, 544.

SCANNING ELECTRON MICROSCOPIC STUDY OF THE ORGAN OF CORTI IN NORMAL AND SOUND-DAMAGED GUINEA PIGS

Eduard R. Soudijn, MD

Groningen, The Netherlands

With the collaboration of

J. D. Bleeker, MD

P. E. Hoeksema, MD

I. Molenaar, MD

J. P. van Rooyen, MSc

R. J. Ritsma, PhD

From the Departments of Otolaryngology (Professor Dr. P. E. Hoeksema), Medical Electron Microscopy (Professor Dr. I. Molenaar) and Audiology (Professor Dr. R. J. Ritsma), University of Groningen, Oostersingel 59, Groningen, The Netherlands.

This study will be submitted as a doctoral thesis at the University of Groningen, The Netherlands. It was supported by grants from the Dutch Heinsius Houbolt Foundation and the Dutch National Prevention Fund.

ACKNOWLEDGMENTS

The author is indebted to the following:

Messrs. J. A. Oosterbaan, I. Stokroos, H. de Weerd and E. H. Blaauw for their valuable assistance in preparing the specimens: Dr. W. L. Jongebloed for sharing his knowledge on scanning electron microscopy; Messrs. D. Huizinga, H. R. A. Meiborg, M. Goslinga, J. M. Martens and H. Wierenga for the photographic work: Messrs. K. Kuitert, G. T. Prins and G. Kors for their technical assistance; Messrs. F. van Til and J. H. van Dijk for their audiological assistance; Messrs. L. Kop and C. J. Baarveld for their assistance in pathology (Professor Dr. H. N. Hadders); Messrs. J. Berens, J. Louwes, A. A. van Veenen and L. Vijfschaft who took care of the laboratory animals.

The English translation was made by Mr. Th. van Winsen. Mrs. Marianne Jeuring carefully typed the manuscript.

Last but by no means least, my wife, Ann, is thanked for her unfailing patience.

ANATOMICAL TERMINOLOGY

In the Cochlea

Apical – in the direction of the helicotrema

Basal – in the direction of the round and oval windows

The four turns are designated or numbered:

first or basal turn
second or upper basal turn
third or lower apical turn
fourth or apical turn

In the Cochlear Duct (Scala Media) According to Iurato[1]

Longitudinal or spiral	– parallel to the axis of the cochlear duct and therefore perpendicular to the fibers of the basilar membrane
Transverse or radial	– perpendicular to the axis of the cochlear duct and therefore parallel to the fibers of the basilar membrane
Inner or internal	– towards the modiolus
Outer or external	– towards the spiral ligament
Upper or vestibular	– towards Reissner's membrane
Lower or tympanic	– towards the tympanic surface of the basilar membrane

CONTENTS

Page

INTRODUCTION 1

CHAPTER I. A BRIEF DESCRIPTION OF THE COCHLEA 4

CHAPTER II. MATERIALS AND METHODS 6

CHAPTER III. SCANNING ELECTRON MICROSCOPY OF THE ORGAN OF CORTI 16

CHAPTER IV. ACOUSTIC TRAUMA CAUSED BY PURE TONES 35

CHAPTER V. OTOLOGIC DRILLS — A POSSIBLE ACOUSTIC DANGER 43

CHAPTER VI. ACOUSTIC TRAUMA CAUSED BY DRILL NOISE 47

SCANNING ELECTRON MICROSCOPIC STUDY OF THE ORGAN OF CORTI IN NORMAL AND SOUND-DAMAGED GUINEA PIGS

EDUARD R. SOUDIJN, MD

GRONINGEN, THE NETHERLANDS

SUMMARY — A method was evolved by which the organ of Corti could be examined in its entirety with the scanning electron microscope, the organ meanwhile retaining its spiral form. This made it possible to assess traumatic effects on the cochlea and qualify lesions in terms of extent, localization and pattern. It was also found possible eventually to cut the same specimen into sections for cellular and subcellular studies. The number of guinea pigs examined totalled 91, divided into three groups. The first group was used to study the anatomy of the organ of Corti with special reference to normal variations and artifacts. Unmistakable indications were found that the longest stereocilia of the inner hair cells are linked to the tectorial membrane. The animals of the second group were exposed to pure tones of high intensity, whereupon, lesions of the organ of Corti were described according to intensity, time, and frequency. Three different types of otologic drills were used to perform mastoidectomies on temporal bones and on the cadaver. The noise produced was analyzed as to intensity and frequency range. It was found that the drill with the lowest rpm (and highest torque) produced the highest noise intensities, at levels which can be traumatic to the human organ of hearing. The animals of the third group were exposed to the amplified noise produced by otologic drills of three different types. The resulting lesions in the organ of Corti were examined by the method described for scanning electron microscopy and compared. In spite of the wide variation in individual lesions, patterns of degeneration of three different types could be distinguished. The high-speed and the very-high-speed drill inflicted less damage on the organ of Corti than the low-speed drill. It is therefore advised to refrain from using the latter drill in prolonged operations.

INTRODUCTION

It has long been known that sounds of high intensity can inflict damage on the organ of hearing. As early as 1831 this was described in the *Lancet* by Fosbroke,[2] who already differentiated between hearing loss following exposure to the sound of big guns, and that after years of work in a forge. In 1890, Habermann[3] tested the hearing of 20 boilermakers, all of whom were found to suffer from perceptive hearing defects. An autopsy was later performed on one of them, and microscopic examination of the cochleae revealed that both organs of Corti showed degeneration in the basal turn. Rather than ascribing this to old age, Habermann[3] explained it by the chronic exposure to noise in the forge.

Anatomical and pathological studies of the cochlea have always played an important role in the investigation of the cause of this sensorineural hearing loss. However, these studies encountered four obstacles: the minute dimensions necessitated microscopy; the position deep in the skull impeded rapid fixation; the enveloping bone required decalcification; and the complexity of structure called for serial sections. It was therefore not until 1851 that Corti[4] described the structure of the organ of hearing with such accuracy that his name remained attached to it. The results of studies of the cochlea have since been more or less determined by the advances in microscopic technique. One investigator has made an astonishing exception to this rule: in 1881 and 1884, Retzius[5] published an atlas of the organ of hearing in vertebrates. His atlas presented marvelous drawings of the macroscopy and microscopy of the inner ear, and has so far remained peerless (see Fig. 34, Chapter III). We cannot but feel the greatest admiration for the way in which Retzius,[5] using the dissection techniques of his day and simple optical aids, managed to show details which modern investigators are today recording photographically with the aid of sophisticated electron microscopic equipment.

In the early years of the 20th century Wittmaack,[6] Yoshii,[7] Marx,[8] and Röhr[9] performed extensive experiments in various animal species to test the traumatic effect of loud sounds on the cochlea. Yoshii[7] established that the first degenerative changes occurred in the organ of Corti, more specifically in the sensory cells. Röhr[9] described the great variability of auditory damage in various test animals, even when the same sound was offered, of the same intensity and during the same period of time. These observations have stood up as correct to this day.

With improved means to regulate intensity and pitch of sounds, there was an increasing interest in further investigation of the traumatic effect of loud sounds on the cochlea and in comparison of results. A standard work in this field, *Das akustische Trauma,* was published in 1947 by Rüedi and Furrer.[10]

Other methods of investigation have evolved, such as behavior audiometry in test animals, and methods to study the electrophysiology and histochemistry of the cochlea. Anatomy and pathological anatomy, however, continued to be dependent on material cut into sections. With the improved resolving power made available by the transmission electron microscope, subcellular structures could be examined, but investigators were still dependent on (be it ultrathin) sections.[1,11-13]

Although a treasury of data was obtained with the various above mentioned methods, and an enormously more profound understanding of the function and structure of the cochlea was attained, yet a morphological study of the organ of Corti in its totality remained impossible. Engström *et al*[14] have evolved a method which made this possible by cutting the organ of Corti into sectors. Thus, large parts of the organ of Corti can be visualized with the phase-contrast microscope. The regular arrangement of sensory and supporting cells forms a characteristic pattern on the vestibular surface of the organ of Corti. In a damaged organ, the degenerative changes manifest themselves in particular on the vestibular surface. Resulting changes in the pattern become visible even at a fairly low power. The great advantage lies in the fact that hundreds of sensory and supporting cells in a single specimen can be examined. The surface specimen technique of Engström *et al*[14] has been successfully used by numerous investigators.[15-27] However, it is interesting to note that, according to his drawings, Retzius[5] must already have been using the principles of such a method.

This method was eventually adapted to the use of the scanning electron microscope. Barber and Boyde[28] were the first to study the inner ear of octopi in this way, while Lim and Lane[29] studied the mammalian inner ear. This method of investigation, too, was soon widely used.[30-48] An invaluable advantage of using a scanning electron microscope is its much higher depth of field.[33,49] Magnifications from 20 to 20,000 times are possible. But a disadvantage of this method is that the organ of Corti has to be divided into sectors, which entails the risk that parts of the organ are lost.

To ensure complete elimination of this risk, efforts should be made to evolve a method whereby the organ of Corti could be visualized in its entirety. The need for such a method is apparent from the publications of Bohne[50] and Spoendlin and Brun,[51] who described a method to study the entire organ in surface preparation. But in these procedures, too, the cochlear duct has to be divided into half turns. These are difficult to handle because of their tiny dimensions, and cannot always be examined in a true horizontal plane.[50] In the method of Spoendlin and Brun,[51] the use of the circular saw entails a loss of nearly 5% of the entire sensory cell population.

The value of this method is obvious, because it enables the investigator to study the same specimen also from sections. In this way sensory cell loss can be quantitatively determined, and the site and extent of the lesion can be accurately delineated, whereupon qualitative determinations can be made.

In view of the above-mentioned problems, a method was developed for the study of the organ of Corti *in toto* with the scanning electron microscope. To illustrate the validity of this method a comparative study was made of the traumatic effects of pure tones and of otologic drills. It is not generally known that sanitary ear surgery can be followed by sensorineural hearing loss, particularly for high-pitched sounds. The cause of this hearing loss is to be sought in the loud noise which accompanies removal of bone tissue during the operation. In the past this was done with hammer and chisel, but today otologic drills are used. Sensorineural hearing defects have been described after both.[52-56]

The first chapter gives a description of the cochlea on the basis of light-microscopic findings. Materials and methods are discussed in the next chapter. The third chapter describes the normal anatomy of the organ of Corti on the basis of scanning electron microscopic photographs, and discusses variations in the hair cell pattern and artifacts. A chapter on acoustic trauma caused by pure tones is followed by an analysis of the noise of otologic drills of three different types. The final chapter discusses acoustic trauma caused by drill noise.

CHAPTER I

A BRIEF DESCRIPTION OF THE COCHLEA

Cochlear Structure Studied with the Light Microscope

"Because of its very complex shape, the inner ear is called the labyrinth."[1] It can be divided into a membranous and a bony part or, in functional terms, into a vestibular and a cochlear part. The mammalian cochlea is indeed shaped like a snail shell. The guinea pig cochlea has slightly more than four turns. The central axis or modiolus contains the cochlear nerve and the spiral ganglion. The turns contain the cochlear duct or scala media, which encloses the actual sense organ of Corti (Fig. 1). The cochlear duct bisects a turn and separates the scala vestibuli on the apical side from the scala tympani on the basal side.

The cochlear duct is bounded on the outside by the upper portion of the spiral ligament, the inside of which is covered by the stria vascularis. In the direction of the modiolus the duct is bounded by the bony spiral lamina on which the spiral limbus rests. The upper boundary is formed by Reissner's membrane, which extends between the spiral limbus and the spiral ligament. The lower boundary is formed by the basilar

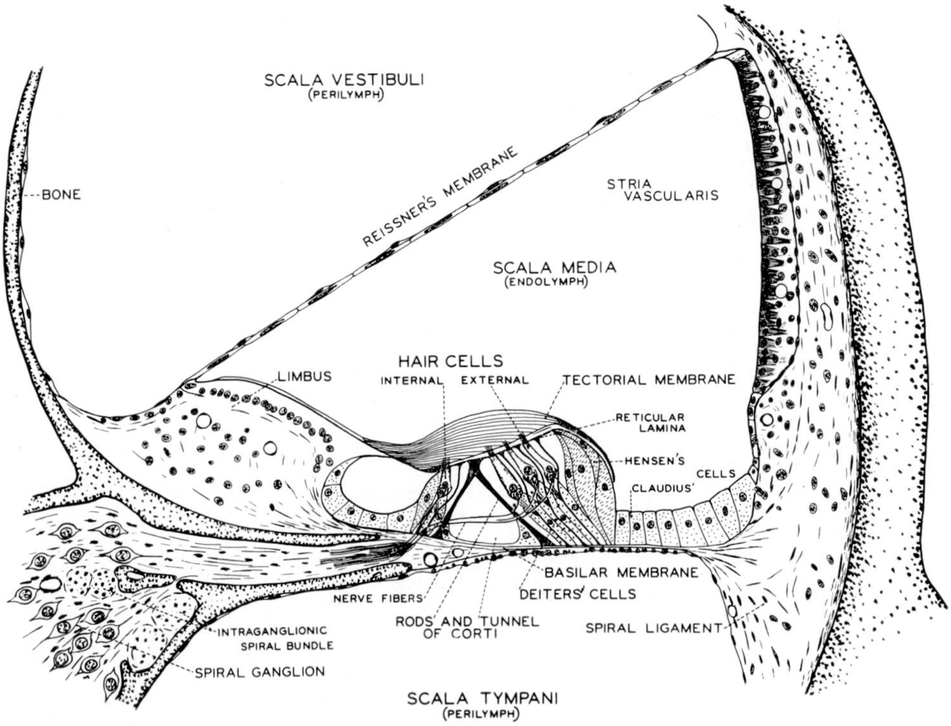

Fig. 1. Drawing of a cross section of the cochlear partition of a guinea pig in the lower part of the second turn. The organ of Corti is bounded on the inside by the inner sulcus, and on the outside by the outer sulcus. The space around the external hair cells is called Nuel's space. The under surface of the basilar membrane is covered with basilar membrane cells. (By courtesy of Davis *et al.*[57] J Acoust Soc Am 25:1182, 1953.)

membrane, which extends between the spiral ligament and the bony spiral lamina and is covered by basilar membrane cells on the side of the scala tympani. The organ of Corti rests on the basilar membrane and is spiral shaped.

On the outside the spiral limbus ends in two sharp extremities: the vestibular lip and the tympanic lip. These lips enclose the inner sulcus. From the vestibular lip the tectorial membrane extends across and is partly attached to the sensory cells and supporting cells of the organ of Corti. From the inside out, the following component parts of the organ of Corti can be designated: to begin, the inner sulcus, which is lined with a layer of cubical epithelial cells known as inner sulcus cells. Next comes a single row of border cells lying against the inner wall of the inner hair cells. The inner hair cells in turn are supported by the inner phalangeal cells, which rest against the inner pillar cells. The latter show an unmistakable fiber structure and constitute the inner boundary of the tunnel of Corti, of which the outer pillar cells form the outer boundary.

Towards the spiral ligament one finds three rows of sensory cells: the outer hair cells, contained in Nuel's space and resting on Deiters' cells. Each Deiters' cell has a phalangeal process which angulates and extends to the upper surface of the organ of Corti, where it broadens into a phalangeal plate. The surface of the sensory cells, jointly with that of the surrounding supporting cells, forms a thin, firm layer: the reticular membrane. Rows of stereocilia can be visualized near the hair cells by the surface specimen technique. The W-configuration of the stereocilia of the outer hair cells can also be distinguished (Fig. 2A). After the third row of outer hair cells and the last row of Deiters' cells, comes a ridge of supporting cells, the Hensen cells. Even further externally, the epithelium becomes cubical again, and much lower, the Claudius cells, which line the outer sulcus and continue in the spiral ligament.

CHAPTER II

MATERIALS AND METHODS

Materials

"We can probably assume with some confidence that the organ of Corti in man has about the same mechanical strength that it has in the guinea pig. Size and structure are very similar, particularly if we compare the corresponding regions that are most sensitive to the same frequency," wrote Davis in 1953.[57] This is why young guinea pigs weighing 250-500 g were used as test animals. Guinea pigs have several other advantages as well. They are easily obtained and kept, and the cochlea is contained in an ample tympanic bulla, which facilitates dissection. The cochlea is of sufficient size to process the various turns separately under the preparation microscope. Young animals are less liable to otitis than mature animals, and presbycusis is avoided. Nearly all animals used were laboratory bred and healthy. The noise level measured in the rooms where the animals were accommodated rarely exceeded 65 dB. It was taken into account that the organ of hearing in very young guinea pigs (up to eight days old) is more vulnerable to sound damage than that in mature animals.[25] The test animals used were therefore at least four weeks old.

The 91 guinea pigs used were divided into three groups. The first group (n = 42) was not exposed to auditory stress. The second group (n = 19) was exposed to pure tones. The third group (n = 30) was exposed to otologic drill noise. The organs of Corti of both cochleae from all the animals, except two which died in the course of the experiments, were examined with the scanning electron microscope. A few specimens were also used for the surface specimen technique or for transmission electron microscopy. Spiral ganglion and acoustic nerve were not systematically examined, although this was certainly possible by this method (Fig. 2B).

Methods

To gain a general impression of the guinea pig's hearing, Preyer's auricle reflex was always tested at the start of the experiment. This reflex, also known as acoustic reflex, is an involuntary movement of the anterosuperior edge of the pinna in response to an auditory stimulus of high intensity.[58] For this test the animal was held about 10 cm away from a hand audiometer* with which brief tones of 500, 1,000, 2,000 and 4,000 Hz can be produced. The sound level on the dial was 80 dB. The true sound level at these frequencies and at this distance was 100 dB as measured with a sound level meter at the same distance. Some animals failed to respond to repeated efforts to provoke the reflex. They were found to suffer from bilateral otitis media, and were eliminated from further experiments, which were confined to animals with a distinct positive Preyer's reflex.

Sound. The guinea pigs used in sound tests were submitted to the following procedure. Anesthesia was induced by inhalation of some halothane, whereupon the auditory meatus was examined and cleansed if necessary. The normal guinea pig ear drum shows the same reflex as the human ear drum. Only animals with intact ear drums and an unmistakable light reflex were used in the experiments. During the inhalation anesthesia, thiopental sodium (30 mg/kg body weight) was injected intraperitoneally,[59] which ensured continuation of the anesthesia for about two hours. In some cases, additional injections were required during the experiment. During anesthesia an insert telephone was used to offer a pure tone or drill noise, as a

*Alfred Peters and Sons, Ltd., Sheffield, England.

rule, only to the right ear. The anesthesia served to suppress the protective effect of the stapedius and tensor tympani muscles on the cochlea.[57,60-65] The situation thus created corresponded with that of a patient undergoing mastoidectomy under general anesthesia (in such cases, too, the effect of the middle ear muscles is suppressed).

The pure tones were produced by means of an oscillator* and amplified with a power amplifier.** The insert telephone*** is normally used in hearing aids. The sound level was repeatedly standardized with the aid of an impulse precision level meter.**** The telephone was fixed to the right auricle with dual adhesive tape in such a way that the telephone aperture was free in the cavum conchae. The distance between telephone and drum was thus always about the same.

The noise produced by three different types of otologic drills was recorded, analyzed and reproduced. The reproduced drill noise was offered only to the right ear, in the same way as the pure tones.

Nearly all sound experiments lasted two hours; only a few drill noise experiments continued for three hours. Except for the animals used in the time experiment, all guinea pigs exposed to sounds of high intensity were sacrificed after three to seven weeks. It was assumed that degeneration of sensory and supporting cells, if any, would be complete after three weeks.[66] Before sacrificing the animals, another attempt was made to provoke a Preyer's reflex; this was usually positive. However, in a few animals submitted to unilateral sound tests and, with a negative reflex, bilateral otitis media was found. This infection must have occurred after exposure to sound of high intensity. The tympanic bullae were filled with pus, and adjacent bone had thickened markedly. Nevertheless, these animals' cochleae were also examined with the scanning electron microscope, on the presumption that brief otitis media as a rule does not damage the organ of Corti.

Fixation. Two different fixation techniques were used. First of all, fixation of the cochlea by perfusion. This technique (although with different fixatives) has been used for decades in fixation of the inner ear for light microscopy, with good results.[7,67] Since perfusion fixation has been increasingly used for transmission electron microscopy in recent years, this technique was employed also for scanning electron microscopic examination of the cochlea.

Deep anesthesia was effected by intraperitoneal injection of 60 mg sodium thiopental per kg body weight. The abdomen was opened and the diaphragm incised, causing collapse of the lungs and giving an excellent view of the still-beating heart. A venipuncture needle was introduced into the left ventricle and the right atrium was incised, while at the same time the inferior vena cava and abdominal aorta were clamped. For optimal fixation the vascular bed to be perfused had to be dilated. This was achieved by injection of 75 ml 0.4% $NaNO_2$ in 0.1 M phosphate buffer at pH 7.35 $\pm$ 0.05 through the needle,† followed by introduction of the fixative: 500 ml 2% glutaraldehyde in the same buffer at the same pH. The total osmolarity amounted to 430 mOsm $\pm$ 20 mOsm. The fluids were contained in bottles kept at room temperature, suspended one meter above the guinea pig, to be perfused and connected to the venipuncture needle by plastic tubing. This arrangement ensured an equal hydrostatic pressure throughout all experiments. The procedure took about 30 minutes. During perfusion the neck and front paws stiffened, signifying a proper course of fixation. The perfusion fixation technique has the advantage of giving ample time for resection of the temporal bones and opening of the tympanic bullae.

*Hewlett-Packard Co., Palo Alto, CA. Type 209A.

**Philips Electronic Instruments, Inc., Mount Vernon, NY. Code PM 5175.

***Robert Bosch Gmbh., Berlin, West Germany. Type TML 47.

****B & K Instruments, Inc., Cleveland, OH. Type 2204.

†Personal communication from PFA Martinez-Martinez and H. De Weerd.

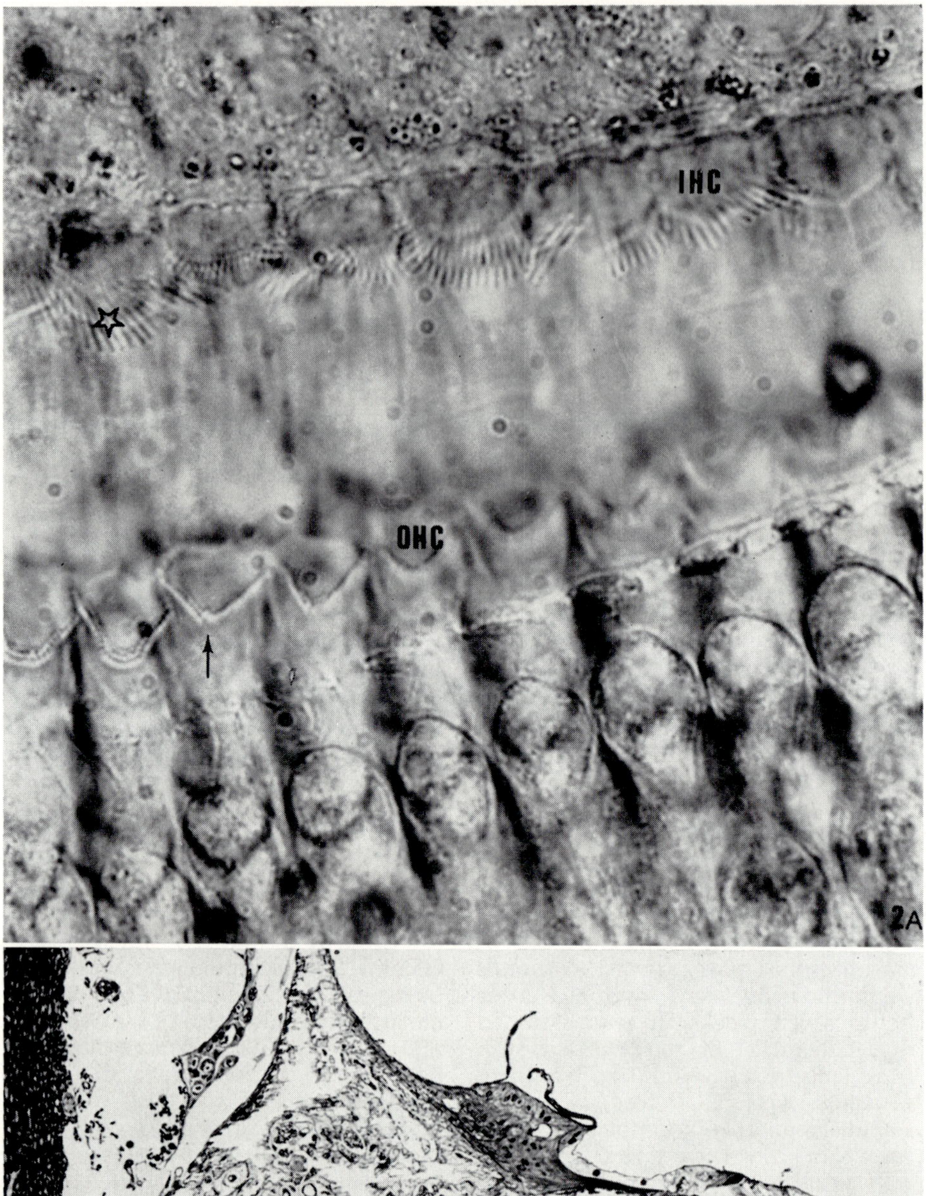
IHC
OHC
2A
SG
AN
2B

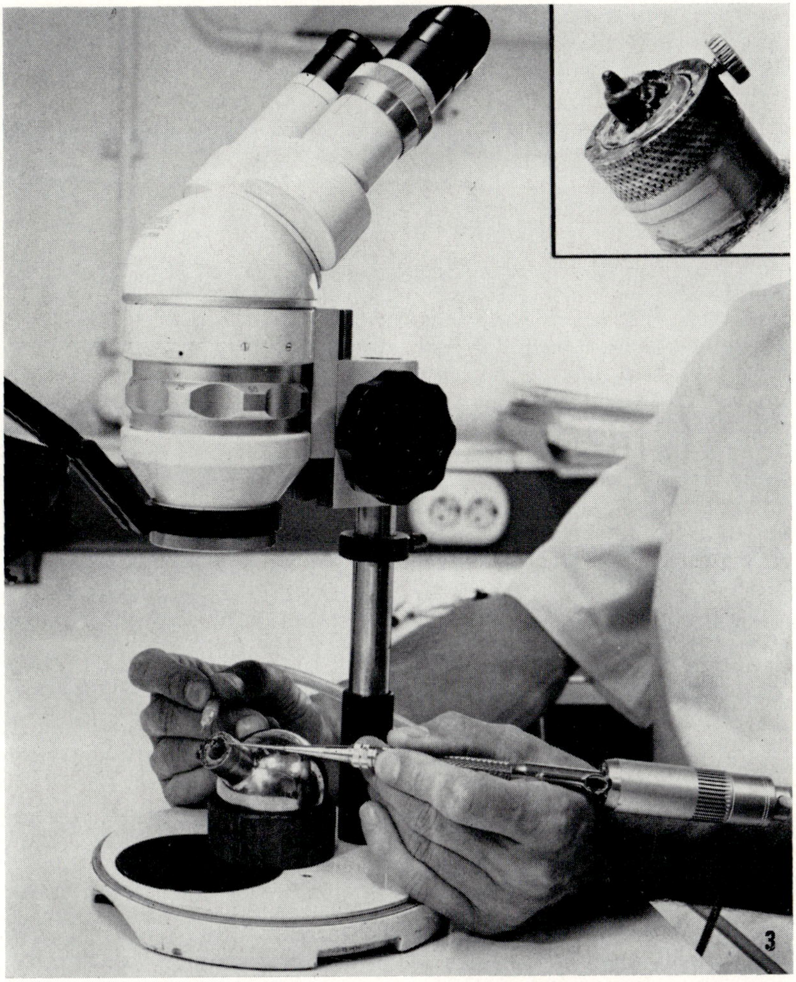

Fig. 3. Preparation of a cochlea using a binocular preparation microscope. The specimen is glued to an aluminum disk and clamped in a holder (inset). By turning the massive metal sphere the specimen is made accessible from all sides. The bony capsule is ground down with a modern drill, hand-piece and diamond burrs, as used in ear microsurgery. A thin jet of nitrogen blows the bone dust away and at the same time cools the specimen.

The second fixation technique is known as labyrinthine fixation. It was used in fixation of about one-third of the total number of cochleae. The same intraperitoneal anesthesia was used. The animal was decapitated and the temporal bones were quickly resected from the skull and cut open to expose the cochlea. A slender hook was used to open the cochlea at the apex and perforate the round and oval windows.[14] This took only a few minutes. The coch-

Fig. 2. A) Surface specimen of the organ of Corti of a guinea pig. The stereocilia (asterisk) of the inner hair cells (IHC) are angulated because the specimen was slightly compressed. Of the three rows of outer hair cells (OHC), only the first is in focus because the specimen is not entirely flat. The stereocilia of the OHC show a W-configuration (arrow) (Phase-contrast microscope (PCM) 1,560 X). B) Upper basal turn. Cross section through the acoustic nerve (AN), the spiral ganglion (SG) and the organ of Corti of a specimen which has first been studied with a scanning electron microscope (SEM) (LM 180 X).

leae were then immersed in 2% glutaraldehyde in 0.1 M phosphate buffer at pH 7.35 ± 0.05.

Both techniques ensure rapid fixation, thus minimizing postmortal changes. The second technique gives slightly less shrinkage of the specimen but has the disadvantage that the surface of the organ of Corti is occasionally obscured by a precipitate, probably from endolymphatic protein.

Preparation, Dehydration and Drying. The bone was cut a few millimeters below the basal turn of the cochlea, with the modiolus virtually perpendicular to the cut surface. The temporal bone was further trimmed down so as to fit in its entirety in the specimen holder for later scanning electron microscopy. The tissue must not be allowed to dry up during this processing. The specimen was kept in a 2% glutaraldehyde solution at 4 C for four hours. It was then washed five times in 0.9% NaCl and five times in distilled water. Dehydration was effected through an acetone series of increasing concentration, starting with a 30% acetone solution and increasing by 10% steps to absolute acetone. Some specimens were washed and dehydrated with the aid of an EM tissue processor.* The results thus obtained proved to be superior to those obtained by the conventional nonautomated method. In absolute acetone the specimens were placed in a critical point drying apparatus** and dried by means of Freon 13®.*** Although in a critical point apparatus the shrinkage of biological material is much less than that as compared with air-drying, it can nevertheless still amount to as much as 10%.[68] The advantage of the critical point apparatus over freeze-drying is that the biological material becomes firmer.[69] This is of great importance in dissecting the entire organ of Corti.

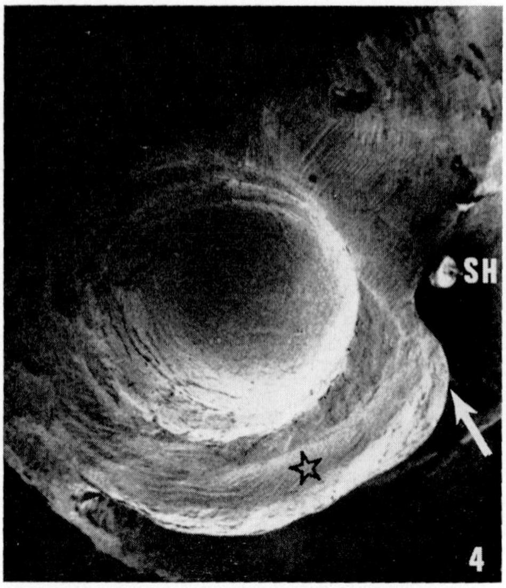

Fig. 4. A left cochlea viewed from above. The stapes head (SH) is just visible. An arrow indicates the round window. The bone has been ground down as far as possible, particularly on the medial side. The otic capsule is intact. The groove milled in the basal turn is identifiable (asterisk) (SEM 10 X).

The cochlea with some fragments of the temporal bone was then glued to an aluminum disk with the aid of two-component epoxy resin. For optimal fixation of the specimen to the disk, the latter was beveled out so that the glue would find some lateral support. The disk with the specimen was then placed in OsO_4 vapor for about six hours. The vapor invaded the specimen, thus improving conduction for electrons and facilitating the image formation of the scanning electron microscope. A specimen kept in the vapor for more than six hours can become fragile so that the organ of Corti is readily damaged and severed from the modiolus during dissection.

Microdissection. The aluminum disk was clamped in a holder especially designed for this purpose, and under a binocular preparation microscope**** the specimen was processed at magnifications of 6, 12 and 25 times. The holder consists of a metal sphere which fits

*American Optical Corp., Buffalo, NY. Model 9000933. Made for C. Reichert, Optische Werke A. G., Vienna, Austria.

**Polaron Equipment, Ltd., London, England. Type E 3000.

***E. I. du Pont de Nemours & Co., Inc., Wilmington, DE.

****Wild Heerbrugg Instruments, Inc., Farmingdale, NY.

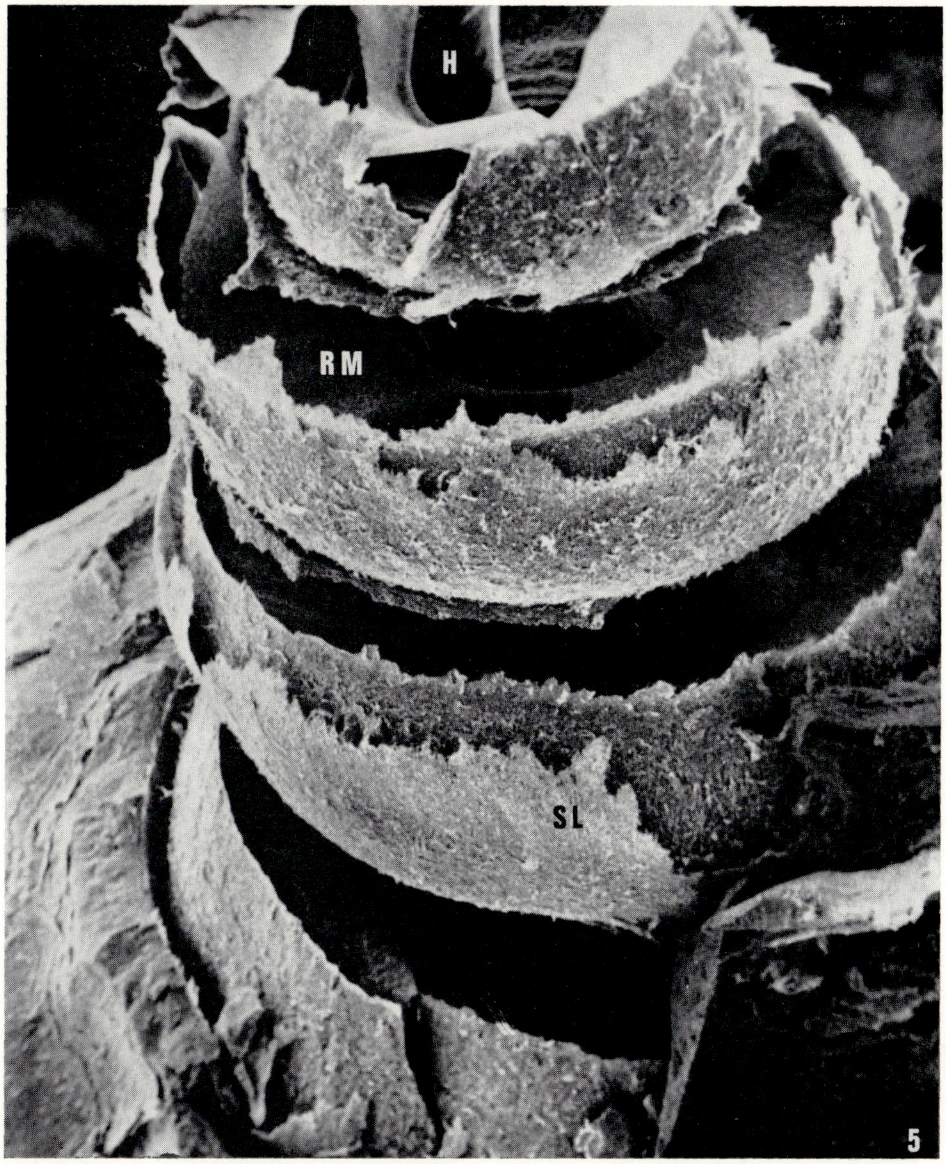

Fig. 5. The otic capsule of a left cochlea has been cut away over nearly three turns. The thinner the capsule, the more easily this is done. The spiral ligament (SL) and Reissner's membrane (RM) are visible. H — Helicotrema. The spiral ligament seems to consist of two parts, the innermost of which is the stria vascularis (SEM 68 X).

in a cup. This makes it possible to turn the specimen as required to work under various angles. Another advantage is that focusing rarely needed to be done with the control knob of the microscope but could be effected by slight adjustments of the position of the sphere. For dissection of the organ of Corti in its entirety, enveloping bone tissue first had to be ground down to minimal thickness. A modern drill with diamond burrs proved to be very effective for this purpose (Fig. 3). Using burrs of decreasing diameter, particularly the medial part of the osseous cochlea, and most of the bone of the basal turn were

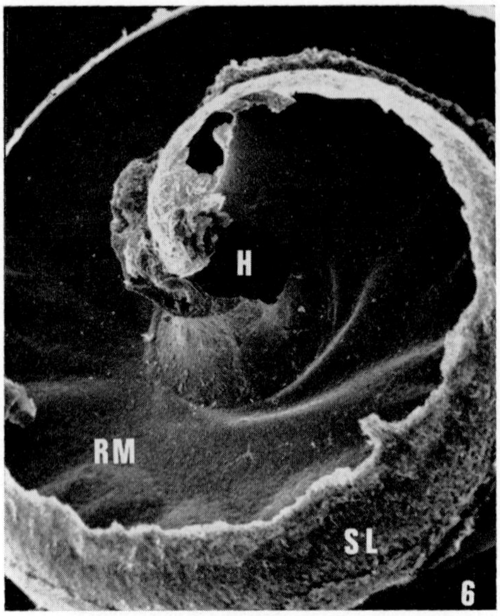

Fig. 6. The apical turn of a right cochlea after removal of the bony capsule. H — Helicotrema; RM — Reissner's membrane; SL — Spiral ligament. The aperture next to the helicotrema is artificial (SEM 73 X).

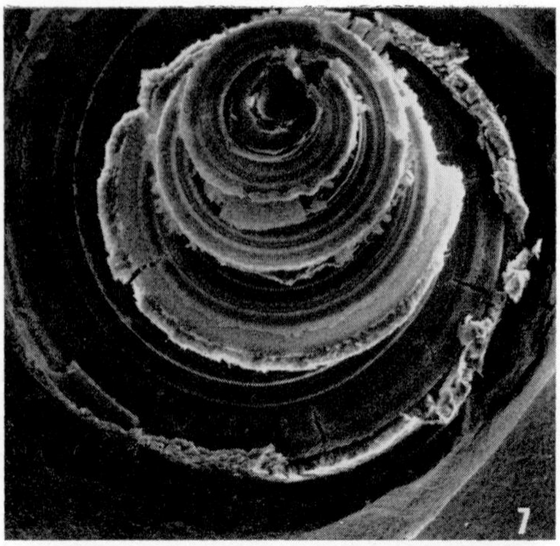

Fig. 7. A right organ of Corti ready for examination. The bony capsule and spiral ligament have been successively removed from the three apical turns. From the basal turn only part of the enclosing bone and part of the spiral ligament were removed to spare the organ of Corti, which is very vulnerable at this level. Reissner's membrane was blown away. The tiny radial ruptures and the longitudinal rupture are artifacts (SEM 25 X).

ground down (Fig. 4). Efforts were made to keep the cochlea completely closed in order to avoid damage to the organ of Corti. Continuous removal of the bone dust was ensured by a thin jet of nitrogen blown through an injection needle with a diameter of 0.5 mm, which at the same time served to cool the specimen.

To open the cochlea, a short hook or scalpel of the type used in micro ear surgery was used to cut the bone away in a circular pattern, starting at the apex and following the turns. Viewed from above, the turns of a right cochlea are clockwise, while those of a left cochlea are counterclockwise. The membranous part of the cochlea was left intact so far as possible (Figs. 5, 6). The basal turn offered difficulties in this respect because at this level the spiral ligament and the organ of Corti could be readily impinged on when the otic capsule was broken away. To prevent this, a tiny groove was fraised in the bone of the basal turn from the round window, above the level of the basilar membrane (Fig. 4). This was easily done with a 3 x 0 diamond burr. When the bone was then removed, it broke exactly on the groove, leaving spiral ligament and organ of Corti intact.

A delicate hook or watchmaker's tweezers were then used to detach the spiral ligament from the three upper turns. The basilar membrane ruptured at the level of the outer sulcus with the exception of the ligament at the basal turn, which remained intact; only the apical edge of the spiral ligament was removed. Although an oblique view of the organ of Corti in the basal turn thus becomes impossible, it could nevertheless be clearly visualized from above in the scanning electron microscope, because the basal turn has a much larger diameter than any of the other three turns.

Only the tectorial membrane and the Reissner's membrane could at this stage still obstruct the view on the upper surface of the organ of Corti. However, the tectorial membrane proved to have so shrunken due to fixation, dehydration or drying that it did not obstruct

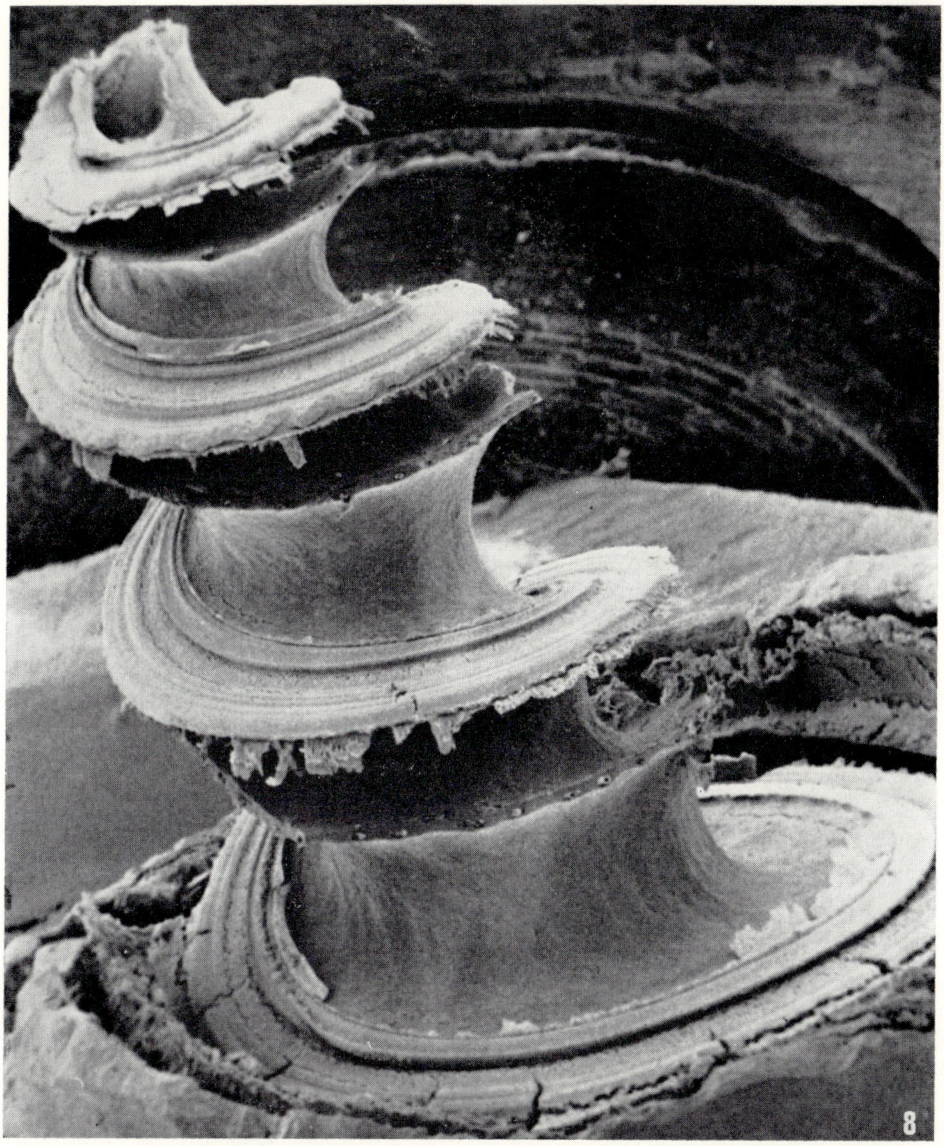

Fig. 8. Lateral view of the entire organ of Corti (SEM 55 X).

the view. As a rule it was found curled in. The fragility of Reissner's membrane made it possible to blow it away from all turns with the thin jet of nitrogen. The organ of Corti was thus exposed from helicotrema to round window (Figs. 7, 8, 9).

Before the specimen could be placed in the scanning electron microscope, conduction had to be further improved. For this purpose a thin coating of colloidal graphite was applied to the surface of the glue. Immediately after, the disk with the specimen was coated in high vacuum with subsequently thin films of carbon, gold and carbon. The total thickness of the coating was estimated on the basis of the color (green), and amounted to about 300 Å. The specimen was then ready for investigation in the scanning electron microscope. By slightly altering the angle of the spec-

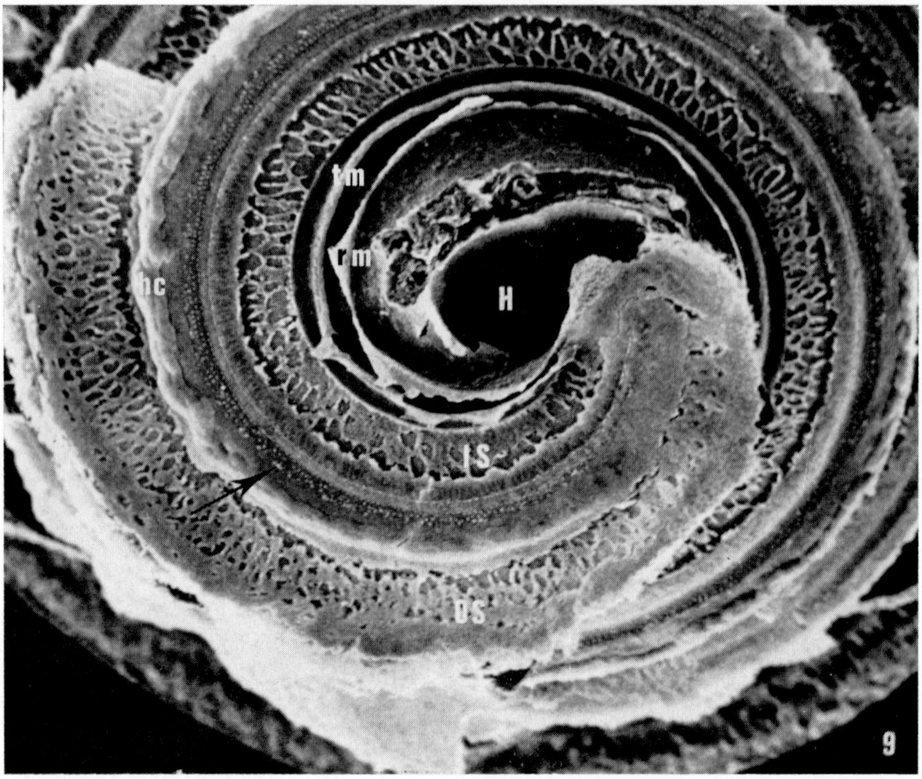

Fig. 9. The apical turn of a right cochlea. The turns are clockwise. H — Helicotrema; RM — Remnants of Reissner's membrane; TM — Markedly shrunken tectorial membrane; IS — Inner sulcus; arrow indicates sensory cells; HC — Undulating dam of Hensen's cells; OS — Outer sulcus (SEM 100 X).

imen again and again, the sense organ could be examined on the TV screen turn by turn, following the spiral. Higher magnifications were used to visualize the characteristic pattern, and for detailed examination of the surface of individual hair cells and supporting cells. The only part of the organ of Corti not in direct view was the small, extremely basal part (at this point the organ of Corti slopes steeply down). This part could be made accessible by detaching the specimen from the disk, rotating it 90° and remounting it.

In an exsiccator, the specimens could be kept for months. The above described method of dry dissection was made possible by a combination of a degree of toughness of the tissue resulting from the cross-linking during glutaraldehyde fixation and slight shrinkage caused by dehydration and drying. As a result, the organ of Corti remained attached to its natural support, the modiolus, and the other parts could be removed. The procedure of drilling and dissection took about 45 minutes per cochlea. Nearly all micrographs were made with a scanning electron microscope at 15 kV acceleration voltage.*

It is also possible that after using this method for examining the surface of the organ of Corti, the same specimen is used to study the organ from sections. For this purpose the entire organ of Corti with the modiolus was embedded and cut. The light microscope or transmission electron microscope could then be used to study cellular or intracellular structures at any site, selected with the scanning electron microscope, in the organ of Corti (Fig. 10).

*Jeol USA, Medford, MA. Model JSM-U3 or -35R.

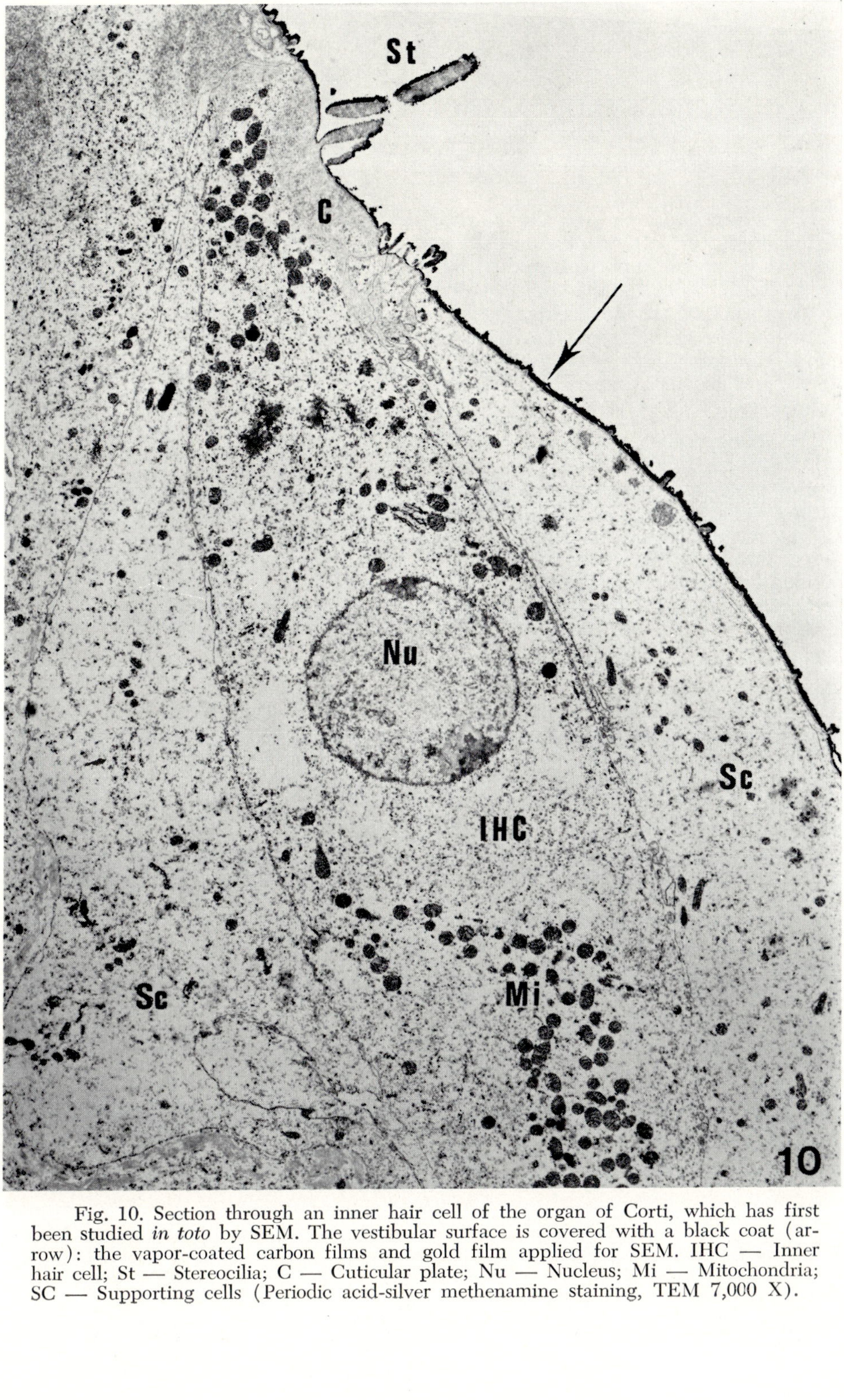

Fig. 10. Section through an inner hair cell of the organ of Corti, which has first been studied *in toto* by SEM. The vestibular surface is covered with a black coat (arrow): the vapor-coated carbon films and gold film applied for SEM. IHC — Inner hair cell; St — Stereocilia; C — Cuticular plate; Nu — Nucleus; Mi — Mitochondria; SC — Supporting cells (Periodic acid-silver methenamine staining, TEM 7,000 X).

CHAPTER III

SCANNING ELECTRON MICROSCOPY OF THE ORGAN OF CORTI

Anatomy

The surface and part of the interior of the organ of Corti were examined in the first group of 40 normal guinea pigs (Figs. 11-27). For detailed information on the structure of the cochlea we refer to the literature of previously mentioned authors[1,4,5,11-14,16,19,29-31,34,36,38-41,43,46-48] and to the work of Held[70] and Kolmer.[71]

The sensory cells, or hair cells, are divided by the pillar cells into a single row of inner, and usually three rows of outer hair cells (Fig. 11). The vestibular surface of these cells bears hairs or stereocilia. The pillar cells are likewise divided into an inner and outer row. Together they form Corti's tunnel (canal of Corti).

On the inside of the inner hair cells lies a row of slender supporting cells whose surface is characterized by numerous microvilli. These cells are otherwise known as border cells.[1,43] The inner hair cells are separated from each other by inner phalangeal cells. Closer to the modiolus lies a row of oblong cells which are part of the inner sulcus. These cells are clearly demarcated by the presence of microvilli. The other cells of the inner sulcus are flatter and of more variable shape. Their nucleus is often visible on the surface. The inner sulcus cells are partly concealed by the shrunken tectorial membrane. Even closer to the modiolus, interdental cells form the surface of the spiral limbus, and Reissner's membrane inserts here.

The inner pillar cells are virtually rectangular at the top, and on the surface separate the inner hair cells from the outer hair cells. The outer pillar cells are pear-shaped on the surface and separate the outer hair cells of the first row from each other and partly from those of the second row.[5] Over most of the length of the organ of Corti there are three rows of outer hair cells, characterized by their regular arrangement and the W-configuration of their stereocilia. The outer hair cells are not only separated from each other by the heads of outer pillar cells, but also by the phalangeal plates of the first and the second row of Deiters' cells. These phalangeal plates are knuckle-shaped. Those of the third row of Deiters' cells are polygonal and form a continuous row on the outside of the organ of Corti. This pro-

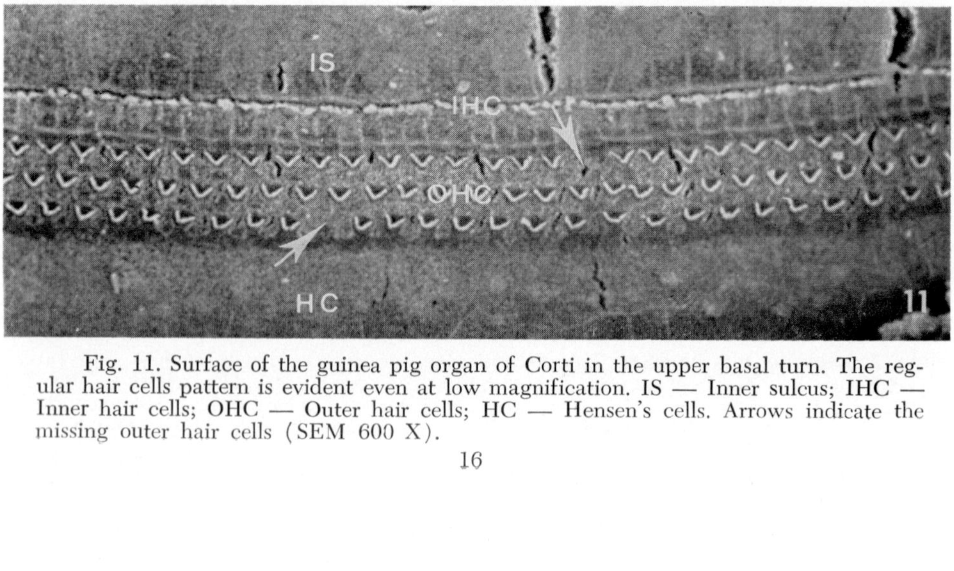

Fig. 11. Surface of the guinea pig organ of Corti in the upper basal turn. The regular hair cells pattern is evident even at low magnification. IS — Inner sulcus; IHC — Inner hair cells; OHC — Outer hair cells; HC — Hensen's cells. Arrows indicate the missing outer hair cells (SEM 600 X).

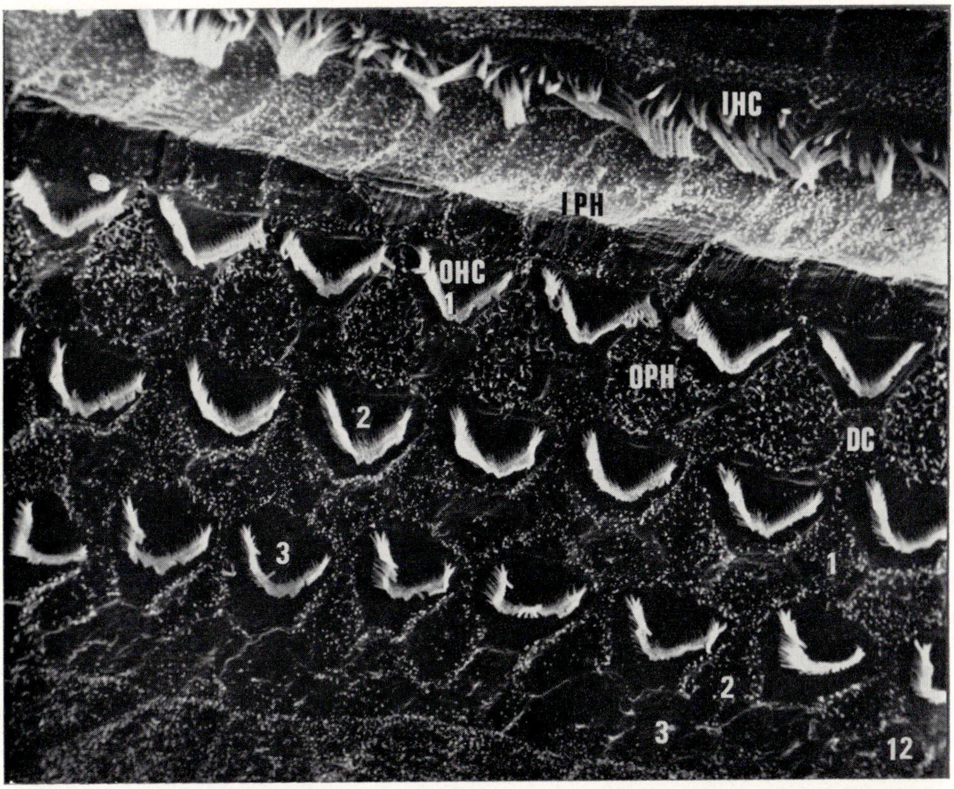

Fig. 12. Upper basal turn. The inner hair cells (IHC) are separated from the three rows of outer hair cells (OHC 1,2,3) by the inner pillar heads (IPH), which show some slight distortion. This indicates the site at which the outer pillar heads are still localized beneath the inner pillar heads. The outer hair cells of the first row are separated from each other by the pear-shaped outer pillar heads (OPH). There are three rows of Deiters' cells (DC 1,2,3). The phalangeal plates of Deiters' cells are knuckle-shaped in the first two rows, and polygonal and closely packed in the third row. The stereocilia of the OHC show a W-configuration. Unlike the surface of the sensory cells, that of the supporting cells shows an abundance of microvilli (SEM 2,500 X).

vides a sharp demarcation from the Hensen's cells. Unlike the sensory cells, the phalangeal plates and pillar heads show an abundance of microvilli (Fig. 12). In the apical turn the Hensen's cells constitute a high dam, which gradually loses height in the direction of the round window. At the apex this dam takes an undulating course, and this also diminishes in basal direction (Fig. 8). This undulating shape is a constant finding. More externally lies the outer sulcus, lined with Claudius' cells; these are lower than Hensen's cells and resemble those of the inner sulcus. The outer sulcus changes into the spiral prominence.

The stereocilia of an inner as well as of an outer hair cell of the guinea pig stand in three rows of varying lengths, like organ pipes. In the apical part, there are interconnections between the longest stereocilia of an inner hair cell (Fig. 13). These were also observed by Bredberg *et al.*[41] However, the longest stereocilia of the outer hair cell also seem to be interconnected, at least in the upper two-thirds (Figs. 14, 15). The stereocilia of the inner and the outer hair cells are arranged in a W-configuration, this showing a much wider angulation in the inner than in the outer hair cells.[71,73] The shortest stereocilia of the inner hair cell are evidently thinner than the others, whereas the stereocilia

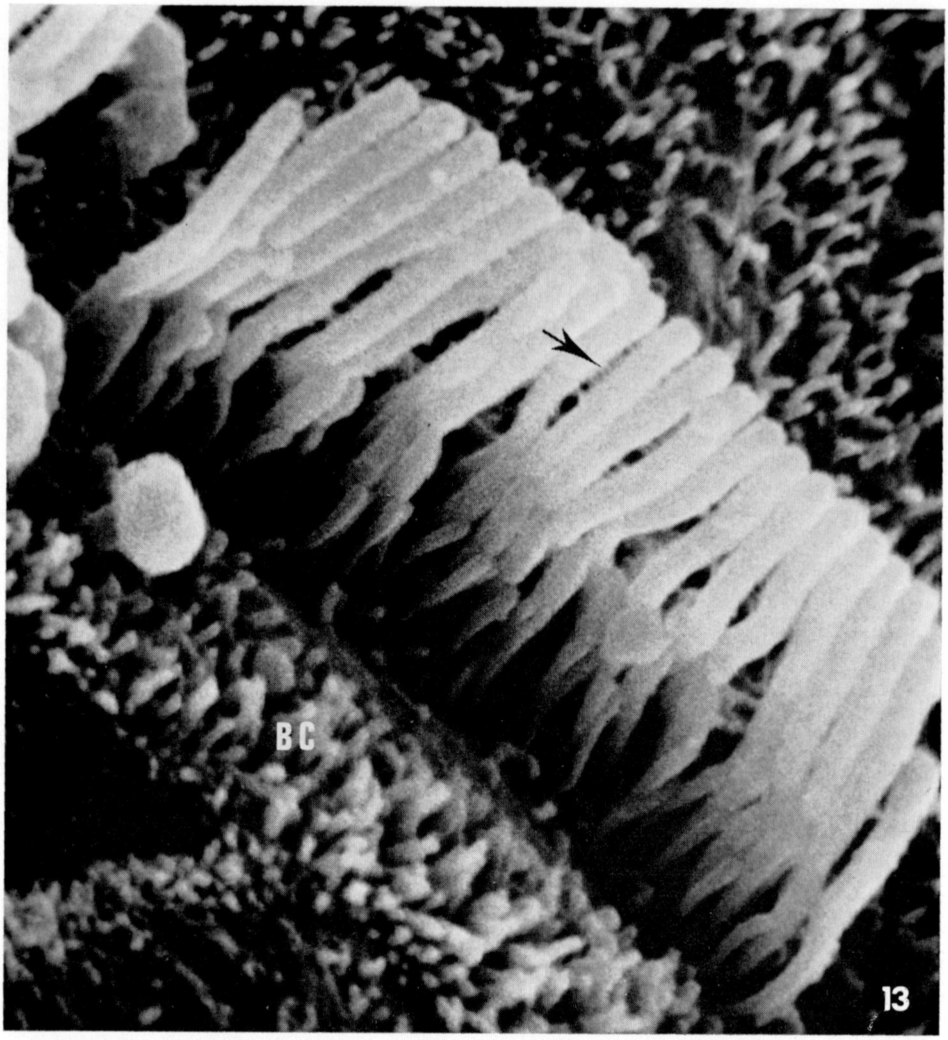

Fig. 13. Lower apical turn. Inner hair cell viewed from the inside. Three rows of stereocilia of different lengths. Some of the longest are interconnected (arrow); the shortest are thinner than the others. The many microvilli in the foreground stand on the surface of a border cell (BC). The mushroom-shaped bulge between the two sensory cells may be from an inner phalangeal cell (SEM 15,300 X).

of the outer hair cell all seem to be of the same thickness.[41] The ends of the stereocilia of the outer cells are clubbed and packed close together, seemingly supporting each other and forming a single unit.[73] All stereocilia are slightly thinner at the base, and the different rows stand at different angles (Fig. 16).

The combination of the stereocilia of a hair cell is reminiscent of a leaf spring design. It may be assumed that only the longest connect with the tectorial membrane, and that a bending of the stereocilia stimulates the sensory cell. The stereocilia of different lengths represent the spring leaves. When the longest stereocilia are bent in by a sound wave, their resistance will increase progressively and displacement will be only small; when they are bent out, their resistance will be considerably less owing to the presence of the shorter ones. This

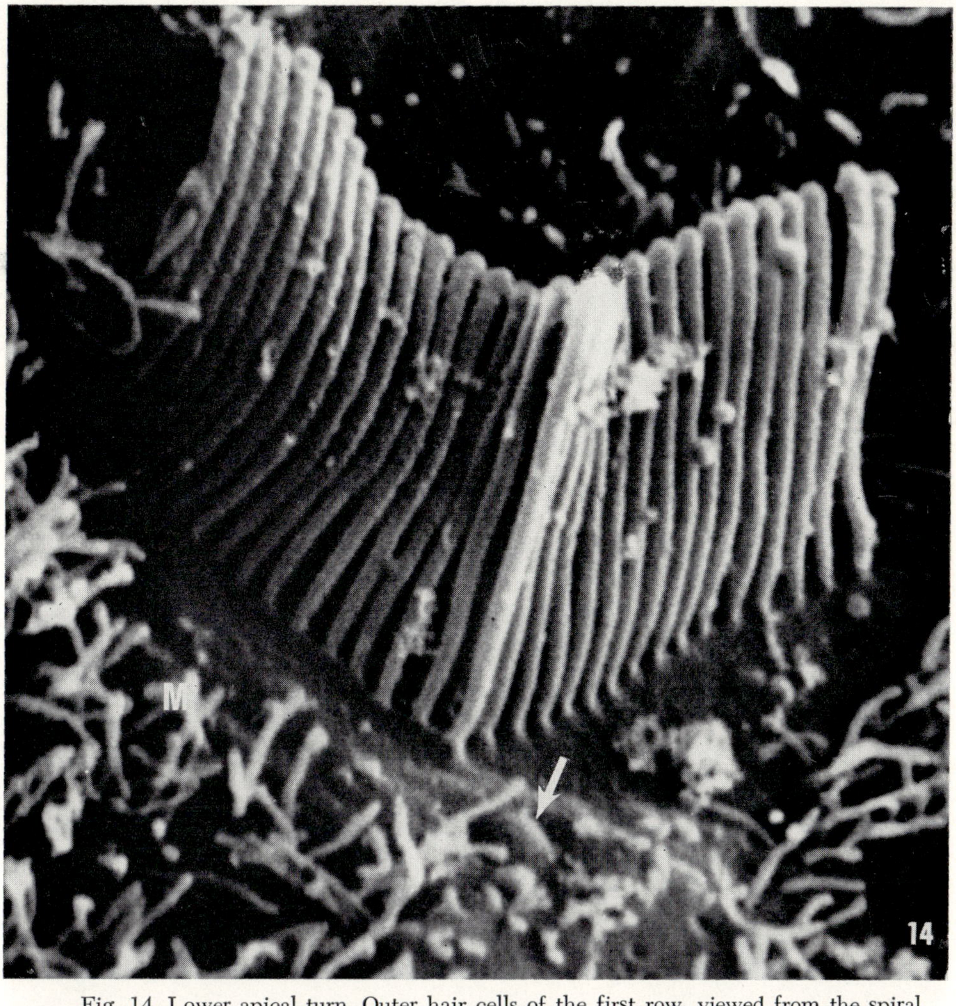

Fig. 14. Lower apical turn. Outer hair cells of the first row, viewed from the spiral ligament. The ends of the longest hairs are clubbed. The stereocilia are apart at the base, but come together at a higher level. The arrow indicates an elevation of the cell surface caused by the basal body. M — Microvilli of the supporting cells (SEM 15,400 X).

is entirely in accordance with reports by Flock *et al*[72] and von Békésy,[74] who on the basis of other morphological and electrophysiological findings established an unmistakable predilection of the outer hair cells for radial movement, towards the spiral ligament. This is in the direction of the basal body, which is regarded as the site of maximum sensitivity of the cell membrane. The localization of the basal body is visible by a slight thickening of the surface of the outer hair cells.[34,72,75]

When the organ of Corti ruptures in the course of dissection, other parts can become visible. For instance, it can then be seen that the surface of the outer pillars is granular. Similar granular surfaces of the outer pillars are shown in photographs by Iurato,[1] and Angelborg and Engström.[47,48] Nerve fibers extend through Corti's tunnel: the radiating tunnel fibers which ramify and extend between the outer pillars to the outer hair cells (Fig. 17). These fibers are believed to be part of the efferent system, the

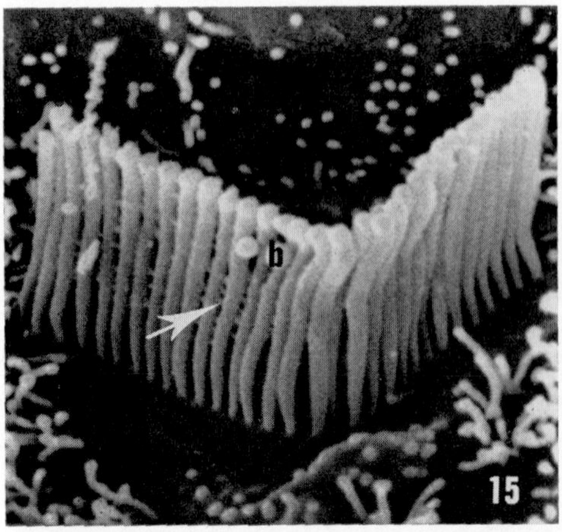

Fig. 15. Apical turn. Outer hair cell of the first row viewed from the outside. Due to slight outward displacement of the longest stereocilia, interconnections between the longest hairs are visible in the upper two-thirds (arrow). The blebs (b) on the stereocilia are observed in normal as well as in sound-damaged cochleae (SEM 8,400 X).

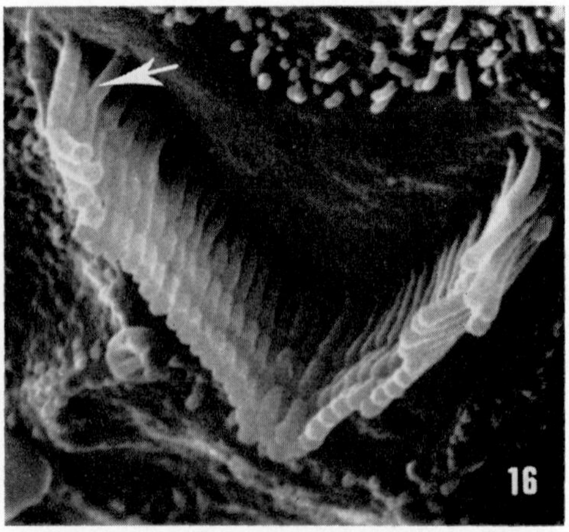

Fig. 16. Basal turn. Outer hair cell of the first row viewed from the inside. The longest stereocilia are shorter than those in more apical turns. The three rows of stereocilia of different lengths are of equal thickness and closely packed to form what seems to be a single unit. The lower parts of the stereocilia slightly angulate from each other (arrow) (SEM 8,400 X).

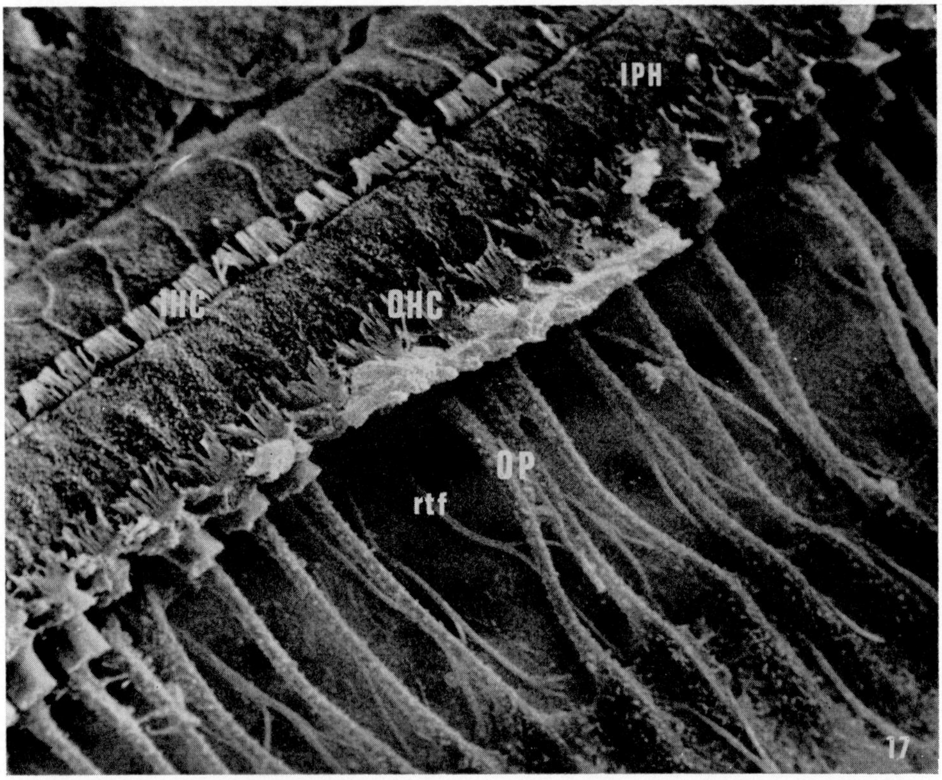

Fig. 17. Upper basal turn. Part of the organ of Corti with view into Corti's tunnel. Only the inner hair cells (IHC), inner pillar heads (IPH) and outer pillars (OP) as well as the first row of disrupted outer hair cells (OHC) are visible. Nerve fibers extend through the tunnel and ramify: the radiating tunnel fibers (rtf). The surface of the outer pillars is granular (SEM 1,260 X).

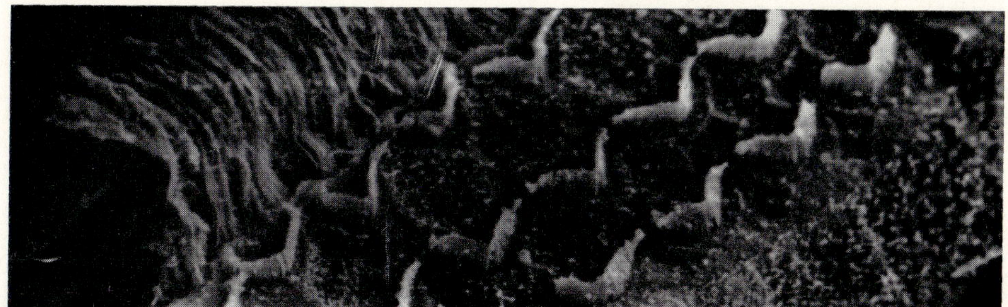

Fig. 18. Basal turn. Nuel's space becomes visible when parts of the organ are broken away. Three rows of outer hair cells (OHC) with their cell bodies. These rest on Deiters' cells (DC), each of which has a phalangeal process (Ph). At the surface this broadens to become a phalangeal plate (SEM 2,800 X).

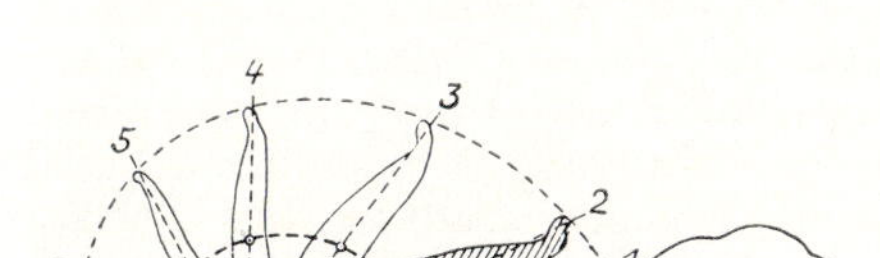

Fig. 19. Upper basal turn. Diagram of the organ of Corti and tectorial membrane of the guinea pig. Due to transverse and longitudinal shrinkage the membrane is loosened and finally reversed on the spiral limbus. Stages 2 and 6 (hatched) were taken from specimens. (After Werner,[86] Monatsschr Ohrenheilkd Laryngorhinol 17:1017, 1937. With permission of Georg Theime Verlag, Stuttgart, West Germany.)

bundle of Rasmussen.[76] The outer hair cells are localized in Nuel's space and rest on the Deiters' cells. Each Deiters' cell has a phalangeal process which broadens at the surface to form a phalangeal plate, always skipping every other cell so that the outer hair cells seem to be optimally separated (Fig. 18).

The tectorial membrane seems to play an important role in excitation of the sensory cells.[77-79] The mechanism of action has been a subject of discussion for decades.[1,38,43,46,72,73,75,80-85] One of the reasons undoubtedly lies in the difficulty to produce a reproducible morphology, because this membrane is subject to marked distortion when fixed, dehydrated and dried for morphological examination. As early as 1937, Werner[86]

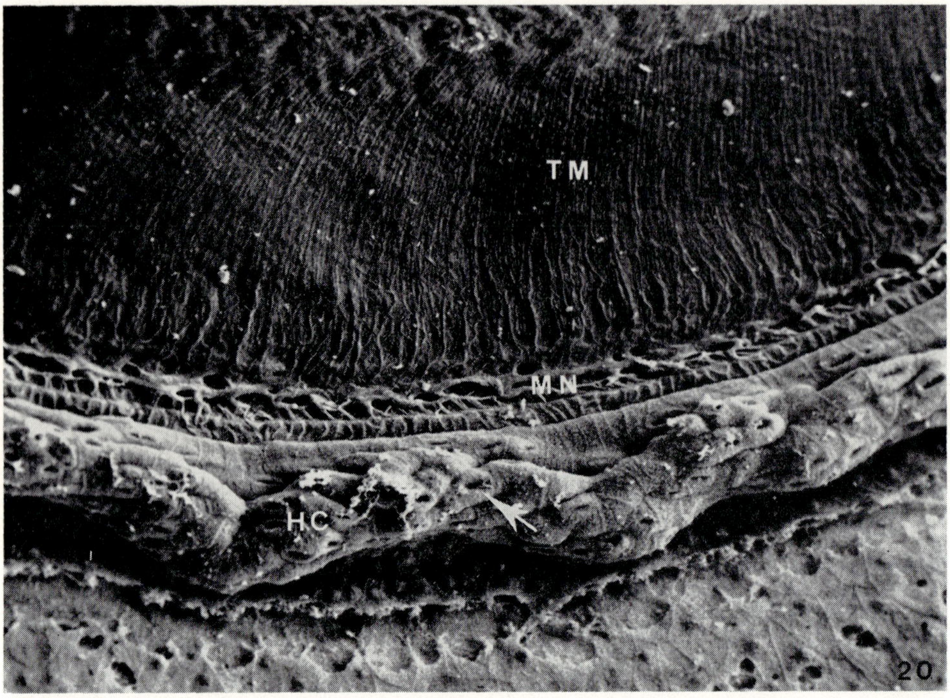

Fig. 20. The tectorial membrane (TM) of the apical turn viewed from above. The fiber course is not radial but slightly angulates from the radius and is more or less S-shaped. Attached to the third row of Deiters' cells are processes of the tectorial membrane which form the marginal net (MN). The dam of Hensen's cells (HC) here takes an undulating course. The depressions in the Hensen's cells (arrow) are artifacts (SEM 380 X).

mentioned these changes and explained why the tectorial membrane is rarely, if ever, fixed in its natural position. He described how this membrane can shrink in three directions: in height, in width, and longitudinally, *i.e.*, parallel to the axis of the cochlear duct (Fig. 19). It is precisely this shrinkage that has been utilized in the present study to visualize the surface of the organ of Corti. The tectorial membrane is made up of fibrillae and ground substance,[83] and can be divided into three zones: the limbal, the middle, and the marginal zone. The latter ends externally in a network known as marginal net. Although in guinea pigs this is not highly developed,[43] this net was often found visible in our specimens, especially in the apical turn. It is quite conceivable that the above mentioned shrinkage causes the network to stretch before it breaks, as a result of which it seems much larger than it really is. We observed on several occasions that the marginal net was attached to the outer row of phalangeal plates of Deiters' cells, sometimes exactly at the boundary with the Hensen's cells. The fibrillae of the tectorial membrane are not radially arranged but angulate slightly from the radius and are more or less S-shaped (Fig. 20).

It has been repeatedly demonstrated that the longest stereocilia of the outer hair cells are firmly attached to the tectorial membrane.[36,43,73,87] Using the scanning electron microscope, Kosaka *et al*,[36] Lim[43] and Tanaka *et al*,[46] were in fact able to demonstrate imprints. In our specimens we observed hyperextension or fracture of the longest stereocilia of the outer hair cells several times (Fig. 21). This artifact would seem to suggest a firm connection.

The question whether the longest stereocilia of the inner hair cells are also

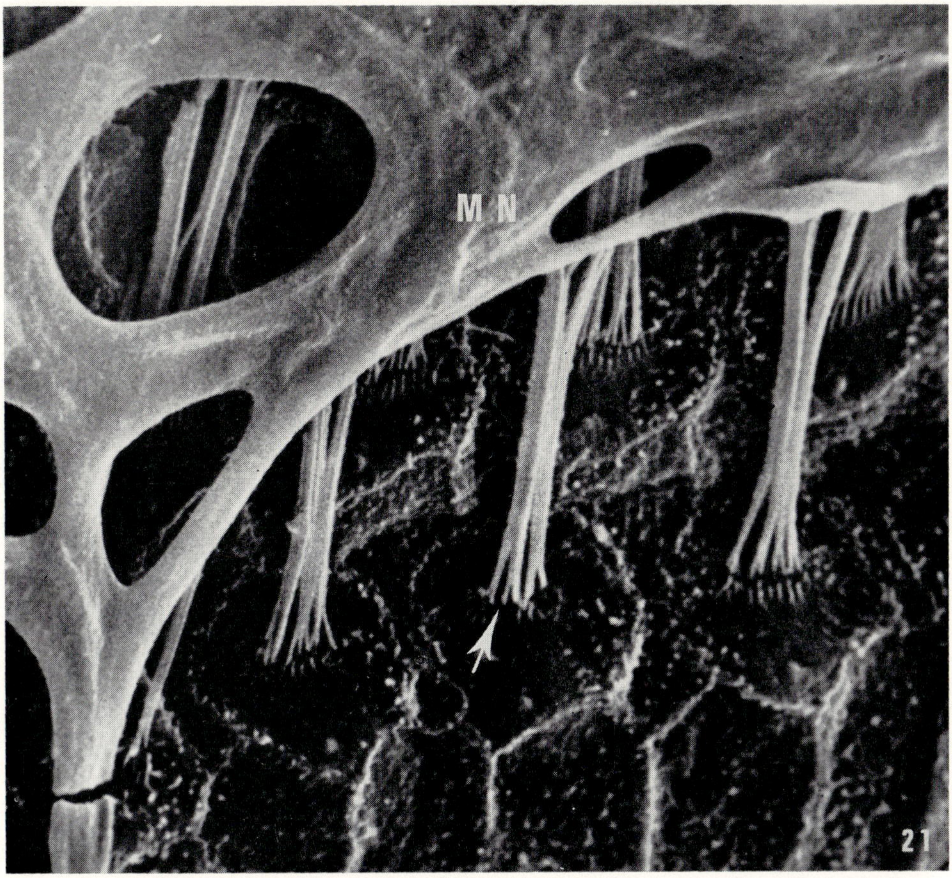

Fig. 21. Lower apical turn. Contact between outer hairs and tectorial membrane. Hyperextended and partly disrupted stereocilia (arrow) of outer hair cells are visible through defects in the marginal net (MN). This is undoubtedly an artifact caused by shrinkage of the tectorial membrane, but it does indicate a firm connection between stereocilia and this membrane (SEM 4,200 X).

connected with the tectorial membrane has, so far, remained moot. In any case, it is certain that the connection between inner hair cell stereocilia and the tectorial membrane is weaker than that between outer hair cell stereocilia and the membrane.[73] Nevertheless, our study has revealed unmistakable indications of a connection between inner hair cell stereocilia and the tectorial membrane. In Figure 22 some of the longest stereocilia of the inner hair cells are obviously hyperextended, and in Figure 23 at least two have broken and are still attached to the tectorial membrane. Both phenomena are suggestive of an existing connection. A more detailed knowledge of this connection is essential to theorization on the excitation of the organ of Corti. Does it involve activation by a flow of fluid or displacement of the tectorial membrane relative to the basilar membrane?

On the tympanic surface of the tectorial membrane five lines can be distinguished (Fig. 24). Three of these take an undulating course and mark the sites of insertion of the longest stereocilia of the outer hair cells. The remaining two lines are slightly curved. The outermost of the two is localized at the level of the inner hair cells, and may be another indication that the longest inner hair cell stereocilia are here connected

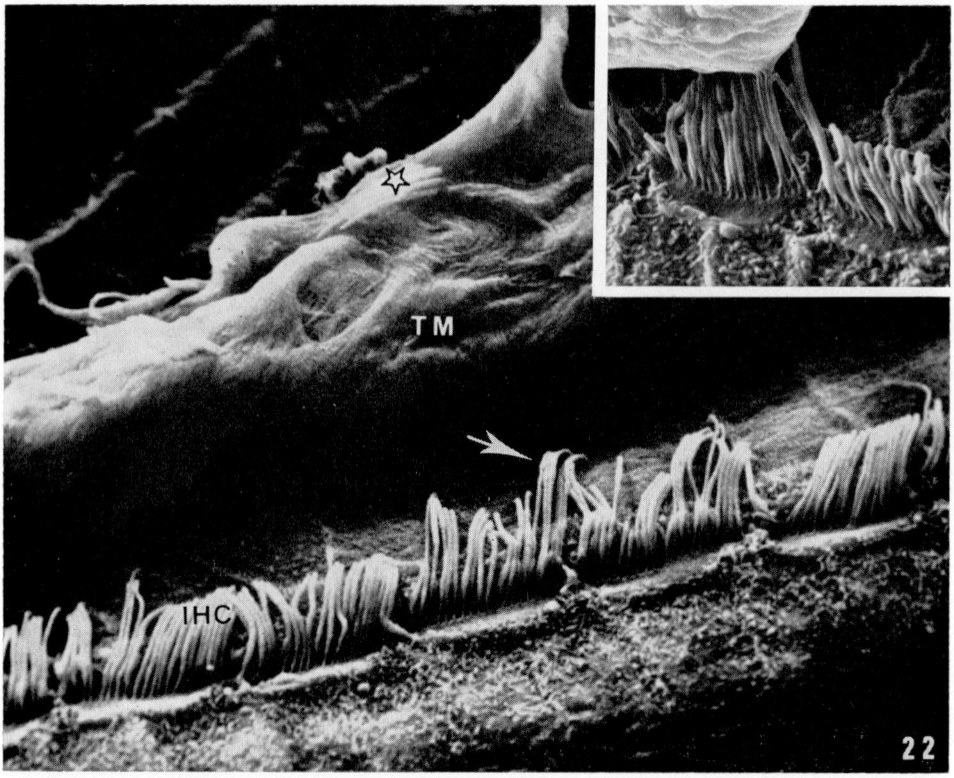

Fig. 22. Apical turn. Partly curled-up tectorial membrane (TM). Some of the longest stereocilia of the inner hair cells (IHC) are hyperextended (arrow). This may indicate a former connection between these stereocilia and the tectorial membrane, to which stereocilia of outer hair cells are still attached (asterisk) (SEM 2,500 X). Inset: some stereocilia of the inner hair cell are hyperextended and still attached to the tectorial membrane (SEM 2,800 X).

with the tectorial membrane. The fifth line may mark the site of the connection between this membrane and the border cells, as described by Lim,[43] although no trabeculae are observed here. The area between the two slightly curved lines is sometimes called Hensen's stripe.

The vestibular surface of the basilar membrane becomes visible when the organ of Corti is accidently removed. The surface is relatively smooth between the remnants of the inner and outer pillars. The former site of the Deiters' cells, too, is identifiable only by three rows of points (Fig. 25). The tympanic surface of the basilar membrane is more readily visualized than the vestibular surface. To achieve this, the specimen is broken at the basal turn, rotated 180° and reglued, whereupon it is again coated with carbon and gold. The basilar membrane cells form a compact layer in the basal turn which, towards the apex, gradually loosens and assumes the features of a network.[13,47] The fibrillae of the basilar membrane are clearly visible through the meshes of this network. They take a radial course in relation to the modiolus and are more or less perpendicular to the course of the pattern of the basilar membrane cells (Fig. 26). Angelborg and Engström[47] observed kinocilia on these cells.

Variations in the Hair Cell Pattern

Before degenerative characteristics can be distinguished in the organ of Corti, the normal variations in the hair cell pattern should be thoroughly known. Each normal cochlea has some sensory cells missing.[5,14] The missing cells are

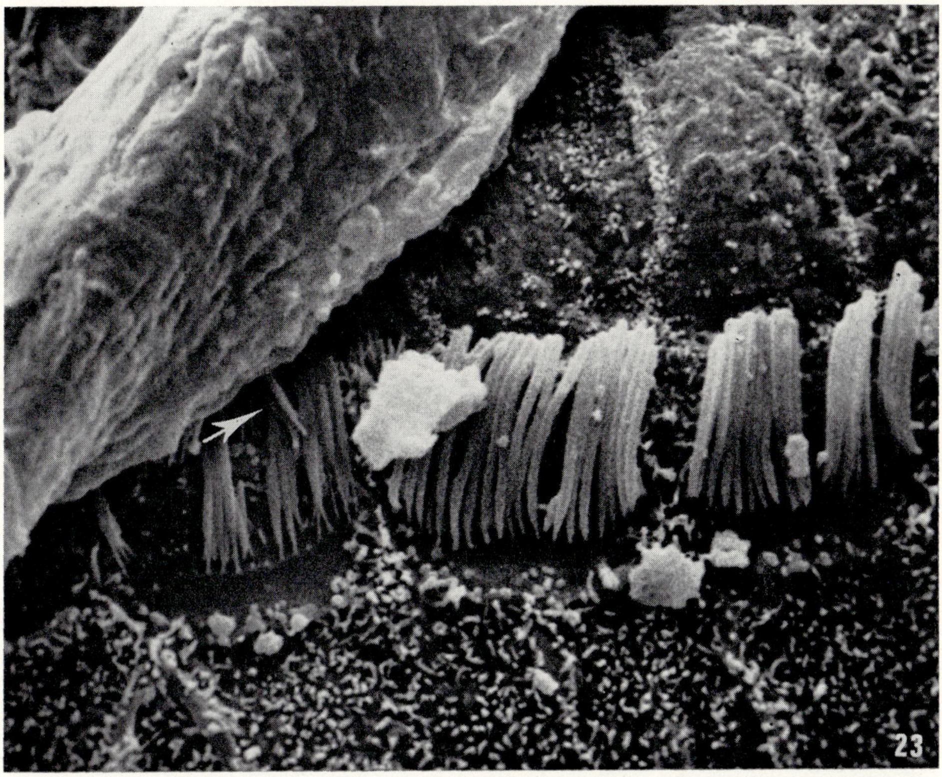

Fig. 23. Basal half apical turn. The tectorial membrane is partly curled up, and stereocilia of inner hair cells are visible as a result. At least two stereocilia seem to have broken off from the cell surface and to be still attached to the tectorial membrane (arrow). This is likewise an artifact, but it is indicative of a connection (SEM 4,600 X).

usually outer and rarely inner hair cells. In normal test animals, apart from missing single hair cells, sporadically small groups of hair cells were found to be missing, producing the effect of a cicatrix in the surface of the organ of Corti. The number of missing sensory cells in the normal pattern of the basal, upper basal, lower apical, and basal half of apical turns totals about 100. Whether these cells have always been absent or were lost during the relatively short lives of the test animals, is unknown.

When more than eight cells per scar were missing, it was assumed that acoustic trauma was involved.

The apical turn occupies a special position in the hair cell pattern. In the apex, the organ of Corti begins with virtually only inner hair cells. Pillar heads and outer hair cells are totally absent, as is also the Hensen's cell dam. At this level, inner and outer sulcus merge in a semicircular arch. Following the turn, a variable number of inner hair cells are succeeded by the first outer hair cells, which show a rather chaotic pattern. The typical W-configuration of the stereocilia is still lacking, as is the regular hair cell pattern. It is only in the course of the apical turn that the regular pattern gradually emerges (Figs. 27, 28), beginning with the first row of outer hair cells and continuing with the second and third rows.[17,46] The rectangular shape of the inner pillar heads also emerges. It is often not until the basal quarter of the apical turn that the organ of Corti assumes its characteristic regular pattern. Consequently, it is hardly possible to demonstrate degenerative changes in the apical half turn. For this reason, Bohne *et al*[88] did not include the apical half turn in her sound damage

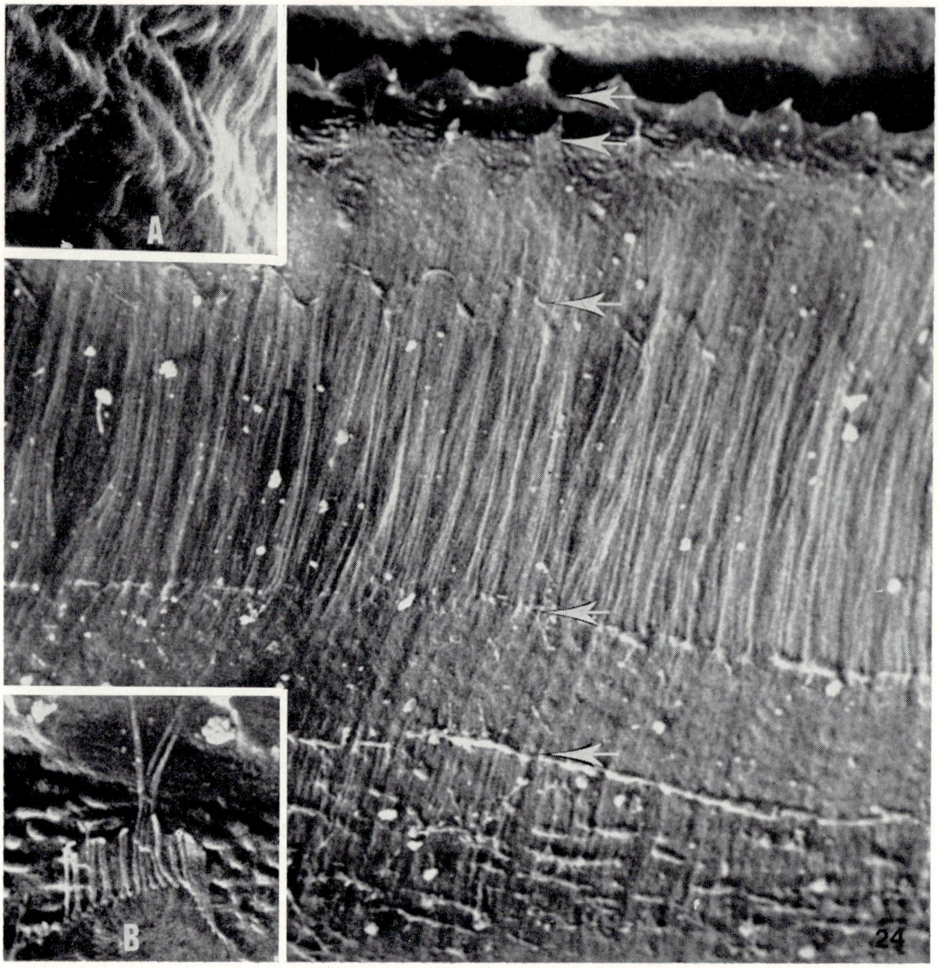

Fig. 24. Basal turn. Tympanic surface of tectorial membrane. Five lines are visible (arrows); the first three take an undulating course and form the sites of insertion of the longest stereocilia of the outer hair cells. The remaining two lines are slightly curved. The fourth line is seen at the level of the inner hair cells and probably marks the site of attachment of the longest stereocilia of these cells to the tectorial membrane. The fifth line is probably the site at which border cell trabeculae are attached to the tectorial membrane (SEM 1,660 X). Inset A) Imprints of stereocilia of an outer hair cell in the tectorial membrane (SEM 7,500 X). Inset B) Detail of second undulating line; some stereocilia have remained attached to the tectorial membrane, and a few of these are hyperextended (SEM 5,200 X).

studies. In the present study the same policy was adopted.

The site of a missing sensory cell on the surface is occupied by several hypertrophied supporting cells. Not only is their surface larger but their microvilli also seem more numerous.[44] A certain system can be discerned in the occupation of missing cell sites. The site of a cell missing from the first row of outer hair cells is occupied by the two adjacent outer pillar heads[18] (Fig. 29). In the second row it is both the outer pillar heads and the phalangeal plates of Deiters' cells that reconstruct the reticular membrane (Fig. 30), but in the third row it is only the phalangeal plates. Not infrequently the pattern of the Hensen's cells changes simultaneously. Engström *et al*[14] described the replacement

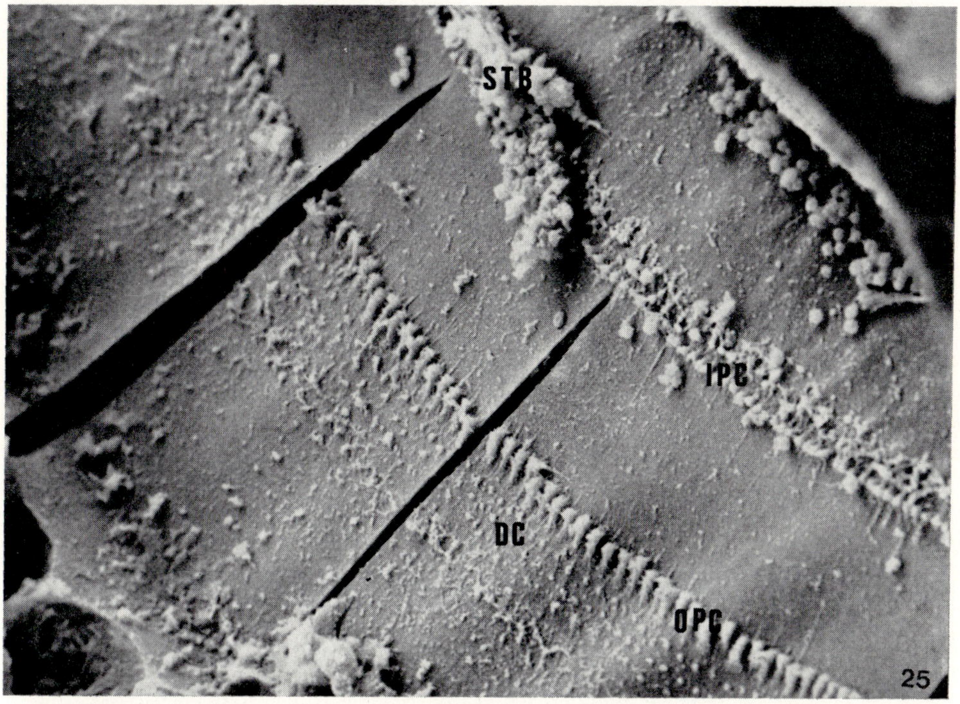

Fig. 25. Basal turn. The basilar membrane viewed from above after removal of the organ of Corti. Between the sites of insertion of the inner (IPC) and outer pillar cells (OPC), the surface is relatively smooth. The three rows of dots indicate the former sites of Deiters' cells (DC). At the level of the missing inner pillar cells a bundle of nerve fibers is observed: the spiral tunnel bundle (STB). The two ruptures are radial artifacts (SEM 380 X).

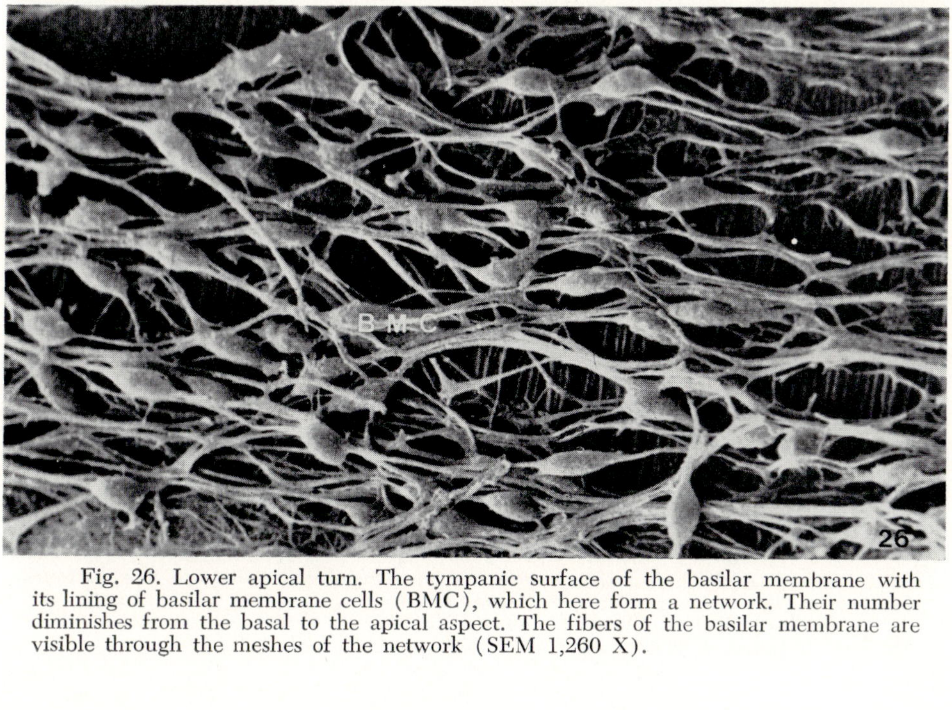

Fig. 26. Lower apical turn. The tympanic surface of the basilar membrane with its lining of basilar membrane cells (BMC), which here form a network. Their number diminishes from the basal to the apical aspect. The fibers of the basilar membrane are visible through the meshes of the network (SEM 1,260 X).

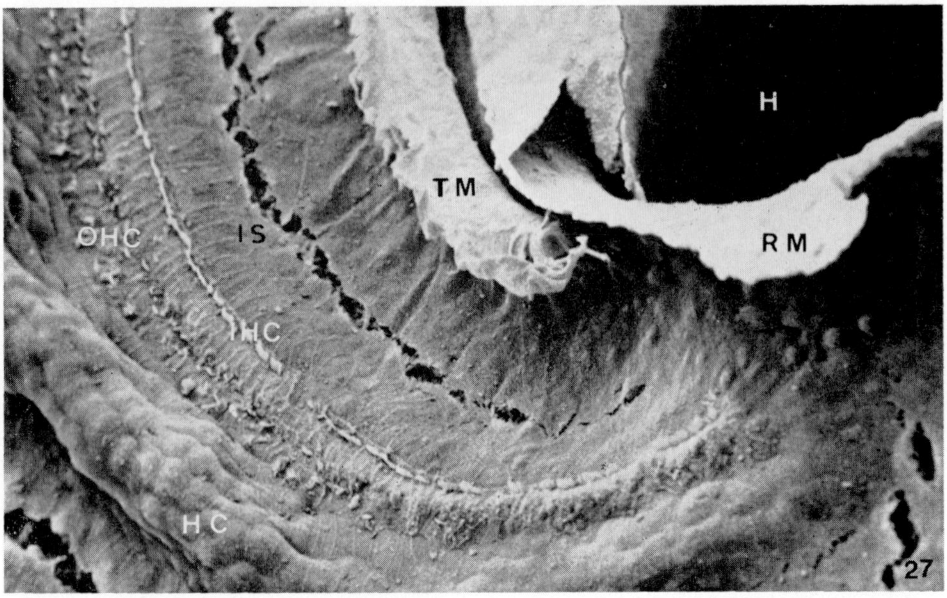

Fig. 27. The extremely apical part of the organ of Corti near the helicotrema (H). The inner hair cells (IHC) are arranged in a row in which a few are missing. Apically there are no outer hair cells. Following the turn in basal direction they are arranged in an exceedingly irregular pattern. Where the first outer hair cells (OHC) become visible, the dam of Hensen's cells (HC) begins. RM — Reissner's membrane; TM — Tectorial membrane; IS — Inner sulcus (SEM 380 X).

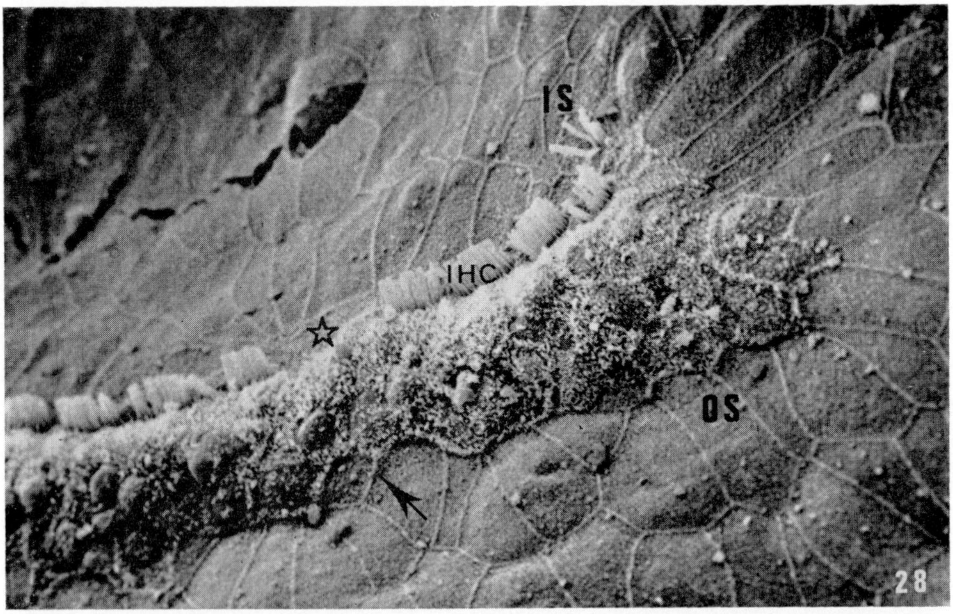

Fig. 28. Detail of Figure 27. The extremely apical part of the organ of Corti. The inner hair cells (IHC) are arranged in a row. A zone of cells with irregular contours (arrow) and covered with microvilli is seen at the site where pillar cells and outer hair cells appear further down. The inner sulcus (IS) merges with the outer sulcus (OS). An asterisk marks the sites of some missing sensory cells (SEM 1,260 X).

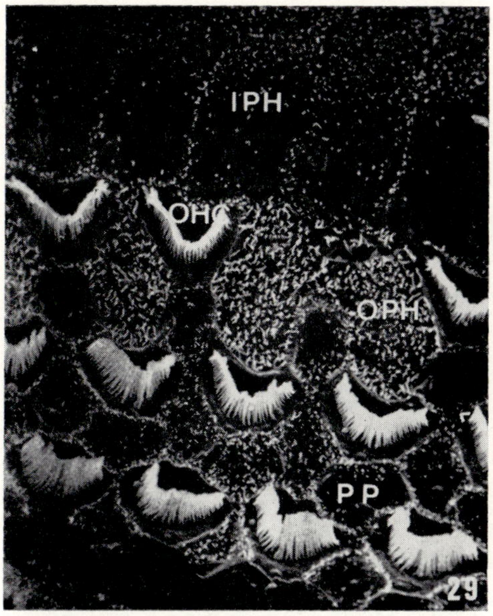

Fig. 29. Basal turn. Missing cell in the first row of outer hair cells (OHC), the site being occupied by two hypertrophied outer pillar heads (OPH). The small tear in the surface at this site is an artifact, possibly due to diminished strength of the reticular membrane. IPH — Inner pillar heads; pp — Phalangeal plate of Deiters' cell (SEM 2,400 X).

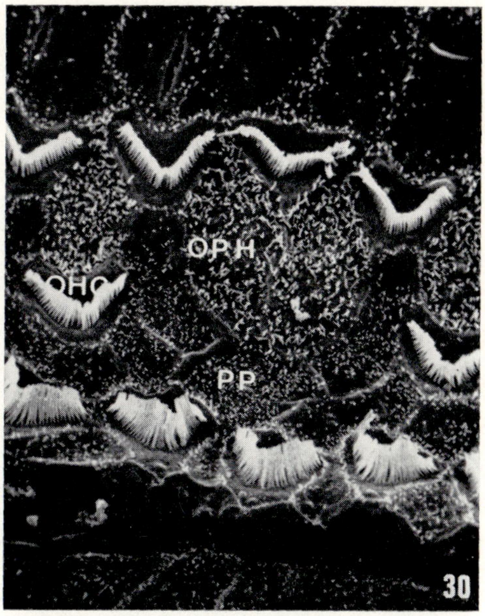

Fig. 30. Basal turn. Two missing outer hair cells (OHC) in the second row. Their sites in the reticular membrane are occupied by hypertrophied outer pillar heads (OPH) and phalangeal plates (pp) of Deiters' cells (SEM 2,400 X).

of a sensory cell by supporting cells as "phalangeal scar." Changes in the regular pattern are discernible at magnifications of 400 times and up.

Missing inner hair cells, much less common in the normal cochlea, are also replaced by supporting cells, covered with numerous microvilli. Spoendlin[13] demonstrated this by transmission electron microscopy. It is difficult to judge from the surface whether the inner pillar cell, border cell, inner sulcus or inner phalangeal cell replaces the missing inner hair cell. A combination of these supporting elements may be involved. Unlike the cell boundaries of outer hair cells, those of the inner hair cells warrant no conclusion in this respect (Fig. 31). Not infrequently, however, an enlarged inner sulcus cell was observed. The supporting cells apparently have a secondary function: closure of the reticular membrane after degeneration of a sensory cell. After all, a defect in the reticular membrane could entail ion leakage.

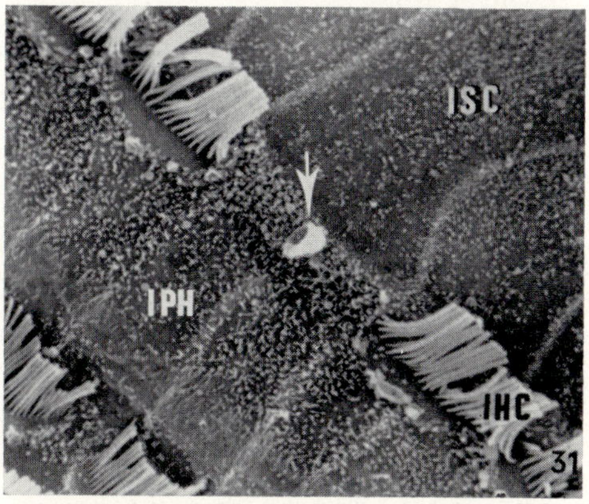

Fig. 31. Apical turn. Missing inner hair cell (IHC). Its site shows an abundance of microvilli. The boundaries between the individual supporting cells are ill-defined. The structure in the exact center (arrow) could not be interpreted but has been observed in other specimens as well. ISC — Inner sulcus cell; IPH — Inner pillar head (SEM 2,400 X).

Frequently, tiny ruptures were ob-

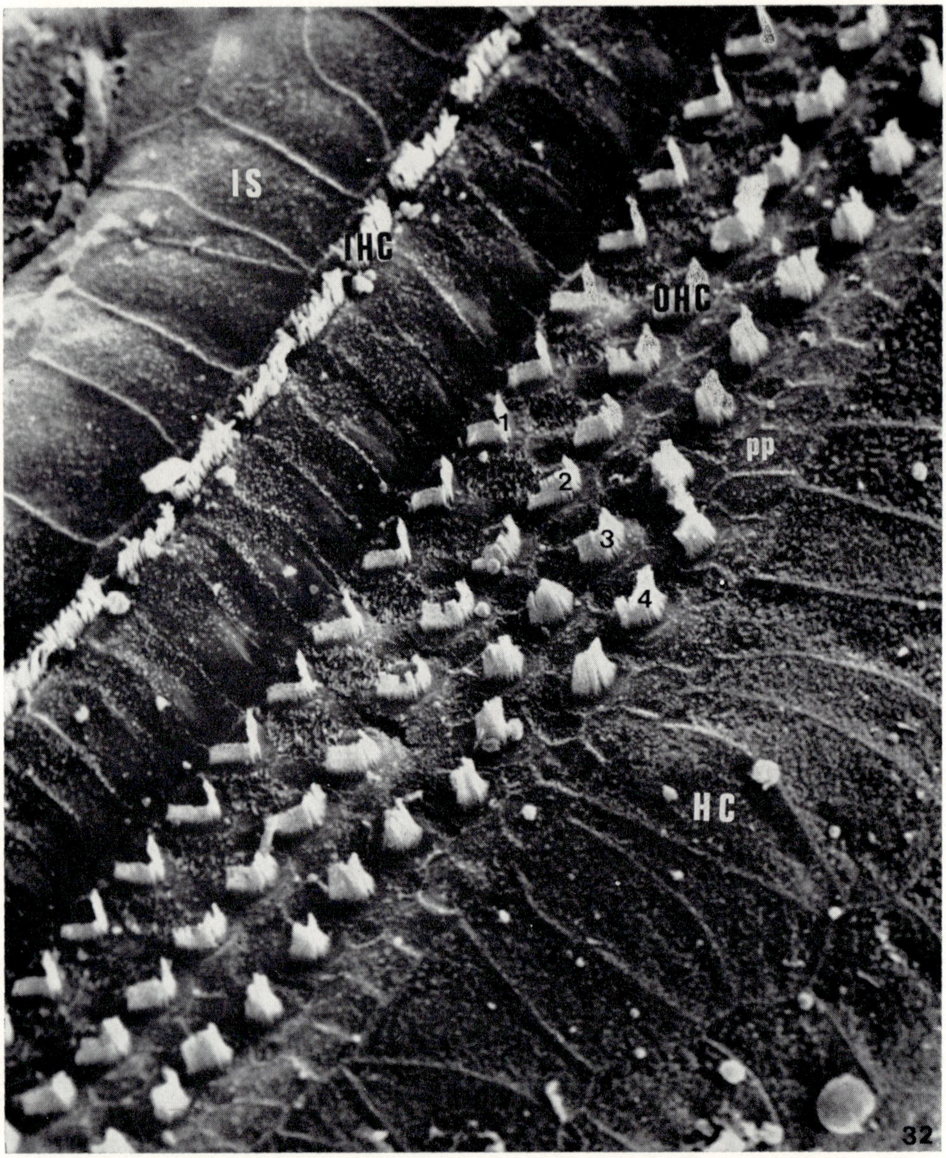

Fig. 32. Upper basal turn. The outer row of outer hair cells shows duplication. At this site the pattern of Deiters' cells and Hensen's cells has also slightly changed. IS — Inner sulcus; IHC — Inner hair cell; OHC 1,2,3,4 — Four rows of outer hair cells; pp — Phalangeal plate of Deiters' cells; HC — Hensen's cells (SEM 1,530 X).

served in the surface where scars were seen. These were doubtless artifacts, which could have been caused by the frailty of the reticular membrane and slight shrinkage of the specimen.

The normal hair cell pattern is characterized not only by missing sensory cells but also by duplications, more frequently of outer than of inner hair cells. Sometimes there are four rows of outer hair cells; this is mostly observed in the basal and the upper basal turn (Fig. 32). The duplication here seemed to have been effected by opposite movements of sensory cells until they were lying abeam. Inner hair cell duplication

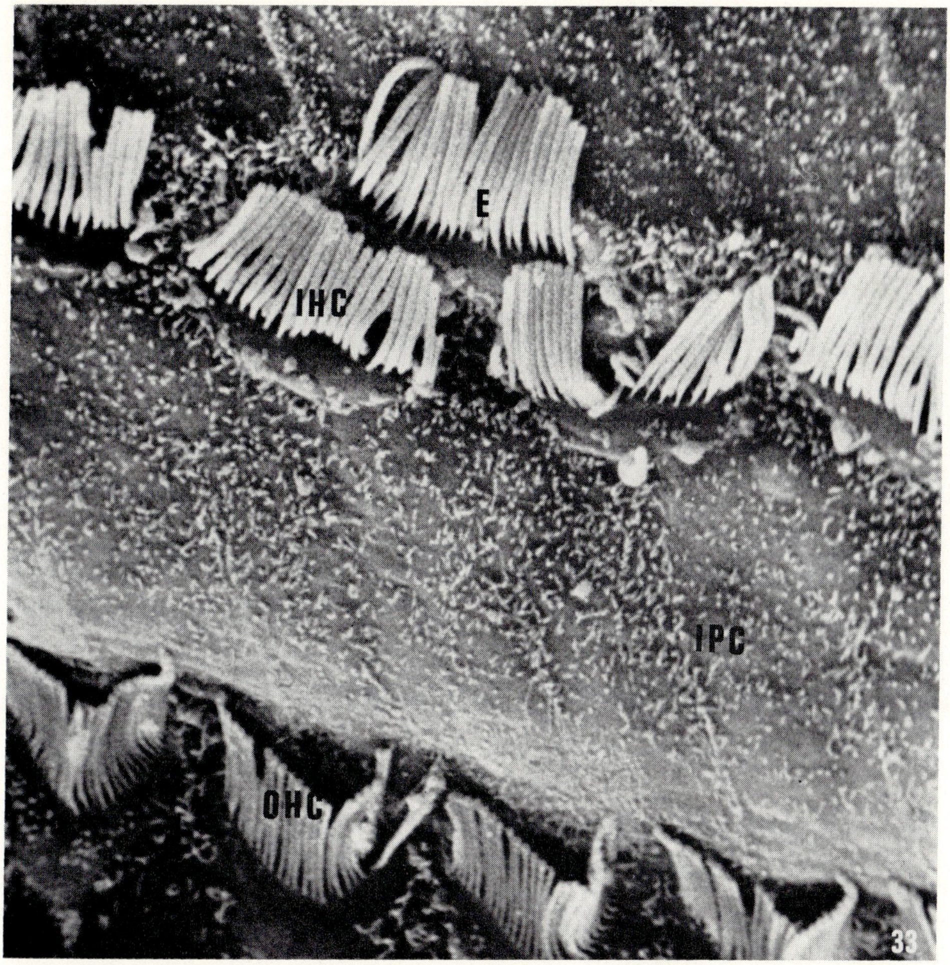

Fig. 33. Apical turn. Duplication of an inner hair cell (IHC). The extra cell (E) is localized on the inside of the row, centrally in front of two others. The first row of outer hair cells (OHC) is still visible. Slight artificial irregularity in the arrangement of the stereocilia. IPH — Inner pillar head (SEM 4,600 X).

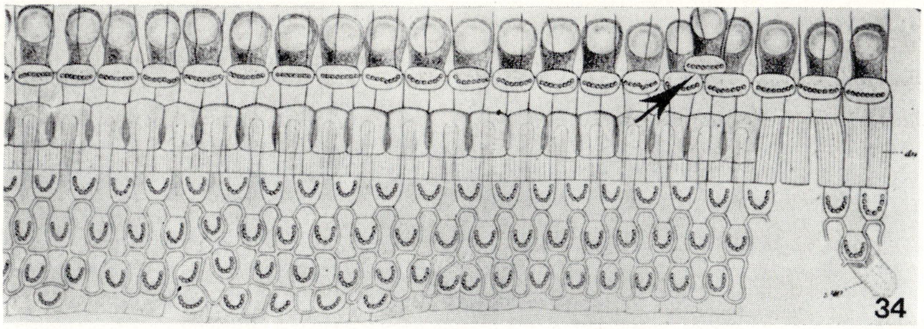

Fig. 34. Organ of Corti of a rabbit. Nearly a century ago Retzius drew a similar duplication of an inner hair cell, likewise in the apical turn, and similarly placed in relation to two other cells (arrow) (600 X). From: Das Gehörorgan der Wirbeltiere, part II, 1884.[5]

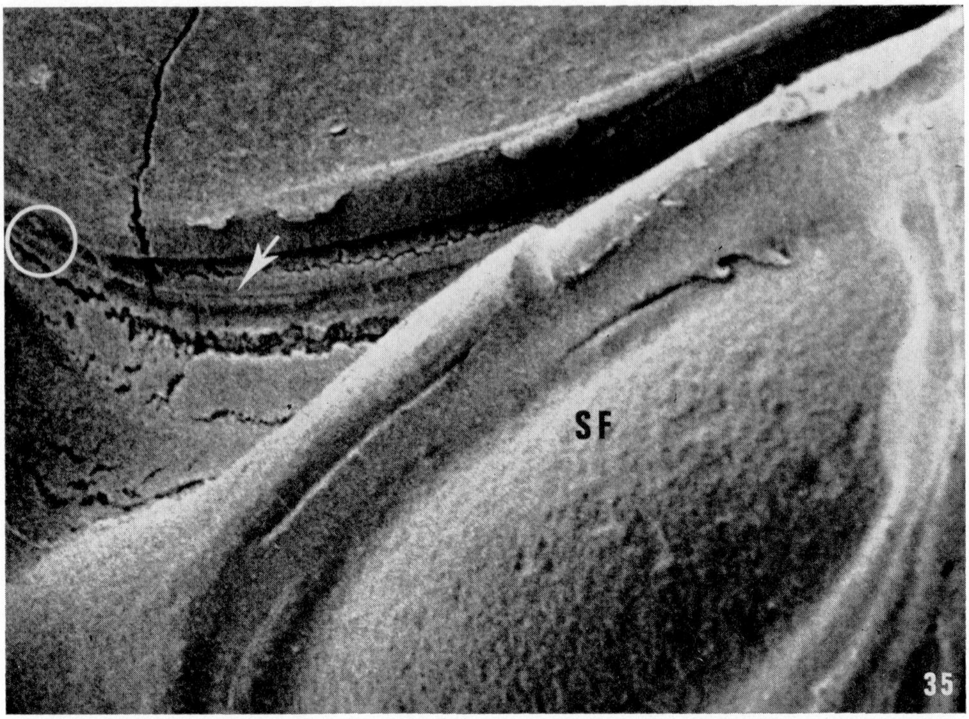

Fig. 35. The basal end of the organ of Corti. In the oval window the stapes footplate (SF) is visible from the inside. The arrow indicates the site of the organ of Corti, which here has its minimal width and extends past the oval window. The circle indicates the basal end, see Figure 36 (SEM 100 X).

is rare, and not confined to a given turn (Fig. 33). Yet Retzius[4] observed it in his early studies of rabbits (Fig. 34).

The regularity of the cell pattern of the organ of Corti gradually increased from the apical to the basal turn, that at the apex being negligible and that at the base being maximal.

In guinea pigs, the basal part of the organ of Corti passes the round and the oval window (Fig. 35). The surface of the outer hair cells is kidney-shaped at this level, and the legs of the W-configuration of these cells are farther apart. The stereocilia are shortest here. The dam of Hensen's cells is quite absent, inner and outer sulcus merging as they do in the apex. The regularity of the hair cell pattern is maintained down to the basal end (Fig. 36).

Artifacts

Apart from a knowledge of the normal variations in the hair cell pattern, it is of great importance to be able to identify artifacts. Normal changes and artifacts alike are to be differentiated from acoustic damage to the organ of Corti.

It is astonishing that only relatively few artifacts are seen in the preparation of this delicate organ. Artifacts could be caused by fixation, dehydration and drying, but also by variations in temperature in the critical point apparatus or by vibrations during the grinding down of the otic capsule. That the sense organ tolerates all these traumatic processes is explained by a combination of factors. First of all, the organ of Corti has a degree of firmness due to its numerous supporting cells. Some of these cells derive their strength from fibrillar structures,[70] as was found especially with the transmission electron microscope.[1,11-14] Second, the reticular membrane has a high degree of stiffness. Third, the use of glutaraldehyde as fixative enhanced firmness. Finally, dissecting was facili-

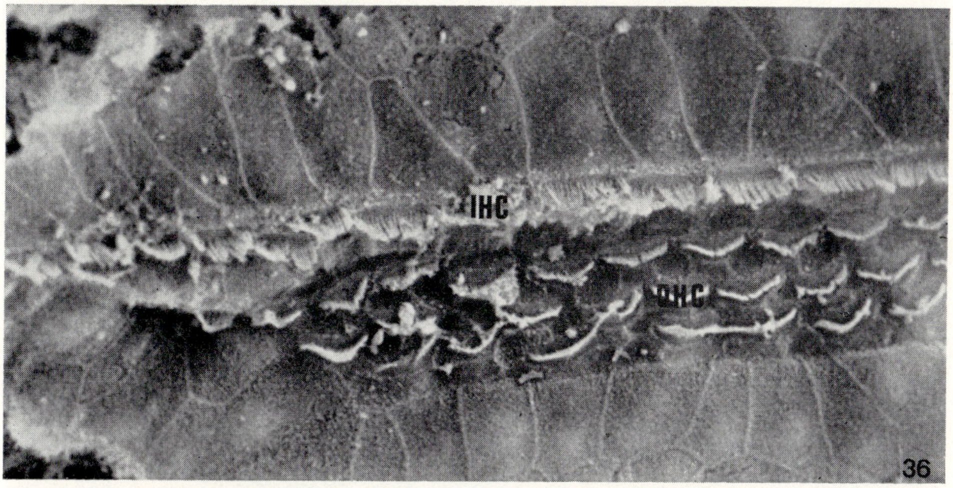

Fig. 36. Detail of Figure 35. The basal end of the organ of Corti. After no more than five inner hair cells (IHC) the organ assumes its "classic" pattern. The organ has its minimal width here. The W-configuration of the outer hair cells (OHC) is less pronounced because the angle between the long legs is wide. The surface of the outer hair cells is kidney-shaped at this level (SEM 1,600 X).

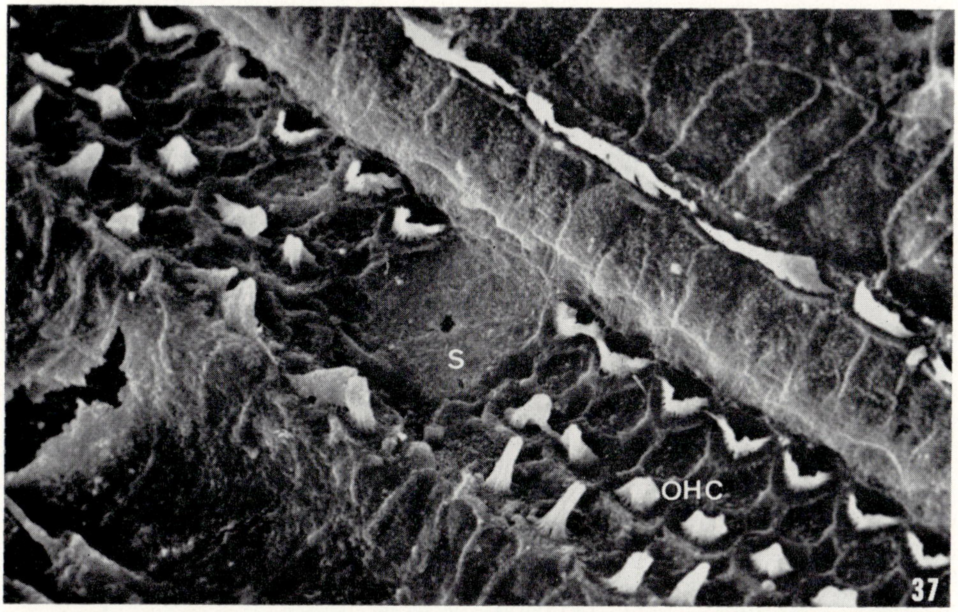

Fig. 37. Lower apical turn. This specimen was accidentally air-dried. It shows marked shrinkage, as a result of which the outer hair cells (OHC) are pronounced, while the supporting cells are depressed. The cell boundaries are emphasized, whereas details become vague. The stereocilia are stuck together. In the reticular membrane, some outer hair cells are missing (normal variation). An opening is seen in the scar (S). The Hensen's cells show a tear (SEM 1,260 X).

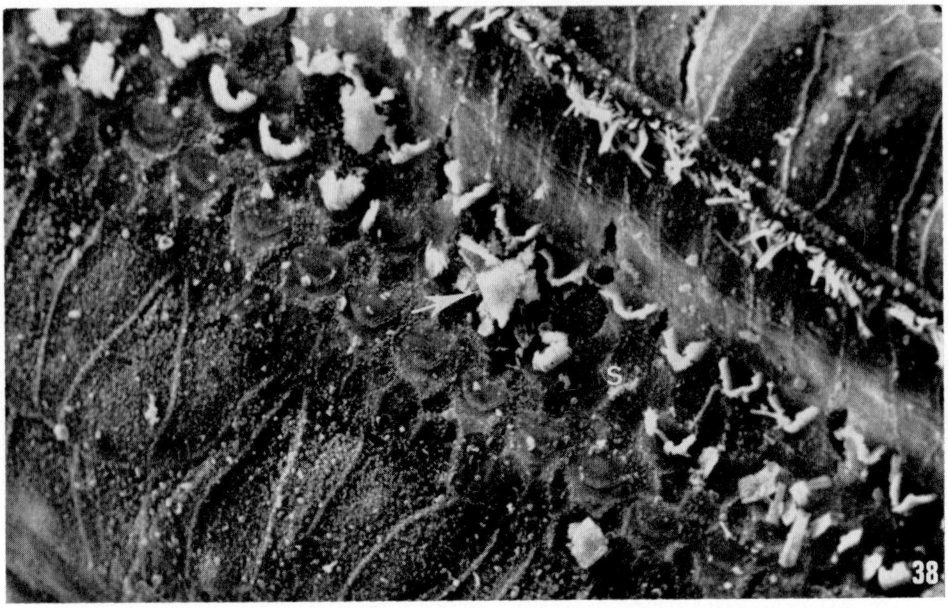

Fig. 38. Upper basal turn. Preparation damage to the organ of Corti. The hairs of the third and some of those of the second row of outer hair cells have broken off. Some are completely detached (arrow). The second row shows a phalangeal scar (S) because phalangeal plates of Deiters' cells have replaced the sensory cell. The surface shows several ruptures and is covered with debris (SEM 1,260 X).

tated by the fact that the cochlea was dry. This made it feasible to break away the otic capsule while leaving the membranous part of the cochlea attached to the modiolus. This became possible by slight shrinkage during drying, as a result of which the spiral ligament was loosened from the enveloping bone.

Yet shrinkage was the artifact which posed the greatest problems in the course of this study. When during the dehydration procedure in the acetone series the specimen was accidentally air-dried, shrinkage was enormous and all details were lost (Fig. 37). This risk was greatest when the specimen was in the absolute acetone at a high room temperature.

In the basal turn, where the basal membrane and the organ of Corti are much smaller and seemingly more fragile, spiral ruptures sometimes occurred between inner and outer hair cells, precisely in the area of Corti's tunnel. In such cases, the inner hair cells were still connected with the spiral limbus, and the outer hair cells with the spiral ligament. However, missing cells or cell groups could still be localized without difficulty. It was found that ruptures and defects in the reticular membrane generally showed a predilection for sites from which sensory cells or sensory and supporting cells had been lost.

Occasionally, a ropy precipitate was found on the organ of Corti in labyrinthine fixation. This was possibly caused by precipitation of protein from the endolymph. In some cases, part of the organ of Corti was found to curl in, due to causes so far unknown. Parts of the organ can break off during dissection under the binocular microscope. The relative grossness of these lesions facilitated identification of these artifacts (Fig. 38). The layers applied to the specimen by vacuum-coating should not be too thick, lest the specimen be "snowed under" and details be lost.[68]

In view of these findings, the tautness of the cell surface was taken as the principal criteria of the quality of the specimen. The less shrinkage and tearing, the closer its resemblance to its natural state.

CHAPTER IV

ACOUSTIC TRAUMA CAUSED BY PURE TONES

Study of the Factors: Intensity, Time Lapse and Frequency

In an effort to obtain information which might be useful in studying acoustic trauma caused by otologic drills, a study was first made of the traumatic effect of pure tones on the organ of Corti. Three series of guinea pigs were used for this purpose. In the first series the intensity of a pure tone of a given frequency and duration was varied. In the second series a pure tone of a given frequency, duration and intensity was offered, but the interval between the end of the tone and the sacrifice of the animal was varied. In the third series the frequency of a pure tone of given duration and intensity was varied. In this way an attempt was made to obtain information on the localization, time of occurrence and degree of damage to the organ of Corti.

The literature agrees to some extent on the order in which cellular elements of the organ of Corti are damaged in the case of an acoustic trauma. As early as 1909 Yoshii[7] described, on the basis of sectioned material, degeneration of the outer hair cells as the first evidence of acoustic trauma in the cochlea. With increasing duration or intensity of the tone offered, the inner hair cells were damaged next, and finally the entire supporting apparatus. After complete degeneration of the organ of Corti only a low dam of cubical epithelium remained. These findings were corroborated in the course of subsequent decades, not only from sectioned material but also by the surface specimen technique and with the scanning microscope.[10,13,14,17,37,41,57,67,89-93]

Lurie *et al*,[94] found detachment of the basilar membrane cells as a first sign of degeneration caused by acoustic trauma, but others were unable to confirm this.[10] In their book, Rüedi and Furrer[10] formulated important conclusions which have retained their validity and may therefore be repeated here:

1. A pure tone is more traumatic than a noise of the same intensity and duration.

2. When a pure tone of sufficient duration and intensity is offered, degeneration of sensory and supporting cells can extend over several turns, preferably in apical direction.

3. The site and extent of a given acoustic trauma show marked interindividual variations; nevertheless, the maximum of the lesion is usually localized in the basal end of the upper basal turn.

4. It is impossible to demonstrate a frequency localization in the cochlea with an acoustic trauma.

5. The cause of the 4,000-6,000 Hz dip in the audiogram is still obscure.

Degenerative changes of the outer hair cells become apparent in an early stage from a disarrangement of the stereocilia.[14] Lim and Melnick[37] and Bredberg *et al*[41] found blebs on the stereocilia with the scanning electron microscope. This bleb formation can be one of the first signs of acoustic trauma, but has also been found in normal test animals. Other early signs are probably fusion of hairs with formation of giant stereocilia.[13,41,44,93] Sensory cells showing these abnormalities can hardly be considered able to function normally. The high differentiation of the sensory cells limits their regenerative possibilities, and a return to a normal structure is consequently unlikely.[95,96] The cell disappears completely, being discarded into the endolymphatic space, and the supporting elements fill the opening, thus closing the defect in the surface of the sensory organ.[13]

Results

For each cochlea, a cochleogram of

TABLE I

COCHLEOGRAMS OF GUINEA PIGS EXPOSED TO 2,000 HZ FOR TWO HOURS AT VARIOUS INTENSITIES

Animal No.	*Intensity*	*Right Cochlea* — *Turn 1*, 2, 3, 4
1	96 dB SPL	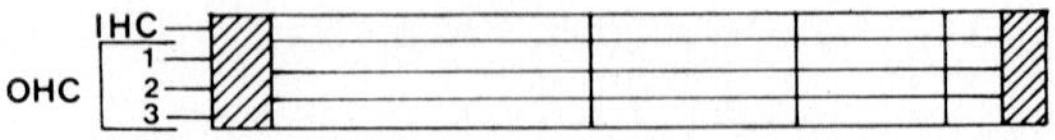
2	106 dB SPL	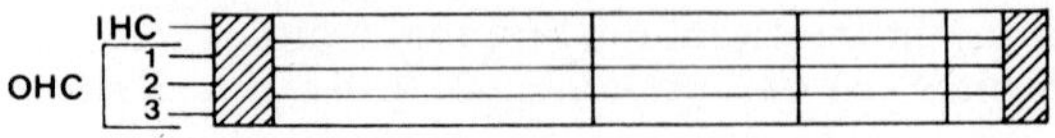
3	116 dB SPL	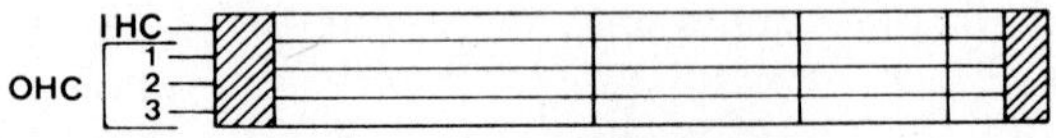
4	126 dB SPL	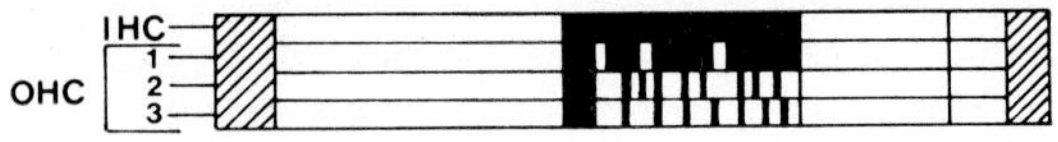
5	Control	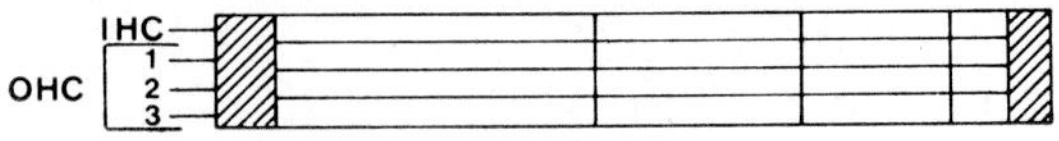

Simplified cochleograms of guinea pigs exposed to a pure tone of 2,000 Hz for two hours, applied to the right ear at different intensities. Black areas indicate damaged or missing hair cells and hatched areas indicate parts of the organ of Corti not included in assessment. Only acoustic lesions are indicated. The relative lengths of the various turns of the cochlea were calculated from scanning electron microscopic photographs. Only at 126 dB SPL were extensive lesions found in the apical quarter of the basal turn and throughout the upper basal turn. In particular, the inner hair cells and the first-row outer hair cells were damaged.

the entire organ of Corti was made in which the missing hair cells and scars were registered per turn, as distributed over the inner hair cells and three rows of outer hair cells. This provided a detailed record of the extent, localization, and pattern of the cellular degenerations found. The apical half of the apical turn and the extremely basal part of the basal turn were not assessed. The former was excluded in view of its constant irregularity, and the latter because it rarely shows any abnormalities, and microdissection of this part of the organ of Corti is very time consuming.

In the first series of five guinea pigs the intensity of the pure tone was varied. Four animals were exposed to a tone of 2,000 Hz for two hours. The fifth served as control; the animal was anesthetized, and the usual telephone was taped to its right ear, but no tone was supplied. The first guinea pig was exposed to 96 dB sound pressure level (SPL), the second to 106 dB SPL, the third to 116 dB SPL and the fourth to 126 dB SPL. The animals were sacrificed three to four weeks after exposure to the tone. In the simplified cochleogram, the number of normally missing cells, scattered over a turn, were excluded by subtraction as follows: from the basal turn 50 inner and/or outer hair cells, from the upper basal turn 25, from the lower apical turn 20, and from the basal half of the apical turn, five sensory cells (Table I).

Only the right cochlea of the fourth guinea pig (126 dB SPL) showed unmistakable degeneration of sensory cells in the apical quarter of the basal turn and throughout the upper basal turn. Scars indicating collapse of the organ of Corti were not seen. In the upper basal turn it was especially the inner hair cells and the outer hair cells of the first row that had degenerated. Some inner hair cells had disappeared completely; others were still present but had lost all or nearly all their stereocilia. Outer hair

TABLE II

COCHLEOGRAMS OF GUINEA PIGS EXPOSED TO 2,000 HZ FOR TWO HOURS AT 130 dB SPL AT VARIOUS INTERVALS

Animal No.	*Interval*	*Right Cochlea* — *Turn 1*, *2*, *3*, *4*
1	5 min	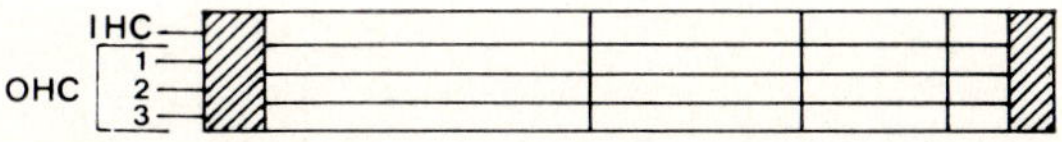
2	5 min	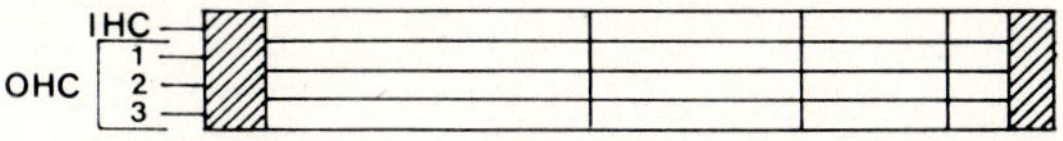
3	24 hr	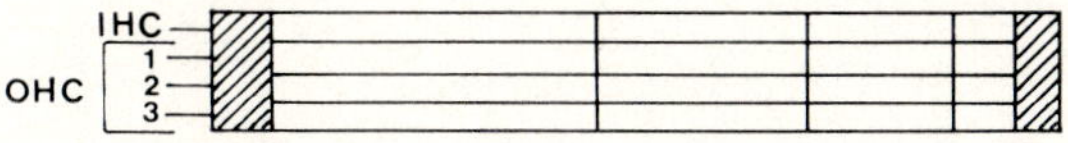
4	24 hr	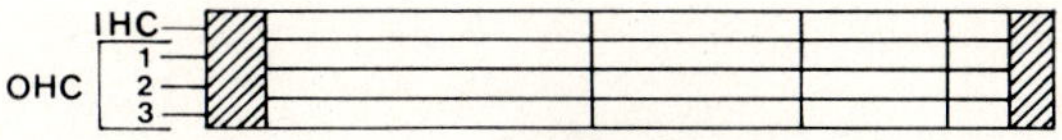
5	1 wk	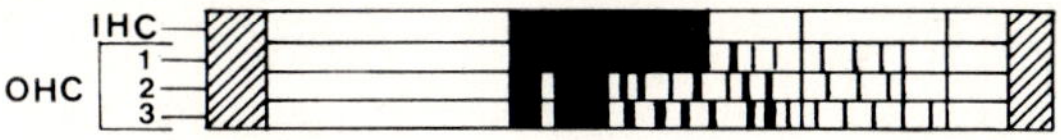
6	1 wk	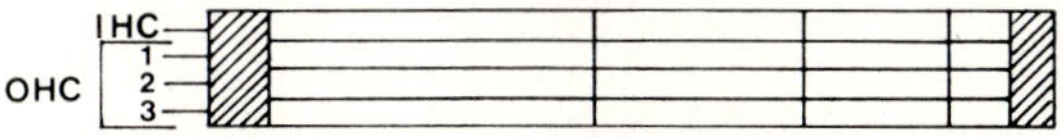
7	3 wk	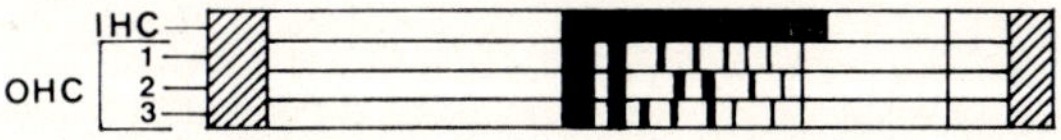
8	3 wk	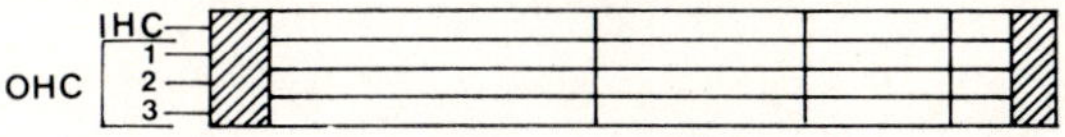
9	3 mo	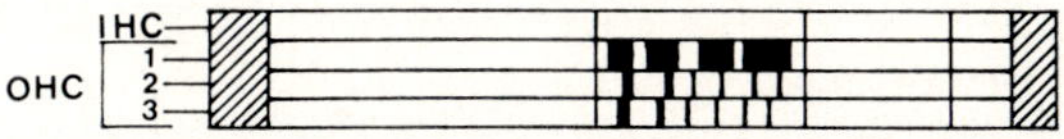
10	3 mo	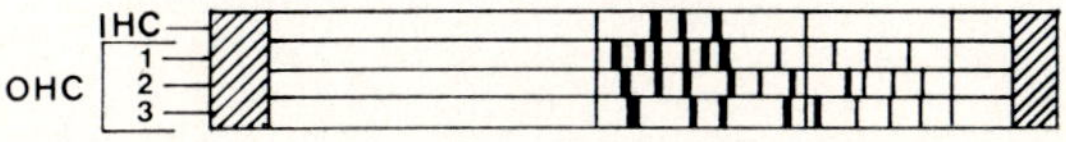

cells in the second and third rows also showed a decrease in number but this decrease was less pronounced (Table I).

The remaining nine cochleae (three exposed and six controls) showed no evidence of acoustic trauma. This means that the cochleae of the control animal did not differ from the other seven either. The left cochlea of the fourth guinea pig had not suffered from the 126 dB SPL applied to the right ear. The protective effect of the head had apparently been sufficient, and the left cochlea could be used as control.[22]

In the second series the interval between exposure to the tone and the time of sacrifice of the animal was varied. If an acoustic trauma of the organ of Corti were of a purely mechanical nature, it could be assumed to be visible in the specimen immediately after the infliction. If it is based on a metabolic process, changes are not likely immediately to become visible on the vestibular surface of the sensory cell. After all, the cuticular plate is characterized by considerable stiffness. When a sensory cell is persistently irritated until it degenerates due to an excess of metabolites, then evidence of this should be more readily

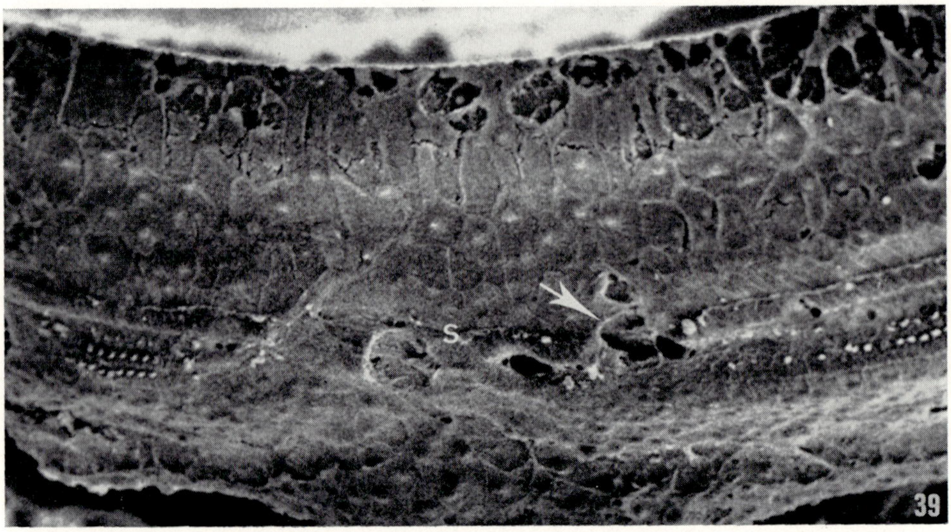

Fig. 39. Transition from basal to upper basal turn. The right ear was exposed to a tone of 2,000 Hz for two hours at 130 dB SPL, the animal being sacrificed one week after exposure. Slightly more than 0.2 mm of the organ of Corti have been lost completely. To the left of the scar (S) there are a few outer hair cells of normal appearance of the second and third row. On the extreme left a second scar is just visible. The defects in the surface (arrow) are probably artifacts (SEM 320 X).

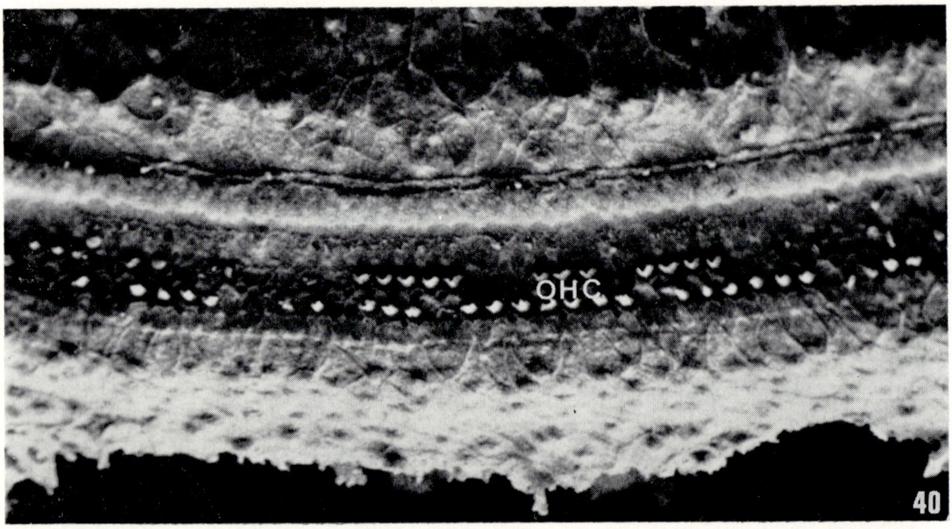

Fig. 40. Upper basal turn of the cochlea shown in Figure 39, exposed to 2,000 Hz for two hours at 130 dB SPL. All inner and outer hair cells of the first row have been lost. Some of the outer hair cells (OHC) of the second and most of those of the third row are intact. The number of cells of normal appearance increases from the inside out (SEM 480 X).

visualizable in the cell body, *e.g.*, by transmission electron microscopy.[13,88]

This series consisted of ten guinea pigs, divided into five pairs. They were all exposed to the same tone: 2,000 Hz for two hours with an intensity of 130 dB SPL, applied to the right ear. The first two guinea pigs were submitted to intravital perfusion five minutes after exposure to the tone. The second pair after

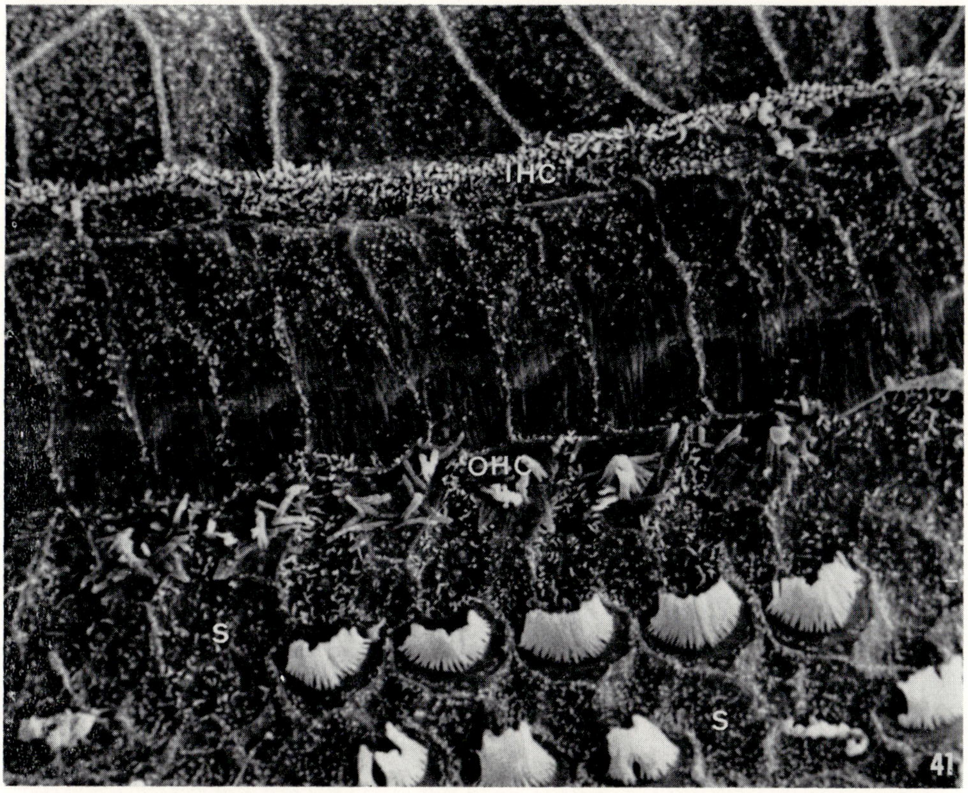

Fig. 41. Detail of Figure 40. Inner hair cells (IHC) and first-row outer hair cells (OHC) show degenerative features. Some inner hair cells seem to have been completely replaced by supporting cells whose surface is covered with microvilli (arrow). In others the oval contours of the sensory cell are still visible, and only the stereocilia seem to have disappeared (asterisk). The first-row outer hair cells show extensive clumping of stereocilia. Phalangeal scars (S) indicate missing outer hair cells. The other sensory cells appear to be quite normal (SEM 2,500 X).

24 hours, the third pair after one week, the fourth pair after three weeks and the fifth pair after three months. The first two pairs (five minutes and 24 hours) showed no abnormalities. In the pair sacrificed after one week, three of the four cochleae were normal but the right cochlea of one animal showed extensive lesions in the organ of Corti. The damage extended from the apical quarter of the basal turn to the basal quarter of the lower apical turn (Table II). More than two turns showed abnormalities. A striking finding was that three-quarters of the basal turn showed an entirely regular hair cell pattern, whereas the fourth quarter showed a scar measuring more than 0.2 mm due to complete degeneration of the organ of Corti and its replacement by a layer of polygonal epithelium. More apically there were some 15 outer hair cells of normal appearance in the second and third row, which were followed by another scar of approximately the same size (Fig. 39). This was localized in the basal part of the upper basal turn. Following the upper basal turn in apical direction, signs of degeneration were seen mainly in the inner hair cells and the first row of outer hair cells. But the second and third rows of outer hair cells also showed missing cells or groups of cells (Fig. 40). In the lower apical turn the number of damaged cells gradually diminished, and a regular pattern was resumed in the start of the apical turn.

In the upper basal and lower apical

TABLE III

COCHLEOGRAMS OF GUINEA PIGS EXPOSED FOR TWO HOURS AT 4,000 AND 1,000 HZ FOR 110 AND 134 dB*

Animal No.	*Tone (Hz)*	*Cochlea*	*dB SPL*	*Turn 1 2 3 4*
1	4,000	R	110	
2	4,000	R	110	
3	1,000	R	134	
4	1,000	L	134	
5	1,000	R	134	
6	1,000	L	134	
7	1,000	R	134	

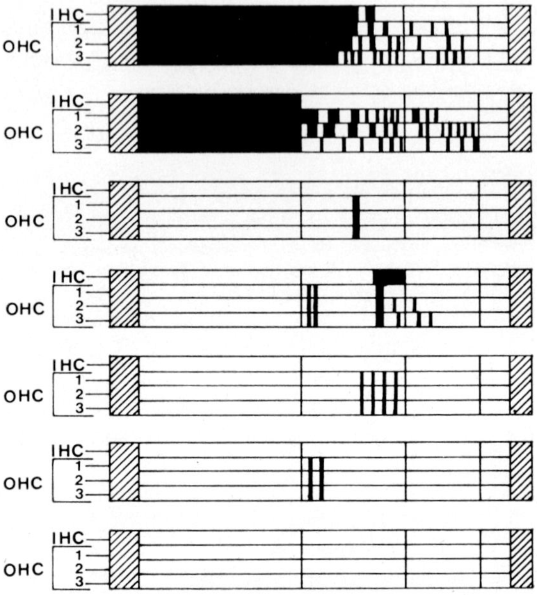

turns, some inner hair cells were entirely missing and had been replaced by supporting cells which were characterized by an abundance of microvilli on the surface. From other inner hair cells only the stereocilia seemed to have disappeared. Some of the stereocilia of the outer hair cells of the first row had fused. This is to be interpreted as a consequence of the acoustic trauma (Fig. 41).

In the pair sacrificed after three weeks, one right cochlea was found to show evidence of an acoustic trauma, which was less extensive (from the apical quarter of the basal turn through the apical end of the upper basal turn). Again the largest scars were found at the transition from basal to upper basal turn, and again there were two sites at which the entire organ of Corti had been replaced by an epithelial zone. And again the number of missing sensory cells diminished in apical direction. This applied to the inner as well as to the outer hair cells. At the sites of degenerated sensory cells the surface was often covered with debris: discarded cell contents. Apparently the degenerative process was still unfinished after three weeks.

Both guinea pigs sacrificed after three months showed signs of degeneration in the right cochlea. In one, these signs were found in the upper basal turn, and in the other in the upper basal and lower apical turns. The supporting apparatus of the organ of Corti was found intact throughout. The scars were small and numerous, but mainly confined to the outer hair cells.

In the third series, which consisted of five guinea pigs, two different frequencies were studied at different intensities. Two animals were exposed to a pure tone of 4,000 Hz applied to the right ear for two hours at an intensity of 110 dB SPL. The remaining three were exposed to a tone of 1,000 Hz at an intensity of 134 dB SPL, likewise, for two hours; two were bilaterally exposed, and of the third, only the right ear was exposed. The bilateral exposures were carried out in an effort to establish possible right/left differences. The animals were sacrificed after three to four weeks.

The two right cochleae exposed to 4,000 Hz showed extensive lesions: large parts of the organ of Corti had degenerated and been replaced by low polygonal epithelium. The multiple lesions in one case encompassed the entire basal turn and the basal half of the upper basal turn; size and number of scars gradually diminished in apical direction. In the other cochlea the degeneration likewise started in the basal turn, with a maximum at the transition from basal to upper basal turn. Again the lesions diminished in size towards the apex, but they extended slightly further into the lower apical turn (Table III).

Of the five cochleae exposed to 1,000 Hz at 134 dB SPL, four showed fairly small scars in the organ of Corti. One showed no acoustic lesions. Although the scars were small, they were nevertheless either larger (more than eight sensory cells) or more numerous (more than six scars) than would be compatible with normal variations in the hair cell pattern. As already stated, this was accepted as a criterion for acoustic damage. Most lesions were localized in the upper basal turn. In three of the four damaged cochleae the lesions were confined to the outer hair cells. No distinct left/right difference was demonstrable; nor could it be excluded with certainty. In view of the smallness of the lesions the duration or the intensity of the pure tone of 1,000 Hz had apparently been marginal for the causation of visible lesions on the surface of the organ of Corti (Table III). The three left cochleae not exposed to pure tones showed no abnormalities.

DISCUSSION

It was confirmed in this study that the sensory cells of the organ of Corti are the elements most vulnerbale to acoustic trauma. The guinea pigs of the first series were exposed to a pure tone of 2,000 Hz at varying intensities. Only at 126 dB SPL were distinct lesions of the organ of Corti observed. Lower intensities produced no visible changes on the surface of the organ of Corti. It is possible, however, that changes occurred in hair cells and nerve fibers which can be morphologically demonstrated only with the transmission electron microscope.[88] This need not preclude further investigation, for it was found possible first to scan the entire organ and then to embed it, cut it into sections and study the sections with the transmission electron microscope.

In the second series, in which the interval between exposure to the tone and sacrifice of the animal was varied, lesions were found after one week, three weeks and three months. The fact that the organ of Corti showed no visible degenerative changes after five minutes and after 24 hours would seem to suggest that the trauma involves a disturbance in the metabolism of the sensory cells as a result of strain on perceptive function. It is more likely, however, that a combination of metabolic and mechanical factors is involved.[17,97] It is an obvious inference that mechanical damage, specifically of the cell membrane, should play a more important role as the intensity of the tone increases.

In the third series, with varied frequencies and intensities, a tone of 4,000 Hz at 110 dB SPL proved to be much more traumatic than one of 1,000 Hz at 134 dB SPL. The maximum lesion was found in the basal turn at 4,000 Hz, and in the upper basal turn at 1,000 Hz. The fact that only minor lesions occurred at a frequency of 1,000 Hz is in agreement with the findings reported by Stockwell *et al.*[17] We are unable to explain the extensiveness of the enormous lesions after exposure to 4,000 Hz at 110 dB SPL.

Some common characteristics were observed in the three series. The largest lesions, involving all rows of sensory cells, were invariably found in the basal turn or at the transition from basal to upper basal turn. They generally started abruptly and the number of degenerated hair cells gradually diminished in the direction of the apex, along the turns. On two occasions, duplication of the scar was observed at the site of the largest lesion, the scars being separated by a number of hair cells of normal appearance. This duplication was likewise observed by Stockwell *et al*,[17] using the phase-contrast microscope. In the upper basal turn proper, we occasionally observed a pattern of degeneration in which a combination of inner hair cells and first row outer hair cells proved to show lesions. This is worthy of note because the outer hair cells are presumed to be most vulnerable to acoustic trauma. One might therefore expect all outer hair cells to degenerate first while inner hair cells remain intact. This proved not always to be the case.

Beagley[91,92] observed a separation in the organ of Corti exactly on the boundary between Deiters' cells and Hensen's cells after a pure-tone acoustic trauma. We were unable to corroborate this finding. Beagley, however, applied a tone of 500 Hz vs frequencies of 1,000, 2,000 and 4,000 Hz in our study.

Fused stereocilia and giant stereocilia of outer and inner hair cells, missing stereocilia of inner hair cells, and the presence of cellular debris on the surface of the organ of Corti, are evidence of as yet incomplete sensory cell degeneration. These features were no longer visible three months after the acoustic trauma. Giant stereocilia might be an artifact of dissection due to hyperextension of the stereocilia fused as a result of the acoustic trauma, upon removal of the tectorial membrane.

In the test animal showing acoustic trauma of the right cochlea, the left cochlea invariably showed a normal hair cell pattern with the variations described earlier. At these intensities and frequencies, therefore, the left cochlea could be used as control.

CHAPTER V

OTOLOGIC DRILLS – A POSSIBLE ACOUSTIC DANGER

Sensorineural hearing loss is undoubtedly among the most serious complications of an ear operation. If this loss is total, the term, "dead ear" applies; if it is partial, then the audiogram usually reveals a loss of high tones (over 2,000 Hz). The causes of this hearing loss have been sought in excessive manipulation on the stapes and damage to the round window.[98,99] Paparella[100] and Helms[101] demonstrated that the cochlea can be injured when the chain of auditory ossicles is made to vibrate by an otologic drill, as a result of which the sacculus and the organ of Corti can be totally or partially destroyed. On the other hand, suction on the aditus can also cause excessive movements of the chain of ossicles.

Occasionally, operations not involving the ossicles and the middle ear, *e.g.*, a simple mastoidectomy, can also be followed by loss of hearing for high tones. Rüedi and Furrer[10] were able to demonstrate a temporary threshold shift in an experiment in which the mastoid was submitted to hammering in volunteers. Arnold[52] and Schuknecht and Tonndorf[54] published a case report in this context. They ascribed the hearing loss to the use of hammer and chisel to remove bone during the operation. According to De Montmollin,[53] the sound which this produces can attain values up to 143 dB. And such noise levels are indubitably injurious to the organ of Corti.

Hammer and chisel have been virtually obsolete in these operations, electric drills and turbine drills have almost entirely superseded them. But the risk of high-tone hearing loss has not disappeared.[53,55,56] An obvious inference is that the cause of this hearing loss is to be found in the noise produced by the otologic drill used to remove the bone. Schuknecht and Tonndorf,[54] however, were unable to demonstrate any cochlear damage in an experiment on cats. But the feline skull cannot be compared with the human skull as to thickness and composition of bones. The extensive series of patients examined by these authors likewise showed no sensorineural type hearing loss following ear operations with electrically driven burrs. De Montmollin[53] analyzed drill noise intensities and found values up to 116 dB, dependent on burr size and location of the microphone. Unfortunately, he did not specify the type of drill used. Paulsen[102] compared the drill noise of three otologic drills with different speeds. He concluded that the sound pressures were about the same for the three drills, being up to 100 dB and more.

In view of uncertainties in the relevant literature, a comparative study was made of the frequency patterns and noise levels of normal, high-speed and very-high-speed drills during drilling on human temporal bones and on the cadaver.

METHODS AND MATERIALS

The three types of otological drill investigated (Fig. 42) were:

1. The now almost classic low-speed Kaltenbach-Voigt drill,* with an idle electromotor speed of 12,000 rpm.

2. The high-speed Ritter-Kerr Tympano-Torque drill,** with an idle electromotor speed of 20,000 rpm.

3. The very-high-speed Hall air drill,*** compressed nitrogen-driven turbine motor with an idle speed of 100,000 rpm.

The burrs used were the spherical as

*Kaltenbach and Voigt, Biberach, West Germany. Type 530.

**Ritter A. G., Karlsruhe, West Germany. Type MD 5000.

***Hall International, Inc., Santa Barbara, CA. Type 100.

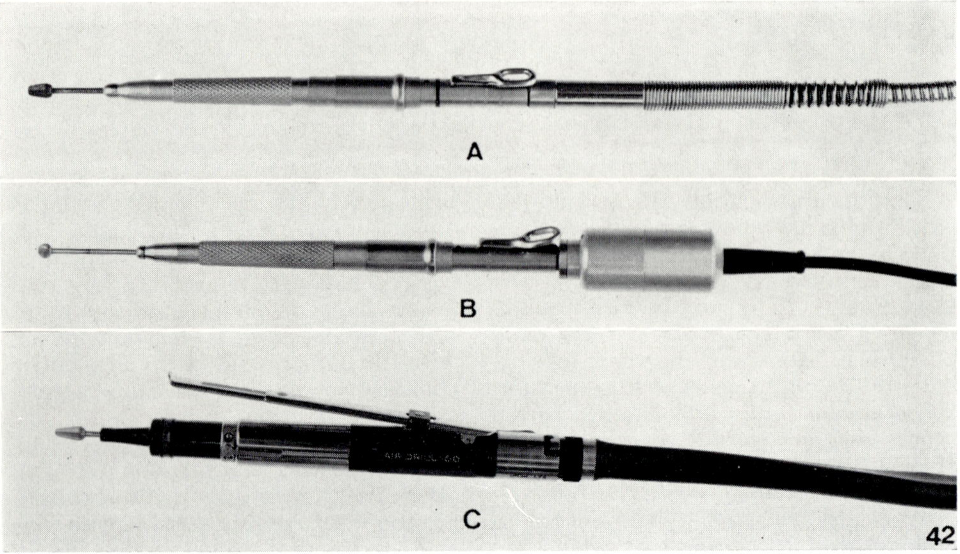

Fig. 42. The hand pieces of the three drill types whose noise was analyzed. A) The hand piece is linked to the Kaltenbach-Voigt drill type 530 (not shown) via a transmission cable enclosed in flexible tubing. The idle speed of the electromotor is 12,000 rpm. B) The hand piece is continuous with the Ritter Kerr Tympano-Torque type MD 5000 micromotor, which weighs 100 g and has an idle speed of 20,000 rpm. The flexible tubing encloses power wires. C) The hand piece of the Hall air drill type 100 contains the turbine motor. It weighs 170 g and operates on compressed nitrogen. Its idle speed is 100,000 rpm at a nitrogen consumption of 170 l/min. The flexible tubing enclosed nitrogen supply line and exhaust.

well as the conical cutting type, with a diameter of 4-7 mm. Straight hand pieces were used throughout.

In order to establish whether removal of bone with the above mentioned drills could damage the organ of Corti, animal experiments seemed a reliable and direct method.[54,100] It seemed questionable, however, whether a mastoidectomy on a test animal could be regarded as an equivalent in terms of acoustic stress to an operation on a patient. Both the duration and the noise levels, after all, would differ widely. A similar objection could be raised to experimenting exclusively on human temporal bones. The air conduction noise would not be very different, but the bone conduction noise caused by drilling would be quite different owing to absence of the entire head. This is why cadaver mastoidectomies were performed, imitating the situation present during surgery on a patient.

Noise generated by drilling reaches the cochlea by two routes: air conduction, and bone conduction. The air conduction noise was measured directly with the aid of a condenser microphone.* To measure the bone conduction noise, an accelerometer** was screwed into the bone of the skull slightly cranial to the temporal line. In order to determine the relation between accelerometer output and equivalent air conduction noise, the accelerometer was standardized with the aid of an audiometer*** and a bone conductor. The latter was placed on the cadaver's forehead. Narrow-band noise was used as a signal in order to avoid phase influences.

The audiometer reading in decibels reflects, so to speak, the intensity of the

*B & K Instruments, Inc., Cleveland, OH. Type 4134 with probe UA 0040.

**B & K Instruments, Inc., Cleveland, OH. Type 4334.

***Alfred Peters and Sons, Ltd., Sheffield, England. Type SPD 5.

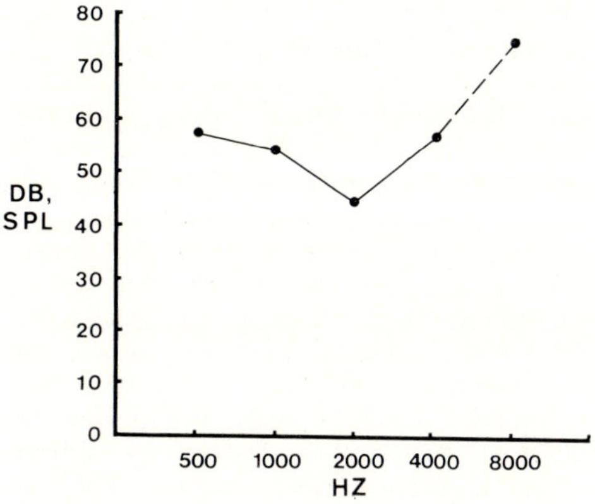

Fig. 43. Accelerometer output RE 1 μV as a function of the frequency when a vibration corresponding with 60 dB SPL is applied via the bone conductor.

noise which would have to be offered by air conduction in order to produce the same stimulation in the cochlea as that caused by the bone conductor. Figure 43 shows the accelerometer output as a function of the frequency at a constant equivalent air conduction noise of 60 dB SPL. Control experiments on temporal bones and on the artificial mastoid disclosed a linear relation between accelerometer output and equivalent air conduction noise. During drilling, both the bone conduction noise and the air conduction noise were recorded on an instrumentation recorder.* A diagram of

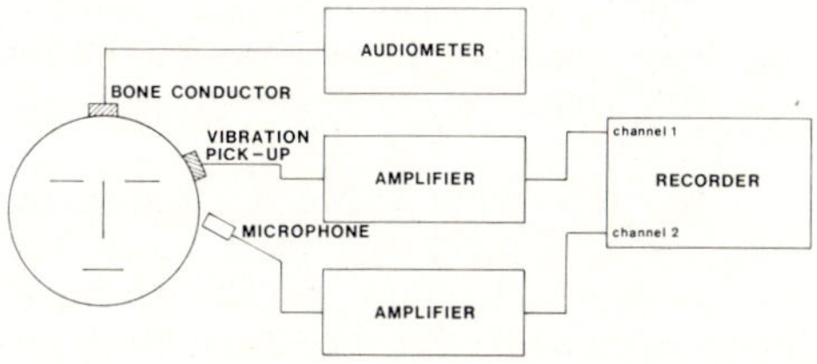

Fig. 44. Diagram showing the setup for recording drill noise. The bone conductor placed in the center of the forehead is connected with the audiometer. The accelerometer is screwed into the skull bone just above the temporal line, and is connected with the recorder via an amplifier. The probe microphone is placed close to the ear and is connected with the recorder via another amplifier.

TABLE IV

DRILL NOISE OF THREE OTOLOGIC DRILLS

		Decibels		
		Hz 1,000	*Hz 2,000*	*Hz 4,000*
Kaltenbach-Voigt drill				
Conical burr	90%	92	105	85
	50%	102	115	94
	10%	107	119	99
	max	110	125	105
Spherical burr	90%	80	92	71
	50%	89	106	90
	10%	97	113	95
	max	115	120	105
Ritter-Kerr drill				
Conical burr	90%	80	93	71
	50%	87	101	78
	10%	92	109	87
	max	95	115	90
Spherical burr	90%	71	82	68
	50%	78	90	77
	10%	85	100	82
	max	95	110	90
Hall air drill				
Conical burr	90%	62	80	64
	50%	73	93	76
	10%	83	102	84
	max	95	105	90
Spherical burr	90%	65	80	59
	50%	75	92	75
	10%	82	100	82
	max	90	105	90

For each drill the values obtained with the largest conical burr (7 mm ø) and with the largest spherical burr (7 mm ø) are given. The noise levels are given in dB in octave bands with center frequencies of 1,000, 2,000 and 4,000 Hz. The upper three figures of each frequency indicate the levels exceeded during 90%, 50% and 10% of the drilling time, respectively. The bottom figure indicates the maximum value measured.

the experimental setup is presented in Figure 44.

RESULTS

The records of the noise of the three drills with spherical as well as conical burrs were analyzed. In all cases, the intensity of the air conduction noise was found to be 20-30 dB less than that of the bone conduction noise. Bearing in mind the purpose of this study, only the bone conduction noise was therefore

*Philips Electronic Instruments, Inc., Mount Vernon, NY. Analog 7.

analyzed further. A frequency analysis in octave bands was made of the bone conduction noise recorded. The results of this analysis are presented in Table IV. Because the low frequency plays no important role in acoustic trauma, only the octave bands with a central frequency of 1,000 Hz and over were studied. The octave around 8,000 Hz was not included in the table because standardization in this range proved to be unreliable. However, the results in this range were used for quantitative comparison of the three drills. Per frequency, four numerical values are given for each situation. The first indicates the noise level which was exceeded during 90% of the drilling time; the second indicates the noise level exceeded during 50% of the drilling time; the third indicates the level exceeded during 10% of the drilling time; the fourth indicates the maximum noise level recorded (which was usually no more than 10 dB above the 10% level).

The difference between the 90% level and the maximum level recorded never exceeded 35 dB. This difference expresses such factors as the difference in burr pressure and the difference in bone structure. Efforts were always made to drill at maximum burr pressure. It was also found that, for all situations, the noise levels produced were maximal in the octave band around 2,000 Hz.

It was found that the Hall air drill produced substantially less noise than the two electrically driven drills. The difference from the Ritter-Kerr drill was about 5-10 dB, while that from the Kaltenbach-Voigt drill was as much as 20-30 dB. The conical burr produced more noise than the spherical. Additional determinations showed that both types produced as much more noise as the diameter was larger. The larger burr-bone contact surface apparently played an important role. The values found in the octave band around 8,000 Hz showed similar features. Again the Hall air drill was less noisy than the other two, and the conical burr more noisy than the spherical.

DISCUSSION

The noise levels measured in the octave band around 2,000 Hz all exceeded 105 dB. It is to be noted that the values pertain to drilling in a normal, *i.e.*, adequately pneumatized mastoid. Drilling in a sclerotic mastoid might well produce higher values. The question can be raised whether these noise levels can give rise to permanent acoustic trauma. It seems that the time of exposure should be considerably longer than that during an operation in order to produce acoustic trauma with certainty. However, not every human individual is equally (in)-sensitive to noise. Actual practice has shown that only a minority of patients show high-tone hearing loss. This observation was earlier confirmed by De Montmollin,[53] who found temporary or permanent perceptive hearing loss after 21 out of 265 radical mastoidectomies, *i.e.*, 7.9%. He ascribed this loss to the use of drill and chisel.

With the Hall air drill, acoustic trauma can therefore be expected to be rare, but with the Ritter-Kerr and especially with the Kaltenbach-Voigt drill the noise level can rise to values at which acoustic trauma is a definite possibility. One of the reasons for the superiority of the Hall air drill in this respect is undoubtedly the fact that the drill stops as soon as the burr is pressed hard against the bone. This was confirmed by the finding that the difference between conical and spherical burrs was minimal with this drill.

CONCLUSIONS

1. The bone conduction noise in drilling was found to have a much higher intensity than the air conduction noise, the difference being 20-30 dB.

2. Of the three drills analyzed, the Hall air drill produced least noise, and the Kaltenbach-Voigt produced most. The difference between these two was 20-30 dB.

3. Conical burrs were generally more noisy than spherical burrs, and larger diameters were more noisy than smaller.

4. With all drills, levels of 105 dB or over were measured in the range around 2,000 Hz. Prolonged drilling in the human temporal bone therefore entails a risk of an acoustic trauma of the organ of hearing even with the relatively noiseless Hall air drill.

CHAPTER VI

ACOUSTIC TRAUMA CAUSED BY DRILL NOISE

It was demonstrated in the preceding chapter that noise produced by drills of three different types can attain intensity levels which can have an injurious effect on the human organ of hearing. In a comparative study of the traumatic effects on the organ of Corti, therefore, test animals were submitted to drill noise. Since it was quite conceivable that the true noise level rarely causes lesions, the drill noise was reproduced with 10 dB amplification, permitting us to limit the number of test animals used.

A total of 33 guinea pigs were used in three groups of 11 animals each. The first group was exposed to the noise of the low-speed drill, the second to that of the high-speed drill, and the third to that of the very-high-speed drill. In each group, eight guinea pigs were exposed to drill noise applied to the right ear for two hours under anesthesia, and two were exposed to the same noise for three hours (again using the right ear). One animal served as control: it was anesthetized for two hours and a telephone was taped to the right ear, but no noise was applied.

All left cochleae served as additional controls. The insert telephone was taped to the auricle, as already described for the experiment with pure tones. The guinea pigs were in general anesthetized in order to approximate the situation of an ear operation, *e.g.*, a mastoidectomy, as closely as possible. Since it was technically impracticable to offer the noise by bone conduction, air conduction was used. As described in the preceding chapter, the standard curve of the accelerometer was used for this purpose (Fig. 43). The audiometer reading in dB reflects, so to speak, the intensity of the sound which would have to be offered by air conduction in order to produce in the cadaver cochlea the same state of stimulation now caused by the bone conductor. Inversely, it is possible to determine the sound which would have to be offered by air conduction in order to produce the same effect as the burr would produce by bone conduction (air conduction sound equivalent). With the aid of a multi-octave filter* and an amplifier it proved possible to convert the recorded drill noise to an air conduction sound equivalent.

The so converted noise of three different drill types was recorded on endless tapes.** Using a tape recorder,*** amplifier,** and telephone,** the noise was reproduced and offered to the right ear of the guinea pig (Fig. 45). The noise of the low-speed and the high-speed drill was offered in 30-second periods alternating with ten-second "silent" intervals. With the very-high-speed drill this was impossible. When the highest possible pressure was applied, this drill stopped after about ten seconds. The noise of this drill was therefore offered in ten-second periods alternating with ten-second "silent" intervals. The total duration of the first two drills' noise exceeded the total duration of the noise of the very-high-speed drill. This was a true reflection of reality, for a mastoidectomy performed with a very-high-speed turbine drill takes substantially less time than an operation using a lower-speed drill.

Since the experiments with pure tones had shown that lesions could not be expected until after at least one week, the guinea pigs were sacrificed three to seven weeks after exposure to the drill

*Peekel Division, Rotterdam, The Netherlands. Type TF 824.

**Philips Electronic Instruments, Inc., Mount Vernon, NY. Type CE tapes, PM 5175 amplifier, Q 11 telephone.

***Sony Corp. of America, Long Island City, NY. Type TC 105.

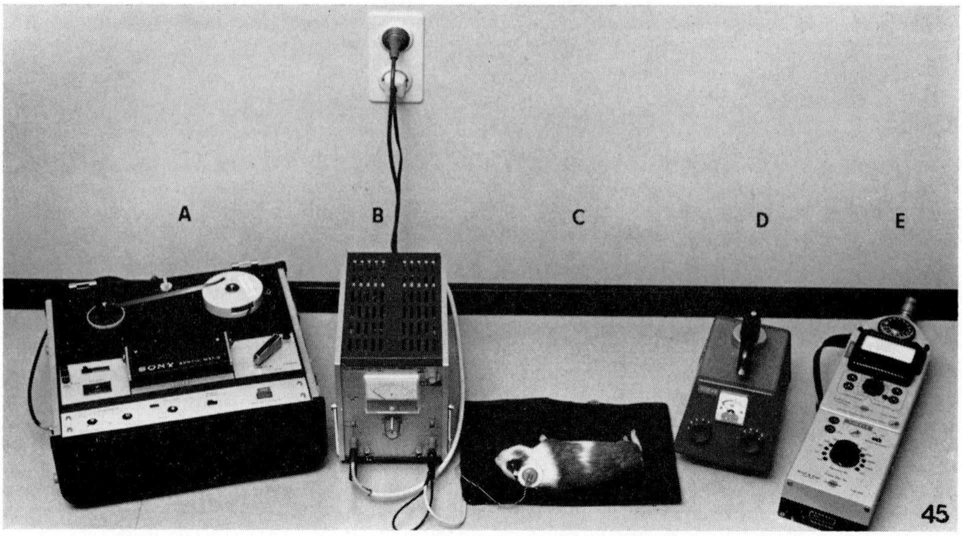

Fig. 45. Setup used to offer the drill noise to the guinea pig. A) tape recorder with endless tape; B) amplifier; C) guinea pig under general anesthesia, the telephone taped to the auricle; D) hand audiometer to determine Preyer's reflex; E) impulse precision sound level meter used to standardize the noise.

TABLE V

COCHLEOGRAMS OF GUINEA PIGS EXPOSED FOR TWO HOURS TO THE NOISE OF A LOW-SPEED DRILL, AMPLIFIED BY 10 dB

Animal No.	*Right Cochlea* — *Turn 1*, 2, 3, 4
1	
2	
3	
4	
5	
6	
7	
8	

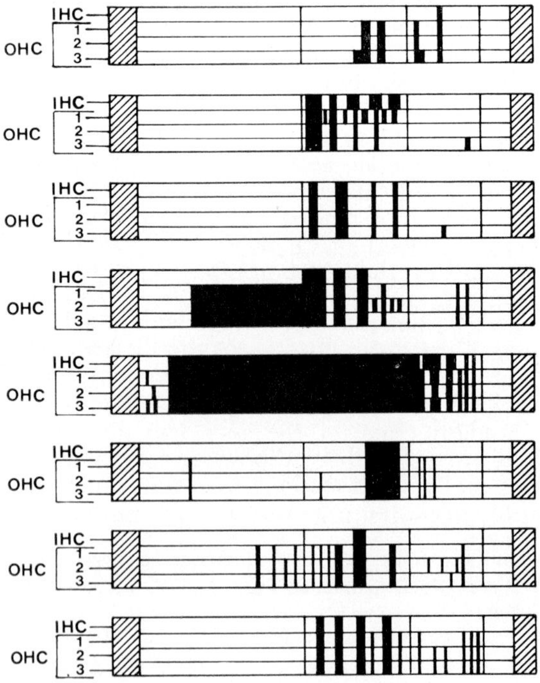

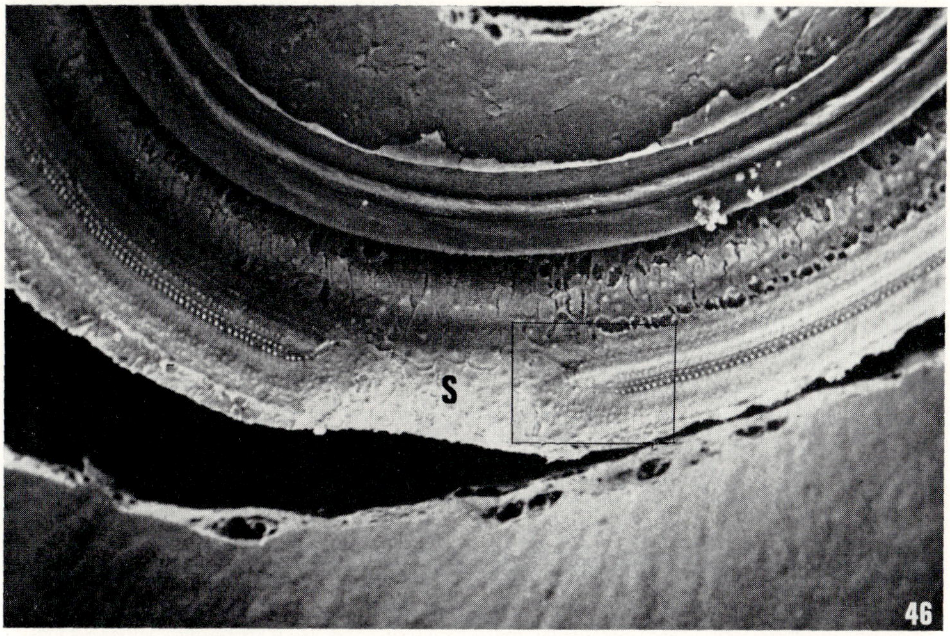

Fig. 46. Basal half of upper basal turn. Cochlea exposed for two hours to intermittent noise of low-speed drill, amplified by 10 dB. Animal sacrificed after six weeks. A circumscribed scar (S) indicates the site of maximal damage. Even at this low power it is evident that all sensory cells at the site of the lesion have disappeared (SEM 125 X).

noise. Both organs of Corti were examined in their entirety with the scanning electron microscope. The procedure has been described in Chapter II. An evaluation of lesions in the organ of Corti was recorded in a cochleogram.

RESULTS

In the first group, the eight guinea pigs exposed for two hours to the noise of the low-speed drill, amplified by 10 dB, all showed unmistakable lesions in the right organ of Corti (Table V). None of the eight left organs of Corti showed any lesion but this group showed the normal pattern with a score of missing outer and a few missing inner hair cells. Apparently again the protective effect of the skull had been sufficient to prevent visible damage to the surface in the left organ of Corti.

Again the apical half of the apical turn of the organ of Corti was excluded because of its variable number of missing sensory cells. The extremely basal part up to the round window was not considered. The extent of the various lesions in the organ of Corti varied widely. The least damaged cochlea showed four small scars in the area of the outer hair cells, only one of which was accompanied by degeneration of some of the inner hair cells as well. The scars were found in the upper basal and lower apical turns. In the most severely damaged cochlea the lesion extends over basal, upper basal and lower apical turns, both inner and outer hair cells having degenerated. In the remaining six cochleae the largest lesions were found in the upper basal turn (Figs. 46, 47). In four cochleae, the surface of the basal turn was entirely intact. Following the turns in apical direction the number of missing and degenerated sensory cells gradually diminished and a normal hair cell pattern was almost casually resumed. Giant stereocilia were occasionally seen in the apical turn. Clumping of stereocilia and dumping of cell contents were often in evidence (Fig. 48). The presence of apparently normal sensory cells among extensive lesions formed a striking appearance.

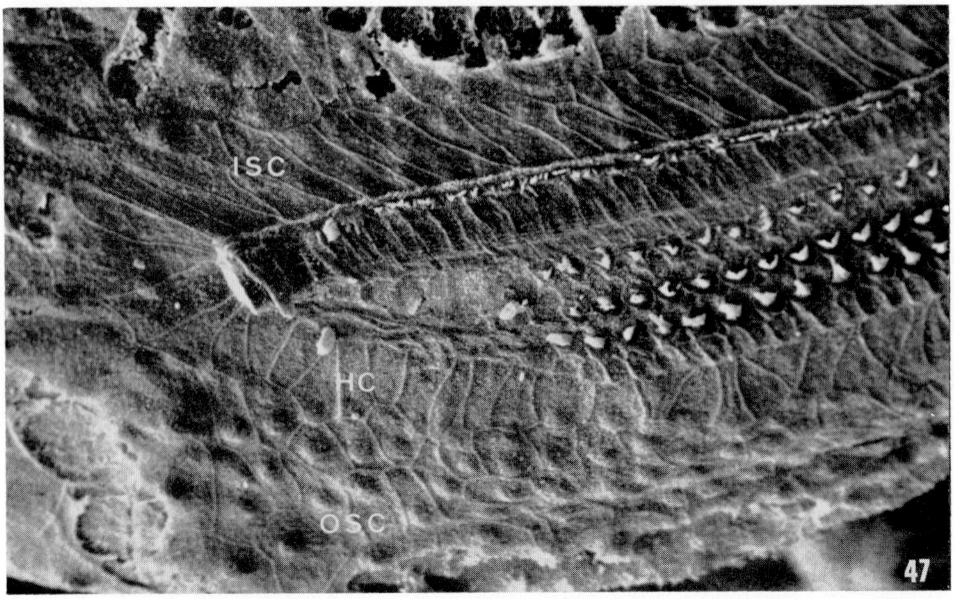

Fig. 47. Detail of Figure 46. The organ of Corti is discontinued fairly abruptly; the inner sulcus cells (ISC) with their oblong cell surfaces seem to merge into the Hensen's cells (HC) and the polygonal outer sulcus cells (OSC) (SEM 760 X).

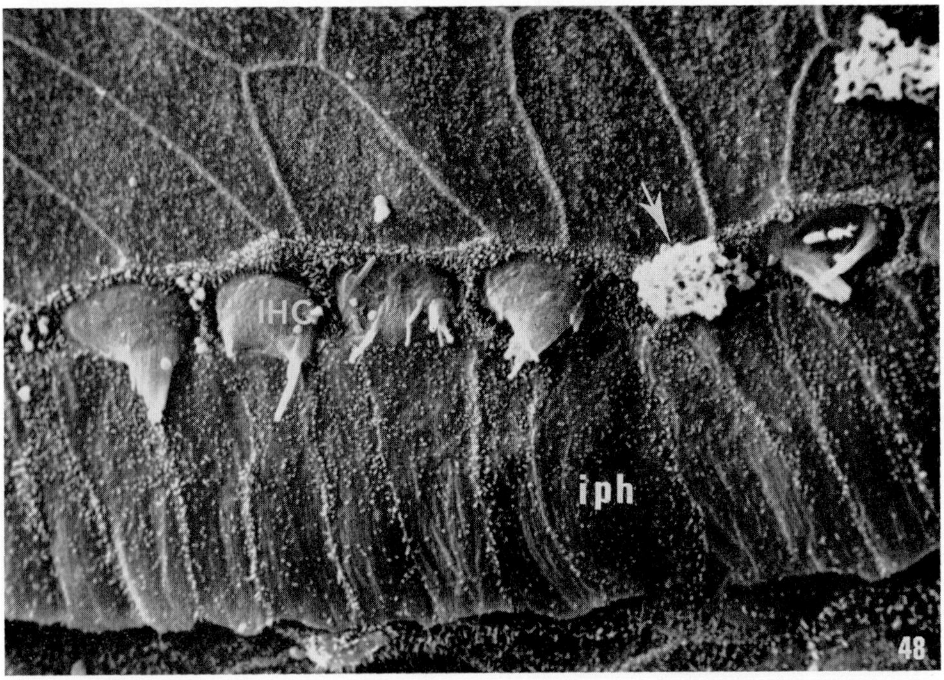

Fig. 48. Detail of lower apical turn. This cochlea was exposed for three hours to the intermittent noise of a low-speed drill, amplified by 10 dB. The animal was sacrificed after three weeks. Lesions extend over the lower apical, upper basal and basal turns, where only the inner hair cells (IHC) and inner pillar heads (IPH) are still identifiable. The stereocilia of the inner hair cells have fused almost completely. The sensory cells are about to be or have been discarded (arrow) (SEM 3,800 X).

TABLE VI

COCHLEOGRAMS OF GUINEA PIGS EXPOSED FOR TWO HOURS TO THE NOISE OF A HIGH-SPEED DRILL, AMPLIFIED BY 10 dB

Animal No.	*Right Cochlea* — *Turn 1* · *2* · *3* · *4*
1	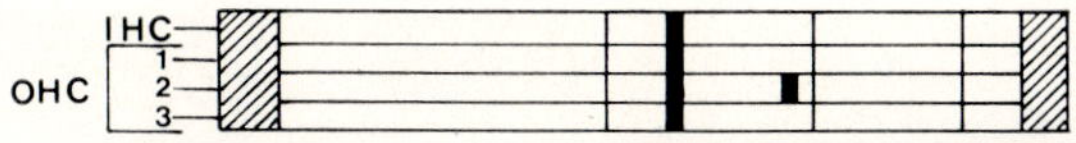
2	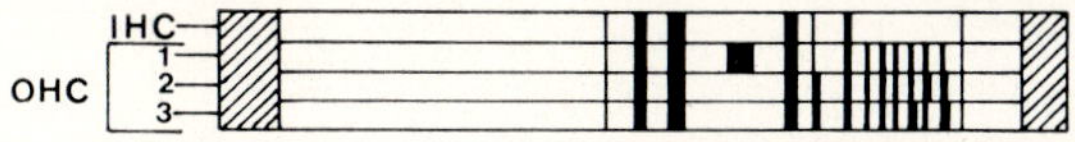
3	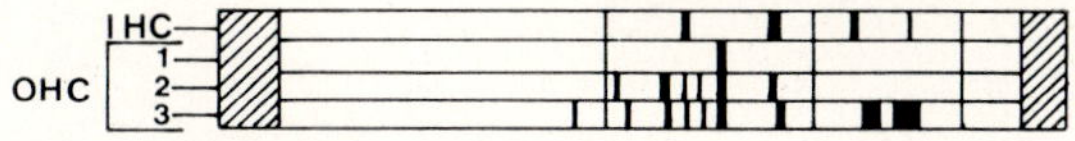
4	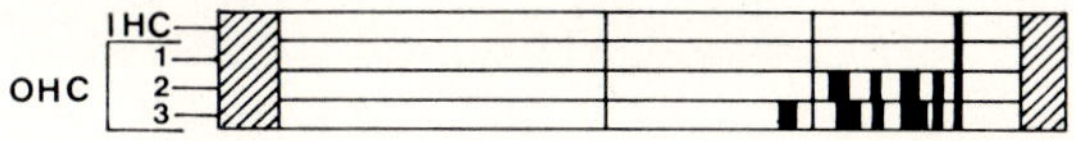
5	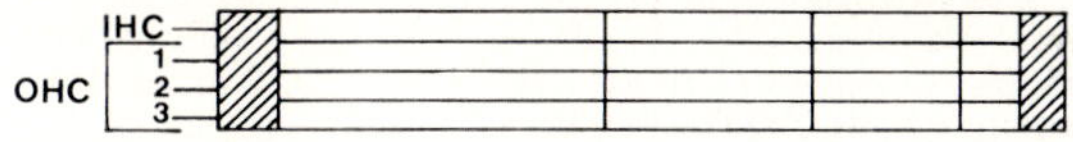
6	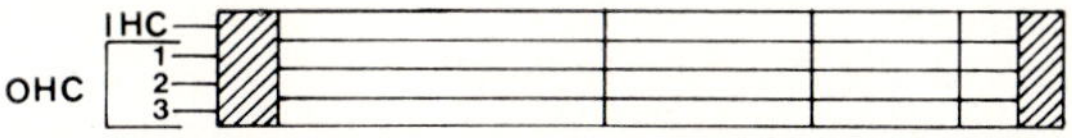
7	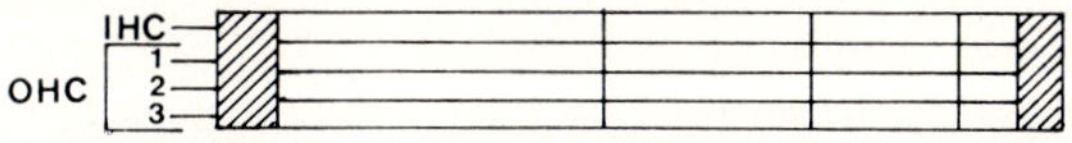
8	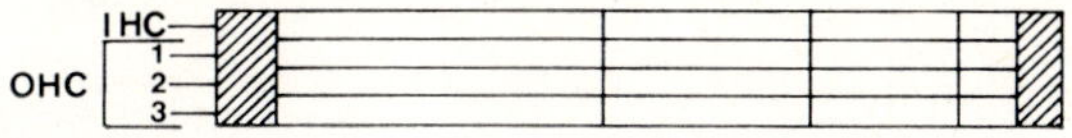

Of the two guinea pigs exposed to three hours of low-speed drill noise applied to the right ear, one showed an enormous lesion of the right organ of Corti. Only in the basal part of the basal turn and in the basal part of the apical turn was a more or less regular hair cell pattern identifiable in small areas. Most of the remainder of the organ of Corti had been destroyed. The other animal showed scars in the last quarter of the basal turn and in three-quarters of the upper basal turn. The damage evidently also involved the inner hair cells. In the basal half of the lower apical turn, another scar was observed, which was confined to the outer hair cells. The control animal showed no lesion on either side. The left cochleae of the two exposed animals were also quite normal.

In the second group, unmistakable lesions of the organ of Corti were found in four of the eight right cochleae exposed for two hours to the noise of the high-speed drill (Table VI). In three of these four, the lesions were localized in the lower apical and upper basal turns. In one, they were confined to the upper basal turn. Most lesions involved only the outer hair cells. In only one cochlea did the organ of Corti show collapse over a short distance. A conspicuous finding was that outer hair cells, particularly in the second and third rows, were missing (Fig. 49). The remaining four right cochleae and the two cochleae of the control animal showed no lesions. Of the eight left cochleae, seven were normal. One left cochlea showed extensive lesions in the lower apical turn: numerous scars, with missing inner hair cells also. The cause of these lesions has remained obscure. However, a purulent secretion was found to fill the tym-

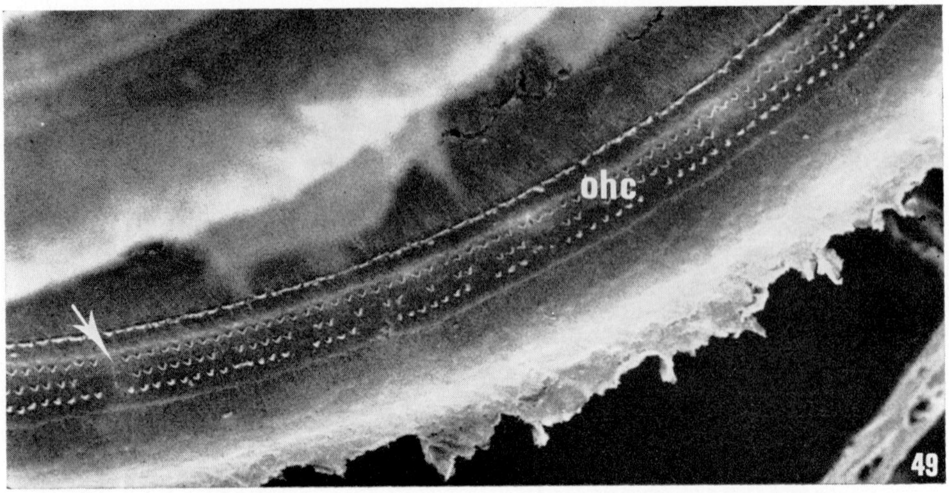

Fig. 49. Upper basal turn of a right cochlea exposed for two hours to the intermittent noise of a high-speed otologic drill. The animal was sacrificed after five weeks. The drill noise was amplified by 10 dB. A few outer hair cells (OHC) are occasionally missing from the second and third rows. The arrow indicates a small scar in the three rows of outer hair cells (SEM 260 X).

panic bulla. Yet a correlation between the otitis and the loss of sensory cells is not very likely. The two right cochleae exposed for three hours to drill noise amplified by 10 dB, showed lesions through three turns of the organ of Corti. In the apical half of the basal turn, the upper basal turn and the basal half of the lower apical turn, there was scattered loss of outer hair cells with many small scars. The two left cochleae were normal.

In the third group, one of the eight guinea pigs exposed for two hours to the noise of the very-high-speed drill amplified by 10 dB and applied to the right ear, showed labyrinthitis: the cochlea was entirely filled with connective tissue interspersed with leucocytes (Figs. 50, 51, 52). The tympanic bulla and middle ear also showed inflammatory changes. Of the remaining seven right cochleae, five showed acoustic trauma (Table VII). The distribution of lesions differed widely in different cochleae, ranging from the apical half of the basal turn to the basal half of the apical turn. The scars were usually of limited size, alternating with normal areas of the organ of Corti. Lesions were most numerous in the upper basal turn. Inner hair cells were often damaged in

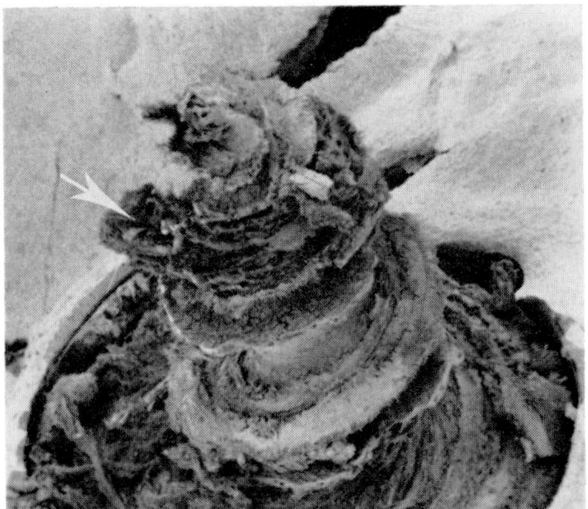

Fig. 50. Right cochlea of a guinea pig exposed for two hours to the noise of a very-high-speed otologic drill. The animal was sacrificed after three weeks. The bony capsule has been removed. There is a labyrinthitis with destruction of the entire organ of Corti. Connective tissue is visible between the turns (arrow) (SEM 22 X).

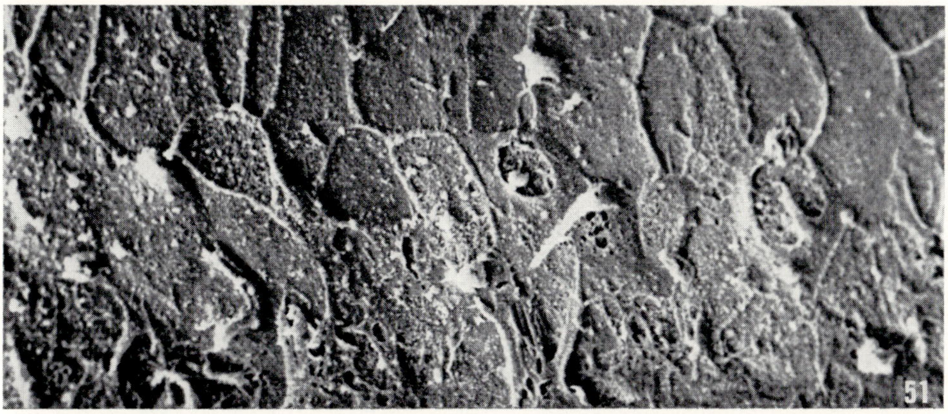

Fig. 51. Detail of Figure 50. This is probably all that has remained of the organ of Corti (SEM 1,260 X).

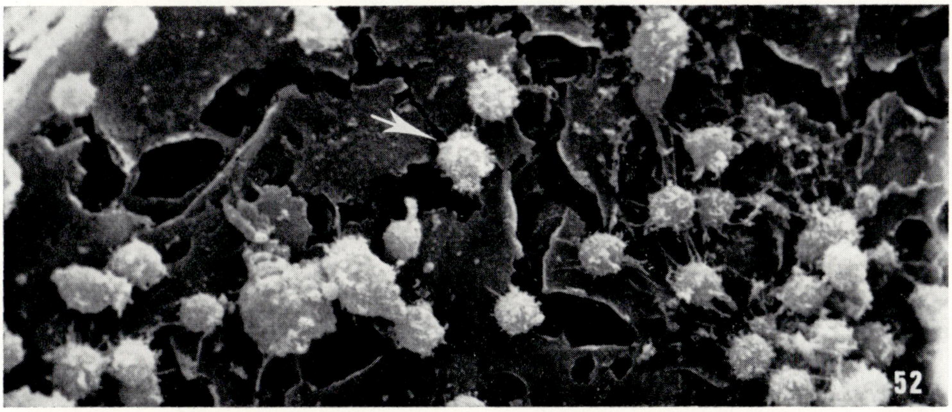

Fig. 52. Detail of Figure 50. Leucocyte accumulations are visible at several sites in the cochlea (arrow) (SEM 1,260 X).

lesions which did or did not involve first-row outer hair cells. In some instances the loss involved only outer hair cells (Fig. 53). Two of the eight left cochlea showed extensive cell loss in the upper basal and lower apical turns (cause unknown); the remaining six were normal. In the two right cochleae exposed to the same noise for three hours, the organs of Corti showed extensive lesions, which in both involved mostly the upper basal and lower apical turns. The corresponding left cochleae were normal.

DISCUSSION

The findings of this study have confirmed that identical acoustic traumas can produce widely different lesions in the organ of Corti; different both in extent and in localization. But the changes in the hair cell pattern were not constant either. Yet certain patterns of degeneration were observed again and again in the experiments. To begin with, there was the large circumscribed lesion, which involved total destruction of the organ of Corti over several tenths of millimeters, leaving only a low crest of epithelium. Second, there was the combination of lesions of a row of inner hair cells with lesions of first-row outer hair cells, a combination also found in the experiments with pure tones. Finally, there was a scattered loss of hair cells, solitary or in small groups, which involved the outer hair cells of the second and third rows more than those of the

TABLE VII

COCHLEOGRAMS OF GUINEA PIGS EXPOSED FOR TWO HOURS TO THE NOISE OF A VERY-HIGH-SPEED DRILL, AMPLIFIED BY 10 dB

Animal No. — *Right Cochlea*: *Turn 1*, 2, 3, 4

1

2

3

4

5

6

7

8

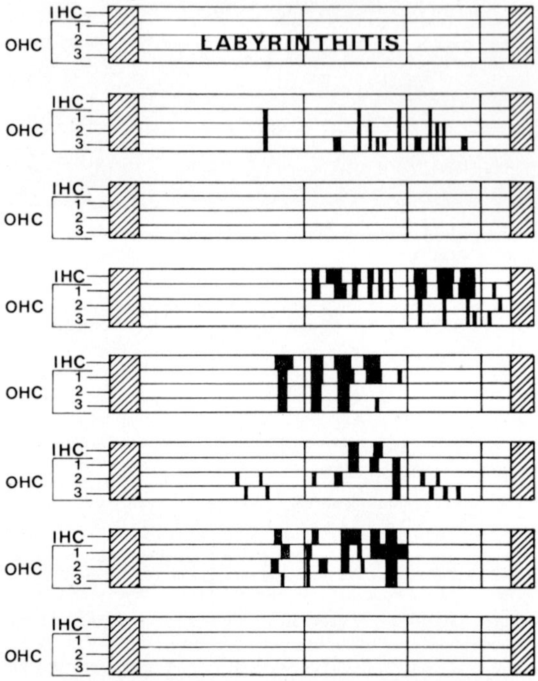

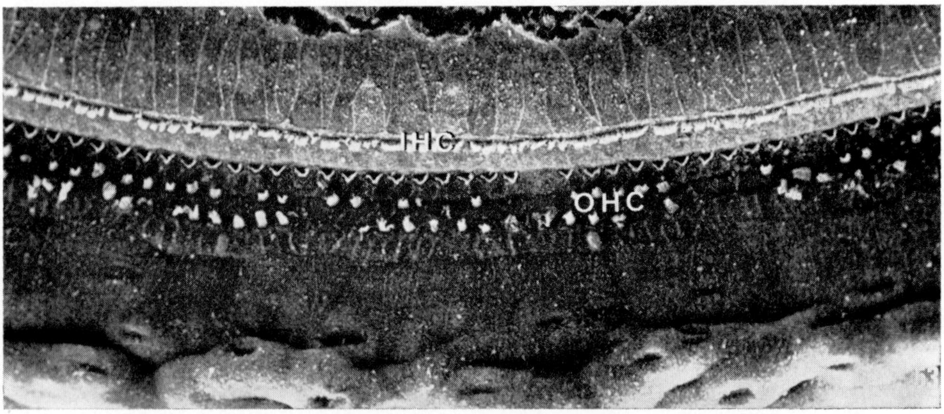

Fig. 53. Lower apical turn. Cochlea exposed for two hours to the intermittent noise of a very-high-speed drill, amplified by 10 dB. The animal was sacrificed after five weeks. The inner hair cells (IHC) are intact. The outer hair cells (OHC) have partly disappeared, the cell loss in the second and third rows exceeding that in the first row (SEM 440 X).

first row, leaving the inner hair cells entirely intact.

As expected from the drill noise analysis, the low-speed drill proved to be most traumatic. The analysis also showed that the high-speed drill produced up to 10 dB more noise than the very-high-speed drill, but this was not confirmed by the cochleograms obtained. The very-high-speed drill produced more extensive and more numerous lesions than the high-speed drill. A conspicuous finding was that, after exposure to the amplified noise of the three drills tested during more than two hours, the lesions were very much larger and often extended through three turns.

Had the noise of the drills been offered at true intensity, no, or only minimal, lesions might have occurred in the organ of Corti in these guinea pigs. In human mastoidectomies, however, the mastoid is often sclerotic and requires longer and harder drilling than the cadaver mastoid. The noise intensities can then attain values in excess of the values we measured; and the risk of acoustic damage to the organ of Corti increases accordingly. The drill noise was offered intermittently in order to imitate the actual situation during an operation. Intermittent noise is believed to be less injurious than continuous noise, because the metabolism of the sensory cells has time to recover during the "silent" intervals.

It is not known why the lesions in the organ of Corti in these experiments varied so widely in localization, extent and pattern, whereas, in the audiogram of an acoustically traumatized patient the dip is invariably found at 4,000-6,000 Hz. Further experiments with supplemental behavior audiometry and electrocochleography might well provide an answer to this question. Whether the highly individual sensitivity of the test animals to acoustic trauma has played a role in this respect is difficult to establish. In any case, this individual sensitivity is a factor also in human individuals.

Extrapolating our results to ear surgery, the following can be stated. Any operation on the ear entails a risk of development or exacerbation of sensorineural hearing loss, and individual sensitivity certainly plays a role in this respect. In ear operations involving the use of an otologic drill, one takes an additional acoustic risk by exposing the diseased ear to sound intensities which can have a traumatic effect on the organ of Corti. This risk increases by as much as the bone involved is more sclerotic, for this requires longer drilling and an increased pressure of the burr against the bone, by which duration and intensity of drill noise increase. Of course, this applies specifically to sanitizing ear operations in which a considerable amount of sclerotic bone must be removed. On the other hand, the type of drill and the shape and size of the burr are also of importance. The low-speed drill produces more noise than the high-speed or the very-high-speed drill. This is due not so much to the difference in rpm as to the difference in torque. The higher torque of the low-speed drill permits of greater pressure of the burr on the bone, and this involves an increased intensity of noise. Conical burrs were found to be more noisy than spherical burrs of the same diameter. All burrs of larger diameter were noisier than burrs of smaller diameter.

CONCLUSIONS

1. The noises of three different types of otologic drills, amplified by 10 dB, produced discernible lesions in the organ of Corti in the guinea pig.

2. Although there were marked interindividual variations in the extent, localization and pattern of the lesion, it was, nevertheless, possible to distinguish patterns of degeneration of three different types.

3. The use of otologic drills of the types investigated entails an acoustic risk.

4. The high-speed and the very-high-speed drills tested were acoustically safer than the low-speed drill.

5. Prolonged continuous drilling is inadvisable, and the same applies to the frequent use of a conical burr.

REFERENCES

1. Iurato S: *Submicroscopic Structure of the Inner Ear.* Oxford, Pergamon Press, 1967, p XI

2. Fosbroke J: Practical observations on the pathology and treatment of deafness. Lancet I:645-648, 1831

3. Habermann J: Ueber die Schwerhörigkeit der Kesselschmiede. Arch Klin Exp Ohren Nasen Kehlkopfheilkd 30:1-25, 1890

4. Corti A: Recherches sur l'organe de l'ouie des mammifères. Z Wiss Zool 3:109-169, 1851

5. Retzius G: *Das Gehörorgan der Wirbeltiere. I & II.* Stockholm, Samson & Wallin, 1881, 1884

6. Wittmaack K: Über Schädigung des Gehörs durch Schalleinwirkung. Z Ohrenheilkd 54:37-80, 1907

7. Yoshii U: Experimentelle Untersuchungen über die Schadigung des Gehörorgans durch Schalleinwirkung. Z Ohrenheilkd 58: 201-251, 1909

8. Marx H: Untersuchungen über experimentelle Schädigungen des Gehörorganes. Z Ohrenheilkd 59:333-343, 1909

9. Röhr H: Ergebnisse experimenteller Schallschädigungsversuche bei Tieren. Beitr Anat Phys Pathol Ther Ohres 16:14-31, 1921

10. Rüedi L, Furrer W: *Das akustische Trauma.* Basel, Karger Verlag, 1947

11. Engström H, Wersäll J: Structure of the organ of Corti I. Acta Otolaryngol (Stockh) 43:1-10, 1953

12. Engström H, Wersäll J: Structure of the organ of Corti II. Acta Otolaryngol (Stockh) 43:323-334, 1953

13. Babel J, Bischoff A, Spoendlin H: *Ultrastructure of the Peripheral Nervous System and Sense Organs.* Stuttgart, Georg Thieme Verlag, 1970

14. Engström H, Ades HW, Andersson A: *Structural Pattern of the Organ of Corti.* Stockholm, Almqvist & Wiksell, 1966

15. Kohonen A: Effect of some ototoxic drugs upon the pattern and innervation of cochlear sensory cells in the guinea pig. Acta Otolaryngol [Suppl] (Stockh) 208, 1965

16. Bredberg G: Cellular pattern and nerve supply of the human organ of Corti. Acta Otolaryngol [Suppl] (Stockh) 236, 1968

17. Stockwell CW, Ades HW, Engström H: Pattern of hair cell damage after intense auditory stimulation. Ann Otol Rhinol Laryngol 78:1144-1168, 1969

18. Watanuki K, Kawamoto K, Katagiri S: Repair pattern in the reticular lamina of the organ of Corti after hair cell loss. Ann Otol Rhinol Laryngol 78:1210-1219, 1969

19. Johnsson LG: Reissner's membrane in the human cochlea. Ann Otol Rhinol Laryngol 80:425-438, 1971

20. Pye A: Effect of exposure to intense pure tones on the hearing organ of animals. Rep Inst Laryngol Otol 20:245-252, 1971

21. Gonzales G, Miller N, Wasilewski V: Progressive neuro-ototoxicity of kanamycin. Ann Otol Rhinol Laryngol 81:127-131, 1972

22. Hunter-Duvar IM, Elliott DN: Effects of intense auditory stimulation: hearing losses and inner ear changes in the squirrel monkey I. J Acoust Soc Am 52:1181-1192, 1972

23. Voldrich L: Experimental acoustic trauma. Acta Otolaryngol (Stockh) 74:392-397, 1972

24. Hunter-Duvar IM, Elliott DN: Effects of intense auditory stimulation: hearing losses and inner ear changes in the squirrel monkey II. J Acoust Soc Am 54:1179-1183, 1973

25. Falk SA, Cook RO, Haseman JK, *et al*: Noise induced inner ear damage in newborn and adult guinea pigs. Laryngoscope 84: 444-453, 1974

26. Henderson D, Hamernik RP, Sitler R: Audiometric and anatomical correlates of impulse noise exposure. Arch Otolaryngol 99:62-64, 1974

27. Hunter-Duvar IM, Bredberg G: Effects of intense auditory stimulation: hearing losses and inner ear changes in the chinchilla. J Acoust Soc Am 55:795-801, 1974

28. Barber VC, Boyde A: Scanning electron microscopic studies of cilia. Z Zellforsch Mikrosk Anat 84:269-284, 1968

29. Lim DJ, Lane WC: Cochlear sensory epithelium. Ann Otol Rhinol Laryngol 78: 827-841, 1969

30. Lim D: Three dimensional observation of the inner ear with the scanning electron microscope. Acta Otolaryngol [Suppl] (Stockh) 255:5-38, 1969

31. Bredberg G, Lindeman HH, Ades HW, *et al*: Scanning electron microscopy of the organ of Corti. Science 170:861-863, 1970

32. Engström H, Ades HW, Bredberg G: *Sensorineural Hearing Loss.* London, J & A Churchill, 1970, p 127-156

33. Marovitz WF, Arenberg IK, Thalmann R: Evaluation of preparative technique for the scanning electron microscope. Laryngoscope 80:1680-1700, 1970

34. Marovitz WF, Thalmann R, Arenberg IK: Scanning electron microscopy of freeze-dried guinea pig organ of Corti. Proc Third Annu Scan Elect Micr Symp (Chicago), 1970, p 273-280

35. Thalmann R, Thalmann I, Comegys TH: Dissection and chemical analysis of substructures of the organ of Corti. Laryngoscope 80:1619-1645, 1970

36. Kosaka N, Tanaka T, Takiguchi T, *et al*: Observation on the organ of Corti with scanning electron microscope. Acta Otolaryngol (Stockh) 72:377-384, 1971

37. Lim DJ, Melnick W: Acoustic damage of the cochlea. Arch Otolaryngol 94:294-305, 1971

38. Lindeman HH, Ades HW, Bredberg G, *et al*: The sensory hairs and the tectorial membrane in the development of the cat's organ of Corti. Acta Otolaryngol (Stockh) 72:229-242, 1971

39. Lundquist PG, Flock A, Wersäll J: Raster- und Elektronen Mikroskopie des menschlichen Labyrinths. Monatsschr Ohrenheilkd Laryngorhinol 105:285-300, 1971

40. Marovitz WF, Thalmann R, Arenberg IK: Specialized extracellular structures of the inner ear. Proc Fourth Annu Scan Elect Micr Symp (Chicago), 1971, p 313-320

41. Bredberg G, Ades HW, Engström H: Inner ear studies. Acta Otolaryngol [Suppl] (Stockh) 301:3-60, 1972

42. Crysdale WS, Stahle J: Ultrasonic irradiation of the guinea pig cochlea. Ann Otol Rhinol Laryngol 81:87-98, 1972

43. Lim DJ: Fine morphology of the tectorial membrane. Arch Otolaryngol 96:199-215, 1972

44. Lindeman HH, Bredberg G: Scanning electron microscopy of the organ of Corti after intense auditory stimulation: Effects on stereocilia and cuticular surface of hair cells. Arch Klin Exp Ohren Nasen Kehlkopfheilkd 203:1-15, 1972

45. Stahle J, Högberg L, Engström B: The laser as a tool in inner-ear surgery. Acta Otolaryngol (Stockh) 73:27-37, 1972

46. Tanaka T, Kosaka N, Takiguchi T, *et al*: Observation on the cochlea with S.E.M. Proc Sixth Annu Scan Elec Micr Symp (Chicago), 1973, p 428-433

47. Angelborg C, Engström B: The tympanic covering layer. An electron microscopic study in guinea pig. Acta Otolaryngol [Suppl] (Stockh) 319:43-56, 1974

48. Engström B: Scanning electron microscopy of the inner ear structure of the organ of Corti and its neural pathways. Acta Otolaryngol [Suppl] (Stockh) 319:57-66, 1974

49. Arenberg IK: Scanning electron microscopy in otorhinolaryngologic research, 1970. Arch Otolaryngol 95:477-483, 1972

50. Bohne BA: Location of small cochlear lesions by phase contrast microscopy prior to thin sectioning. Laryngoscope 82:1-16, 1972

51. Spoendlin H, Brun JP: The block-surface technique for evaluation of cochlear pathology. Arch Oto Rhino Laryng (Berlin) 208:137-145, 1974

52. Arnold GE: Beitrag zur Kenntnis der Lokalisation der beginnenden Cochlearis affektion II. Monatsschr Ohrenheilkd Laryngorhinol 73:673-686, 1939

53. De Montmollin D: Etude du traumatisme acoustique opératoire dans les interventions de l'oreille. Pract Otorhinolaryngol (Basel) 22:81-92, 1960

54. Schuknecht HF, Tonndorf J: Acoustic trauma of the cochlea from ear surgery. Laryngoscope 70:479-505, 1960

55. Massena-Lacerda S, Bebear JP: Etude des variations de la conduction osseuse après tympanoplastie par la voie transmastoidienne. Rev Laryngol Otol Rhinol (Bord) 91:517-525, 1970

56. Kupperman R: Iatrogene lawaaibeschadigingen van de cochlea. Ned Tijdschr Geneeskd 118:984, 1973

57. Davis H, and Associates: Acoustic trauma in the guinea pig. J Acoust Soc Am 25:1180-1189, 1953

58. Preyer W: *Specielle Physiologie des Embryo*. Leipzig, Grieben's Verlag, 1885, p 481

59. Van der Gulden WJI, Van Hooydonk CL, de Jong P, *et al*: Proefdierkunde I en II. Nijmegen, Drukkerij van Mameren, 1972

60. Kato T: Zur Physiologie der Binnenmuskeln des Ohres. Pfluegers Arch 150:569-625, 1913

61. Wever EG, Lawrence M: *Physiological Acoustics*. Princeton, Princeton University Press, 1954, p 195-196

62. Galambos R, Rupert A: Action of the middle ear muscles in normal cats. J Acoust Soc Am 31:349-355, 1959

63. Hilding DA: The intratympanic muscle reflex as a protective mechanism against loud impulsive noise. Ann Otol Rhinol Laryngol 69:51-60, 1960

64. Wersäll R: The tympanic muscles and their reflexes. Acta Otolaryngol [Suppl] (Stockh) 139:41-42, 1958

65. Borg E, Møller AR: Effects of ethylalcohol and pentabarbital sodium on the acoustic middle ear reflex in man. Acta Otolaryngol (Stockh) 64:415-426, 1967

66. Eldredge DH, Covell WP, Davis H: Recovery from acoustic trauma in the guinea pig. Laryngoscope 67:66-84, 1957

67. Hoessli H: Weitere experimentelle Studien über die akustische Schädigung des Säugetierlabyrinths. Z Ohrenheilkd 64, 65: 101-145, 1912

68. Boyde A, Wood C: Preparation of animal tissues for surface scanning electron microscopy. J Microsc (Oxf) 90:221-249, 1969

69. Boyde A: Freeze drying in the preparation of animal tissue and cell specimens for electron microscopy. Publication NoP 1/1: p 1-22, 1973

70. Held H: *Die Cochlea der Säuger und*

der Vögel, ihre Entwicklung und ihre Bau. Handb Norm Pathol Physiol. Berlin, Springer Verlag, 1926, XI, p 467-526

71. Kolmer W: *Gehörorgan. Handb Mikrosk Anat Mensch.* Berlin, Springer Verlag, 1927, III, p 250-478

72. Flock A, Kimura R, Lundquist PG, *et al*: Morphological basis of directional sensitivity of the outer hair cells in the organ of Corti. J Acoust Soc Am 34:1351-1355, 1962

73. Kimura RS: Hairs of the cochlear sensory cells and their attachment to the tectorial membrane. Acta Otolaryngol (Stockh) 61: 55-72, 1966

74. von Békésy G: Microphonics produced by touching the cochlear partition with a vibrating electrode. J Acoust Soc Am 23: 29-36, 1951

75. Engström H, Ades HW, Hawkins JE: Structure and functions of the sensory hairs of the inner ear. J Acoust Soc Am 34:1356-1363, 1962

76. Spoendlin H: Innervation patterns in the organ of Corti of the cat. Acta Otolaryngol (Stockh) 67:239-254, 1969

77. Ter Kuile E: Die Uebertragung der Energie von der Grundmembran auf die Haarzellen. Pfluegers Arch 79:146-157, 1900

78. Ter Kuile E: Die richtige Bewegungsform der Membrana basilaris. Pfluegers Arch 79:484-509, 1900

79. De Vries H, Bleeker JDJW: The Microphonic activity of the labyrinth of the pigeon. Acta Otolaryngol (Stockh) 37:298-306, 1949

80. Shambaugh GE: Die membrana tectoria und die Theorie der Tonempfindung. Z Ohrenheilkd 59:159-168, 1909

81. De Vries H: Struktur und Lage der Tectorialmembran in der Schnecke, untersucht mit neueren Hilfsmitteln. Acta Otolaryngol 37:334-338, 1949

82. Borghesan E: Tectorial membrane and organ of Corti considered as a unique anatomic and functional entity. Acta Otolaryngol (Stockh) 42:473-486, 1952

83. Iurato S: Submicroscopic structure of the membranous labyrinth. Z Zellforsch Mikrosk Anat 52:105-128, 1960

84. Wever EG: The mechanics of hair-cell-stimulation. Ann Otol Rhinol Laryngol 80:786-804, 1971

85. Zwicker E: Investigation of the inner ear of the domestic pig and the squirrel monkey with special regard to the hydromechanics of the cochlear duct. Symp Hearing Theory, IPO Eindhoven, Holland, 1972

86. Werner CF: Ueber artifizielle Veränderungen des Innenohres und ihre Beziehungen zu den pathologischen Vorgängen. Monatsschr Ohrenheilkd Laryngorhinol 17: 1017-1044, 1937

87. Hilding AC: Studies on the otic labyrinth I. On the origin and insertion of the tectorial membrane. Ann Otol Rhinol Laryngol 61:354-370, 1952

88. Bohne BA, Eldredge DH, Mills JH: Cochlear potentials and electron microscopy applied to the study of small cochlear lesions. Ann Otol Rhinol Laryngol 82:595-608, 1973

89. Spoendlin H: Submikroskopische Veränderungen am Corti'schen Organ des Meerschweinchens nach akustischer Belastung. Pract Otorhinolaryngol (Basel) 20:197-214, 1958.

90. Engström H, Ades HW: Effect of high-intensity noise on inner ear sensory epithelia. Acta Otolaryngol [Suppl] (Stockh) 158:219-229, 1960

91. Beagly HA: Acoustic trauma in the guinea pig I. Acta Otolaryngol (Stockh) 60: 437-451, 1965

92. Beagly HA: Acoustic trauma in the guinea pig II. Acta Otolaryngol (Stockh) 60: 479-495, 1965

93. Ward WD, Duvall AJ: Behavioral and ultrastructural correlates of acoustic trauma. Ann Otol Rhinol Laryngol 80:881-896, 1971

94. Lurie MH, Davis H, Hawkins JE: Acoustic trauma of the organ of Corti in the guinea pig. Laryngoscope 54:375-386, 1944

95. Schuknecht HF: Presbyacusis. Laryngoscope 65:402-419, 1955

96. Von Schulthess G: *Innenohr und Trauma. Fortschr Hals Nasen Ohrenheilkd.* Basel, Karger Verlag, 1961, p 1-152

97. Spoendlin H: Primary structural changes in the organ of Corti after acoustic overstimulation. Acta Otolaryngol (Stockh) 71:166-176, 1971

98. Sataloff J: *Hearing Loss.* Philadelphia, J. B. Lippincott Co, 1966, p 154-155, 192-193

99. Von Beickert P: *Hals- Nasen- Ohren Heilkunde.* Berends J, Link R, Zöllner F (eds). Stuttgart, Thieme Verlag, 1966, Bd III, Teil 2, p 1331-1332

100. Paparella MM: Acoustic trauma from the bone cutting burr. Laryngoscope 72:116-126, 1962

101. Helms J: Die Bewegung der Stapes fussplatte bei Bohrtraumen an der Kette. Arch Klin Exp Ohren Nasen Kehlkopfheilkd 202:559-563, 1972

102. Paulsen K: Vor- und Nachteile hochtouriger Bohrmachinen bei der Knochenpräparation. Arch Klin Exp Ohren Nasen Kehlkopfheilkd 196:123-126, 1970

SURVEY OF THE DEVELOPMENT OF LARYNGEAL EPITHELIUM

John A. Tucker, MD
Philadelphia, Pennsylvania

Branislav Vidic, SD
Washington, DC

Gabriel F. Tucker, Jr., MD
Chicago, Illinois

Jeffrey Stead, BS
Philadelphia, Pennsylvania

From the Institute of Laryngology and Human Communication, Hahnemann Medical College and Hospital, Philadelphia, Pennsylvania; the Department of Anatomy, Georgetown University, Washington, DC; and the Division of Otolaryngology-Communicative Disorders, the Children's Memorial Hospital, Chicago, Illinois.

Presented at the meeting of the American Broncho-Esophagological Association, Palm Beach, Florida, April 27-28, 1976.

SURVEY OF THE DEVELOPMENT OF LARYNGEAL EPITHELIUM

JOHN A. TUCKER, MD
PHILADELPHIA, PENNSYLVANIA

GABRIEL F. TUCKER, JR., MD
CHICAGO, ILLINOIS

BRANISLAV VIDIC, SD
WASHINGTON, DC

JEFFREY STEAD, BS
PHILADELPHIA, PENNSYLVANIA

SUMMARY — An overview of the developing laryngeal epithelium has been presented to establish the norm. The sequential relationships of the formation of the protective laryngeal covering, cellular and glandular, have been reviewed. The topographical distribution of the epithelial elements in the human larynx are illustrated in the adult and contrasted in the child. Unique and previously undescribed cellular ultrastructure and transition areas have been identified. Biological integration of form and function is again well illustrated in the epithelium of the human larynx.

Various techniques of studying the epithelium of the human larynx have been employed. Classic isolated histologic study was done as early as the mid-1800s.[1] The technique of Epstein,[2] in 1958, employed longitudinal sectioning of the gross specimen into strips. Each strip was then serially sectioned. Whole organ sectioning was applied in a three-dimensional picture by Tucker in 1961.[3] With this three-dimensional principle, one not only studied depth in the larynx, but coronal section offered a comparison of contrast, one hemilarynx to the other. Since then large collections of whole organ studies have been internationally developed, with specific reference to carcinoma of the larynx.[4]

A relatively rapid and simple technique of defining laryngeal epithelium was described by Zilliacus[5] in 1905, with the use of dyes for staining the entire gross specimen. This technique permitted differentiation of the two types of epithelium. Stell *et al*[6] in 1972 utilized Tyronin dye, a basic red dye, to stain the ribonucleic acid. The various gross staining methods have been shown to depend largely upon the "differential permeability of the two types of the epithelium."[6]

This presentation will be divided into two parts, Developmental Considerations, consisting of observations made mainly by standard light microscopy, and Laryngeal Topographical Cellular Considerations, including observations made mainly by scanning and transmission electron microscopy.

DEVELOPMENTAL CONSIDERATIONS — PART A

The protocol objective was to compare by standard light microscopy, scanning electron microscopy and transmission electron microscopy, normal laryngeal epithelium in a survey of mucosal laryngeal development.

Further, the intent was to correlate, in a three-dimensional standard and ultrastructural perspective, the general pattern of mucosal cellular distribution throughout the larynx.

Not since 1955, with the article of Hopp,[7] has the development of the epithelium of the larynx been closely studied. Hopp reviewed in great detail the existing literature, historically and scientifically. In addition, he studied 25 prenatal specimens. Two probable embryos, six fetal, as well as two adult specimens were studied in serial section. He specifically noted that "few really good microscopic sections of adult larynges were available at that time."

The present authors are indeed fortunate to have access to an extensive resource of prenatal, embryologic and fetal, as well as postnatal, child and adult material from which to draw selected specimens.

Of interest was Hopp's note of the

then existing conflict and diverse scientific opinions in the literature. Only two points will be reviewed.

A controversy existed in the late 1880s over whether the squamous epithelium of the larynx was the result of gradual differentiation (physiologic metaplasia) from the embryo,[8] or whether islands of squamous epithelium appeared because of functional pathologic changes (pathologic metaplasia).[9] Heymann proposed that the developmental characteristics of the larynx were predetermined by its strategic anatomical location. Essentially, he subscribed to the "demonstration of Ganghofner," 1897, as quoted by Hopp,[7] that the larynx developed from two areas, supraglottically the base of the tongue and subglottically the trachea. This is similar in some respects to Frazer's[10] 1910 concept of the importance of the "transverse cavity" — the pharyngeal floor — and that the supraglottic larynx results from "secondary inclusion of the part of the cavity of the pharynx by an upward growth of its floor, while the saggital (median) part of the larynx (infraglottic) is the drawn out proximal end of the pulmonary diverticulum."[10]

Heymann[11] (1898) noted the normal variable thickness of the epithelium from point to point and individual to individual. "This implied little or no significance to the numerical mucosal diameters, as described by Henle and Luschka."[11] Finally, Heymann described two completely different types of epithelium, ciliated cylindrical and stratified squamous epithelium, and recognized goblet cells, the latter considered to be derived from ciliated cells.

Hopp's own observations on the 25 specimens noted, agreed with those of Soulie and Bardier,[12] Kanthack,[8] and Kallius,[13] "that the differentiation of the epithelium of the larynx is always an orderly process, with a definite pattern throughout embryonic life to achieve its adult appearance." This process was called "physiologic metaplasia."[7] The authors concur with these observations.

TABLE I
ANATOMIC DEVELOPMENTAL MATERIAL

Material	*Stage (S) or Age (A) ca-wk*	*Specimen No.*	*Plane of Section*
Prenatal	*S 14	8308	S
Embryo	*S 16	6511	S
	*S 20	460	H
	*S 23	9226	H
Fetus	A 10	LIA-420	C
	**A 12	LIA- 8	C
	A 14	LIA-413	S
	**A 16	LIA- 15	S
	A 20	LIA-254	S
	**A 24	LIA- 4	C
	**A 28	LIA- 27	C
	**A 34	LIA- 20	C
	A 36	LIA-256	H
Postnatal	**A 42 (term)	LIA- 52	C
	**A 12	LIA- 29	C

*Carnegie Collection (U. of California at Davis); **Johns Hopkins Collection (Baltimore); S — Sagittal; H — Horizontal; C — Coronal. All specimens were studied by standard light microscopy.

Observations. The importance of employing a recognized staging system throughout a developmental study cannot be overstressed. Only by the use of a method such as the Carnegie staging system which divides the embryonic period proper, approximately the first eight weeks, into 23 levels of development, can a step-by-step tracing of development be accomplished.[14] The inaccuracy inherent in time and length measurement in the embryonic period makes such terminology as "the 7 mm stage" not acceptable. Accordingly, all embryonic material studied and literary references are made to staged human material (Table I).

Unfortunately, to date no such staging system for the larynx exists in the fetal period and estimates of time, weight and measurements of crown-rump and crown-heel length are used in approximate levels of development.[15]

Established standard light microscopy specimens were reviewed in the embryo, fetal, infant, adolescent, and adult periods to confirm a perspective of laryngeal epithelial development.

The early development of the larynx in staged human embryos has been specifically outlined in the recent literature,

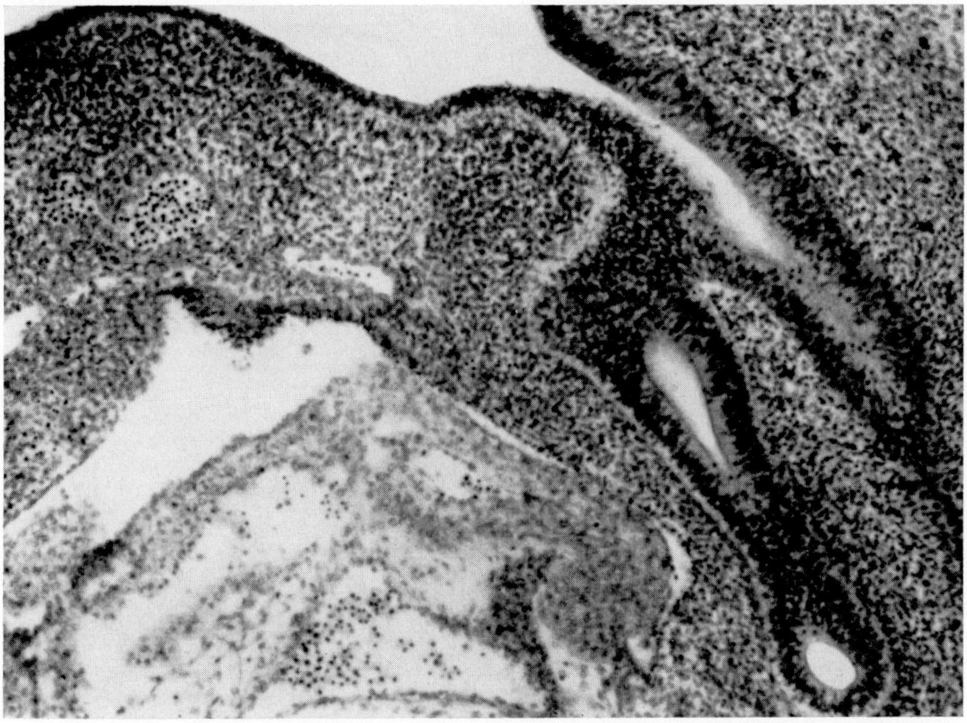

Fig. 1. At Stage 14, Carnegie collection specimen 8308 (5.85 mm) saggital section near the median plane. Respiratory tube, ventral to the digestive canal in the site of the inlet of the embryonic larynx is ascertainable. The lamina and epithelial plate extending ventrally from the laryngeal epithelium in the median plane, are still quite small.

by Tucker and O'Rahilly[16] and O'Rahilly and Tucker.[17] As noted by Walander,[18] "the primordium of the laryngeal epithelium is to be sought in the epithelial lamina." The latter has been identified as first appearing in the 14th stage[17] (ca 5-7 mm – ca 32 days), as a cellular mass in the median plane between the arytenoid swelling (Fig. 1).

At Stage 16 the epithelial lamina is present in relationship to the vestibulotracheal and pharyngotracheal canals which are variable in patency.[16]

At the end of the embryonic period proper, Stage 23, most all structures of the larynx are present.[16] The epithelium of the larynx is rudimentary in form. Stratified, somewhat cuboidal cells are present but without cilia. No glandular development is seen.[7,15] The mucosa of the epiglottis is multicellular in depth and the laryngeal surface of the epiglottis is interestingly convoluted. The glottis still shows varying degrees of patency.

In the third month of prenatal development, ciliated cells, and vibratile cilia appear for the first time (47/60 mm) in the fetus,[12] but are sparse, quite short in length, and are on the epithelium of ventricular bands and within the ventricle (Fig. 2). The epithelium is 3-4 cells thick and columnar in structure.[12] The true cord, on its medial aspect, has only a single columnar epithelial layer.[4] The glottis and infraglottic larynx is now patent.[19] Specimens reviewed were at 10 and 12 weeks. "Glandular buds" have been observed at the end of the third month.[12]

In the fourth month, cilia are present within the larynx and the esophagus,[20] as well as noted in the postcricoid larynx. In the fifth month, glandular development is clearly defined,[12,15] and stratified, cylindrical, ciliated epithelium covers the ventricular bands.

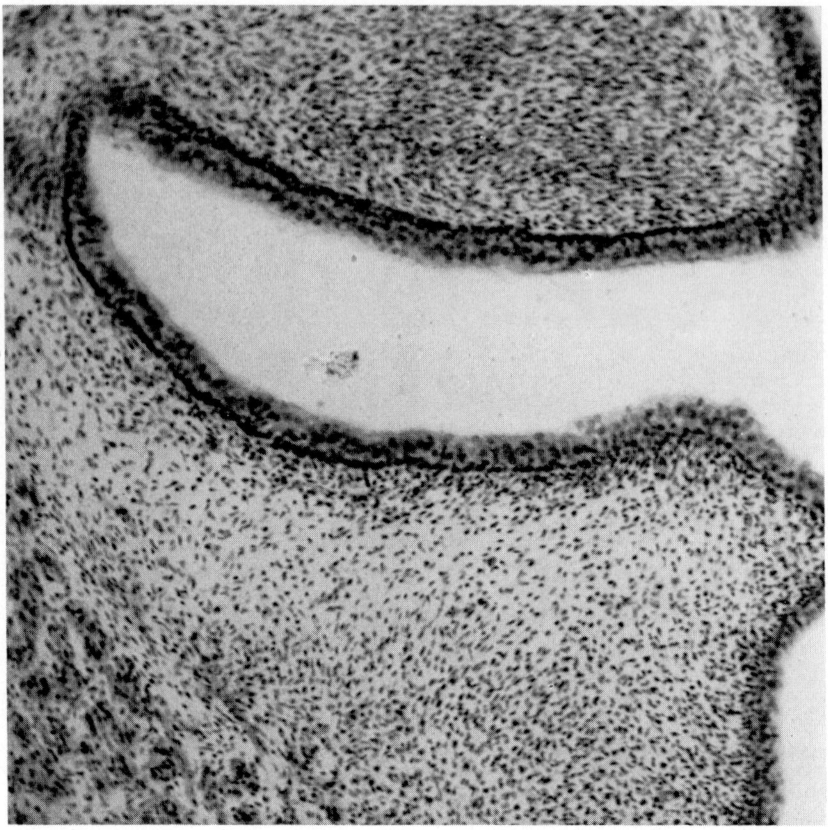

Fig. 2. Fetal specimen, 12 weeks, Laryngeal Institute Acquisition (LIA) 8, coronal section. The glottis and infraglottic larynx are now patent. High power view of the laryngeal ventricle, ventricular band and true vocal cord. Cilia are sparse and short in length. They are present on the epithelial cells of the ventricular bands and within the ventricle.

From six months to term there is little change in the characteristics of the laryngeal epithelium. The stratified squamous epithelium of the vocal cords diminishes in height with desquamation.

At 40-42 weeks, term, mature, stratified, squamous epithelium is present on the true cord as well as on the ventricular band, within the medial aspect of the ventricle and on the medial laryngeal surface of the epiglottis (Fig. 3). Well-ciliated respiratory epithelium is seen on the laryngeal surface of the epiglottis, in the ventricle, the infraglottic larynx and trachea.

At three months postnatal, the squamous epithelial elements of the larynx, ventricular band and true cord are appreciably more mature in characteristics. Again, little growth change is noted epithelially other than in mass density of ciliated cells between the epithelium of the 3-month-old and that of the adult.[21]

A special note should be made to areas of cell transition. Classically laryngeal cellular transition is most prominent on the superior surface of the true vocal cord within the ventricle and on the under surface of the true cord, the infraglottic larynx.[7,12] Cellular transition appears to be rather abrupt in two distinct cellular types, that of stratified squamous epithelium and columnar ciliated epithelium,[22] as observed by standard light microscopy (Figs. 4, 5).

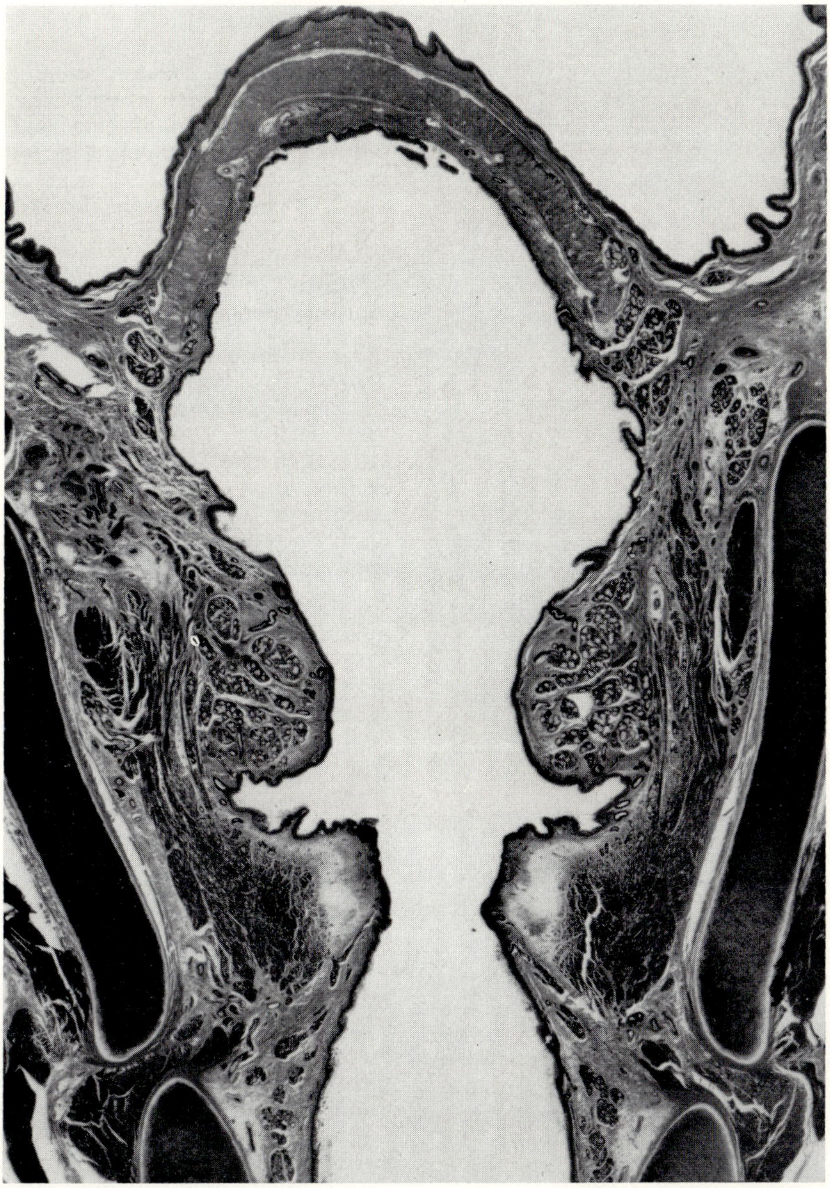

Fig. 3. Term, 40 weeks, specimen LIA 52, coronal section. Stratified squamous epithelium is present on the true cord and ventricular band. Deep glandular structures are submucosally present.

LARYNGEAL TOPOGRAPHICAL CELLULAR CONSIDERATIONS — PART B

Scanning Electron Microscopy and Transmission Electron Microscopy Considerations of Laryngeal Epithelium. Published reviews of the normal electron microscopic anatomy of the human larynx have been limited.[23,24] This is in contrast to the repeated detailed studies of the epithelium of the trachea.[25-27] Previous descriptions of transmission electron microscopy and standard light microscopy have been reported but without scanning correlation of the same

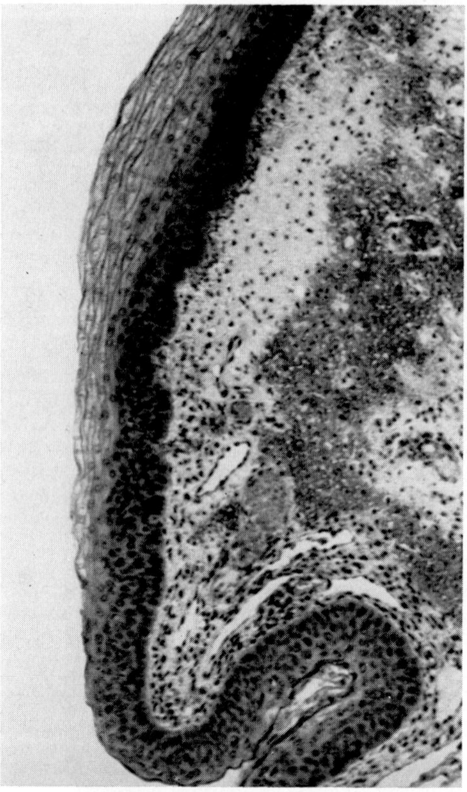

Fig. 4. Postnatal specimen, 3 months, coronal section, LIA 29. Epithelial surfaces of the larynx are appreciably more mature in character. Shown is mature stratified squamous nonkeratinized epithelium of the true vocal cord.

larynx. Further, prior scanning electron microscopy studies have only been reported in the cancerous larynx and again without transmission electron microscopy, standard light microscopy correlation,[28] or indication of discrete cellular topographical distribution.

No reference has been made to the functional aspects of the mucociliary apparatus as suggested by anatomical cellular distribution.[29] The established function of the ciliated cell is relative to secretory activity and transport. The secretory activity of the respiratory tract is a constantly changing dynamic phenomenon. The mucus producing cell (goblet cell) produces to protect the entire epithelium by providing a physiologic base, the surface mucus blanket (the gel phase).[30]

The general pattern of the respiratory epithelium is a functional integration of pseudostratified, ciliated, columnar epithelial cells together with the goblet cell, the mucus producing and serous producing secretory cell. The latter provides a (lipid water) secretion (sol phase) which is mechanically supportive, much as an interciliary lubricant to ciliary activity. These cells are closely related to the brush border cell and multifunctional basal cell.

The ultrastructure of cilia and ciliogenesis has been well documented.[31] Reference will only be made to the fact that respiratory cilia is made up of rather constant 9-segmental, plus 2, microtubular couples or pairs. These microtubules are synthesized within the basal body as polypeptide tubular protein structures.[32]

Ciliary motion is a highly dynamic, multidirectional, two-stage phenomenon. These "hair-like" organelles move liquids over fixed cells. "The cilia beat when the microtubules, powered by adenosine triphosphate (ATP), slide past one another."[33]

The neural elements of respiratory epithelium and cilia are sensory, autonomic to mucus production and secretion, and respond to various stimuli, temperature, bacterial activity, and antigens, *etc.*

Objectives. This study relates specifically to three adult human specimens. Electron microscopic observations were made to ascertain the general characteristics of different epithelia related to the topographical locations of the epithelial territories within the larynx. Also, particular attention was directed towards delineation of the transitional zones from one type of epithelium to another. In addition, the adult laryngeal epithelia was compared with a neonatal subject at corresponding levels of organ section (Table II).

Method. The classic pathology technique of splitting the cricoid lamina and opening the larynx from its posterior (dorsal) aspect, creates a pattern of symmetrical laryngeal halves. This symmetry makes possible a controlled com-

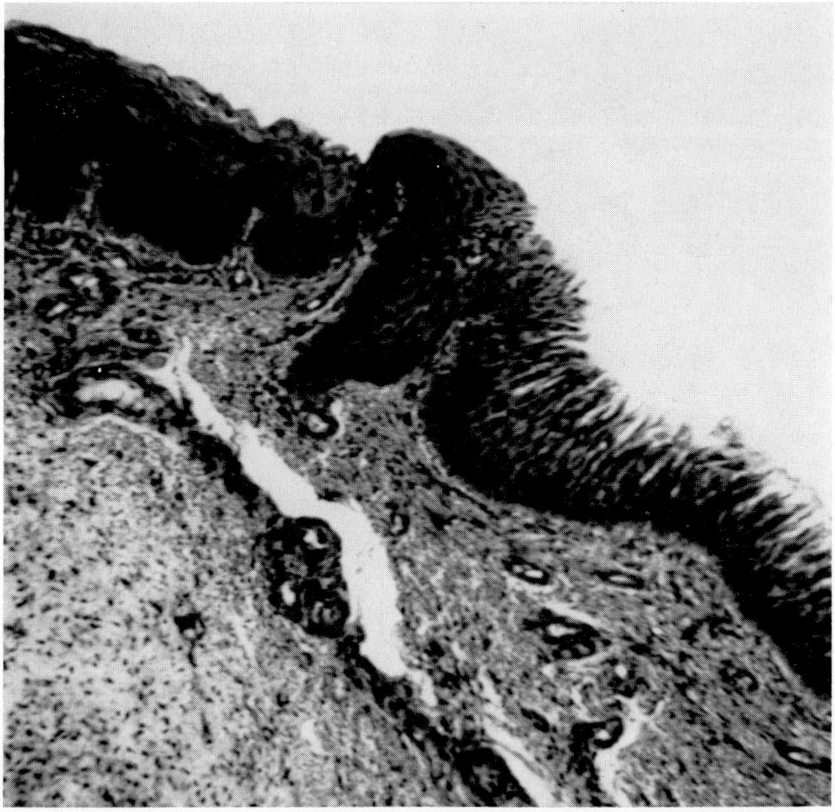

Fig. 5. Specimen same as in Figure 4, LIA 29. Transition of the squamous epithelium to pseudostratified columnar epithelium is illustrated.

parison of one side to the other by varying histological techniques.

Accordingly, the adult male larynx was studied by standard light microscopy, scanning electron microscopy and transmission electron microscopy. The adult female larynx was studied by scanning electron microscopy and transmission electron microscopy. The infant larynx was studied by scanning electron microscopy and transmission electron microscopy.

Figure 6 illustrates, in saggital section, the ipsilateral study pattern. Coding represents the following:

1. lingual surface of the epiglottis (ventral)

2. laryngeal surface of epiglottis (dorsal)

TABLE II

ELECTRON MICROSCOPY ANATOMICAL MATERIAL

Hahnemann Georgetown Specimen	*Age*	*Sex*	*Standard Light Microscopy*	*Scanning Electron Microscopy*	*Transmission Electron Microscopy*
I	73	M	+	+	+
II	51	F	0	+	+
III	60	M	0	+	+
IV	New Born	F	+	+	+

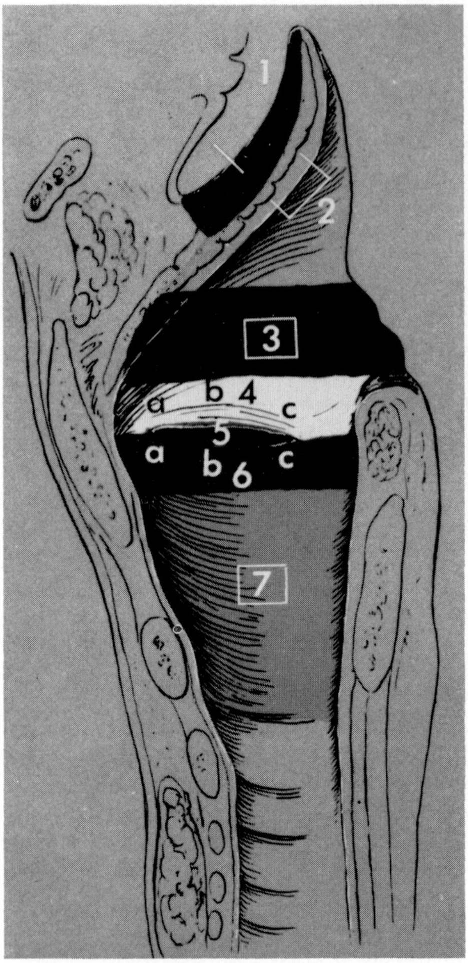

Fig. 6. Sagittal section of larynx, illustrating the ipsilateral study pattern. Coding represents the following: (1) lingual surface of the epiglottis (ventral); (2) laryngeal surface of epiglottis (dorsal); (3) aryepiglottis fold — vestibule; (4) ventricular band — a, anterior; b, mid; c, posterior; (5) ventricle; (6) true vocal cord — a, anterior; b, mid; c, posterior; (7) subglottic larynx.

3. aryepiglottic fold – vestibule

4. ventricular band – a, anterior; b, mid; c, posterior

5. ventricle

6. true vocal cord – a, anterior; b, mid; c, posterior

7. subglottic larynx

In addition, Figure 7 shows a wedge section (a) of the adult larynx which permitted study of the intact anterior commissure by scanning electron microscopy. Resulting mirror sections, (b) and (c), were then available for comparative transmission electron microscopy and standard light microscopy. Specifically, the infant larynx was sectioned in a frontolateral aspect, Figure 7, permitting scanning electron microscopy of the greatest portion, including the anterior commissure (a′), with transmission electron microscopy study of the remaining specimen. Areas of the adult pyriform sinus and postcricoid larynx were also surveyed by scanning electron microscopy.

Specimens were carefully screened for minimal trauma. All cases of endotracheal intubation and manipulation were excluded. Further, no tissue with gross mucosal disease, such as leukoplakia, hyperkeratosis or carcinoma were included. The object was to establish as close as possible a description of the norm and not the pathological. Specimens were secured with minimal postmortem delay.

Observations. The lingual surface of the epiglottis, (Figs. 6, 8) and the adital level of the larynx, are lined with stratified squamous epithelium. The cells of this epithelium, especially those located towards the basal lamina, are associated with the neighboring cells with junctional complexes. In many locations, the adjacent cells are interlocked by extensive trilaminar plasmalemmal foldings. These specializations of the epithelial cells are less pronounced towards the surface, where the cells flatten and lose their typical intracellular substructure. Scanning observations identify many cells that seem to be in different phases of desquamation. Excretory ducts of the submucosal glands may open at all levels within this epithelium.

The laryngeal surface of the epiglottis, Figure 6 (2), shows another variety of epithelium that is uniformly covered by a columnar-appearing cell. It is interesting to note that the latter cells are relatively free at their apices, without obvious junctional complexes between cells. The profile view of this epitheli-

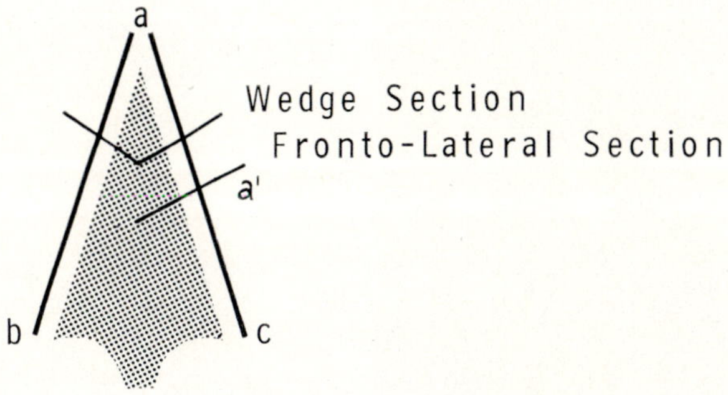

Fig. 7. Wedge section of the adult human larynx (a); comparative mirror images of the true vocal cord (b, c); frontolateral section of the infant human larynx (a′).

um demonstrates a stratified character. It is apparent that these cells, starting from the basal lamina, are interlocked with the adjacent cells by numerous plasmalemmal projections. In addition, a columnar shape of the most superficial layer of cells is clearly demonstrated.

The lower vestibule is lined by a heavily ciliated epithelium, Figure 6 (3), with possibly other cell types of nonciliated and/or goblet-like cell type variety dispersed throughout. On an average the length of cilia at this level measures approximately 4 mμ. Nonciliated columnar cells of this epithelium are presumably of the same variety as

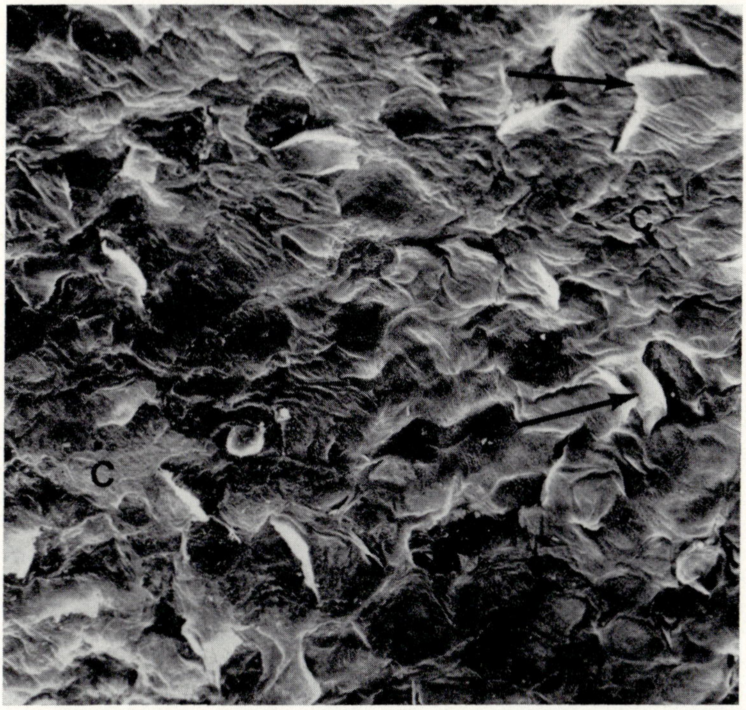

Fig. 8. The surface of the stratified squamous epithelium characteristic of territories 1 and 2 is demonstrated. Some cells (C) of the superficial layer are flat and presumably adhere tightly to the underlying cells. Many other cells (arrows) are fixed at different stages of desquamation. Tissue was fixed in aldehydes, dehydrated, dried by critical point method and coated with a 200 Å thick layer of gold palladium. (X300)

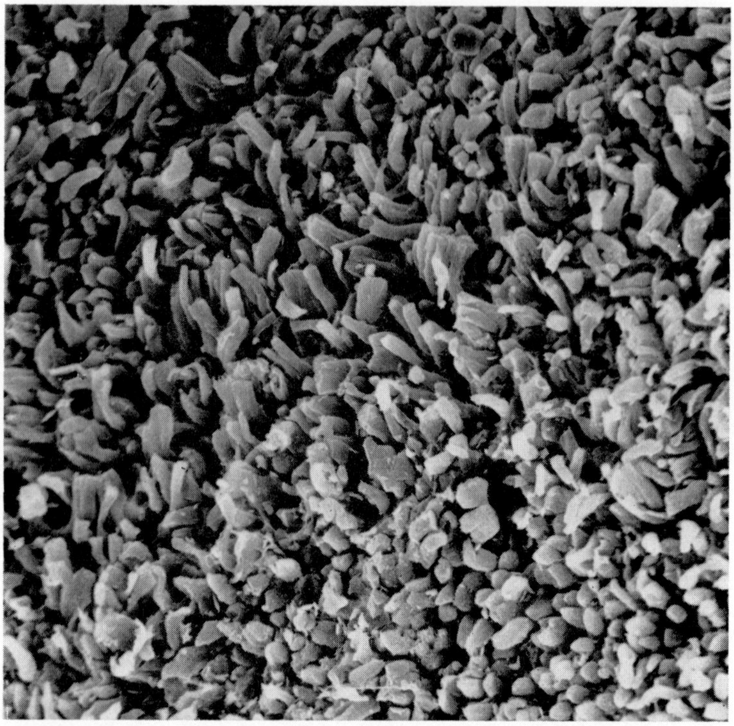

Fig. 9. The surface of the stratified nonsquamous epithelium characteristic of territory 3 is shown in this illustration. The surface cells appear cuboidal to columnar in shape, and their apices present no characteristic junctional complexes with the neighboring cells. Tissue was fixed with aldehydes, dehydrated, dried by critical point method and coated with a 200 Å thick layer of gold palladium. (X300)

those found at the transitional level between the ciliated and nonciliated cells of the ventricular band, Figure 9.

The anterior part of the ventricular band, Figure 7 (4) a,b,c shows an abrupt transition from the stratified squamous epithelium of the vestibule to a columnar, presumably stratified epithelium. However, in addition to squamous and columnar cells, occasional ciliated cells and cells with villus-like projections, or short cilia, are also observed on the surface. One particular cell type incorporated in this epithelium has the surface characteristics (polygonal apical surface, tight junctions with neighboring cells, short apical projections) resembling a goblet cell elsewhere in the respiratory system. The transmission microscopy of these cells indeed reveals in the apical cytoplasm numerous secretory granules. The substructure of the latter (fibrillar network embedded in an electron-translucent matrix) suggests a long-chain molecule of a mucosubstance-like composition. The remaining segment of the vestibular fold shows a more or less typical epithelium of the respiratory tract. This is pseudostratified columnar ciliated epithelium.

The ventricular epithelium, Figure 6 (5), is of a respiratory variety. However, it abruptly undergoes a transition towards the level of the vocal cord. This transition is characterized by a modification of the ciliary apparatus. Where the individual cilium becomes indistinguishable, Figure 10, the apical portion of these columnar cells appears to be covered by an amorphous layer of material which we have as yet no criteria to characterize on the basis of its surface properties. Transmission electron microscopy views should enable one to detect whether or not the amorphous material represents a deposit over the cells or a

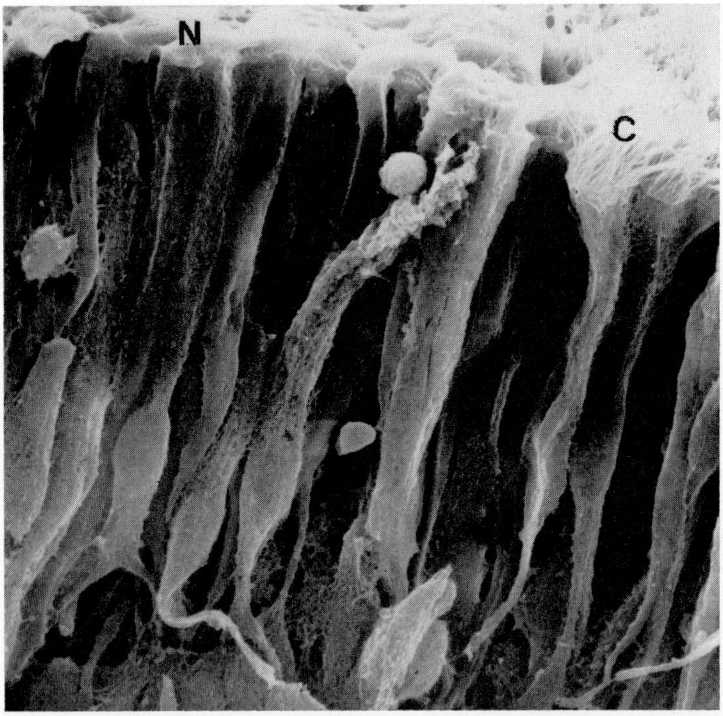

Fig. 10. This is a lateral aspect of transitional cells found between the ciliated epithelium (C) of the laryngeal ventricle and the nonciliated epithelium (N) of the ventricular surface of vocal cord. All cells are columnar in shape with a basal enlargement containing the nucleus. The apical parts of these cells are typically narrow and they represent characteristic junctional complexes with neighboring cells. The luminal surface of these cells is covered with either cilia or an amorphous appearing and electron-dense material respectively, in the ventricle and on the vocal cord. Tissue was fixed with aldehydes, dehydrated, dried by critical point method and coated with a 200 Å thick layer of gold palladium. (X1200)

part of apical projections. Light microscopy sections, however, indicate that the general structure of cells along the transitional zone is the same, despite an abrupt disappearance of cilia from the ventricle towards the vocal cord.

The anterior commissure, Figure 7, is lined by a modified type of ciliated cells. The main property of these cells is a uniform surface structure of ciliary apparatus consisting of slender and short individual projections. The anterior part of the vocal cord is covered with a squamous epithelium, Figure 11. The cells are polygonal in shape and measure to 22 mμ in radius. While some cells display a flat and smooth surface, others are covered with small or medium-size villus projections. In the infolded portions of the middle segment of the cord, in addition to the squamous cells, the apices of apparently some other cells or projections of squamous cells are observed. The latter variety shows a lower electron-opacity and surface characteristics resembling a villus coat. A similar relation between the squamous and protruding cells is found on the posterior segment of the vocal cord. Here, however, the predominate location of the protruding cells within the infoldings of the cord is not obvious. These cells are rather randomly distributed among the squamous cell territories.

The subglottic part, Figure 6 (7), of the larynx is lined by a typical ciliated epithelium. In this epithelium the cells other than the ciliated, *e.g.*, nonciliated cuboidal, secretory, brush border, *etc*, are rare.

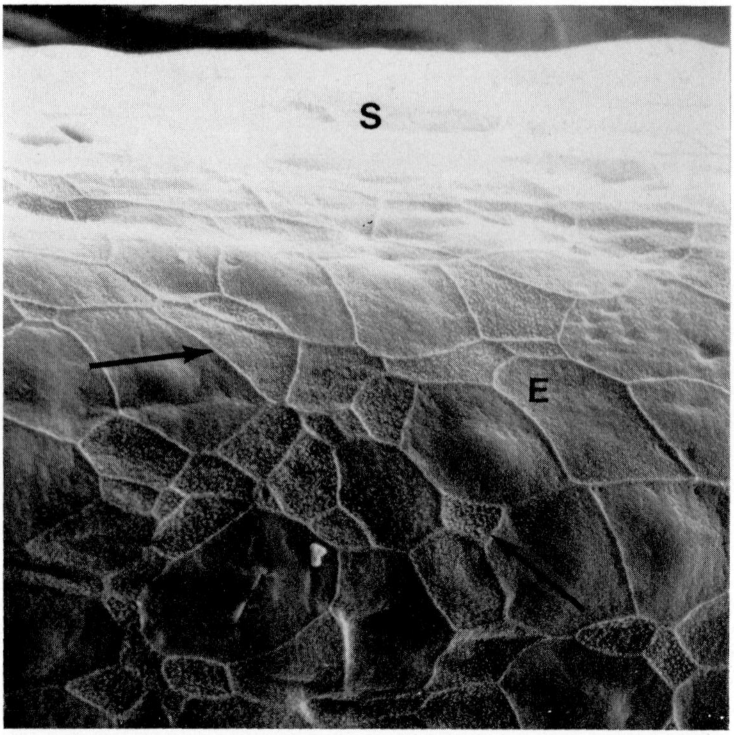

Fig. 11. The surface of the edge (E) and the subglottic aspect (S) of the anterior third of the vocal cord is demonstrated. Although in this instance the superficial cells appear as flat and squamous, the junctional complexes between the neighboring cells (arrows) are evident as prominent ridges. Some of these cells are covered by short projections, or microvilli. Tissue was fixed with aldehydes, dehydrated, dried by critical point method and coated with a 200 Å thick layer of gold palladium. (X900)

The epithelium of neonatal larynx, in general terms, resembles that described for the adult. The most striking difference is in the distribution of ciliated territories. The infantile epithelium is more restricted in its ciliary area. Also in the neonate the vestibule and the adjacent cords show much less of the ciliated epithelium. Along the vocal cords, the stratified squamous epithelium is modified as the ventricle is approached to become columnar rather than ciliated, as in the adult subjects. Further, the transition of stratified squamous epithelium from the vocal cord to the ciliated epithelium of the subglottic region takes place at a more inferior level than in the adult. Although the length of cilia measures ca 4 mμ, these organelles are thinner in the neonatal epithelium in comparison to the adult cells.

CORRELATION — PARTS A AND B

The topographical distribution of the observed cellular elements of laryngeal epithelium are as follows. In the adult, the ciliated epithelium covers the lower vestibule, part of the vestibular cord, ventricle, and the entire subglottic space immediately from the sharp margin of the inferior surface of the vocal cord. The differences in the child are most strikingly seen in the distribution of ciliated territories, which are more restricted than in the adult.

The transition areas, particularly within the ventricle and in the subglottic larynx, are identified and need further study.

The classically accepted description by standard light microscopy of a sharp demarcation between pseudostratified columnar epithelium to squamous epithelium is not upheld by scanning electron microscopy and transmission electron microscopy. Current observations suggest a more gradual graduation of cellular structure with loss of cilia. The continuity and maintenance of a stratified columnar epithelial cell is recognized to then evolve ultimately into a truly stratified squamous cellular structure.

REFERENCES

1. Stricker S: *Manual of Human and Comparative Histology*. H Power (trans), London, New Sydenham Society, 1872, p 38

2. Epstein SS: A stripping technique for the examination of the total epithelial surface of the larynx. J Pathol Bacteriol 75:472-473, 1958

3. Tucker GF Jr: A histological method for the study of the spread within the larynx of carcinoma. Ann Otol Rhinol Laryngol 70: 910-921, 1961

4. Tucker GF Jr: The anatomy of laryngeal cancer. Can J Otolaryngol 3:413-431, 1974

5. Zilliacus W: Die Ausbreitung der verschiedenen Epithelarten im menschlichen Kehlkopfe und eine neue Methode, dieselbe festzustellen. Anat Anz 26:25-30, 1905

6. Stell PM, Gregory I, Watt J: Techniques for demonstrating the epithelial lining of the larynx. J Laryngol Otol 38:589-594, 1972

7. Hopp ES: The development of the epithelium of the larynx. Laryngoscope 65: 475-499, 1955

8. Kanthack AA: Studien uber die Histologie der Larynxschleimhaut. Arch Pathol Anat 118:137-147; 273-294; 326-342, 1889

9. Heymann R: Beitrage z kenntniss d epithels u d drusen d menschliches kehlkopfes im ges u krank zustande. Virchows Arch 118: 320-348, 1889

10. Frazer JE: The development of the larynx. J Anat Physiol (Paris) 44:156-191, 1910

11. Heymann J: Die Histologie der Schleimhaut des Kehlkopfes und der Luftrohre. Handb Laryngol Rhinol: 1:134-164, 1898

12. Soulie A, Bardier E: Recherches sur le developpement du larynx chez l'homme. J Anat Physiol (Paris) 43:137-240, 1907

13. Kallius E: Beitrage zur entwickelungsgeschichte des kehlkopfes. Anat 9:303-363, 1897

14. Shikinami J: Detailed form of the Wolffian body in human embryos of the first eight weeks. Contr Embryol Carneg Instn 18:46-61, 1926

15. Tucker JA, Tucker GF: Some aspects of fetal laryngeal development. Ann Otol Rhinol Laryngol 84:49-55, 1975

16. Tucker JA, O'Rahilly R: Observations on the embryology of the human larynx. Ann Otol Rhinol Laryngol 81:520-523, 1972

17. O'Rahilly R, Tucker JA: The early development of the larynx in staged human embryos. Part 1: Embryos of the first five weeks (to Stage 15). Ann Otol Rhinol Laryngol (Suppl 7) 82:3-27, 1973

18. Walander A: Prenatal development of the epithelial primordium of the larynx in the rat. Acta Anat, Suppl 13 (Suppl 2 ad vol 10): 1-140, 1950

19. Tucker GF, Smith HR: A histological demonstration of the development of laryngeal connective tissue compartments. Trans Am Acad Ophthalmol Otolaryngol 66:308-318, 1962

20. Patten BM: *Human Embryology*. New York, McGraw-Hill, 1968

21. Tucker GF: *Human Larynx Coronal Section Atlas*. Washington, DC, Armed Forces Institute of Pathology, 1971

22. Holliday JA: Light and electron microscopy of the epithelium of the human true vocal cord. Laryngoscope 81:1596-1601, 1971

23. Sugár J: An electron microscopic study of early invasive growth in human skin tumors and laryngeal carcinoma. Eur J Cancer 4:33-38, 1968

24. Sugár J, Faragó L: Ultrastructure of laryngeal precanceroses. Acta Otolaryngol (Stockh) 62:319-332, 1966

25. Rhodin J, Dalhamn T: Electron microscopy of the tracheal ciliated mucosa in rat. Z Zellforsch Mikroskip Anat 44:345-412, 1956

26. Hilding DA, Hilding AC: Ultrastructure of tracheal cilia and cells during regeneration. Ann Otol Rhinol Laryngol 75:281-294, 1966

27. Barber VC, Boyde A: Scanning electron microscopic studies of cilia. Z Zellforsch Mikrosk Anat 84:269-284, 1968

28. Biondi S, Biondi-Zappala M: Surface of laryngeal mucosa seen through the scanning electron microscope. Folia Phoniatr 26: 241-248, 1974

29. Friedmann I, Bird ES: Ciliary structure, ciliogenesis, microvilli. Electron microscopy of the mucosa of the upper respiratory tract. Laryngoscope 81:1852-1868, 1971

30. Dulfano MJ (ed): *Sputum; Fundamentals and Clinical Pathology*. Springfield, Ill, C C Thomas, 1973

31. Fawcett DW, Porter KR: A study of the fine structures of ciliated epithelia. J Morphol 94:221-281, 1954

32. Fawcett D: *The Cell.* Philadelphia, Pa, Saunders, 1966

33. Satir P: How cilia move. Sci Am 231 (4):44-52, 1974

REPRINTS — John A. Tucker, MD, Institute of Human Communications and Laryngology, Hahnemann Medical College and Hospital, 230 North Broad Street, Philadelphia, PA 19102.

FINE STRUCTURES OF THE NORMAL MUCOSA IN DEVELOPING RAT MIDDLE EAR

SHOICHI MAEDA, MD

GORO MOGI, MD MOTOW OH, MD

UBE, JAPAN

SUMMARY — Forty-two fetal and 90 developing young rats were studied electron microscopically to obtain a normal cellular distribution pattern of middle ear mucosa. The results showed that while ciliated columnar or cuboidal cells interspersed with secretory cells were predominantly distributed around the tympanic orifice and transitional zone, cuboidal or squamous nonciliated cells without secretory granules were numerous in the remaining part of the bulla. Development of ciliated cells started at the 17th or 18th fetal day, paralleling that of secretory cells. The number of ciliated and secretory cells increased rapidly after birth. Glands were not found in the osseous tube, tympanic orifice, or other portions of the middle ear cavity in fetal, newborn, or suckling rats, while they are abundant in the cartilaginous portion of the tube. The findings of this study indicate that both secretory and ciliated cells are normal components of middle ear mucosa although these cells are restricted to the tympanic orifice and transitional zone, and that the mucociliary defense system starts to develop during the fetal stage.

Little is known about the etiology and pathogenesis of chronic middle ear diseases, such as serous or mucoid otitis media, chronic otitis media and mastoiditis, and cholesteatosis. The establishment of the anatomical constitution of normal mucosa covering the middle ear cleft in animals and human beings will help to understand the etiopathogenesis of these disorders.

Formerly, it was believed that the lining membrane of the normal middle ear cavity is a flat nonfunctional endothelium-like membrane with no secretory activity.[1-4] In 1955, Friedmann[5] observed that a normal flat endothelium-like lining was converted into a columnar respiratory-type epithelium forming gland-like structures in guinea pig middle ears in which experimental otitis media had been induced. Senturia *et al*[6] demonstrated the progressive development of secretory glands in the middle ears of dogs following the production of middle ear effusions. Ojala[7] had previously made similar findings. These investigators considered that in the presence of mild inflammation, metaplasia of the endothelium-like middle ear epithelium into a pseudostratified columnar epithelium with secretory cells took place. However, Sadé,[8] after studying 80 temporal bones from patients without any otological diseases, found goblet cells and glands among or beneath the ciliated epithelium of the tympanic cavity. He considered the secretory cells to be a normal component of the mucosa lining the middle ear cavity and further demonstrated the presence of a mucociliary transportation system in the human middle ear.[9] In 1967, Lim *et al*[10] studied, using electron microscopy, the tympanic orifice of the Eustachian tube and middle ear mucosa in guinea pigs. They found that the mucosal layer of the middle ear adjacent to the tympanic orifice was characterized by the presence of a ciliated columnar epithelium and granulated secretory cells. Kawabata and Paparella[11] investigated the mucoperiosteal lining of the normal human middle ear cleft by electron microscopy. Although no goblet cells were found, it was shown that the epi-

From the Departments of Otolaryngology and Anatomy, Yamaguchi University School of Medicine, Ube, Japan.

thelium consisted of ciliated, nonciliated and basal cells as seen in the respiratory mucosa. Hentzer,[12] in his electron microscopic observation of normal human middle ear mucosae, demonstrated the existence of five types of cells in the epithelium. These were the nonciliated cell without secretory granules, the nonciliated cell with secretory granules, the ciliated cell, the intermediate cell and the basal cell. Results of many subsequent studies[13-20] have accumulated evidence indicating that the epithelium lining the middle ear cavity and Eustachian tube in both animals and humans is the respiratory type of mucosa. Moreover, recent immunologic studies[21-25] on middle ear effusions have confirmed this evidence from the viewpoint of immunochemistry. However, Tos and Bak-Pedersen,[26-29] in their studies on the middle ear epithelium and Eustachian tube in human beings, using the PAS-alcian blue whole mount method, suggested that the existence of glands or the increase of goblet cell density and distribution are the sequelae of previous pathological action upon the middle ear and Eustachian tube. This supposition conflicts with the assumption that the glands and goblet cells are normal components of middle ear mucosa.

This investigation was designed to determine the cellular distribution of the middle ear epithelium in fetal and suckling rats, to obtain a better understanding of the function of middle ear mucosa.

METHODS AND MATERIALS

A total of 90 healthy suckling rats and young rats (Sprague Dawley) ranging from one day postnatal to generative age, and of 42 fetal rats from 15 to 21 days fetal, were used. Sexually mature female rats were placed with males overnight. The next morning was designated day zero of a 21-day period of gestation. All animals were decapitated and their temporal bones were removed immediately. One third of them were prepared for scanning electron miscroscopy (SEM), one third for transmission electron microscopy (TEM) and the remainder for light microscopy (LM). Specimens with inflamed middle ear mucosa detected by stereomicroscopy were excluded from this investigation. Eighty-eight bullae were fixed in 4 C 2.5% cacodylate buffered glutaraldehyde for two to three hours, and opened with a horizontal section under a stereomicroscope. Then they were thoroughly rinsed in 4 C 0.1 M cacodylate buffer at pH 7.4 using a pipette before postfixation in 4 C 1% osmic acid for one to two hours. The specimens were dehydrated in graded ethanol from 50% to 100%, soaked in isoamyle acetate and dried using the CO_2 critical point drying method. The surface of the mucous membrane was coated with carbon and gold (200-300 Å) in a vacuum evaporator on a rotating stage, and examined with SEM* at an accelerating voltage of 10 kv and 10-20° of tilt angle.

For TEM observations, 88 bullae were prefixed in 4 C buffered 1% glutaraldehyde for two to three hours and postfixed in 4 C 1% osmic acid in cacodylate buffer for one to two hours after being rinsed in 4 C 0.1 cacodylate buffer. The mucous membrane was dissected from the bony wall while immersed in the glutaraldehyde solution. After fixation, the mucous membrane was dehydrated in graded alcohols, embedded in Epon 812®,** trimmed, and remounted for ultratome thin sectioning. The specimen was sectioned with a microtome,† stained both by uranyl acetate and lead citrate, and examined with a TEM.††

For light microscopic observations, the remainder were fixed in 10% neutral formalin and prepared with routine histological techniques. A series of sections were stained with H. and E., PAS, alcian blue and PAS-alcian blue.

RESULTS

Since the topography of the rat middle ear resembles that of the guinea pig, names for parts in the tympanic cavity were adopted as described by Lim *et al*[10] and Hussl and Lim.[30]

Cell Distribution Pattern

It was apparent from SEM and TEM observations that, as a rule, the epithelium of the bullae and Eustachian tube in all postnatal rats and 21 day-fetal rats, was composed of four different types of cells: these were nonciliated cells without secretory granules, nonciliated cells with secretory granules, ciliated cells, and basal cells. The pattern of cell distribution in the middle

---

*Model JSM-S1 (SEM). JEOL Ltd., Tokyo, Japan.
**Shell Chemical Co., New York, N. Y.
†Model MT-1. Nissei Industrial Co., Tokyo, Japan.
††Model JEM 100B. JEOL Ltd., Tokyo, Japan.

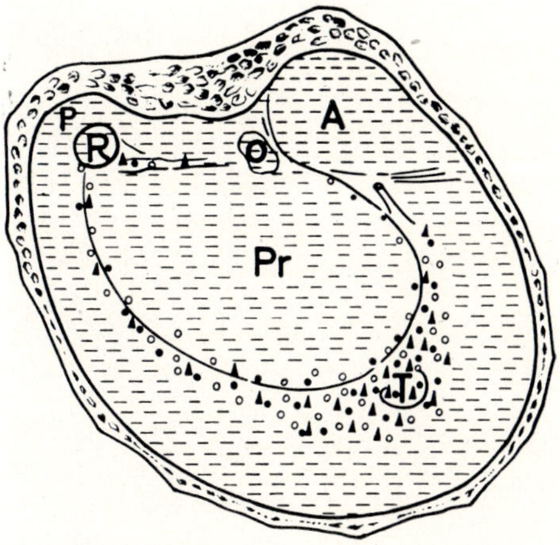

Fig. 1. Schematic drawing of a horizontal section of the bulla in suckling rats showing an average distribution of ciliated cells, nonciliated cells with secretory granules, nonciliated cells without secretory granules and squamous nonciliated cells. ▲ - Ciliated cells; ● - Cuboidal and columnar nonciliated cell with secretory granules; o - Cuboidal and columnar nonciliated cell without secretory granules; "–" - Squamous nonciliated cell; T - Tympanic orifice of the Eustachian tube; Pr - Promontory; A - Anterior recess; P - Posterior recess; R - Round window; O - Oval window.

ear mucosae of suckling rats was similar to that of adult rats. Figure 1 is a schematic picture summarizing the cellular distribution of the middle ear cavity in suckling rats. The epithelium of the tympanic orifice and transitional zone contains numerous ciliated cells and secretory cells (Fig. 2A). The number of ciliated and secretory cells diminished toward the distal margin of the transitional zone, where cuboidal cells become squamous (Fig. 2B). In the promontory, nonciliated cells with microvilli are abundant (Fig. 2C), while secretory cells are not present in this area except for in the marginal portion where only a few secretory cells are scattered throughout the nonciliated epithelium. As seen in Figure 2B, in the margin of the transitional zone, there are a few ciliated cells, which seem to be islands, surrounded by nonciliated cells. The surfaces of the nonciliated cells were flat in most cases, but were elevated near the ciliated cells. Cells with an elevated surface were perhaps secretory cells. The epithelium of the anterior and posterior recesses and the bulla proper consist of simple squamous cells with microvilli (Fig. 2D). Most cells of the mucosa covering the round window membrane and the adjacent area are nonciliated cells (Fig. 3A), but a few ciliated and secretory cells are observed in this portion in some cases (Fig. 3B). Cells seen in the ossicles and footplate are flat, having few microvilli (Fig. 3C). The mucosal epithelium of the eardrums consists of simple squamous cells with or without microvilli (Fig. 3D). The epithelium of the bony portion of the Eustachian tube was composed of pseudostratified columnar cells. The cells were ciliated, and secretory cells existed among these ciliated cells.

Glands were consistently found in the cartilaginous portion of the tube in all newborn and suckling rats, as well as adult rats, while their presence in the bony portion was very rare. Figure 4 exhibits glands from which a duct opens into the tubal lumen of the cartilaginous portion in a 12-day postnatal rat. These glandular cells were usually positive for PAS-alcian blue staining. The number of glands increased rapidly after birth. The gland formation seemed to spread from the pharyngeal orifice toward the tympanic orifice. However, no glands were detectable in the mucosa covering the tympanic orifice, transitional zone and other portions of the middle ear.

In fetal and newborn rats, both ciliated and secretory cells were rare in the mucosa of the tympanic orifice and transitional zone. Figure 5 shows pictures of SEM, TEM and PAS-alcian blue staining of the mucosa covering the transitional zone in a 21-day fetal rat. Although the cell distribution pattern was similar to that of suckling rats, secretory cells in the active phase were rarely observed, and only in the tympanic orifice and transitional zone. In Figure 5A, a mucous substance is seen on the surface of a nonciliated cell. Both ears from each of three rats aged

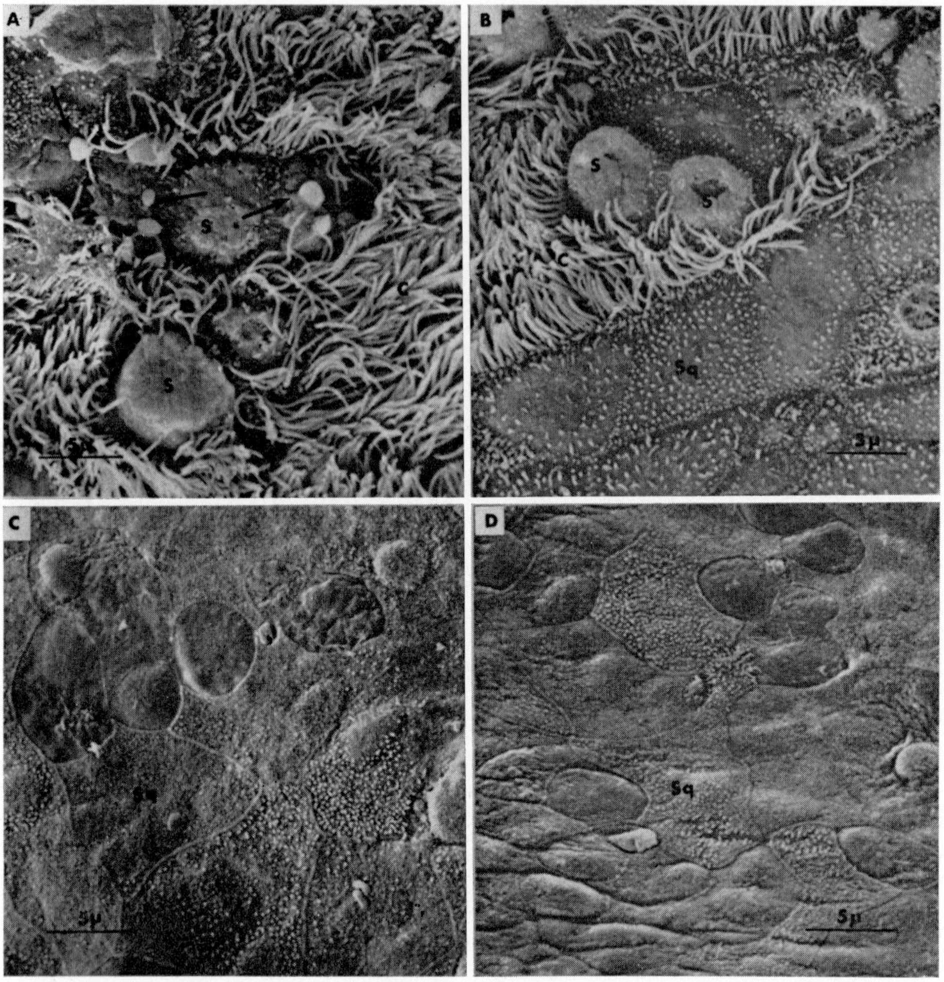

Fig. 2. Scanning electron micrograph of the luminal surface in 5-day postnatal rats. A) Transitional zone. There are numerous ciliated (C) and scattered secretory cells (S) which are protruded. Arrows indicate secretory extrusions with expanded tips of microvilli. (X2200) B) The distal margin of the transitional zone. The number of secretory (S) and ciliated cells (C) diminishes. There are elevated nonciliated cells near the ciliated cells. (X2100) C) The mucous membrane of the promontory. Squamous nonciliated cells (Sq), some with numerous and some with few microvilli, are widespread in this area. (X2400) D) The anterior recess. The epithelium consists of squamous nonciliated cells (Sq). (X2400)

19, 20, and 21 days fetal were examined for glands by serial sections and PAS-alcian blue staining. A few glands were present only in the pharyngeal orifice and cartilaginous portion of the tube in specimens from 20 and 21 days fetal. However, these glandular cells were not stained with PAS-alcian blue.

Fifteen Days Fetal. Because of immature bullae in this stage, the surface preparation of the middle ear for SEM was not made. One litter was examined by TEM and LM. The epithelium covering the middle ear was mainly composed of a few cell layers of the squamous type, but cells near the tympanic orifice were cuboidal. As shown in Figure 6A, most cuboidal cells have a relatively large ovoid or round nucleus, a few mitochondria and rough-surfaced

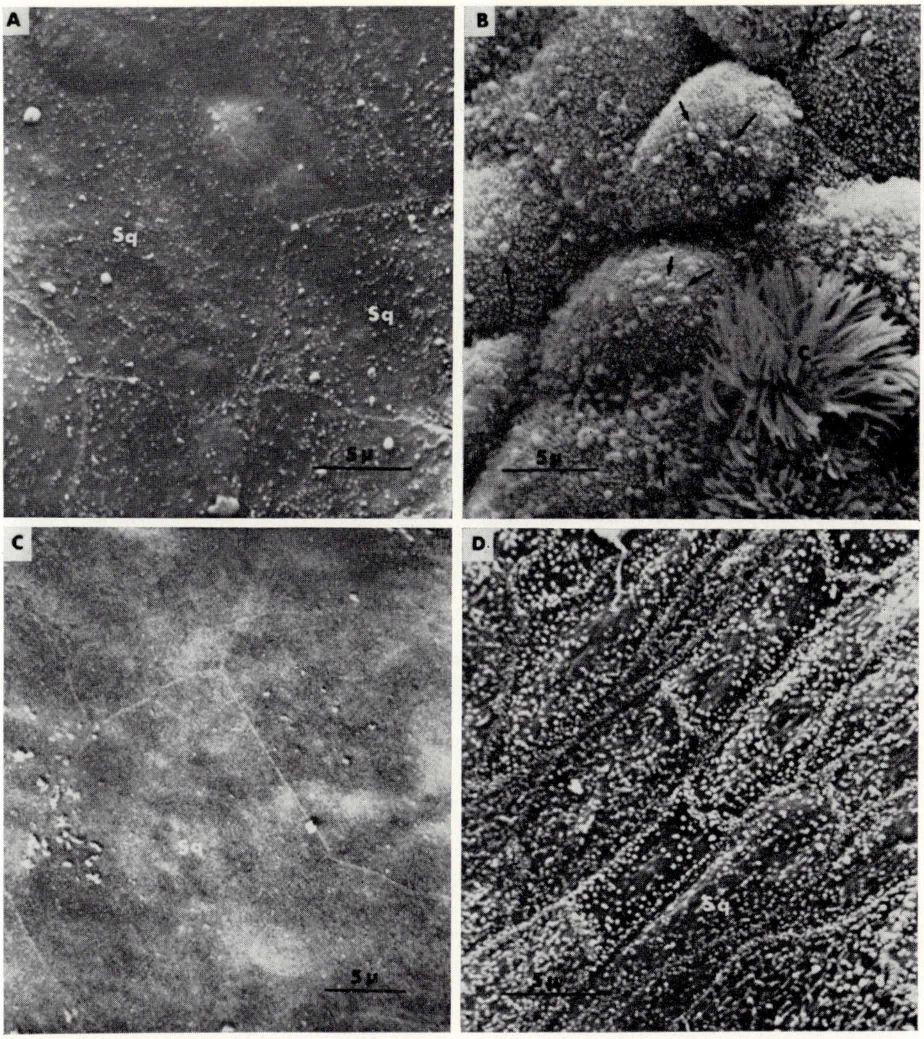

Fig. 3. A) The mucosal surface of round window in a 20-day postnatal rat. Most cells are squamous nonciliated (Sq), with or without microvilli. (X2400) B) The margin of the round window membrane with a few ciliated (C) and secretory cells (S) in a 13-day postnatal rat. Arrows show secretory extrusions with expanded tips of microvilli. (X2400) C) Scanning micrograph of the footplate in a 10-day postnatal rat, showing squamous nonciliated cells (Sq) without microvilli. (X2200) D) The mucosal surface of the eardrum in a 1-day postnatal rat. Squamous nonciliated cells (Sq) with numerous microvilli are seen. (X2800)

endoplasmic reticula (rER), and numerous clusters of ribonucleoprotein (RNP) granules scattered throughout the cytoplasm. The Golgi elements are small, and the apical plasma membrane is simple, having no microvilli or cilia. Cells with "primary cilia,"[31,32] as shown in Figure 6B, are rarely detected. The cell has several aggregations of glycogen particles and various sized mitochondria in the supranuclear portion of the cytoplasm. However, very rarely, some cuboidal cells possessed well-developed organelles, such as a well-developed Golgi complex with various sized small vesicles and cisternae, containing an amorphous substance, various sized mitochondria, elongated rER

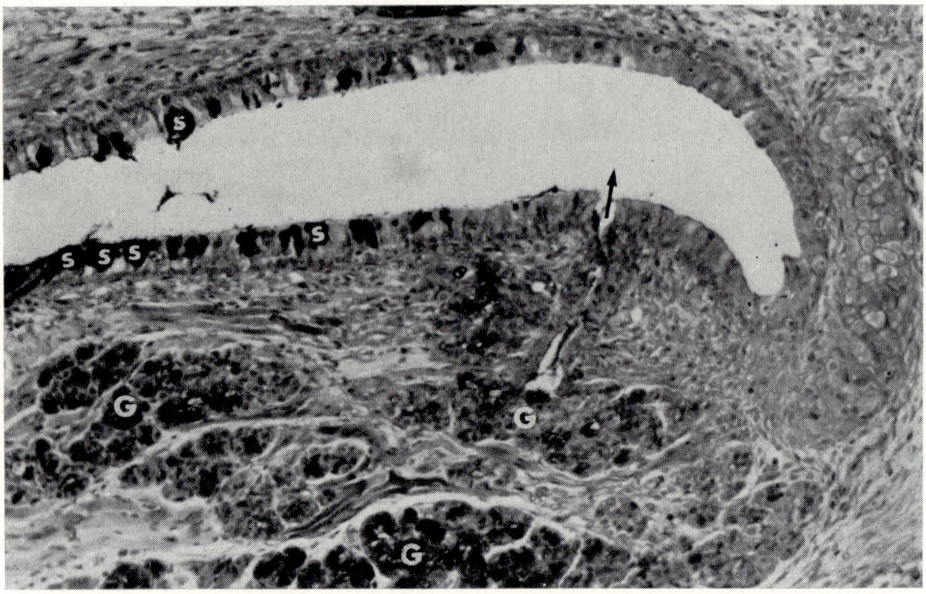

Fig. 4. Cross-sectional view of the cartilaginous portion of the Eustachian tube in a 12-day postnatal rat, showing PAS-AB positive secretory cells (S) and glands (G) from which a duct opens into the tubal lumen (arrow). (X300)

filled with an amorphous substance, numerous clusters of RNP granules scattered throughout the cytoplasm, and a centriole.

Sixteen Days Fetal. Four ears were examined by SEM. This observation revealed no cilia or secretory droplets. Most cells had no cilia, but had microvilli near the cell boundary. Hemispherical protrusions of the nuclei were observed (Fig. 7). Four ears were examined by TEM. The fine structure of the mucosal cells at this stage was very similar to that at 15 days fetal. However, the number of the cells with well-developed organelles increased slightly.

Seventeen Days Fetal. Both ears from each of two rats were examined by SEM and TEM. Most cells of the middle ear cavity were squamous, but cuboidal and columnar cells in the tympanic orifice and transitional zone were more common than in 15 and 16 days fetal. A few of these cuboidal and columnar cells apparently had immature cilia. Figure 8A,B,C shows a "primary cilium,"[31,32] demonstrating nine outer ciliary fibers and the absence of the central pair (9 + 0 arrangement). A few shorter cilia (0.5 to 2.0μ in length) in a 9 + 2 arrangement are visible adjacent to the primary cilium. Many basal bodies and mitochondria occur in the supranuclear portion of the cytoplasm in the same cell. A few immature secretory cells (probably goblet cells) were detected in the tympanic orifice. These cells had light secretory granules which were partially enclosed by a fine limiting membrane and partially fused together in the apical portion of the cytoplasm. These secretory granules were surrounded by elongated rER which contained amorphous substances, and numerous clusters of free RNP granules. A well-developed Golgi complex and a few mitochondria are arranged at the periphery of the cytoplasm (Fig. 8D). However, cells stained with PAS-alcian blue were not found in serial sections of the middle ear of a fetal rat obtained from the same litter as examined by SEM and TEM.

Eighteen Days Fetal. Both ears from each of two rats were observed by SEM and TEM. As seen in Figure 9A, in general, cilia become quite apparent

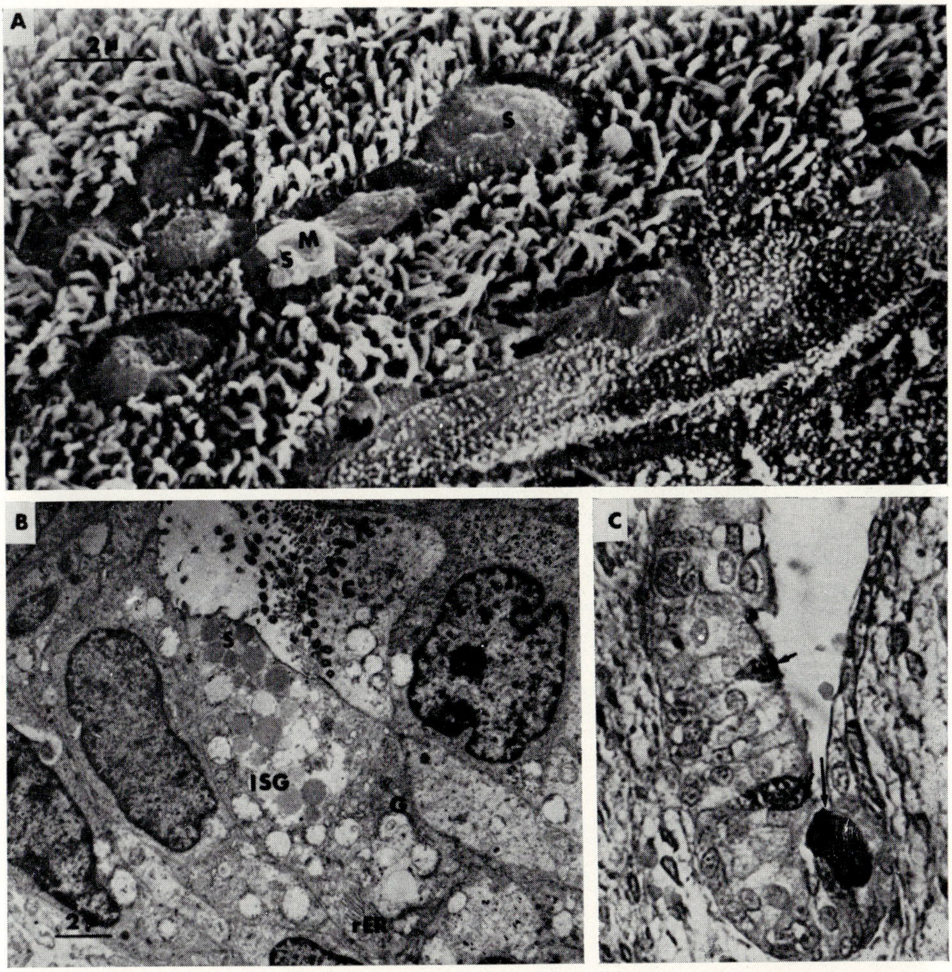

Fig. 5. A) Surface view of the mucous membrane of the transitional zone near the tympanic orifice in a 21-day fetal rat. There are many ciliated (C) and secretory (S), and a few squamous nonciliated cells (Sq). Surfaces of the secretory cells are granular and convex, covered with a mucous substance (M). The lower right corner is adjacent to the promontory. (X6800) B) Transmission electron micrograph of a similar region. Mature ciliated (C) and secretory cells (S) are visible. The secretory cells contain light secretory granules (lSG) which aggregate and partially fuse to each other in the supranuclear portion. They are surrounded by rough endoplasmic reticuli (rER), free ribosomes and mitochondria. A developed Golgi complex (G) is seen at the periphery of the cytoplasm. (X3800) C) A light microscopic photograph of a similar area showing cuboidal and columnar PAS-AB positive cells (arrow) interspersed with ciliated cells. (X1000)

among numerous microvilli, and the number of ciliated cells increased. However, the distribution of ciliated cells was restricted to the tympanic orifice and transitional zone. In the TEM observation, immature secretory cells were still rare. The organelles of both ciliated and immature secretory cells were well-developed, whereas those of nonciliated cells in 17 and 18-day fetal rats were still in a state of poor development.

Nineteen Days Fetal. Both ears from each of four rats were examined by SEM and TEM. Cells with short and immature cilia are more abundant than

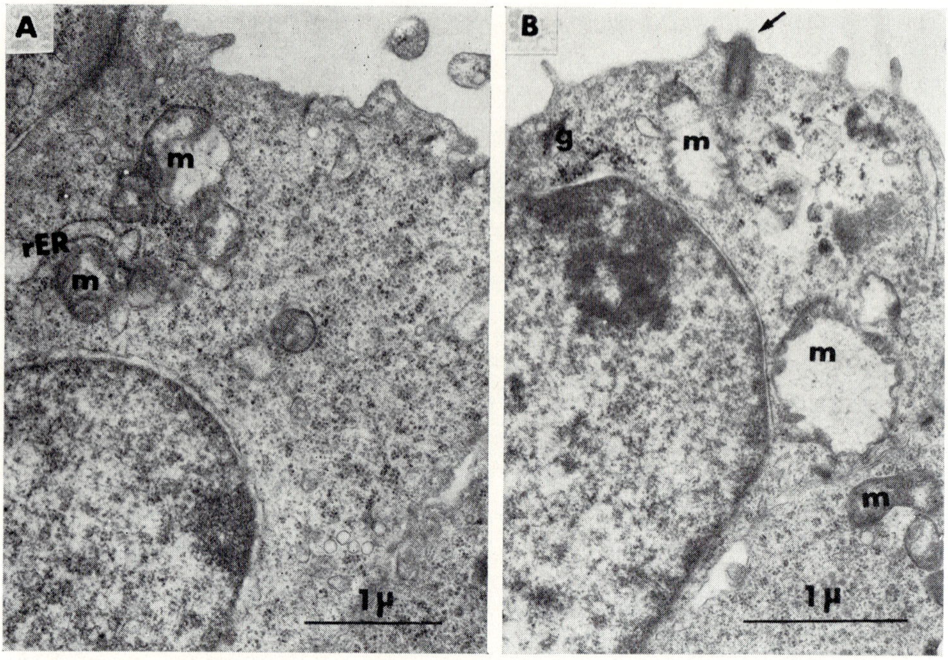

Fig. 6. A) Electron micrograph of the mucosa lining of the transitional zone in a 15-day fetal rat. A cuboidal nonciliated cell has only a few mitochondria (m), rER, and numerous clusters of free ribosomes. (X16,000) B) A cuboidal cell has a "primary cilium" (arrow), various sized mitochondria (m) and glycogen particles (g). (X19,000)

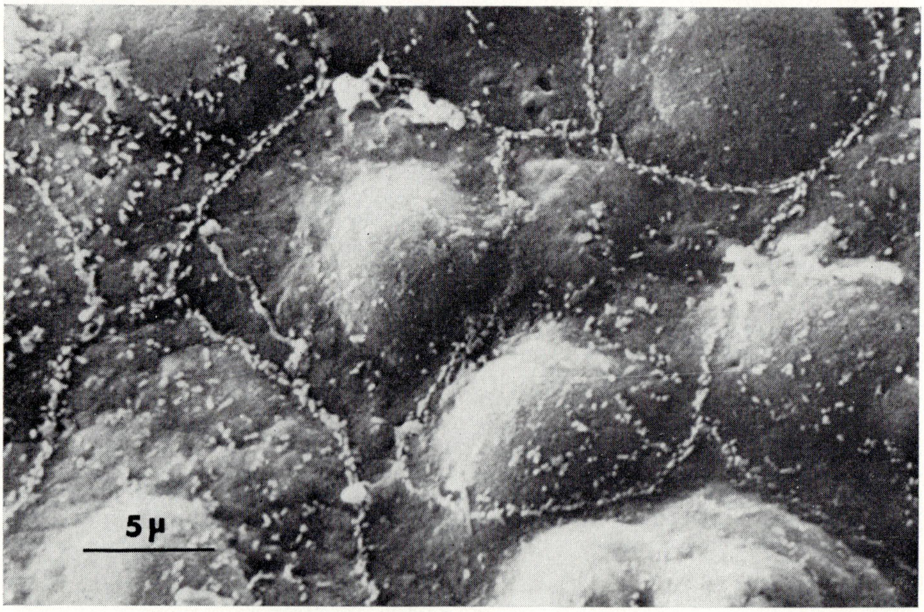

Fig. 7. Scanning micrograph of the transitional zone in a 16-day fetal rat. Nonciliated cells have hemispherical protrusions of the nuclei and a few microvilli. (X3000)

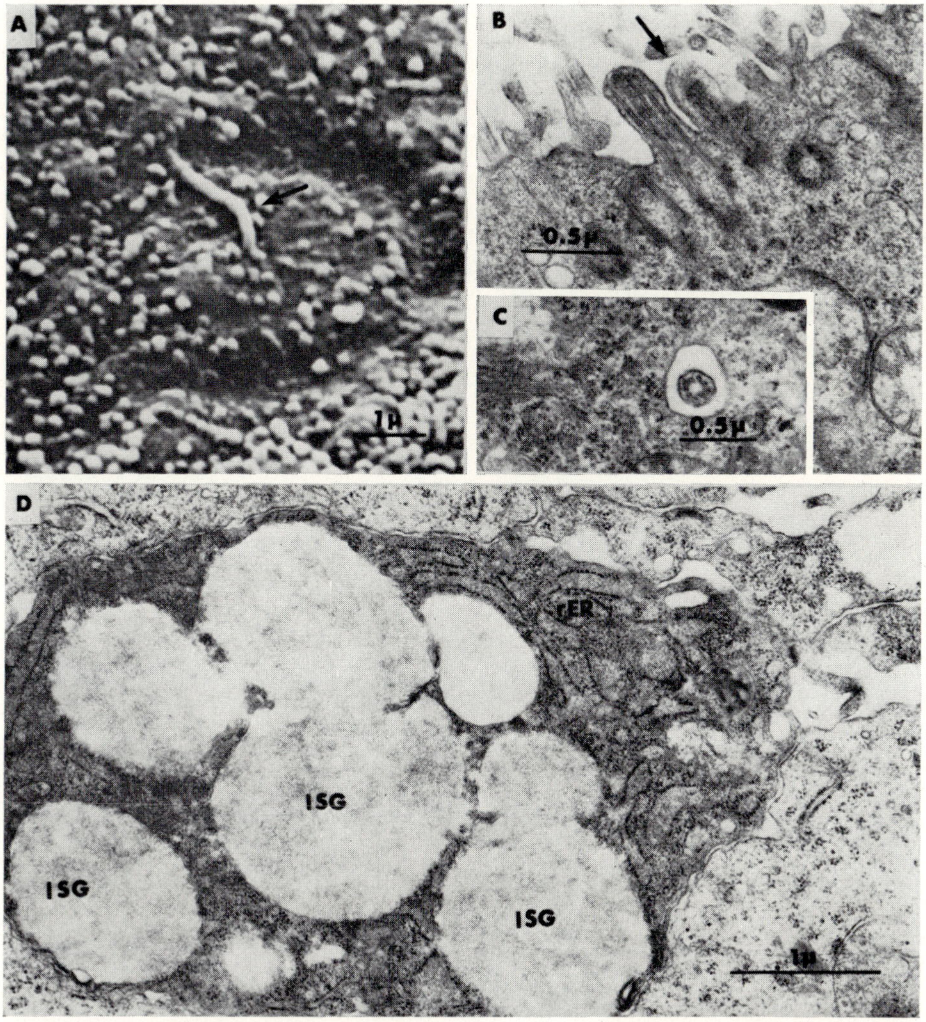

Fig. 8. A) SEM photograph of the transitional zone in a 17-day fetal rat exhibiting a primary cilium (arrow). (X9500) B) TEM photograph showing the vertical section of a primary cilium (arrow). A cilium with 9 + 2 arrangement is present adjacent to the primary cilium. (X26,000) C) Cross-section of a primary cilium. The peripheral doublet fibers are present, but the central pair is not developed. (X20,000) D) An immature secretory cell (probably a goblet cell) in the tympanic orifice of a 17-day fetal rat. The cell has a few light secretory granules (lSG) which are partially enclosed by a fine membrane and partially fused. These secretory granules are surrounded by abundant elongated rER which contain an amorphous substance, and by quite numerous clusters of free ribosomes. (X20,000)

in specimens from earlier stages (Fig. 9B). As seen in Figure 9C, most nonciliated cells contain many elongated rER containing amorphous substances and aggregations of glycogen particles adjacent to the various sized mitochondria at the supranuclear portion. Free ribosomes were profuse throughout the cytoplasm. The apical plasma membrane seemed to be coated with fine filamentous substance, and swollen tips of various sized microvilli were visible.

Twenty Days Fetal. Both ears from each of four rats were observed by SEM and TEM. Fully formed cilia with the characteristic nine peripheral

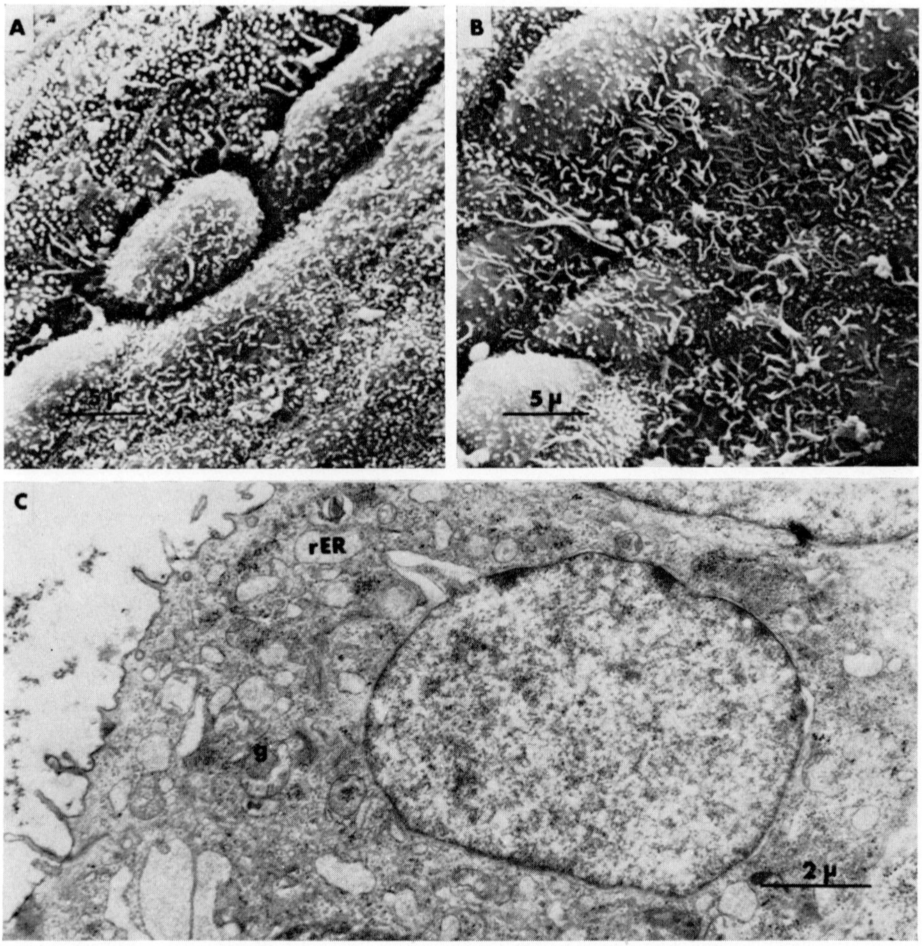

Fig. 9. A) Surface view of the transitional zone in an 18-day fetal rat. Many short and immature cilia are present among numerous microvilli. (X2200) B) Scanning view of the luminal surface of the transitional zone in a 19-day fetal rat. (X2200) C) TEM photograph of the cuboidal nonciliated cells in the transitional zone of a 19-day fetal rat. Many elongated rER, which contain amorphous substances, and aggregations of glycogen particles (g) adjacent to mitochondria are seen in the supranuclear portion. (X7000)

and two central filaments on the ciliated border of the epithelium were frequently observed at this stage (Fig. 10A). As seen in Figure 10B, there are many basal bodies in the light layers just beneath the free cell surface, and many various sized mitochondria in the adjacent area. As shown in Figure 10C,D, two types of secretory cells can be distinguished. One of them has light granules which are partially enclosed by fine limiting membranes and partially fused in the supranuclear portion. The other has dark granules, which are solitary and even in size, and many free ribosomes in the supranuclear portion. The former was found in the tympanic orifice and the latter in the transitional zone.

Twenty-one Days Fetal. Both ears from each of four rats were examined by SEM and TEM. Figure 5A shows the surface structure of the epithelium covering the tympanic orifice and transitional zone in a 21-day fetal rat. The epithelium consisted of many ciliated

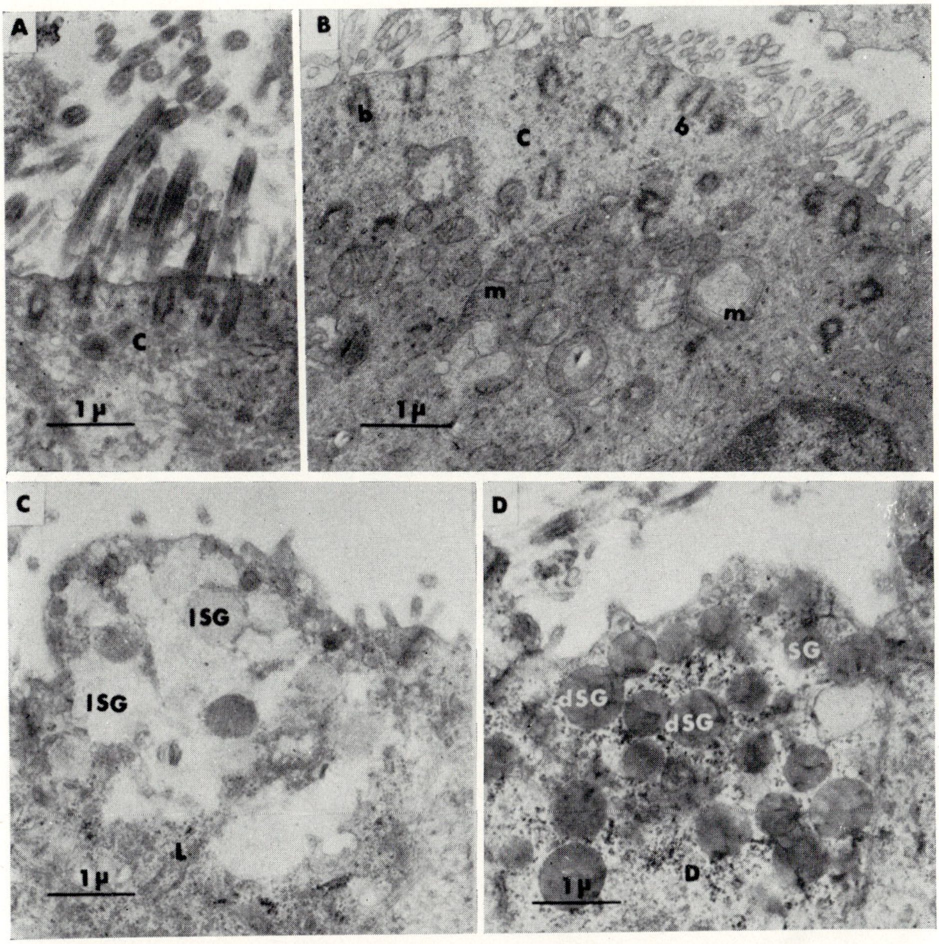

Fig. 10. TEM pictures of ciliated cells (C) and the secretory epithelium (S) of the transitional zone in 20-day fetal rats. A) Fully-formed cilia with the characteristic nine peripheral and two central filaments. (X12,000) B) Many basal bodies and various sized mitochondria (m) in the supranuclear portion of a ciliated cell. (X12,000) C) A light secretory cell (L). Light secretory granules (lSG) are partially enclosed by fine limiting membranes and partially fused to one another to form a large mass in the supranuclear portion. (X12,000) D) A dark secretory cell (D). Dark secretory granules (dSG) are solitary and even in size. (X12,000)

and nonciliated cells. However, as a rule, at this stage cilia were 0.7 to 2.5μ in length and 0.1 to 0.2μ in diameter. Nonciliated cells with convex and granular surfaces were scattered in the ciliated epithelium. A mucous droplet was seen on occasional nonciliated cells present in the tympanic orifice and transitional zone. Figure 5B is a TEM picture of an area similar to that of Figure 5A, showing light granulated secretory and ciliated cells. The light secretory granules were aggregated and partially fused in the supranuclear portion. They were surrounded by rER with amorphous substances, several mitochondria, and free ribosomes. A developed Golgi complex was found at the periphery of the cytoplasm. As observed in Figure 5C, some epithelial cells in this area were positive for PAS-alcian blue. These cells were stained blue with alcian blue and purplish magenta with PAS-alcian blue stain.

One Day Postnatal. Both ears from

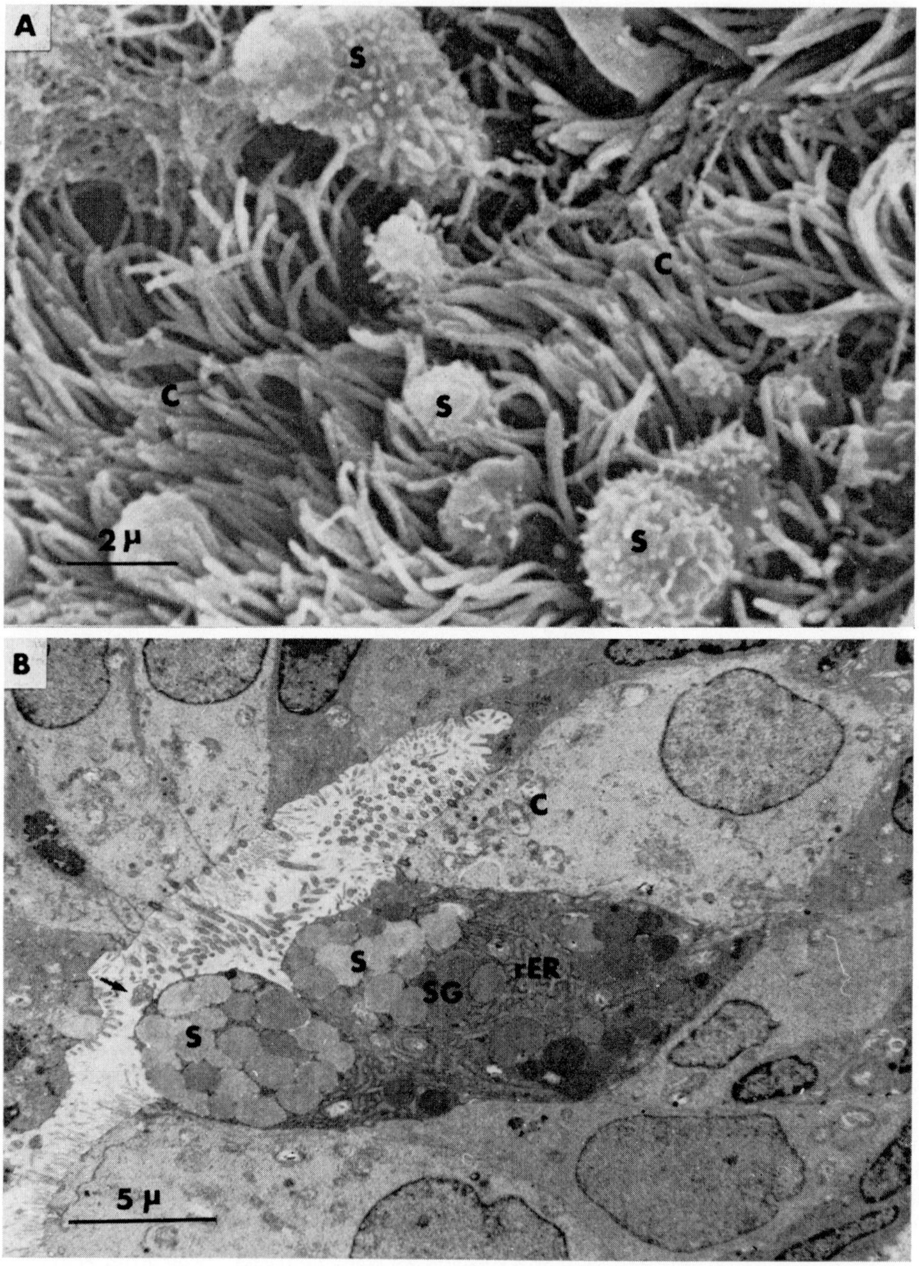

Fig. 11. Mucosal surface of the transitional zone in a 1-day postnatal. A) Many protruding secretory (S) and ciliated cells (C) are present. (X6000) B) Electron micrograph of the mucous membrane in a similar region. Secretory cells (S), which have secretory granules (SG) with varying electron densities, and numerous dilated rER which protrude among the ciliated cells (C). The arrow indicates a microapocrine projection. (X3200)

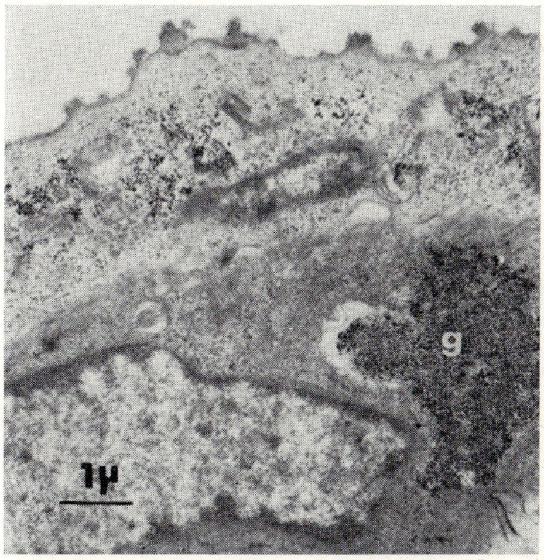

Fig. 12. The lining membrane of the promontory in a 2-day postnatal rat (Alcian blue staining for electron microscope). The surface of the mucosa is coated with filamentous substances increased in electron density by alcian blue. Aggregations of glycogen particles (g) are seen. (X11,000)

each of four rats were examined by SEM and TEM. Numerous protruding secretory cells are visible among many motile cilia in the mucosa of the tympanic orifice and transitional zone (Fig. 11A). As shown in Figure 11B, secretory cells are filled with light secretory granules which are partially fused in the apical portion. The limiting membranes of a few secretory granules were partially fused with the apical plasma membrane. They were surrounded by dilated rER with amorphous substances similar to those of the secretory granules. Occasionally, secretory cells which contained light and dark secretory granules were detectable. These granules differed in size and density. Ciliated cells had fully-formed motile cilia and many various sized mitochondria in the light layers beneath the free cell surface. The other nonciliated and basal cells contained aggregations of glycogen particles. The central portion of the promontory was covered with a simple squamous cell layer. On the cell surface of this area, there were seen numerous and various sized tips of microvilli which were coated with fine filamentous substances. Many glycogen aggregations were detected throughout the cytoplasm. However, no ciliated or granulated cells were found in this area. The number of PAS-alcian blue positive cells increased in the tympanic orifice and transitional zone at this stage.

Two Days Postnatal. Both ears from each of four rats were examined by SEM and TEM. Figure 12 shows the mucosa lining of the promontory which was treated with alcian blue for TEM. The surfaces of the microvilli were coated with fine filamentous substances whose electron density was increased by alcian blue staining. These substances seemed to be a mucopolysaccharide which is called the "glycocalyx."[33,34] Glycogen particles could be seen in squamous nonciliated cells and basal cells, but not in ciliated and secretory cells.

Six Days Postnatal (Eight Ears for SEM and TEM). Mature ciliated cells and secretory cells were abundant in the tympanic orifice and transitional zone. The distribution pattern was very similar to that of adult rats. In other words, the number of ciliated and secretory cells and PAS-alcian blue positive cells had increased to that observed in adult rats. It was also evident that the number and size of many ciliated cells were almost the same as in adult rats. These findings suggest that the development of middle ear mucosa of newborn rats is accomplished at this stage. Lengths of cilia were between 2.5 and 4.3μ. The diameters are about 0.1 to 0.2μ (Fig. 13A). Figure 13B shows protrusions of light secretory granules, with and without dark cores, to the luminal surface. While many secretory cells with light granules existed, dark granulated cells and mixed granulated cells were rarely found.

Modes of Secretion

The most common secretory cells present in the epithelium covering the middle ear cavity and Eustachian tube of fetal (at the terminal stage), newborn, suckling, and adult rats were those characterized by their distinct

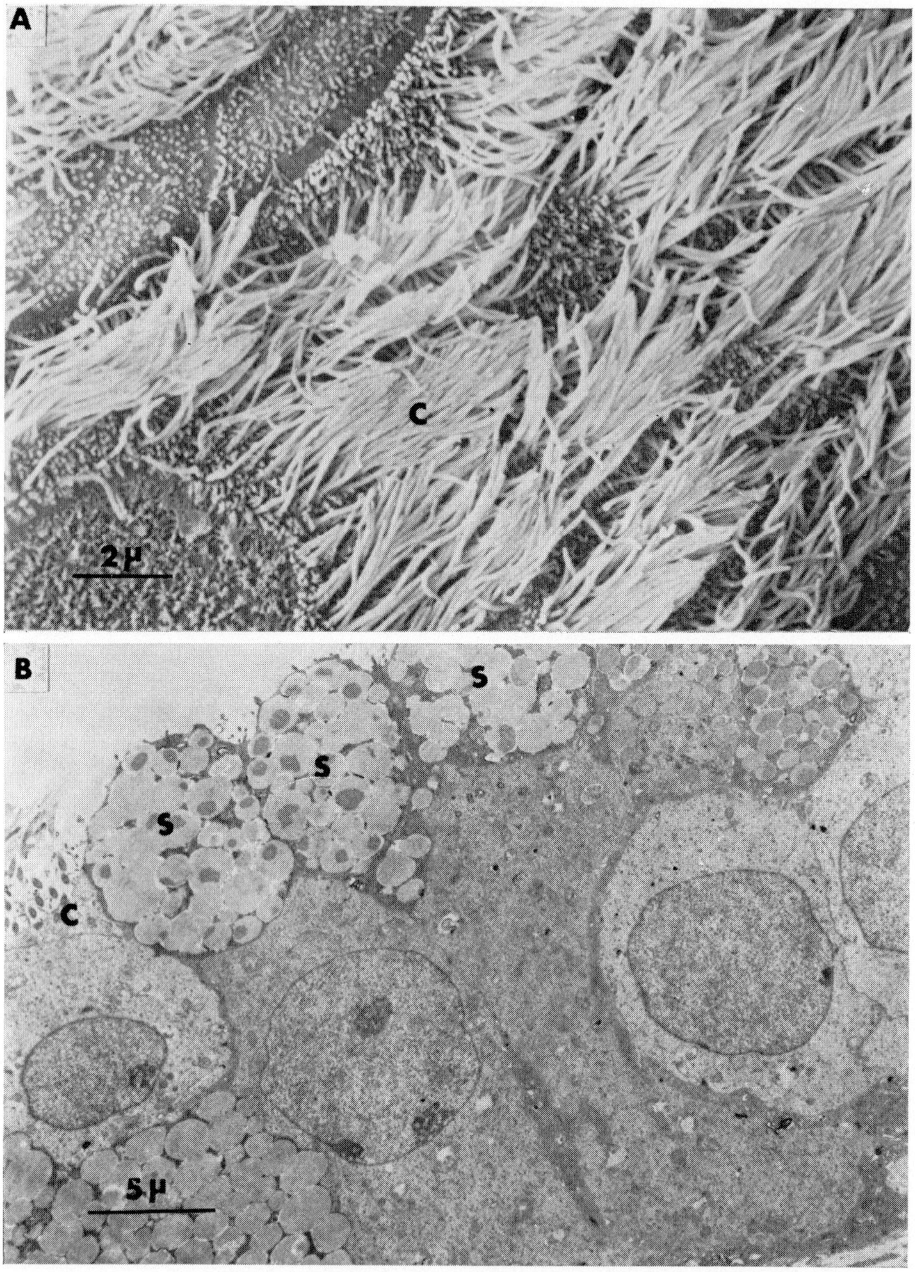

Fig. 13. A) Scanning view of the transitional zone in a 6-day postnatal rat. Mature ciliated cells (C) are present. (X5500) B) TEM of secretory cells (S) in the transitional zone of a 6-day postnatal rat. Some light secretory granules with and without dark cores are fused with the apical plasma membrane. (X2800)

light granules. The appearance of cells with dark granules was rare and the mixed granulated cells were more common, although not as common as those characterized by light granules. However, signs of the active secretory phase were seen in specimens taken from 21-day fetal rats and postnatal rats. Four

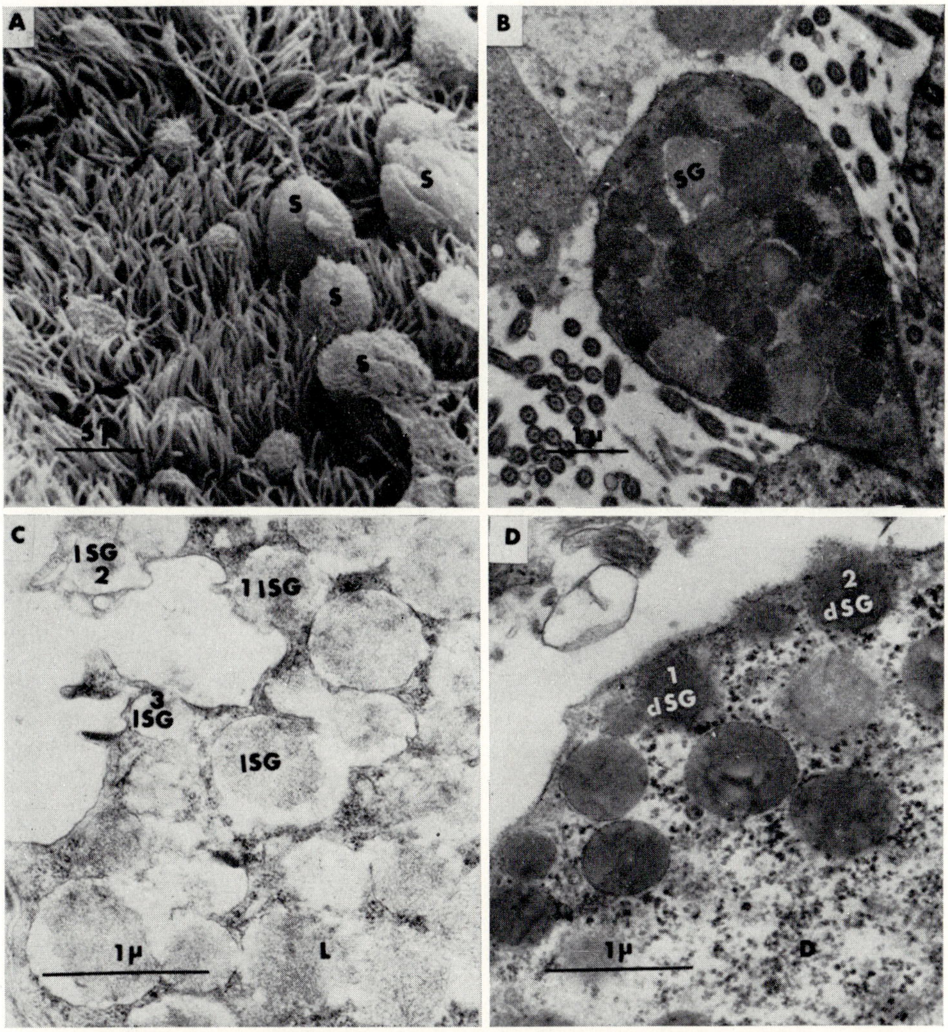

Fig. 14. A) Scanning micrograph of macroapocrine secretion (type II) in the transitional zone near the tympanic orifice of a 3-day postnatal rat. Apocrine projections of secretory cells (S) are seen among ciliated cells. (X2400) B) TEM micrograph of the similar region shows pinching off of the upper portion of the mixed granulated cell (type II). Secretory granules (SG) join to form a large mass in the cytoplasm. (X11,000) C) TEM of eccrine secretion (type IV) in the transitional zone of a 3-day postnatal rat, showing the different stages of secretory granule extrusion in the light granulated cell (L); initial contact (1), protrusion of the membrane (2), and final opening of the cell membrane and extrusion (3). (X22,000) D) TEM of eccrine secretion (type V) in the transitional zone of a 2-day postnatal rat, depicting the different stages of secretory granule extrusion in the dark granulated cell (D): initial contact (1), and protrusion of the membrane by lesis (2). (X19,000)

different modes of secretion were recognized. According to Kurosumi's classification,[35] these were macroapocrine (type II), microapocrine (type III) and eccrine (types IV and V) secretions. Type IV is characterized by the fact that the cell membrane allows the escape of secretory granules without disturbing the integrity of secretory cells, while in the secretory mode of type V, secretory substances diffuse out to the lumen without breaking the cell membrane. Types II and IV appeared to be the most common in the mixed and light granulated cells. Type V was seen in dark granulated cells. As seen in Figure 14A, "'apocrine projections" or "secretory extrusions" are common in the tympanic orifice and transitional zone of postnatal rats. This secretory extrusion was specific for type II. Figure 14B is a TEM picture of this secretion, illustrating the fact that secretory granules join together to form a large mass inside the cytoplasm, separate from the cell and become a secretory droplet. In Figures 2A and 3B, arrows indicate secretory extrusions with expanded tips of microvilli in suckling rats. We considered this mode to be the microapocrine secretion. Figure 14C represents the type IV secretory mode, in which aggregations of light granules are seen in the apical zone of the cytoplasm. Some granules fused to each other and to the surface plasma membrane. A small part of the cell membrane allowed the emergence of secretory granules. Figure 14D is a TEM photograph of a dark granulated secretory cell in the 2-day postnatal rat, exhibiting type V eccrine secretion. Molecular diffusion of the granules to the lumen without interrupting the cell membrane was observed. This mode was found exclusively in dark granulated cells.

DISCUSSION

Although it is generally believed that the middle ear mucosa is a respiratory epithelium with secretory and mucociliary properties, there is controversy concerning the cell distribution, particularly the presence of secretory cells. Schwarzbart[2] and Buch and Jorgensen[4] found no glands or goblet cells in the middle ear in a study of serial sections of a large number of human temporal bones obtained from fetuses, newborn babies, infants, and adults. However, Bendek[36] reported that secretory epithelia with glands were present in 30% of the biopsy specimens of the oval window niche mucosa obtained from ten patients undergoing operations for otosclerosis. Sadé[8] reported the existence of mucous glands and goblet cells in the middle ear mucosa of patients with no otological diseases. In a postmortem study of normal temporal bones using electron microscopy, Hentzer[12] and Lim and Shimada[15,17] confirmed the presence of both secretory and ciliated cells. They also found glands in a few cases. Lim *et al*[18,19] further demonstrated that the distribution of the ciliated cells in the middle ear unequivocally parallels that of the secretory cells. They found numerous secretory cells in the bony portion of the Eustachian tube and hypotympanum and small numbers were found in the antrum and promontory.

As Bak-Pedersen and Tos[27] pointed out, divergent results concerning the cell distribution of the normal human middle ear are probably due to differences in method and previous diseases of the middle ear unknown to the investigators. To avoid the latter problem, fetal, newborn and suckling rats were employed in this study.

The results of this study show that, in general, the cellular distribution patterns in the middle ear mucosa and tympanic bulla in suckling rats and adult rats were similar, even though the distribution of ciliated and secretory cells varied to a certain extent from one adult rat to another. The tympanic orifice of the tube and the transitional zone were covered with ciliated cells and secretory cells, but the density of both types was higher in the tympanic orifice than in the transitional zone. The number of ciliated and secretory cells diminished near the margin of the transitional zone, where the cuboidal cells became squamous cells. A similar cell distribution pattern was observed in guinea pig middle ears by Lim *et al.*[10,18] They emphasized that the distribution of the secretory cells was exactly parallel to that of the ciliated cells. In the present investigation the same finding was demonstrated in rat middle ear mucosae. Lim *et al*[18] clearly demonstrated a mucociliary transportation pathway to the tympanic orifice from the transitional zone by showing that carbon particles placed in the transitional zone were moved to the tympanic orifice and cleared through the tube. Our results revealed that the development of ciliated cells started at 17 or 18 fetal days, paralleling that of secretory cells, even though the incidence of these cells was very low. This finding suggested that ciliated and secretory cells (though limited to the tympanic orifice and transitional zone) are normal components of the middle ear mucosa and that the middle ear starts to provide for the mucociliary system in the fetal stage.

It is important to note that, whereas at 21 fetal days PAS-alcian blue positive epithelial cells and mucous droplets on the mucosal surface appeared rarely, the number of ciliated and secretory cells and PAS-alcian blue positive cells increased rapidly after the birth. At six postnatal days the incidence of these cells and the number and size of the cilia of many ciliated cells equalled that of the adult rats. Apparently, therefore, the development of middle ear mucosa of newborn rats is accomplished by the sixth postnatal day. In the middle ear mucosa of suckling rats ranging in age from six to ten days, the distribution of secretory and ciliated cells was limited to the tympanic orifice, transitional zone, and the tube. These functional cells were not detected in other portions of the middle ear, such as the promontory, anterior and posterior recesses, oval and round window niches, ossicles or tympanic membrane. However, in more advanced suckling rats and adult rats, islands of ciliated and secretory cells were rarely found in areas where a simple squamous epithelium was usually present. The mechanism involved in the appearance of ciliated and secretory cells in areas where the squamous epithelium is present is not clear. However, it is likely that some pathological stimuli upon the middle ear mucosa cause this, since the middle ear cavity is open to air through the Eustachian tube and since several experimental studies[5,6,37-39] have indicated that flat epithelial cells can be induced to become either ciliated or secretory cells.

In this study, glands were not found in the osseous tube, tympanic orifice, or other areas of the middle ear cavity in fetal, newborn, and unadvanced suckling rats, while true glands were common in the cartilaginous portion of the tube. Ladman and Mitchell[40] reported that seromucous glands are located only in the cartilaginous portion of the tube in mice. Contrarily, several authors[8,12,18,26,36] have demonstrated glands in presumably normal middle ears of human beings. However, Lim *et al*[18] stated, from results of animal experiments,[39] that glands observed in both the human and animal ears are most likely derived from postinflammatory healing. They observed that the lamina propria are extremely thick when these glands (cystic formations) are numerous. Therefore, they suggested that these gland formations are the sequelae of inflammatory reactions. On the basis of their findings that no mucous glands were present in the middle ear mucosa covering the osseous tube and middle ear cavity of premature and newborn infants, Bak-Pedersen and Tos[26,29] claimed that mucous glands are probably not a normal component of the middle ear mucosa. Findings of the present investigation also supported this assumption.

Lim *et al*[10,13,15,18,19,37] have identified the presence of several morphologically different secretory cells in both animal and human middle ear mucosae; these were light granulated (goblet cells), dark granulated, mixed granulated, and lamellar-granulated cells. According to them, the light granulated cells were most common while the dark or mixed granulated cells were less common. The lamellar-granulated cells were found only in a few specimens of the presumably normal middle ear epithelium. The present investigation clearly demonstrated all these secretory cells except for the lamellar-granulated cells. It is generally accepted that the light granulated cells secrete mucus. Lim *et al*[13,15,18,19] have suggested that the dark granulated cells synthesize and secrete enzymes or proteins, opposing the supposition that the diverse ultrastructural and cytochemical characteristics of the light granulated, mixed granulated, and dark granulated cells are only expressions of different phenotypes of the same secretory cells. In this study no evidence was obtained to indicate the nature of the dark granules. However, it is interesting to note that the type V (Kurosumi's classification)[35] secretory mode was exclusively seen in the dark granulated cells, while types II and IV were most common in the light granulated and mixed granulated cells, and that these two secretory cells could be distinguished from each other at 20 fetal days. At this stage, signs of active secretion were still absent.

Recent studies have suggested three possible defense mechanisms in the middle ear mucosa—mucociliary,[8,9,17-19] immunologic,[19,21-25,41] and enzymatic.[19,42] Results of the present study showed that the middle ear mucosa and Eustachian tube start to provide for the mucociliary defense system at the fetal stage. The mucosal immunity of the middle ear was also studied. Further studies may clarify the course of development of the immunologic defense system in the middle ear.

REFERENCES

1. Graves GO, Edwards LF: The Eustachian tube. Arch Otolaryngol 39:359-399, 1944

2. Schwarzbart A: A reappraisal of the clinical and morphological classification of the tympanic spaces and the Eustachian tube. Ann Otol Rhinol Laryngol 67:241-245, 1958

3. Bloom W, Fawcett P: *A Textbook of Histology*, ed 8. Philadelphia, WB Saunders Co, 1962, p 668

4. Buch NH, Jørgensen MB: Eustachian tube and middle ear. Arch Otolaryngol 79: 472-480, 1964

5. Friedmann I: The comparative pathology of otitis media—Experimental and human. II. The histopathology of experimental otitis of the guinea pig with particular reference to experimental cholesteatoma. J Laryngol Otol 69:588-601, 1955

6. Senturia BH, Carr CD, Ahlvin RC: Middle ear effusions: pathologic changes of the mucoperiosteum in the experimental animal. Ann Otol Rhinol Laryngol 71:632-648, 1962

7. Ojala L: Contribution to the physiology and pathology of mastoid air cell formation. Acta Otolaryngol (Stockh) (Suppl) 86:1-134, 1950

8. Sadé J: Middle ear mucosa. Arch Otolaryngol 84:137-143, 1966

9. Sadé J: Ciliary activity and middle ear clearance. Arch Otolaryngol 86:128-135, 1967

10. Lim DJ, Paparella MM, Kimura RS: Ultrastructure of the Eustachian tube and middle ear mucosa in the guinea pig. Acta Otolaryngol (Stockh) 63:425-444, 1967

11. Kawabata I, Paparella MM: Ultrastructure of normal human middle ear mucosa. Preliminary report. Ann Otol Rhinol Laryngol 78: 125-137, 1969

12. Hentzer E: Ultrastructure of the normal mucosa in human middle ear, mastoid cavities, and Eustachian tube. Ann Otol Rhinol Laryngol 79:1143-1157, 1970

13. Lim DJ: Protein secreting cells in the normal middle ear mucosa of the guinea pig. An autoradiographic investigation. Ann Otol Rhinol Laryngol 79:82-94, 1970

14. Hilding DA, Heywood P: Ultrastructure of middle ear mucosa and organization of ciliary matrix. Ann Otol Rhinol Laryngol 80: 306-312, 1971

15. Lim DJ, Shimada T: Secretory activity of normal middle ear epithelium: Scanning and transmission electron microscopic observations. Ann Otol Rhinol Laryngol 80:319-329, 1971

16. Sadé J: Cellular differentiation of the middle ear lining. Ann Otol Rhinol Laryngol 80:376-383, 1971

17. Shimada T, Lim DJ: Distribution of ciliated cells in the human middle ear. Electron and light microscopic observations. Ann Otol Rhinol Laryngol 81:203-211, 1972

18. Lim DJ, Shimada T, Yoder M: Distribution of mucus-secreting cells in normal middle ear mucosa. Arch Otolaryngol 98:2-9, 1973

19. Lim DJ: Functional morphology of the lining membrane of the middle ear and Eustachian tube. An overview. Ann Otol Rhinol Laryngol 83 (Suppl 11: 5-22) 1974

20. Maeda S, Honjo S, Mogi G: Surface structure of the normal mucosa in developing rat middle ear. Scanning Electron Micros part III, 565-572, 1974

21. Bernstein JM, Buffalo NY, Tomasi TB Jr, *et al*: A histopathologic and immunochemical report. Am Acad Ophthalmol Otolaryngol 76:1305-1318, 1972

22. Mogi G, Honjo S, Maeda S, *et al*: Secretory immunoglobulin A (SIgA) in middle ear effusions. Observation of 160 specimens. Ann Otol Rhinol Laryngol 82:302-310, 1973

23. Mogi G, Honjo S, Maeda S, *et al*: Secretory immunoglobulin A (SIgA) in middle ear effusions. A further report. Ann Otol Rhinol Laryngol 83:92-101, 1974

24. Ogra PL, Bernstein JM, Yurchak AM,

et al: Characteristics of secretory immune system in human middle ear: Implications in otitis media. J Immunol 112:488-495, 1974

25. Mogi G, Honjo S, Maeda S, *et al*: Quantitative determination of secretory immunoglobulin A (SIgA) in middle ear effusions. Ann Otol Rhinol Laryngol 83:239-246, 1974

26. Bak-Pedersen K, Tos M: Mucous glands in the middle ear and osseous Eustachian tube. Ann Otol Rhinol Laryngol 82:80-88, 1973

27. Bak-Pedersen K, Tos M: Distribution and density of goblet cells in the normal adult human middle ear. Ann Otol Rhinol Laryngol 82:240-247, 1973

28. Tos M: Production of mucus in the middle ear and Eustachian tube. Embryology, anatomy, and pathology of the mucous glands and goblet cells in the Eustachian tube and middle ear. Ann Otol Rhinol Laryngol 83:44-58, 1974

29. Bak-Pedersen K, Tos M: Middle-ear mucosa in newborn infants. Ann Otol Rhinol Laryngol 83:168-173, 1974

30. Hussl B, Lim DJ: Secretory cells in the middle ear mucosa of the guinea pig. Cytochemical and ultrastructural study. Arch Otolaryngol 89:691-699, 1969

31. Stubblefield E, Brinkley BR: Cilia formation in Chinese hamster fibroblasts in vitro as a response to colcemid treatment. J Cell Biol 30:645-652, 1966

32. Sorokin SP: Reconstructions of centriole formation and ciliogenesis in mammalian lungs. J Cell Sci 3:207-230, 1968

33. Bennet HS: Morphological aspects of extracellular polysaccharides. J Histochem Cytochem 11:14-23, 1963

34. Yamada E: The fine structure of the gall bladder epithelium of the mouse. J Biophys Biochem Cytol 1:445-457, 1955

35. Kurosumi K: Electron microscopic analysis of secretion. Int Rev Cytol 11:1-124, 1961

36. Bendek GA: Histopathology of transudatory-secretory otitis media. Arch Otolaryngol 78:33-38, 1963

37. Lim DJ, Hussl B: Tympanic mucosa after tubal obstruction: An ultrastructural observation. Arch Otolaryngol 91:585-593, 1970

38. Paparella M, Hiraide F, Juhn S, *et al*: Cellular events involved in middle ear fluid production. Ann Otol Rhinol Laryngol 79:766-779, 1970

39. Lim DJ, Klainer A: Cellular reactions in acute otitis media. Laryngoscope 81:1772-1786, 1971

40. Ladman A, Mitchell AJ: The topographic relations and histological characteristics of the tubulo acinar glands of the Eustachian tube in mice. Anat Rec 121:167-185, 1958

41. Hussl B, Lim DJ: Experimental middle ear effusions: an immunofluorescent study. Ann Otol Rhinol Laryngol 83:332-342, 1974

42. Veltri RW, Sprinkle PM: Serous otitis media–Immunoglobulins and lyzozyme levels in the middle ear fluid and serum. Ann Otol Rhinol Laryngol 82:297-301, 1973

Acknowledgment–The authors wish to thank Dr. David J. Lim (Columbus, Ohio) for his kind review and suggestions to this manuscript.

Reprints–Shoichi Maeda, MD, Department of Otolaryngology, Yamaguchi University School of Medicine, Ube-City, Yamaguchi Pref., Japan.

SPIRAL MIGRATION THEORY OF ORGAN OF CORTI DEVELOPMENT

WILLIAM F. MAROVITZ, PhD

JOEL M. A. SHUGAR, MDCM KHALID M. KHAN, MS

NEW YORK, NEW YORK

SUMMARY – A mitotic zone has previously been demonstrated on the luminal surface of the posteromedial wall of the otocyst in the plane of the endolymphatic duct and at the junction of cochlea with primitive saccule. In this experiment the application of fluorodeoxyuridine (FudR) (an antimitotic agent) demonstrates the existence of a discrete synthetic zone for the otocyst which lies nearby to the otic zone of mitosis. Cells labeled by FudR and, therefore, in the mitotic synthetic (S) phase are always found away from the lumen (antiluminal surface) when the animals are sacrificed soon after injection. Cellular migration from synthetic zone through the luminal mitotic area and beyond is hypothesized. Once cellular division is completed the cells appear to follow a spiral course (from medial to lateral) over the anterior wall of the otocyst. The cells continue their spiral course entering the thin side of the cochlear base. From this strategic location the cells migrate around the sides of the cochlea to reach and to form the pseudostratified wall and complete the thin side of the cochlear duct. The pitch of this migration pattern is similar to the helical pitch of the mature cochlear duct and may be responsible for the adult configuration.

In rats a single zone of mitotic activity has been shown to be responsible for the production of the entire cochlea.[1] This zone is situated in the plane of the endolymphatic duct at the junction of the cochlea with saccule and was first visualized by the application of the antimitotic drug, colchicine. Colchicine stops mitosis in metaphase by the inhibition of spindle fiber formation.[2,3] The morphologic effect of the drug is to render cells conspicuous by the scattered pattern of their condensed metaphase chromosomes; producing the so-called C-metaphase.[2] Colchicine is, therefore, able to mark the process of chromosomal separation (M-phase) but does not allow visualization of cells involved in the predivision synthetic (S) phase or in a pre- or postmitotic resting phase (G_2 and G_1, respectively).

Fluorodeoxyuridine (FudR) was used in this experiment to identify the otic zone of mitotic synthesis and to investigate the possibility of cellular migration. FudR blocks DNA synthesis by inhibiting the enzyme thymidilate synthetase and, thus, preventing the conversion of deoxyuridylic acid to thymidilic acid.[4-6] The drug has been shown to be incorporated during the synthetic (S) phase of division, and its effect is observable after this time.[7] The result of FudR treatment is nuclear pyknosis, chromatolytic degeneration and cellular death.[7-10] In the central nervous system it has been shown that the migration pattern of cells is not hindered by FudR and that pyknotic nuclei trace the normal postmitotic migration pattern.[8] Because of the possibility of cellular migration in the otocyst, the time at which the animal is sacrificed after the administration of FudR becomes paramount. If the animal is sacrificed soon after incorporation of FudR, pyknotic nuclei do not have a chance to migrate and are distributed uniformly throughout the antiluminal synthetic zone. If the animal is allowed to live for longer intervals of time after the injection, migration (if present) of the labeled cells

---

From the Department of Otolaryngology, Mount Sinai School of Medicine, New York, New York. Supported in part by a grant from the Deafness Research Foundation.

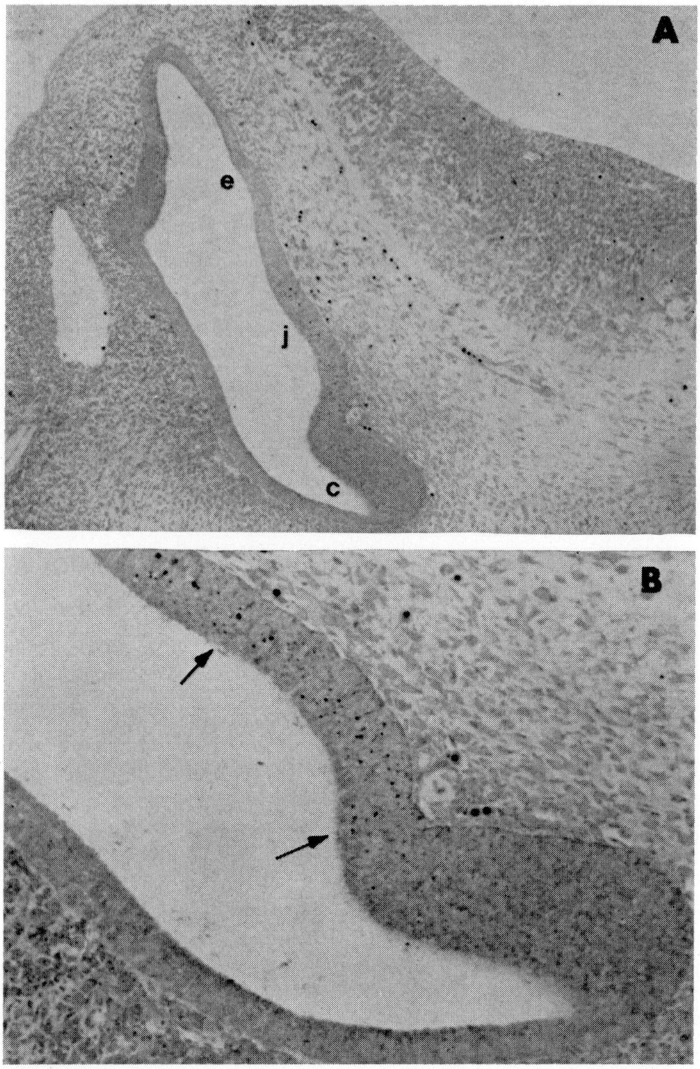

Fig. 1. Thirteen day otocyst, FudR - treated for four hours. A) (X75). B) J zone (between arrows) displays cellular degeneration. Note that cochlear duct distal to j zone is free of drug effect (X180). e - Endolymphatic duct. c - Cochlear duct. j - Junction of saccule and cochlear duct. This illustration and all subsequent photomicrographs were stained with 1% Toluidine blue.

should occur. By noting the location of pyknotic nuclei at various time intervals after injection, the migration pattern of cells forming the cochlear duct can be detected and reconstructed. On day 13 the cochlea is actively and rapidly growing[9] and the spatial location of mitotic cells is known.[1] For these reasons the day 13 animal was studied to localize the synthetic zone and to determine any migrational pattern. The application of an antimitotic drug at any time during the growth of the cochlea should only affect its mitotic zone, sparing any distal segment which has already been completed. The location of cellular destruction by FudR should, therefore, be similar in a day 13,14,15 or 16 animal; however, the length of cochlea spared the effect of FudR should be greater with increasing age. FudR also was administered to a day

14 and 16 animal to test the migration hypothesis and add further credibility to the proposed growth zone.

METHODS AND MATERIALS

Six pregnant female rats on day 13 of gestation were injected intraperitoneally with 200 mgm/kg of FudR dissolved in saline. The rats were then sacrificed at 4,6,8,10 and 24 hours from the time of injection. The rats were anesthetized with ether and a midline abdominal incision was carried down through peritoneum exposing the bicornate uterus, which was removed and placed in cold 4 C 0.1 M cacodylate buffer at pH 7.4. The fetuses were individually removed from their embryonic sac and put into 4 C, 2% glutaraldehyde in 0.1 M cacodylate buffer, dehydrated in graded ethanol, cleared in propylene oxide, and left overnight in 1:1 propylene oxide: epon. The next day the tissues were put in epon for 2 hours and embedded in fresh epon at 60 C for 24 hours. The head of the fetus was oriented so that vertical cuts at 5μ intervals were made in an anteroposterior direction through the otocyst. This gave us two otocysts per animal to study. The second part of the experiment consisted of day 14 and 16 animals injected with 200 mg/kg FudR intraperitoneally and sacrificed eight hours later.

The pups of uninjected mothers of the same conception age were sacrificed and served as controls. Serial sections of fetuses were made on glass knives on either an LKB ultramicrotome or LKB prymitome. Sections were picked up and transferred to drops of water on a glass slide. When the slide was filled with sections they were placed on a hot plate to evaporate the water, causing the epon sections to adhere to the slide. The hot slides were stained with 1% toluidine blue in 1% borax for about ten seconds. The slides were rinsed in distilled water, dried and covered.

RESULTS

Four hours after treatment antiluminal cells on the medial wall of the otocyst in the region of the primitive saccule and cochlea were found to contain vacuoles, many of which contained dark staining metachromatic granules (Figs. 1, 2). The nuclei of the affected cells did not have a normal smooth contour and contained aggregates of darkly stained material. Severely affected cells demonstrated nuclear fragmentation. This circumscribed zone of cellular degeneration extended for a greater distance anterior to the plane of the endolymphatic duct than behind. The segment of cochlea which had been formed before injection of the drug did not exhibit the effect of FudR. There was also a conspicuous decrease in cellular division in the region of the mitotic zone. Samples removed six hours after injection yielded essentially the same information, except that the cellular degeneration had progressed to the extent that most nuclei had fragmented (Figs. 3, 4). On the eighth hour after injection, the distribution of the metachromatic granules and nuclear debris had changed. They were now also located laterally in the wall of the saccule and thin wall of the base of the cochlea (Fig. 5).

Ten hours following the injection the location of labeled cells was essentially the same as at eight hours, but the amount of labeling laterally was increased (Fig. 6). At 24 hours the labeled cells were still found in the cochlear base, but they were now localized in the pseudostratified wall which represents the analogue of the organ of Corti (Figs. 7, 8). Day 14 and 16 animals, eight hours after injection, gave essentially the same distribution pattern as the day 13 animal at eight hours (Figs. 9-11). The only difference between these data points was a longer segment of cochlea free from the effect of the drug as a factor of fetal age.

In the day 13 control animal on the antiluminal aspect of the wall of the otocyst at the junction of saccule with cochlea, there is a zone of metachromatic granules and nuclear fragmentation (Fig. 12). This zone is qualitatively similar to the otic disruption caused by FudR, but it is quantitatively much less extensive and restricted to a very precise region. This zone became less pronounced in the zone of mitosis previously described.[1]

Control animals on day 14 and 16 consistently exhibit a small zone of cellular destruction identical to the nuclear degeneration in FudR treated animals (Figs. 13-15). Degenerating cells remain localized in this area and in contradistinction to FudR treatment, never migrate.

DISCUSSION

The cytoplasm of cells affected by FudR had many vacuoles, most of

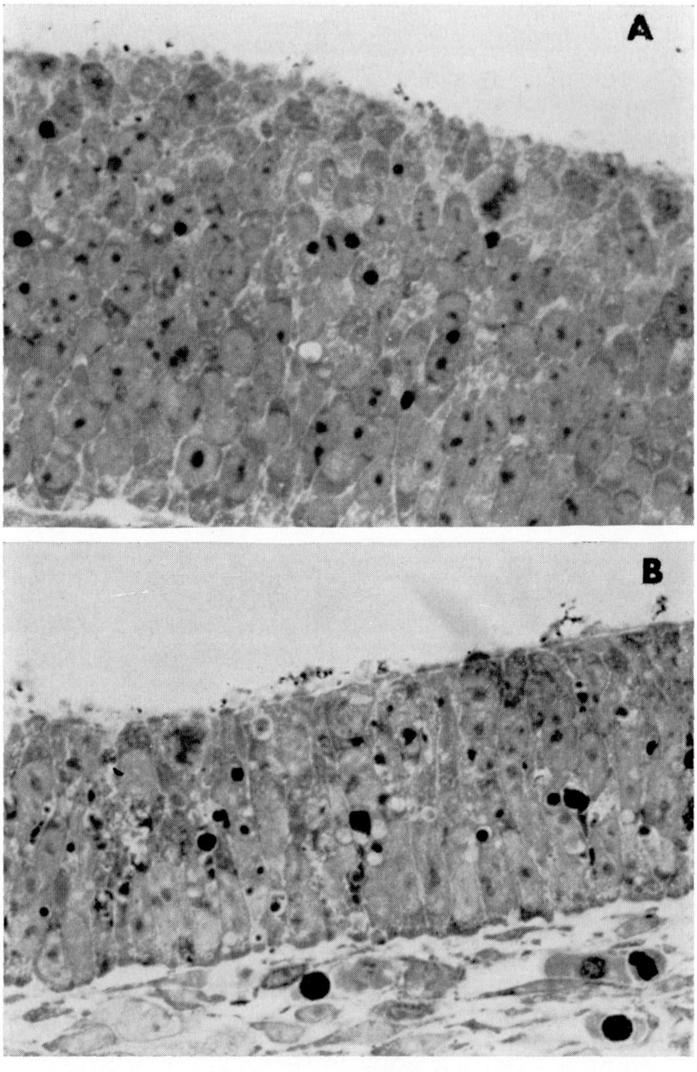

Fig. 2. A) Thirteen day control otocyst (X750). B) Thirteen day otocyst treated with FudR for four hours (X750).

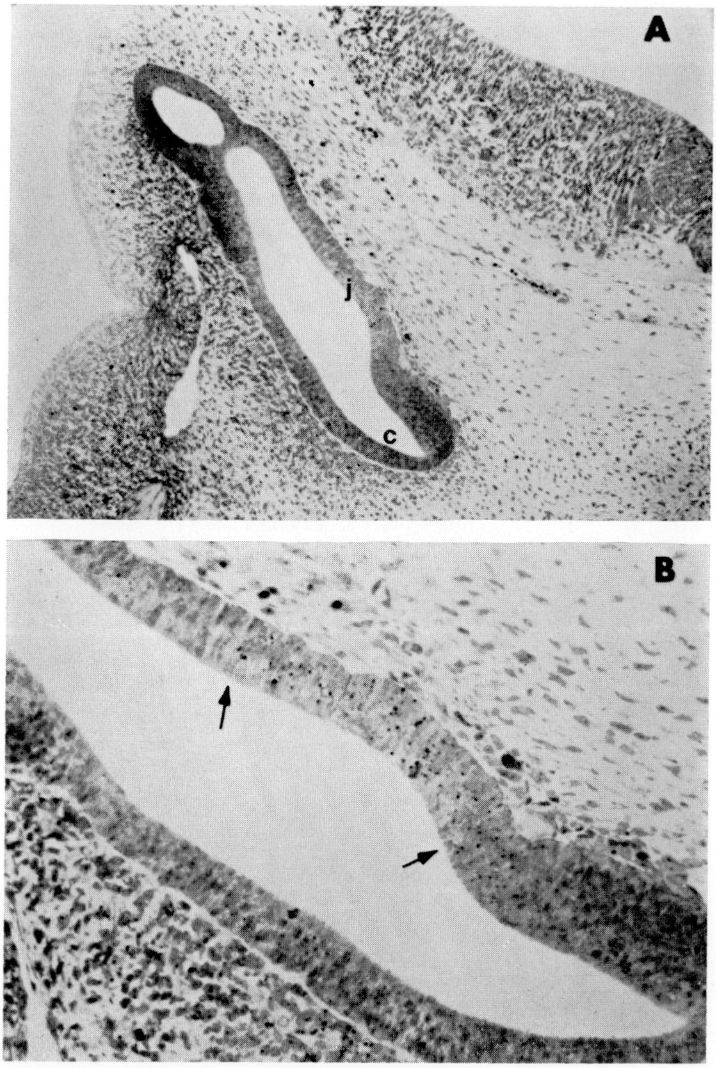

Fig. 3. Thirteen day otocyst treated for six hours by FudR. A) (X75). B) j zone (between arrows) displays cellular degeneration. Note that the cochlear duct distal to j zone is free of drug effect (X180).

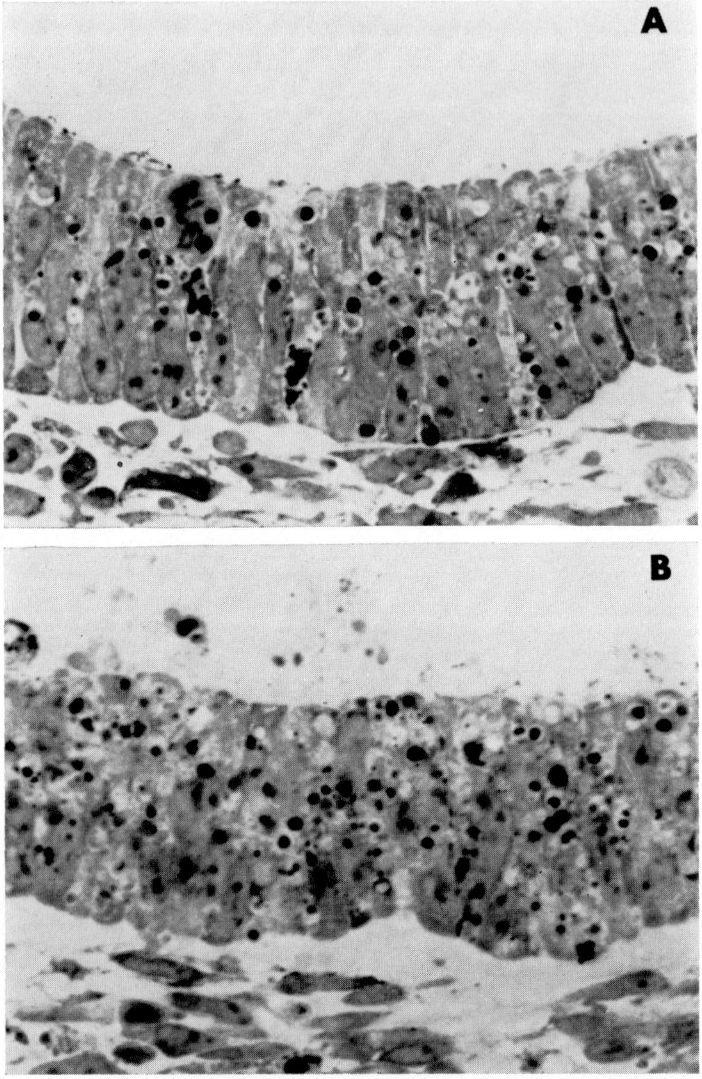

Fig. 4. A) Thirteen day otocyst treated for six hours by FudR (X750). B) Thirteen day otocyst treated for ten hours by FudR (X750).

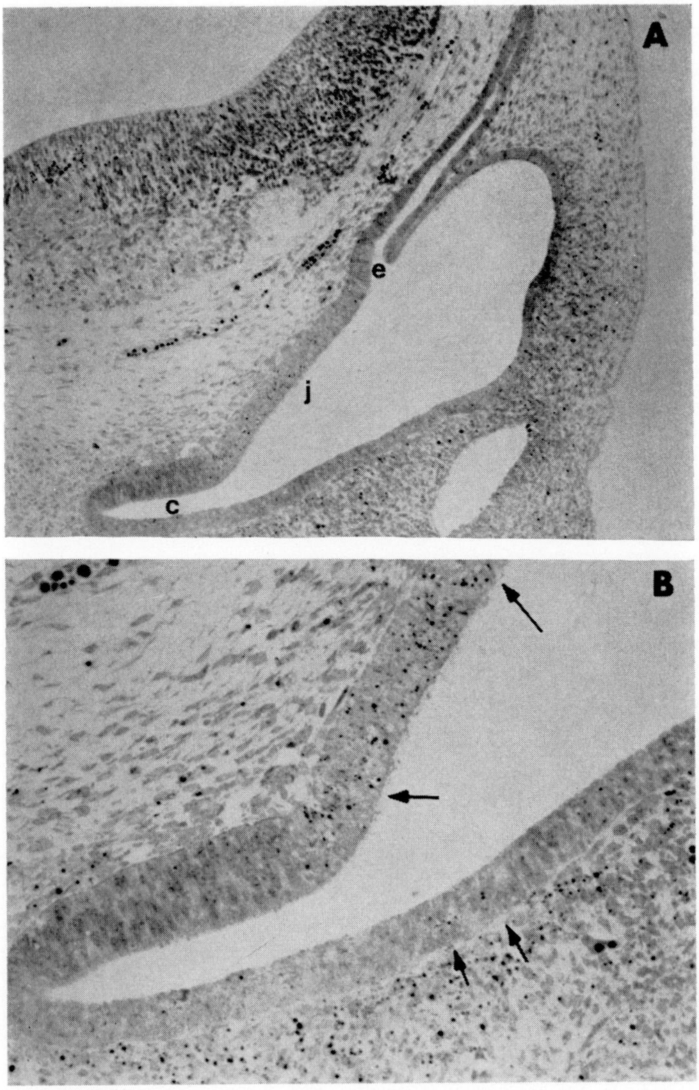

Fig. 5. Thirteen day otocyst treated for eight hours by FudR. A) (X75). B) j zone (between arrows) on medial wall of otocyst displays cellular degeneration. Note migration of products of cellular degeneration to lateral wall of otocyst as indicated by short arrows (X180).

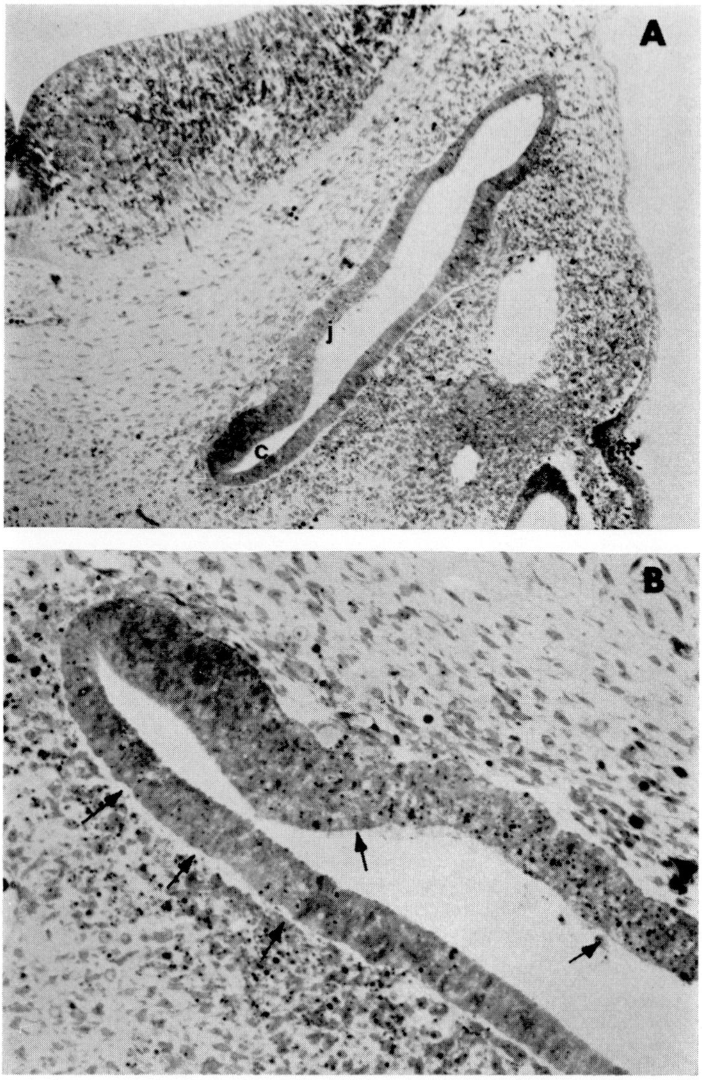

Fig. 6. Thirteen day otocyst treated for ten hours by FudR. A) (X75). B) j zone (between arrows) on medial wall of otocyst displays cellular degeneration. Note migration of products of cellular degeneration to thin wall of base of cochlear duct (X180).

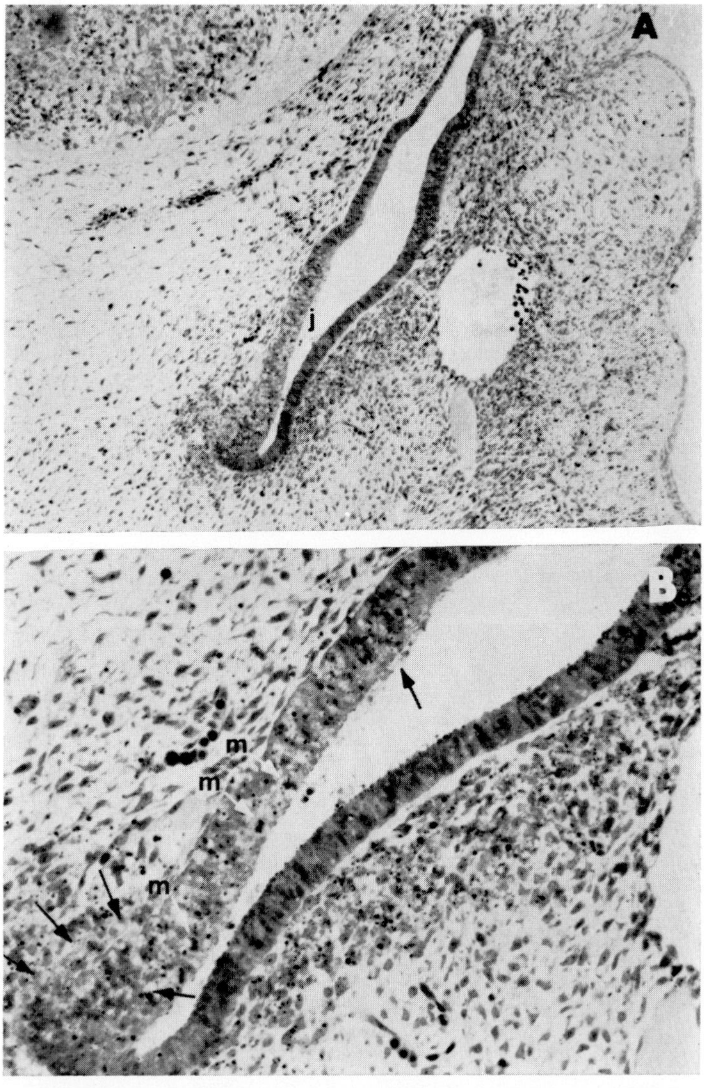

Fig. 7. Thirteen day otocyst treated for 24 hours by FudR. A) (X75). B) j zone (between arrows) on medial wall of otocyst displays cellular degeneration. Note migration of products of cellular degeneration to thick wall of base of cochlear duct as indicated by arrows. Note recovery of mitosis (M) (X180).

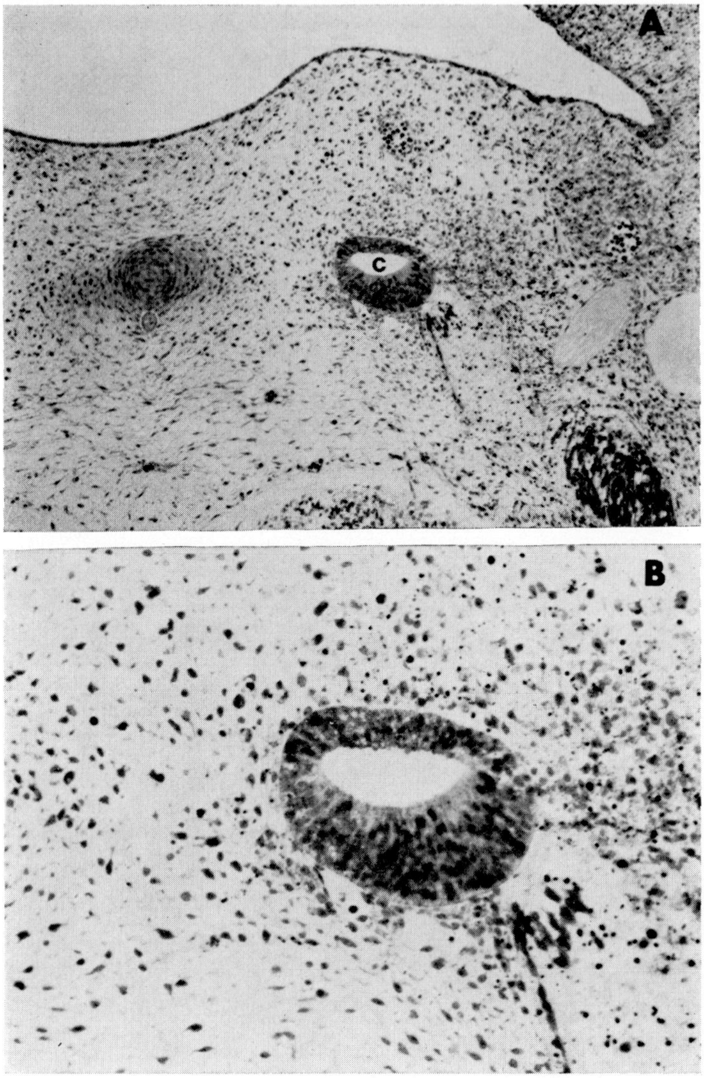

Fig. 8. Thirteen day otocyst treated for 24 hours by FudR. This is a section through a more distal segment of cochlea than in Figure 7. Note absence of drug effect. A) (X75). B) (X180).

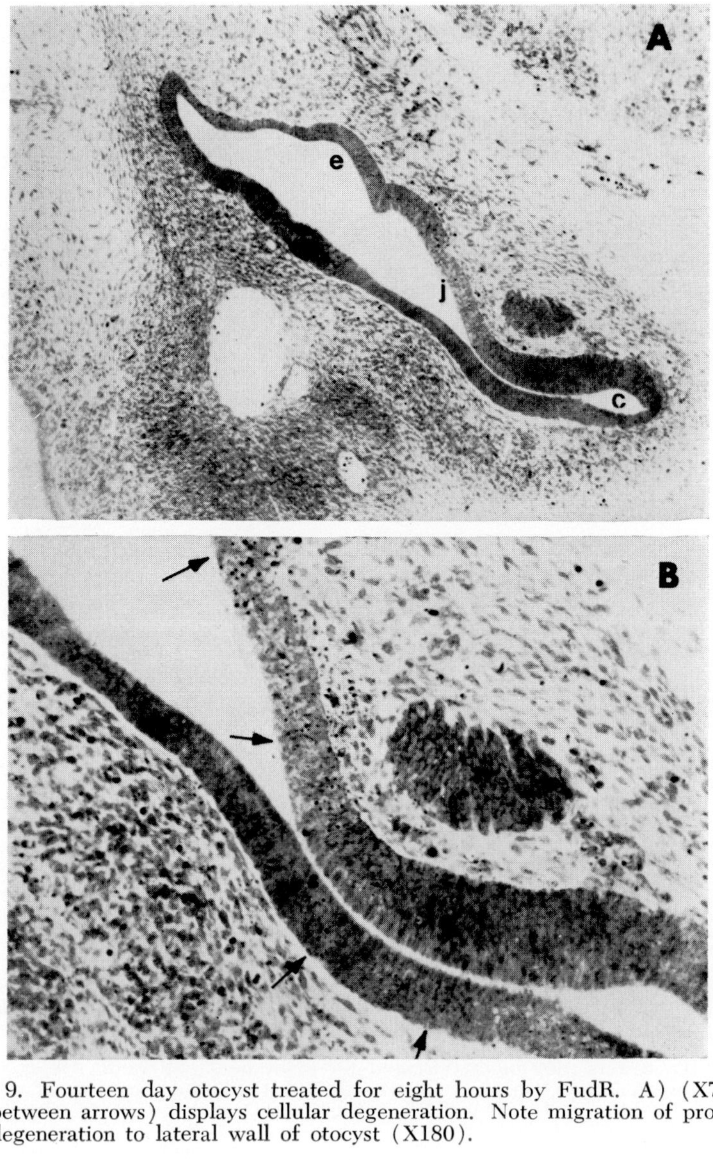

Fig. 9. Fourteen day otocyst treated for eight hours by FudR. A) (X75). B) j zone (between arrows) displays cellular degeneration. Note migration of products of cellular degeneration to lateral wall of otocyst (X180).

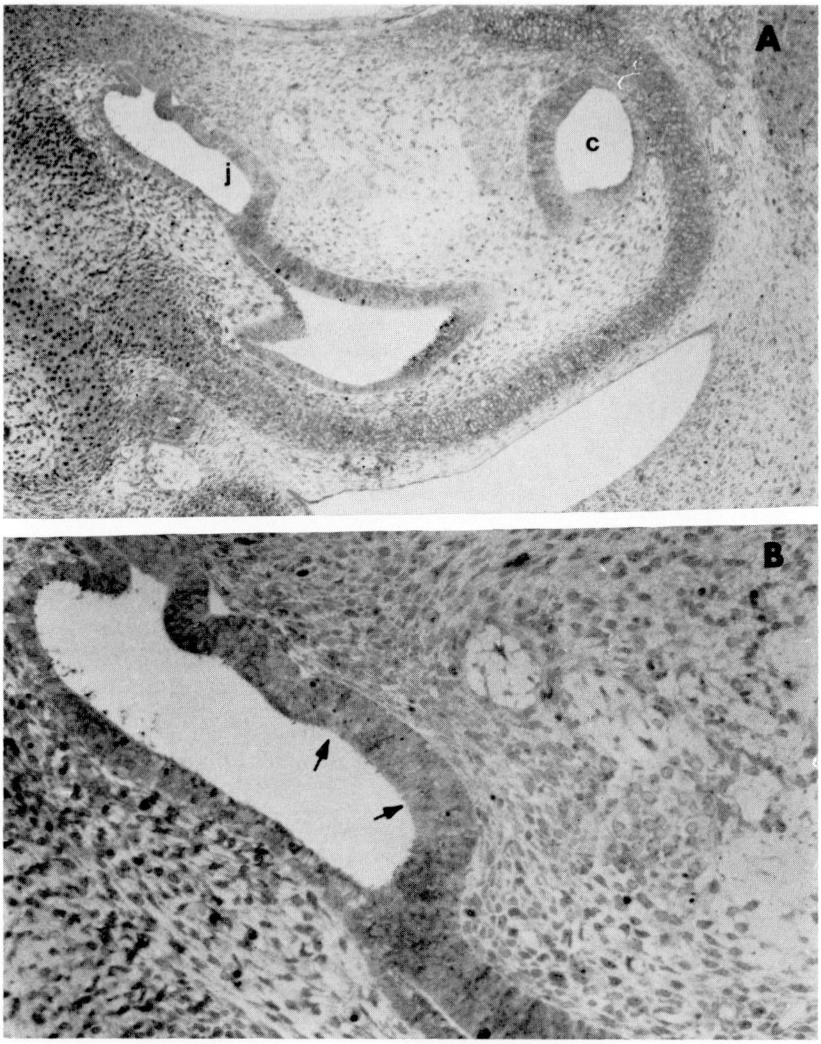

Fig. 10. Sixteen day otocyst treated for eight hours by FudR. A) (X75). B) j zone (between arrows) displays cellular degeneration. Not migration of products of cellular degeneration to lateral wall of otocyst (X180).

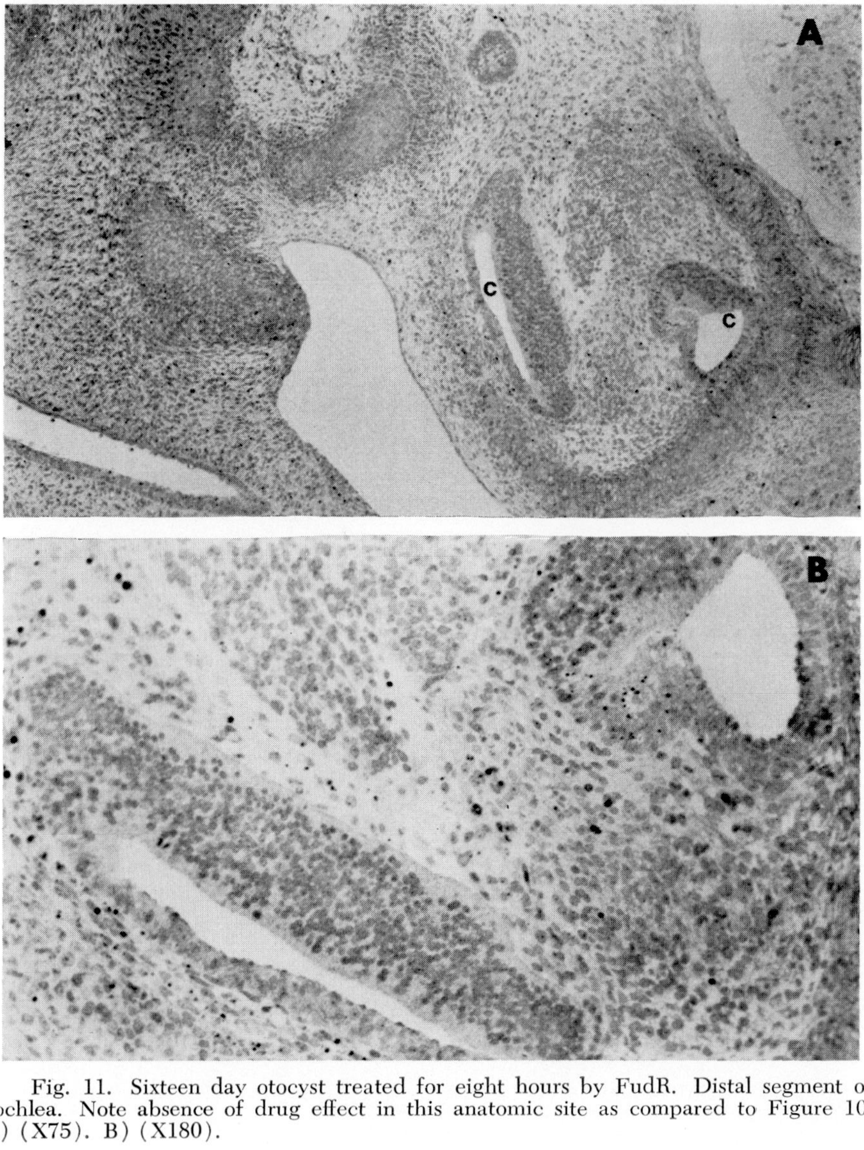

Fig. 11. Sixteen day otocyst treated for eight hours by FudR. Distal segment of cochlea. Note absence of drug effect in this anatomic site as compared to Figure 10. A) (X75). B) (X180).

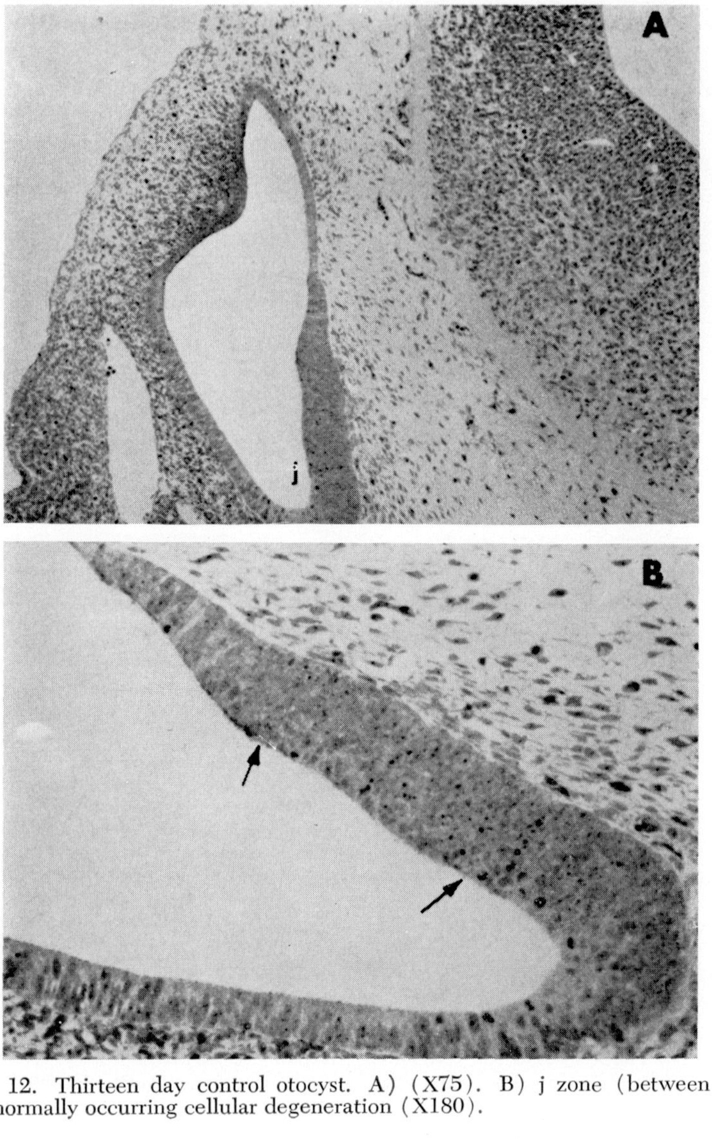

Fig. 12. Thirteen day control otocyst. A) (X75). B) j zone (between arrows) displays normally occurring cellular degeneration (X180).

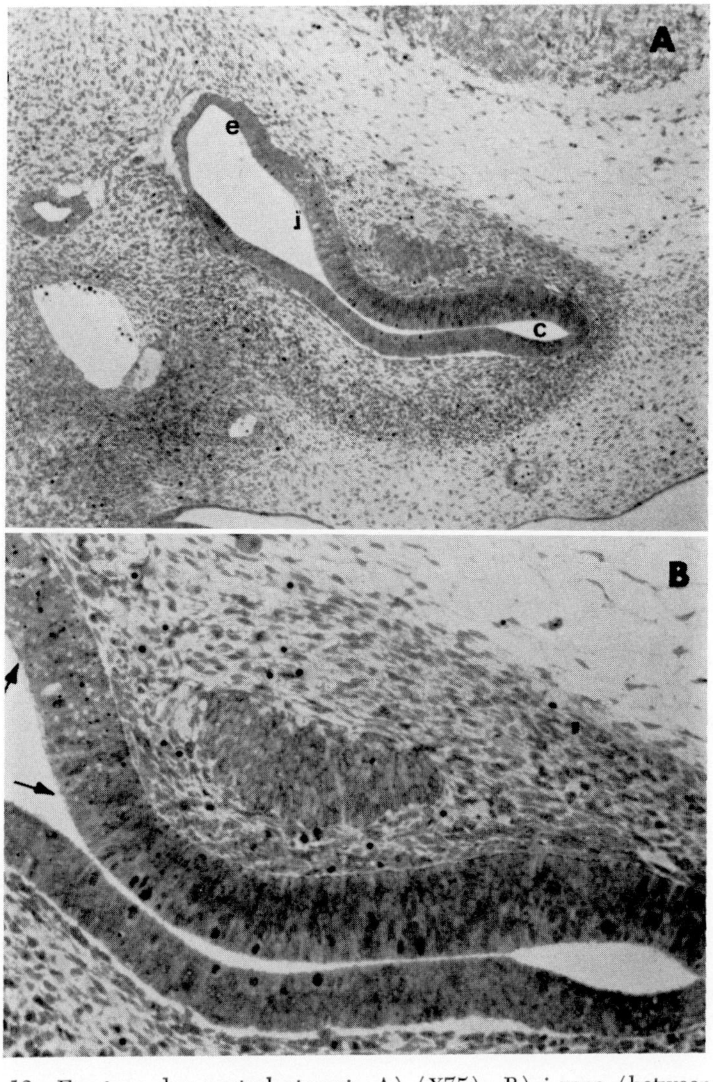

Fig. 13. Fourteen day control otocyst. A) (X75). B) j zone (between arrows) displays normally occurring cellular degeneration (X180).

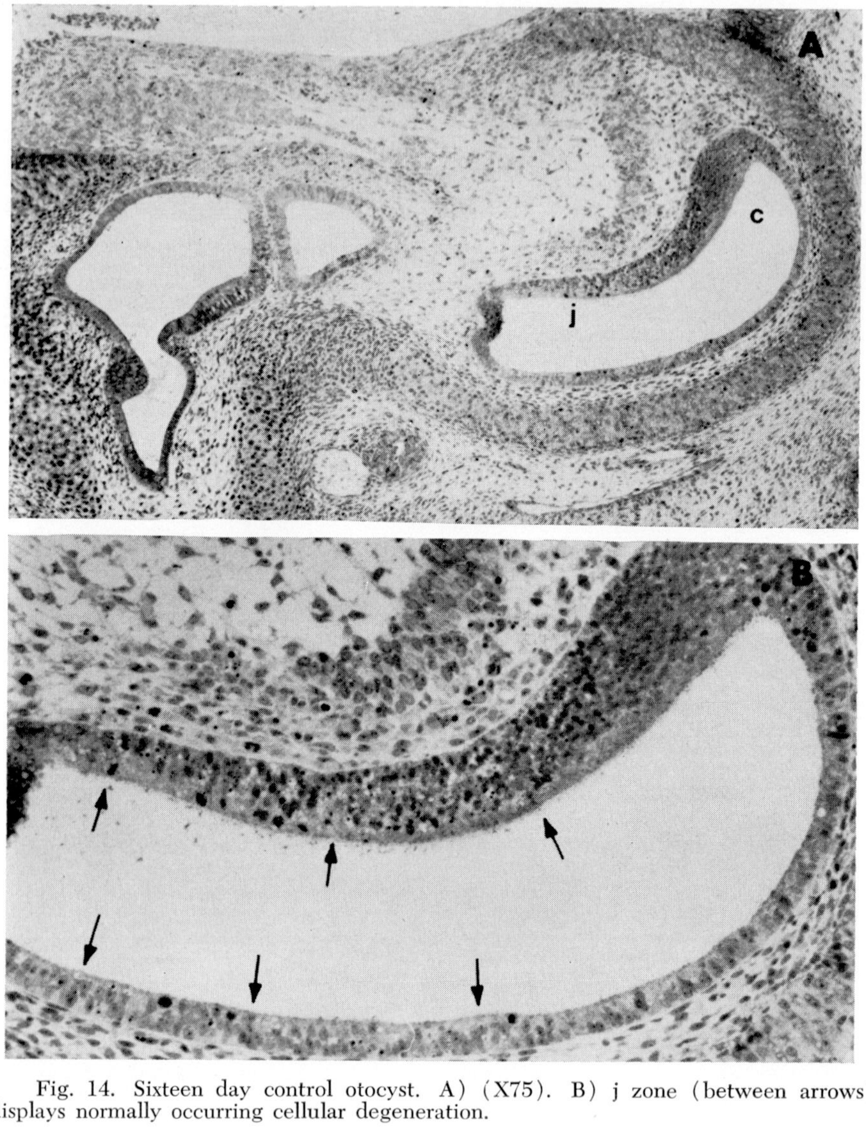

Fig. 14. Sixteen day control otocyst. A) (X75). B) j zone (between arrows) displays normally occurring cellular degeneration.

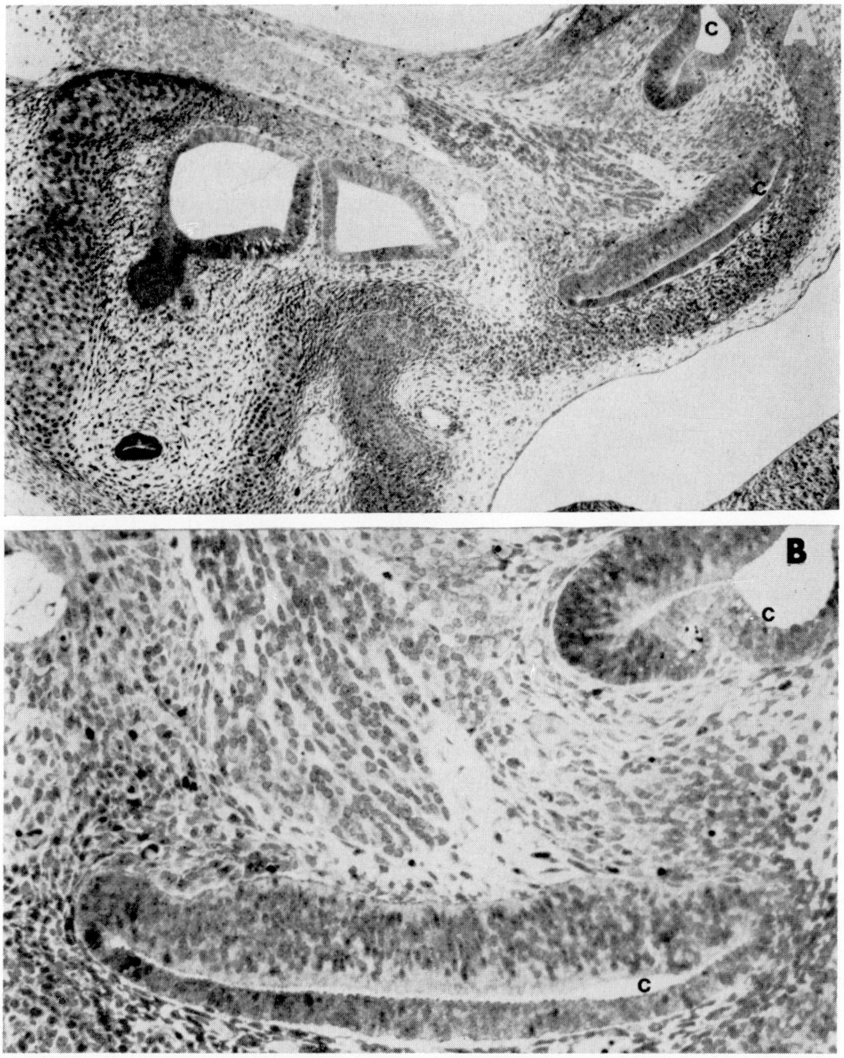

Fig. 15. Sixteen day control otocyst. Distal segment of cochlea. A) (X75). B) (X180).

which contained dark staining metachromatic granules (Figs. 2, 4). The nuclei of these cells were of irregular contour and contained aggregates of darkly stained material. The nuclei of the most severely affected cells were fragmented. These observations of the fetal otocysts were in agreement with the effect seen in developing rat brain.[8,10] The number of affected cells increased for approximately ten hours following FudR injection. By 24 hours the number of cells containing pyknotic nuclei had decreased and occasional mitotic figures again were observed (Fig. 7). Apparently not all synthetic cells were equally affected. It may be that while cells just beginning synthesis are severly affected and die, those nearer the end of their synthetic phase are less likely to be altered and are able to recover.

The majority of cells labeled at four hours were antiluminal and near the basement membrane, which is the area shown by Ruben[11] to be the synthetic

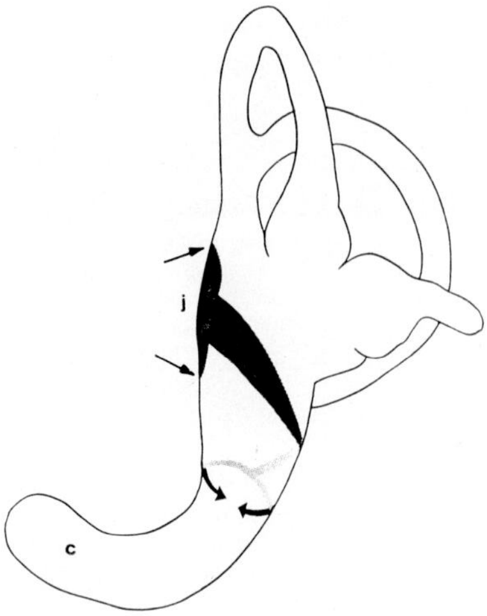

Fig. 16. Schematic representation of the spiral migration theory of cochlear duct formation. Cells formed at a mitotic center on the medial wall of the otocyst between saccule and cochlear appendage migrate first to lateral wall and then back toward medial. For a complete description, please consult the discussion section of the text.

zone of the otocyst. This finding, together with the conspicuous absence of mitosis in the growth zone previously demonstrated by Marovitz and Shugar,[1] support the mode of action of FudR as blocking DNA synthesis.

Four and six hours after injection, pyknotic cells were located primarily on the medial wall of the otocyst at the junction of saccule and cochlea. At eight to ten hours, pyknotic nuclei continue to be observed in the medial wall. They are also found more anteriorly in the wall of the otocyst and laterally at the junction of saccule and cochlea. At 24 hours, pyknotic cells were located in the medial wall of the otocyst and in the base of the cochlea on the thick convex wall.

The changing distribution of pyknotic cells following FudR treatment most probably represents the migrational pattern of postsynthetic (G_2) cells of normal rat otocyst.

Based on these results, the following descriptive picture of development is hypothesized: cells undergo synthesis away from the lumen in the medial wall of the otocyst at the junction of cochlea and saccule. This zone overlaps the zone of mitotic activity demonstrated with colchicine, but is slightly more extensive; (occupying more of the medial wall anterior to the plane of the endolymphatic duct). The cells then leave this antiluminal synthetic zone, migrating to the lumen in the region of the mitotic zone. From this position they follow a spiral course from medial to lateral until the thin base of the cochlea is reached. From that location the cells travel laterally around the sides of the cochlear duct to form the thick pseudostratified wall. The pitch of this hypothesized spiral migration pattern is similar to the helical pitch of the mature cochlear duct, and may help explain how the cohclear duct attains its mature arrangement (Fig. 16).

The observed migration pattern is based on the assumption that pyknotic nuclei follow a normal postmitotic course of migration. There is support for this contention in the work of Webster *et al.*[8] In those experiments, pyknotic neuroblasts produced as the result of FudR treatment follow the same migration pattern as normal cells. A similar study on the fate of otic cells, using tritiated thymidine and autoradiography, is currently in progress.

On days 14 and 16, the distal cochlea which was formed prior to injection was not labeled. Only the medial wall of the otocyst demonstrated the drug effect eight hours after injection. This tells us, without regard to injection date, that the portion of cochlear duct already formed is not affected. Only the growth zone and area into which these cells normally migrate demonstrate the nuclear label. This supports the contention that the cochlea grows from a single generative zone located at its junction with the saccule.

The effect of FudR on the growth zone of experimental animals caused us to focus our attention on the corresponding region of the control otocyst. Much to our surprise, this area in untreated control animals also demonstrated a similar morphologic picture of cytoplasmic granules and chromatolysis. This supports the contention that cell death in embryonic tissue might have a limited expression, even though causative factors are different.[12] While the corresponding zones of experimental and control fetuses were qualitatively similar, they were quantitatively markedly dissimilar. The zone of degeneration in normal controls was considerably smaller than in experimental animals and, most importantly, cells were never seen to migrate from this zone. Perhaps the normal cellular degeneration is easily taken care of by some reparative system. The FudR, by causing an increase in cellular death, might overwhelm this system so that migration could subsequently be observed. This area in the normal otocyst apparently represents a region of high mitotic activity where cells are actively undergoing synthesis of DNA and later division. As in other organs of the body, cellular degeneration could be a part of the process of differentiation.[12,13] It might be then, that more cells are produced than needed and the cell death represents a remodeling process. It is also possible that this zone represents an embryonic elimination of unwanted cellular organelles (such as endoplasmic reticulum, Golgi, and mitochondria) as a prelude to further cellular differentiation. The mechanism of such cellular or intracellular destruction at this moment is speculative and a more detailed electron microscope evaluation of this region is currently being undertaken to elucidate the mechanism.

REFERENCES

1. Marovitz WF, Shugar J: Single mitotic center for rodent cochlear duct. Ann Otol Rhinol Laryngol 85:225-233, 1976

2. Deysson A: Antimitotic substances. Int Rev Cytol 24:99-148, 1968

3. Dustin P Jr: New aspects of the pharmacology of antimitotic aspects. Pharmacol Rev 15:449-480, 1963

4. Bosch L, Harber E, Heidelberger C: Studies on fluorinated pyrmidines, V. Effects on nucleic acid metabolism *in vitro*. Cancer Res 18:335-343, 1958

5. Hartman KU, Heidelberg C: Studies of fluorinated pyrmidines XIII. Inhibition of thymidylate synthetase. J Biol Chem 236: 3006-3013, 1961

6. Cohen SS, Fluks JA, Barner HD, *et al*: The mode of action of 5 fluorouracil and its derivatives. Proc Natl Acad Sci USA 44: 1004-1012, 1958

7. Ruecker RR, Mueller GC: Studies of unbalanced growth in tissue culture. I. Induction and consequences of thymidine deficiency. Cancer Res 20:1584-1591, 1969

8. Webster W, Shimada M, Langman J: Effect of fluorodeoxyuridine, colcemid, and bromodeoxyuridine of developing neocortex of the mouse. Am J Anat 137:67-86, 1973

9. Sher AE: The embryonic and postnatal development of the inner ear of the mouse. Acta Otolaryngol (Stockh) Supp 285, 1971

10. Maruyama S, Chiga M, D'agostino AN: Selective necrosis in the fetal rat central nervous system produced by 5-fluoro-2′-deoxyuridine. A morphologic study. J Neuropathol Exp Neurol 27:96-107, 1968

11. Ruben RJ, Van de Water T, Poresky A: Cell kinetics of the 11 and 12 day mouse otocysts. Laryngoscope 81:1709-1718, 1971

12. Marayama S, D'agostino AN: Cell necrosis in the central nervous system of normal rat fetuses. An electron microscopic study. Neurology (Minneap) 17:550-558, 1967

13. Kullen B: Cell degeneration during normal ontogenesis of the rabbit brain. J Anat 89:153-160, 1955

ACKNOWLEDGMENT—The authors wish to express their gratitude to Ms. Barbara Carter for her assistance in the preparation of this manuscript.

REPRINTS—William F. Marovitz, PhD, Dept. of Otolaryngology, Mount Sinai School of Medicine, Fifth Ave. and 100th St., New York, NY 10029.

ABBREVIATIONS USED IN ILLUSTRATIONS

FIGURES 1-19

A - Ampulla of a semicircular canal

CD - Cochlear duct

Ga - Statoacoustic ganglion

Gs - Acoustic portion of ganglion

G - Stato (vestibular) portion of ganglion

L - Lumen

N - Neuron of statoacoustic ganglion

nf - Nerve fiber

PI - Pars inferior

PL - Perilymphatic space

PR - Primary ridge of anterior and posterior semicircular canals

PS - Pars superior

SC - Semicircular canal

SH - Tuft of sensory hairs

*Asterisk is used to denote the cupula of a crista or the tectorial membrane of an organ of Corti.

>Arrowhead is used to denote the luminal surface of organ of Corti formations.

EFFECTS OF REMOVAL OF THE STATOACOUSTIC GANGLION COMPLEX UPON THE GROWING OTOCYST

THOMAS R. VAN DE WATER, PhD

BRONX, NEW YORK

SUMMARY — An experiment was designed to answer the question as to whether or not the neural elements of the statoacoustic ganglion complex have a trophic effect upon the histodifferentiation of the sensory structures of the embryonic mouse inner ear anlage as it develops *in vitro*. The embryonic inner ear anlage with associated otic mesenchyme and statoacoustic ganglion complex was excised from 11, 12, and 13-day CBA/C57 mouse embryos. The inner ear explants of each gestational age group were further divided into two groups: the first group "A" (with) statoacoustic ganglion was explanted to the organ culture system without further surgical intervention; the second group "B" (without) statoacoustic ganglion underwent further surgical manipulation during which their statoacoustic ganglion complexes were dissected away prior to explantation to *in vitro*. The explanted embryonic inner ears were allowed to develop in organ culture until the equivalent of gestation day 21 *in vivo* was reached for each group; then all cultures were fixed and histologically processed and stained by a nerve fiber stain, in combination with a stain for glucoprotein membranes. Each specimen was code labeled and scored for histodifferentiation of sensory structures. Light microscopic observations confirmed that in group "A" cultures, statoacoustic ganglion neurons and their nerve fibers were present in association with the developed sensory structures; neither ganglion cell neurons nor their nerve fibers were found to be present in the sensory structures that developed in the group "B" organ culture specimens. Quantification revealed no consistent trend of greater occurrence of any sensory structure in the groups of explants analyzed. The presence of such a trend would have signified the probable existence of a trophic effect of the statoacoustic ganglion neural elements upon development of inner ear sensory structures in the group "A" explants of the 11, 12, and 13-day embryo inner ear organ culture specimens when compared to the aganglionic group "B" cultures. Microscopic comparison of the sensory structures and their sensory hair cells that developed in the organ cultures revealed no differences in the quality of the histodifferentiation of either group "A" or group "B" explants. A base to apex pattern of histodifferentiation of the organ of Corti sensory structures, which has been described to occur *in vivo*, was noted to occur in the *in vitro* developed cochlear ducts of all of the explanted inner ears without respect to whether neural elements were present ("A") or absent ("B") during development. It was concluded from the quantification of histodifferentiation data and the above observation on the pattern of differentiation of Corti's organ that no trophic effect of neural elements of the statoacoustic ganglion complex influencing the histodifferentiation of sensory structures of 11, 12, and 13-gestation day mouse embryo inner ear explants as they differentiate *in vitro* could be demonstrated.

Trophic effects are best defined as interactions between nerves and other cells which initiate or control molecular modification in the other cells and/or the neuron. The theory that nerves exert a trophic influence upon the structures with which they are associated dates back to the observations of Todd, 1823,[1] in limb regeneration of amphibians, and Ranvier, 1875,[2] in his observations that taste buds lost their structural integrity after denervation.

Spiedel, in 1948,[3] and in a later publication[4] reported the effects of chronic denervation upon the regeneration of lateral line organs of regenerating tails in *Rana catesbiana* tadpoles. He found that nerveless lateral line sense organs

From the Department of Otorhinolaryngology, Albert Einstein College of Medicine, Yeshiva University, 1300 Morris Park Avenue, Bronx, New York. The experimental work described in this paper was aided by grants from National Institutes of Health No. NS08365, National Foundation — March of Dimes, Deafness Research Foundation, and Nebur Foundation.

Presented at the meeting of the American Otological Society, Inc., Palm Beach, Florida, April 25-26, 1976.

could regenerate and obtain the configuration of a mature lateral line sensory structure, but lateral line sense organs that did not have neural connections for extended periods (19 months) did eventually degenerate. Spiedel[3,4] also noted that the number of lateral line sensory structures of chronically denervated tail regenerates was less and the distance between the occurrence of these sensory structures was greater than observed in tails that regenerated with uninterrupted neural relationships. Flock *et al*[5] recently repeated the short term portion of the chronic denervation experiments of Spiedel[3,4] in regenerating tails of *Amblystoma mexicanum* tadpoles. Their results reaffirmed the original observations of Spiedel on an ultrastructural level. Flock *et al*[5] showed electron micrographs of sensory hair cells of denervated regenerates that had assumed a normal doublet orientation and whose basal portions contained numerous synaptic bodies surrounded by synaptic vesicles. Long term observations were not made on the regenerated tails of the *A mexicanum* tadpoles.

There have been several reports on the relationship between the statoacoustic ganglion and the developing sensory hair cells of the membranous labyrinth. Kaan[6] stated, in her observations on the development of inner ears of amphibian tadpoles, that contact with the auditory ganglion stimulated the formation of macular epithelium. Knowlton[7] in her anatomical analysis of the development of sensory structures in the chick membranous labyrinth reported a relationship between the time of occurrence of neural innervation and maturation of sensory structures. Ruben[8] and later Sher[9] in their respective studies on the development of the mouse inner ear suggested a relationship between the pattern and onset of afferent innervation and the base to apex pattern of histodifferentiation of Corti's organ. Friedmann[10] observed that the inclusion of large portions of neural elements in explants of chick embryo otocysts enhanced the development of sensory structures in these otocysts as they developed *in vitro*. Orr[11] performed dissociation/reaggregation experiments with extirpated 3½-day chick embryo otocysts. She observed in organ cultures of the reaggregated tissues that there was a relationship between the level of histodifferentiation of reformed sensory hair cell membrane structures and the proximity of neural elements. Orr suggested from these observations a relationship between the presence of neural elements and the degree of histodifferentiation of the reformed sensory structures in these organ cultures. Thornhill,[12] in his ultrastructural study on the development of the membranous labyrinth of the lamprey, observed that individual sensory cells appeared to be autonomous and apparently intrinsically polarized with respect to orientation within the sensory structure and differentiation up to the ciliary bud stage of development. He further stated that at the ciliary bud stage of development neuronal contact appeared to be necessary to stimulate further differentiation of individual sensory hair cells. The preceding articles have supported the hypothesis that some form of neuronal interaction is essential for complete histodifferentiation of sensory hair cells and their sensory structures. The following articles support the opposite conclusion. Fell[13] in her original experiments with extirpation and culture of the chick embryo otocysts *in vitro* reported excellent differentiation of sensory structures but made no mention of the inclusion of the VIII cranial nerve ganglion or the inclusion of any other neural elements. Hoadley[14] explanted four-day chick otocysts to chorioallantoic membranes and reported differentiation of chick inner ear sensory structures with no mention of neural elements. Evans[15] repeated some of Hoadley's original experiments of grafting chick otocysts to chorioallantoic membranes. Evans specifically employed a Bodian protargol stain to detect nerve fibers and reported that none were observed in the developed inner ear explants. Waterman[16] explanted 10 and 11-day rabbit embryo otocysts to chorioallantoic membrane preparations of chicken eggs. He claimed to have obtained differentiation of membranous labyrinth sensory areas independent of neural innervation.

In all of the above articles, there was no mention of a specific effort to exclude elements of the VIII cranial nerve ganglion from the explants at the time of explantation. Instead, the reports are based on microscopic observations of sensory areas that appear to have developed with no apparent neural elements; this does not rule out a possible trophic effect of transient neural interaction during the developmental period prior to the fixation of the explanted otocyst.

Recent observations by Van De Water and Ruben[17] on quantification of the development of sensory structures in organ cultures of mouse embryo otocysts have shown an uncoupling of the relationship between the presence of neuronal elements and differentiation of inner ear sensory structures. The frequency of occurrence of sensory structures was 30% greater than the frequency of sensory structures with associated neural elements of statoacoustic ganglion cells. Altman reported in 1933[18] a naturally occurring human malformation in which histological analysis of the temporal bone specimen yielded a normally developed crista and ampulla of the posterior semicircular canal and a total lack of the posterior ampullar nerve or its canal. The *in vitro* observations of Van De Water and Ruben,[17] coupled with the congenital malformation reported by Altman,[18] still did not rule out possible neural interaction at some period in development prior to the time when the specimen was microscopically analyzed.

It had been reported by Farbman[19] that the trophic effect of gustatory nerve ganglion primordia upon the development of taste buds in fetal tongue explants can be demonstrated to occur in organ culture.

When all of the evidence that has been presented above is examined, the question of whether the statoacoustic ganglion complex exerts a trophic influence upon the morphogenesis and histodifferentiation of sensory structures of the developing inner ear is still an open question with no definitive evidence proving or disproving the existence of a trophic interaction phenomenon. A trophic interaction between a developing sensory receptor structure and its ganglion primordia has been demonstrated[19] to occur in an organ culture environment. An organ culture system which promotes the development of mouse inner ear sensory structures has been demonstrated[20] and ultrastructural evidence of developing synaptic junctions between hair cells and neuronal elements of these cultures has been reported.[21]

Van De Water and Ruben[17] have presented a system of analysis whereby the *in vitro* organogenesis of the membranous labyrinth that occurs in these organ cultured explants of mouse embryo otocysts can be quantified and the data compared, as demonstrated in the analysis of the development of the kreisler mutant *in vitro*.[22] Because trophic influences can be demonstrated to occur in organ culture and organogenesis of the mouse inner ear does occur *in vitro* and is accessible to quantification procedures, an experiment was designed to definitively provide data to answer the question as to whether or not statoacoustic ganglion neural elements exert a trophic effect upon the organogenesis of the mouse inner ear as it develops *in vitro*.

An experiment has been devised where both aspects, the statoacoustic ganglion complex and the absence of these neural elements, are represented during the critical period of development of the sensory structures of the membranous labyrinth, with the resultant data being subjected to quantification.

MATERIAL AND METHODS

Experimental Plan. The scoring system that has been used in the quantification of *in vitro* development[20,22] was utilized to evaluate the consequences of surgical manipulation of explanted mouse embryo otocysts (Group A) with respect to explanted unmodified otocysts (Group B). Otocysts were excised from mouse embryos on gestation days 11, 12 and 13. These three respective gestational age groups of excised otocysts were further subdivided into two groups for each gestational age group. The "B" groups underwent further surgical manipulation, during which their statoacoustic ganglion complexes were dissected free from the otocysts and its adhering cephalic mesenchyme and were then explanted into the organ culture dishes. The "A" groups were explanted into the organ culture dishes with their statoacoustic ganglion complexes intact and without any further surgical manipulation other than the original surgical extirpation from the embryo. Eleven, 12 and 13-day otocyst explants of both groups A and B developed for 10, 9 and 8 days respectively *in vitro* so that on the day of fixation all cultures attained a common day of comparable *in vivo* development, day 21. Each group of organ cultured otocysts was composed of 30 specimens. The organ cultured otocysts were fixed and prepared for histological quantification with a combination of nerve and glycoprotein staining techniques. Scoring was done on code labelled specimens to rule out the factor of experimenter bias and the code was not broken until all specimens were scored for quantification of development.

Organ Culture System. Falcon organ culture dishes were used as they provide an optimal environment for the growth of the otocyst while enabling the researcher to obtain a photographic record of the development of the mouse otocyst *in vitro*. The culture dishes were No. 3010, 60 x 15 mm, plastic organ culture dishes with an absorbent ring of filter paper. The outer chamber was moistened with sterile, pyrogen free, distilled water, while the inner dish depression was filled with 0.15 ml of organ culture medium. The organ culture medium was prepared by supplementing Neuman and Tytell serumless medium with 20% fetal calf serum, 1% glutamine and 100 units of penicillin per ml of medium. The organ culture medium was made fresh at the beginning of each week and discarded at the end of each week. A continuous ring of sterile unbleached vaseline was placed on the inner surface of the organ culture dish top so that a sterile gas tight closure could be made when the top was closed. All organ cultures were incubated at 34.5 C. The organ culture medium was changed every two days.

Any glassware used in the experiments was washed in 7X biodegradable detergent, rinsed ten times in running tap water, three times in glass distilled water and then sterilized in a steam autoclave.

Surgical Procedure. The experimental animal was the CBA/C57 hybrid mouse.* The gestation period was timed by the vaginal plug method, the date of observation of the mucoid plug being designated as day one of gestation. Gravid females were sacrificed by cervical dislocation on days 11, 12 and 13 of gestation. The uterus was removed intact and placed in a Felsen dish containing prewarmed organ culture media and the embryos removed as needed.

The Felsen dish was placed on the stage of a dissecting microscope** and the embryos were held to the bottom of the dish with a pair of No. 3 watchmaker's forceps. The surface skin of the embryo was removed with No. 5 watchmaker's forceps. Dorsal-ventral incisions were made on the anterior and posterior aspect of the otocyst. An incision was completed over the dorsal aspect of the otocyst at a level just above the dorsal aspect of the endolymphatic projection and the otocyst with its associated mesenchyme and statoacoustic ganglion complex was gently separated from the rhombencephalon. At this time the nerve connection of the ganglion complex was teased out of the area acoustica of the brain stem.

While the otocyst was still held in place by its cephalic mesenchyme at the base, the statoacoustic ganglion complex was dissected free by separating the complex from its close association with the medial wall of the otocyst and hooking it out with a fine bent tungsten probe. The ventral incision was then made and the otocyst was picked up, using two pairs of slightly open No. 5 watchmaker's forceps and holding the otocyst in the groove of the forceps with the surface tension of the media. Operative procedures varied with gestational age, the 11-day embryo had a slightly ventromedial and anterior relationship of ganglion complex to otocyst. The 12-day embryo's ganglion complex was associated with the ventromedial aspect of the otocyst, whereas the 13-day embryo's ganglion complex was in a close medial relationship and could be seen as two joined parts, stato and acoustic.

One ear of each embryo was excised with its ganglion complex intact while the contralateral inner ear underwent surgical excision of its statoacoustic ganglion complex prior to explantation. The explanted ears were placed in their respective Falcon dishes, marked "A," with ganglion, and "B," without ganglion, for holding. When all of the surgical procedures had been completed, the specimens were examined for operative trauma and, if any was discovered, that otocyst was discarded. The otocysts were now transferred to organ culture dishes and oriented with their medial surfaces in contact with the plastic surface of the dish, lateral sides facing up. Anatomical and surgical controls were taken from each gestational age group with the otocysts of every fourth embryo excised being fixed immediately after excision in 2.5% glutaraldehyde for two hours at 4 C and then processed for histology according to the method described by Van De Water *et al.*[20]

Histology. Specimens were fixed in 2.5% glutaraldehyde and processed for histology. The processed specimens were cut at 7μ and stained, using Rasmussen's modification of

*Obtained from Jackson Memorial Laboratories.

**E. Leitz, Rockleigh, NJ.

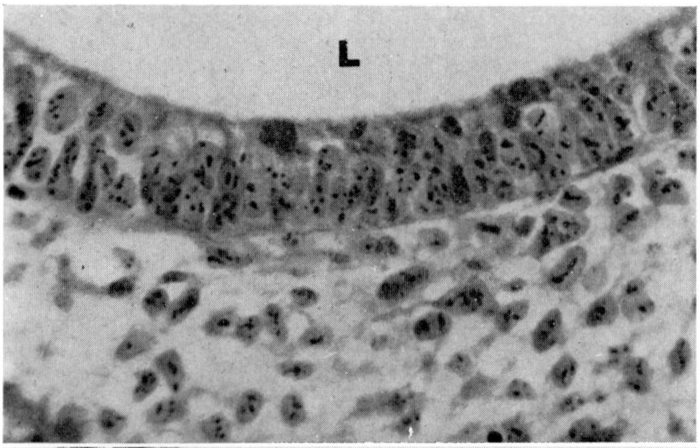

Fig. 1. Ventromedial wall of an 11-day mouse embryo otocyst at the time of explantation to *in vitro*. No nerve fibers are present. (X500)

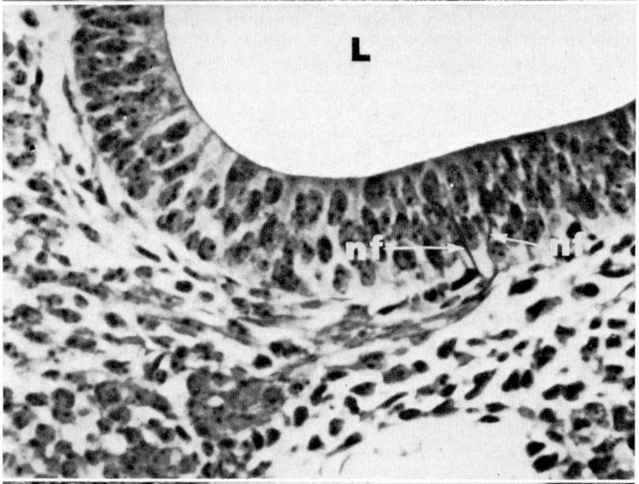

Fig. 2. Ventromedial wall of a 12-day mouse embryo inner ear anlage at the time of explantation to *in vitro*. A few pioneering nerve fibers are present in the wall of the inner ear anlage. A portion of the statoacoustic ganglion is present. (X500)

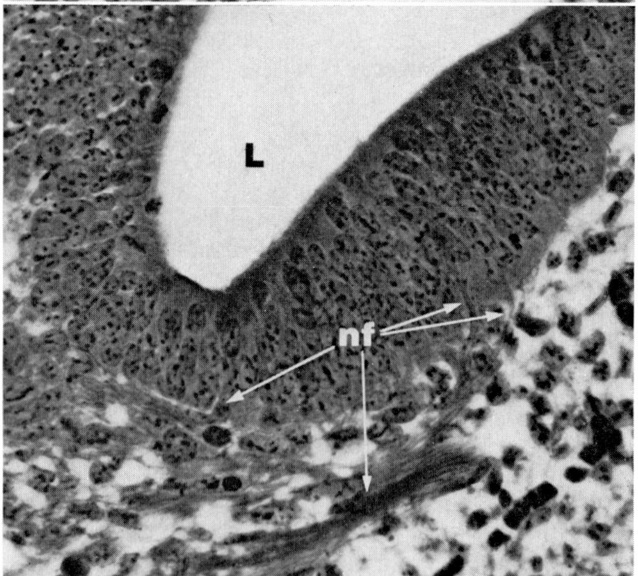

Fig. 3. Ventromedial wall of a 13-day mouse embryo inner ear anlage at the time of explantation to *in vitro*. Several fascicles of nerve fibers are penetrating into presumptive sensory areas of the inner ear anlage. A portion of the statoacoustic ganglion is present. (X500)

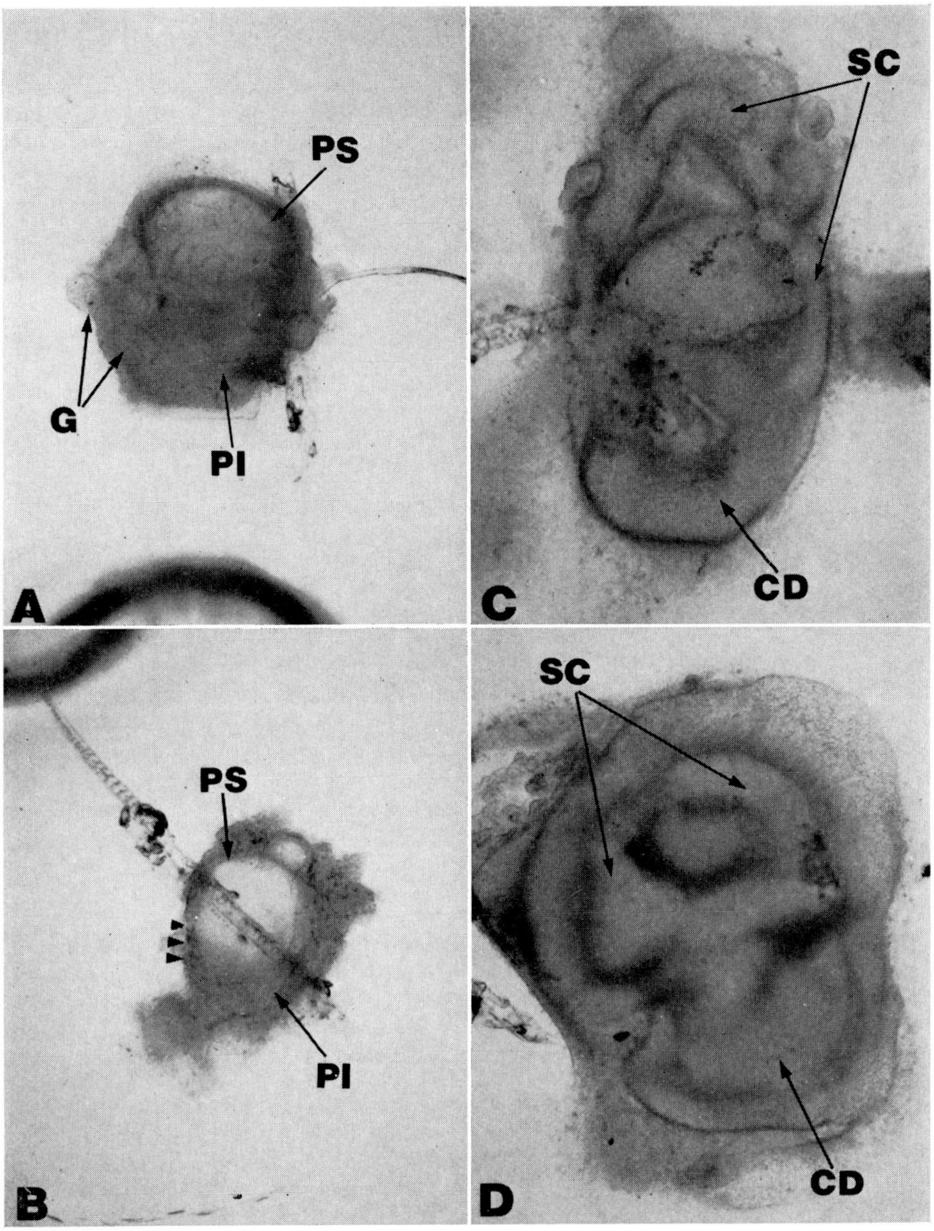

Fig. 4. Microphotographs of living explants of 11-day mouse embryo otocysts after 0 hours *in vitro* (A and B); ten days *in vitro* (C and D). Cultures A and C have an intact statoacoustic ganglion complex. Cultures B and D have had their statoacoustic ganglion complex excised prior to explantation to *in vitro*. Three arrowheads in B denote the site of excision of the ganglion complex. (X50)

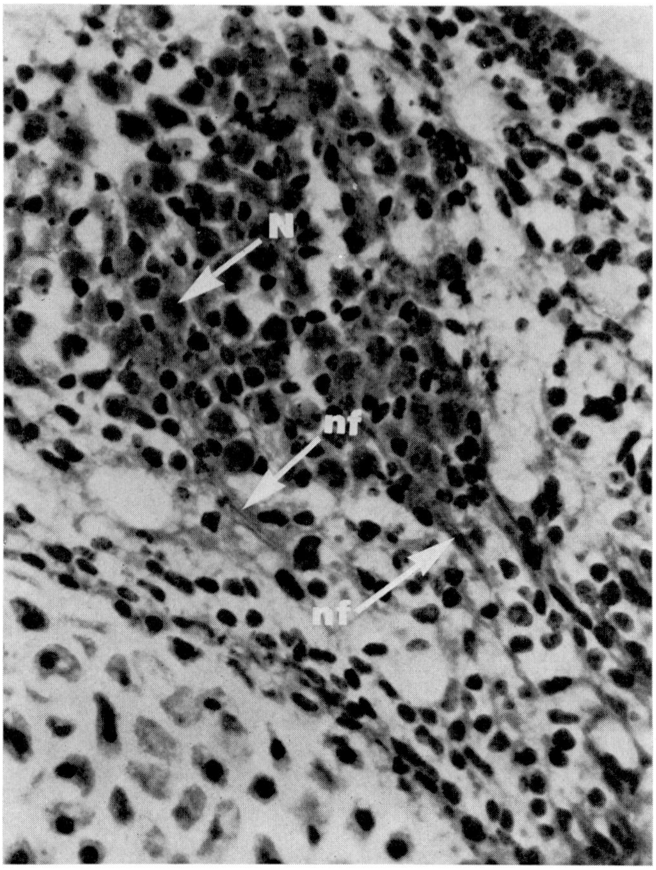

Fig. 5. Eleven-day otocyst — ten days *in vitro*. Statoacoustic ganglion cells and nerve fibers from a "with ganglion" explant. (X500)

Bodian's silver protargol method with gold toning in combination with Schiff's periodic acid technique.[20]

Microphotography of Live Cultures. Specimens were photographed while in the Falcon plastic organ culture dishes on the day of explantation and on the day of fixation, to provide a permanent record of morphogenesis of the organ culture specimens. A stereozoom photographic microscope,* with a green filter using 35 mm high contrast copy film, provided the photographic system.

RESULTS

Otocyst Innervation at Time of Explantation to In Vitro. Representational photomicrographs of sections through inner ear presumptive sensory areas of 11, 12 and 13-day CBA/C57 mouse embryos are seen in Figures 1, 2 and 3 respectively. The 11-day mouse embryo otocyst is seen in Figure 1. The statoacoustic ganglion complex is rostral to the anteromedial wall of the otocyst. It is not seen in this micrograph. No nerve fibers were observed to penetrate the basement membrane of this developing otocyst in any of the microscopically analyzed serial sections. The 12th gestation day mouse otocyst, as seen in Figure 2, has few nerve fibers that originate from the statoacoustic ganglion complex (G) and penetrate the basement membrane; these nerve fibers then assume a pioneering fiber configuration (see arrows). Many pioneering fibers forming nerve fasicles (see arrows) of the statoacoustic ganglion complex are seen as-

*Model 7-S, Wild-Heerbrugg Instruments, Inc., Farmingdale, NY.

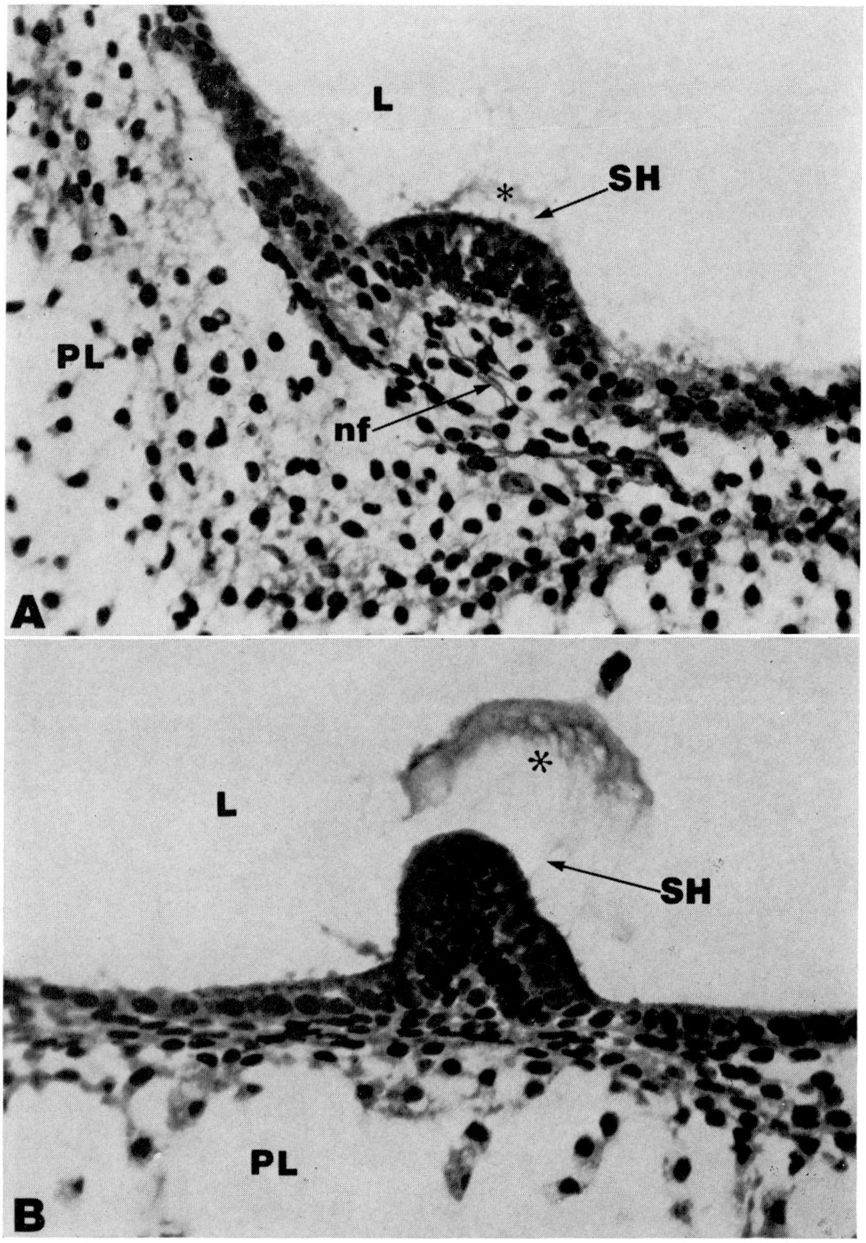

Fig. 6. Eleven-day otocyst — ten days *in vitro*. A) With ganglion explant; a crista with neural elements. B) Without ganglion explant; a crista without neural elements. (X500)

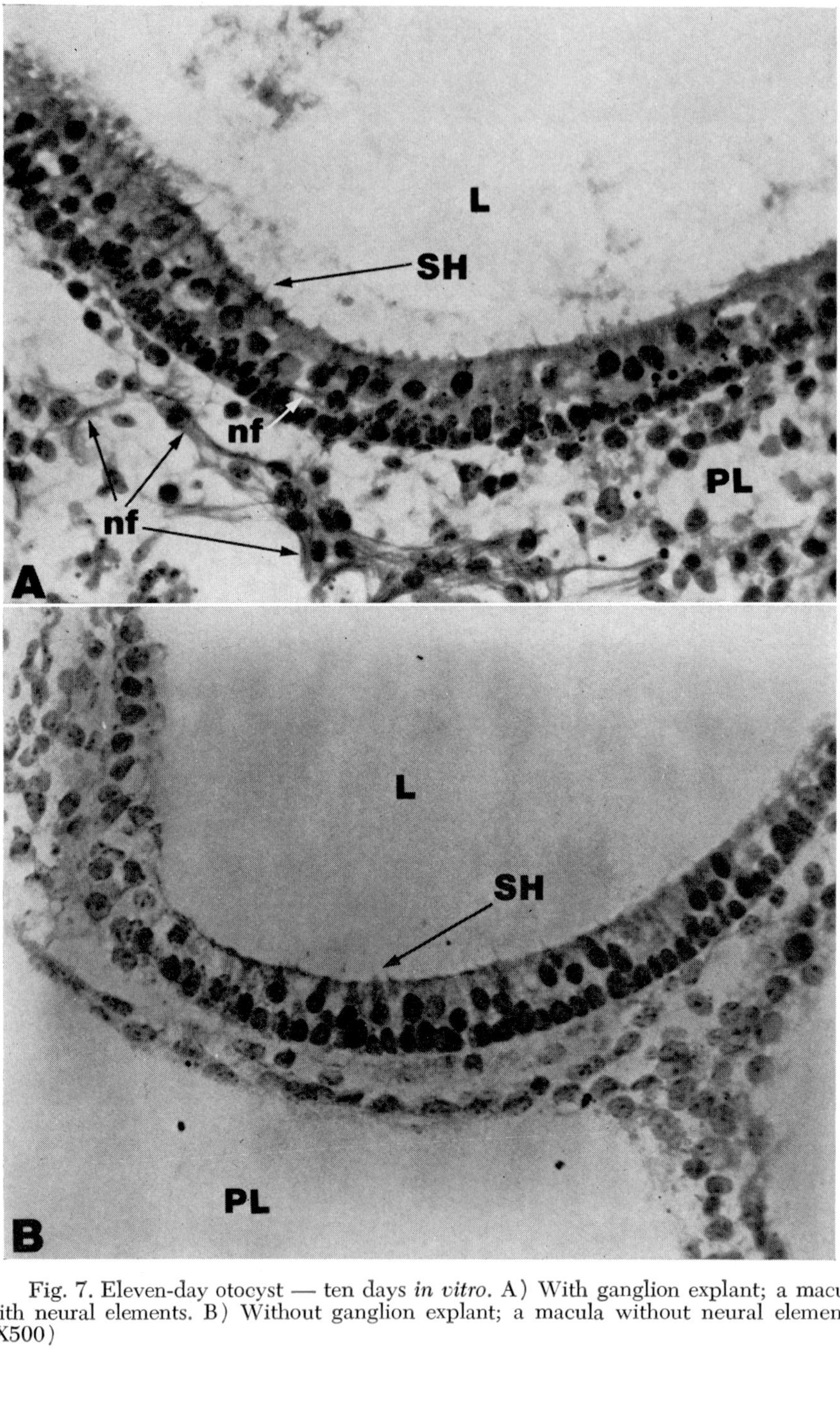

Fig. 7. Eleven-day otocyst — ten days *in vitro*. A) With ganglion explant; a macula with neural elements. B) Without ganglion explant; a macula without neural elements. (X500)

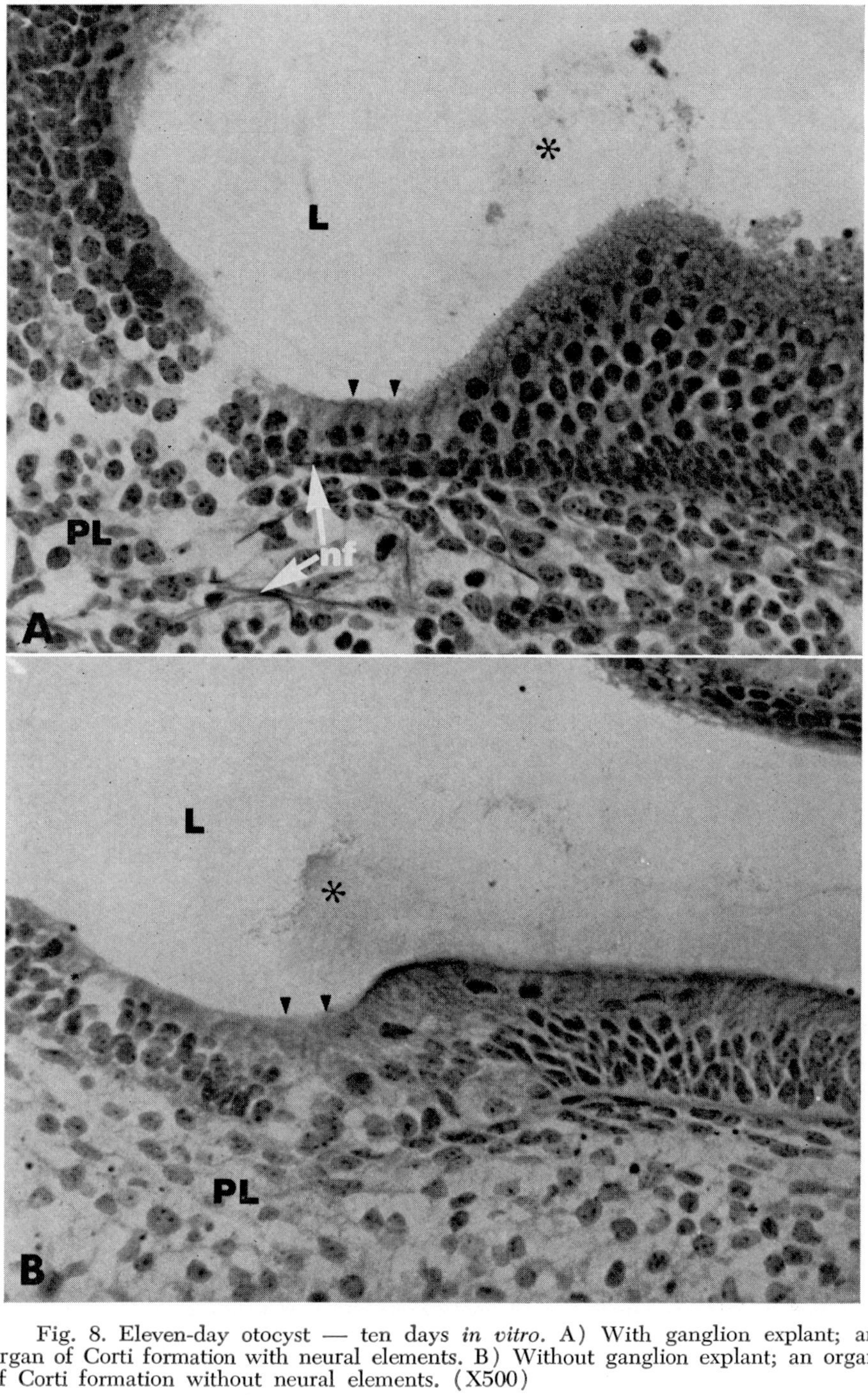

Fig. 8. Eleven-day otocyst — ten days *in vitro.* A) With ganglion explant; an organ of Corti formation with neural elements. B) Without ganglion explant; an organ of Corti formation without neural elements. (X500)

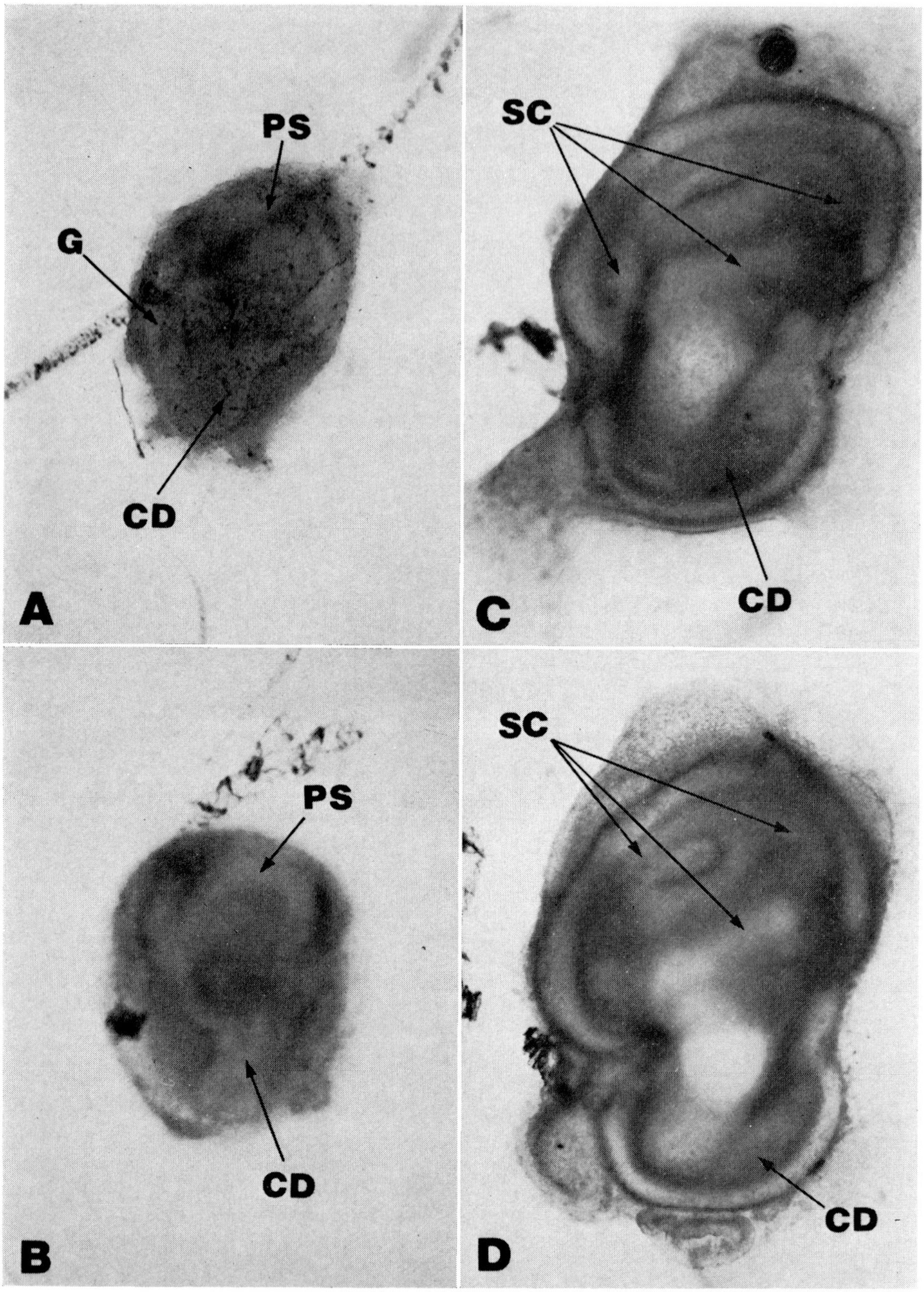

Fig. 9. Microphotographs of living explants of 12-day mouse embryo inner ear anlage after: 0 hours *in vitro* (A and B); nine days *in vitro* (C and D). Cultures A and C have an intact statoacoustic ganglion complex. Cultures B and D have had their statoacoustic ganglion complex excised prior to explantation to *in vitro*. (X50)

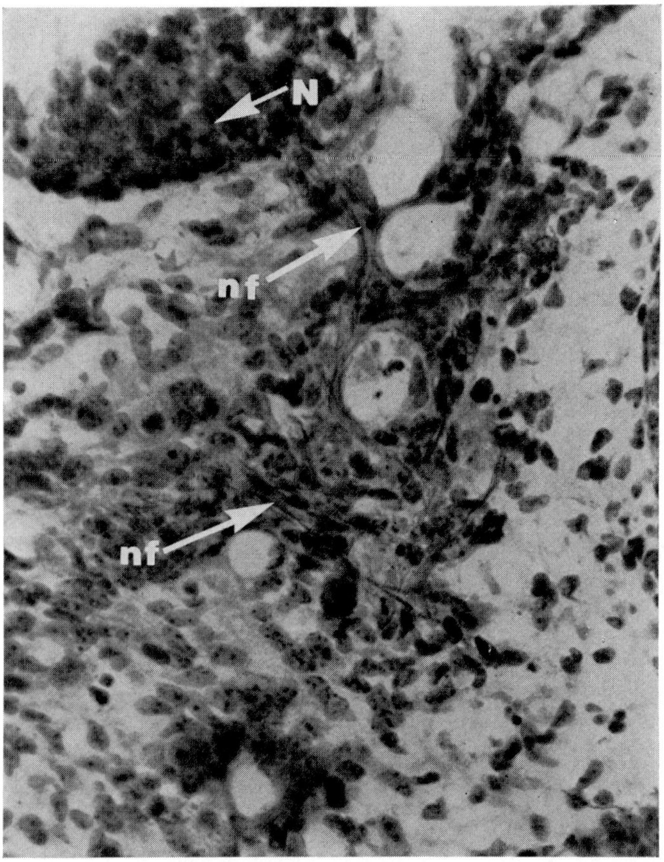

Fig. 10. Twelve-day inner ear anlage — nine days *in vitro*. Statoacoustic ganglion cells with nerve fibers from a with ganglion explant. (X500)

sociated with presumptive areas of sensory epithelial cells in the 13-gestation day mouse embryo inner ear. A demonstration of this (arrows) is seen in the photomicrograph of the section of the 13-day embryo inner ear in Figure 3. This series of microphotographs confirms and extends the observations of Sher[9] in his description of the development of the inner ear of the CBA-J normal mouse. The serial section analysis of protargol stained series of 11, 12 and 13-gestation day CBA/C57 mouse embryo inner ears showed that no nerve fibers were observed in association with the epithelium of the 11-day otocyst. Pioneering fiber behavior of nerve fibers of the statoacoustic ganglion complex was observed to begin on the 12th day of gestation and selective fasciculation was observed on the 13th gestational day in relationship with the developing epithelium of the inner ear.

Morphogenesis In Vitro. The 11-day mouse otocyst at the time of explantation is a hollow, shield-shaped organ with its statoacoustic ganglion complex located on the ventrorostral aspect of its anterior wall. Microphotographs of living specimens at the time of explantation are seen in Figures 4-8. The 11-day otocyst with its ganglion complex intact is seen in Figure 4A. An 11-day otocyst that has had its ganglion complex surgically extirpated (see arrow heads) at the time of explantation is shown in Figure 4B. A micrograph of a live 11-day mouse embryo otocyst, with an intact statoacoustic ganglion that de-

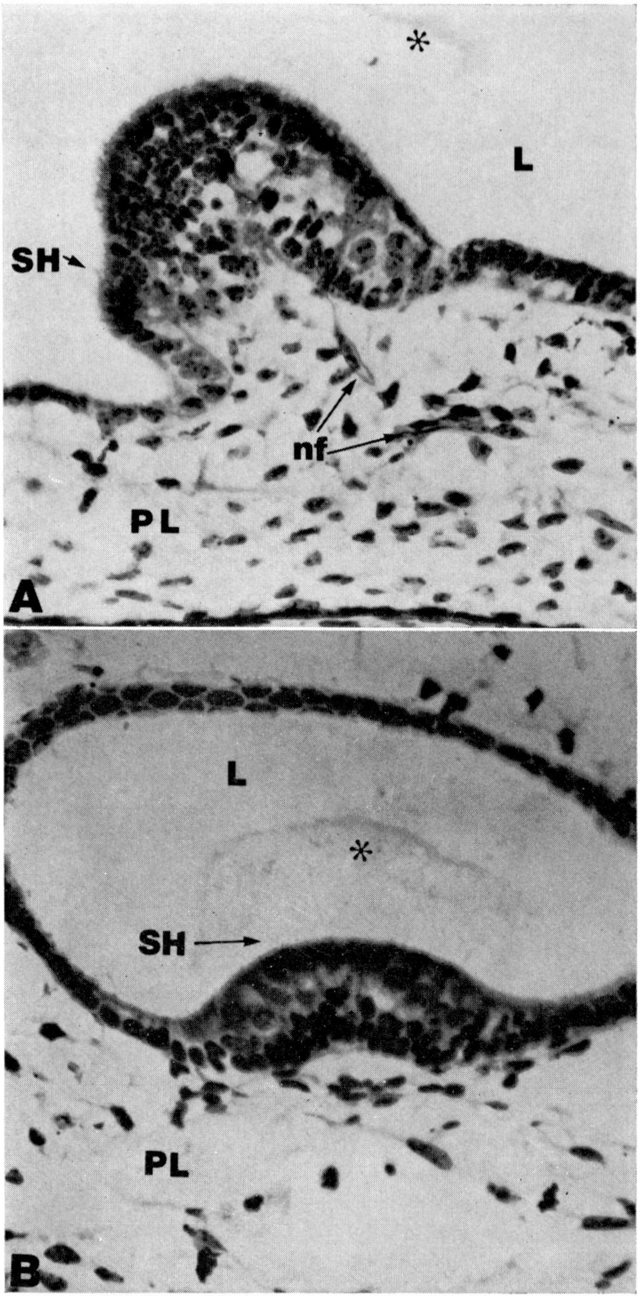

Fig. 11. Twelve-day inner ear anlage — nine days *in vitro*. A) With ganglion explant; a crista with neural elements. B) Without ganglion explant; a crista without neural elements. (X500)

veloped for ten days in organ culture, is illustrated in Figure 4C. An 11-day otocyst specimen that had its statoacoustic ganglion excised at time of explantation to *in vitro* and then was grown in organ culture for ten days, is represented in Figure 4D. Both organ cultured specimens (Fig. 4C, D) developed slightly hooked cochlear ducts (CD) and two rudimentary semicircular canals (SC). Both of these organ cultured specimens appear to have undergone a

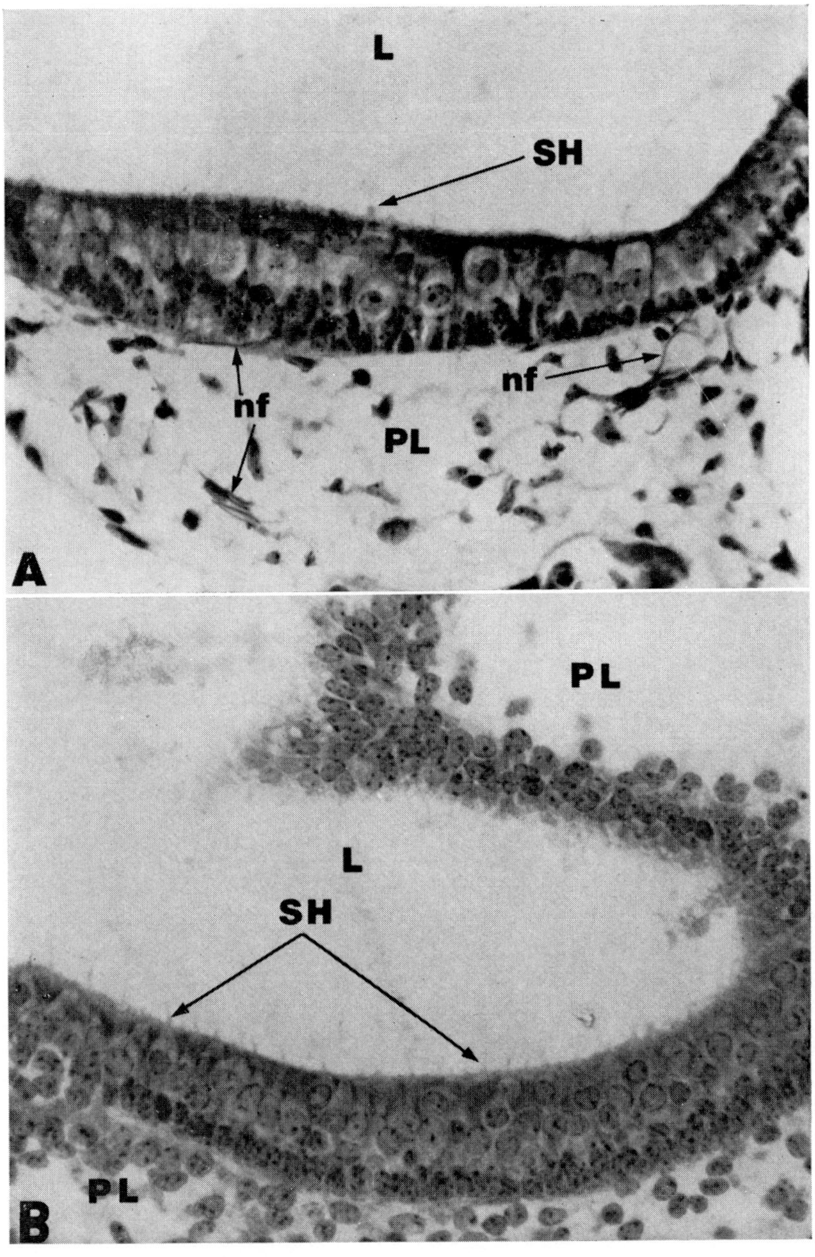

Fig. 12. Twelve-day inner ear anlage — nine days *in vitro*. A) With ganglion explant; a macula with neural elements. B) Without ganglion explant; a macula without neural elements. (X500)

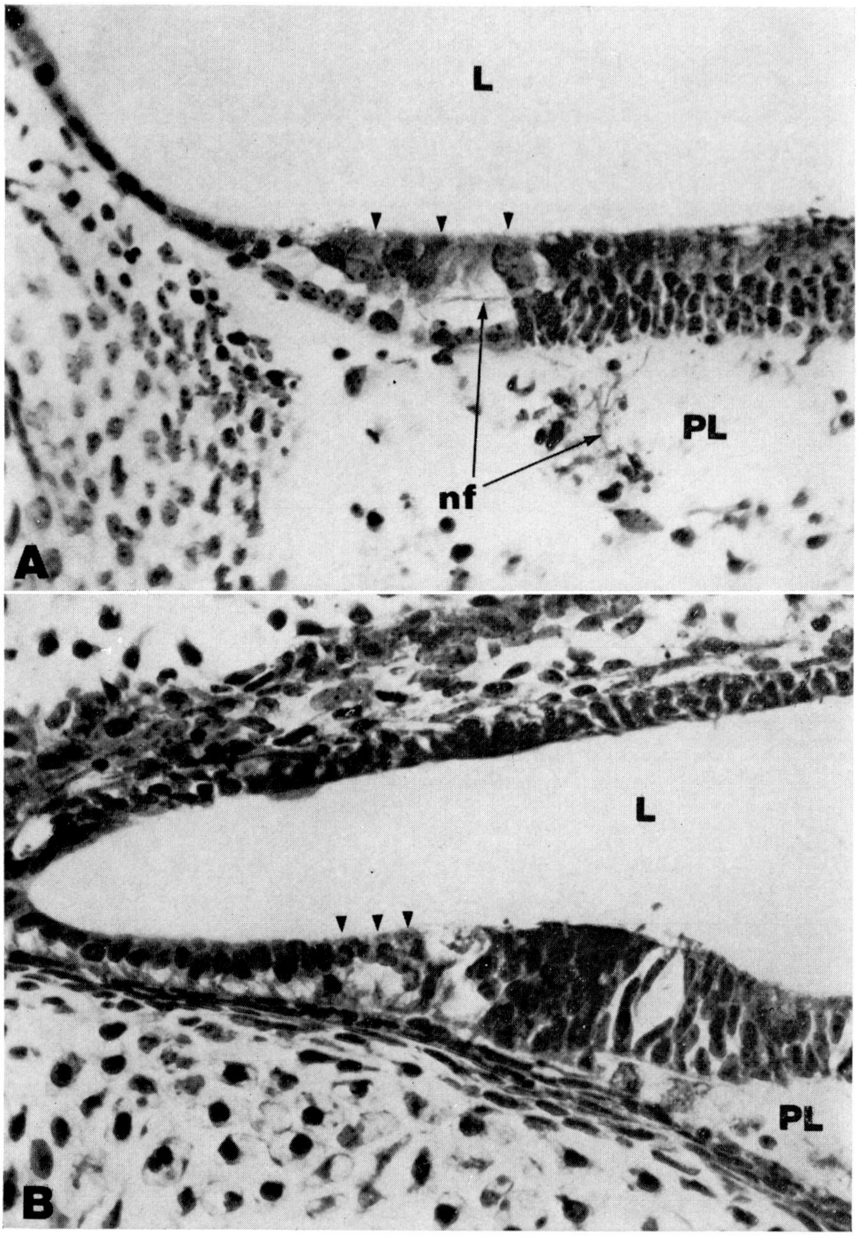

Fig. 13. Twelve-day inner ear anlage — nine days *in vitro*. A) With ganglion explant; an organ of Corti formation with neural elements. B) Without ganglion explant; an organ of Corti formation without neural element. (X500)

comparable amount of morphogenesis *in vitro.*

Twelve-day mouse embryo otocysts at the time of explantation to *in vitro* are shield-shaped with a ventral elongation that is the anlage of the cochlear duct. The statoacoustic ganglion complex has now assumed a more medial location with respect to the otocyst. Twelve-day otocysts *in vitro* are seen in the photomicrographs of Figures 9-13. Figure 9A is an explanted otocyst with its ganglion complex intact and Figure 9B is an otocyst that has had its ganglion complex surgically extirpated prior to being placed in organ culture. Twelve-day otocysts that have developed for nine days in vitro are seen in Figures 9C, D and are with and without statoacoustic ganglion cultures respectively. Well defined cochlear ducts that have completed approximately one full turn in coiling and three semicircular canals are present in both specimens shown in Figures 9 C, D. A morphological form comparable to the end state development obtained in the neonate *in vivo* was not obtained in these cultures but the basic pattern of *in vivo* morphogenesis was followed. The *in vitro* morphogenesis observed to have occurred in both specimens, 9C and 9D, appears equal in development.

By the 13th gestation day, the mouse embryo inner ear has begun to differentiate its morphological structure prior to explantation into organ culture. The primary ridge (PR) of the anterior and posterior semicircular canals is evident and the beginning cochlear elongation of the 12-day otocyst is now a definite cochlear projection (CD) and is beginning to hook anteriorly as it extends in a ventromedial direction. Figure 14 A, B respectively show 13-gestation day embryo inner ears as they are explanted with and without their statoacoustic ganglion complexes. The statoacoustic ganglion complex is now easily differentiated into its component vestibular (Gs) and acoustic (Ga) divisions. The vestibular division is very closely associated with the rostral medial wall at the level of the entry of the endolymphatic duct into the medial wall of the otocyst, and the acoustic division is intimately associated with the anterior and medial aspect of the developing cochlear projection (Fig. 14A). Thirteen-day embryo inner ears that have developed for eight days in organ culture are seen in the microphotographs of Figure 14 C, D. The specimen in Figure 14C developed with the influence of its statoacoustic ganglion complex present, whereas the inner ear seen in Figure 14D developed without the influence of its ganglion complex. Both organ cultured inner ears (14C, D) developed well formed cochlear ducts that coiled and three well defined semicircular canals. The morphogenesis of these specimens did not differ significantly from each other or from the normal end state morphogenesis that occurs in the *in vivo* neonate of comparable age.

There appears to be a progressive acquisition of the morphological pattern of development of the inner ear that develops *in vitro* and a complete *in vivo* pattern of morphogenesis is not present in explanted embryonic inner ears until the 13th day of gestation. Each earlier stage, day 12 and day 11, has its own basic *in vitro* pattern of morphogenesis which is progressively more limited with decreasing embryo age. These earlier *in vitro* patterns of morphogenesis are similar to what occurs *in vivo* at earlier stages but never progresses to the final end state form as seen in the *in vitro* morphogenesis of the 13-day inner ear explants.

All 180 explanted inner ears were observed daily with a dissecting microscope and no consistent deviation in the *in vitro* morphogenesis patterns of these 11, 12 and 13-gestation day otic explants was noted between the "A" (with ganglion) and the "B" (without ganglion) groups of organ cultures.

Histodifferentiation In Vitro. The morphogenesis of 11-day otocyst explants of "A" and "B" groups is depicted in Figure 4. A photomicrograph of statoacoustic ganglion cells that developed in the group "A" cultures of the 11-day embryo otocysts after ten days of organ

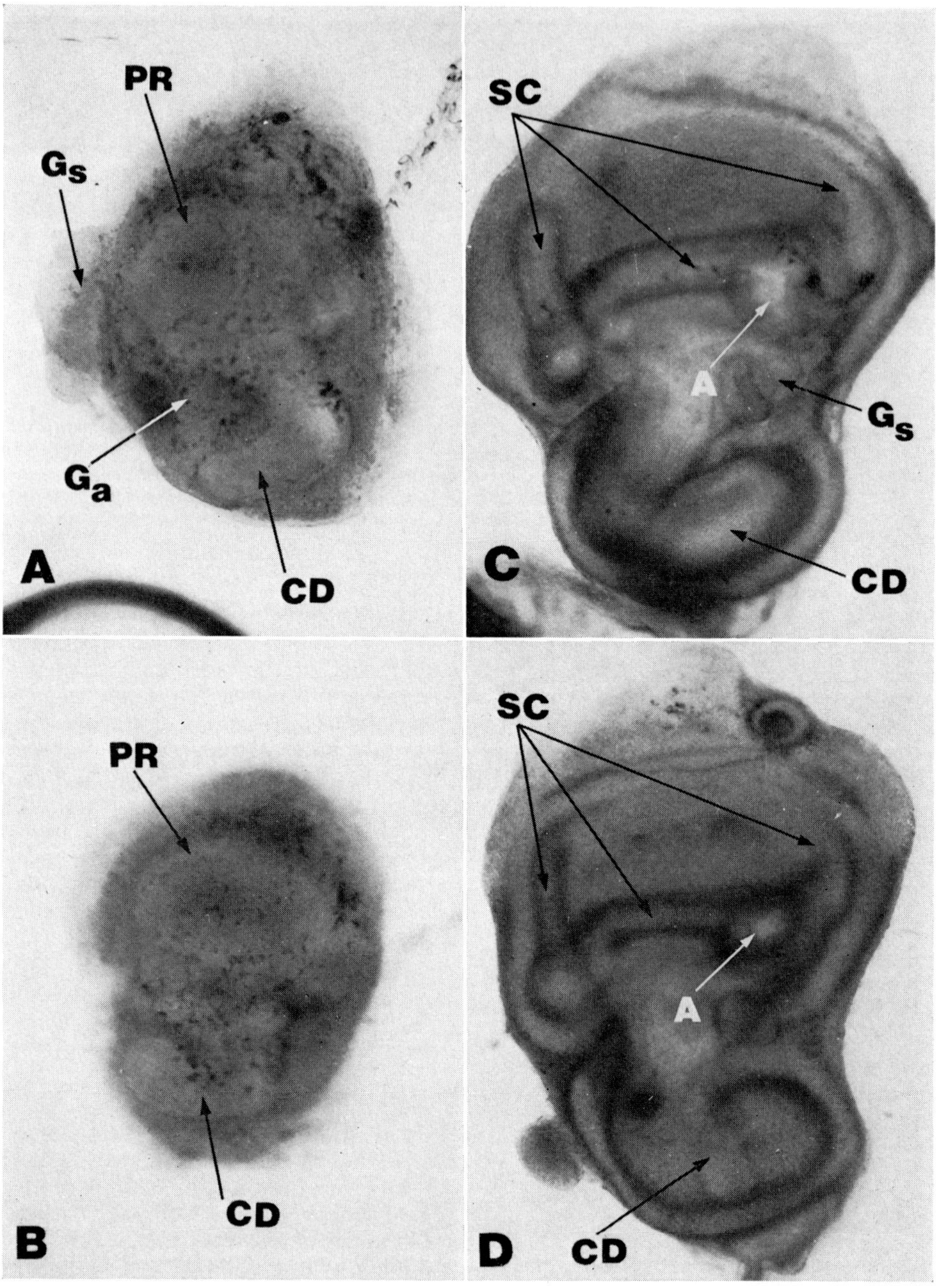

Fig. 14. Microphotographs of living explants of 13-day mouse embryo inner ear anlage after: 0 hours *in vitro* (A and B); eight days *in vitro* (C and D). Cultures A and C have an intact statoacoustic ganglion complex. Cultures B and D have had their statoacoustic ganglion complex excised prior to explantation to *in vitro*. (X50)

culture is presented in Figure 5. Many neuron cell bodies (N) that are characterized by large pale nuclei, each containing several prominent nucleoli, are present in Figure 5. These statoacoustic ganglion neurons were observed to send out fascicles of nerve fibers (nf) that terminated in the immediate areas of the sensory structures that had developed in the organ cultures. A side by side comparison of the three major types of sensory structures that develop in the mammalian inner ear is presented in the following series of microphotographs from cultures of 11-day otocysts that developed with, "A", and without, "B", their statoacoustic ganglion complexes for ten days *in vitro*. Figures 6A and 6B are two cristae that developed in explanted mouse otocysts. The top 6A photomicrograph is a crista with neuronal elements present (nf) and the bottom 6B is a crista that developed without the benefit of nerve fibers (white arrow). The histological development observed in these two cristae is comparable, both possess sensory hair cells with their tufts of sensory hairs (SH) projecting out into the lumen (L) of the developed inner ears and both specimens also possess cupulae which are marked with asterisks (*). Maculae of sensory hair cells of both ganglionic and aganglionic otocyst cultures are presented in Figure 7. Both specimens (7A, B) show comparable histological development of sensory hair cells with their associated tufts of sensory hairs (SH) but only the top photomicrograph (7A) presents a network of nerve fibers (nf) associated with the macular sensory structure. Organ of Corti formations (Fig. 8) were observed to differentiate in both groups, "A" and "B," of cultures of 11-day otocysts but only the otocysts explanted with their statoacoustic ganglion complexes intact (group "A") developed nerve fibers that were associated with the sensory hair cells of Corti's organ (Fig. 8A). The sensory hair cell areas of these organs of Corti are indicated on their luminal surfaces by two arrowheads. Forming tectorial membranes are indicated by asterisks (*). The histological development of the sensory structures of the cochlear duct (organ of Corti) was comparable in groups "A" and "B" of these ten-day cultures of 11-day mouse embryo otocysts.

The morphological advances of the 12th gestation day mouse embryo otocysts *in vitro* of explants of group "A" and group "B" is shown in the photomicrographs in Figure 9. An area of statoacoustic ganglion cells that developed during the nine days *in vitro* culture period of a 12th gestation day explant with an intact statoacoustic ganglion complex is seen in Figure 10. These neurons (N) were observed to give off fascicles of nerve fibers that invaded the supporting and sensory cell layers of the sensory structures of group "A" explants. Two cristae of comparable levels of histodifferentiation are presented in Figure 11. The top crista (11A) developed in a 12-day otocyst culture that was explanted with an intact ganglion complex ("A") and nerve fibers are seen penetrating the layer of supporting cells of this sensory structure. The lower crista (11B) developed in a without ganglion explanted otocyst ("B") and no nerve fibers were present. Both specimens possess well developed sensory hair tufts and cupulae. Maculae of sensory hair cells that differentiated in 12th gestation day organ culture specimens are presented in the photomicrographs in Figure 12. Nerve fibers are seen penetrating the layer of supporting cells of the macula (12A) of an organ culture specimen that was explanted with its statoacoustic ganglion intact ("A"). Well differentiated sensory hair cells with their ciliary tufts of sensory hairs are seen in both maculae (12A, B) irrespective of the presence of nerve fibers. No nerve fibers were detected in the organ culture specimen ("B") of Figure 12B. Figure 13 presents two photomicrographs of organ of Corti formations that developed in the cochlear ducts of the 12-day mouse otocysts that developed *in vitro*. The area of Corti's organ is indicated on the luminal surface of both specimens by arrowheads. Both specimens presented a well differentiated organ of Corti with inner and outer hair cells. Nerve fibers were seen only in Figure 13A which is the otocyst

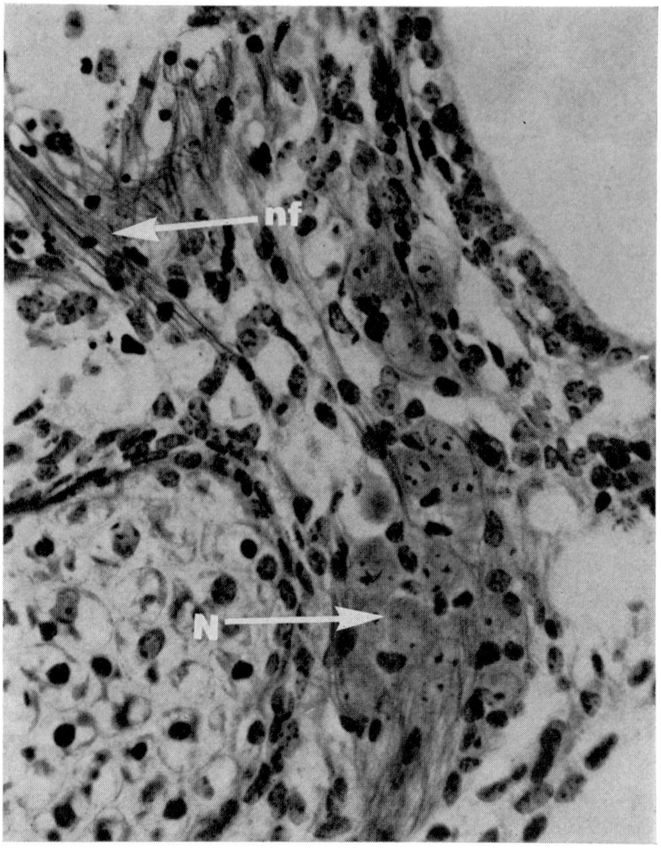

Fig. 15. Thirteen-day inner ear anlage — eight days *in vitro*. Statoacoustic ganglion cells with nerve fibers from a with ganglion explant. (X500)

that was explanted with its statoacoustic ganglion complex ("A").

Figure 14 illustrates the *in vitro* morphogenesis of the explanted 13th gestation day inner ear that developed for eight days in organ culture. Statoacoustic ganglion neurons (N) with nerve fibers are present in 13-day (group "A") explants (Fig. 15) that included the statoacoustic ganglion complex at the time of explantation to *in vitro*. Cultures where the statoacoustic ganglion complex was excised prior to explantation (group "B") did not develop neuronal elements. A crista from an organ culture specimen that did not possess any neuronal elements (Fig. 16B) appears to be comparable in histological differentiation to a crista that developed with statoacoustic ganglion neurons and nerve fibers (Fig. 16A). Both cristae have well defined supporting cell layers and sensory hair cells with tufts of sensory hairs on their luminal surfaces. Cupulae were also noted to be well formed in both specimens. Maculae of sensory hair cells developed in explanted inner ears of 13-day mouse embryos. Photomicrographs of these sensory structures with (group "A") and without (group "B") neural elements are seen in Figure 17A and B respectively. The cultures with intact statoacoustic ganglia had nerve fibers penetrate through their layers of supporting cells and terminate in the area of the sensory hair cell bases. The maculae that developed in 13-day group "A" and group "B" cultures appeared equal in histodifferentiation. Two photomicrographs of organ of Corti sensory structures (ar-

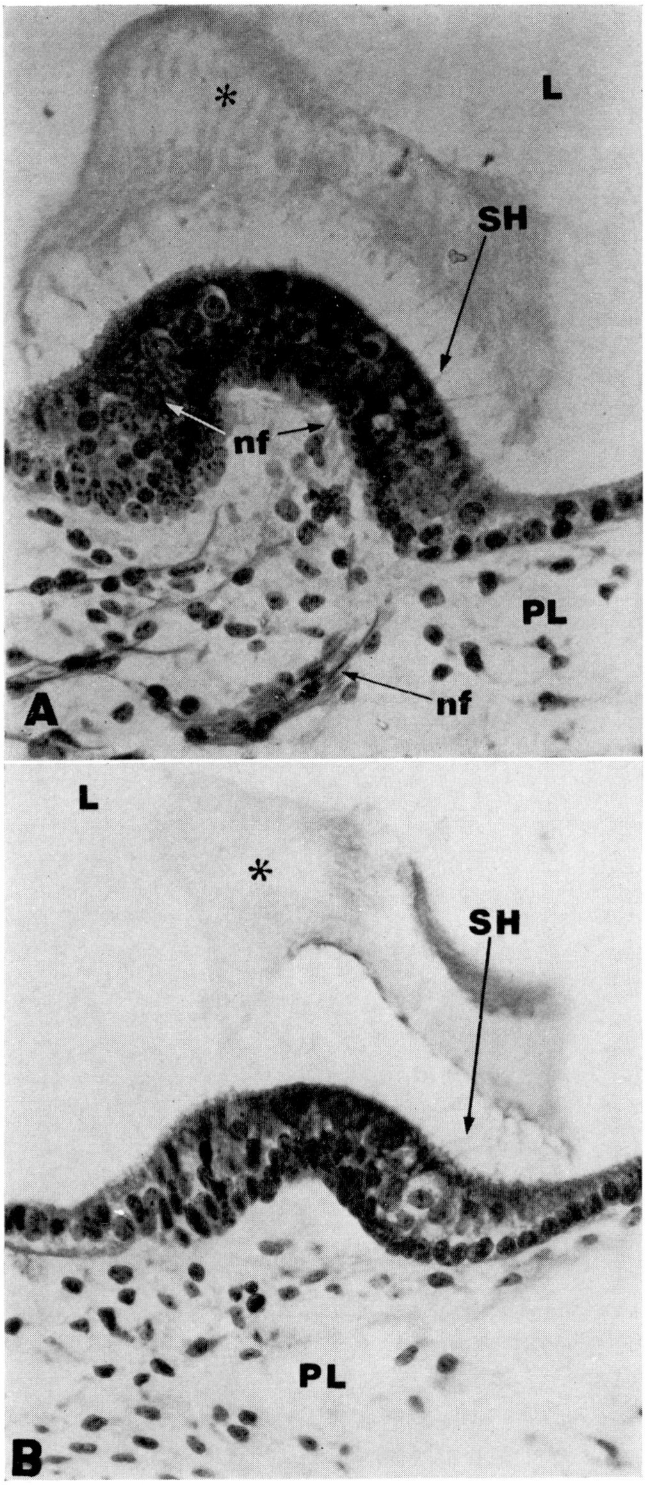

Fig. 16. Thirteen-day inner ear anlage — eight days *in vitro*. A) With ganglion explant; a crista with neural elements. B) Without ganglion explant; a crista without neural elements. (X500)

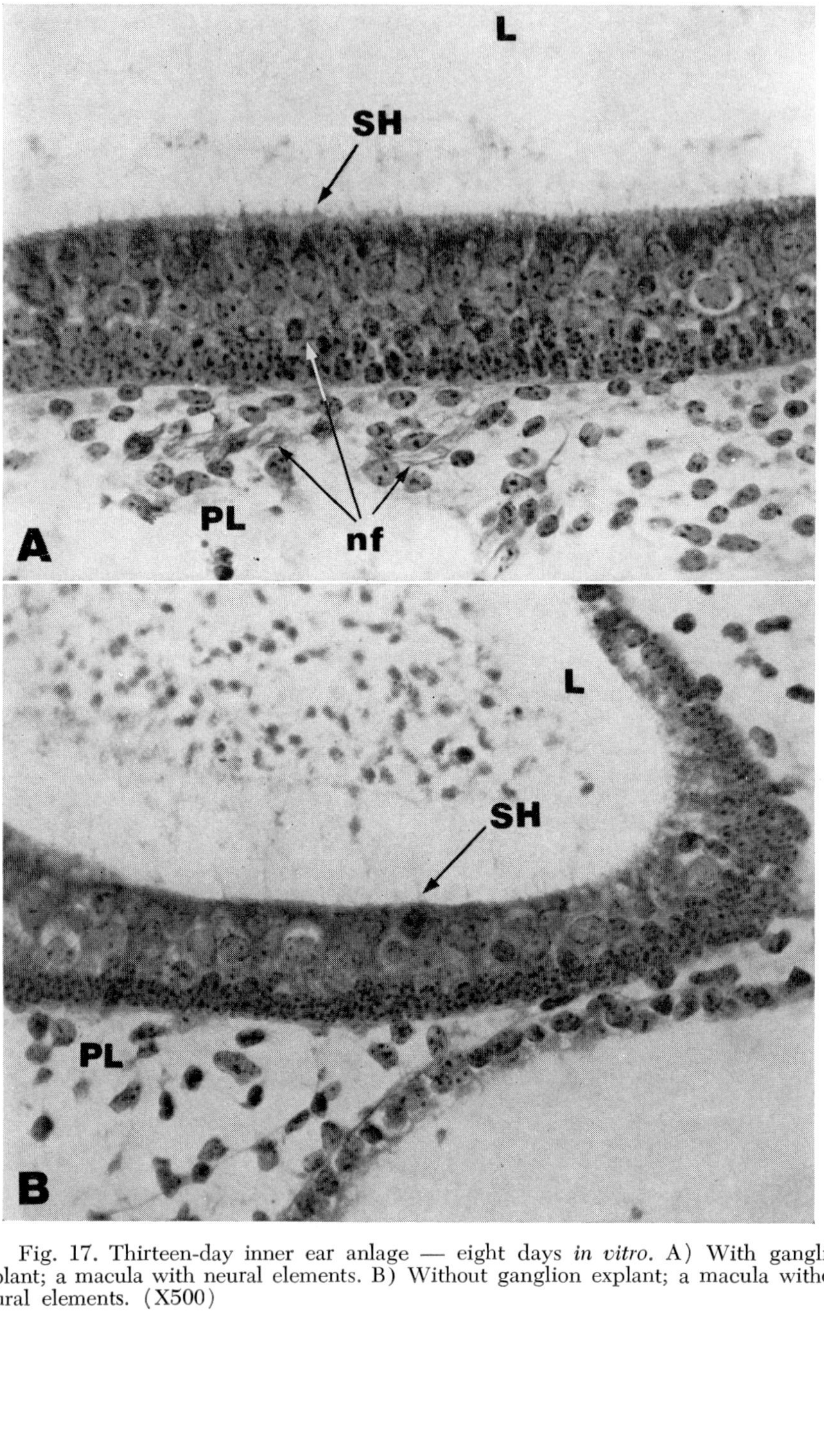

Fig. 17. Thirteen-day inner ear anlage — eight days *in vitro.* A) With ganglion explant; a macula with neural elements. B) Without ganglion explant; a macula without neural elements. (X500)

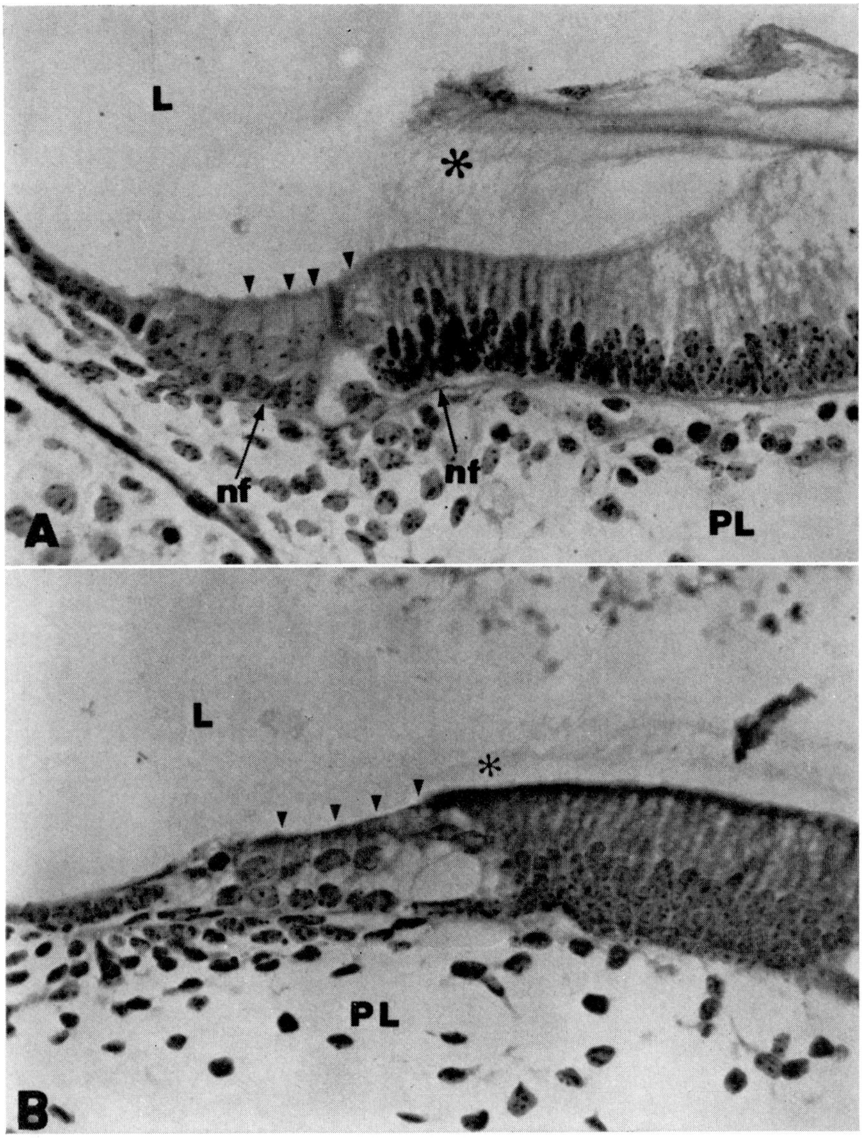

Fig. 18. Thirteen-day inner ear anlage — eight days *in vitro.* A) With ganglion explant; an organ of Corti formation with neural elements. B) Without ganglion explant; an organ of Corti formation without neural elements. (X500)

rowheads) from the cochlear ducts of *in vitro* developed 13-day embryonic inner ears are present in Figure 18. These sensory structures appear equivalent in histodifferentiation, both possess inner hair cells, outer hair cells, supporting cells, Deiters' cells, inner and outer pillar cells, Hensen's cells and tectorial membranes (*). The Corti's organ of the "A" group specimen has associated nerve fibers while the "B" group specimen does not have any neural elements present.

The series of photomicrographs presented in Figures 4-18 show a side by side comparison of the histological structure of all the major sensory structures that differentiated in the *in vitro* devel-

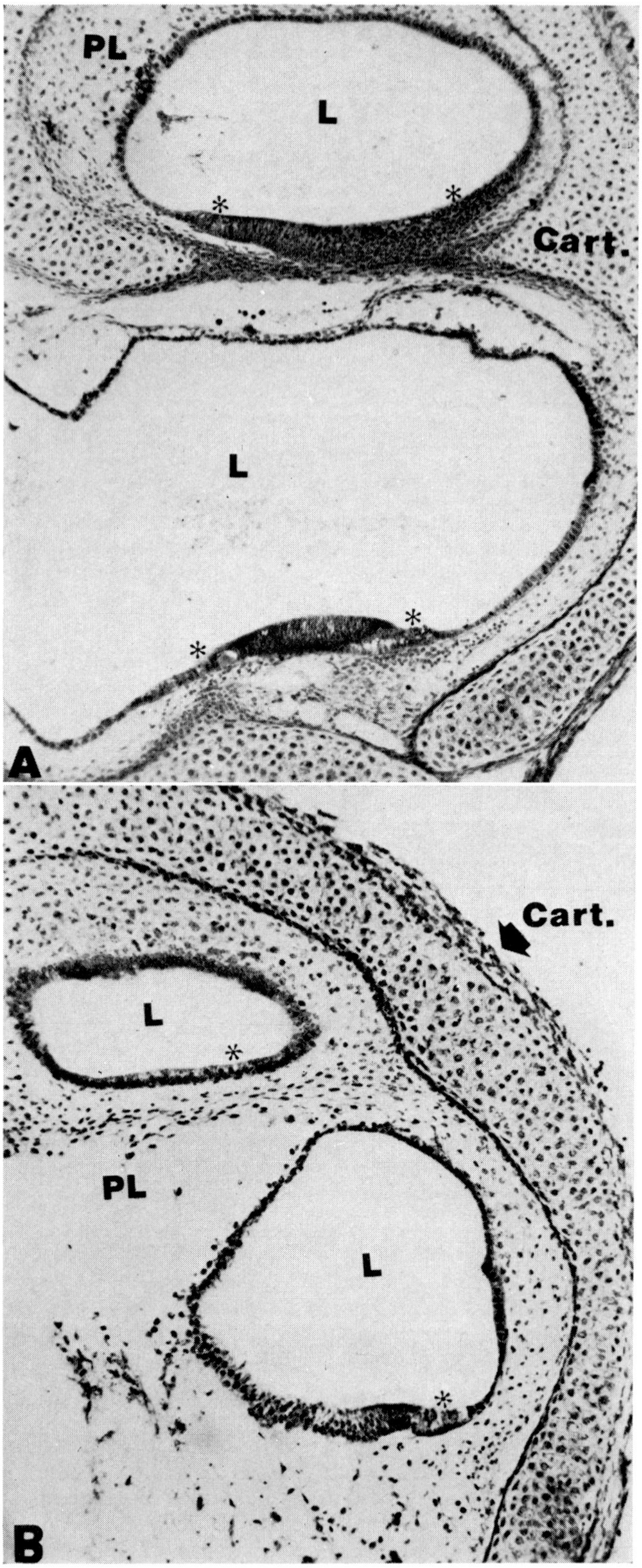

Fig. 19. Twelve-day otocysts — nine days *in vitro*. A) With ganglion explant; a section through the cochlear duct showing base to apex pattern of differentiation. B) Without ganglion explant; a section through the cochlear duct showing base to apex pattern of differentiation. Sensory structures are indicated on their luminal surface by an asterisk. (X350)

TABLE I
HISTOLOGICAL QUANTIFICATION RESULTS WITH (A) AND WITHOUT (B) STATOACOUSTIC GANGLION STUDY

	Gestation Day of Explant					
	11th		*12th*		*13th*	
Histological Features	A	B	A	B	A	B
Cartilaginous otic capsule	100%	100%	100%	100%	100%	100%
Perilymphatic spaces	100%	100%	100%	100%	100%	100%
Statoacoustic ganglion cells	100%	0	100%	0	100%	0
Nerve fibers associated with sensory structures	100%	0	100%	0	100%	0
Utriculosaccular space	100%	100%	100%	100%	100%	100%
Maculae: one only	0	7%	9%	12%	3%	15%
two	97%	93%	91%	84%	93%	85%
Total	97%	100%	100%	96%	96%	100%
Semicircular canals: one only	33%	30%	0	12%	0	11%
two only	50%	70%	58%	52%	14%	27%
three	10%	0	42%	36%	86%	62%
Total	93%	100%	100%	100%	100%	100%
Cristae: one only	3%	4%	3%	0	0	8%
two only	20%	18%	18%	24%	10%	23%
three	77%	78%	79%	76%	90%	69%
Total	100%	100%	100%	100%	100%	100%
Cochlear duct	97%	100%	94%	96%	100%	100%
Organ of Corti	93%	93%	94%	96%	100%	96%
Stria vascularis	90%	93%	94%	92%	100%	96%
Tectorial membrane	71%	93%	85%	76%	86%	73%
Endolymphatic duct	87%	96%	88%	96%	100%	92%
Endolymphatic sac	87%	96%	88%	92%	100%	88%
Total number of specimens analyzed	30	30	30	30	30	30

"A" - with statoacoustic ganglion complex
"B" - without statoacoustic ganglion complex

oped mouse embryo inner ear explants. These sensory structures were grouped by embryonic age at the time of explantation to *in vitro*. These gestational age groups were further subdivided into two groups which are "A," explanted *with* statoacoustic ganglion complex, and "B," explanted *without* the statoacoustic ganglion complex. Neurons with nerve fibers were seen to develop in the inner ear explants of the "A" groups of each gestational age that was explanted and allowed to develop *in vitro*. The nerve fibers present could be identified (serial section analysis) as originating from the statoacoustic ganglion neurons and were associated with the sensory structures that had developed in the group "A" cultures. The group "B" sensory structures that developed *in vitro* did not have any neural elements associated with them.

In the analysis of histodifferentiation *in vitro* each sensory structure of group "A" and "B" of each gestational age group was observed with oil immersion for structure of the hair cells. The following histologic qualities were observed: cell morphology, staining characteristics of nucleus and cytoplasm; morphology of sensory hair tufts and relationships of sensory structure and their membranes. In each gestational age group observed, no meaningful differences were found between "A" and "B" groups in any of the above mentioned histologic characteristics. The histodifferentiation of cupulae and maculae was found to be equal in all cultures. The organ of Corti was observed to attain a more advanced state of histodifferentiation in the 12 and 13-day explants than in the 11-day explanted otocysts. There was no correlation found in this advanced histodifferentiation of Corti's organ and whether this sensory receptor had formed in either a group "A" or group "B" series within its gestational age group. The organ of Corti was observed to histologically differentiate in a base to apex pattern (Fig. 19) as has been observed in organogenesis of the mouse cochlear duct that develops *in vivo*.[9,23] This base to apex pattern of differentiation was observed in both group "A" (Fig. 19A) and group "B" cultures (Fig. 19B) of all gestational age explants. The sensory structures and the cell types that composed these sensory structures (Table I) observed in group "A" and "B" explants did not show any significant differences in histodifferentiation at the three gestational ages tested for *in vitro* development.

Quantification of In Vitro Histodifferentiation. The serially sectioned specimens were examined under low power for the development of specific sensory structures and under dry and oil immersion for the development of sensory hair cells and the association of any neural elements with the developed sensory structures. Each sensory structure was examined and recorded on the quantification sheet for that particular code labeled specimen. After all 180 specimens had been rated for development of sensory structures, the code was broken and each quantification sheet was put into the group to which it belonged: 11-day "A"; 11-day "B"; 12-day "A"; 12-day "B"; 13-day "A" and 13-day "B." The data for each group was gathered and was converted into a percentage of occurrence when compared to the total number of specimens (30 organ cultures) analyzed for that group. The following results were obtained: A cartilaginous otic capsule always developed in all of the groups of explanted inner ears; the formation of perilymphatic spaces was also noted to occur in 100% of the explants. Neurons of the statoacoustic ganglion complex and their nerve fibers which invaded the supporting and sensory hair cell area of the sensory receptor structures were present in all of the group "A" culture specimens and in none of the group "B" explants. A utriculosaccular space developed in all explants. Two maculae sensory receptors developed in 97% of the 11-day group "A" explants with no explants observed to form only one macula. Ninety-three percent of the 11-day group "B" cultures developed two maculae and 7% developed only one macula. In the 12-day group "A" series, 91% developed two maculae and 9% developed only one macula. Eighty-four percent of the 12-day group "B" presented two maculae and 12% presented only one macula. Thirteen day-group "A" explants had two maculae in 93% and one macula in 3% of the specimens. Eighty-five percent of the 13-day group "B" specimens differentiated two maculae while only one macula was seen in the remaining 15%. The normal number of semicircular canals that differentiate *in vivo* is three. The following results were obtained *in vitro*. In the 11-day explants semicircular canals developed at the following rates: group "A" cultures — three canals in 10%, two only in 50%, and one only in 33%; group "B" cultures — three canals in none, two in 70%, and one only in 30%. Twelve-day organ cultures showed the following rate of semicircular canal development: group "A" specimens — three canals in 42% and two only in 58%; group "B" cultures — three canals in 36%, two only in 52% and one only in 12%. Organ cultures of 13-day otic explants developed semicircular canals as follows: group "A" specimens — three canals in 86% and two only in 14%; group "B" explants — three in 62%, two only in 27% and one only in 11%. The normal number of cristae to develop *in vivo* is three, one found in each semicircular canal ampulla. In the *in vitro* development system the following number of cristae developed in each group: 11-day organ cultures, group "A"

— three cristae in 77%, two only in 20% and one only in 3%; and in group "B" — three cristae in 78%, two only in 18% and one only in 4%; 12-day organ cultures, group "A" — three cristae in 79% and two only in 18% and one only in 3%; and in group "B" — three cristae in 76% and two only in 24%; 13-day organ culture specimens presented in group "A" — three cristae in 90% and two only in 10%; in group "B" — three cristae in 69%, two only in 23% and one only in 8%. Cochlear ducts developed in 97% of the group "A" 11-day explants and in 100% of the group "B" cultures. Organ of Corti formation was observed in 93% of both group "A" and "B" 11-day specimens. Stria vascularis tissue was found in 11-day group "A" and "B" cultures to be 90% and 93% respectively. Tectorial membrane formations were present in 71% of the group "A" and 93% of the group "B" 11-day organ cultures. In the 12-day specimens 94% of the group "A" and 96% of the group "B" cultures exhibited advances in cochlear duct formation and developed organ of Corti sensory structures. Stria vascularis tissue was observed to form in 94% of the "A" and 92% of group "B" 12-day explants. Tectorial membranes formed in 85% of the group "A" and 76% of group "B" 12th gestation day organ culture specimens. Thirteen day-explanted inner ears developed a cochlear duct in all of the group "A" and group "B" cultures. Organ of Corti sensory structures and stria vascularis tissue were observed to develop in 100% of the group "A" and 96% of the group "B" 13-day explants. Tectorial membranes formed in 86% of the group "A" and 73% of the group "B" 13-day specimens. Endolymphatic ducts and sacs formed in 87% of the group "A" and 96% of the group "B" 11-day otocyst explants. Eighty-eight percent of the group "A" 12-day cultures formed endolymphatic ducts and sacs. In the 12-day group "B" cultures, 96% formed endolymphatic ducts and 92% endolymphatic sacs. All of the 13-day group "A" cultures formed endolymphatic ducts and sacs. Thirteen-day group "B" explants showed development of endolymphatic ducts in 92% and 88% had endolymphatic sac formations.

TABLE II

HISTOLOGICAL QUANTIFICATION SUMMARY

		Stato-Acoustic Ganglion *A*	*B*
Cartilaginous otic capsule		100%	100%
Perilymphatic spaces		100%	100%
Statoacoustic ganglion		100%	0
Nerve fibers associated with sensory structures		100%	0
Utriculosaccular space		100%	100%
Maculae: one only		4%	11%
two		94%	87%
	Total	98%	98%
Semicircular canals: (Rudimentary)	one only	11%	17%
	two only	41%	50%
	three	46%	33%
	Total	98%	100%
Cristae: one only		2%	4%
two only		16%	22%
three		82%	74%
	Total	100%	100%
Cochlear duct		97%	99%
Organ of Corti		96%	95%
Stria vascularis		95%	94%
Tectorial membrane		81%	81%
Endolymphatic duct		92%	95%
Endolymphatic sac		92%	92%
Total number of specimens analyzed		90	90

"A" — with statoacoustic ganglion complex
"B" — without statoacoustic ganglion complex

A side by side comparison of this data is presented in Table I. Group "A" is represented by the "With" column and group "B" is represented by the "Without" column in each of the three gestational ages employed in the experiment. This data from Table I was then grouped into two general categories of "With" (group A) and "Without" (group B) statoacoustic ganglion complex and presented in Table II. The summarized data of Table II was then converted into a histogram form so that the significance of the data would be

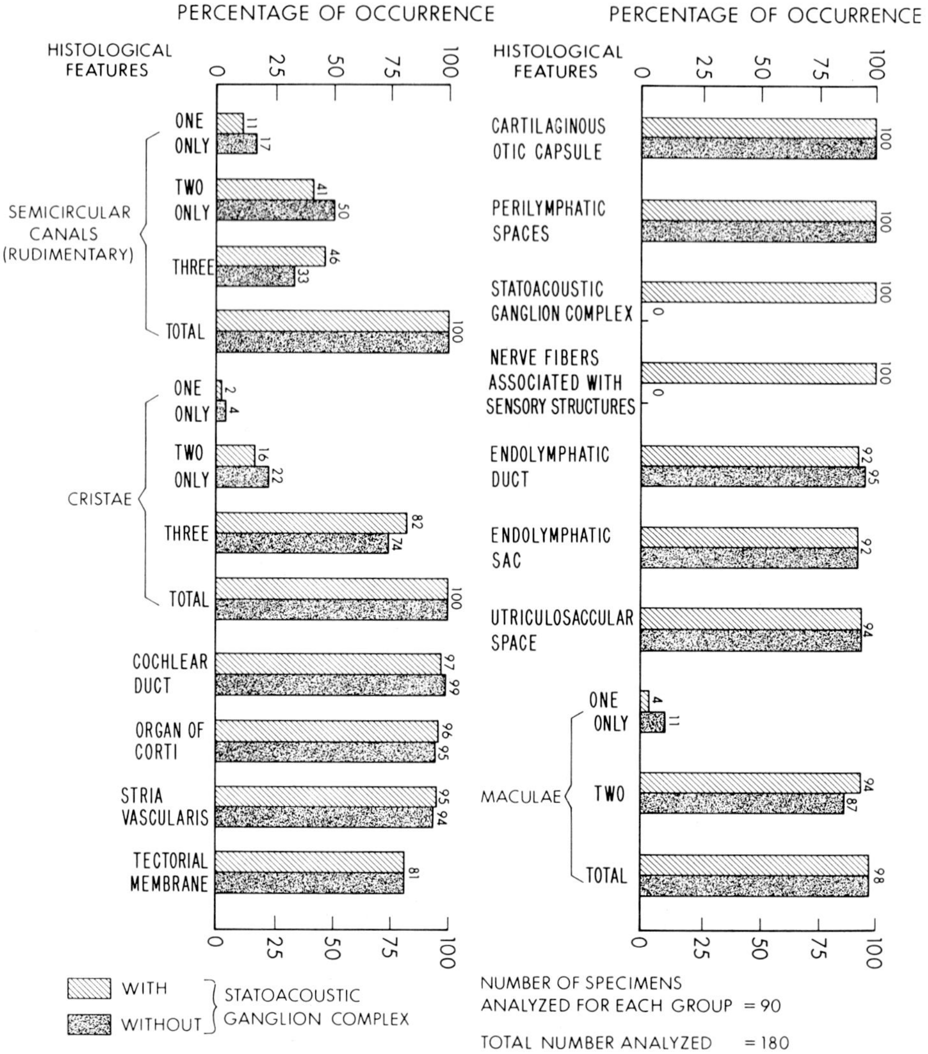

Fig. 20. Histological quantification summary.

better visualized. This is presented in Figure 20. With this treatment of the data, generalized differences become more apparent between the "with" and "without" statoacoustic ganglion complex otic explants; cartilaginous otic capsules, perilymphatic spaces, utriculosaccular spaces, tectorial membrane formations and endolymphatic sacs occurred with equal frequency in both group "A" and group "B" cultured inner ears. Cochlear duct, organ of Corti sensory structures, stria vascularis tissue and endolymphatic duct structures occurred with a difference of 3% or less between group "A" and group "B" and this was considered an insignificant difference in rate of occurrence. Maculae occurred with an overall equal frequency in both group "A" and "B" cultures, but two maculae occurred with 7% greater frequency in the group "A" cultures. A similar pattern was noted with the occurrence of semicircular canals and cristae of the group "A" cultures. Three semicircular canals occurred at 13% greater frequency in "A" cultures and three cristae occurred with 8% greater frequency in the "A" cultures when compared to the "B" cultures, although the overall frequency of occurrence of cristae and maculae was similar for both groups "A" and "B."

DISCUSSION

The three different embryonic ages chosen for this study of trophic effects of neural elements upon differentiation of inner ear sensory structures represent three distinct phases of the relationship between the differentiating neural elements of the statoacoustic ganglion and the presumptive ectodermal cells of inner ear sensory structures. The 11-day otocyst did not show any relationship between its statoacoustic ganglion neural elements and the ectodermal cells that compose the otocyst. Ruben *et al*[24] have found the 11-day otocyst to be composed of a population of homogenous, asynchronously dividing cells. Tritium labeled thymidine studies by Ruben[8] of the tenth gestation day mouse otocyst did not reveal any cells undergoing terminal mitosis and entering into a differentiative course of development. The 11th gestation day mouse otocyst was not included in this study by Ruben.[8] The 12-day otocyst has a few statoacoustic ganglion nerve fibers assuming a pioneering fiber configuration and penetrating the basement membrane and growing in around the ectodermal cells, some of which are destined to become sensory cells. Ruben *et al*[24] found that the 12-day otocyst does not behave as a homogenous, asynchronously dividing group of cells but that many cells are leaving the proliferative phase. Ruben[8] has previously reported that on this 12th day of gestation some of the cells are undergoing their terminal mitoses and entering into a course of histodifferentiation. In the 13-day specimen the relationship of nerve fibers to areas of presumptive sensory epithelial cells is well established and selective fasciculation is occurring at specific areas. Ruben[8] found many cells undergoing their terminal mitoses on this gestation day and large numbers of cells entering into a course of histodifferentiation. To simplify the above, the three phases represented could be designated as: 11-day — no contact; 12-day — sparse contact; and 13-day — frequent contact. If a trophic effect of statoacoustic ganglion neural elements is responsible for triggering or influencing the quality or quantity of differentiation of sensory structures of the developing inner ear *in vitro,* then when these presumptive sensory structure areas are deprived of this trophic influence by surgical extirpation of the ganglion prior to explantation to *in vitro*, a graded effect on the development of inner ear sensory structures would be expected. The presumptive sensory cells that had the least contact with neural elements would be expected to be the greatest affected and vice versa.

The results of the histological quantification of the occurrence of sensory structures in the three different categories of neuronal contact as represented by gestational age is presented in Table I. No consistent trend of greater occurrence of any sensory structure that developed in the *in vitro* developed explants that would signify the existence of a trophic effect of the neuronal elements on the development of sensory structures is present in either the group "A" or group "B"" explants. There are some differences in the frequency of occurrence of two classes of sensory structures. These are the occurrence of maculae and cristae. There is a reduction in the frequency of occurrence of a second macula in the "B" group explants of 12 and 13-day inner ear explants. A decrease in the occurrence of a third semicircular canal and its associated crista in 13-day explants is also noted. No such similar results are evident for the cochlear duct structures. These results may possibly be explained by the following observations. The statoacoustic ganglion complex is dissected with relative ease from the 11-day inner ear but by the 12th day of development the ganglion complex is more closely associated with the medial wall of the otocyst (Fig. 2) and care must be taken not to tear the medial wall, for during dissection this wall shows a mild pulling distortion when the ganglionic mass is dissected. This situation is even more aggravated by the 13th day and extreme care must be taken to dissect free the stato portion of the ganglionic complex. The medial and anterior wall is moderately distorted when the stato portion of the ganglion is dissected free. This increasing difficulty of dissection is most probably due to the nerve fibers that have penetrated the otocyst (Fig. 3) which are pulled free. It can be assumed that some mechanical damage would result at the site from where the nerve fibers are pulled. The acoustic portion of the ganglion which supplies the cochlear duct is still loosely associated with this structure at the time of dissection, and although it is difficult to dissect by the 13th day of gestation it does not cause a pulling distortion on the developing cochlear duct when dissected. The differences in occurrence of these sensory structures is also too small to be suggestive of a trophic phenomenon. This becomes evident when the three gestational age groups are grouped together under two common headings of group "A" (with) and group "B" (without) as seen in Table II. This can be done because although the inner ears were explanted on different days of embryonic development they were cultured *in vitro* for a compensating number of days; the end result being that all of the inner ear explants on their day of fixation reached an equivalent day of *in vivo* development, which is gestation day 21, the approximate day of birth in this mouse strain. No major differences are seen in the *in vitro* development of sensory structures in the summary of Figure 20.

Another observation that supports the concept that the neural elements of the statoacoustic ganglion complex do not exert a trophic effect upon the differentiation of sensory structures of the inner ear is the observation that the base to apex pattern of histodifferentiation of the organ of Corti of the cochlear duct occurred in both group "A" and group "B" explants (see Figures 19A and B respectively). Tello[23] had noted that innervation of the mouse organ of Corti proceeds from base to apex. Most studies (Retzius;[25] Boettcher;[26] Wade;[27] Bast and Anson;[28] Weibel;[29] and Sher[9]) have shown that the cytological maturation of the organ of Corti begins at the basal end and proceeds to the apex. Ruben[8] and Sher[9] have suggested that innervation of the organ of Corti could play a role in initiating (trophic effect) the differentiation of the cells of Corti's organ. This base to apex pattern of differentiation of the organ of Corti was present in the explants that developed without neural elements (Fig. 19B), as well as the cultures that developed with neural elements (Fig. 19A); therefore, this pattern of cytological differentiation of Corti's organ can no longer be ascribed to be initiated by a trophic interaction with neuronal elements of the statoacoustic ganglion.

Orr[11] suggested that the complete cytodifferentiation of hair cells in sensory membranes of the *in vitro* developed chick inner ear is dependent on innervation. Orr's hypothesis of a trophic effect of nerves on hair cell differentiation was based on her observations of histogenesis of sensory membranes in reaggregates of chick otocysts that had developed in organ culture. She always found neural elements associated with sensory structures that contained well differentiated sensory hair cells, and in those sensory structures that contained incompletely differentiated hair cells it was noted that no neural elements were present. Orr concluded her hypothesis from this experimental data. An alternate interpretation to explain the results of Orr[11] is presented here. In her reaggregation experiments, Orr[11] used trypsin to dissociate the cells of the embryonic chick otocysts. It has been shown by Hodges *et al*[30] that tritium labeled trypsin is taken up into the cell and there may be an effect on cellular structural components (Revel *et al*,[31] 1974). This intracellular presence and action of trypsin could damage some of the cells that are in a critical stage of differentiation at the time of trypsinization and thereby inhibit the expression of full differentiation. Ruben[8] has shown that some cells of the 12-day mouse otocyst that are destined to differentiate into sensory hair cells are leaving the proliferative phase and entering a differentiative phase. The four-day chick otocyst appears to be at a similar stage of differentiation as the 12-day mouse embryo otocyst. Since some of the presumptive sensory hair cells may be going through the stages of differentiation together, they may sort out in reaggregation (Curtis,[32] 1961, and Steinberg,[33] 1970) and form a sensory area in the reaggregate. If the differentiating undamaged hair cells exert a trophic effect on the axon outgrowth and orientation of the differentiating statoacoustic ganglion cells and the trypsin damaged hair cells did not, then nerve fibers would be found associated with the sensory membranes that contained fully differentiated hair cells and vice versa. Coughlin[34,35] (1975), has shown that in the *in vitro* morphogenesis of the mouse submandibular gland, it is the glandular epithelium that exerts a possible chemotactic (trophic) effect upon the axon outgrowth and orientation of its parasympathetic nerve ganglion. A similar situation was alluded to by Spiedel[4] in the regenerating lateral line of the frog tadpole. The hypothesis which states that differentiating hair cells attract nerve fibers by chemotaxis, if proven, would constitute a trophic effect. Chemotaxis as defined by Jacobson[36] is the directed growth of nerve fibers along a concentration gradient toward the source of some diffusable substance. The trophic effect would be the action of the differentiating hair cell upon the axon outgrowth and orientation of the differentiating statoacoustic ganglion cells. This hypothesis would also explain why innervation precedes cytodifferentiation of the organ of Corti as has been previously noted in this discussion. Chemodifferentiation of presumptive sensory hair cells could precede cytodifferentiation of these developing hair cells and the trophic effect of nerve fiber attraction by a chemotactic mechanism mediated by the chemodifferentiated hair cells. The observation of chemotaxis and inductive effect has been shown to be active in other systems and mediated by a single biochemical cell product, most notably in the slime mold system where Bonner[37] has shown cyclic AMP to be both a cell attractant (acrasin) and an inducer of stalk cell differentiation.

The observation that no trophic effect of the statoacoustic ganglion neural elements upon the differentiation of sensory structures of the mouse embryo inner ear that developed *in vitro* is supported by VIII nerve section experiments of Ruben *et al*,[38] Spoendlin and Gacek,[39] and Spoendlin.[40,41] These experiments showed no effect on inner ear morphology or function as a peripheral sensory end-organ in mature animals with chronic sectioning of the VIII nerve for extended periods of time.

REFERENCES

1. Todd JR: On the process of reproduction of the members of the aquatic salamander. Q J Sci Lit Arts 16:84-96, 1823

2. Ranvier L: *Traite Technique d'Histologie*. Paris, F. Savy, 1875 (Footnote, pp 948-949)

3. Speidel CC: Nerves in vivo. Sci Mon 67:178-185, 1948

4. Speidel CC: In vivo studies of myelinated nerve fibers. Int Rev Cytol 16:174-186, 1964

5. Flock A, Jorgensen M, Russell I: Physiology of individual hair cells and their synapses, in Moller AR (ed): *Basic Mechanisms in Hearing*. New York, Academic Press, 1973

6. Kaan HW: Experiments on the development of the inner ear in *Amblystoma punctatum*. J Exp Zool 46:13-61, 1926

7. Knowlton VY: Correlation of the development of membranous and bony labyrinths, acoustic ganglia, nerves and brain centers of the chick embryo. J Morphol 121:179-208, 1967

8. Ruben RJ: Development of the inner ear of the mouse: A radioautographic study of terminal mitosis. Acta Otolaryngol (Stockh) Suppl 220, 1967

9. Sher A: Embryonic and postnatal development of the inner ear of the mouse. Acta Otolaryngol (Stockh) Suppl 285, 1971

10. Friedmann I: In vitro culture of the isolated otocyst of the embryonic fowl. Ann Otol Rhinol Laryngol 65:98-103, 1956

11. Orr MF: Histogenesis of sensory epithelium in reaggregates of dissociated embryonic chick otocysts. Dev Biol 17:39-44, 1968

12. Thornhill RA: Development of the labyrinth of the lamprey. Proc R Soc Lond (Biol) 181:175-198, 1972

13. Fell HB: Development "in vitro" of the isolated otocyst of the embryonic fowl.

Arch Exp Zellforsch Besonders Gewebezuecht 7:69-81, 1928

14. Hoadley L: The independent differentiation of isolated chick primordia in chorioallantoic grafts. The eye, nasal region, otic region and mesencephalon. Biol Bull 46:281-297, 1924

15. Evans HJ: The independent differentiation of the sensory areas of the avian inner ear. Biol Bull 84:252-262, 1943

16. Waterman AJ: The development of the inner ear rudiment of the rabbit embryo in a foreign environment. Am J Anat 63:161-219, 1938

17. Van De Water TR, Ruben RJ: Quantification of the "in vitro" development of the mouse embryo inner ear. Ann Otol Rhinol Laryngol (Suppl 4:19-21) 1973

18. Altmann F: Zur anatomie und formalin Genese der Atresis auris congenita. Monatsschr Ohrenheilkd Laryngorhinol 67:765, 1933

19. Farbman AI: Taste bud regeneration in organ culture. Ann NY Acad Sci 228:350-354, 1974

20. Van De Water TR, Heywood P, Ruben RJ: Development of sensory structures in organ cultures of the twelfth and thirteenth gestation day mouse embryo inner ears. Ann Otol Rhinol Laryngol 82 (Suppl 4:1-18) 1973

21. Van De Water TR, Heywood P: The in vitro development of innervated sensory hair cells of a mammal. Acta Otolaryngol (Stockh), to be published

22. Van De Water TR, Ruben RJ: Symposium: New data for noise standards. (III) Organ culture of the mammalian inner ear — A tool to study inner ear deafness. Laryngoscope 84:738-749, 1974

23. Tello JR: Le reticule des cellules cillies du labyrinthe chez la souris et son independance des terminaisons nerveuses de la VIII paire. Tran de lab de recherces biol. de l'Univ. de Madrid 27:151-186, 1931

24. Ruben RJ, Van De Water TR, Polesky A: Cell kinetics of the eleven and twelve day mouse otocysts. Laryngoscope 81:1708-1718, 1971

25. Retzius MG: *Das Gehororgan der Wirbelthiere,* 2 vol. Stockholm, Samson and Wallin, 1881-1884

26. Boettcher A: *Uber Entwicklung und Bau des Gehorlabyrinths.* Dresden, Blockman, Soba and Schultze, 1869

27. Wada T: Anatomical and physiological studies on the growth of the inner ear of the albino rat. Wistar Inst Anat Biol Memoirs 10: 1-174, 1923

28. Bast TH, Anson BJ: *Temporal Bone and the Ear.* Springfield, Illinois, Charles C. Thomas, 1949

29. Weibel ER: Zur Kenntnis der Differenzierungsvorgange in Epithel des Ductus Cocholearis. Acta Anat (Basel) 29:53-90, 1957

30. Hodges GM, Livingston DC, Franks CM: The localization of trypsin in cultured mammalian cells. J Cell Sci 12:887-902, 1973

31. Revel JP, Hoch P, Ho D: Adhesion of culture cells to their substratum. Exp Cell Res 84:207-218, 1974

32. Curtis ASG: Timing mechanisms in the specific adhesion of cells. Exp Cell Res Suppl 8:107-122, 1961

33. Steinberg MS: Does differential adhesion govern the self-assembly of tissue structure: Equilibrium configurations and the emergence of a hierarchy among populations of embryonic cells. J Exp Zool 173:395-434, 1970

34. Coughlin MD: Early development of parasympathetic nerves in the mouse submandibular gland. Dev Biol 43:123-139, 1975

35. Coughlin MD: Target organ stimulation of parasympathetic nerve growth in the developing mouse submandibular gland. Dev Biol 43:140-158, 1975

36. Jacobson M: *Developmental Neurobiology.* New York, Holt, Rinehart and Winston, 1970

37. Bonner JT: Induction of stalk cell differentiation by cyclic AMP in the cellular slime mold *Dictyostelium discoideum.* Proc Natl Acad Sci USA 65:110-113, 1970

38. Ruben RJ, Hudson W, Chiong A: Anatomical and physiological effects of chronic section of the eighth nerve in cat. Acta Otolaryngol (Stockh) 55:473-484, 1962

39. Spoendlin H, Gacek R: Survival of the peripheral dendrites after section of the cochlear nerve. Proc Int Congr Neuropathol 5th Excerpta Med Found Int Congr, Ser. No. 100:926-934, 1965

40. Spoendlin H: Degeneration behavior of the cochlear nerve. Arch Klin Exp Ohren Nasen Kehlkopfheilkd 200:275-291, 1971

41. Spoendlin H: Innervation densities of the cochlea. Acta Otolaryngol (Stockh) 73: 235-248, 1972

REPRINTS — Thomas R. Van De Water, PhD, Department of Otorhinolaryngology, Albert Einstein College of Medicine, 1300 Morris Park Ave., Bronx, NY 10461.

SOME UNRESOLVED PROBLEMS CONCERNING THE COCHLEAR NERVE

R. LORENTE DE NÓ, MD

LOS ANGELES, CALIFORNIA

SUMMARY — Three types of afferent fibers innervate the hair cells of the organ of Corti: 1) specific radial fibers which establish contacts with a very few neighboring internal hair cells; 2) spiral fibers, each one of which establishes contact with a number of external hair cells distributed throughout long segments of the cochlea; and 3) unspecific radial fibers which are collaterals arising radially at irregular intervals from fibers of the ganglionic spiral bundles and which establish contact with internal hair cells. The existence of spiral ganglionic bundles of fibers oriented apicalward has long been described, and the fact that a number of ganglionic spiral fibers give off radial collaterals to innervate internal hair cells was illustrated by Cajal and by Lorente de Nó. However, those structural details are not mentioned in the modern literature. In the ventral nucleus there are neurons with efferent axons which join the trapezoid body and cells with short axons ramified within the ventral nucleus itself. Two types of cells with efferent axons are illustrated and described, the spherical or bushy cell and the basket cell; and it is shown that branches of division of the two types of efferent axons form association tracts which end in the tuberculum acusticum. Also, the fact is illustrated that fibers having their cells of origin in that tuberculum form association paths which end in the ventral nucleus by means of extensive ramifications which form numerous synaptic endings. The dendritic and fibrillar plexuses in the ventral nucleus are described, an analysis is made of the relationships between the two plexuses and of the synaptic junctions that mediate transmission of nerve impulses. The synaptic junctions belong to a considerable number of types and in all illustrations the important fact repeatedly appears that one and the same fiber may form synaptic endings of widely different sizes and shapes located either on the same neuron or, more frequently, on different neurons. The intimate structure of each type of synaptic ending cannot be revealed by light microscopy, but only light microscopy can reveal to which kind of fiber the synaptic endings do belong. The presentation is concluded with a brief and preliminary discussion of physiological corollaries of certain general features of the anatomy of the acoustic system.

For a number of years and working in several scientific institutions, but chiefly from 1931 to 1936 in the Central Institute for the Deaf in St. Louis, Missouri, a systematic analysis was carried out of the endings of the cochlear nerve in the primary acoustic nuclei and of the structure of those nuclei. A brief survey of the plan of the structure of the nuclei was published in 1933,[1] and a brief description of the endings in the cochlea was published shortly thereafter.[2]

In this essay, the complete publication of the results obtained is begun by presenting data on the structure of the anterior or ventral nucleus, and by reviewing the existing knowledge of the cochlear endings.

From the extensive and excellent literature on the acoustic nuclei that has collected in the past few years, reference is being made here only to those papers immediately related to the problems that are discussed in this essay. A more detailed analysis will be made in later essays. For simplicity, the nucleus ventralis is divided only in two parts, caudal, *n.v. I* and rostral, *n.v. II*.

The presentation of the anatomical information will be made in five sections. In the first, data are presented on the

---

From the Departments of Surgery and Anatomy, U.C.L.A. Medical School, Los Angeles, California. This study was supported by grants from the Deafness Research Foundation, The Ahmanson Foundation, and Hope for Hearing Foundation, U.C.L.A.

Presented at the meeting of the American Otological Society, Inc., Palm Beach, Florida, April 25-26, 1976.

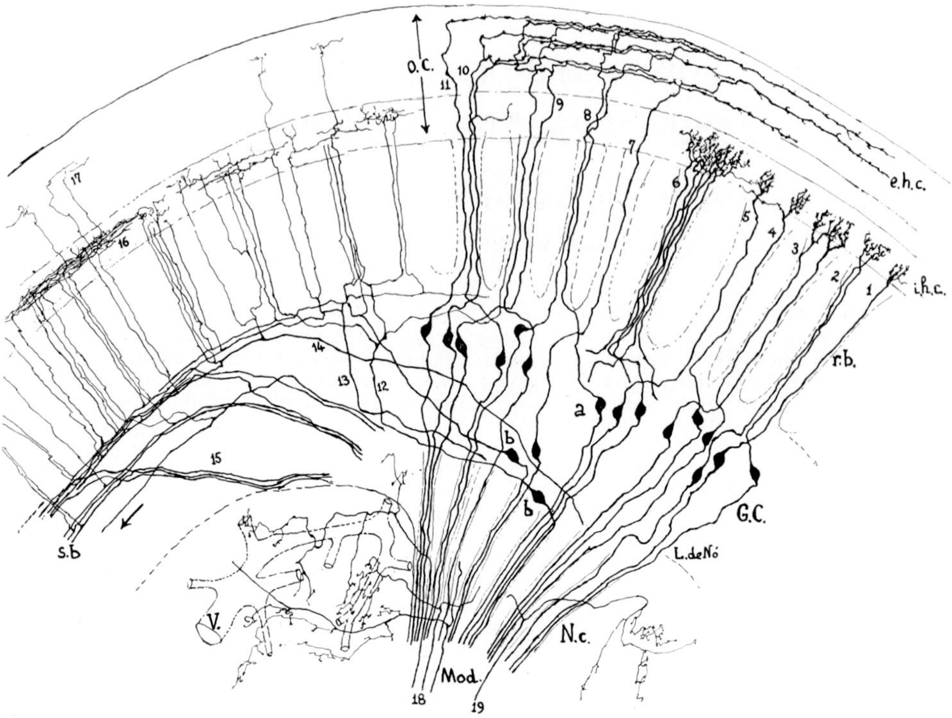

Fig. 1. Except for the blood vessel *V* and accompanying nerve fibers, the drawing reproduces cells and fibers found in a single section passing through the basal spiral turn of the cochlea. Eight-day old mouse. Golgi rapid method. *G.C.* — Ganglion of Corti; *Mod.* — Modiolus; *N.C.* — Cochlear nerve; *O.C.* — Organ of Corti; *a, b* — Cells of the ganglion of Corti; *e.h.c* — External hair cells; *i.h.c* — Internal hair cells. The ganglion cells labeled *a* give rise to the specific radial fibers for internal hair cells and to the external spiral fibers. The ganglion cells labeled *b* give rise to unspecific radial fibers for internal hair cells (notice ramified fibers *12, 13,* and *14*). The bundles labeled *15, sb, 16* and *17* undoubtedly belong to Rasmussen's efferent system. (By permission of *Laryngoscope.*[2])

(peripheral) endings of the acoustic fibers in the cochlea; in the second, a description is made of the (central) endings of the cochlear fibers in the ventral or anterior nucleus; in the third, a brief description is made of selected types of neurons with efferent axons and of neurons with axons ramified within the acoustic nuclei themselves, and illustrations are presented of the dendritic and fibrillar plexuses; in the fourth, the establishment of contacts (synapses) between those two plexuses is analyzed. Finally, in the fifth section, a brief discussion is made of theoretical questions arising, among others, from the fact that in the ventral nucleus the number of branches of fibers of endogenous origin is about as great as the number of branches of cochlear fibers.

ENDINGS OF THE ACOUSTIC FIBERS IN THE COCHLEA

At the Symposium on the "Neural Mechanism of Hearing" held 39 years ago, during the 70th meeting of the American Otological Society, I presented a diagram illustrating what at that time was believed to be known about the innervation of the hair cells of the cochlea (Fig. 1).[2]

At that time the existence of Rasmussen's efferent system of fibers[3-5] was not known, and it was believed that the radial bundles of fibers in Corti's ganglion were formed by afferent fibers which innervated regions of the organ of Corti located at some distance from the ganglion cells of origin. The situation changed, and indeed in a radical form, when Rasmussen's bundle was identified as an aggregate of efferent fibers and at present it seems to be generally believed that all the fibers having a radial course within the ganglion are efferent. This belief, however, is erroneous. It stands in contradiction with available evidence.

On the basis of the information presented in Figure 1 it is obviously permissible to believe that the bundles of thin fibers labeled *16* and *17* belong to Rasmussen's efferent system.* However, the fibers that arise from the ganglion cells labeled *b, b,* one of which has been labeled *12,* as well as the similar fiber *13* and probably also *14,* must necessarily be afferent fibers. As can readily be noted, the afferent fibers of type *b* divide into several thinner branches which, after having formed an irregular horizontal plexus at the outer surface of the ganglion, bend sharply at right angles to penetrate into Corti's organ and establish contacts with internal hair cells. It is important to note that the inner hair cells innervated by branches of a single afferent fiber of type *b* are located at considerable distances from one another.

The existence of cochlear afferent fibers of type *b* was not described for the first time by me in 1937! As a matter of fact, Cajal[6] described the existence of radial ganglionic fibers having their origin in Corti's ganglion cells as well as the existence of afferent radial fibers which within the ganglion give off several branches for the organ of Corti.

Thus, after the existence of Rasmussen's efferent system has been taken into account, Figure 1 shows that the organ of Corti receives three types of afferent fibers, which may be called 1) specific radial fibers (*1* to *6*) each fiber innervating only one or a very few neighboring inner hair cells, 2) unspecific radial fibers (branches of ganglion cells labeled *b* and probably also *13* and *14*), which give off a number of radial branches innervating internal hair cells located at significant distances from one another, and 3) external spiral fibers which innervate the external hair cells.

Between the three types of afferents there must be important physiological differences. The specific radial fibers must carry impulses accompanied by a strong "local sign" indicating the point of the organ of Corti at which excitation of the internal hair cell has occurred, while activity of the unspecific radial fibers can show only that stimulation within a rather wide zone of the organ of Corti has taken place.

Remarkably enough, even though each external spiral fiber innervates a number of hair cells located in a wide zone of the organ of Corti, it is quite likely that the nerve impulses carried by the external spiral fibers are accompanied by a definite "local" sign, the evaluation of which in the acoustic centers must depend upon the number of active fibers. For the sake of the argument, let it be assumed that each spiral fiber has synaptic contacts with five hair cells, *1* to *5*. Assume that a weak sound has mildly activated external hair cells. In view of the great rapidity with which electrotonic decrement of subliminal stimuli takes place in thin fibers, the distances between individual synapses in each spiral fiber are undoubtedly too long for effective summation of subliminal disturbances. If, however, the sound is strong enough to initiate at ending *5* a small nerve impulse, this impulse will propagate itself with progressively decreasing size toward ending *4* where it will be reinforced; *i.e.*, its magnitude will be increased; further reinforcements will take place at endings *3, 2* and *1* with the result that the impulse will acquire that size which is required for uniform conduction; consequently the impulse will be able to reach the acoustic nuclei.[7] Of course, if the stimulation is produced by a strong sound it is quite possible that endings *2* and *1* will be sufficient to initiate a full-sized nerve impulse. But since in such a case a large

*In all probability the two thin fibers to the left of the arrows labeled *O.C.* in Figure 1, like the fibers labeled *17,* belong to the efferent system for the external hair cells.

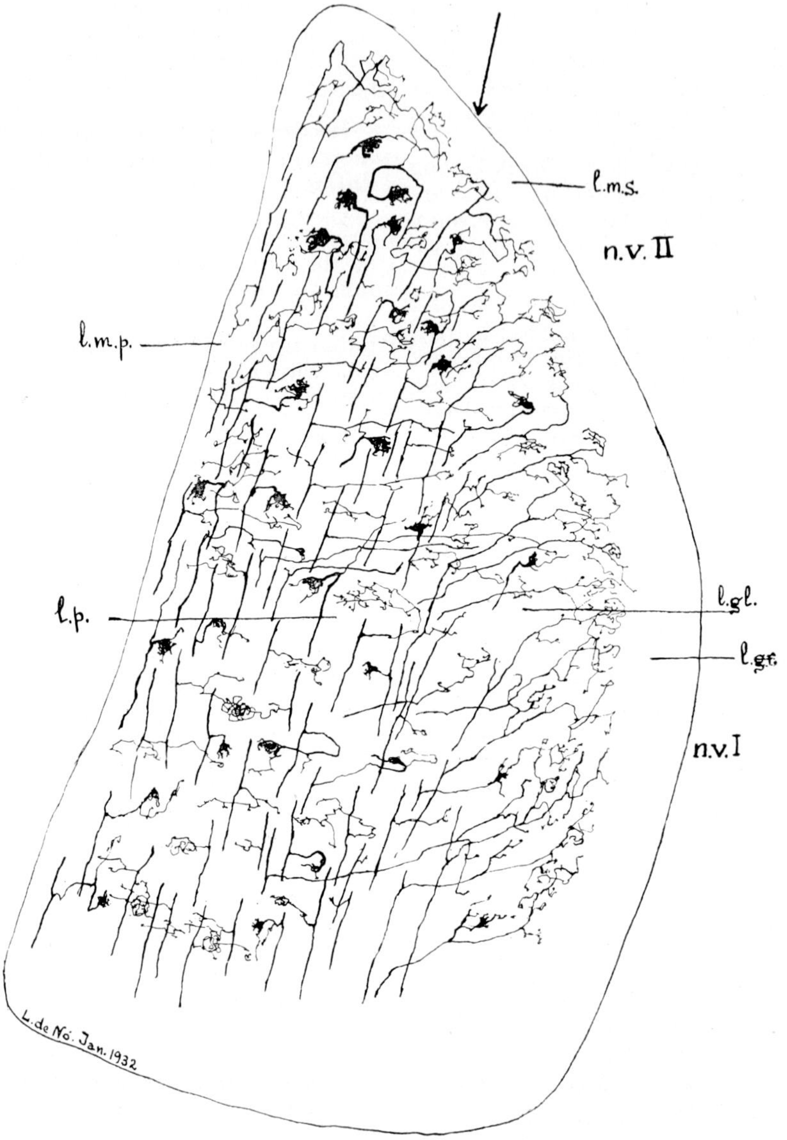

Fig. 2. Oblique frontal section through the *nucleus ventralis*. *n.v. II* — Rostral, *n.v. I* — Caudal part of the *ventral nucleus*. *l.m.p.* — *lamina medullaris profunda*; *l.p.* — *lamina principalis*; *l.m.s.* — *lamina marginalis superficialis*; *l.gl.* — *lamina glomerularis*; *l.gr.* — *lamina granularis*. The arrow on top of the drawing indicates the direction of the section reproduced in Figure 3. Golgi rapid method.

number of external spiral fibers will have become simultaneously active, the position and the number of active fibers will yield to the acoustic nuclei information sufficient to ascertain where in the organ of Corti the maximum of stimulation has been produced.

It should be noted that, as far as I can see, at the present status of nerve physiology the outlined hypothesis of the mechanism of stimulation of the external spiral fibers seems to be the only one possible. The hypothesis has an important consequence, namely, that effective

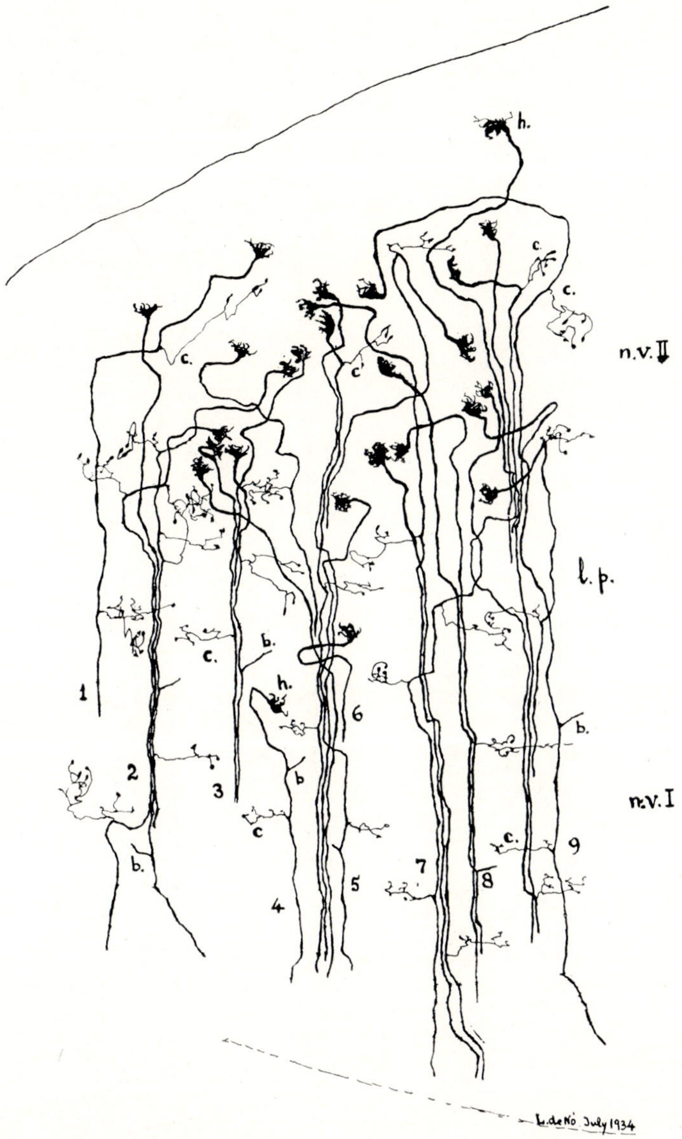

Fig. 3. Endings of specific radial acoustic fibers in the magnocellular system of *n.v. I. h* — Chalices of Held; *b* — Long collaterals for the lamina glomerularis; *c* — Short collaterals. Golgi rapid method.

stimulation of external spiral fibers is unidirectional. A small impulse initiated at or near the end of the spiral fiber will grow while traveling toward the parent fiber and will eventually reach the acoustic centers, while an impulse that might grow while traveling in an opposite direction will die out at the end of the spiral fiber.

ENDINGS OF THE COCHLEAR FIBERS IN THE VENTRAL OR ANTERIOR NUCLEUS

An important problem is to ascertain whether different types of central endings correspond to the three different types of cochlear afferents. An attempt to solve the problem can be best made in the ventral nucleus where the anterior fibers of division of the cochlear

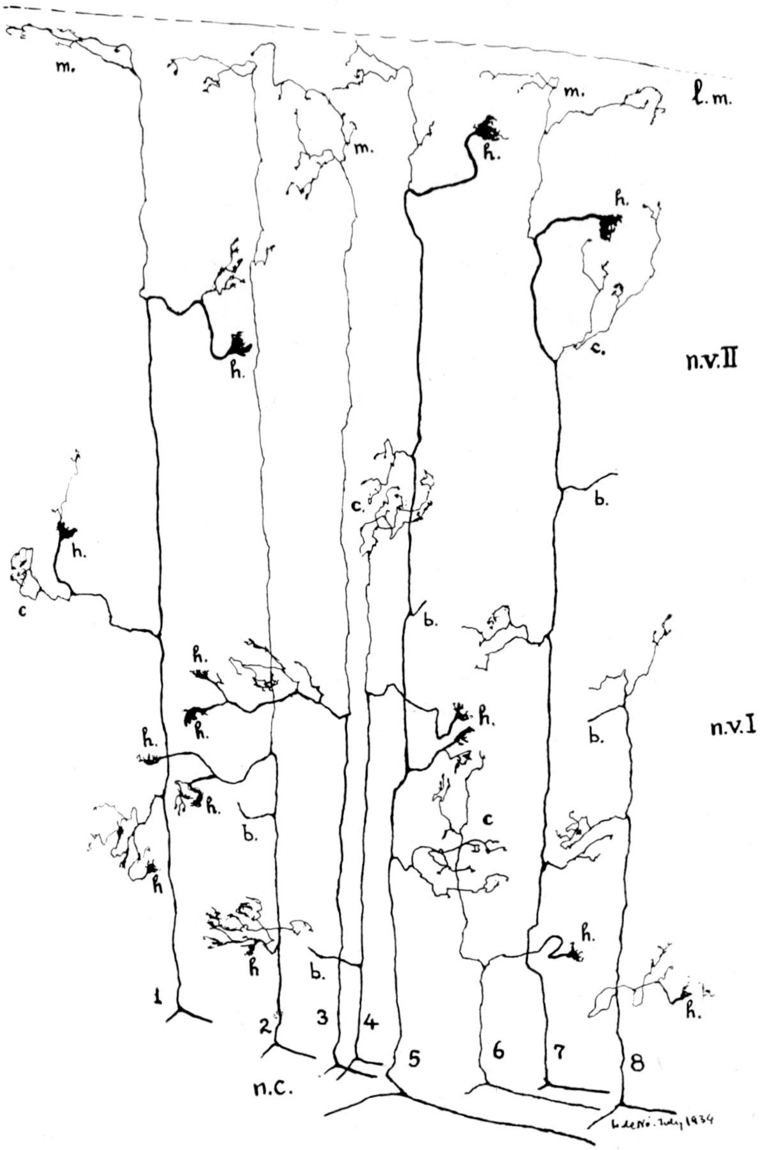

Fig. 4. Endings of specific radial fibers (*1, 5, 7*) and of external spiral fibers (*2, 3, 4, 6, 8*) in the ventral nucleus. *n.c.* — Division of the cochlear fiber into anterior and posterior branches.

nerve are arranged in more or less parallel bundles. Although much attention was dedicated to the problem and, in fact, three different types of central cochlear fibers were found to exist, the correspondence of the three central to the three peripheral systems still is somewhat problematic.

The most numerous types of central fibers include those which reach the magnocellular system of spherical cells in the oral part of the anterior or ventral nucleus. Fibers of this type are illustrated by Figure 3 and by fibers 5 and 7 of Figure 4. There can be hardly, if any doubt that those fibers are the central branches of the specific radial fibers of the cochlea. The second type of cen-

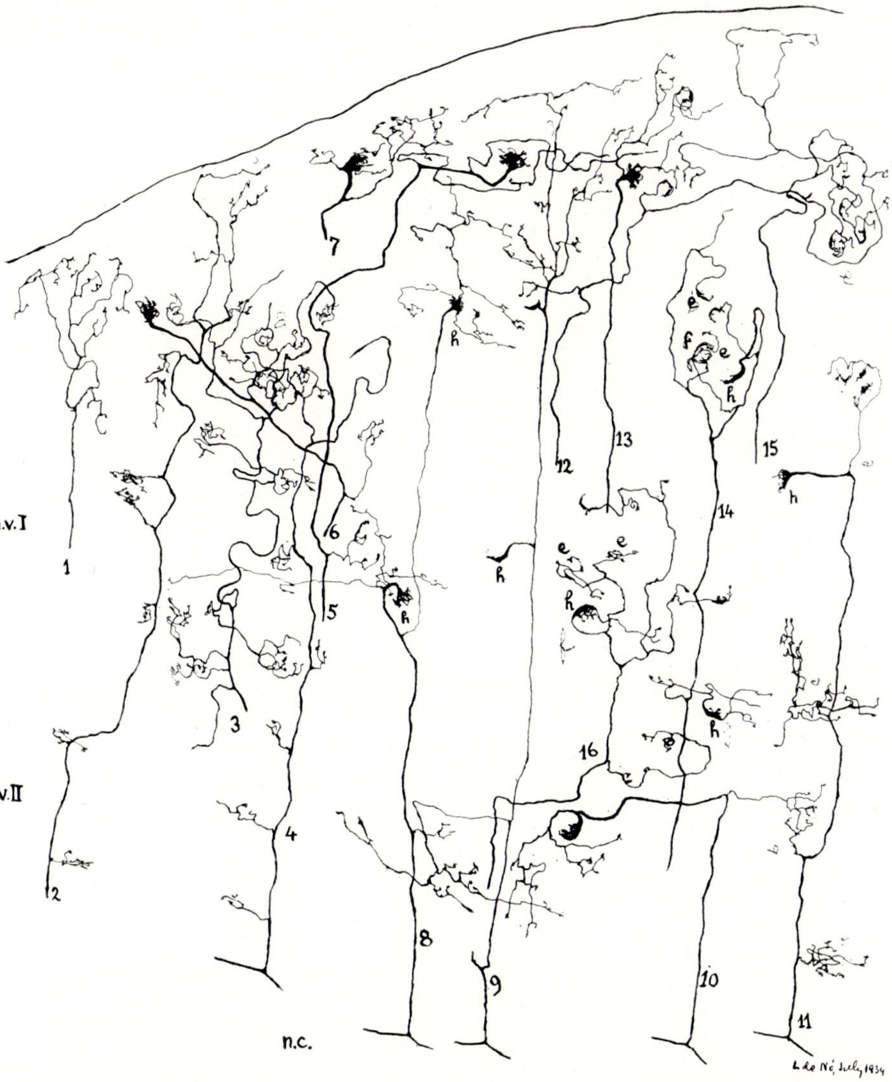

Fig. 5. Oblique section through the ventral nucleus showing endings of cochlear fibers and of endogenous fibers (further explanation in the text). Golgi rapid method.

tral cochlear branches is much less numerous; it is illustrated by fibers *2, 3, 6* and *8* in Figure 4. The main branches of those fibers have not been seen reaching the magnocellular system of spherical cells although they may send thin collateral branches into it. A logical assumption is that the second type of central fibers corresponds to the external spiral fibers of the cochlea, since according to Spoendlin[8] and to Morrison *et al*[9] the number of spiral fibers is not more than 10-15% of the number of radial fibers. A third type, also composed of a relatively small number of fibers, ends mainly by means of diffuse ramifications located in the internal or medial marginal lamina (Fig. 6). A possible assumption is that the third system of central fibers belongs to the unspecific radial fibers. However, only future research may solve this problem.

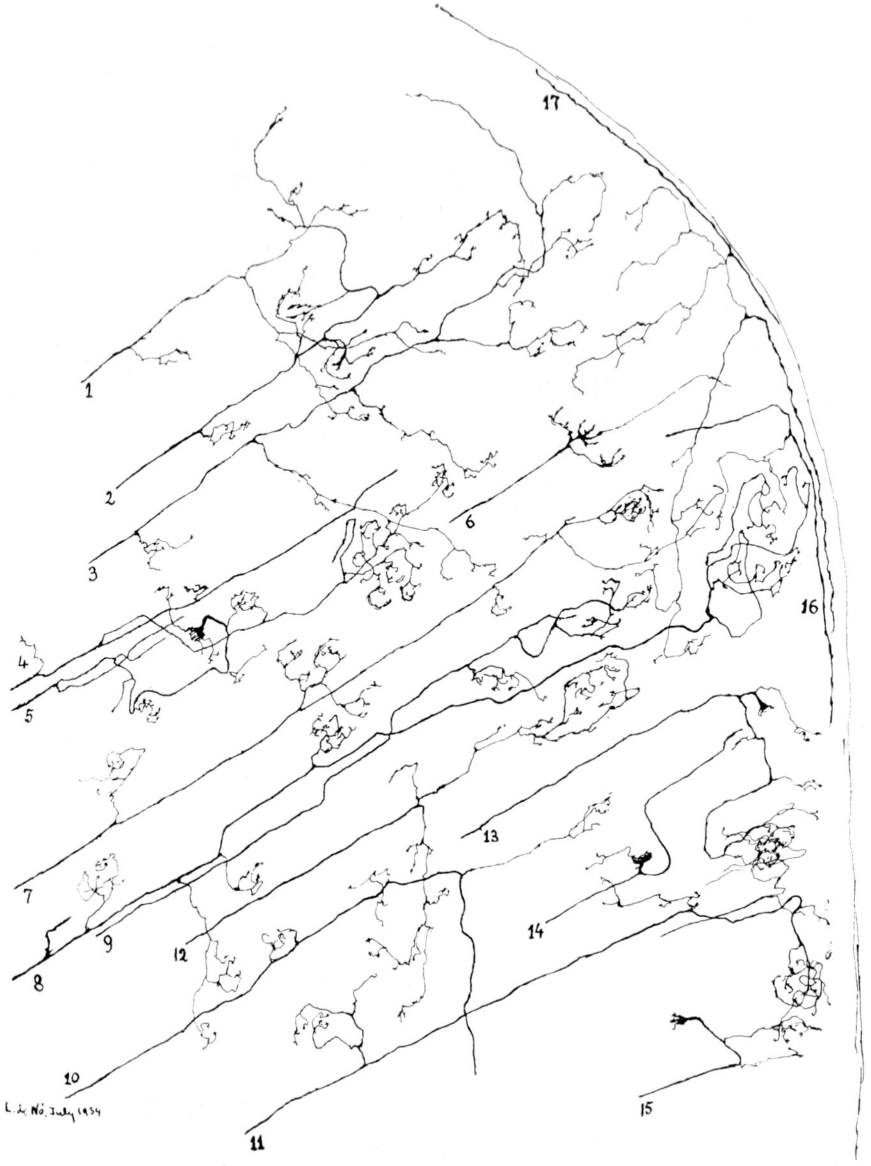

Fig. 6. Longitudinal section passing through the *lamina medullaris interna*. *16* and *17* are endogenous fibers. The rest are, in all probability, endings of unspecific radial fibers. Golgi rapid method.

Figure 2 reproduces an oblique frontal section of the ventral nucleus which presents the cochlear fibers cut into relatively long segments. As in this particular section, only a limited number of cochlear fibers were stained without admixture of other elements, it may easily be observed that the ascending or anterior cochlear branches run in more or less parallel bundles through the *lamina principalis* of *nucleus ventralis I* (*n.v. I*) giving off Held endings and long and short collaterals terminated by single or by clusters of synaptic knobs. Of particular interest are the long collaterals ending in the zone labeled *l.gl.* The anatomical purpose of the long system of collaterals will be analyzed elsewhere.

As can readily be observed in Figure 2, the cochlear fibers are arranged in three different streams. The central stream invades the magnocellular system of spherical cells, establishing synaptic endings which are called Held's chalices or bulbs. As was first observed by Cajal,[6] the Held endings in the posterior part of the ventral nucleus have smaller sizes. At times it will be convenient to call the large endings Held chalices and the smaller endings Held bulbs. In the caudal end of the anterior nucleus the Held bulbs are hardly larger than ordinary synaptic knobs. The central stream in Figure 2 undoubtedly corresponds to the radial cochlear fibers.

It can also be seen in Figure 2 that the lateral stream does not quite reach the zone of the ventral nucleus occupied by the largest spherical cells and that in addition to profusely ramified collateral fibers it gives off only small Held bulbs. As was postulated above, the lateral stream corresponds to the spiral cochlear fibers.

In Figure 2 only a small part of the medial stream has been reproduced, namely, the two lax ramifications at the level of the line *l.m.p.* (Fig. 6). As was assumed above, those lax or diffuse ramifications are probably formed by the unspecific radial fibers.

As was first described by Osen[10] the largest cells which have spherical shape and which also have been called bushy cells by Brawer and Morest[11] form a definite system in the oral pole of the ventral nucleus. Figure 3 reproduces part of a very successful Golgi stain of cochlear fiber endings with large Held chalices in that magnocellular system. It will be noted that no collaterals arise from the chalices themselves and that during their course the cochlear fibers give off only a moderate number of short collaterals *c* as well as a few somewhat thicker branches *b* which undoubtedly reach the zone labeled *l.gl.* in Figure 2.

It is important to mention that no fiber of the type illustrated by Figure 3 forms more than one Held chalice. Conversely, in the magnocellular system of spherical cells, each cell receives one, and only one Held chalice. Clearly, therefore, transmission of acoustic impulses through the magnocellular system of spherical cells must be accompanied by a very definite "local sign."

Figure 4 presents a number of fibers found on the lateral part of the central stream in a parasagittal section, having approximately the orientation indicated by the vertical arrow on Figure 2. Fibers 5 and 7 undoubtedly belong to the same type as the fibers in Figure 3, even though fiber 5 has a large synaptic ending in the caudal part of the ventral nucleus.

Fibers *1, 2, 3, 4, 6, 8* (Fig. 4) clearly belong to a different type. In the first place they form only Held bulbs (*i.e.*, small Held chalices) and ramified collateral branches. Some fibers (*4, 6, 8*) form only one Held bulb but other fibers form a number of Held bulbs. All the fibers of this type are short and do not reach the magnocellular part of the nucleus ventralis, even though some of them (*2, 3*) have long, thin collaterals that may even reach the *lamina marginalis* (*l.m.*).

It should be noted that, although the details illustrated by Figures 3 and 4 have remained unpublished and consequently unknown for over 40 years, very recently Brawer and Morest,[11] also using Golgi's method, have made accurate descriptions of a number of the types of cochlear endings in the anterior nucleus. In their noteworthy paper, Brawer and Morest emphasize the all-important point (and to me a well-known fact) that Held endings (chalices or bulbs) come in contact only with cells of spherical type (bushy cells in Brawer and Morest's terminology). The other main type of cell with efferent axon, the stellate cell of Brawer and Morest, have never been seen in contact with a Held ending neither in my old investigations nor in the recent one by Brawer and Morest.

Owing to the technique of reproduction they used, the figures published by Brawer and Morest present with great clarity a fact which is not so easy to observe in Figures 3 and 4. From a point 200 or 300μ or even more from a large Held ending, the diameter of the nerve fiber increases progressively to become at the chalice at least twice as large as it had initially been. Such a progressive increase in diameter can hardly serve to increase the speed of conduction because the thickening increases the amount of membrane that has to be activated per unit length, but when the impulse reaches the margin of the chalice the amount of active membrane behind the margin certainly is large enough to prevent delay in the activation of the chalice.

The drawings in Figures 2 to 4 present the anatomy of the cochlear endings as an exceedingly simple matter. The true complexity of the situation begins to appear in Figure 5, which reproduces part of an oblique parasagittal section of the ventral nucleus, the orientation of the knife being such that only a small part of the magnocellular system was included in the section. The position of this system is given by the four large Held chalices which are formed by fibers *5, 6, 7* and *13* in the uppermost part of the drawing.

In the drawing in Figure 5 endogenous fibers have been included, *i.e.,* fibers which are branches of axons of cells of the acoustic nuclei themselves. The manner in which fibers *1* and *3* ramify themselves leaves no doubt whatever that *1* and *3* are endogenous fibers. As can readily be noted, the arborization formed by fiber *3* interlaces with the arborizations formed by collateral branches of acoustic fibers *2, 4, 5* and *6.* Judging by the shape of their terminal arborization, fibers *12* and *15* are endogenous fibers but the rest of the fibers included in the drawing, *8, 9, 10, 14* and *16* undoubtedly are cochlear fibers ramified in the zone of the anterior or ventral nucleus which lies caudal to the magnocellular system (*nucleus ventralis II*; *n.v. II*). All those fibers, *8, 9, 10, 14* and *16* probably are central branches of external spiral fibers. It should be noted that in the case of fiber *9* after the initial division of the parent cochlear fiber, the anterior division again divided into two branches, only one of which, *9,* was included in the plane of the section.

Finally, in addition to the endogenous fibers *16* and *17,* Figure 6 presents 15 cochlear afferent fibers which were stained quite completely in a parasagittal section passing through the deep marginal lamina (*i.e.,* near the medial border) of the ventral nucleus. As was mentioned above, in all probability those cochlear fibers are the endings of the unspecific radial fibers. A few of the fibers in Figure 6 display Held bulbs of small size but in the main the fibers end, forming profuse ramifications with terminal branches possessing either single or bunches of synaptic knobs. Although the number of fibers of the type illustrated by Figure 6 seems to be relatively small, the existence of those fibers must play an important role since their branches establish contact with the marginal cells which are mainly cells of Golgi type II and which, as will appear below, give rise to endogenous fibers which ramify themselves and end within the ventral nucleus itself.

EFFERENT AND ENDOGENOUS NEURONS IN THE VENTRAL OR ANTERIOR NUCLEUS

The published knowledge of the cell population of the ventral nucleus is rather limited because in the work published in the recent literature, histological methods were used which do not disclose the distribution of the axons and dendrites of the neurons.

The problem can be well-defined by means of Figure 7, which was prepared with the use of frontal sections almost normal to the anterior branches of division of the cochlear nerve, which passed through or near to the caudal margin of the magnocellular system of spherical cells. In the drawing have been included cells with long axons (Golgi type I) giving rise to the efferent fibers of the ventral nucleus, which form the trapezoid body. Cells with efferent axons are *2, 3, 4, 5, 6,* and *9.* Figure 7 also contains cells with short axons (Golgi type II), *i.e.,* with axons which form endo-

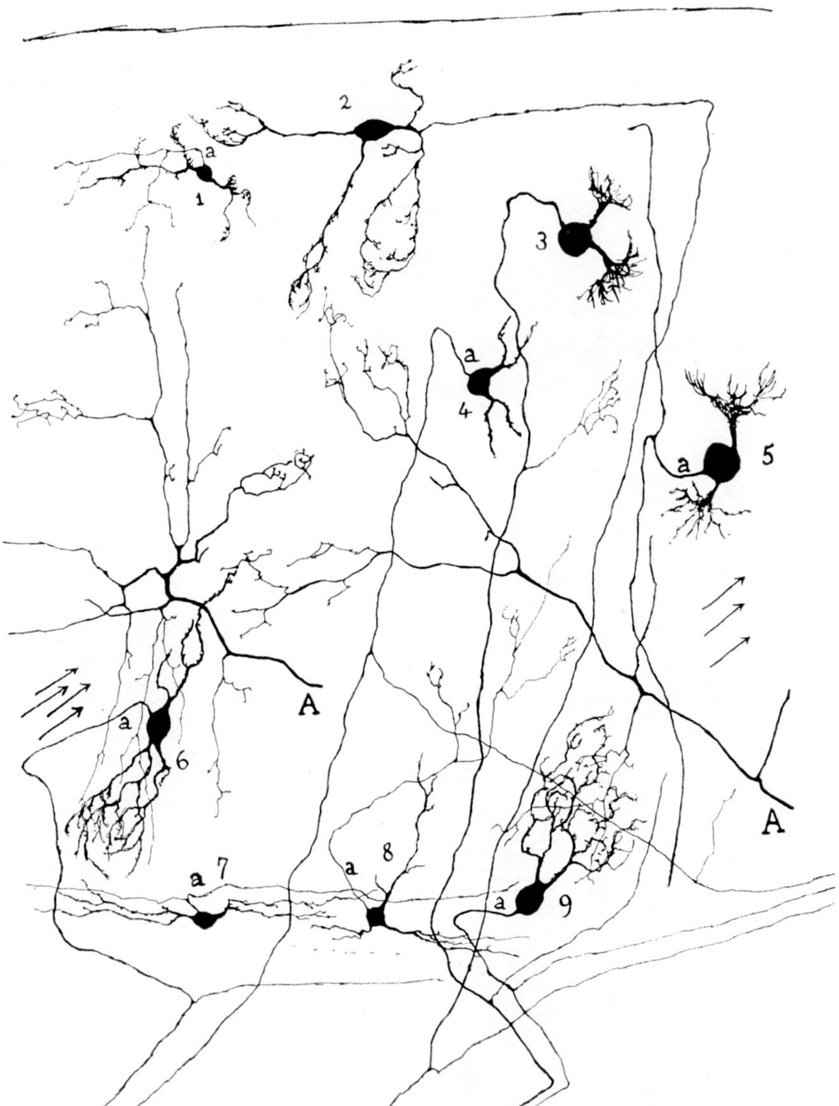

Fig. 7. Cells with long axons (*2, 3, 4, 5, 6, 9*) and cells with short axons (*2, 7, 8*). The ramifications labeled *A, A*, are of endogenous origin. Golgi rapid method.

genous arborizations, which ramify themselves entirely within the ventral nucleus itself. In Figure 7 cells *1, 7* and *8* are cells with short axons and *A, A* are parts of the endogenous arborizations of cells of Golgi type II of large magnitude (Fig. 9, *5, 6*).

The neurons of the anterior nucleus may be classified into three main types.

Type S

The cells of this type have a spherical body and were called "spherical" by Osen.[10] They also may be called brush cells in reference to their dendrites. They correspond to one of the types of cells with efferent axons described by Cajal.[6] Each cell has a limited number of dendrites, usually two or three, but oc-

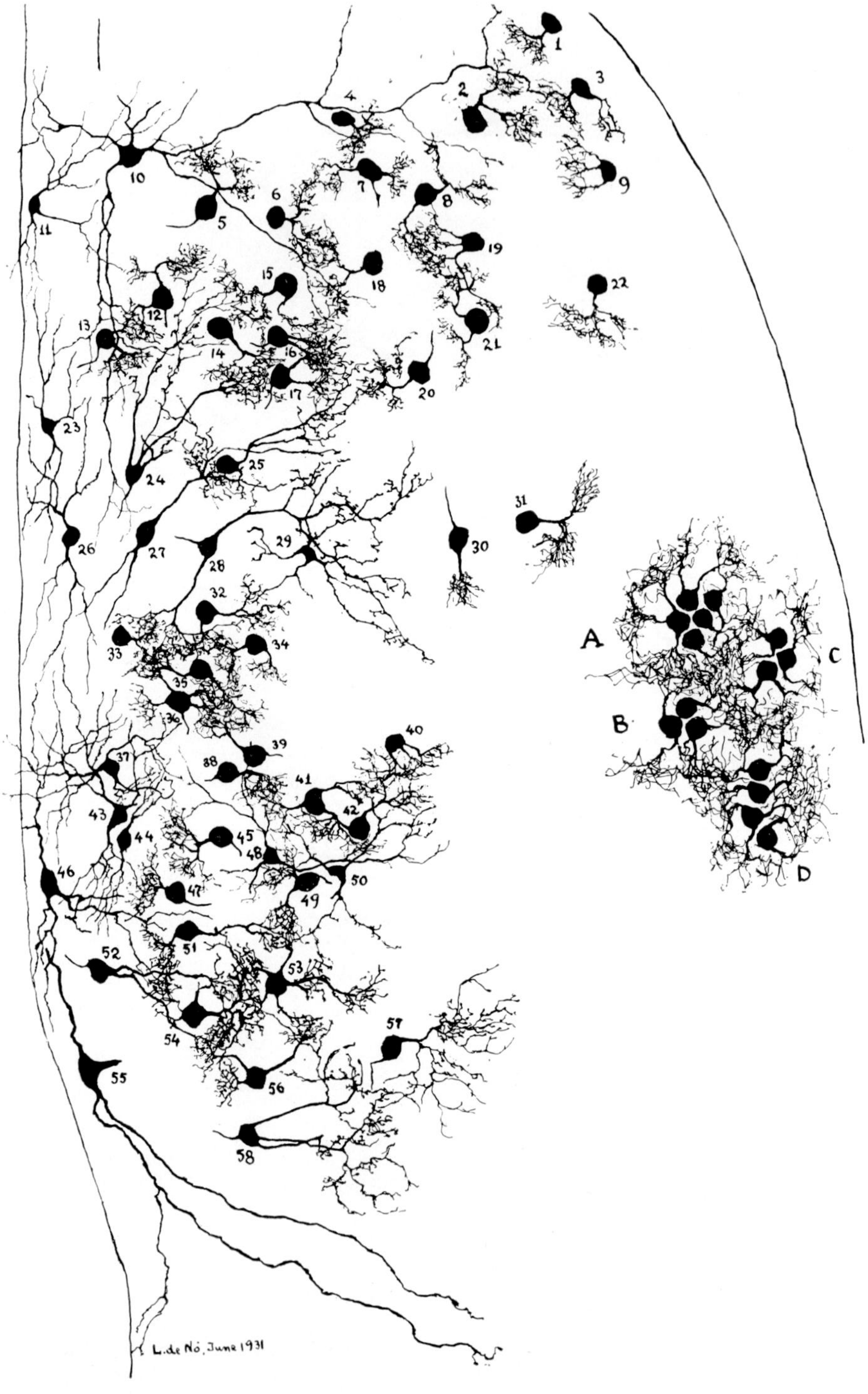

Fig. 8. Dendritic plexus in the magnocellular complex of *n.v. I*, as demonstrated by Golgi-Cox method. Adult cat.

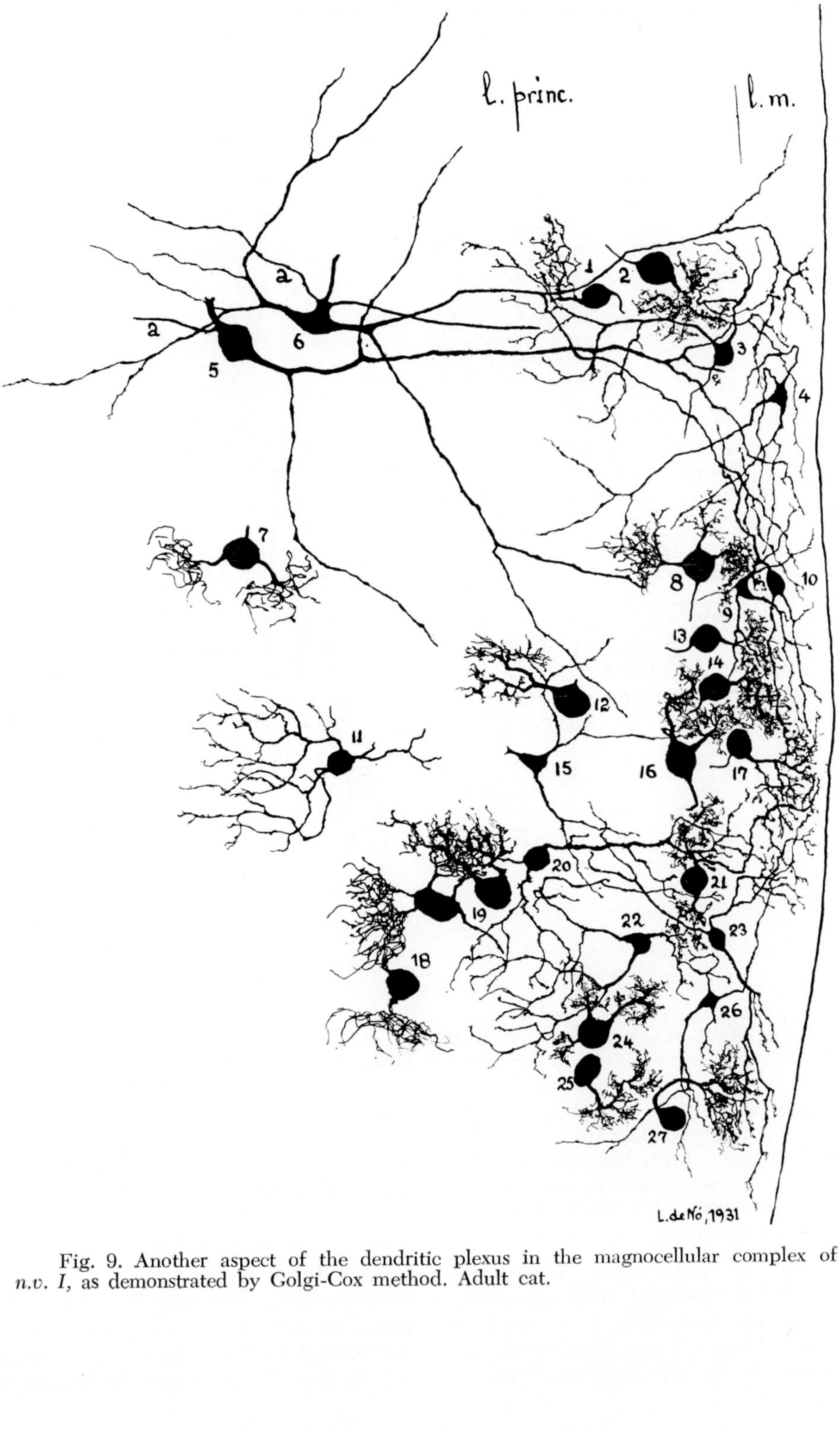

Fig. 9. Another aspect of the dendritic plexus in the magnocellular complex of *n.v. I,* as demonstrated by Golgi-Cox method. Adult cat.

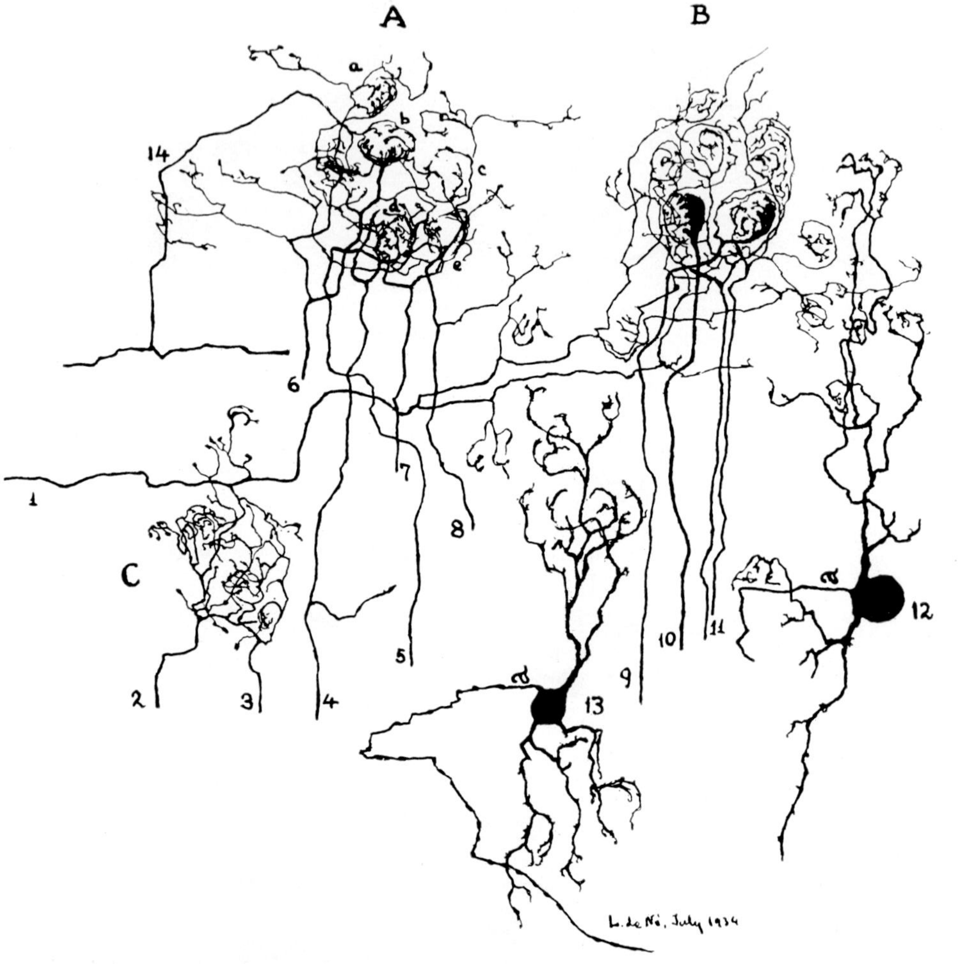

Fig. 10. Partial illustrations of the fibrillar plexus in *n.v. I*. Globular cells *12* and *13* have been taken from a different section. Golgi rapid method.

casionally, they have only one dendrite. Each dendrite divides into numerous interlaced thin branches which gives rise to a dense dendritic ramification having the aspect of a bush or a brush (see also Fig. 17).

In this part of the ventral nucleus the axons of the spherical cells may (Fig. 7, *3*) or may not (Fig. 7, *5*) give off collateral branches ramified within the nucleus, but in all cases the axon always divides to give a branch to an association path for the tuberculum acusticum. In some cases (Fig. 7, *3*) the association branch arises after the axon has reached the trapezoid body, in which case the association branch joins the *tractus ventrotubercularis ventralis*. In other cases, however, the axon of the spherical cell (Fig. 7, *5*) divides within the ventral nucleus, one branch descending to join the trapezoid body and the

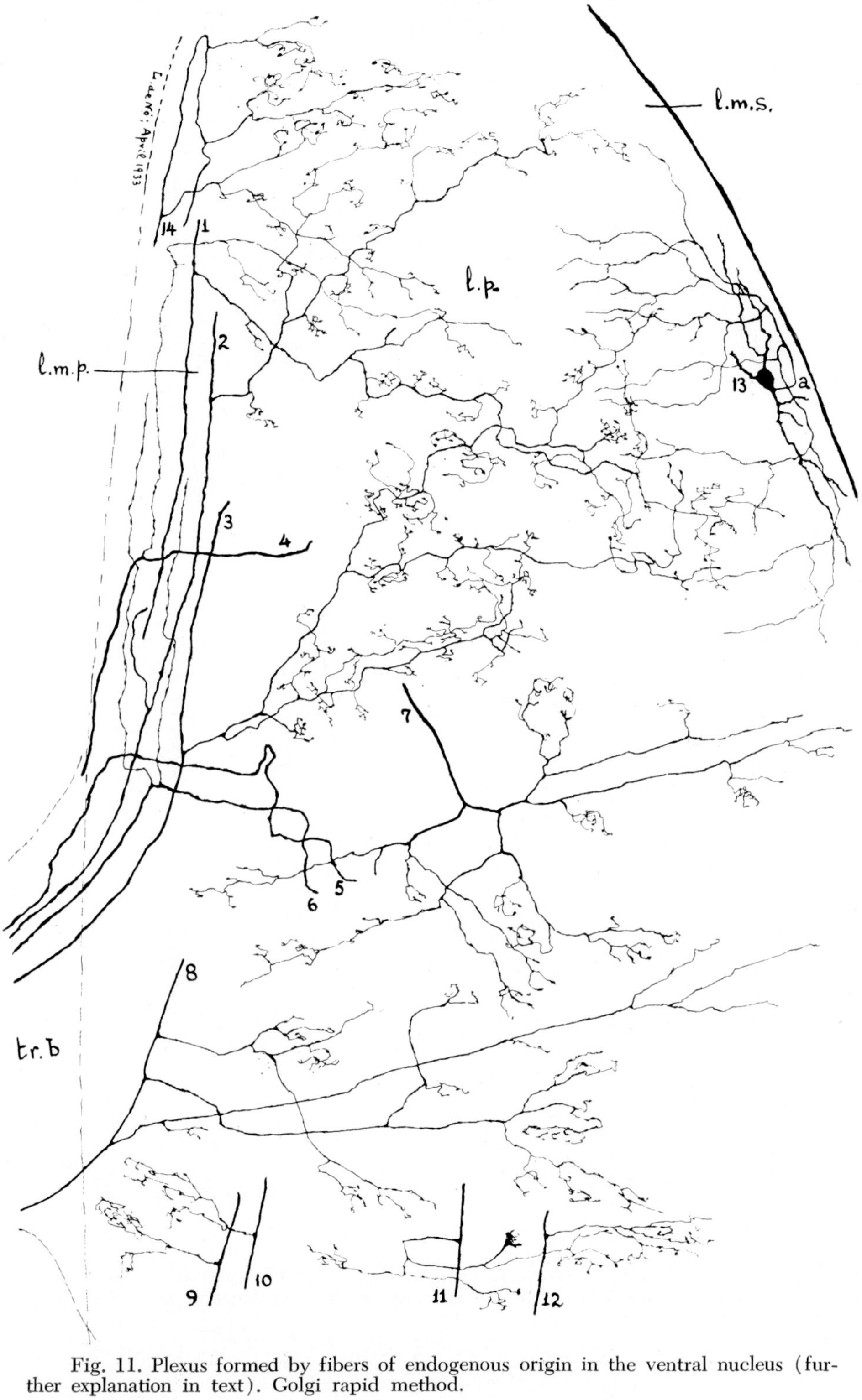

Fig. 11. Plexus formed by fibers of endogenous origin in the ventral nucleus (further explanation in text). Golgi rapid method.

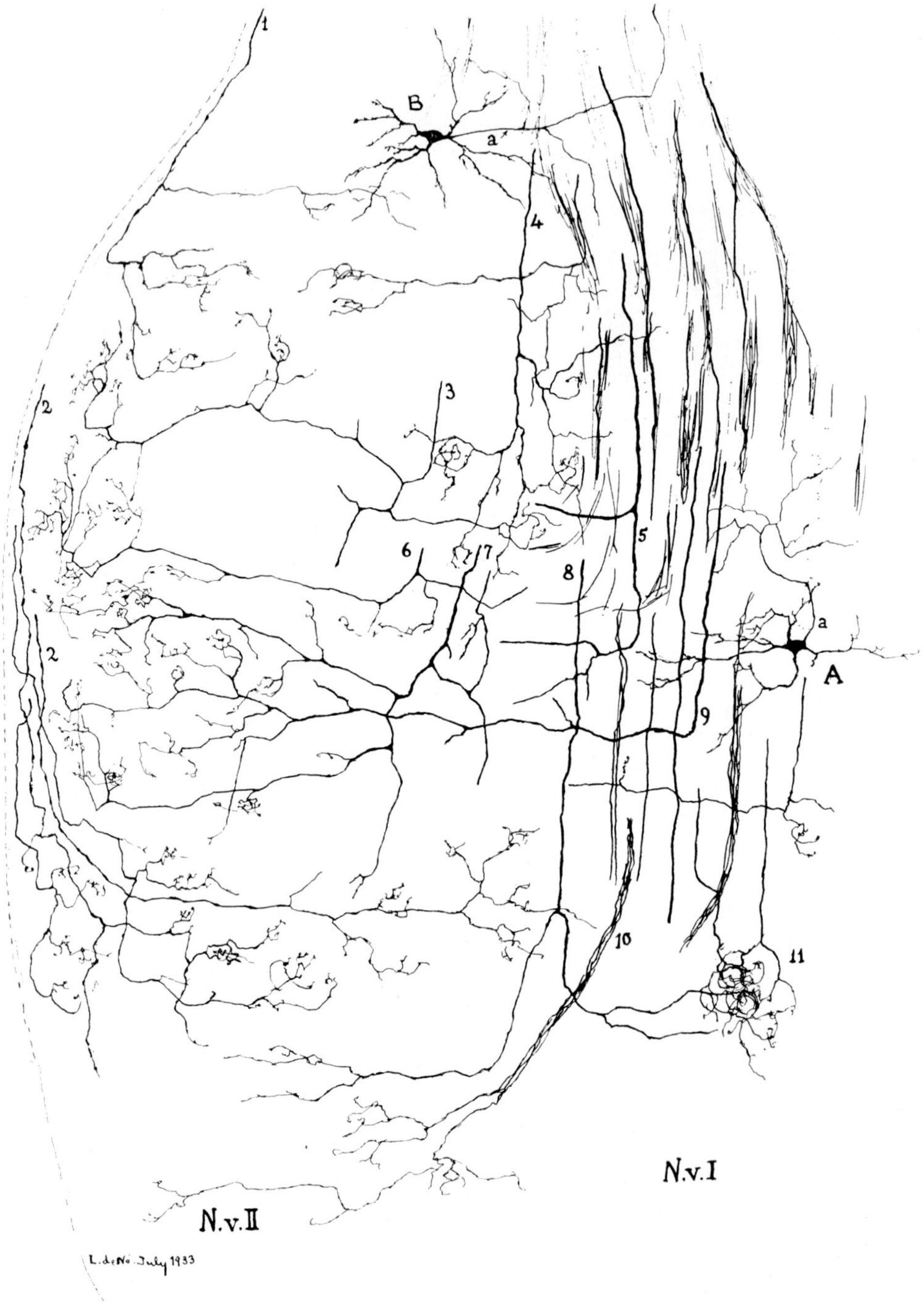

Fig. 12. Plexus formed by fibers carried to the ventral nucleus by an association tract originated in the tuberculum acousticum (further explanation in text). Golgi rapid method.

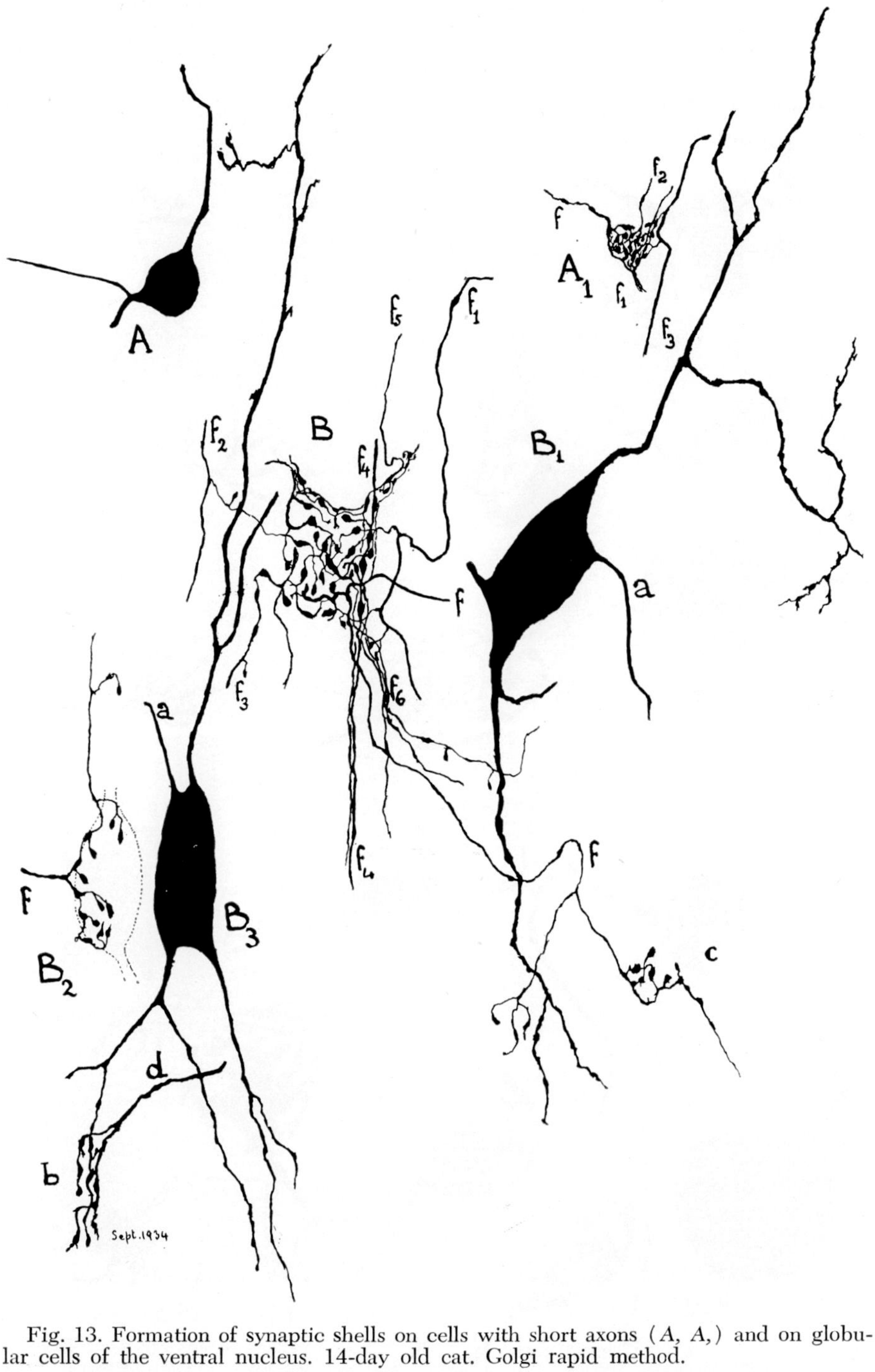

Fig. 13. Formation of synaptic shells on cells with short axons (A, A,) and on globular cells of the ventral nucleus. 14-day old cat. Golgi rapid method.

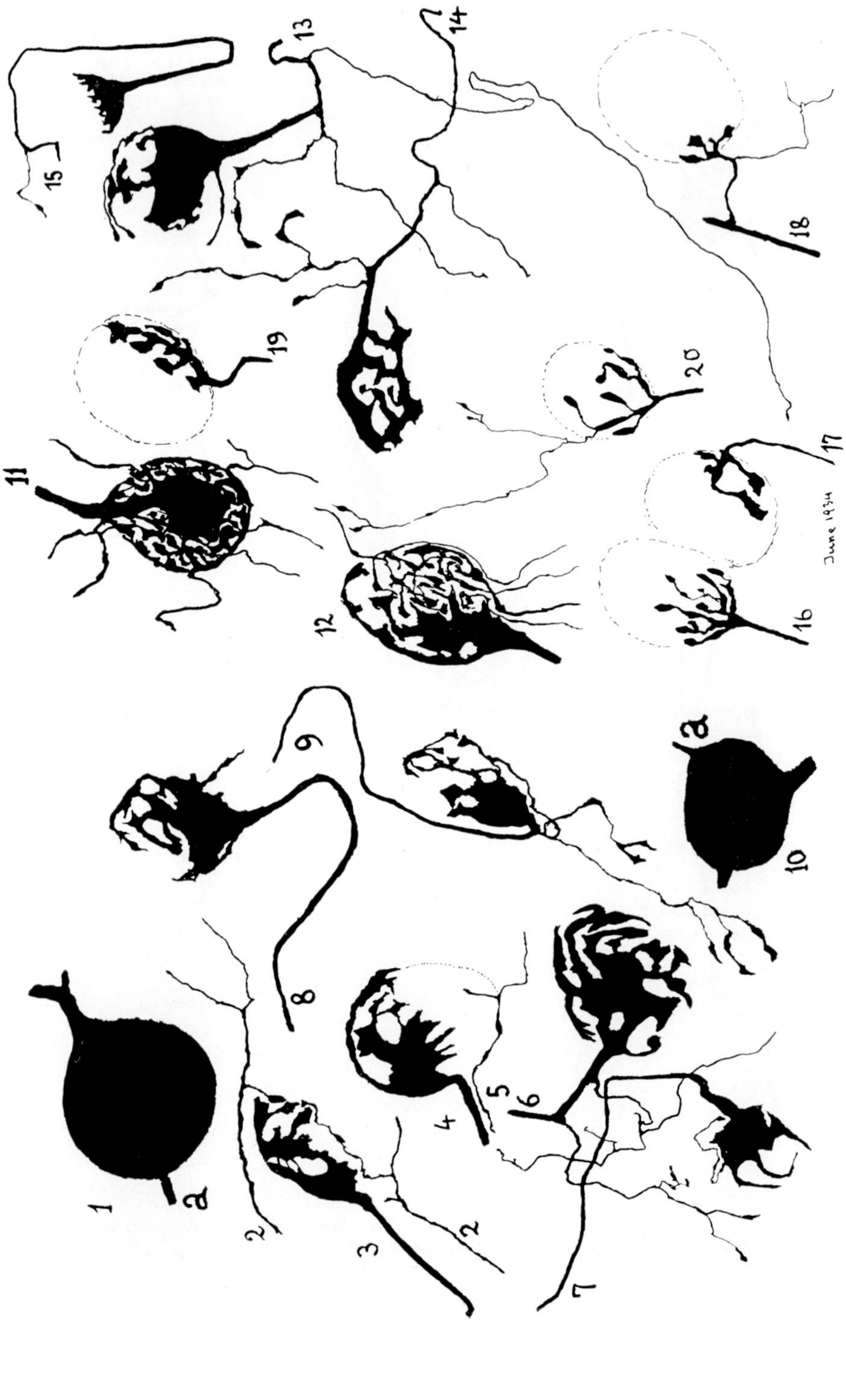

Fig. 14. Types of chalices of Held in the ventral nucleus. Taken from several slides prepared by Golgi rapid method.

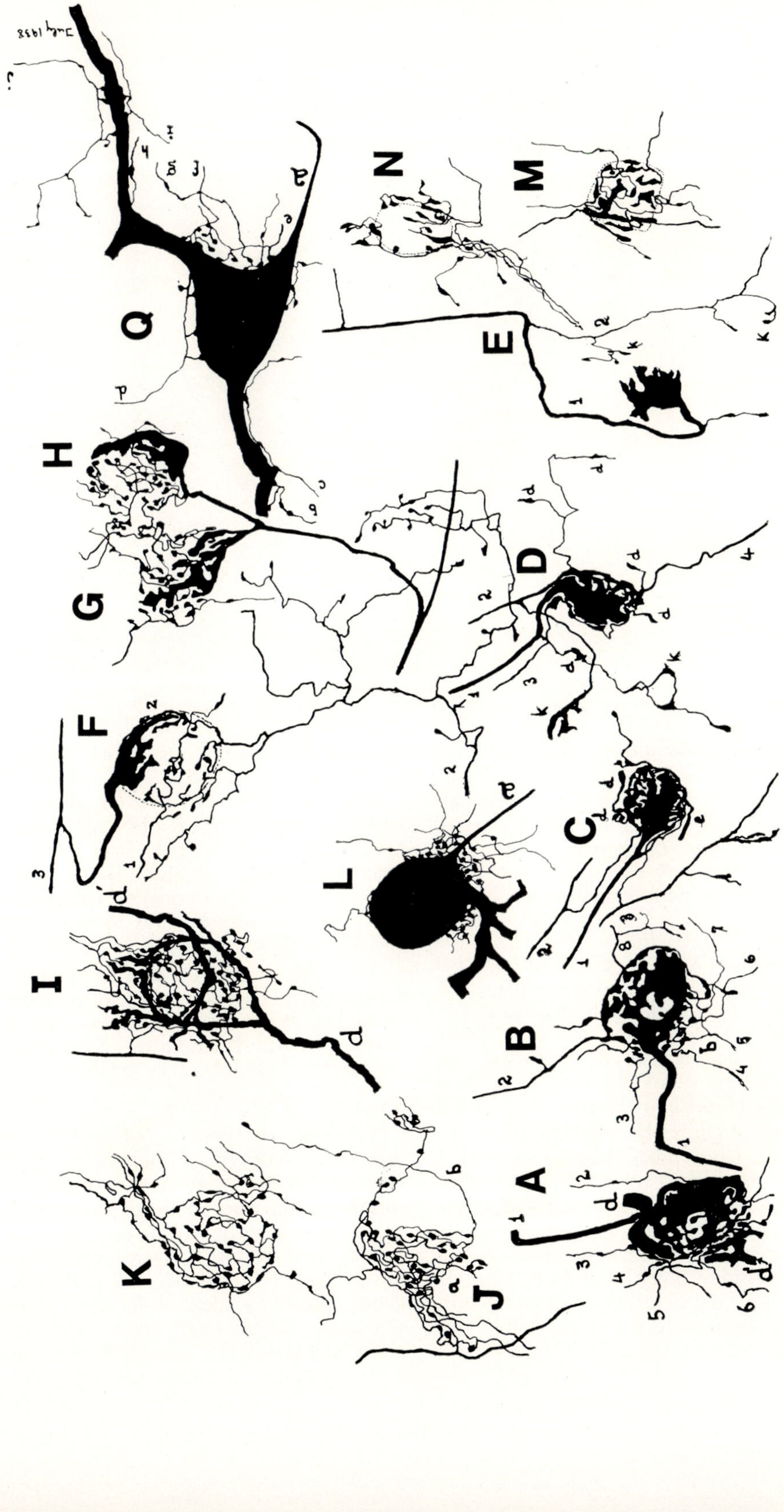

Fig. 15. Chalices of Held and other types of synaptic endings in the ventral nucleus. Golgi rapid method.

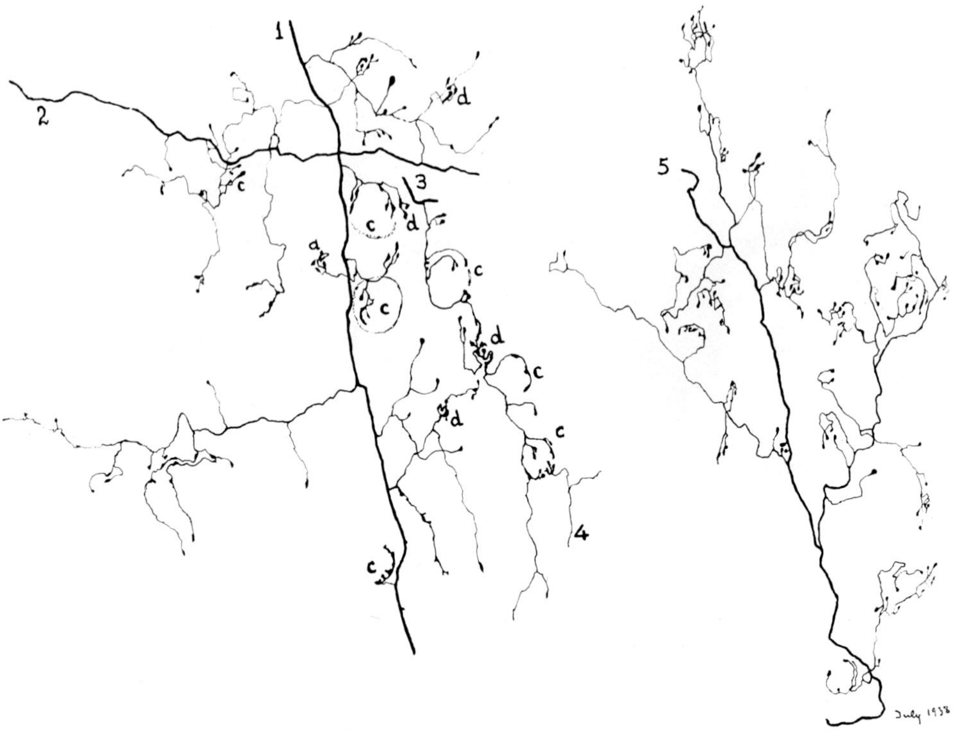

Fig. 16. Ramifications of endogenous fibers in the ventral nucleus.

other branch ascending to reach the *tractus ventrotubercularis dorsalis.* Each spherical cell receives one and only one Held chalice but in the caudal part of the nucleus (*n.v. II*) it may happen that one brush cell may receive two or three Held bulbs, as was described by Cajal.[6]

TYPE M (MULTIPOLAR)

The second type of cell with efferent axon includes all those cells with efferent axons which do not establish contact with a Held chalice or a Held bulb. To the cells of type *M*, acoustic impulses can be delivered only by synaptic knobs of ordinary type.

Cells *2, 4* (only the initial parts of the dendrites have been drawn) *6* and *9* (Fig. 7; see also Fig. 10, *12, 13*) illustrate the multiplicity of shapes that the efferent cells of type *M* may have. In the part of the ventral nucleus that is under consideration the cells of type *M* have only one detail in common; during their branching the dendrites of one or more cells tend to form "baskets" enclosing the bodies of other neurons, chiefly spherical cells. Any attempt to classify the cells of type *M* according to their morphology is obviously impossible. For example, cell *6* in Figure 7 may be called "bipolar" while cell *9* which has all its dendrites oriented in one direction may be said to be an "octopoid" cell.

The cells of types *S* and *M* belong to Golgi type I because they have a long axon that is an efferent fiber, *i.e.*, one that leaves the boundaries of the acoustic nuclei to reach other centers.

TYPE G

The cells of type *G* (of which there are many subtypes) belong to Golgi type II because they have axons which ramify within the acoustic nuclei themselves at a distance from the cell body, which may be very short or relatively long. Figure 7 presents one cell with a short axon (*1*) located in the external marginal lamina and two cells with short axons (*7, 8*) located in the inter-

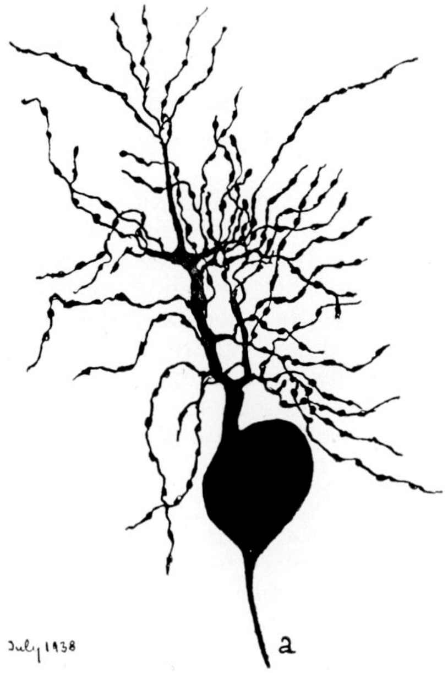

Fig. 17. Cell body and dendritic arborization of a cell of spherical type. Adult cat. Golgi-Cox method.

nal marginal lamina. In the *lamina principalis* of the anterior nucleus there also are numerous cells with short axons even though it is difficult to obtain simultaneous stains of the cell body and dendrites together with an important part of the axonal arborization. Figure 7 presents two arborizations *A, A* which probably belong to axons of cells such as *5* and *6* in Figure 9. It is also possible that the arborization *A* on the left side is the end of the arborization of an association fiber having its origin in a large neuron of the nucleus centralis of the tuberculum acusticum.

Figure 8 presents the plexus formed by the cell bodies and dendrites in a frontal section through the magnocellular system of the anterior or ventral nucleus. All the cells that have been included in the drawing were present in a single 120μ-thick histological section stained after Golgi-Cox, but in order to avoid repetitiousness blank spaces have been left in the drawing. Complete identification of all the cell types is not possible because as a rule Golgi-Cox method fails to stain the axons of the neurons, but on the basis of the experience acquired with Golgi's osmic acid methods, it is possible to make highly probable statements concerning the majority of the cells in Figure 8. Within the *lamina marginalis interna* there is a large number of cells (*10, 11, 23, 26, 37, 46* and *55*) which undoubtedly are cells with short axons. Cells *29* (almost at the center of the drawing) and *50* undoubtedly are small cells with short axons. Cells *24, 27, 28, 48, 57* and *58* are basket cells having widely different body shapes. Finally, all the other cells in the drawing are spherical (bushy) cells.

Important properties of the dendritic plexus formed by the spherical cells are illustrated on the right-hand side of Figure 8. It will be seen that, as is often the case, the cells are grouped in glomeruli, *A, B, C, D*, seemingly empty spaces surrounding the cells of each glomerulus, and the dendrites come together to form dense plexuses in the spaces between glomeruli. The kind of elements that are present in those seemingly empty spaces will be mentioned below during the discussion of Figure 10.

The drawing in Figure 9 was also prepared from a single Golgi-Cox section through the oral magnocellular system, but in this particular section a considerable number of neurons of the external marginal zone were stained. Cells *3, 4, 9, 10, 23* and *26* undoubtedly are cells with short axons similar to cell *1* in Figure 7 and cell *13* in Figure 12. From the four cells near the top of the drawing, cells *1* and *2* (Fig. 9) are spherical cells of different sizes and cells *5* and *6* are large cells with short axons and exceedingly extensive dendritic ramification. Cells *11* and *22* are of type M. All the other neurons in the drawing are spherical neurons.

Given the great reliability of the Golgi-Cox method, Figures 8 and 9 may be taken as evidence that in the magnocellular system and in general in the oral half of the anterior or ventral nucleus (*n.v. I*) the spherical cells greatly outnumber all other types. In another paper it will be shown that the relative number of multipolar cells greatly increases as the points of division of the primary cochlear fibers are approached. Nevertheless, spherical cells of small size are found even between the undivided primary cochlear fibers.

Except for basket cells *12* and *13*, which were taken from other sections, Figure 10 was drawn from a single frontal section passing slightly rostral to the caudal margin of the magnocellular system. It represents an attempt to illustrate how the fibrillar plexuses are formed which articulate themselves with the dendritic plexuses.

In Figure 10 the manner in which the fibers branch out leaves no doubt that the fibers labeled *1* to *8* and *14* are endogenous fibers, *i.e.*, fibers which have their origin in the acoustic nucleus themselves. *C* shows that coincidence of branches of three endogenous fibers are sufficient to form a rather dense plexus but in this particular sample of the fibrillar plexus no particular arrangement of fibrils can be discerned. However, by fortunate, but wholly unknown circumstances, at *A*, the coincidence of branches from endogenous fibers *4, 5, 6, 7, 8,* and *14* resulted in a plexus having empty spaces *a, b, c, d, e* in which, undoubtedly, bodies of spherical cells were located (some of the spherical cells were faintly stained in yellow). On the other hand, at *B*, four cochlear fibers *9* to *11*, together with branches of endogenous fibers, form a plexus in which spaces are left for spherical cells and their Held chalices. The chalices supplied by fibers *9* and *10* are included in the drawing while the chalices supplied by fibers *11* either were not stained or were not included in the section.

If plexuses *A* and *B* (Fig. 10) are thought of being superposed, and to the result of the superposition dendritic plexuses are added, such as those in Figure 8 *A* to *D*, and if to the new result dendritic branches are added of cells such as *12* and *13* (Fig. 10), then an approximate idea of the complexity of the structure of the magnocellular system of the cochlear anterior nucleus is obtained, and one cannot fail to realize that in each small volume of that fraction of the acoustic nuclei each neuron establishes in its body and dendrites an exceedingly large number of synapses with nerve fibers which in part arrive from the cochlea, but which to a large extent have their origin in the acoustic nuclei themselves.

Ramifications of axons of cells of Golgi type II constitute only one type of endogenous fibers. A second type of endogenous fiber, which is particularly important in the magnocellular system, is illustrated by Figure 11, which reproduces observations made in a slightly oblique frontal section, the upper part of which passed almost through the oral end of the magnocellular system.

All the fibers in Figure 11 are identifiable; *a* is the short axon of marginal cell *13*. Fibers *9* to *12* (below) are segments of cochlear fibers and fiber *7* in all probability is the end ramification of a fiber of the *tractus ventrotubercularis.* All the other fibers including fiber *8* are axons of spherical (bushy) cells. Fiber *14* (Fig. 11) has an initial upward course, and after having given off two profusely ramified collaterals it goes toward the trapezoid body (*tr.b*). Fibers *1, 2, 3* and *8* also give off profusely ramified collaterals. Fibers *4* and *6* do not give collaterals within the nucleus but after reaching the white matter they give off branches which have an ascending course and form *U* fibers which penetrate into the nucleus to become ramified. The collaterals of fiber *5* were probably not included in the histological section.

If consideration is given to the fact that only a few axons of spherical cells are present in Figure 11, it becomes obvious that the totality of collaterals of such axons must constitute an exceedingly dense plexus or, otherwise stated, it becomes obvious that each spherical cell must receive numerous synapses from their companion spherical cells in the magnocellular system of the anterior nucleus.

Consideration of the behavior of the axons of the spherical cells readily shows that the anterior (oral) and the posterior (caudal) parts of the anterior cochlear nucleus have widely different properties.

As it appears in Figure 7 in the part of the ventral nucleus caudal to the magnocellular system (*i.e.,* in *n.v. II*) the axons of the spherical cells give off none or only a few collaterals which are poorly ramified within the nucleus, but the axons divide into two branches, one branch which joins the trapezoid body and reaches upper acoustic centers while the other branch joins a ventrotubercular tract. Since the axons of the numerous cells of type M also send a branch to the ventrotubercular tract it may be said that only the caudal half of the ventral nucleus (*n.v. II*) is the locus of origin of the ventrotubercular association tracts. However, in the dorsal ventrotubercular tract there is an important stream of rather coarse fibers which run in the opposite direction, *i.e.,* which run from the tuberculum acusticum toward the ventral nucleus, where they end precisely in the magnocellular system of spherical cells (*n.v. I*).

Whether fibers *1* and *2* in Figure 12 had their origin in the tuberculum acusticum is not known, but it lies beyond doubt that fibers *3* to *10* (Fig. 12) had their origin in the tuberculum acusticum, perhaps, or rather, probably, in the nucleus centralis and that they ended in the magnocellular system (*n.v. II*), their end arborizations being intermixed with the arborizations of the collaterals of the axons of spherical cells (Fig. 11).

Thus we reach an interesting conclusion. If the cochlear afferents are said to be fibers of the first order, the collaterals of spherical cells are fibers of the second order, while the fibers that arrive from the tuberculum acusticum to the magnocellular complex of the ventral nucleus are fibers of third and fourth order. Since all those fibers have synaptic contacts with spherical cells it is clear that during stimulation of the cochlea with a pure tone the spherical cells of *n.v. I* must receive simultaneously in their different synapses, impulses of various orders and that the constellation of impulses reaching the spherical cells must be different during the first few instants after the stimulation has been started and at a later time during constant delivery of the pure tone. Clearly, simple assumptions are hardly permissible as to the manner in which acoustic impulses are transmitted through the primary acoustic nuclei.

SYNAPSES IN THE ANTERIOR NUCLEUS

Figures 13 to 17 illustrate the manner in which synaptic contacts are established in the acoustic nuclei. The cells presented in Figure 13 were taken from the caudal part of the anterior nucleus (*n.v. I*). Cell *A* is undoubtedly a small cell with a short axon. As it appears in A_1 the clusters of synaptic knobs formed by four fibers, *f* to f_3 were sufficient to form a practically complete synaptic shell or scale on the surface of the cell.

The cells labeled B are large multipolar neurons. Cell B_2 was stained faintly in yellow and it received a single stained cluster of synaptic knobs. Although cell *B* was not stained, an important part of the fibers and knobs forming its synaptic shell were intensely stained. As can readily be noted, each one of the seven or eight stained fibers contributed interlacing clusters of knobs to the synaptic shell. The manner in which the synaptic shells A_1 and *B* (Fig. 13) are formed is also typical for all multipolar neurons (motoneurons and interneurons) of the medulla and spinal cord.[12] Short segments of some thick dendrites may also be provided with a continuous shell but, as a rule, the synaptic endings on dendrites are established, at least in the acoustic nuclei, usually in discrete short dendritic zones separated by relatively long distances (about several microns). For example, fiber *f* (Fig. 13) after having left a cluster of knobs on scale *B* continued and ended forming a cluster of synaptic knobs *c*, each one of which was destined to establish contact with dendrites of a group such as that which is presented in *b* (Fig. 14). Clearly, therefore, each dendrite establishes contacts with a large number of fibers but each fiber supplies to the dendrite only one or a small cluster of knobs, the individual synaptic zones in each dendrite being separated by distances which may be a number of microns long.

Under conditions such as these it is

quite clear that at the cell bodies at which convergence of a large number of synaptic knobs takes place, full-sized nerve impulses can be readily established, while in the dendrites small nerve impulses will be initiated which will reach the cell body and the axon only if during conduction in the dendrite the small impulse is reinforced by stimulation effected at a new synaptic zone or by summation with another small impulse provided by a collateral dendritic branch.[7]

As was described above, the acoustic fibers form special endings (Held chalices or bulbs) on the spherical cells. Figure 14 presents a number of types of Held endings (the relative scale in Figure 14 is undoubtedly correct; for the absolute scale Figures 3 to 7 of the excellent paper by Brawer and Morest[11] should be consulted). The Held chalices are laminar structures perhaps 2 or 3μ thick and as a rule they are provided with a number of "holes." In part, as was stated by Cajal,[6] the holes allow dendrites to pass, but in the main the holes serve for the surface of the cell to establish contacts with small or large synaptic knobs supplied by fibers of small caliber; in this manner, the synaptic shell of the spherical cells becomes complete.

Even the chalices of the largest size (Fig. 14, *4, 6, 8, 11, 12* do not cover more than one-half of the surface of the spherical cell. When the Held endings are small (Fig. 14, *7, 9*) thin branches may arise from the border of the chalice to form synaptic knobs in contact with other spherical cells or with dendrites. When the Held endings are as small as those in Figure 14, *15* to *20* only a small part of the spherical cell is covered with such endings unless a number of several Held endings are present in the same cell in the manner that was described by Cajal[6] (Fig. 15 *A* to *D*).

Additional details on the synaptic scale or shell of spherical cells is presented in Figure 15. In the cases of cells *J* and *K* only the part of the synaptic scale made out of small synaptic knobs was stained, the stain being not complete but uniform enough to show that approximately one-half of the surface of the synaptic shell is covered with small synaptic knobs to which those must be added which are located in the "holes" of the Held chalices. In the case of cell *I* it can be seen how dendrites *d* and *d′* belonging to basket cells branch out tending to form a basket surrounding the spherical cell and its synaptic shell. In the case of cell *L* a number of synaptic knobs were found in the proximity of the axon *a*, many of them making synaptic contact with the cell body. No contact, however, was observed between the axon and one synaptic knob.

Cells *L, J, K,* and *I* were located in the oral part of *n.v. II* in the proximity of the magnocellular complex. All the other structures reproduced in Figure 15 were located in the caudal part of *n.v. I* in the proximity of the points of division of the acoustic fibers. In the case of cell *A* the presence of dendrites *d* and *d′* would have required the use of half-tones to present with clarity the synaptic shell. In the case of cell *B* however, it is obvious that the visible half of the synaptic shell is formed by a rather large Held chalice belonging to fiber *1*, a series of large knobs (actually a small Held bulb) belonging to fiber *2* and a number of small synaptic knobs belonging to fibers of smaller size. In the drawing of shell *C* the only detail that appears with clarity is the presence in the shell of contributions of a number of fibers. However, in the case of cell *D* it can readily be seen that when viewed from above, the shell included a large Held bulb supplied by fiber *1* and a smaller Held bulb supplied by fiber *2* and synaptic knobs supplied by fibers *3* and *4*. It should be noted that all those fibers gave off branches having synaptic terminals for dendrites (*d*) or cell bodies of other neighboring cells. In the case of cell *F* only three fibers participating in the synaptic shell were stained. Fiber *3* formed a small Held bulb and fiber *1* supplied a few synaptic knobs; synaptic knobs for cell *F* were also supplied by an extensively ramified fiber, the cut end of which is labeled *2* (immediately above the letter *a*, which denotes the axon of cell L), the knobs supplied by this fiber being located chiefly near the lower and lateral margin of the cell *F* next to the repeated numeral *2*.

Cells *G* and *H* illustrate an exceptional occurrence, the ascending or anterior branch of an acoustic fiber ended near the point of bifurcation by forming two small Held chalices applied to two neighboring small spherical cells. *M* and *N* are cells of the interstitial nucleus making contact with an unusually large number of knobs of acoustic origin. Finally *Q* is a large multipolar neuron (undoubtedly a cell of Golgi type II) in the body and dendrites of which a number of fibrils formed synaptic endings.

DISCUSSION

It hardly needs be emphasized that the manner in which acoustic sensation is ultimately created depends primarily upon the manner in which the nerve impulses initiated in the cochlea are transmitted through the primary acoustic nuclei. Such a transmission cannot be a simple matter since, as was clearly shown in 1933, the primary acoustic nuclei have an exceedingly complex structure and contain numerous types of neurons which are interconnected by powerful association tracts.

The complexity of the problem appears clearly when consideration is given to the system brush or spherical cells — Held chalices. At first sight it seems that such a system should serve for faithful one-to-one transmission of the cochlear impulses to the upper acoustic centers. The situation, however, has proven to be far more complex. The amount of surface of the cell body covered by a Held chalice is not greater, on the contrary it is smaller than the amount which is covered by small synaptic knobs which, in part, are supplied by collaterals of cochlear fibers and in part by endogenous fibers having a variety of origins. In addition, a large number of synaptic connections must be established in the dendrites of the brush cells.

Figure 17 reproduces a drawing that was prepared, with great care with the help of a projection apparatus, of a brush cell of the simplest type, since it possessed only one dendrite. Of course, from the more or less cylindrical tree only those dendritic branches could be reproduced, which were included in the 120μ section. The maximum width of the cell body was approximately 50μ.

In view of the existence of synapses on the dendrites as well as small synapses in the holes of the chalices of Held it is evident that transmission of impulses cannot depend solely on the acoustic impulses carried by the chalices. The possibility, of course, exists that some of the small synapses are inhibitory and that their action may go so far as to prevent activation of the brush cell by the chalice. At least, inhibitory synapses may serve to cause a delay in the initiation of the impulse in the brush cell. On the other hand, some of the small synapses may be excitatory and consequently, they may shorten the synaptic delay of the impulse initiated by the chalice of Held. Of course, even if the small synapses should serve only to modify the effect of the chalices of Held, their role would be quite important, since in the acoustic system timing plays an exceedingly important role and time differences measured in microseconds may be sufficient to prevent the exact localization of sound. Similarly, errors in the timing of transmission of acoustic impulses would seriously interfere with true perception of speech or music.

Although exact figures cannot be given, no significant error will be committed if it is assumed that within the magnocellular system of spherical cells in the ventral nucleus the number of endogenous fibers is at least as great and probably greater than the number of fibers resulting from branching of primary (cochlear) acoustic fibers. The endogenous fibers are of multitudinous origins: 1) Collateral branches of axons of brush cells. Figure 11 shows how important this system is. In this system there are also included collaterals of the sparse multipolar cells included in the magnocellular system. 2) Collaterals and end ramifications of association tracts such as the branches of the ventrotubercular tract presented in Figure 12. 3) Centrifugal fibers arising from upper acoustic centers. The existence of

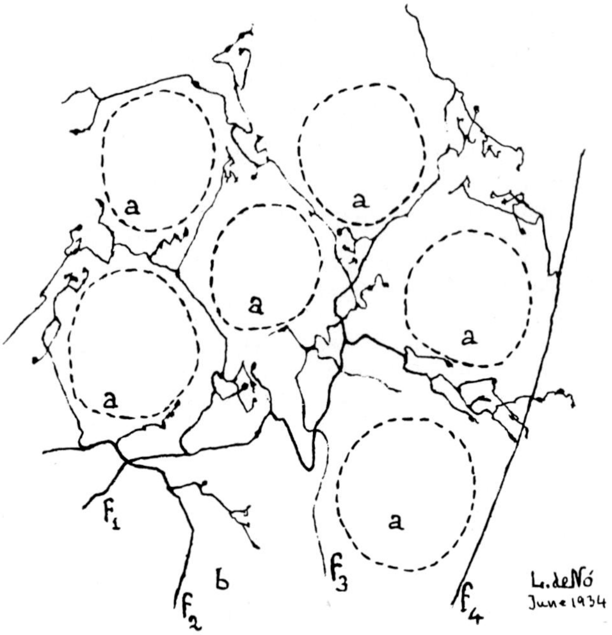

Fig. 18. Fibers f_1 to f_4 form synaptic endings which come in contact exclusively with dendrites located in the spaces between the spherical cells *a, a*. Golgi rapid method.

such fibers was demonstrated by Rasmussen but the fibers themselves have not been identified yet with Golgi's method. 4) Ramifications of the axons of cells with short axons (Golgi type II) (Fig. 7 *1, 7, 8*; Fig. 11, *13*).

In order to show how large the number of cells innervated by an endogenous fiber may be, Figure 16 presents parts of the arborizations of five large endogenous fibers of unknown origin, all of them characterized by the fact that giving off branches did not result in an appreciable decrease of the diameter of the fiber. In the case of the fibers labeled *1* and *3* it was possible to ascertain whether the synaptic contacts were established with cell bodies (*c*) or with dendrites (*d*).

Reference must also be made to the peculiar type of synaptic endings reproduced in Figure 18. As is often the case, many cells of the spherical type were stained in light yellow. The contours of those cells (*a, a*) are given by the dotted lines. It will be noted that in the spaces between spherical cells there were fibers f_1 to f_4 that gave off branches having synaptic endings in the seemingly empty spaces between the *a* cells. Therefore, it must be concluded that among the endogenous fibers there are fibers of a certain type which establish contacts exclusively with dendrites. The origin of the fibers of this peculiar type is unknown.

In preparing the drawings *A, A* of endogenous fibers in Figure 7, only that number of branches have been included which were sufficient to illustrate the general features of the arborizations. In the case of Figure 19 the part of the arborization of a short axon included in the 120μ-section has been reproduced completely with extreme care. The arborization was located in the central part of *n.v. I* and the height of the oval cell *a* on the left of the drawing was approximately 50μ. The cell of origin of the short axon was either not stained or not included in the section.

It will be noted that in its upward course the axon undergoes a decrease in diameter whenever it gives off a branch.

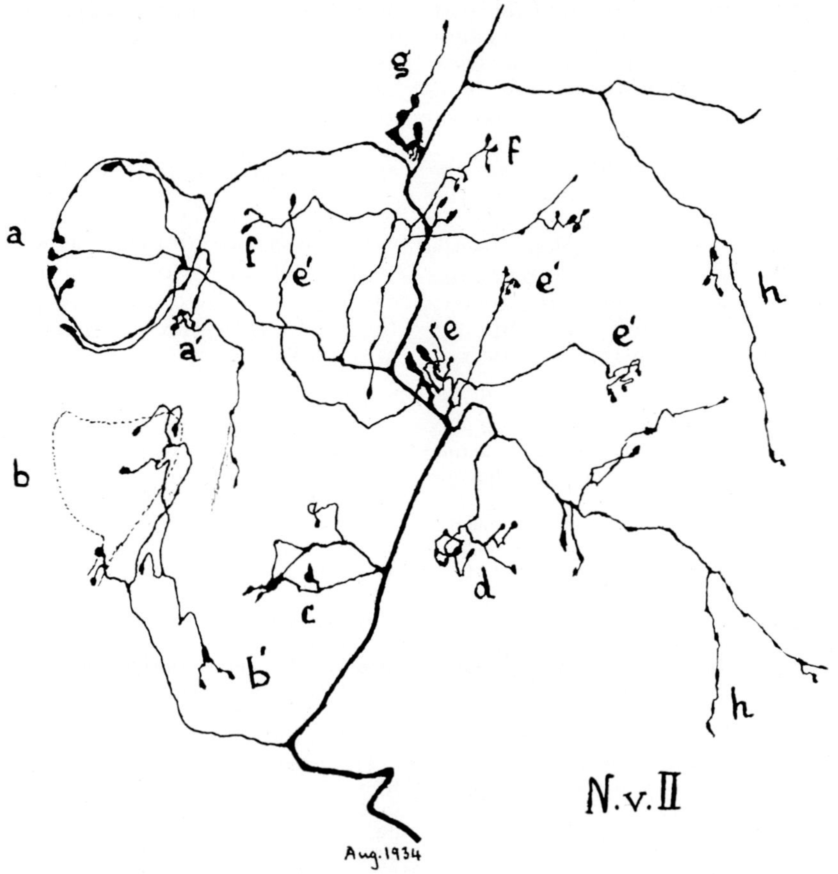

Fig. 19. Ramification reproduced with greatest possible accuracy of an endogenous fiber (short axon) of *n.v. II.* Golgi rapid method.

The large synaptic knobs *e* and the smaller knobs *e'* and *f* arise from the same point of the fiber; but in view of the length and caliber of the fibrils it is obvious that knobs *e'* and *f* will be reached by the nerve impulse considerably later than knobs *e*. Similarly, the large knobs *c* and *g* will be reached at an early time, while the smaller knobs *d* and *h* will be reached considerably later. It should also be noted that the globular cell *c* receives endings *a* and a_1, having their origin at different parts of the same branch of the short axon. Finally, attention will be called to the frequently observed fact that the various synaptic knobs may be at considerable distance apart, which are given to the same cell by a single fiber *b*.

In 1933, while discussing the significance of the plan of the structure of the acoustic nuclei, the general conclusion was reached that those nuclei are made out of two types of neurons; "effector" neurons which transmit the acoustic impulses to higher centers and "regulator" neurons which contribute in essential manner to determining the mode of operation of the effector neurons. At present that general conclusion may be stated in a more definite form.

In the first place it has become known that all acoustic pathways contain both ascending or afferent and descending or centrifugal fibers, a set of circumstances that makes a unit out of the entire acoustic system, since ultimately the activity in a part of the system must depend to a greater or lesser degree upon the happenings at all other parts of the system. Moreover, it is known from electrical studies that the acoustic system is in constant activity, which, as was shown by the important work of Koerber *et al*,[13] is largely independent from the cochlea. In fact, those authors showed that after destruction of the cochlea the activity in the ventral nucleus ceases while the activity in the tuberculum acusticum is modified but little. It may therefore be concluded that although spontaneous activity in the acoustic system fails to produce a conscious sensation of sound, it serves to determine the physiological state of the various parts of the acoustic system in such a manner that, in spite of varying conditions, inside and outside the brain, actual sounds may be perceived with fidelity.

The extensive work required to restore the original drawings as well as the writing of the manuscript have been made possible by a generous grant from the Deafness Research Foundation, New York, NY.

REFERENCES

1. Lorente de Nó R: Anatomy of the eighth nerve. III. General plan of structure of the primary cochlear nuclei. Laryngoscope 43:327-350, 1933

2. Lorente de Nó R: The neural mechanism of hearing. I. Anatomy and physiology. b) The sensory endings in the cochlea. Laryngoscope 47:373-377, 1937

3. Rasmussen GL: Efferent fibers of the cochlear nerve and cochlear nuclei, in Rasmussen GL, Windle WS (eds): *Neural Mechanisms of the Auditory and Vestibular Systems.* Springfield, IL, C C Thomas, 1960, pp 105-115

4. Rasmussen GL: Efferent connections of the cochlear nucleus, in Graham AB (ed): *Sensorineural Hearing Processes and Disorders.* Boston, Little, Brown and Co, 1967, pp 61-75

5. Rasmussen GL: Anatomic relationship of the ascending and descending auditory systems, in Fields WS, Alford BR (eds): *Neurological Aspects of Auditory and Vestibular Disorders.* Springfield, IL, C C Thomas, 1966, pp 5-19

6. Cajal SR: *Histologie du Système Nerveux.* Paris, A. Maloine, 1909, vol 1

7. Lorente de Nó R, Condouris GA: Decremental conduction in peripheral nerve. Integration of stimuli in the neuron. Proc Natl Acad Sci USA 45:592-617, 1959

8. Spoendlin H: Innervation densities of the cochlea. Acta Otolaryngol (Stockh) 73: 235-248, 1972

9. Morrison D, Schindler RA, Wersäll J: A quantitative analysis of the afferent innervation of the organ of Corti in guinea pig. Acta Otolaryngol (Stockh) 79:11-23, 1975

10. Osen KK: Cytoarchitecture of the cochlear nuclei in the cat. J Comp Neurol 136: 453-484, 1969

11. Brawer JR, Morest DK: Relations between auditory nerve endings and cell types in the cat's anteroventral nucleus seen with the Golgi method and Nomarski optics. J Comp Neurol 160:491-506, 1975

12. Lorente de Nó R: Synaptic stimulation of motoneurons as a local process. J Neurophysiol 1:195-206, 1938

13. Koerber KC, Pfeiffer RR, Warr WR, *et al*: Spontaneous spike discharges from single units in the cochlear nucleus after destruction of the cochlea. Exp Neurol 16:119-130, 1966

REPRINTS — R. Lorente de Nó, MD, Departments of Surgery and Anatomy, 32-34 Rehabilitation Center, Los Angeles, CA 90024.